Principles and Practice of Medical Genetics

Principles and Practice of Medical Genetics

Volume 2

Editors

Alan E. H. Emery MD, PhD, DSc, FRCP(E), FRS(E)

Professor and Chairman
University Department of Human Genetics
Western General Hospital
Edinburgh

David L. Rimoin MD, PhD

Professor of Pediatrics and Medicine
UCLA, School of Medicine
Chief, Division of Medical Genetics
Harbor-UCLA Medical Center
Los Angeles

Assistant Editor

Jeffrey A. Sofaer BDS, PHD

Editorial Assistant

A. P. Garber MS

Foreword by
Victor A. McKusick MD
William Osler Professor of Medicine,
The Johns Hopkins University School of Medicine
Baltimore

CHURCHILL LIVINGSTONE
EDINBURGH LONDON MELBOURNE AND NEW YORK 1983

CHURCHILL LIVINGSTONE
Medical Division of Longman Group Limited

Distributed in the United States of America by Churchill
Livingstone Inc., 1560 Broadway, New York, N. Y. 10036,
and by associated companies, branches and representatives
throughout the world.

First published 1983

ISBN 0 443 02129 5

British Library Cataloguing in Publication Data
Principles and practice of medical genetics.
 1. Medical genetics.
 I. Emery, Alan E. H.   II. Rimoin, David L.
 III. Sofaer, Jeffrey A.
 616'.042   RB155

Library of Congress Cataloging in Publication Data
Principles and practice of medical genetics.
 Bibliography: p.
 Includes index.
 1. Medical genetics.   I. Emery, Alan E. H.
 II. Rimoin, David L., 1936–   .   [DNLM: 1. Genetics,
Medical.   2. Hereditary disease.   QZ 50 P957]
 RB155.P694   1983   616'.042   82–23613

Printed and bound in Great Britain by
William Clowes (Beccles) Limited, Beccles and London

Foreword

The Principles and Practice of Medicine was the title of Osler's landmark textbook, first published in 1892. It is significant that the Emery-Rimoin textbook of medical genetics takes basically the same title. In its own way, it too is a landmark, a milestone in the development of human genetics as a clinical discipline in the last quarter century.

Establishment of the correct chromosome count of man (1956) and of abnormal chromosome numbers in three congenital disorders, namely, the Down, Klinefelter and Turner syndromes (1959), were made possible by simple improvements in technique, particularly hypotonic treatment of the cells for study. In the years that followed, extensive studies of the pathologic anatomy of the chromosomes, combined since 1970 with equally extensive studies of the genic anatomy of the chromosomes ('chromosome mapping'), provided a neo-Vesalian basis for clinical genetics. These advances gave the clinical geneticist 'his organ,' which he could biopsy and the disorders of which he could analyze and attempt to repair just as the cardiologist has the heart, the neurologist the nervous system, and so on. Thus, in about a quarter of a century, clinical genetics has gone from being able to get the chromosome count correct to being a recognized medical specialty in some countries.

The last two decades have seen a confluence of cytogenetics, biochemical genetics, immunogenetics and population genetics to constitute the field of clinical genetics as we now know it. Indeed, in the last few years even molecular genetics has joined the clinical genetics stream, as 'recombinant DNA' and 'restriction enzyme' technologies have provided means of diagnosing genetic disease at the level of DNA itself. Thus in a quarter of a century, medical genetics has gone from a primitive state in which the specific enzyme deficiency was known for only a very few inborn errors of metabolism, to being able to recognize the presence of the sickle cell mutation in the DNA of an unborn human being, for example, by the change of a single nucleotide (from CTC to CAC) in the sixth codon of the gene for the beta-chain of hemoglobin.

Human genetics, medical genetics, clinical genetics – these terms deserve definition. *Human genetics* is an academic discipline that is concerned with all aspects of biologically inherited variation in man. *Medical genetics* is that, and much more, since it also involves – indeed has as its main focus – heritable variation in the range that it is 'abnormal,' representing 'disease.' *Clinical genetics* is that aspect of medical genetics concerned with diagnosis, prognosis, management and prevention in individual patients and their families.

Osler's *Principles and Practice of Medicine* was a 'one-man book' for the first seven editions (and 20 years) of its existence. By its very nature, human genetics as a clinical specialty cuts across all other specialties; infectious disease and immunology, as clinical disciplines, have the same characteristic. Because of the peculiar nature of the field of the genetics, multiple authorship of this definitive and authoritative textbook of medical genetics is a necessity.

The breadth of the field of medical genetics is increased further by the fact that, just as 'genetics is the science of variation,' medical genetics is the science of pathologic variation; because of the interplay between genetic and non-genetic factors in determining that variation, exogenous influences either as simulators or as collaborators in etiology and pathogenesis must be kept in mind. Teratology is, thus, an aspect of medical genetics, and much of epidemiology must be encompassed as well.

The medical geneticist is the last of the generalists; he is a general specialist. For many of us the very breadth of the field of medical genetics is one of its most exciting and attractive features. Another is represented by its deep roots in the fundamental aspects of molecular, cellular, and even social biology. Both the breadth and the depth of medical genetics are admirably presented by the Emery-Rimoin textbook.

1983   Victor A. McKusick MD

Preface

Medical Genetics has come of age as a unique specialty in medicine. All practitioners of medicine regardless of their individual specialty, encounter numerous patients with genetic disorders or conditions strongly influenced by hereditary factors and must be aware of their aetiology, pathogenesis, natural history and prognosis, as well as current approaches to their treatment and prevention. Unlike most other medical specialties, which are limited to a body system, age range or diagnostic modality, medical genetics has no such limits, involves all bodily systems and utilizes all manner of diagnostic and therapeutic modalities. In addition, the recent spectacular advances in cellular, biochemical and molecular genetics have been quickly translated into clinical applicability, and thus there are unique diagnostic tools available in modern genetics to which most practitioners of medicine have never been exposed.

There is a vast array of information available relating to genetic disease, which is found not only in genetics or general medical journals but appears throughout the many speciality and subspecialty medical journals and basic science journals as well. Although there are excellent textbooks and reference books dealing with the basic principles of medical genetics, or specific areas of medical genetics and broad catalogues of syndromes, inherited diseases and chromosomal diseases, there is no up-to-date reference source which attempts to cover all areas of medical genetics, from basic principles, to specific diseases, to therapy and prevention. Since most medical geneticists will encounter patients with a wide variety of genetic diseases and since most medical specialty text books do not pay a great deal of attention to the principles of genetics or genetic diseases, it was felt that a broad reference book in medical genetics, ranging from basic principles to applied genetics would be useful. The editors have undertaken the difficult task of trying to compile all of this information under one cover.

This task might have been easier 20 years ago when both of the editors were fellows and doctoral students at the Moore Clinic at Johns Hopkins Hospital with Dr Victor McKusick. At that time medical genetics was a relatively new specialty and the number of authors who could have contributed to this text was quite limited. The explosion of knowledge in genetics has been so great over the last two decades that complete coverage of all aspects of medical genetics is clearly impossible. Rather than ask relatively few individuals to contribute sections covering broad areas, such as the genetics of ophthalmology or the genetics of the endocrine glands, we have elected to conscript over 100 authors, each of whom has been asked to contribute to a relatively well defined area related to their own field of expertise. Thus each of the chapters is written by an individual who has had personal experience in the area in which he has been asked to write. The danger of this type of compilation is that there will be areas of medical genetics that have been excluded because they fell between the lines of the individual experts. We hope that our readers will bring these areas of omission to our attention so that they can be corrected in the next edition. We feel that we have included an outstanding group of international experts who have attempted to bring their current area of expertise to this readership in a relatively brief but complete form, with much of the information in useful tabular form and a fairly complete bibliography. We wish to thank these many individuals for their excellent contributions and apologize for the harassment they may have received from us.

In addition we would like to thank the individuals who contributed in a clerical and editorial fashion to this book including Margaret Fairbairn, Rita Anand, Dorothy Rivera, Toni Armstrong and Elena Hanson. We should also like to thank the publishers themselves especially Andrew Stevenson and Claire McLeod for their encouragement and much helpful advice. Finally, we should especially like to offer our gratitude to Dr Victor McKusick, who kindly agreed to write the foreword to this book. Dr McKusick's teaching, inspiration and encouragement were the prime factors in the development of both of our careers in medical genetics and thus we are doubly grateful to him.

Edinburgh and Los Angeles, 1983
A.E.H.E
D.L.R.

Contributors

Dharam P. Agarwal *PhD*
Professor of Human Genetics
Institute of Hamburg
FRG

Grace E. S. Aherne *BSc MBBS DCH*
Clinical Assistant
University Department of Ophthalmology
Royal Victoria Infirmary
Newcastle upon Tyne
UK

Chester A. Alper *AB MD*
Scientific Director
Center for Blood Research;
Professor of Pediatrics at the Childrens Hospital
Harvard Medical School
Boston, Massachusetts
USA

Ingrun Anton-Lamprecht *ScD*
Director of the Institute for Ultrastructure Research
of the Skin
Hautklinik
Ruprecht-Karls-Universität Heidelberg
FRG

Felicia B. Axelrod *MD*
Associate Professor, Pediatrics
New York University School of Medicine
New York
USA

Howard P. Baden *MD*
Professor of Dermatology
Harvard Medical School;
Dermatologist, Massachusetts General Hospital
Boston, Massachusetts
USA

Robin M. Bannerman *DM FRCP FACP*
Professor of Medicine and Pediatrics;
Head of Divisions of Medical and Human Genetics
State University of New York at Buffalo
USA

Gregory S. Barsh *BS*
Predoctoral Fellow
Department of Pathology
University of Washington
Seattle, Washington
USA

Peter Beighton *MD PhD FRCP DCH*
Professor of Human Genetics
Medical School
University of Cape Town
South Africa

Rosemary Biggs *BSc PhD MD FRCP MA*
Director (Retired)
Oxford Haemophilia Centre
Oxford
UK

D. Timothy Bishop *BSc PhD MSc*
Assistant Professor
Department of Biophysics and Computing
University of Utah
Salt Lake City, Utah
USA

Gerry R. Boss *MD*
Assistant Professor of Medicine
School of Medicine
University of California, San Diego
La Jolla, California
USA

Walter G. Bradley *DM FRCP*
Chairman and Professor of Neurology
University of Vermont College of Medicine
Burlington, Vermont
USA

Peter H. Byers *MD*
Associate Professor
Departments of Pathology and Medicine (Medical
Genetics)
University of Washington
Seattle, Washington
USA

C. O. Carter *DM FRCP*
Professor Emeritus of Clinical Genetics
University of London
London
UK

Ann C. Chandley *PhD DSc*
Senior Research Scientist
MRC Clinical and Population Cytogenetics Unit
Western General Hospital
Edinburgh
UK

Albert de la Chapelle *MD MScD*
Professor and Chairman
Department of Medical Genetics
University of Helsinki
Finland

Joel Charrow *BS MD*
Assistant Professor of Pediatrics
Northwestern University Medical School;
Attending Physician, Division of Genetics
Children's Memorial Hospital
Chicago, Illinois
USA

M. Michael Cohen Jr *DMD PhD*
Professor of Oral Pathology
Faculty of Dentistry;
Professor of Pediatrics
Faculty of Medicine
Dalhousie University
Halifax, Nova Scotia
Canada

David R. Cox *MD PhD*
Assistant Professor of Pediatrics
Department of Pediatrics
University of California
San Francisco, California
USA

David Miles Danks *MD BS FRACP*
Professor of Paediatrics
University of Melbourne;
Director, Birth Defects Research Institute
Royal Children's Hospital Research
Foundation
Melbourne
Australia

A. Davie *PhD*
S.E.R.C. Research Fellow
Department of Mathematics
University of Edinburgh
Edinburgh
UK

John H. DiLiberti *MD*
Associate Professor of Pediatrics
Oregan Health Sciences University;
Chief of Pediatrics
Emanuel Hospital
Portland, Oregon
USA

George N. Donnell *MD*
Winzer Professor and Chairman
Department of Pediatrics
USC School of Medicine;
Pediatrician-in-Chief
Childrens Hospital of Los Angeles
Los Angeles, California
USA

Victor Dubowitz *MD PhD FRCP DCH*
Professor of Paediatrics
Department of Neonatal Medicine;
Co-director
Jerry Lewis Muscle Research Centre
Royal Postgraduate Medical School
London
UK

Roswell Eldridge *MD*
Head, Clinical Neurogenetic Studies
NES, NINCDS, National Institutes of Health
Bethesda, Maryland
USA

Richard Emanuel *MA DM FRCP FACC*
Senior Cardiologist
The Middlesex Hospital;
Physician to the National Heart Hospital;
Lecturer, Cardiothoracic Institute
London
UK

Alan E. H. Emery *MD PhD DSc FRCP FRS*
Professor and Chairman
University Department of Human Genetics
Western General Hospital
Edinburgh
UK

Charles J. Epstein *MD*
Professor of Pediatrics and Biochemistry
University of California
San Francisco, California
USA

Richard W. Erbe *MD*
Associate Professor of Pediatrics
Harvard Medical School;
Chief, Genetics Unit
Massachusetts General Hospital
Boston, Massachusetts
USA

D. A. Price Evans *MD DSc PhD FRCP*
Professor of Medicine;
Chairman, Department of Medicine;
Director, Nuffield Unit of Medical Genetics
University of Liverpool;
Honorary Consultant Physician
Royal Liverpool Hospital and
Broadgreen Hospital
Liverpool
UK

Gerald M. Fenichel *MD*
Professor and Chairman
Department of Neurology;
Professor, Department of Pediatrics
School of Medicine
Vanderbuilt University
Nashville, Tenessee
USA

Delbert A. Fisher *MD*
Professor of Pediatrics and Medicine
UCLA School of Medicine
Harbor-UCLA Medical Center
Torrance, California
USA

Uta Francke *MD*
Associate Professor of Human Genetics and Pediatrics
Yale University School of Medicine
New Haven, Connecticut
USA

Jeffrey Friedman *MD*
Clinical Affiliate
Children's Hospital of Philadelphia;
Associate Director, Clinical Investigation
Wyeth Laboratories
Philadelphia, Pennsylvania
USA

Ingrid Gamstorp *MD*
Professor of Child Neurology
Department of Pediatrics
University Hospital
Uppsala
Sweden

Tobias Gedde-Dahl Jr *MD PhD*
Senior Geneticist
Department of Genetics
The Norwegian Radiumhospital
Oslo
Norway

Park S. Gerald *MD*
Chief, Clinical Genetics Division
Children's Hospital Medical Center;
Professor, Department of Pediatrics
Harvard Medical School
Boston, Massachusetts
USA

H. Werner Goedde *MD*
Professor and Director
Institute of Human Genetics
University of Hamburg
Hamburg
FRG

Lowell A Goldsmith *MD*
James H. Sterner Professor of Dermatology;
Chief, Dermatology Unit (Medicine)
University of Rochester School of Medicine and
Dentistry
Rochester, New York
USA

Richard M. Goodman *MD*
Professor of Human Genetics
Sackler School of Medicine
Tel Aviv University
The Chaim Sheba Medical Center
Tel Hashomer
Israel

Stephen I. Goodman *MD CM*
Professor of Pediatrics
University of Colorado School of Medicine
Denver, Colorado
USA

Jean de Grouchy *MD*
Directeur de Recherche CNRS-Paris-France;
Directeur de Laboratoire de
Cytogénétique Humaine et Comparée
Hôpital Necker-Enfants-Malades,
Paris
France

Kevin Grumbach *BS*
Research Assistant
Cornell University Medical College
New York
USA

Judith G. Hall *MD*
Professor of Medical Genetics
University of British Columbia
Vancouver, British Columbia
Canada

James W. Hanson *MD*
Associate Professor of Pediatrics;
Chairman, Division of Medical Genetics
University of Iowa Hospitals and Clinics
Iowa City, Iowa
USA

A. E. Harding *MD MRCP*
Registrar in Neurology
The National Hospital for Nervous Diseases,
Queen Square
London
UK

Peter S. Harper *MA DM FRCP*
Professor of Medical Genetics
Welsh National School of Medicine;
Consultant in Medical Genetics;
Consultant Physician
University Hospital of Wales
Cardiff
UK

Rodney Harris *BSc MD FRCP FRCPath DTM&H*
Professor of Medical Genetics
University of Manchester
St Mary's Hospital
Manchester
UK

John R. Heckenlively *AB MD*
Assistant Professor
Department of Ophthalmology;
Associate Member
Jules Stein Eye Institute
UCLA School of Medicine
Los Angeles, California
USA

John Z. Heckmatt *MBChB MRCP*
Nattrass Memorial Lecturer in Paediatric Neurology
Department of Paediatrics and Neonatal Medicine
Royal Postgraduate Medical School
London
UK

Kurt Hirschhorn *MD*
Herbert H. Lehman Professor of Medicine;
Chairman, Department of Pediatrics
Mount Sinai Medical Center
New York
USA

Rochelle Hirschhorn *MD*
Professor of Medicine
New York University School of Medicine
New York
USA

Karen A. Holbrook *PhD*
Associate Professor
Departments of Biological Structure and Medicine
University of Washington
Seattle, Washington
USA

J. J. Hoo *MD*
Research Associate
Institute of Human Genetics
University of Hamburg
Hamburg
FRG

Phillip A. Hooker *MD PhD*
Department of Dermatology
Harvard Medical School
Massachusetts General Hospital
Boston, Massachusetts
USA

William A. Horton *MD*
Associate Professor of Medicine and Pediatrics
University of Kansas Medical Center
College of Health Sciences
Kansas City, Kansas
USA

Paul S. Ing *PhD*
Clinical Genetics Associate
Boys Town Institute for Communication
Disorders in Children
Omaha, Nebraska
USA

Sherwin J. Isenberg *BA MD*
Associate Professor and Vice-Chairman
Department of Ophthalmology
UCLA School of Medicine;
Pediatric Ophthalmologist
Jules Stein Eye Institute;
Chief of Ophthalmology
Harbor/UCLA Medical Center
California
USA

Charles E. Jackson *MD*
Chief, Clinical Genetics Division
Department of Medicine
Henry Ford Hospital, Detroit;
Clinical Professor, Department of Medicine
University of Michigan School of Medicine
Ann Arbor, Michigan
USA

Kenneth Lyons Jones Jr *MD*
Associate Professor, Department of Pediatrics
University of California, San Diego
School of Medicine
La Jolla, California,
USA

Marilyn C. Jones *MD*
Assistant Professor of Pediatrics
University of California, San Diego;
Director, Dysmorphology and Genetics
Children's Hospital
San Diego, California
USA

Michael M. Kaback *MD*
Professor, Departments of Pediatrics and Medicine
UCLA School of Medicine;
Associate Chief, Division of Medical Genetics
Harbor-UCLA School of Medicine
Torrance, California
USA

Haig H. Kazazian Jr *MD*
Professor of Pediatrics
Johns Hopkins University School of Medicine
Johns Hopkins Hospital
Baltimore, Maryland
USA

John Kelemen *MD*
Director, Neuromuscular Service
Nassau County Medical Center;
Assistant Professor of Neurology
S.U.N.Y. at Stony Brook
New York
USA

Dennis K. Kinney *PhD*
Lecturer on Psychology
Department of Psychiatry
Harvard Medical School;
Assistant Psychologist,
McLean Hospital,
Belmont, Massachusetts,
USA

Hans-Reinhard Koch *MD*
Professor
Universitäts-Augenklinik
Venusberg
Bonn
FRG

Ralph S. Lachman *MD*
Professor of Radiology and Pediatrics
UCLA School of Medicine;
Chief, Division of Pediatric Radiology
Harbor-UCLA Medical Center
Torrance, California
USA

Michael Laurence *MA DSc MBChB FRCP FRCPath*
Professor of Paediatric Research
Welsh National School of Medicine;
Hon. Consultant Clinical Genetics
South Glamorgan Health Authority
Heath Park, Cardiff
UK

Claire O. Leonard *MD*
Assistant Professor of Pediatrics
University of Utah
Salt Lake City, Utah
USA

Jules G. Leroy *MD PhD*
Professor of Genetics and Medical Genetics
Antwerp University Medical School
Wilryk
Belgium

Lenore S. Levine *MD*
Professor of Pediatrics;
Program Director, Pediatric Clinical Research Center;
Associate Director, Pediatric Endocrinology
Cornell University Medical College
New York
USA

Jack Lieberman *MD*
Chief, Respiratory Disease Section
Sepulveda Veterans Administration Medical Center;
Professor of Medicine,
UCLA School of Medicine
Los Angeles, California
USA

Herbert A. Lubs *MD*
Professor of Pediatrics;
Director Genetics Division
University of Miami School of Medicine
Miami, Florida
USA

W. Morrice McCrae *MBChB FRCP*
Consultant Physician
Royal Hospital for Sick Children;
Senior I ecturer, Department of Child Life and Health
University of Edinburgh
Edinburgh
UK

Virginia Michels *MD*
Assistant Professor – Genetics
Mayo Clinic
Rochester, Minnesota
USA

Michael E. Miller *MD*
Professor and Chairman,
Department of Pediatrics
University of California, Davis
School of Medicine
Davis, California
USA

Orlando J. Miller *BS MD*
Professor of Human Genetics and Development;
Professor of Obstetrics and Gynecology
College of Physicians and Surgeons
Columbia University;
Attending Obstetrician and Gynecologist,
Columbia Presbyterian Medical Center
New York
USA

Hugo W. Moser *MD*
Director, John F. Kennedy Institute;
Professor of Neurology and Pediatrics
Johns Hopkins University
Baltimore, Maryland
USA

Byron Myhre *MD PhD*
Professor of Pathology
UCLA School of Medicine
Los Angeles, California
USA

Henry L. Nadler *MD*
Dean and Professor of Pediatrics,
Wayne State University School of Medicine
Detroit, Michigan
USA

Maria I. New *MD*
Professor and Chairman, Department of Pediatrics;
Division Head, Pediatric Endocrinology;
Associate Program Director, Pediatric Clinical Research Center;
Harold and Percy Uris Professor of Pediatric Endocrinology and Metabolism
Cornell University Medical College
New York
USA

Won G. Ng *PhD*
Associate Professor of Research Pediatrics
University of Southern California
School of Medicine
Los Angeles, California
USA

Reijo Norio *MD*
Docent of Clinical Genetics
University of Helsinki;
Director, Department of Medical Genetics
Väestölitto, the Finnish Population and
Family Welfare Federation
Helsinki
Finland

Marlene Otter *PhD*
Department of Medicine
University of Chicago
Chicago, Illinois
USA

Eberhard Passarge *MD*
Professor of Human Genetics
Department of Human Genetics
University of Essen
FRG

John H Pearn *AM MD PhD FRCP FRACP DCH*
Reader in Child Health
Royal Childrens Hospital
Brisbane, Queensland
Australia

Alan K. Percy *MD*
Associate Professor of Pediatrics (Neurology)
Baylor College of Medicine
Houston, Texas
USA

John A. Phillips III *MD*
Associate Professor of Pediatrics
Johns Hopkins University
School of Medicine
Johns Hopkins Hospital
Baltimore, Maryland
USA

Reed E. Pyeritz *MD PhD FACP FABMG*
Assistant Professor of Medicine and Pediatrics;
Director of Clinical Services
Medical Genetics
Johns Hopkins University School of Medicine,
Baltimore, Maryland
USA

J. A. Raeburn *MBChB PhD FRCP*
Senior Lecturer
Department of Human Genetics
University of Edinburgh;
Honorary Consultant
Lothian Health Board
Edinburgh
UK

Craig T. Ramey *PhD*
Professor of Psychology and Director of Research
Frank Porter Graham Child Development Center
University of North Carolina
Chapel Hill, North Carolina
USA

Vincent M. Riccardi *MD*
Associate Professor of Medicine, Pediatrics and Ob-Gyn
Baylor College of Medicine,
Houston, Texas
USA

David L. Rimoin *MD PhD*
Professor of Pediatrics and Medicine
UCLA School of Medicine;
Chief, Division of Medical Genetics
Harbor-UCLA Medical Center
Torrance, California
USA

D. F. Roberts *ScD*
Professor of Human Genetics,
University of Newcastle upon Tyne;
Hon. Consultant in Genetics to the Royal
Victoria Infirmary
Newcastle
UK

Pauline E. Robertson *MBChB DObst RGOG*
Registrar
Department of Human Genetics
Western General Hospital
Edinburgh
UK

Thomas F. Roe *MD*
Associate Professor, Clinical Pediatrics
University of Southern California
School of Medicine
Los Angeles, California
USA

Fred S. Rosen *MD*
James L. Gamble Professor of Pediatrics
Harvard University Medical School
Cambridge, Massachusetts
USA

Jerome I. Rotter *MD*
Assistant Professor of Medicine and Pediatrics
UCLA School of Medicine
Division of Medical Genetics
Harbor-UCLA Medical Center
Torrance, California
USA

Janet D. Rowley *MD*
Professor, Department of Medicine
University of Chicago
Chicago, Illinois
USA

R. Neil Schimke *MD*
Professor of Medicine and Pediatrics,
Division Director, Metabolism, Endocrinology and
Genetics
College of Health Sciences and Hospital
Kansas City, Kansas
USA

Eveline E. Schneeberger *MD*
Department of Pathology
Massachusetts General Hospital;
Associate Professor, Department of Pathology
Harvard Medical School,
Cambridge, Massachusetts,
USA

C. Ronald Scott *MD*
Professor, Department of Pediatrics,
University of Washington,
Seattle, Washington
USA

J. Edwin Seegmiller *MD*
Professor of Medicine
Department of Medicine
University of California, San Diego
La Jolla, California,
USA

Larry J. Shapiro *MD*
Associate Professor of Pediatrics
UCLA School of Medicine,
Division of Medical Genetics
Harbor-UCLA Medical Center
Torrance, California
USA

David O. Sillence *MD FRACP*
Senior Lecturer in Human Genetics,
University of Sydney;
Visiting Physician, Genetics Clinic,
Royal Alexandra Hospital for Children
New South Wales
Australia

Marcel Simon *MD*
Professeur de Clinique Médicale
Clinique Médicale B
Hôpital Sud,
Rennes
France

Joe Leigh Simpson *MD*
Professor of Obstetrics and Gynecology;
Head, Section of Human Genetics
North Western University Medical School
Chicago, Illinois
USA

Rosalind Skinner *MB BS MD*
Clinical Lecturer
University Department of Human Genetics
Western General Hospital
Edinburgh
UK

Håvard Skre *MD*
Director, Department of Neurology
Akershus Central Hospital;
Associate Professor of Neurology,
University of Oslo
Oslo
Norway

Jeffrey A. Sofaer *BDS PhD*
Senior Lecturer, Department of Oral Medicine and Oral
Pathology and Department of Human Genetics
University of Edinburgh
Edinburgh
UK

J. Spranger *MD*
Professor of Pediatrics
Children's Hospital
University of Mainz
Mainz
FRG

Joel Sugar *BA MD*
Associate Professor of Ophthalmology;
Director, Cornea Service
University of Illinois Hospital
Eye and Ear Infirmary
Chicago, Illinois
USA

Graham Sutton *MBChB PhD*
Registrar in Community Medicine
Lothian Health Board
Edinburgh
UK

P. K. Thomas *DSc MD FRCP*
Professor of Neurology
University of London
Royal Free Hospital School of Medicine
and the Institute of Neurology
London
UK

Catherine Turleau *MD*
Chargé de Recherche CNRS – Paris – France;
Laboratoire de Cytogénétique Humaine et Comparée
Hôpital Necker-Enfants-Malades
Paris
France

Gerd Utermann *MD*
Institut für Humangenetik und
Genetische Poliklinik
Philipps-Universität Marburg
Marburg
FRG

Demetris Vassilopoulos *MD PhD*
Reader in Neurology
Department of Neurology
University of Athens
Athens
Greece

Arthur M. O. Veale *MBChB PhD FRACP MCCMNZ*
Professor of Human Genetics and Community Health
University of Auckland,
Auckland
New Zealand

Friedrich Vogel *MD*
Professor of Human Genetics;
Director, Institut für Anthropologie und Humangenetik
University of Heidelburg
FRG

Mette Warburg *MD*
Consulting Ophthalmologist
Gentofte Hospital
Department for the Multiple Handicapped
Gentofte
Denmark

Alfred Wegener *Dip Biol*
Universitäts-Augenklinik
Venusberg
Bonn
FRG

L. N. Went *DSc*
Professor of Human Genetics
University of Leiden
Leiden
The Netherlands

Robert Williamson *PhD FRCPath*
Professor of Biochemistry
St Mary's Hospital Medical School
University of London
London
UK

R. F. J. Withers *MSc AKC*
Senior Lecturer in Human Genetics
Middlesex Hospital Medical School
London
UK

Carl J. Witkop Jr *BS DDS MS*
Professor and Chairman, Division of Genetics
Department of Oral Pathology and Genetics
School of Dentistry;
Professor of Dermatology
School of Medicine
University of Minnesota
Minneapolis, Minnesota
USA

Jonathan Zonana *MD*
Associate Professor of Medical Genetics,
Pediatrics and Crippled Children's
Division
Oregon Health Sciences University;
Director of Regional Services
Crippled Children's Division
Eugene, Oregon
USA

Contents *Volume 2*

Contents *Volume 1*

The chondrodysplasias

D. L. Rimoin and R. S. Lachman

The skeletal dysplasias are a heterogeneous group of disorders associated with abnormalities in the size and shape of the limbs, trunk and/or skull which frequently result in disproportionate short stature. Until the 1960's, most disproportionate dwarfs were considered to have either achondroplasia (those with short limbs) or Morquio disease (those with short trunk). It is now apparent that there are over 80 distinct skeletal dysplasias which have been classified primarily on the basis of their clinical or roentgenographic characteristics (Appendix and General References).

CLASSIFICATION AND NOMENCLATURE

Current nomenclature for these disorders is most confusing and is based on the part of the skeleton that is affected roentgenographically (e.g., the epiphyseal dysplasias, the metaphyseal dysplasias), on a Greek term that describes the appearance of the bone or the course of the disease (e.g., diastrophic [twisted] dysplasia, thanatophoric [death-seeking] dysplasia), on an eponym (e.g., Kniest dysplasia, Ellis van Creveld syndrome), or by a term that attempts to describe the pathogenesis of the condition (e.g., achondroplasia, osteogenesis imperfecta). The extent of the heterogeneity in these disorders and the variety of methods used for their classification have resulted in further confusion. Clinical classifications have divided the skeletal dysplasias into those with short-limbed dwarfism, and those with short-trunk dwarfism. The short-limbed varieties have been further subdivided on the basis of the segment of the long bones that is most severely involved. Other clinical classifications have been based on the age of onset of the disorder: those disorders that manifest themselves at birth (achondroplasia) versus those that first manifest in later life (e.g., pseudoachondroplasia). Associated clinical abnormalities have also been used in subdividing these disorders. Examples are the myopia of spondyloepiphyseal dysplasia congenita, the cleft palate of Kniest dysplasia, the fine hair of cartilage-hair hypoplasia, and the polydactyly and congenital heart disease of the Ellis van Creveld syndrome. Still other disorders have been classified on the basis of their apparent mode of inheritance; for example, the dominant and X–linked varieties of spondyloepiphyseal dysplasia.

The most widely used method for differentiating the skeletal dysplasias has been the detection of skeletal radiographic abnormalities. Radiographic classifications are based on the different parts of the long bones that are abnormal (epiphyses, metaphyses or diaphyses) (Fig. 51.1 and 51.2). Thus, there are epiphyseal and metaphyseal dysplasias which can be further divided depending on whether or not the spine is also involved (spondyloepiphyseal dysplasias, spondylometaphyseal dysplasias). Furthermore, each of these classes can be further divided into several distinct disorders based on a variety of other clinical and radiographic differences.

In an attempt to develop a uniform nomenclature for these syndromes, an International Nomenclature of Constitutional Diseases of Bone was proposed in 1970

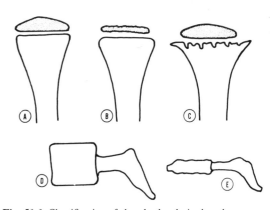

Fig. 51.1 Classification of chondrodysplasias based on radiologic involvement of long bones (A,B,C) and vertebrae (D,E).

Involvement	Disease category
A+D	Normal
B+D	Epiphyseal dysplasia
C+D	Metaphyseal dysplasia
B+E	Spondyloepiphyseal dysplasia
C+E	Spondylometaphyseal dysplasia
B+C+E	Spondyloepimetaphyseal dysplasia

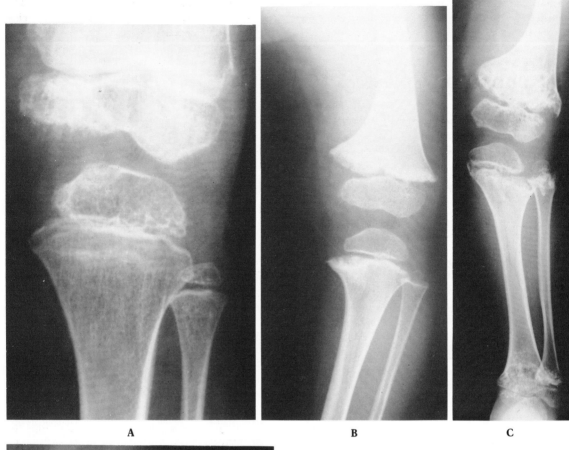

A   B   C

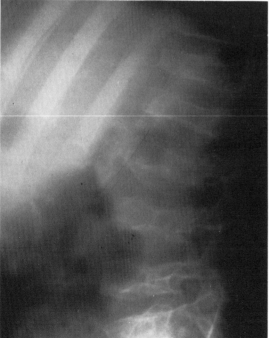

D

Fig. 51.2 Radiographs of knee (A,B,C) and spine (D) from patients with a variety of chondrodysplasias.
A. Epiphyseal dysplasia – note the small irregular epiphyses and normal metaphyses, from a patient with spondyloepiphyseal dysplasia congenita
B. Metaphyseal dysplasia – note the irregular and widened metaphyses with normal epiphyses, from a patient with metaphyseal dysplasia, type Schmid.
C. Epimetaphyseal dysplasia – note the abnormal epiphyses and metaphyses from a patient with spondyloepimetaphyseal dysplasia – type Strudwick.
D. Platyspondyly – note the flat and irregular vertebrae from a patient with spondylometaphyseal dysplasia, type Kozlowski.

and updated in 1977 (See Appendix). This International Nomenclature divides the constitutional disorders of the skeleton into five major groups: the osteochondrodysplasias (abnormal growth or development of cartilage and/or bone), the dysostoses (malformations of individual bones, singly or in combination), (Chapter 54), the idiopathic osteolyses (a group of disorders associated with multifocal resorption of bone), the skeletal disorders associated with chromosomal aberrations and primary metabolic disorders.

The osteochondrodysplasias are further divided into: 1) defects of growth of tubular bones and/or spine (e.g., achondroplasia), which are frequently referred to as chondrodysplasias (this Chapter); 2) disorganized development of cartilage and fibrous components of the skeleton (e.g., multiple cartilagenous exostoses) (Chapter 53); and 3) abnormalities of density or cortical diaphyseal structure and/or metaphyseal modelling (e.g., osteogenesis imperfecta) (Chapter 52).

The chondrodysplasias are further subdivided into those disorders manifest at birth as opposed to those that first become apparent in later life. This division may be purely artificial, since identical pathogenetic mechanisms of differing degrees of severity may occur in allelic disorders resulting in differences in the age of manifestation. For example, both congenital and infantile presentations of osteogenesis imperfecta are seen within the same families manifesting dominant inheritance. On the other hand, many disorders which share common radiographic features and have thus been classified into one group, such as the spondyloepiphyseal dysplasias, almost certainly result from different pathogenetic mechanisms.

As short stature is a frequent finding in these disorders, the term 'dwarfism' has been historically used for them. However, 'dwarfism' is thought to result in stigmatization and is popularly unappealing, and for these and other reasons, the term 'dwarfism' has been dropped from the current nomenclature and replaced by the term 'dysplasia'. This latter term, which means 'disordered growth,' reflects the probable pathogenesis of the majority of the chondrodysplasias. In contrast, malformations of single bones or groups of bones, which presumably do not reflect a generalized disorder of the skeleton, have been referred to as 'dysostoses'.

Although the International Nomenclature provides a uniform standard for referring to specific disorders, so that the same disease is called the same thing by all authors, many of the names are inaccurate. For example, achondroplasia and achondrogenesis are inaccurate terms in defining the pathogenesis of these conditions, but are so well entrenched in the literature that they persist. As the morphology, pathogenesis, and especially the basic biochemical defect in each of these disorders is unraveled, this nomenclature should be changed to refer to the specific pathogenetic or metabolic defect. The aetiologic or pathogenetic nomenclature is now being used for certain skeletal dysplasias, such as the mucopolysaccharidoses, mucolipidoses and disorders of mineralization (e.g., β-glucuronidase deficiency, fucosidosis, hypophosphatasia).

CLINICAL EVALUATION

The osteochondrodysplasias are syndromes which represent generalized disorders of the skeleton and usually result in disproportionate short stature. Affected individuals usually present with the complaint of disproportionate short stature and the abnormality in stature must first be documented by the use of the appropriate growth curves with adjustment for ethnic background and parental heights (Rimoin & Horton, 1978). In general, patients with disproportionate short stature have skeletal dysplasias, whereas those with relatively normal body proportions have endocrine, nutritional, prenatal or other nonskeletal defects. There are exceptions to these rules, as cretinism can lead to disproportionate short stature, and a variety of skeletal dysplasias, such as osteogenesis imperfecta and hypophosphatasia may result in normal body proportions.

A disproportionate body habitus may not be readily apparent on casual physical examination. Thus anthropometric measurements, such as upper to lower segment ratio, sitting height and arm span must be obtained before the possibility of a mild skeletal dysplasia, such as hypochondroplasia or multiple epiphyseal dysplasia can be excluded. Although sitting height is a more accurate measure of head and trunk length, it requires special equipment for consistent accuracy. Upper to lower segment ratios (U/L), on the other hand, provide a fairly accurate measure of body proportions and can be easily obtained. The lower segment measure is taken from the symphysis pubis to the floor at the inside of the heel, and the upper segment is obtained by subtracting the lower segment value from the total height. McKusick (1972), has published standard U/L curves for both Caucasian and Black Americans which are quite useful for rapid assessment of proportion. For example, a Caucasian infant has an upper/lower segment ratio of approximately 1.7; it reaches 1.0 at approximately 7–10 years, and then falls to an average U/L of 0.95 as an adult. Blacks, on the other hand, have relatively long limbs, and reach a U/L of approximately 0.85 as adults. Another index of limb versus trunk length is based on the arm span measurement, which usually falls within a few centimeters of total height. These measurements are most useful in determining whether or not an abnormally short individual is proportionate or not, and the type of disproportion present. For example, a short-limbed

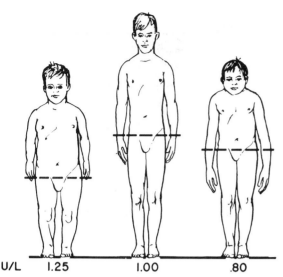

U/L   1.25   1.00   .80

Fig. 51.3 Upper-Lower segment ratios in 8 to 10 year old individuals with short limb dwarfism, proportionate stature and short trunk dwarfism (from left to right respectively). The child on the left has short limbs and short stature with an elevated U/L, whereas the child on the right has a short trunk and short stature with a reduced U/L. U/L equals upper segment length/lower segment length.

dwarf will have an abnormally high U/L ratio and an arm span which is considerably shorter than his height (Fig. 51.3).

As in the differential diagnosis of most other disorders, an accurate history, family history and physical examination may lead one to the correct diagnosis. As the International Nomenclature indicates, certain skeletal dysplasias have prenatal onset and manifest at birth, whereas others may not manifest until late infancy or early childhood. Thus a child who was normal until 2 years of age and then develops disproportionate short-limbed dwarfism is more likely to have pseudoachondroplasia or multiple epiphyseal dysplasia than achondroplasia or SED congenita. As has already been pointed out, classification on the basis of age of onset may not be totally accurate, as in certain disorders marked variability in expression is seen with both prenatal and postnatal onset of the disease in the same family (e.g., osteogenesis imperfecta type I). Furthermore, many parents may not notice short stature until one or two years of age, whereas, in reality, it existed from the time of birth.

A detailed physical examination may reveal the correct diagnosis or point to the likely diagnostic category (Table 51.1). First, one must establish whether the disproportionate shortening affects primarily the trunk or the limbs, and if the latter, whether it is proximal (rhizomelic), middle segment (mesomelic), or distal

(acromelic), or a combination of these (Figure 51.4). A disproportionately *large head* with frontal bossing and flattening of the bridge of the nose suggests achondroplasia or thanatophoric dysplasia. *Clover-leaf skull* is sometimes associated with thanatophoric dysplasia and rarely with campomelic dysplasia and a variety of malformation syndromes. *Congenital cataracts* suggest chondrodysplasia punctata. *Myopia* may be found associated with Kniest dysplasia or spondyloepiphyseal dysplasia congenita. Complete or partial *cleft palate*, bifid uvula or high-arched palate may be found in Kniest dysplasia, spondyloepiphyseal dysplasia congenita or diastrophic dysplasia. The *upper lip* is short and tethered in chondroectodermal dysplasia. Acute swelling of the *pinnae of the ears* in the newborn period, followed by cauliflower ears, is characteristic of diastrophic dysplasia.

Postaxial *polydactyly* is characteristic of chondroectodermal dysplasia and of the lethal short rib-polydactyly syndromes, and may also be seen in asphyxiating thoracic dysplasia (Fig. 51-5). Preaxial polydactyly is frequently observed in chondroectodermal dysplasia, short rib-polydactyly syndrome II (Majewski) and rarely in short rib-polydactyly syndrome I (Saldino-Noonan). In diastrophic dysplasia the *hands* are short and broad, the thumbs are hypermobile, proximally inserted and abducted leading to the 'hitch-hiker thumb' configuration, and flexion creases in the fingers are frequently absent (Fig. 51.5). In achondroplastic children, the hand has a trident appearance (Fig. 51.5). Hypoplastic *nails* are characteristic of chondroectodermal dysplasia, whereas the nails may be short and broad in the McKusick type of metaphyseal dysplasia (cartilage-hair hypoplasia). *Club feet* may be seen in infants with Kniest dysplasia, SED congenita, osteogenesis imperfecta, but are most characteristic of diastrophic dysplasia. Multiple *joint dislocations* suggest Larsen syndrome, Ehlers-Danlos syndrome type VII, or otopalatodigital syndrome; less severe degrees of joint laxity, particularly of the hands, may be seen in other types of skeletal dysplasia (e.g., cartilage-hair hypoplasia and pseudoachondroplasia). Bone *fractures* may occur in all of the osteogenesis imperfecta syndromes and several types of hypophosphatasia, osteopetrosis, dysosteosclerosis and achondrogenesis type I (Parenti-Fraccaro).

In the neonate or infant, a long, narrow *thorax* suggests asphyxiating thoracic dysplasia, chondroectodermal dysplasia or metatropic dysplasia. A very small thorax is also seen in thanatophoric dysplasia, the short rib-polydactyly syndromes and homozygous achondroplasia. In some neonates with spondyloepiphyseal dysplasia congenita, the sternum and neck is short and the chest may be small with pectus carinatum producing early respiratory distress. In the child or adult, *scoliosis* is frequently seen in metatropic dysplasia and diastrophic dysplasia, whereas a short, broad thorax with

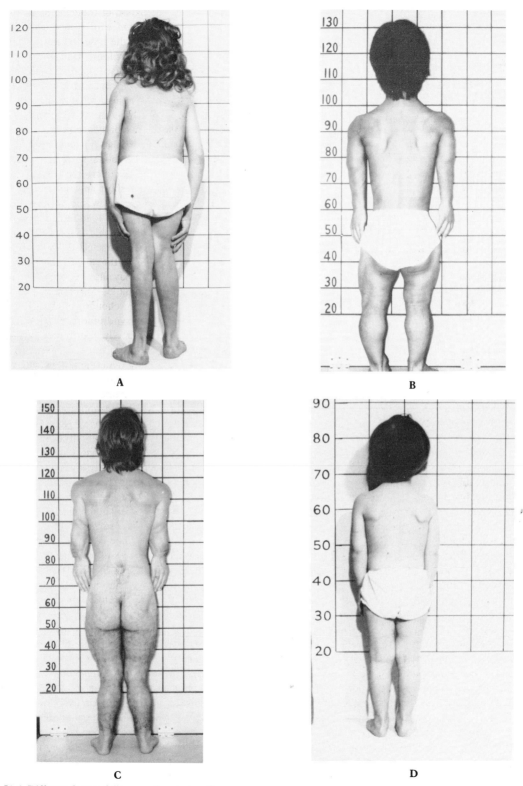

Fig. 51.4 Different forms of disproportionate dwarfism.
A. Short trunk dwarfism in a girl with Dyggve-Melchior-Clausen syndrome.
B. Short limb dwarfism of the rhizomelic type in a boy with achondroplasia.
C. Short limb dwarfism of the mesomelic type in a boy with mesomelic dysplasia, Langer type.
D. Short limb dwarfism of the acromelic type in a girl with peripheral dysostosis.

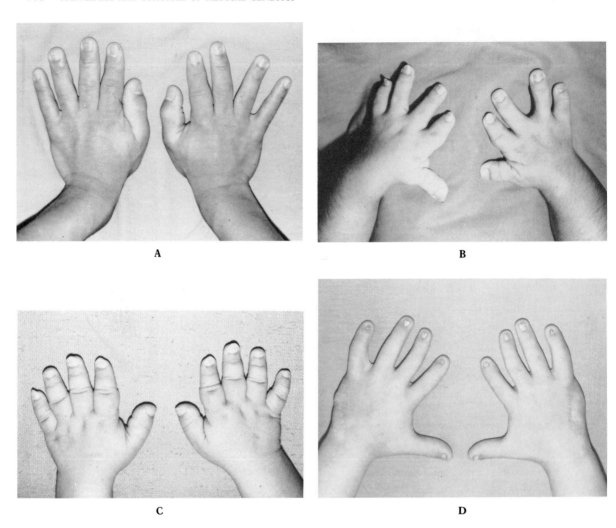

Fig. 51.5 Characteristic hand abnormalities in different types of chondrodysplasia.
A. Achondroplasia – note the trident appearance of the hand and generalized brachydactyly.
B. Diastrophic dysplasia – note the hitch hiker thumb and synphalangism.
C. Metaphyseal chondrodysplasia type McKusick – note the short hypermobile hands with squared off terminal phalanges.
D. Chondroectodermal dysplasia – note the repaired post axial polydactyly and the nail dysplasia.

Harrison's grooves is a frequent manifestation in various metaphyseal dysplasias.

Congenital *cardiac defects* are seen in several of the skeletal dysplasias. In chondroectodermal dysplasia, the most common lesion is an atrial septal defect with a common atrium. In short rib-polydactyly syndrome I (Saldino-Noonan), a variety of very complex lesions involving the great vessels, transposition or double outlet right or left ventricle and ventricular septal defect have been reported, whereas in short rib-polydactyly syndrome II (Majewski), the most common cardiac defect is transposition of the great vessels.

Gastrointestinal manifestations are not common in the skeletal dysplasias, but congenital megacolon can be seen in cartilage-hair hypoplasia, malabsorption in the Schwachman-Diamond syndrome, and anorectal anomalies in short rib-polydactyly syndrome.

In the older child or adult, the complications associated with specific disorders may aid in the diagnosis. For example, *spinal stenosis* with symptoms of spinal cord claudication are characteristic of achondroplasia, whereas *odontoid hypoplasia* and C-1-C-2 subluxation are frequently seen in Morquio disease and spondyloepiphyseal dysplasia. *Genu varum* is seen in a number of skeletal dysplasias, but in achondroplasia it is associated with lateral curvature primarily of the middle seg-

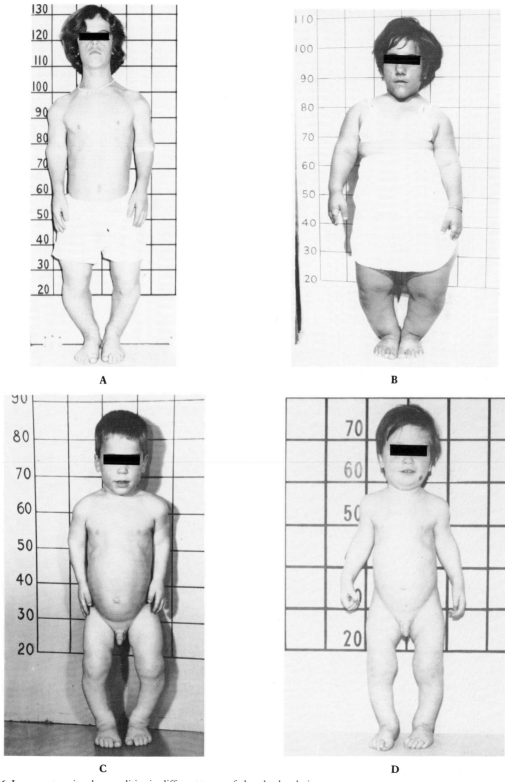

Fig. 51.6 Lower extremity abnormalities in different types of chondrodysplasia.
A. Achondroplasia – note the genu varum with marked proximal over growth of fibula
B. Metaphyseal chondrodysplasia, type McKusick – note the genu varum with marked distal over growth of the fibula.
C. Pseudoachondroplastic dysplasia – note the marked genu varum involving the entire lower extremity.
D. Metatropic dysplasia – note the genu varum with prominence of the knees and ankles.

ment of the limb with overgrowth of the fibula proximally, whereas in cartilage-hair hypoplasia, there is generalized bowing with marked overgrowth of the fibula distally (Fig. 51.6). In pseudoachondroplasia, genu varum, valgum or a windswept abnormality may be seen, but it is associated with severe instability and ligamentous laxity at the knees (Fig. 51.6). Thus, careful physical examination with delineation of all of the skeletal and nonskeletal abnormalities can be quite helpful in arriving at a diagnosis.

A complete family history, details of stillborn children and parental consanguinity should be obtained. Parents should always be closely examined, looking for evidence of a dysplasia in a partially expressed form. This is especially important in dominantly inherited disorders with wide variability of expressivity, where a parent may be mildly affected without knowing it (e.g., osteogenesis imperfecta). The health of parental sibs, especially male sibs and male relatives of the mother, should be questioned, as some conditions are inherited in an X–linked fashion. Since each of the skeletal dysplasias most frequently present as an isolated case in the family, an isolated instance of a skeletal dysplasia in a family cannot provide information as to the mode of inheritance of the particular disorder. However, the type of familial aggregation, when it occurs, can be most helpful. For example, affected sibs with normal parents indicates a recessive type of disease and, for the most part, rules out autosomal dominant disorders, such as achondroplasia and hypochondroplasia. If two achondroplastic parents produce a severely affected offspring, it is most likely homozygous achondroplasia, rather than thanatophoric dysplasia. However, different modes of inheritance have been observed in disorders that cannot be distinguished clinically, such as the X–linked and certain autosomal forms of spondyloepiphyseal dysplasia.

RADIOLOGICAL EVALUATION

The next step in the evaluation of the disproportionately short patient is to obtain a full set of skeletal radiographs. A full series of skeletal views including anterior and posterior, lateral and Towne views of the skull, anterior – posterior and lateral views of the spine, anterior – posterior views of the pelvis and extremities, with separate views of the hands and feet is usually required. Lateral views of the foot are particularly helpful in identifying punctate calcification of the calcaneous which may be a clue to the diagnosis of the milder forms of chondrodysplasia punctata, confirming the absence of hypoplasia of calcaneus and talus in newborns with SED congenita, and in delineating the double ossification centers of the calcaneus in the Larsen syndrome. Skele-

tal radiographs alone will often be sufficient to make an accurate diagnosis, since the classification of skeletal dysplasias has been based primarily on roentgenology (Table 51.1). Attention should be paid to the specific parts of the skeleton which are involved (spine, limbs, pelvis, skull) and within each bone, to the location of the lesion (epiphysis, metaphysis, diaphysis) (Figures 51.2 and 51.3). The skeletal radiographic features of many of these diseases change with age and it is usually beneficial to review radiographs taken at different ages when possible. In some disorders, the radiographic abnormalities following epiphyseal fusion are nonspecific, so that the accurate diagnosis of an adult disproportionate dwarf may be impossible unless prepubertal films are available.

Radiologic diagnosis is also based upon recognition of unique patterns of abnormal skeletal ossification, such as the total lack or marked reduction of ossification of the vertebral bodies in the achondrogenesis syndromes (Figure 51.7). Some radiographic features characterize certain disorders. For example, in achondroplasia the acetabulae are flat with tiny sacrosciatic notches, rather square iliac wings with rounded corners and an oval translucent area in the proximal femora and humeri in infants. In Kniest dysplasia and metatropic dysplasia, the long bones, and femora in particular, have a dumbbell shaped appearance in the newborn period. Bowing of the limbs (campomelia) is observed in campomelic dysplasia, osteogenesis imperfecta, congenital hypophosphatasia, thanatophoric dysplasia and a heterogenous group of disorders with broad bent long bones.

There are calcified projections or spikes on the lateral borders of the metaphyses of the femorae in thanatophoric dysplasia, the achondrogeneses (both types) and short rib-polydactyly syndrome type I (Saldino-

Fig. 51.7 Radiographs of different forms of lethal neonatal dwarfism.

A. Achondrogenesis, type I (Parenti type) – note the irregular shortened ribs with anterior flare, abnormal iliac bones with some suggestion of ischial development, no ossification of vertebral bodies and the widened, extremely short femurs.

B. Achondrogenesis type II (Langer-Saldino type) – note the almost entire lack of ossification of the vertebral bodies, the short ribs, the lack of ossification of the pubic and ischial bones, the characteristic ilia and shortened tubular femurs with cupped ends.

C. Thanatophoric dysplasia – note the curved short long bones with metaphyseal spikes, short ribs, and inverted U shaped vertebrae in the lumbar area.

D. Short rib polydactyly syndrome, type I (Saldino-Noonan type) – note the marked rib shortening and flaring, the apparently long trunk, characteristic femurs with pointed ends and a hypoplastic abnormal pelvis.

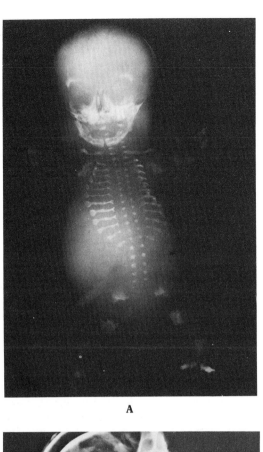

A

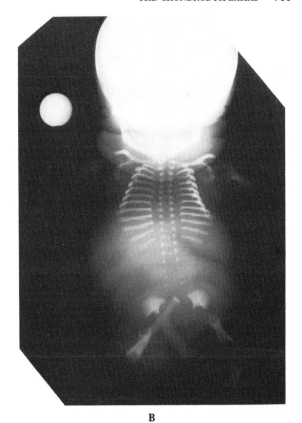

B

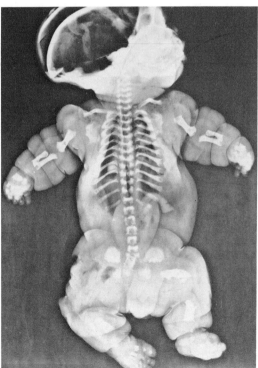

C

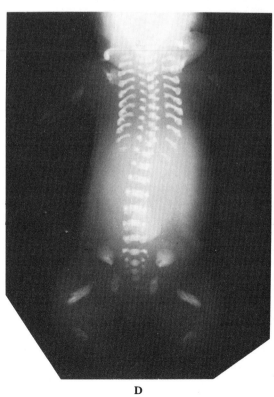

D

Noonan) (Fig. 51.7). Cupping of the ends of the ribs and the long bones and metaphyseal flaring are features of a large number of dysplasias, including achondroplasia, the metaphyseal dysplasias, asphyxiating thoracic dysplasia and chondroectodermal dysplasia.

While fractures in the newborn suggest one of the osteogenesis imperfecta syndromes, fractures may also be seen in congenital osteopetrosis and severe hypophosphatasia. In achondrogenesis type I (Parenti-Fraccaro), the ribs are thin and wavy with beading suggesting fractures, but the long bone and vertebral findings readily distinguish this from osteogenesis imperfecta. In the older individual, fractures may also be seen in a variety of osteopetrotic syndromes, including dysosteosclerosis and pyknodysostosis.

Retarded ossification, manifest by absence of epiphyseal centers or marked delay in their ossification, is found in spondyloepiphyseal dysplasia congenita, Kniest dysplasia and other spondyloepimetaphyseal and multiple epiphyseal dysplasias. Stippling of the epiphyses is characteristic of the various forms of chondrodysplasia punctata, but may also be seen with cerebral-hepato-renal syndrome, Warfarin-related embryopathy and occasionally with chromosomal trisomy, lysosomal storage diseases, diphenylhydantoin-induced embryopathy, the Smith-Lemli-Opitz syndrome and congenital infections.

Rib shortening is most severe in the short rib-polydactyly syndromes and thanatophoric dysplasias, but may also be marked in patients with asphyxiating thoracic dysplasia, chondroectodermal dysplasia and metatropic dysplasia, and in some cases of metaphyseal dysplasia.

Marked decrease in ossification of the vertebral bodies suggests a diagnosis of achondrogenesis (Fig. 51.7). Marked reduction in ossification of the cervical, upper thoracic and lumbosacral vertebral bodies may also be seen in spondyloepiphyseal dysplasia congenita, Kniest dysplasia and other types of spondyloepiphyseal dysplasias. Severe platyspondyly is characteristic of metatropic dysplasia, congenital lethal hypophosphatasia, lethal perinatal osteogenesis imperfecta type II, thanatophoric dysplasia, Morquio disease and spondylometaphyseal dysplasia (Kozlowski type), among others. In thanatophoric dysplasia, the vertical bodies have a characteristic ossification defect so that they appear U-shaped in the thoracic spine, but with an inverted U-shape in the lumbar spine (Fig. 51.7). In spondylometaphyseal dysplasia (Kozlowski type), the AP view of the spine is characteristic with a central core and widely separated platyspondylic bodies which overhang the pedicles, reminiscent of an open staircase. Coronal clefts of the vertebrae can be seen in Kniest dysplasia, Rolland-Desbuquois syndrome, Weisenbach-Zweymuller syndrome, short rib-polydactyly syndrome type I and the various types of chondrodysplasia punctata.

These examples are representative of but a few of the many typical radiographic features seen in the skeletal dysplasias (Table 51-1). In many instances, an accurate diagnosis can be made by simply examining the skeletal radiographs, but in other disorders, only the general type of dysplasia, such as spondyloepiphyseal dysplasia, can be readily classified, and further information may be required to diagnose its exact form. Furthermore, only part of the heterogeneity of the skeletal dysplasias has been delineated to date and there are many disorders that will require morphologic or biochemical studies for their exact delineation.

CHONDRO-OSSEOUS MORPHOLOGY

In recent years, morphological studies of chondro-osseous tissue have revealed specific abnormalities in many of the skeletal dysplasias, (Rimoin, 1975; Sillence et al, 1979; Stanescu et al, 1977; Yang et al, 1976; Rimoin & Sillence, 1981) (Table 51.1). In certain of these disorders, histologic examination of chondro-osseous tissue may be useful in making an accurate diagnosis of the specific skeletal disorder. In other disorders, no histopathological alterations are present, or they are nonspecific, and in these cases pathologic examination is useful only in ruling out a diagnosis.

On morphologic grounds, the chondrodysplasias can be broadly divided into: (1) those disorders which show no qualitative abnormality in endochondral ossification, (2) those in which there are abnormalities in cellular morphology, (3) those with abnormalities in matrix morphology, and (4) those in which the abnormality is primarily localized to the area of chondro-osseous transformation. In certain disorders, abnormalities in two or more of these areas can be seen.

Conditions with minimal disturbance of endochondral ossification include achondroplasia and hypochondroplasia, where endochondral ossification is qualitatively normal, but where there are abnormalities in the height and arrangement of proliferative columns, particularly in the center of the large growth plates. Ultrastructural studies show an increased number of dead chondrocytes and increased cytoplasmic glycogen. In asphyxiating thoracic dysplasia, where several workers have shown prominent lipid inclusions in chondrocytes, the growth plate organization is essentially normal.

In the achondrogenesis syndromes, defects in cellular morphology, matrix and/or chondro-osseous transformation can be seen. In achondrogenesis I (Parenti-Fraccaro) the chondrocytes are large and contain prominent PAS-positive inclusions. Endochondral ossification is markedly disturbed with absence of columns of proliferative cells and lack of cellular hypertrophy. In achondrogenesis II (Langer-Saldino) there is complete disruption of endochondral ossification with large ballooned chondrocytes and little intervening matrix (Fig. 51.8). These changes would suggest a metabolic defect leading to reduced synthesis of a matrix component.

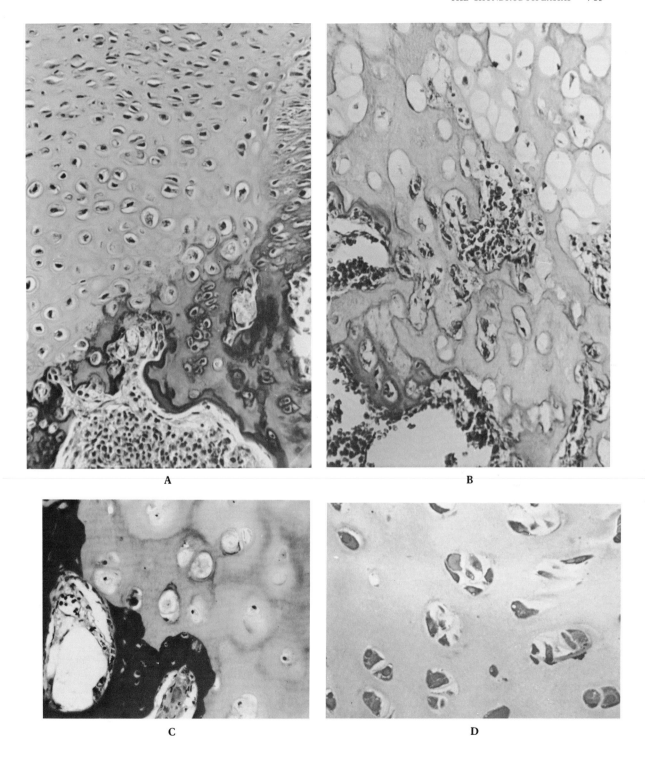

Fig. 51.8 Histological abnormalities in chondro-osseous tissue from various chondrodysplasias.
A. Thanatophoric dysplasia – note the lack of cellular columns and the abnormal broad trabeculae in the lower right hand corner.
B. Achondrogenesis, type II (Langer-Saldino) – note the large chondrocytes with little intervening matrix and the incorporation of chondrocytes into the cartilaginous spicules in the lower left hand corner.
C. Diastrophic dysplasia – note the large chondrocytes surrounded by whorls of collagen and the intracartilaginous ossification (black)
D. Pseudoachondroplasia – note the clusters of chondrocytes containing large greyish inclusion bodies.

Table 51.1 Clinical, radiographic, morphologic and genetic features in the chondrodysplasias (Associated with defects of growth of tubular bones and/or spine)

Dysplasia	Clinical features				
	Head and neck	Chest and trunk	Limbs	Other	Skull
A. Identifiable at birth					
1. Achondrogenesis I (Parenti-Fraccaro)	round or oval face, membranous skull; short neck	short, round	very short	congenital heart defects	poorly mineralized, multiple bone islands; proportionate face and skull
2. Achondrogenesis II (Langer-Saldino)	round, flat face; short neck	short barrel-shaped	very short	distended abdomen; fetal hydrops	
3./4. Thanatophoric dysplasia ± cloverleaf skull	large, bulging forehead; prominent eyes, depressed nasal bridge; wide fontanelles & sutures; ± cloverleaf skull	small, narrow, pear-shaped thorax	markedly short	± hydrocephalus; congenital heart and CNS defects	large calvarium, short base, small foramen magnum
5. Short rib-polydactyly syndrome type I (Saldino-Noonan)	round, flattened face	hydropic appearance, narrow thorax, protuberant abdomen	markedly short hands & feet; post axial polydactyly	± defects of heart, kidneys, lungs, and GI tract	
6. Short rib-polydactyly syndrome type II (Majewski)	short flat nose; low set ears, ± cleft lip or palate	hydropic appearance; narrow thorax; protuberant abdomen	moderately short; pre or post-axial polydactyly	± PDA, dysplastic kidneys, respiratory tract anomalies	
7a. Chondrodysplasia punctata; rhizomelic type	flat face, depressed bridge & tip of nose		proximal shortening	cataracts, icthyosiform erythroderma; joint contractures	
7b. Chondrodysplasia punctata; dominant type (Conradi-Hunermann)	flat face, depressed bridge & tip of nose	± scoliosis	asymmetric shortening	cataracts, icthyosiform erythroderma, alopecia, joint contractures	flat facial bones
8. Campomelic dysplasia; long-limbed type	large calvarium, small flat face, low set ears, micrognathia	small, narrow	bowed femora & tibiae with dimple at maximum convexity	respiratory distress, multiple anomalies, sex reversal	enlarged, dolichocephalic; narrow, shallow orbits
9a. Campomelic dysplasia; short-limbed, normocephalic type			all short & bowed		
9b. Campomelic dysplasia; short-limbed, with craniosynostosis	large head, flat face		all short & bowed		cranisoynostosis ± cloverleaf deformity

A.D.	– autosomal dominant	X.D.	– X–linked dominant	RER	– rough endoplasmic reticulum
A.R.	– autosomal recessive	CFE	– capital femoral epiphysis		
X.R.	– X–linked recessive	EM	– electron microscopy		

Radiological features				Chondro-osseous morphology	Inheritance
Ribs	Vertebrae	Pelvis	Limb bones		
thin, short, beaded	absence of centers for vertebral bodies and sacrum	short ilia, no pubic ossification	extremely short; concave ends; multiple spurs	± inclusion bodies in chondrocytes; bulls-eye appearance to chondrocytes; growth plate irregular and hypercellular	A.R.
short	absence of centers for vertebral bodies and sacrum	small ilia with concave inner & inferior margins; absent pubic and ischial bones	short, straight; metaphyseal flaring and cupping	large ballooned chondrocytes with ↓ matrix; growth plate hypercellular and irregular; sclerosed vascular channels	A.R.
short, cupped and splayed anteriorly	hypoplastic, inverted U-shaped (AP); marked flattening with round anterior end (lateral)	small, short; flat spiculated acetabulum; small sacrosciatic notches	short, bowed; metaphyseal flaring with medial spike	generalized disruption of growth plate; poor columns, fibrous bands and fibrous ossification	unknown
very short, horizontal	flat; wide intervertebral disc spaces	small ilia, flat acetabulum	very short; medial and lateral metaphyseal spurs; polydactyly	disorganized growth plate; broad short trabeculae	A.R.
very short, horizontal			short, ovoid tibia; polydactyly, ± premature ossification of epiphyses	irregular columnization	A.R.
	wide coronal clefts	trapezoid ilia; stippling of ischiopubis	stippled calcification in epiphyses, periarticular areas	↑ vascularization of cartilage with dysplastic myxoid or fibrotic areas, irregular growth plate	A.R.
	± coronal clefts; marked stippling of spinal processes & pedicles	stippling of ischopubis	asymmetric shortening; stippled epiphyses & carpal & tarsal centers	cystic myxoid degeneration of cartilage; fibrous scarring at growth plate	A.D.
narrow & wavy; often 11 pairs; hypoplastic scapulae	hypoplastic cervical bodies, others flattened. Increased lumbar interpedicular distance	tall, narrow; increased acetabular angles; vertical ischia, hypoplastic ischiopubic rami	long, slender, bowed femur & tibia	cartilage normal to slightly irregular; periosteal trabeculae converge at point of angulation	?A.R.
11 pairs	mild flattening	mild narrowing	broad, angulated; widened metaphyses		? A.R.
slender		narrow ilia; hypoplastic ischiopubic rami	short, broad, angulated; epiphyseal delay		unknown

Table 51.1 (cont'd)

Dysplasia	Clinical features				
	Head and neck	Chest and trunk	Limbs	Other	Skull
10. Achondroplasia	large head, bulging forehead, low nasal bridge, prominent mandible	slight rib flaring	rhizomelic shortening; fatty folds of skin in infancy; genu varum	early otitis media; spinal stenosis	large calvarium, short base, small foramen magnum
11. Diastrophic dysplasia	acute swelling of pinnae of ears in infancy → cauliflower ears	scoliosis	short with club feet; hitch-hiker thumbs; synphalangism	cleft palate	ossified ear pinnae
12. Metatropic dysplasia		tail-like sacral appendage; trunk appears long & narrow at birth; develop severe scoliosis	short with prominent joints	long in length at birth; appear short limbed in infancy, short trunked later	
13. Chondro-ectodermal dysplasia (Ellis van (Creveld)	± midline puckering of upper lip; ± natal teeth	log narrow chest	post-axial polydactyly of hands, ± of feet; acromesomelic shortening; nail dysplasia	congenital heart disease; epispadius	
14. Asphyxiating thoracic dysplasia (ATD) (Jeune)		long, narrow; prominent rosary; respiratory distress	variable shortening; short, broad hands & feet; ± post-axial polydactyly	respiratory insufficiency, progressive nephropathy	
15. Spondylo-epiphyseal dysplasia congenita; type Spranger-Wiedemann	± round flat face; short neck, prominent eyes, ± cleft palate	short barrel chest, ± pectus carinatum	mild rhizomelic shortening; normal hands ± club feet,	± myopia, retinal detachment, hearing loss, subluxation of CI-C2	
16. Kniest dysplasia	flat face; prominent wide-set eyes; broad mouth ± cleft palate	short trunk	short; prominent knees, joint contractures	myopia, retinal detachment, hearing loss	frontal flattening; maxillary hypoplasia; shallow orbits
17a. Mesomelic dysplasia, type Nievergelt			severe mesomelic shortening; equinovarus club-feet; brachydactyly, clinodactyly		

A.D.	–	autosomal dominant	X.D.	–	X–linked dominant	RER	–	rough endoplasmic reticulum
A.R.	–	autosomal recessive	CFE	–	capital femoral epiphysis			
X.R.	–	X–linked recessive	EM	–	electron microscopy			

Radiological features				Chondro-osseous morphology	Inheritance
Ribs	Vertebrae	Pelvis	Limb bones		
short, cupped anteriorly	decreased lumbosacral interpedicular distance; short pedicles	squared off ilia, small sacrosciatic notches	short, broad; oval radiolucency in proximal femur & humerus in infancy; relative overgrowth of fibula	chondrocytes normal and growth plate regular-periosteal overgrowth	A.D.
precocious ossification of costal cartilages	± scoliosis & lumbar interpedicular narrowing		short with broad metaphyses; delayed epiphyseal ossification; short 1st metacarpal	chondrocytes enlarged, clustered, degenerating; surround by dense collagen; cystic areas with fibrovascular tissue and intracartilagenous ossification	A.R.
short, flared, cupped anteriorly	markedly flattened; wide intervertebral spaces (early); platyspondyly & scoliosis (late)	hypoplastic crescent-shaped ilia; low set anterior iliac spines	short, broad, club-like	chondrocytes vaocuoled with inclusions; growth plate-irregular vascularization	A.R. & A.D.
± short		squared ilia with hook-like spurs at acetabula, similar to ATD	acromesomelic shortening with cone epiphyses; hamate-capitate fusion; slanting proximal tibial metaphyses	variable, ↑ vascularity of cartilage; cartilage islands in metaphysis; irregular columns	A.R.
very short, cupped anteriorly		square, short ilia, flat acetabulum; spurs at ends of acetabulum	premature ossification capital femoral epiphyses; broad proximal femoral metaphyses	variable findings; lipid inclusions in chondrocytes, cartilage islands in metaphysis	A.R.
short	flattened; dorsal wedging (pear-shaped) ± odontoid hypoplasia	retarded ossification of pubic bones	retarded epiphyseal ossification and deformity-hips, knees; retarded ossification of carpal and tarsal centers; coxa vara	dilated RER in chondrocytes, microcysts in prolipherative zone; columns short	A.D.
short	diffuse flattening; coronal clefts	small ilia; increased acetabular angles; irregular acetabular margins	club-like metaphyses; delayed ossification of femoral heads, cloud effect in epiphyseal plate region	swiss cheese cartilage with abnormal vacuolated matrix, perilacunar foaminess; dilated RER	A.D.
			rhomboid-shaped radius, ulna, tibia, fibula; radio-ulnar & tarsal synostosis		A.D.

Table 51.1 (cont'd)

Dysplasia	Clinical features				
	Head and neck	Chest and trunk	Limbs	Other	Skull
17b. Mesomelic dysplasia, type Langer	micrognathia		severe mesomelic shortening		mild mandibular hypoplasia
17c. Mesomelic dysplasia, type Robinow	prominent forehead; hypoplastic mandible; hypertelorism, downslanting palpebral fissures; short, flat nose		mesomelic shortening hypoplastic nails	genital hypoplasia ± cryptorchidism	
17d. Mesomelic dysplasia, type Rheinhardt			moderate mesomelic shortening; radial bowing, ulnar deviation of hands; lateral bowing of legs (cutaneous dimple)		
18. Acromesomelic dysplasia		small thorax, mild truncal shortening	meso and acromelia with mild rhizomelia; square short hands, elbow deformities, upper extremities more severe than lower		
19. Cleido-cranial dysplasia	large, prominent forehead; wide persistant fontanelles & sutures	drooping shoulders & narrow chest, ± scoliosis	hyperextensible, ± coxa vara; fingers short and square	abnormal dentition	decreased ossification; multiple Wormian bones
20. Larsen syndrome	prominent forehead; flattened face; hypertelorism; ± cleft palate or uvula	soft, collapsing thorax	multiple dislocations	severe joint laxity; ± dysraphism of spine → neurologic impairment	craniofacial disproportion
21. Oto-palato-digital syndrome	prominent forehead & supraorbital ridges; hypertelorism, ± cleft palate, small jaw		short, broad thumbs & toes; broad phalanges	± hearing defect; ± mild mental retardation	small mandible with increased angle

A.D.	–	autosomal dominant	X.D.	–	X–linked dominant	RER	–	rough endoplasmic reticulum
A.R.	–	autosomal recessive	CFE	–	capital femoral epiphysis			
X.R.	–	X–linked recessive	EM	–	electron microscopy			

Radiological features				Chondro-osseous morphology	Inheritance
Ribs	Vertebrae	Pelvis	Limb bones		
			short & thick; hypoplastic fibula & distal ulna		A.R. (probably homozygous for dyschondrosteosis gene
	± posterior osseous fusion	+ hemivertebrae	hypoplastic distal ulna, ± radial head dislocation		A.D.
			short radius & ulna; hypoplasia of distal ulna & proximal fubula		A.D.
	infancy & childhood-oval shaped; adult-posterior wedging	hypoplasia of iliac base & irregular acetabulum	progressive shortening with metaphyseal flare, especially acro and mesomelia; mild epiphyseal delay; brachydactyly with cone epiphyses		A.R.
absent or hypoplastic clavicles	± retarded ossification of bodies	retarded ossification and hypoplastic pubis; hypoplasia of ilia	pseudoepiphyses of metacarpals and metatarsals; retarded ossification of carpals and tarsals	mild ↓ in growth plate height; ↓ perosteal ossification	A.D.
	± fusion defects of cervical spine		slender; multiple joint dislocations; duplication of calcaneus		A.D. & A.R.
	narrow pedicles, wide lumbar interpedicular distance	small ilia, ± dislocated hips	hypoplastic distal radius; diffuse hand changes		?XD

Table 51.1 (cont'd)

Dysplasia	Clinical features				
	Head and neck	Chest and trunk	Limbs	Other	Skull
B. Identifiable in later life					
1. Hypochondroplasia	Normal head to slight prominence of forehead	normal-mild lumbar lordosis	Rhizomelic shortening of extremities, short broad hands, limited extension at elbow	mild short stature, muscular appearance	
2. Dyschondrosteosis			Mesomelic shortening; Dorsal subluxation distal end ulna	mild short stature	
3. Metaphyseal dysplasia, type Jansen	prominent forehead		rhizomelic shortening enlarged joints		reticulate pattern in calvarium; sclerosis of base
4. Metaphyseal dysplasia, type Schmid			waddling gait, bowed legs, generalized shortening of limbs		
5. Metaphyseal dysplasia, type McKusick (cartilage hair hypoplasia)	fine sparse lightly pigmented hair, eyebrows		short; lax ligaments; short pudgy hands; telescoping fingers	± megacolon, immune defects, propensity to skin cancer	
6. Metaphyseal dysplasia with pancreatic insufficiency, neutropenia		± small narrow chest	± short	pancreatic insufficiency and malabsorption, neutropenia	
7. Spondylometaphyseal dysplasia, type Kozlowski		kyphoscoliosis; pectus carinatum	waddling gait, knee and hip pain in childhood, limitation of large joints	short trunk short stature	
8a. Multiple epiphyseal dysplasia, type Fairbanks		thoracic kyphosis ± back pain	pain & stiffness in knees, hips & ankles; waddling gait		

A.D.	–	autosomal dominant	X.D.	–	X–linked dominant	RER	–	rough endoplasmic reticulum
A.R.	–	autosomal recessive	CFE	–	capital femoral epiphysis			
X.R.	–	X–linked recessive	EM	–	electron microscopy			

Radiological features				Chondro-osseous morphology	Inheritance
Ribs	Vertebrae	Pelvis	Limb bones		
normal to slightly flaired	lumboscral inter-pedicular narrowing; short pedicle; posterior scalloping	slightly short basilar segments of ilia	rhizomelia with short, wide bones; prominent deltoid tubercle; elongated fibula	normal growth plate, with perhaps widened septa	A.D.
			radius and tibia short in relation to ulna and fibula; Madelung deformity		A.D.
splayed & cupped anteriorly		demineralized	metaphyses wide, splayed, frayed; cortical erosion & sub-periosteal bone formation	chondrocytes large, matrix fibrillar; clusters of hypertropic cells at growth plate; irregular line of ossification with tongues of cartilage in metaphyses	A.D.
			metaphyseal splaying and cupping in all tubular bones; coxa vara, genu varum	same as above	A.D.
splayed & cupped anteriorly			metaphyseal flaring and irregularity, especially knees; long distal fibula	same as above	A.R.
± short, flared			mild metaphyseal irregularity	same as above	A.R.
	platyspondyly with open stair case appearance on AP view	narrow sacrosciatic notches; broad horizontal irregular acetabular roofs	metaphyseal irregularity, widened epiphyseal plate, coxa vara; marked retardation of carpal ossification	↓ proliperative zone, irregular columns, fibrous appearance to matrix; inclusions on EM	A.D.
	end plate irregularity and Schmorl's nodes		small irregularly ossified epiphyses involving all areas, including small bones of the hands and feet	variable-normal to disturbed growth plate, inclusion bodies reported in chondrocytes, dilated RER	A.D.

Table 51.1 (cont'd)

Dysplasia	Clinical features				
	Head and neck	Chest and trunk	Limbs	Other	Skull
8b. Multiple epiphyseal dysplasia, type Ribbing			osteoarthropathy of hips	mild short stature	
9. Arthoro-ophthalmopathy (Stickler)	cleft palate, mandibular hypoplasia, mid face hypoplasia		hypotonia, hyper-extension of joints; later joint pain and morning stiffness	marfanoid habitus, myopia, retinal detachment, conductive hearing loss	
10. Pseudoachondroplastic dysplasia	normal skull and face	trunk appears disproportionately long	very short limbs with genu varum or valgum; hypermotility of joints; small broad hands	not manifested until at least 2 years of age	
11. Spondyloepiphyseal dysplasia tarda		sternal protrusion, back pain,	osteoarthropathy of hips and knees	mild short trunk, short stature	
12. Spondyloepiphyseal dysplasia, other forms (too variable to include)					
13. Dyggve-Melchior-Clausen dysplasia	short neck	thoracic kyphoscoliosis, lumbar lordosis, flared ribs, protruding sternum, short trunk	waddling gait, enlarged joints with restriction; small claw hands	mental retardation (most)	± microcephaly

A.D.	–	autosomal dominant	X.D.	–	X–linked dominant	RER	–	rough endoplasmic reticulum
A.R.	–	autosomal recessive	CFE	–	capital femoral epiphysis			
X.R.	–	X–linked recessive	EM	–	electron microscopy			

Radiological features				Chondro-osseous morphology	Inheritance
Ribs	Vertebrae	Pelvis	Limb bones		
	usually normal but may have early onset of Schmorl's nodes		epiphyseal irregularity and delayed ossification, primarily involving the hips with other epiphyses involved; none-mild involvement of hands and feet		A.D.
	wedging of thoracic vertebra & Schmorl's disease of spine		mild epiphyseal dysplasia especially CFE & distal tibia; irregular articular surfaces; degenerative arthrosis especially of hips		A.D.
	platyspondyly; anterior tongue-like protrusion; end plate irregularity	acetabular irregularity; hypoplastic ischium & pubis	epiphyseal & metaphyseal dysplasia; striking hand involvement with shortening of tubular bones with irregular metaphyses and small round epiphyses; marked CFE dysplasia	prominent inclusions in chondrocytes showing lamellar or granular RER dilatation on EM	A.D. (rarely AR)
	platyspondyly with hump-shaped centra	hypoplastic iliac wings	epiphyseal hypoplasia of large epiphyses and premature osteoarthrosis of hips	fairly normal with clustering of proliferative cells	X.R.
mild flaring	anterior pointed platyspondyly; vertebral notching	lacy iliac crest; hypoplastic ilium, pubis, ischium and acetabular roof; small sacrosciatic notch	small epiphyses, especially CFE; brachydactyly; cone epiphyses; small carpal centers	foci of multiple degenerating chondrocytes surrounded by dense fibrous capsule	A.R.
splayed, bulbous	platyspondyly; pear shaped vertebra; end plate irregularity; scoliosis; C1–C2 subluxation	delayed ischial and pubic ossification	delayed epiphyseal ossification; clubbed shaped femurs (1st year); metaphyseal and epiphyseal changes (after 3 years); dappling of metaphyses with fragmentation; greater involvement of fibula than tibia; ulna than radius	inclusion bodies in chondrocytes, hypocelluar growth plates	?A.R.

Table 51.1 (cont'd)

Dysplasia	Clinical features				
	Head and neck	Chest and trunk	Limbs	Other	Skull
14. Spondyloepimetaphyseal dysplasia, type Strudwick	± cleft palate	pectus carinatum scoliosis	genu valgum	resembles SED congenita at birth	
15. Myotonic chondrodysplasia (Catel-Schwartz-Jampel)	characteristic pinched facial features (expressionless, immobile), narrow palpebral fissures, short neck	protuberant sternum	prominance and limited motion of large joints; coxa vara	microcornea, myopia, juvenile cataracts	large skull with mid-face hypoplasia; platybasia
16. Parastremmatic dysplasia	short neck	stiffness of spine and kyphoscoliosis, increased AP diameter of thorax	abnormal gait, severe deformities of lower extremities, severe genu valgum or varum; multiple joint contractures, short stubby hands	"twisted dwarfs"	
17. Tricho-rhino phalangeal dysplasia, type I	pear-shaped bulbous nose; unusual philtrum; sparse, thin, slowly growing hair		brachydactyly; proximal interphalangeal swelling; thin nails		
18. Acrodysplasia with retinitis pigmentosa and nephropathy (Saldino-Mainzer)			brachydactyly	retinitis pigmentosa; interstitial nephritis; ± cerebellar ataxia	

A.D. – autosomal dominant   X.D. – X–linked dominant   RER – rough endoplasmic reticulum
A.R. – autosomal recessive   CFE – capital femoral epiphysis
X.R. – X–linked recessive   EM – electron microscopy

Radiological features				Chondro-osseous morphology	Inheritance
Ribs	Vertebrae	Pelvis	Limb bones		
neuropathic thorax; downward tilted ribs	platyspondyly; irregular end plates	narrow ilia; acetabular hypoplasia	small epiphyses in proximal femur, humerus, radius, and short tubular bones; knee epiphyses enlarged; slight metaphyseal irregularity		A.R.
slightly splayed; "wooly" changes in scapula and clavicle	biconcave platyspondyly; "flocky or wooly" end plates	large ischial and pubic bones with "wooly" metaphyseal and apophyseal regions	marked wooly changes in carpal centers, metaphyses with hypoplasia of epiphyses, especially CFE; twisted and shortened long bones	lack of columnization; ↓ osteoblasts and osteoclasts	A.D. or X.D.
			type 12 cone epiphyses in hands and feet; shortening of short tubular bones of hands; small CFE associated with Legg Perthes like changes		A.D. (? few A.R.)
			cone epiphyses of hands and feet; metaphyseal widening of femoral necks with sclerosis and hypoplastic appearing CFE		A.R.
					A.R.

In thanatophoric dysplasia (Fig. 51.8), and short rib-polydactyly type I and type II, there appears to be defective maturation of chondrocytes with reduced and disorganized columnization. Consequently, vascular invasion and chondro-osseous transformation are irregular, such that osseous trabeculae are short and deformed with bridging between the trabeculae. Hypertrophic chondrocytes are irregularly arranged at the zone of chondro-osseous transformation and lack columnization.

A group of conditions show dilatation of the chondrocyte rough endoplasmic reticulum, consistent with defective synthesis or abnormal processing of matrix proteins. These include pseudoachondroplasia, where the inclusions are prominent and in some cases show a highly regular RER inclusion (Fig. 51.8), consisting of alternating electron dense and electron lucent lamellae. Dilatation of the rough endoplasmic reticulum is seen also in spondylometaphyseal dysplasia (Kozlowski), autosomal recessive multiple epiphyseal dysplasia and Kniest dysplasia among others. Thus dilatation of the RER is not a diagnostic finding.

The matrix pathology in Kniest dysplasia is striking. Endochondral cartilage with paraffin processing shows dehiscence of matrix leading to the Swiss-Cheese cartilage appearance. With plastic embedding, these are areas of relatively acellular matrix surrounded by attenuated chondrocytes with a bubbly appearance to the perilacunar matrix.

Matrix abnormalities are also seen in diastrophic dysplasia, chondrodysplasia punctata (various types) and the Dyggve-Melchior-Clausen syndrome. In diastrophic dysplasia, the matrix of the reserve zone cartilage develops a particularly fibrillar appearance and shows areas of microscar formation (Fig. 51.8). Chondrocytes both by light microscopy and by electron microscopy are surrounded by dense corona of large collagen fibres. In Dyggve-Melchior-Clausen syndrome, chondrocytes by light microscopy appear to be arranged around a relatively large common lacuna with up to 10 chondrocytes clustered around each lacuna. In chondrodysplasia punctata of both the rhizomelic recessive and dominant Conradi-Hunermann varieties, there appears to be an alteration in epiphyseal and reserve zone cartilage matrix with areas of dystrophic (non-endochondral) ossification, fibrous dysplasia, and even areas of fat deposition.

Since the 1977 International Nomenclature meeting, new chondrodysplasias have steadily been reported. Morphologic studies have often played an integral part in their investigation and nosology. For example, dyssegmental dysplasia and Rolland-Desbuquois syndrome may both represent the spectrum of a unique autosomal recessive syndrome. Preliminary studies reveal matrix pathology very similar to that observed in Kniest dysplasia. Giant cell chondrodysplasia is characterized by a unique pattern of skeletal abnormalities and the morphologic finding of multinucleated giant cells throughout the reserve zone cartilage.

Two new syndromes with striking histopathologic abnormalities have been reported by Stanescu et al (1977), fibrochondrogenesis and hypochondrogenesis. Thus pathological analysis of chondro-osseous tissue can be of great help in the diagnostic evaluation of the chondrodysplasias and can lead to the delineation of new syndromes.

BIOCHEMICAL STUDIES

In recent years, great progress has been made in our knowledge concerning the basic biology and technology of collagen and proteoglycan chemistry and a search for the biochemical defect in certain of the skeletal dysplasias has been performed. Nevertheless, except for the mucopolysaccharidoses and mucolipidoses and certain of the mineralization defects, such as hypophosphatasia, hypophosphataemic rickets and vitamin D dependency rickets, the basic defect has not been uncovered in any of this large group of disorders, although a number of potential abnormalities have been suggested.

Abnormalities in proteoglycan chemistry have been suggested in the Kniest dysplasia and psuedoachondroplasia (Stanescu et al, 1977). The cellular inclusion bodies which have been demonstrated in the chondrocytes in these two disorders would also suggest an abnormality in proteoglycan chemistry. The specific defect in these two disorders, however, remains to be elucidated. Specific abnormalities in cartilage proteoglycans have been demonstrated in several of the mouse chondrodysplasias, however, such as the sulphate donor defect in the brachymorphic mouse and an absence of proteoglycan core protein in the cmd mouse. Similar defects may well exist in certain of their human counterparts.

A specific defect in collagen chemistry has been suggested in numerous of the skeletal dysplasias (Rimoin & Sillence, 1981). Cartilage collagen appears to be qualitatively and quantitatively normal, however, in human achondroplasia. A consistent defect in the electrophoretic migration of cyanogen bromide fragments of type II collagen has been observed in numerous cases of typical thanatophoric dysplasia. However, the amino acid composition of the collagen has been found to be normal and the basis of this electrophoretic defect remains to be elucidated. On the other hand, in two patients with different variant forms of thanatophoric dysplasia, totally different abnormalities in type II collagen have been detected by electrophoretic techniques. Burgeson and Hollister have also found a marked deficiency of hydroxylysine in cartilage and bone collagen in an unusual case of campomelic dwarfism associated with neonatal fractures. Numerous abnormalities in collagen chemistry have now been reported in osteogenesis imperfecta, but these abnormalities have not been consistent, primarily due to the lack of recognition of the heterogeneity in this group of disorders (see Chapter 52).

There are now numerous clues as to possible biochemical defects in several of the skeletal dysplasias. The rapid increase in the knowledge of the basic biology and technology of collagen and proteoglycan chemistry should pave the way for an exciting era in the detection of the basic defect in many of the skeletal dysplasias. However, the biochemical studies must take into account the known and potential heterogeneity in this group of disorders, if a single and consistent defect is to be found in any one disorder. Furthermore, the biochemist should take advantage of the numerous pathogenetic clues suggested by the morphological studies in deciding which disorders might be due to defects in collagen or proteoglycans chemistry, or to other defects in chondrocyte metabolism.

SUMMARY

Thus clinical evaluation of the skeletal dysplasias requires a wide variety of clinical, radiographic and pathologic tools. Diagnosis of the specific form of skeletal dysplasia can be of great importance in the prognosis, prevention and treatment of these disorders, and in the provision of accurate genetic counselling. Since space constraints prevent independent discussion of each of the many chondrodysplasias in this chapter, their salient clinical, radiographic, pathologic and genetic characteristics are outlined in Table 51.1. The reader is referred to the classified bibliography for further details concerning each of these syndromes.

APPENDIX

INTERNATIONAL NOMENCLATURE OF CONSTITUTIONAL DISEASES OF BONE

Revision – May, 1977

INTRODUCTION

The description and separating of new disorders necessitated the creation of an International Nomenclature of Constitutional Diseases of Bone which was first developed in Paris in 1969. Because of the rapid progress in the delineation and classification of these disorders,

the International Nomenclature was revised in May, 1977.

This new list includes the clearly identified forms of a single disease or defect. 'Other forms': mean that other forms of the disorder exist which, as yet, have not been defined well enough to include.

This revision endeavors to modify the previously proposed terms as little as possible and its primary goal has been to introduce the names of a certain number of new conditions which have been defined since the original conference. It is necessary to emphasize that the essential purpose of this nomenclature is to unify the terminology used in this field in different parts of the world. It is not intended to be a classification of skeletal disorders, and the subdivisions proposed are devised only to clarify the presentation of the various disorders.

Among the changes which have been made, attention is directed to the elimination of the term 'dwarfism' which seemed somewhat offensive to the patients or their families. Thus, the term 'diastrophic dwarfism' has been replaced by 'diastrophic dysplasia'.

The constitutional disorders of growth, moreover, have been eliminated from the current list because it seems that they truly do not correspond to constitutional skeletal disorders; it has been proposed that another committee develop a nomenclature of syndromes in which these conditions ought to be included. Among constitutional disorders of growth, only those in which skeletal involvement is predominant as a manifestation have been retained and these are listed among the dysostoses.

Metabolic disorders which involve complex sugars have been designated, insofar as is possible, by the responsible enzymatic defect. By virtue of the pathogenetic uncertainties which surround mucolipidosis II and III, these terms are retained in the nomenclature for the time being.

This nomenclature has been elaborated by a group of Experts who met in Paris in May 1977 at the request of Doctor P. Maroteaux. The meeting was hold under the aegis of the European Society for Pediatric Radiology and the National Fundation – March of Dimes.
List of participants:

Drs J. DORST
    C. FAURE
    A. GIEDION
    J. HALL
    H. J. KAUFMANN
    K. KOZLOWSKI
    L. LANGER
    L. LENZI
    P. MAROTEAUX
    A. MURPHY
    A. K. POZNANSKI

D. RIMOIN
J. SAUVEGRAIN
F. SILVERMAN
J. SPRANGER
R. STANESCU
V. STANESCU

OSTEOCHONDRODYSPLASIAS (abnormalities of cartilage and/or bone growth and development)

I. Defects of growth of tubular bones and/or spine

A Identifiable at birth
1. Achondrogenesis type I (PARENTI-FRACCARO)
2. Achondrogenesis type II (LANGER-SALDINO)
3. Thanatophoric dysplasia
4. Thanatophoric dysplasia with clover-leaf skull
5. Short rib-polydactyly syndrome type I (SALDINO-NOONAN) (perhaps several forms)
6. Short rib-polydactyly syndrome type II (MAJEWS-KI)
7. Chondrodysplasia punctata
   a. Rhizomelic form
   b. Dominant form
   c. Other forms
      Exclude: symptomatic stippling in other disorders (e.g. ZELLWEGER syndrome, Warfarin embryopathy)
8. Campomelic dysplasia
9. Other dysplasias with congenital bowing of long bones (several forms)
10. Achondroplasia
11. Diastrophic dysplasia
12. Metatropic dysplasia (several forms)
13. Chondro-ecto-dermal dysplasia (ELLIS VAN CREVELD)
14. Asphyxiating thoracic dysplasia (JEUNE)
15. Spondylo-epiphyseal dysplasia congenita
    a. Type SPRANGER-WIEDEMANN
    b. Other forms (see B 11–12)
16. Kniest dysplasia
17. Mesomelic dysplasia
    a. type NIEVERGELT
    b. type LANGER (probable homozygous dyschondrosteosis)
    c. type ROBINOW
    d. type RHEINARDT
    e. Others
18. Acromesomelic dysplasia
19. Cleido-cranial dysplasia
20. LARSEN syndrome
21. Oto-palato-digital syndrome

B. Identifiable in later life
1. Hypochondroplasia
2. Dyschondrosteosis
3. Metaphyseal chondrodysplasia type JANSEN
4. Metaphyseal chondrodysplasia type SCHMID
5. Metaphyseal chondrodysplasia type McKUSICK
6. Metaphyseal chondrodysplasia with exocrine pancretic insufficiency and cyclic neutropenia
7. Spondylo-metaphyseal dysplasia
   a. type KOZLOWSKI
   b. Other forms
8. Multiple epiphyseal dysplasia
   a. type FAIRBANKS
   b. Other forms
9. Arthro-ophthalmopathy (STICKLER)
10. Pseudo-achondroplasia
    a. Dominant
    b. Recessive
11. Spondylo-epiphyseal dysplasia tarda.
12. Spondylo-epiphyseal dysplasia, other forms (see A. 15–16)
13. DYGGVE -MELCHIOR-CLAUSEN dysplasia
14. Spondylo-epi-metaphyseal dysplasia (several forms)
15. Myotonic chondrodysplasia (CATEL–SCHWARTZ –JAMPEL)
16. Parastremmatic dysplasia
17. Tricho-rhino-phalangeal dysplasia
18. Acrodysplasia with retinitis pigmentosa and nephropathy (SALDINO – MAINZER)

II. Disorganized development of cartilage and fibrous components of skeleton
1. Dysplasia epiphyseal hemimelica
2. Multiple cartilagenous exostoses
3. Acrodysplasia with exostoses (GIEDION-LANGER)
4. Enchondromatosis (OLLIER)
5. Enchondromatosis with hemangioma (MAFFUCCI)
6. Metachondromatosis
7. Fibrous dysplasia (JAFFE-LICHTENSTEIN)
8. Fibrous dysplasia with skin pigmentation and precocious puberty (McCUNE-ALBRIGHT)
9. Cherubism (familial fibrous dysplasia of the jaws)
10. Neurofibromatosis

III. Abnormalities of density of cortical diaphyseal structure and/or metaphyseal modeling
1. Osteogenesis imperfecta congenita (several forms)
2. Osteogenesis imperfecta tarda (several forms)
3. Juvenile idiopathic osteoporosis
4. Osteoporosis with pseudo-glioma
5. Osteopetrosis with precocious manifestations
6. Osteopetrosis with delayed manifestations (several forms)

7. Pycnodysostosis
8. Osteopoikilosis
9. Osteopathia striata
10. Melorheostosis
11. Diaphyseal dysplasia (CAMURATI-ENGELMANN)
12. Cranio-diaphyseal dysplasia
13. Endosteal hyperostosis
   a. Autosomal dominant (WORTH)
   b. Autosomal recessive (VAN BUCHEM)
14. Tubular stenosis (KENNY-CAFFEY)
15. Pachydermoperiostosis
16. Osteodysplasty (MELNICK-NEEDLES)
17. Fronto-metaphyseal dysplasia
18. Cranio-metaphyseal dysplasia (several forms)
19. Metaphyseal dysplasia (PYLE)
20. Sclerosteosis
21. Dysosteosclerosis
22. Osteo-ectasia with hyperphosphatasia

DYSOSTOSES (Malformation of individual bones, singly or in combination)

I. Dysostoses with cranial and facial involvement.
1. Craniosynostosis (several forms)
2. Cranio-facial dysostosis (CROUZON)
3. Acrocephalo-syndactyly (APERT) and others
4. Acrocephalo-polysyndactyly (CARPENTER) and others
5. Mandibulo-facial dysostosis
   a. type TREACHER-COLLINS, FRANCES-CHETTI
   b. other forms
6. Oculo-mandibulo facial syndrome (HALLERMANN STREIFF-FRANCOIS)
7. Nevoid basal cell carcinoma syndrome

II. Dysostoses with predominant axial involvement
1. Vertebral segmentation defects (including KLIPPEL-FEIL)
2. Cervico-oculo-acoustic syndrome (WILDER-VANCK)
3. SPRENGEL anomaly
4. Spondylo-costal dysostosis
   a. Dominant form
   b. recessive forms
5. Oculo-vertebral syndrome (WEYERS)
6. Osteo-onychodysostosis
7. Cerebro-costo-mandibular syndrome.

III. Dysostoses with predominant involvement of extremities
1. Acheiria
2. Apodia
3. Ectrodactyly syndrome
4. Aglossia-adactyly syndrome
5. Congenital bowing of long bones (several forms) (see also osteochondrodysplasias)
6. Familial radio-ulnar synostosis
7. Brachydactyly (several forms)
8. Symphalangism
9. Polydactyly (several forms)
10. Syndactyly (several forms)
11. Poly-syndactyly (several forms)
12. Camptodactyly
13. POLAND Syndrome
14. RUBINSTEIN-TAYBI Syndrome
15. Pancytopenia-dysmelia syndrome (FANCONI)
16. Thrombocytopenia-radial-aplasia syndrome
17. Oro-digito-facial syndrome
   a. type PAPILLON-LEAGE
   b. type MOHR
18. Cardiomelic syndrome (HOLT-ORAM and others)
19. Femoral facial syndrome
20. Multiple synostoses (includes some forms of symphalangism.)
21. Scapulo-iliac dysostosis (KOSENOW-SINIOS)
22. Hand foot genital syndrome
23. Focal dermal hypoplasia (GOLTZ)

IDIOPATHIC OSTEOLYSES

1. Phalangeal (several forms)
2. Tarso-carpal
   a. including FRANCOIS form and others
   b. with nephropathy
3. Multicentric
   a. HAJDU-CHENEY form
   b. WINCHESTER form
   c. Other forms

CHROMOSOMAL ABERRATIONS

Individual disorders not listed

PRIMARY METABOLIC ABNORMALITIES

I. Calcium and/or phosphorus
1. Hypophosphataemic rickets
2. Pseudo-deficiency rickets (PRADER, ROYER)
3. Late rickets (McCANCE)
4. Idiopathic hypercalcuria
5. Hypophosphatasia (several forms)
6. Pseudo-hypoparathyroidism (normo and hypocalcaemic forms, include acrodysostosis).

II. Complex carbohydrates

1. Mucopolysaccharidosis, type I (alpha-L-iduronidase deficiency)
   a. HURLER form
   b. SCHEIE form
   c. Other forms
2. Mucopolysaccharidosis, type II-HUNTER (sulphoiduronate sulphatase deficiency)
3. Mucopolysaccharidosis, type III – SAN FILIPPO
   type A (Heparin sulphamidase deficiency)
   type B (N-acetyl-alpha-glucosaminidase deficiency)
4. Mucopolysaccharidosis, type IV – MORQUIO (N-acetylgalactosamine-6-sulphate-sulphatase deficiency)
5. Mucopolysaccharidosis, type VI – MAROTEAUX-LAMY (aryl sulphatase B deficiency)
6. Mucopolysaccharidosis, type VII (beta-glucuronidase deficiency)
7. Aspartylglucosaminuria (Aspartyl-glucosaminidase deficiency)
8. Mannosidosis (alpha-mannosidase deficiency)

9. Fucosidosis (alpha-fucosidase deficiency)
10. GM1-Gangliosidosis (beta-galactosidase deficiency)
11. Multiple sulphatase deficiency (AUSTIN, THIEFFRY)
12. Neuraminidase deficiency (formerly Mucolipidosis I)
13. Mucolipidosis II
14. Mucolipidosis III

III. Lipids
1. NIEMANN-PICK disease
2. GAUCHER disease

IV. Nucleic acids
1. Adenosine-deaminase deficiency and others

V. Amino acids
1. Homocystinuria and others

VI. Metals
1. MENKES kinky hair syndrome and others.

REFERENCES

(Modified from Rimoin, D L, Hall, J, Maroteaux, P 1979 International Nomenclature of Constitutional Diseases of Bone with Bibliography. Birth Defects Original Article Series 15 (10)

GENERAL REFERENCES

Beighton P 1978 Inherited Disorders of the Skeleton. Churchill Livingstone, Edinburgh.
Kaufmann A J (ed) 1973 Intrinsic Diseases of Bones. Progress in Pediatric Radiology Vol 4 S Karger, Basel
Maroteaux P 1974 Maladies Osseuses de l'Enfant. Flammarion, Paris
Maroteaux P 1979 Bone Diseases of Children. J B Lippincott, Philadelphia
McKusick V A 1972 Heritable Disorders of Connective Tissue. 4th Ed. C V Mosby, St. Louis
Rimoin D L 1975 The Chondrodystrophies. Advances in Human Genetics 5: 1–118
Rimoin D L (ed) 1976 Symposium on the skeletal dysplasias. Clinical orthopaedics 114: 2
Rimoin D L and Horton W A 1978 Short Stature Part I and Part II. Journal of Pediatrics 92: 523–528 and 697–704
Rimoin D L and Silence D O 1981 Chondro-osseous morphology and biochemistry in the skeletal dysplasias. Birth Defects Original Article Series 17(1): 249–265
Sillence D O, Horton W A and Rimoin D L 1979 Morphologic studies in the skeletal dysplasias. American Journal of Pathology 96: 811
Sillence D, Rimoin D L, Lachman R 1978 Neonatal dwarfism Pediatric Clinics of North America 25: 453
Smith D W 1976 Recognizable Patterns of Human Malformations. 2nd Ed. W B Saunders, Philadelphia
Spranger J W, Langer L O, Wiedemann H R 1974 Bone Dysplasias. An Atlas of Constitutional Disorders of Skeletal

Development. W B Saunders, Philadelphia
Stanescu V, Stanescu R, Maroteaux P 1977 Morphological and biochemical studies of epiphyseal cartilage in dyschondroplasias. Archives Française de Pédiatrie (Suppl 3): 1
Taybi H 1975 Radiology of Syndromes. Year Book Medical Publishers, Chicago
Yang S S, Heidelberger K P, Brough P J, Corbett D P, Bernstein J 1976 Lethal short-limbed chondrodysplasia in early infancy. Perspectives of Pediatric Pathology 3: 1

REFERENCES TO SPECIFIC SYNDROMES

OSTEOCHONDRODYSPLASIAS
Abnormalities of cartilage or bone growth and development or both

I. Defects of growth of tubular bones and/or spine

  A. Identifiable at Birth

1. Achondrogenesis Type I (Parenti-Fraccaro)

1. Houston C S, Awen C F, Kent H P 1972 Fatal neonatal dwarfism. Journal of the Canadian Association of Radiologists 23: 45–61
2. Maroteaux P, Stenescu V, Stanescu R 1976 The lethal chondrodysplasias. Clinical Orthopedics 114: 31
3. Sillence D O, Rimoin D L, Lachman R 1978 Neonatal dwarfism. Pediatric Clinics of North America 25(3): 453–483
4. Yang Sheng-S, Brough A J, Garewal G S, Bernstein J 1974 Two types of heritable lethal achondrogenesis. Journal of Pediatrics 85: 796–801
5. Beluffi G 1977 Achondrogenesis, type I. Fortschritte anf dem Gebiete der Rontgenstrahten und der Nuklear Medizin 127: 341–344

2. Achondrogenesis Type II (Langer-Saldino)

1. Maroteaux P, Stanescu V, Stanescu R 1976 The lethal chondrodysplasias. Clinical Orthopedics 14: 31
2. Saldino R M 1971 Lethal short-limbed dwarfism: achondrogenesis and thanatophoric dwarfism. American Journal of Roentgenology 112: 185
3. Sillence D O, Rimoin D L, Lachman R 1978 Neonatal dwarfism. Pediatric Clinics of North America 25(3) 453–483
4. Yang Sheng-S, Brough A J, Garewal G S, Bernstein J 1974 Two types of heritable lethal achondrogenesis. Journal of Pediatrics 85: 796–801

3. Thanatophoric Dysplasia

1. Horton W A, Rimoin D L, Hollister D W, Lachman R S 1979 Further heterogeneity within lethal neonatal short-limbed dwarfism: The Platyspondylic Types. Journal of Pediatrics 94: 736
2. Maroteaux P, Lamy M, Robert J M 1967 Le nanisme thanatophore. Presse Medicale 75: 2519
3. Saldino R M 1971 Lethal Dwarfism: achondrogenesis and thanatophoric dwarfism. American Journal of Roentgenology 112: 185
4. Langer L O, Spranger J W, Greinacher I, Herdman R C 1969 Thanatophoric dwarfism. Radiology 92: 285–294

4. Thanatophoric Dysplasia with Cloverleaf Skull

1. Partington M W, Gonzales-Crussi F, Khakee S G, Wollin D G 1971 Cloverleaf skull and thanatophoric dwarfism. report of four cases two in the same sibship. Archives of disease in Childhood 46: 656
2. Wiedemann H R, Ostertag B 1974 Kleeblattschädel and Allgemeine Mikromelie: Versuch Einer Nosologischen Zuordnung und Genetischen Elternberatung. Kin Paediatr 186: 261
3. Young R S, Pochaczevsky R, Leonidas J C, Wexler I B, Ratner H 1973 Thanatophoric dwarfism and cloverleaf skull ("Kleeblattschädel"). Radiology 106: 401–405

5. Short Rib-polydactyly Syndrome Type I (Saldino-Noonan) (perhaps several forms)

1. Saldino R M, Noonan C D 1972 Severe thoracic dystrophy with striking micromelia, abnormal osseous development, including the spine and multiple visceral anomalies. American Journal of Roentgenology 114: 257–263
2. Spranger J, Grimm B, Weller M, Weissenbacher G, Herrmann J, Gilbert E, Krepler R 1974 Short rib-polydactyly (SRP) syndromes, type Majewski and Saldino-Noonan. Zeitschrift für Kinderheilkunde 116: 73
3. Verma I C, Bhargava S, Agarwal S 1975 An autosomal recessive form of lethal chondrodystrophy with severe thoracic narrowing, rhizoacromelic type of micromelia, polydactyly and genital anomalies. In: Disorders of Connective Tissue. Birth Defects, Original Article Series XI(16): 167–174
4. Lowry R B, Wignall N 1975 Saldino-Noonan short rib-polydactyly dwarfism syndrome. Pediatrics 56: 121–123
5. Sillence D O 1980 Non-Majewski short rib-polydactyly syndrome. American Journal of Medical Genetics. 7: 223

6. Short Rib-polydactyly Syndrome Type II (Majewski)

1. Majewski F, Pfeiffer R A, Lenz W et al 1971 Polysyndaktylie, Verkurzte Gliedmassen und Genitalfehbildungen: Kennzeichen Eines Selbstandigen Syndromes. Zeitschrift für Kinderheilkunde 111: 118–138
2. Spranger J, Grimm B, Weller M et al 1974 Short rib-polydactyly (SRP) syndromes, types Majewski and Saldino-Noonan. Zeitschrift für Kinderheilkunde 116: 73–94

3. Bido-Lopez P, Ablow R C, Ogden J A, Mahoney M J 1978 A case of short rib-polydactyly. Pediatrics 61: 427–432
4. Chen H, Yang S, Gonzales E, Fowler M and Al Saadi A 1980 Short rib-polydactyly syndrome, Majewski type. American Journal of Medical Genetics 7: 215

7. Chondrodysplasia Punctata

1. Spranger J W, Opitz J M, Bidder U 1971 Heterogeneity of chondrodysplasia punctata. Humangenetik 11: 190–212

a. Rhizomelic Form

1. Spranger J W, Bidder U, Voelz C 1971 Chondrodysplasia punctata (chondrodystrophia calcificans). II der Rhizomele typ. Fortschritte anf dem Gibette der Rontgenstrahlen und der Nuklear Medizin. 114: 327

b. Dominant Form

1. Spranger J W, Bidder U, Voelz C 1970 Chondrodysplasia Punctata (chondrodystrophia calcificans) Type Conradi-Hunermann. Fortschritte anf dem Gebiete der Rontgenstrahken und der Nuklear Medizin. 113: 717–725
2. Theander G, Pettersson J 1978 Calcification in chondrodysplasia punctata. Acta Radiologica Diag Fasc 1: 205–221
3. Kaufman H J, Mahboubi S, Spackman T J, Capitanio M A, Kirkpatrick J 1976 Tracheal stenosis as a complication of chondrodysplasia punctata. Annals of Radiology 19: 203–209
4. Afshani E, Girdany B R 1972 Atlanto-axial dislocation in chondrodysplasia punctata. Radiology 102: 399–401

c. Other Forms. Exclude: Symptomatic stippling in other disorders (eg Zellweger syndrome, warfarin embryopathy)

1. Shaul W L, Emery H, Hall J G 1975 Chondrodyplasia punctata and maternal warfarin use during pregnancy. American Journal of Diseases of Children 129: 360
2. Sheffield L J, Danks D M, Mayne V, Hutchinson L A 1976 Chondrodysplasia punctata-23 cases of a mild and relatively common variety. Journal of Pediatrics 89: 916–923

8. Campomelic Dysplasia

1. Khajavi A, Lachman R, Rimoin D, Schimke R N, Dorst J, Handmaker S, Ebbin A, Perreault G 1976 Heterogeneity in the campomelic syndromes. Radiology 120: 641–647
2. Maroteaux P, Spranger J, Opitz J M, Kucera J, Lowry R B, Schimke R N, Kagan S M 1971 Le syndrome campomelique. Presse Medicale 79: 1157
3. Thurmon T F, DeFraites E B, Anderson E E 1973 Familial camptomelic dwarfism. Journal of Pediatrics 83: 841–843
4. Hoefnagel D, Wurster-Hill D H, Dupree W B, Benirschke K, Fuld G L 1978 Camptomelic dwarfism associated with XY-gonadal dysgenesis and chromosome anomalies. Clinical Genetics 13: 489–499

9. Other Dysplasias with Congenital Bowing of Long Bones (several forms)

1. Khajavi A, Lachman R, Rimoin D, Schimke R N, Dorst J, Handmaker S, Ebbin A, Perreault G 1976 Heterogeneity in the campomelic syndromes. Radiology 120: 641–647
2. Stuve A, Wiedemann H 1971 Congenital bowing of the long bones in two sisters. Lancet 2: 495

10. Achondroplasia

1. Langer L O Jr, Baumann P A, Gorlin R L 1967 Achondroplasia. American Journal of Roentgenology, Radium therapy and Nuclear Medicine 100: 12–26
2. Murdoch J L, Walker B A, Hall J G, Abbey II, Smith K K, McKusick V A 1970 Achondroplasia – a genetic and statistical survey. Annals of Human Genetics 33: 227–244
3. Rimoin D L, Hughes G N F, Kaufman R L, Rosenthal R E, McAlster W H, Silberberg R 1970 Endochondral

ossification in achondroplastic dwarfism. New England
Journal of Medicine 283: 728
4. Scott C I 1976 Achondroplastic and hypochondroplastic
dwarfism. Clinical Orthopaedics 114: 18

11. Diastrophic Dysplasia
1. Hollister D W, Lachman R S 1976 Diastrophic
dwarfism. Clinical Orthopaedics 114: 61–69
2. Horton W A, Rimoin D L, Lachman R S, Skovby F,
Hollister D W, Spranger J, Scott C I, Hall J G 1978 The
phenotypic variability of diastrophic dysplasia. Journal of
Pediatrics 93: 609–613
3. Lamy M, Maroteaux P 1960 La nanisme diastrophique.
Presse Medicale 68: 1977–1980
4. Walker B A, Scott C I, Hall J G, Murdoch J L,
McKusick V A 1972 Diastrophic dwarfism. Medicine 51: 1

12. Metatropic Dysplasia (several forms)
1. Jenkins P, Smith M D, McKinnell J S 1970 Metatropic
dwarfism. British Journal of Radiology 43: 561–565
2. Maroteaux P, Spranger J, Wiedemann H R 1966 Der
Metatropische Zwergwuchs. Archiv für Kinderheilkunde
173: 211–226
3. Rimoin D L, Siggers D C, Lachman R S, Silberberg R
1976 Metatropic dwarfism, the Kniest syndrome and the
pseudoachondroplastic dysplasias. Clinical Orthopedics
114: 70
4. Gefferth K 1973 Metatropic dwarfism. Progress in
Pediatric Radiology 4: 137–151

13. Chondroectodermal Dysplasia (Ellis-van Creveld)
1. Jequier S, Dunbar J S 1973 The Ellis-van Creveld
syndrome. Progress in Pediatric Radiology 4: 167–183
2. Kozlowski K, Szmigiel C, Barylak A, Stropyrowa M 1972
Difficulties in differentiation between chondroectodermal
dysplasia (Ellis-van Creveld syndrome) and asphyxiating
thoracic dystrophy. Australasian Radiology 16: 401–410
3. McKusick V A, Egeland J A, Eldridge R, Krusen D R
1964 Dwarfism in the Amish. I. The Ellis-van Creveld
syndrome. Bulletin of the Johns Hopkins Hospital 115: 306
4. Blackburn M G, Belliveau R E 1971 Ellis-van Creveld
syndrome. American Journal of Diseases of Children
122: 267–270

14. Asphyxiating Thoracic Dysplasia (Jeune)
1. Herdman R C, Langer L O 1968 The thoracic
asphyxiant dystrophy and renal disease. American Journal of
Diseases in Children 116: 192–201
2. Langer L O Jr 1968 Thoracic-pelvic-phalangeal
dystrophy: asphyxiating thoracic dystrophy of the newborn,
infantile thoracic dystrophy. Radiology 91: 447–546
3. Maroteaux P, Savart P 1964 La dystrophie thoracique
asphyxiant; etude radiologique et rapports avec le syndrome
d'Ellis et van Creveld. Annales Radiology 7: 332
4. Oberklaid F, Danks D M, Moyne V, Campbell B 1977
Asphyxiating thoracic dysplasia: clinical, radiological and
pathological information on 10 patients. Archives of Disease
in Childhood 52: 758
5. Koxlowski K, Szmigiel C, Barylak A 1972 Difficulties in
differentiation between chondroectodermal dysplasia
(Ellis-van Creveld syndrome) and asphyxiating thoracic
dystrophy. Australasian Radiology 16: 401–410
6. Cortina J, Beltran J, Olague R, Ceres L, Alonson A,
Lanuza A 1979 The wide spectrum of the asphyxiating
thoracic dysplasia. Pediatric Radiology 8: 93–99

15. Spondyloepiphyseal Dysplasia Congenita

a. Type Spranger-Wiedemann
1. Bach C, Maroteaux P, Schaefer P, Bitan A, Crumiere C
1967 Dysplasia spondylo-epiphysaire congenitale avec
anomalies multiples. Archives Françaises Pediatrie
24: 24–33
2. Spranger J W, Langer L O Jr 1970 Spondyloepiphyseal
dysplasia congenita. Radiology 94: 313–322
3. Spranger J, Wiedemann H R 1966 Dysplasia
spondyloepiphysaria congenita. Helvetica Pediatrica Acta
6: 598–611
4. Kozlowski K, Bittel-Dobrzynska N, Budzynska A 1967
Spondyloepiphyseal dysplasia congenita. Annals of
Radiology 11: 367–375

b. Other Forms (see B 11 and 12)
1. Maroteaux P, Wiedemann H R, Spranger J, Kozlowski
K, Lenzi L 1968 Essai de classification des dysplasies
spondyloepiphysaires. Monographies de Genetique
Medicale. Lyon, France
2. Spranger J, Langer L O 1974 Spondyloepiphyseal
dysplasias. In: Skeletal Dysplasias. Birth Defects Original
Articles Series X(9): 19

16. Kniest Dysplasia
1. Maroteaux P, Spranger J 1973 La maladie de Kniest.
Archives Francaises Pediatrie 30: 735
2. Siggers D, Rimoin D L, Dorst J P, Doty S, Williams B,
Hollister D W, Silberberg R, Cranley R, Kaufman R,
McKusick V A 1974 The Kniest syndrome. In: skeletal
dysplasias. Birth Defects Original Article Series X(9): 193
3. Lachman R S, Rimoin D L, Hollister D W, Dorst J P,
Siggers D C, McAlister W, Kaufman R L, Langer L O 1975
The Kniest syndrome. Radiology 123: 805

17. Mesomelic Dysplasia
1. Kaitila II, Leisti J T, Rimoin D L 1976 Mesomelic
skeletal dysplasias. Clinical Orthopedics 114: 94–106

a. Type Nievergelt
1. Nievergelt K 1944 Positiver Vaterschaftorachivers auf
Grund Erblicher Missbildunger der Extremitäten. Arch
Klaus-Stift Vererb Forsch 19: 157
2. Solonen K A, Sulamaa M 1958 Nievergelt syndrome and
its treatment; a case report. Ann Chir Gynaecol Fenn
47: 142–147

b. Type Langer (probably Homozygous Dyschondrosteosis)
1. Langer L O Jr 1967 Mesomelic dwarfism of the
hypoplastic ulna, fibula mandible type. Radiology
89: 654–660
2. Espiritu C, Chen H, Wooley P V 1975 Mesomelic
dwarfism as the homozygous expression of
dyschondrosteosis. American Journal of diseases of Children
129: 375
3. Silverman F N 1973 Mesomelic dwarfism. Progress in
Pediatrics and Radiology 4: 546–562

c. Type Robinow
1. Kelly T E, Benson R, Temtamy S A, Plotnick L, Levin
S 1975 The Robinow syndrome: an isolated case with a
detailed study of the phenotype. American Journal of
Diseases in Children 129: 383–386
2. Robinow M, Silverman F N, Smith H D 1969 A newly
recognized dwarfing syndrome. American Journal of
Diseases of Children 117: 645–651

d. Type Reinhardt
1. Reinhardt K, Pfeiffer R A 1967 Ulno-fibulare Dysplasie.
Eine autosomal-dominant vererbte Mikromesomelie ähnlich
dem Nievergelts syndrom. Fortschritte anf dem Gebiete der
Rontgenstrahlen und der Nuklear Medizin 107: 379

18. Acromesomelic Dysplasias
1. Campailla E, Martinelli B 1971 Deficit staturale con
micromesomelia. Presentazione di due casi familiari.

Minerva Ortopedica 22: 180

2. Maroteaux P, Martinelli B, Campailla E 1971 Le nanisme acromesomelique. Press Medicale 79: 1839

3. Langer L O, Beals R K, Solomon I L, Bard P A, Baard L A, Rissman E M, Rogers J G, Dorst J P, Hall J G, Sparkes R S, Franken E A 1977 Acromesomelic dwarfism: manifestations in childhood. American Journal of Medical Genetics 1: 87–100

4. Langer L O, Garrett R T 1980 Acromesomelic dysplasia. Radiology 137: 349–355

19. Cleidocranial Dysplasia

1. Faure C, Maroteaux P 1973 Cleidocranial dysplasia. Progress in Pediatrics and Radiology 4: 211

2. Forland M 1962 Cleidocranial Dysostosis. A review of the syndrome. American Journal of Medicine 33: 792

3. Keats T E 1967 Cleidocranial dysostosis: some atypical roentgen manifestations. American Journal of Roentgenology, Radium therapy and Nuclear Medicine 100: 71–74

4. Hawkins H B, Shapiro R, Petrillo C J 1975 The Association of cleidocranial dysostosis with hearing loss. American Journal of Roentgenology, Radium therapy and Nuclear Medicine 125: 944–947

20. Larsen Syndrome

1. Larsen L J, Schottstaedt E R, Bost R C 1950 Multiple congenital dislocations associated with characteristic facial abnormality. Journal of Pediatrics 37: 574

2. Latta R J, Graham B, Aase J, Scham S M, Smith D W 1971 Larsen's syndrome: a skeletal dysplasia with multiple joint dislocations and unusual facies. Journal of Pediatrics 78: 291

3. Steel H H, Kohl J 1972 Multiple congenital dislocations associated with other skeletal anomalies (Larsen's syndrome) in three siblings. Journal of Bone and Joint Surgery 54A: 75

4. Robertson F W, Kozlowski K, Middleton R W 1975 Larsen's syndrome. Clinical Pediatrics 14: 53–60

5. Micheli L J, Hall J E, Watts H G 1976 Spinal instability in Larsen's syndrome. Journal of Bone and Joint Surgery 58A: 562–565

21. Otopalatodigital Syndrome

1. Dudding B A, Gorlin R J, Langer L O 1967 The oto-palato-digital syndrome. American Journal of Diseases of Children 113: 214

2. Gall J C, Stern A M, Poznanski A K, Garn S M, Weinstein E D, Hayward J R 1972 Oto-palato-digital syndromes: comparison of clinical and radiographic manifestations in males and females. American Journal of Human Genetics 24: 24

3. Langer L O 1967 The roentgenographic features of the otopalato-digital (OPD) syndrome. Americal Journal of Roentgenology, Radium Therapy and Nuclear Medicine 100: 63

4. Kozlowski K, Turner G, Scougall J, Harrington J 1977 Oto-palato-digital syndrome with severe X–ray changes in two half brothers. Pediatric Radiology 6: 97–102

B. Identifiable in Later Life

1. Hypochondroplasia

1. Beals R K 1969 Hypochondroplasia. A report of five kindreds. Journal of Bone and Joint Surgery 51A: 728–739

2. Kozlowski K 1973 Hypochondroplasia. Progress in Pediatric Radiology 4: 238–249

3. Walker B A, Murdoch J L, McKusick V A, Langer L O, Beals R K 1971 Hypochondroplasia. American Journal of Diseases of Children 122: 95

4. Frydman M, Hertz M, Goodman R M 1974 The genetic entity of hypochondroplasia. Clinical Genetics 5: 223–229

5. Newman D E, Dunbar J S 1975 Hypochondroplasia. Journal of the Canadian Association of Radiologists 26: 95–103

2. Dyschondrosteosis

1. Langer L O Jr 1965 Dyschondrosteosis: A hereditable bone dysplasia with characteristic roentgenographic features. American Journal of Roentgenology, Radium Therapy and Nuclear Medicine 95: 178–188

2. Kaitila II, Leisti J T, Rimoin D L 1976 Mesomelic skeletal dysplasias. Clinical Orthopaedics 114: 94–106

3. Maroteaux P, Lamy M 1959 La dyschondrosteose. Sem Hôp Paris 35: 3464–3470

4. Felman A H, Kirkpatrick 1970 Dyschondrosteose. American Journal of Diseases of Children 120: 329–331

5. Espiritu C, Chen H, Wooley P V 1975 Mesomelic dwarfism as the homozygous expression of dyschondrosteosis 129: 375–377

6. Carter A R, Currey H L 1974 Dyschondrosteosis (mesomelic dwarfism) – a family study. British Journal of Radiology 47: 634–640

3. Metaphyseal Chondrodysplasia Type Jansen

1. De Haas WHD, DeBoer W, Griffioen F 1969 Metaphyseal dysostosis. A late fellow-up of the first reported case. Journal of Bone and Joint Surgery 51A: 290–299

2. Holt J F 1969 Discussion. In: Skeletal Dysplasias. Part IV, Birth Defects Original Article Series V(4): 73

3. Jansen M 1934 Über atypische Chondrodystrophie (Achondroplasie) und über eine noch nicht beschriebene angeborene Wachstrumstörung des Knochensystems. Metaphysäre Dysostose. Orthopedika Chirgica 61: 253–286

4. Metaphyseal Chondrodysplasia Type Schmid

1. Kozlowski K 1964 Metaphyseal dysostosis. Report of five familial and two sporadic cases of a mild type. American Journal of Roentgenology, Radium Therapy and Nuclear Medicine 91: 601–608

2. Stickler G R, Maher F R, Hunt J C, Burke E C, Rosevaer J W 1962 Familial bone disease resembling rickets (hereditary metaphyseal dysostosis). Pediatrics 29: 996

3. Dent C E, Normand I C 1964 Metaphyseal dysostosis type Schmid. Archives of Disease in Childhood 39: 444

4. Wekselman R 1977 Familial metaphyseal dysostosis. American Journal of Roentgenology, Radium Therapy and Nuclear Medicine 59-A: 690–691

5. Metaphyseal Chondrodysplasia Type McKusick

1. Lux S E, Johnston R B, August C S, Say B, Penchaszhadeh V B, Rosen F S, McKusick V A 1970 Chronic neutropenia and abnormal cellular immunity in cartilage-hair hypoplasia. New England Journal of Medicine 282: 231–236

2. McKusick V A, Eldridge R, Hostetler J A, Ruangwit U, Egeland J A 1965 Dwarfism in the Amish II. Cartilage-hair hypoplasia. Bulletin of the Johns Hopkins Hospital 116: 285–326

3. Ray H C, Dorst J P 1973 Cartilage-hair hypoplasia. Progress in Pediatric Radiology 4: 270–298

6. Metaphyseal Chondrodysplasia with Exocrine Pancreatic Insufficiency and Cyclic Neutropenia

1. Schmerling D H, Prader A, Hitzig W H, Giedion A, Hadorn B, Kuhni M 1969 The syndrome of exocrine pancreatic insufficiency, neutropenia, metaphyseal dysostosis and dwarfism. Helvetica Paediatrica Acta 24: 547

2. Taybi H, Mitchell A D, Friedman G D 1969 Metaphyseal dysostosis and the associated syndrome of pancreatic insufficiency and blood disorders. Radiology 93: 563–571

7. Spondylometaphyseal Dysplasia

a. Type Kozlowski
1. Kozlowski K 1976 Metaphyseal and spondylometaphyseal chondrodysplasias. Clinical Orthopedics 114: 83
2. Kozlowski K, Maroteaux P, Spranger J 1967 La dysotose spondylometaphysaire. Presse Medicale 75: 2769
3. Riggs W, Summit R L 1971 Spondylometaphyseal dysplasia (Kozlowski). Radiology 101: 375
4. Thomas P S, Nevin N C 1977 Spondylometaphyseal dysplasia. American Journal of Roentgenology, Radium Therapy and Nuclear Medicine 128: 89–93
5. Gustavson K H, Homgren G, Probst F 1978 Spondylometaphyseal dysplasia in two sibs of normal parents. Pediatric Radiology 7: 90–96

b. Other forms
1. Rimoin D L 1975 The chondrodystrophies Advances in Human Genetics 5: 1
2. Schmidt B J, Becak W, Becak M L, Soibelman I, Silva Queiroz A, Da Lorga A P, Secaf F, Andrade Carvalho A 1963 Metaphyseal dysostosis. Journal of Pediatrics 63: 106
3. Lachman R, Zonana J, Khajavi A, et al 1978 The spondylometaphyseal dysplasias: clinical, radiologic and pathologic correlation. Annales de Radiologie 22: 125–135

8. Multiple Epiphyseal Dysplasia

1. Spranger J 1976 The epiphyseal dysplasias. Clinical Orthopedics 114: 46

a. Type Fairbank
1. Fairbank H A T 1946 Dysplasia epiphysealis multiplex. Proceedings of the Royal Society of Medicine 39: 315–317
2. Leed N E 1960 Epiphyseal Dysplasia multiplex. American Journal of Roentgenology, Radium Therapy and Nuclear Medicine 84: 506–510
3. Jacobs J 1973 Multiple epiphyseal dysplasia. Progress in Pediatric Radiology 4: 309–324
4. Kozlowski K, Lipska E 1967 Hereditary dysplasia epiphysealis multiplex. Clinical Radiology 18: 330–336

b. Other Forms
1. Juberg R C, Holt J F 1968 Inheritance of multiple epiphyseal dysplasia tarda. American Journal of Human Genetics 20: 549–563
2. Ribbing S 1937 Studien über Heredetaire, Multiple Epiphysenstorungen. Acta Radiologica 35(Suppl): 1–107
3. Hulvey J T, Keats T 1969 Multiple epiphyseal dysplasia. American Journal of Roentgenology, Radium Therapy and Nuclear Medicine CVI: 170–177

9. Arthro-ophthalmopathy (Stickler)
1. Opitz J M, Franc T, Herrmann J 1972 The Stickler syndrome. New England Journal of Medicine 286: 546–547
2. Stickler G B, Belau P G, Farrell F J, Jones J D, Pugh D G, Steinberg A G, Ward L E 1965 Hereditary progressive arthro-opthalmopathy. Mayo Clinical Proceedings 40: 433–455
3. Stickler G B, Pugh D G 1967 Hereditary progressive arthro-ophthalmopathy II. additional observations on vertebral abnormalities, a hearing defect, and a report of a similar case. Mayo Clinical Proceedings 42: 495–500
4. Say B, Berry J, Barbar N 1977 The Stickler syndrome (hereditary arthro-ophthalmopathy). Clinical Genetics 12: 179–182

10. Pseudoachondroplasia

a. Dominant
1. Ford N, Silverman R N, Kozlowski K 1961

Spondylo-epiphyseal dysplasia (pseudo-achondroplastic type) American Journal of Roentgenology, Radium Therapy and Nuclear Medicine 86: 462–472
2. Maroteaux P, Lamy M 1959 Les formes psuedo-achondroplastiques des dysplasies spondylo-epiphysaires. Presse Medicale 67: 383–386
3. Phillips S J, Magsamen B F, Punnett H H, Kistenmacher M L, Campo R D 1974 Fine structure of skeletal dysplasia as seen in pseudoachondroplastic spondyloepiphyseal dysplasia and asphyxiating thoracic dystrophy. In: Skeletal Dysplasias. Birth Defects Original Article Series X(12): 314

b. Recessive
1. Hall J G 1975 Pseudoachondroplasia. In: Disorders of Connective Tissue. Birth Defects Original Article Series XI(6): 187

11. Spondyloepiphyseal Dysplasia Tarda
1. Langer L O Jr 1964 Spondyloepiphyseal dysplasia tarda. Hereditary chondrodysplasia with characteristic vertebral configuration in the adult. Radiology 82: 833–839
2. Maroteaux P, Lamy M, Bernard J 1957 La dysplasie spondyloepiphysaire tardive; description clinique et radiologique. Presse Medicale 65: 1205–1208
3. Bannerman R M, Ingall G B, Mohn J F 1971 X–linked spondylo-epiphyseal dysplasia tarda: clinical and linkage data. Journal of Medical Genetics. 8: 291–301
4. Harper P S, Jenkins P, Laurence K M 1973 Spondylo-epiphyseal dysplasia tarda: a report of four cases in two families. British Journal of Radiology 46: 676–684

12. Spondyloepiphyseal Dysplasia, other forms (see A.15 and 16)

1. Spranger J 1976 The epiphyseal dysplasias. Clinical Orthopaedics 114: 46
2. Spranger J, Langer L O 1974 Spondyloepiphyseal dysplasias. In: Skeletal Dysplasias. Birth Defects Original Article Series X(9): 19–61
3. Maroteaux P, Wiedemann H R, Spranger J et al 1968 Essai de classification des dysplasies spondyloepiphysaires. Simep, Lyon
4. Lachman R S, Rimoin D L, Hall J G, Kozlowski K, Langer L O, Scott C I, Spranger J 1975 Difficulties in the classification of the epiphyseal dysplasias. In: Disorders of Connective Tissue. Birth Defects Original Article Series XI(16): 231–248

13. Dyggve-Melchior-Clausen Dysplasia
1. Naffah J 1976 The Dyggve-Melchior-Clausen syndrome. American Journal of Human Genetics 28: 607
2. Spranger J W, Der Kaloustian J M 1975 The Dyggve-Melchior-Clausen syndrome. Radiology 114: 415
3. Spranger J W, Bierbaum B, Herrmann J 1976 Heterogeneity of Dyggve-Melchior-Clausen dwarfism. Human Genetics 33: 279
4. Kaufman R L, Rimoin D L, McAlister W H 1971 The Dyggve-Melchior-Clausen syndrome. Birth Defects Original Article Series VII: 144–149
5. Bonafede R P, Beighton P 1978 The Dyggve-Melchior-Clausen syndrome. Clinical Genetics 14: 24–30
6. Schorr S, Legum C, Oschshorn M, et al 1977 The Dyggve-Melchior-Clausen syndrome. American Journal of Roentgenology, Radium Therapy and Nuclear Medicine 128: 107–113

14. Spondyloepimetaphyseal Dysplasia (several forms)
1. Arias S, Mata M Pinto-Cisternas J 1976

L'osteochondrodysplasie spondylo-metaphysaire type Irapa: nouveau nanisme over rachis et metatarscens courts. Nouvelle Presse Medicale 5: 319

2. Kozlowski K, Budzinska A 1966 Combined metaphyseal and epiphyseal dysostosis. American Journal of Roentgenology, Radium Therapy and Nuclear Medicine 97: 21

3. Kozlowski K 1974 Micromelic type of spondylo-meta-epiphyseal dysplasia. Pediatr Radiol 2: 61

15. Myotonic Chondrodysplasia (Catel-Schwartz-Jampel)

1. Kozlowski K, Wise G 1974 Spondylo-epi-metaphyseal dysplasia with myotonia. A radiographic study. Radio Diagn (Berl) 6: 817

2. Fowler W M, Loyzer R B, Taylor R G et al 1974 The Schwartz-Jampel syndrome. Its clinical, physiological and histological expressions. Journal of the Neurological Sciences 22: 127

3. Van Huffelen A C, Gabrealo F J M, Van Luypen J S et al 1974 Chondrodystrophic myotonia. Neuropaediatri 5: 71

4. Beighton P 1973 The Schwartz syndrome in Southern Africa. Clinical Genetics 4: 548–555

16. Parastremmatic Dysplasia

1. Langer L O, Petersen D, Spranger J 1970 An unusual bone dysplasia: parastremmatic dwarfism. American Journal of Roentgenology, Radium Therapy and Nuclear Medicine 110: 550–560

2. Rask M R 1963 Morquio-Brailsford osteochondrodystrophy and osteogenesis imperfects: report of a patient with both conditions. Journal of Bone and Joint Surgery 45A: 561–570

3. Horan F, Beighton P 1976 Parastremmatic dwarfism. Journal of Bone and Joint Surgery 58B: 343–346

17. Trichorhinophalangeal Dysplasia

1. Felman A H, Frias J L 1977 Trichorhinophalangeal syndrome – study of 16 patients in one family. American Journal of Roentgenology, Radium Therapy and Nuclear Medicine 129: 631

2. Giedion A, Burdea M, Fruchter Z et al 1973 Autosomal dominant transmission of the trichorhinophalangeal syndrome. Paediatrica Acta 28: 249

3. Poznanski A K, Schmickel R D and Harper H A 1974 The hand in the trichorhinophalangeal syndrome. Birth Defects Original Article Series X(9): 209–219

4. Kozlowski K, Blaim A and Malolepszy E 1972 Trichorhinophalangeal syndrome. Australasian Radiology XVI(4): 411–416

5. Pashayan H M, Solomon L M and Chan G 1974 The trichorhinophalangeal syndrome. American Journal of Diseases of Children 127: 257–261

18. Acrodysplasia with Retinitis Pigmentosa and Nephropathy (Saldino-Mainzer)

1. Saldino R M, Mainzer F 1971 Cone-shaped epiphyses (CSE) in siblings with hereditary renal disease and retinitis pigmentosa. Radiology 98: 39

2. Giedion A 1979 Phalangeal cone-shaped epiphyses of the hands (PhCSEH) and chronic renal disease – the conorenal syndromes. Pediatric Radiology 8: 32

Disorders of bone density, volume and mineralisation

D. O. Sillence

This large group of genetic disorders of the skeleton consists of diseases characterised by abnormalities in the amount, density and remodelling of bone. It can be subdivided into the three following groups: disorders with a net decrease in skeletal tissue, disorders with a net increase of bone, and disorders of mineralisation and mineral metabolism.

DISORDERS WITH DECREASED BONE DENSITY

Decreased bone density may result from reduced production, defective mineralisation, increased breakdown of normal or defective bone, or a combination of these. Osteomalacia (i.e. undermineralised bone) characterises hereditary rickets and other disorders leading to defective mineralisation. Osteopoenia (insufficient bone) characterises the hereditary osteoporoses and a number of other genetic and acquired diseases of childhood. Osteoporosis, i.e. the clinical syndromes resulting from osteopoenia, is characterised by liability to fractures, particularly crush fractures of the vertebrae. The most important numerically of the syndromes with osteoporosis are the osteogenesis imperfecta syndromes.

Osteogenesis imperfecta

The term 'osteogenesis imperfecta' (OI) was advocated by Vrolik in 1840 to explain the origin of an hereditary skeletal condition leading to susceptibility to fracture and severe skeletal deformity. Also known as fragilitas ossium, osteopsathyrosis, Ekman-Lobstein and Vrolik disease, osteogenesis imperfecta is characterized by its variable clinical severity. Until recently this wide variability in severity was explained by the variable expressivity of a single dominant gene. However, recent genetic and epidemiological studies suggest that at least part of the variability in OI can be accounted for by four genetic syndromes, OI types I–IV (Sillence et al, 1979 a, b).

Osteogenesis imperfecta type I
This syndrome is characterised by osteoporosis leading

736

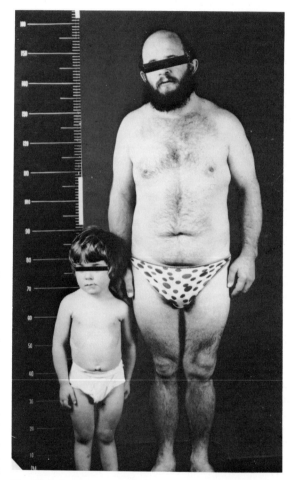

Fig. 52.1 Osteogenesis imperfecta type I. Father and son showing mild shortening of stature. Both have intensely blue sclerae, numerous fractures and mild shortening of stature. Father wears a hearing aid.

to excessive bone fragility, distinctly blue sclerae and susceptibility to presenile conductive hearing loss in adolescents and adults with the disorder (Fig. 52.1).

Inheritance. This is an autosomal dominant trait with variable expressivity. Penetrance for fractures approximates 90% and for blue sclerae 100%. Hearing impairment is age-related (Riedner et al, 1980).

Pathogenesis. This is largely unknown. Biochemical studies of connective tissue and collagens synthesised by cultured fibroblasts suggest that the defect may lie in defective synthesis or defective regulation of the synthesis of the polypeptides of type I collagen, the principal collagen of bone (Sykes et al, 1977).

Natural history. This is the commonest variety of osteogenesis imperfecta and has a birth frequency in the order of 1 per 30 000 live births and a population frequency similarly in the order of 1 per 30 000 (Sillence et al, 1979 a). The sclerae in these patients are generally a deep blue-black. Fractures characteristically result from minimal trauma although despite the tendency to bone fragility, accidental trauma does not always lead to fractures. Some 10% of individuals in families with this trait have fractures at birth, but these are generally few in number, and individuals with fractures at birth subsequently have no more deformity, handicap or number of fractures than individuals who have their first fracture after 1 year of age. Deformities of the limbs in this group are largely the result of fractures, but bowing, particularly of the lower limbs, is common. Other deformities, such as genu valgum and flat feet with a metatarsus varus deformity of the feet, are common. Some 20% of adults have progressive kyphoscoliosis which may be severe. Kyphosis alone is common in older adults but rarely seen in children. There is usually excessive hyperlaxity of ligaments, particularly at the small joints of the hands, feet and knees, but this feature is less marked in adults. There is usually only mild short stature, with body proportions depending on the relative involvement of limbs or spine.

Hearing impairment is a most troublesome complication. It is rarely recognised by 10 years of age. Approximately all affected adults have recognisable hearing impairment by 50 years of age. Almost 40% of adults have severe hearing impairment. This is predominantly conductive, but in some cases both conductive and sensori-neural impairment is found (Riedner et al, 1980).

There is a high frequency of premature arcus senilis in adults with OI type I. No other visual abnormalities are associated with osteogenesis imperfecta.

Hereditary opalescent dentin (dentinogenesis imperfecta) is observed in some families with this trait but not in others (Levin et al, 1980). Opalescent dentin produces a distinctive yellowing and apparent transparency of the teeth, which are often rapidly worn prematurely or broken. Some teeth with opalescent dentin may have a particularly greyish-blue hue. Radiological study of these teeth shows that they have short roots with constricted coronoradicular junction. The fact that opalescent dentin is seen in some families and not in others has been suggested as a feature which may distinguish two hereditary

types of osteogenesis imperfecta with otherwise identical OI type I phenotypes (Levin et al, 1980). It has been proposed that families with normal teeth be designated OI type IA and families with opalescent dentin OI type IB.

Radiographic studies in all patients in this group show generalised osteopoenia, evidence of previous fractures and normal callus formation at the site of recent fractures. Deformities are usually the result of angulation at the site of previous fractures. However, bowing of the femora and tibia and fibula, and deformity in the bones of the feet, particularly metatarsus varus, are observed. Severe osteoporosis of the spine with codfish vertebrae is occasionally seen in these patients, but the majority have normally formed vertebral bodies. Kyphoscoliosis is not usually diagnosed in childhood.

Spontaneous improvement is observed during adolescene with a marked reduction in the frequency of fractures.

Complications. Repeated fractures associated with minimal trauma are a common complication. Ankle sprains and joint dislocations occur rarely.

Differential diagnosis.

1. Juvenile idiopathic osteoporosis. This syndrome has been clearly delineated by Brenton and Dent (1976). The onset of fractures commonly commences in late childhood and the axial skeleton is more severely affected. Spontaneous cure is the rule. The sclerae are not distinctly blue although the normal blueness of the sclerae in childhood must be distinguished from the distinct blueness of the sclerae in OI. Juvenile osteoporosis appears to occur sporadically.

2. Blue sclerae and keratoconus. Greenfield et al, (1973) have summarised the findings in a rare syndrome of blue sclerae with keratoconus, middle ear bone conduction defect and spondylolisthesis. These cases have had no fractures, but did have hyperextensibility of joints, and the syndrome appears to be inherited as an autosomal recessive trait.

3. Blue sclerae, familial nephrosis, thin skin and hydrocephalus. Daentl et al (1978) have delineated this recessive syndrome which is not associated with skeletal fragility.

4. Overlapping connective tissue syndromes

a. Osteogenesis imperfecta with Marfan syndrome. Carey et al (1968) reported a family with 23 cases of OI in four generations. The proband in this family had clinical features of both the Marfan syndrome and of OI, e.g. bone fragility, blue sclerae and deafness in addition to tall stature, arachnodactyly and aortic insufficiency from which he died suddenly at the age of 32 years.

b. Osteogenesis imperfecta and Ehlers-Danlos syndrome. Biering and Iversen (1955) reported a patient with marked joint hyperextensibility, loose wrinkled skin and features of OI, i.e. blue sclerae and osteoporosis leading to fractures.

Therapy. The mainstay of treatment at present is aggressive orthopaedic care with appropriate management of fractures to avoid deformity and unnecessary immobilisation. Magnesium oxide, vitamin C, sodium fluoride, androgenic hormones and calcitonin have been advocated in the medical management of osteogenesis imperfecta but no consistent therapeutic effect has been observed.

Genetic counselling and prenatal diagnosis. For an affected adult marrying a normal partner there is a 50% chance of an affected child. Where two adults with OI type I marry there is a 25% chance for a severely affected infant homozygous for OI type I.

Prenataly ultrasound and radiographic studies are unlikely to differentiate a normal from an affected fetus (Lachman & Hall, 1979). Biochemical prenatal diagnosis is not yet available.

Osteogenesis imperfecta type II

This is a lethal osteogenesis imperfecta syndrome which is characterised by low birth weight and length and the characteristic radiographic finding of crumpled long bones and beaded ribs (Fig. 52.2).

Inheritance. A sufficient number of familial cases with an autosomal recessive pattern of inheritance have been reported to suggest that the majority, if not all, babies with this phenotype result from autosomal recessive inheritance (Sillence et al, 1979 a).

Natural history. Approximately half the cases are stillborn and the remainder die soon after birth due to respiratory insufficiency resulting from the defective thoracic cage. Rarely, infants with this phenotype have survived the newborn period to die within the first year of life from cardiorespiratory complications. Clinically, the skull is soft with multiple palpable bone islands. The face may show beaking of the nose and apparent hypotelorism, and the limbs are extremely short, bent and deformed. The thighs are characteristically broad and fixed at right angles to the trunk. The skin is excessively fragile and thin and maybe torn during delivery. Epidemiological studies suggest that the birth frequency is in the order of 1 per 60 000 births (Sillence et al, 1979 a).

Skeletal radiographs show extreme beading of the ribs due to multiple fractures and a crumpled (accordion-like) appearance of the long bones, especially the femora, with diffuse osteopoenia in the face and skull and multiple bone islands in the vault.

Differential diagnosis.

1. OI with microcephaly and cataracts. Buyse and Bull (1978) have delineated an autosomal recessive syndrome with clinical and radiographic features similar to

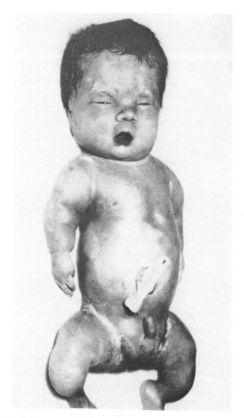

Fig. 52.2 Osteogenesis imperfecta type II. Stillborn infant showing short deformed limbs with broad thighs fixed at right angles to trunk and relatively large head.

those of OI type II, but all affected patients had microcephaly and cataracts.

2. OI with subluxed lenses and coarctation of the aorta. One of the sibs described by Remigio and Grinvalsky (1970) had one dislocated lens, long fingers and coarctation of the aorta. Whether this represents a distinct disorder with other features identical to OI type II or whether it represents variability within OI type II is not yet known.

Treatment. No therapeutic intervention will lead to quality survival.

Genetic counselling and prenatal diagnosis. Even though a dominantly inherited phenocopy of this syndrome is possible, one must counsel effectively as though all cases result from autosomal recessive inheritance, i.e. with a 25% recurrence risk for further affected children.

Prenatal ultrasound and radiographic studies have been used by several groups to detect an affected fetus with short deformed limbs and poor cranial ossification by 20 weeks gestation. In one case the diagnosis has been confirmed by the demonstration of intracellular accumulation of type I procollagen in cultured amniotic cells (Shapiro et al, 1982). O.I. type II is clearly biochemically heterogeneous, so that this technique may not be useful in all pregnancies at risk.

Osteogenesis imperfecta type III

This syndrome is characterised by autosomal recessive inheritance of largely non-lethal OI with severe bone fragility leading to progressive deformity of the skeleton (Sillence et al, 1979 a) (Fig. 52.3).

Inheritance. This is autosomal recessive. The existence of families with varying severity, ranging from newborn lethal OI (but distinct from OI type II) to moderately severe OI compatible with childhood survival suggests that this syndrome may be genetically and biochemically heterogeneous.

Natural history. These individuals present at birth or in infancy with severe bone fragility and multiple fractures leading to progressive deformity of the skeleton. While the sclerae may be particularly blue at birth, observations of several patients with this syndrome suggest that the sclerae become progressively less blue with age. Very few of these patients reach adult life so that it is not known with certainty whether the sclerae are ever completely normal. These infants generally have normal birth weight and often normal birth length, although this may be reduced because of deformities of the lower limbs at birth. Fractures are present in the majority of cases at birth and occur frequently during childhood. Pro-

gressive kyphoscoliosis develops during childhood and progresses into adolescence. Final stature is very short. Hearing impairment has not been reported in children with this syndrome, but it would not be surprising in view of the severe osteopoenia and liability to fractures if there was significant involvement of the ossicular chain leading to hearing defect in some cases. The majority of patients have opalescent dentin with yellowish-brown or grey teeth showing increased wear and chipping. A sizable proportion of cases succumb in infancy or childhood from cardiorespiratory complications.

Skeletal radiographs show generalised osteopoenia with multiple fractures throughout the skeleton. These cases do not show the continuous beading of the ribs or crumpling of all the long bones which is seen in OI type II. There appears to be progressive osteopoenia and a severe degree of platyspondyly with codfish vertebrae in the spine. The skull shows generalised osteopoenia with multiple Wormian bones.

Differential diagnosis.

1. OI with multiple malformations. Saint-Martin et al (1979) have described a syndrome in two male newborns (autosomal or X – linked recessive), quite distinct radiographically from OI type II, with severe osteopoenia of the skull and multiple skeletal deformities and non-skeletal malformations. The latter include syndactyly, cleft palate, omphalocoele and bilateral undescended testes.

Osteogenesis imperfecta type IV

This syndrome is characterised by osteoporosis leading to bone fragility without other features of the classic OI type I syndrome (Sillence et al, 1979 b) (Fig. 52.4).

Inheritance. This type of OI is inherited as an autosomal dominant trait.

Natural history. The sclerae may be bluish at birth but become progressively less blue as the patient matures. Hearing impairment has not been observed in children or adults with this syndrome. On the other hand, opalescent dentin has been observed in some families and not others, suggesting that there may be further heterogeneity within this group. It has been proposed that families with normal teeth be designated OI type IVA and families with opalescent dentin OI type IVB.

The age at onset varies, and fractures may be present at birth or may not occur until adult life; there is variable deformity of the long bones and spine. Significant bowing of the lower limbs may be present at birth as the only feature of this syndrome, and progressive deformity of the long bones and spine has been reported without history of fractures. Several patients in this group have appeared to improve with age in that bowing has lessened. Just as in OI type I, and virtually all patients with osteogenesis imperfecta, these patients appeared to show a spontaneous improvement at the time of puberty, and

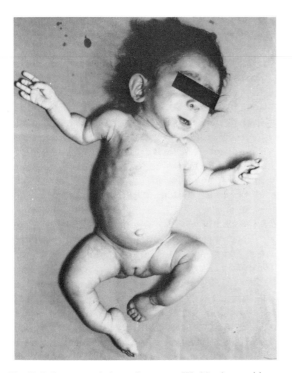

Fig 52.3 Osteogenesis imperfecta type III. Newborn with mild shortening and bowing deformities of the limbs.

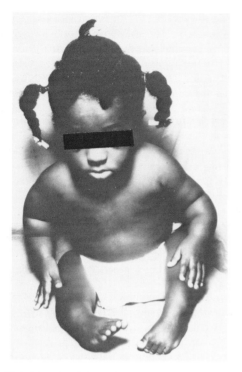

Fig. 52.4 Osteogenesis imperfecta type IV. Patient aged 2 years (not walking) with mild bowing of the lower limbs and sclerae of normal hue; her father is similarly affected.

very few fractures are encountered in adolescents and adults. However, the large majority of patients have short stature of postnatal onset.

Radiographically, this group is defined by generalised osteopoenia. Although multiple fractures may be observed in the skeleton at birth and throughout life, as a group these patients have less osteopoenia and fewer fractures than infants with recessive varieties of osteogenesis imperfecta. The skull shows multiple Wormian bones.

Differential diagnosis.

1. Juvenile idiopathic osteoporosis. This may be distinguished with difficulty from mild forms of OI type IV A, although in the former the onset of fractures is usually late (in the first decade) and there is never a family history (Brenton & Dent, 1976).

2. Osteoporosis with pseudoglimatous blindness(see below).

3. Other Mendelian disorders and inborn errors of metabolism characterised by osteopoenia. Winchester syndrome, Cockayne, Rothmund-Thompson and Fanconi pancytopoenia are all autosomal recessive syndromes in which osteopoenia maybe found. Osteopoenia is also a frequently recognised finding in homocystinuria, methylmalonic acidaemia, dibasic aminoaciduria, prolidase deficiency, glycogen storage disease type I, Menkes syndrome and the Lowe oculocerebrorenal syndrome.

Genetic counselling and prenatal diagnosis. For the offspring of an affected parent by normal mating there is a 50% chance of affected offspring. Prenatal diagnosis by ultrasound and radiography is unlikely to be definitive.

Osteoporosis with pseudogliomatous blindness and mental retardation

This rare syndrome is characterised by generalised osteoporosis leading to fractures and deformities of long bones and spine (Saroux et al, 1967). Ocular pseudogliomata, which may be mistaken for retinoblastoma, develop in infancy. Mild mental retardation has been observed in several of those affected but may be unrelated to the pseudogliomata and osteoporosis (Neuhauser et al, 1976).

DISORDERS WITH INCREASED BONE VOLUME OR DENSITY

Over 20 disorders are known with generalised or localised increase in the density or size of the skeleton or individual skeletal elements.

Osteopetrosis

Several forms have been described with an overlapping spectrum of clinical and radiographic features. Cases which present soon after birth often have a progressive course leading to death at an early age and are described as *osteopetrosis with precocious manifestations*. Cases with dominant inheritance or recessive inheritance of a usually milder disorder are designated *osteopetrosis with delayed manifestations*, sometimes known as osteopetrosis tarda or Albers-Schonberg disease.

Osteopetrosis with precocious manifestations

The precocious form of the disease is most frequently discovered during the first few months of life, but may present as failure to thrive, malignant hypocalcaemia, or anaemia with thrombocytopoenia, or even because of severe, perhaps overwhelming infection. Rarely, fractures lead to medical attention.

Inheritance. Inheritance is generally autosomal recessive, although autosomal dominant inheritance of some cases with newborn presentation is possible.

Pathogenesis. While the exact defect is unknown, it is most likely that osteopetrosis results from either a defect in the maturation of osteoclasts from precursors or a metabolic defect in osteoclasts leading to impairment of bone resorption. Four osteopetrotic disorders have been described in the mouse: grey-lethal (gl), microphthalmic (mi), osteosclerotic (oc) and osteopetrotic (op). Three forms are known in the rat: incisor absent (ia), osteopetrotic (op) and toothless (tl). Which one, if any, is a model for human osteopetrosis is not known. However, the observation that mammalian osteopetrosis can be cured by parabiosis has led to the successful cure with bone marrow transplantation in laboratory animals and in the human disorder (Marks & Walker, 1976; Coccia et al, 1980). Furthermore, some animal osteopetrosis, but not others, can be cured by infusion of monocyte (macrophage) precursors or immunocompetent cells. Milhaud and Labat (1978) have argued that the immuno-deficiency observed in the 'op' rat is primary. This has certain parallels to human osteopetrosis, where Reeves et al (1979) have observed defective monocyte intracell-ular bacterial killing in human newborn osteopetrosis.

Natural history. Generalised hyperostosis maybe recognised at birth but usually develops rapidly following birth and leads to crowding of the marrow cavity with anaemia and extramedullary haemopoiesis, hepatosple-nomegaly and thrombocytopoenia leading to purpura and ecchymosis. Anaemia appears to result not from inadequate erythropoiesis but rather from excessive extracorpuscular haemolysis. A defect in macrophage killing of bacteria may account for a tendency to severe and overwhelming infection. Progressive encroachment on the optic foramina may lead to optic atrophy and blindness. In some cases, evidence of optic nerve encroachment is present at birth. Hypocalcaemia is not an uncommon finding, and serum phosphorus may also be low. Elevated serum alkaline phosphatase is a constant finding. Radiologically, the diagnostic findings are a generalised increase in bone density combined with defective metaphyseal modelling and a 'bone-in-bone' appearance, most marked in the vertebral bodies. Dif-fuse hyperostosis leads to loss of demarcation of the cor-tex and medullary cavities. Irregular condensation of bone at the metaphyses may produce the appearance of parallel plates of dense bone at the ends of the long bones. The skull shows a dense base with normal to increased density of the vault and markedly increased density in the orbital margins.

Treatment. Treatment is aimed at decreasing or arrest-ing progressive hyperostosis, correcting anaemia and thrombocytopoenia, general supportive measures includ-ing prompt and vigorous treatment of infections, and minimising neurological complications, particularly pro-gressive optic atrophy due to encroachment of the optic foramina. It has been reported that a regimen of oral cellulose phosphate, prednisone and low calcium diet has been effective in some patients (Yu et al, 1971). The prednisone arrests the progress of the anaemia. However, this is not useful in all patients. Heparin therapy and parathormone to produce skeletal demineralisation have not produced a remission in patients with osteopetrosis. Neurosurgical unroofing of the optic foramina has been tried in some patients, but the results are difficult to interpret because of the complexities of such surgery and because optic atrophy is often established by the time the

disorder is recognised and surgical intervention is attempted. Bone marrow transplantation of appropri-ately HLA-matched donor marrow has been reported to be curative in several patients, but the long-term success remains to be judged (Ballet et al, 1977; Coccia et al, 1980). Generally, the prognosis for survival is poor and death from complications such as anaemia, bleeding or overwhelming infection is not uncommon in the first few months or years.

Genetic counselling and prenatal diagnosis. For normal parents with one or more infants with congenital osteo-petrosis, the risk approximates 25% for a subsequently affected infant.

Radiographic prenatal diagnosis has been generally unsuccessful in detecting increased bone density during the second trimester, early enough to allow parents the option of therapeutic abortion (Lachman & Hall, 1979).

Osteopetrosis with later onset

Apart from cases with congenital or infantile presentation of osteopetrosis, there are a group of patients in whom the onset of the disease is recognised later (osteopetrosis tarda or Albers-Schonberg disease).

Inheritance. In the majority of cases, this milder pres-entation of osteopetrosis is inherited as an autosomal dominant trait, although families with autosomal reces-sive inheritance have been reported.

Natural history. Patients may present in childhood, adolescence or young adult life because of fractures (10%), mild craniofacial disproportion, mild anaemia, compli-cations arising from neurological involvement or osteitis with osteonecrosis, usually of the mandible. On the other hand, increased bone density maybe discovered inciden-tally on routine radiological study for some non-skeletal problem (Graham et al, 1973).

Skeletal radiographs show generalised increased den-sity of cortical bone with defective metaphyseal modell-ing of the long bones resulting in a club-shaped appearance. There is longitudinal and transverse osteo-dense striation at the ends of the long bones in over half the patients. The vertebral column shows alternating hyperlucent and very dense bands. The base of the skull is usually dense and thickened, but the face and vault are generally less severely involved.

Differential diagnosis.

1. Pycnodysostosis. This is an autosomal recessive trait characterised by generalised hyperostosis and short stature with onset at around 3 years. Distal acro-osteo-lysis and the radiographic pattern of involvement of the skeleton differ from osteopetrosis tarda (see below).

2. Dysosteosclerosis. In this disorder there is major involvement of the spine with flattening of the vertebrae (see below).

Treatment. Therapy should be directed at recognition and treatment of complications. Transfusion maybe required for anaemia, and splenectomy maybe useful in some patients. Frequent testing of visual field and acuity, and baseline radiographs of optic foramina, should be carried out. On the whole, treatment with low-calcium diet, parathormone, calcium cheating agents, corticosteroids and heparin therapy has not shown clear therapeutic advantages.

Pycnodysostosis

This is a rare generalised hyperostotic bone disease recognised from infancy by short limb short stature, characteristic facies and wide anterior fontanelle (Sugiura et al, 1974) (Fig. 52.5).

Inheritance. This disorder is inherited as an autosomal recessive trait.

Natural history. The skull, which appears large, with frontal and occipital bossing and a wide anterior fontanelle, may bring the patient to attention. The hands and feet are short and broad and the nails may be deformed and brittle. The sclerae are often blue, and this, in combination with a tendency to fractures, may lead to confusion with osteogenesis imperfecta.

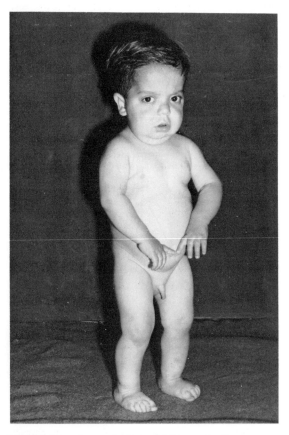

Fig 52.5 Pycnodysostosis. Boy aged 2 years showing short limbs, short stature, large cranium and small chin (courtesy of Dr J. S. Yu, Royal Alexandra Hospital for Children, Camperdown, NSW, Australia).

Radiographically, there is generalised increase in bone density without long bone or metaphyseal striation. The hands characteristically show hypoplasia or aplasia of the distal phalanges. The characteristic findings in the skull are wide sutures and Wormian bones, and in the face, a small mandible with an obtuse mandibular angle.

Genetic counselling. For normal parents there is a 25% risk for further affected offspring. Ultrasound and radiographic prenatal diagnosis is not feasible.

Dysosteosclerosis

This is a rare autosomal recessive skeletal dysplasia characterised by generalised increase in bone density and short stature of postnatal onset. It is differentiated from osteopetrosis and pycnodysostosis by radiological evidence of platyspondyly with superior and inferior irregularity of vertebral ossification and clinical findings of a high incidence of developmental defects of the teeth with delayed eruption of primary dentition, severe hypodontia and early loss of the teeth (Houston et al, 1978). Secondary dentition may fail to erupt. Otherwise, the complications, fractures, visual and hearing loss and recurrent infections of mandible and paranasal sinuses are very similar to those encountered in osteopetrosis.

Osteopoikilosis, osteopathia striata and melorheostosis

These three conditions are most commonly asymptomatic and are usually recognised during routine radiological study including skeletal films. Occasionally, patients are seen with both types of lesions.

In *osteopoikilosis*, numerous small osteo-dense round or oval foci are seen in the skeleton, most commonly in the epiphyses and carpal and tarsal centres. The disorder is inherited as an autosomal dominant trait and maybe associated with joint pain in some 20% of cases and with skin lesions in an unknown proportion. These consist of slightly elevated whitish-yellow fibrocollagenous infiltrations (dermatofibrosis lenticularis disseminata). There is an increased incidence of keloid formation.

In *osteopathia striata*, which is possibly also an autosomal dominant trait, linear regular bands of increased density are seen throughout the skeleton, radiating from the metaphyses and with a fan-like array in the iliac wings. These should be distinguished from similar striations seen in osteopetrosis, which are associated with metaphyseal modelling defects, and transverse bands of osteo-density at the ends of the long bones. Typical changes of osteopathia striata are seen in the syndrome of focal dermal hypoplasia in which linear lesions consisting of dermal hypoplasia with herniation of the adipose tissue and skeletal defects of the limbs (hypoplasia, aplasia and syndactyly) occur.

In *melorheostosis*, irregular linear osteo-dense lesions are seen along the axis of the tubular bones. Single or multiple areas of the skeleton maybe involved. No hereditary basis has been established but the pattern of lesions may be correlated with the sensory sclerotomes. It has been suggested that melorheostosis maybe the late consequence of lesions of the sensory nerve supply to various skeletal elements (Murray & McCredie, 1979). The lesions maybe associated with shortening of certain bones leading to discrepancy in limb length, soft tissue contractures of the joints or palmar and plantar fasciae and intermittently painful swelling of affected joints. The radiological appearance of the osteo-dense lesions has been likened to candle wax flowing down the side of a candle. Management is directed at the orthopaedic complications.

CRANIOTUBULAR REMODELLING DISORDERS

This is a large group of disorders characterised by abnormal modelling as well as increased density of bone. A distinction has been drawn between the craniotubular dysplasias, e.g. cranio-diaphyseal dysplasia, in which modelling abnormalities are prominent (Gorlin et al, 1969) although there is also severe sclerosis of the skull, and the craniotubular hyperostoses, e.g. endosteal hyperostosis (Van Buchem), in which cranial and tubular bones are deformed by overgrowth of osseous tissue rather than by a defect in bone remodelling. This distinction is somewhat arbitrary as all these disorders result from excess bone deposition versus resorption with specifically different patterns of skeletal involvement. In essence, they are all disorders in which there is generally minimum involvement of the spine compared to osteopetrosis, pycnodysostosis and dysosteosclerosis, in which increased osteodensity is seen throughout the spine and rest of the skeleton with minimal changes in the cranial vault.

In diaphyseal dysplasia (Camurati-Englemann), craniodiaphyseal dysplasia, the craniometaphyseal dysplasias, frontometaphyseal dysplasia and pachydermoperiostosis, sclerosis in the region of optic foramina may lead to visual impairment, papilloedema and optic atrophy. Sclerotic narrowing of internal acoustic foramina and the middle ear may lead to various patterns of conductive or sensorineural hearing loss; encroachment on the facial foramina may lead to facial paresis and encroachment on the foramen magnum to long tract signs, hyperreflexia, weakness and even sudden death or paraplegia.

Diaphyseal dysplasia (Camurati-Englemann)
This is a rare craniotubular remodelling disorder (also known as progressive hereditary diaphyseal dysplasia) with significant neuromuscular involvement (Sparkes & Graham, 1972).
Inheritance. Diaphysial dysplasia is inherited as an

autosomal dominant trait with variable penetrance and wide expressivity. There is considerable variation in the signs, symptoms and severity between affected individuals within the same family (Sparkes & Graham, 1972).

Natural history. Symptoms usually begin between 4 and 10 years of age, but the onset of symptoms has been described as early as 3 months and as late as the sixth decade. Failure to thrive or gain weight, fatigability and abnormal gait are frequent presenting symptoms. Pain in the legs of progressively increasing severity may occur. The gait is characteristically wide-based and waddling, with reduced muscle mass and poor muscle tone. Flexion contractures may develop at the elbows and knees. Bow-leg or knock-knee deformity may be seen in the lower limbs, and the feet may be flat and pronated. Deep tendon reflexes in some cases have been hypoactive and in others hyperactive, with occasional ankle clonus. Increased lumbar lordosis and scoliosis may occur with variable degrees of back pain. Symptoms and signs of encroachment on cranial nerves may be present.

The radiographic features include symmetrical fusiform enlargement of the diaphyses of the long bones with normal epiphyses and metaphyses. In the diaphyses, there is enlargement of the cortex by endosteal and periosteal accretion of mottled new bone. The lesions are often first recognised centrally in the long bones and progress proximally and distally with gradual involvement of adjacent normal bone. In the skull, there maybe sclerosis of the frontal areas and base.

Serum calcium, phosphorus and serum alkaline phosphatase are characteristically normal. Muscle histology has been reported to show loss of individual muscle fibres with replacement by adipose tissue, atrophic muscle fibres, and slighly pyknotic sarcolemmal cell nuclei with hyalinisation and decrease in the prominence of cross-striations.

Treatment. Management of this condition should be aimed at maximising the mobility of the patient. Orthopaedic correction of deformity of lower limbs by appropriate osteotomy has been reported to help in the habilitation of these patients. There have been reports of good symptomatic response to low-dose steroid therapy (Allen et al, 1970).

Craniodiaphyseal dysplasia
This is a rare craniotubular remodelling disorder characterised by massive hyperostosis and sclerosis of the skull and facial bones (Fig. 52.6) and hyperostosis and defective remodelling of the shafts of the tubular bones. The epiphyses and metaphyses are only mildly affected or spared. The early symptoms maybe related to respiratory difficulty due to narrowing of the nasal passages (Gorlin et al, 1969; Macpherson, 1974).
Inheritance. This disorder is inherited as an autosomal recessive trait.

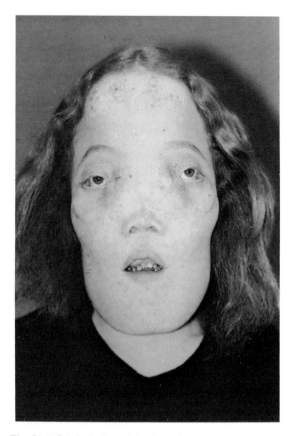

Fig. 52.6 Craniodiaphyseal dysplasia. Boy aged 13 years showing massive hyperostosis of cranium, facial bones and mandible (leontiasis ossea).

Natural history. Flattening of the nasal root maybe noted at birth, and symptoms may occur as early as 3 months of age. Hyperostosis of the cranial and facial bones is progressive in the first years of life, and frank prominence of nasal and adjacent maxillary bones is usually recognised by 1–2 years of age. Symptoms and signs produced by encroachment on cranial foramina are marked.

Skeletal radiographs show massive hyperostosis of the cranial bones developing rapidly during infancy and completely obscuring the detailed structures. The spine, ribs, clavicles and scapulae appear hypermineralised but normal in shape. The metaphyses of the long bones are poorly modelled and there is loss of normal funnelisation and tubulation so that the long bones appear broad and undermodelled. These patients are often of normal to tall stature.

Serum calcium and phosphorus appear to be normal, but serum alkaline phosphatase is markedly increased.

Treatment. There is no effective medical or surgical treatment to prevent the progressive craniofacial hyperostosis and sclerosis and its complications. Special attention should be given to amelioration of hearing and visual impairment and to psychosocial counselling for affected children and their families with this cosmetically disfiguring disorder.

Endosteal hyperostosis and sclereosteosis

This is a group of disorders characterised by marked accretion of osseous tissue at the endosteal (inner) surface of bone, leading to narrowing of the medullary canal or obliteration of the medullary space.

A rare dominantly inherited variety (Worth type) is frequently associated with the presence of a torus palatinus. The torus is a prominent midline ridge of the hard palate in the mouth and is noted in 5% of the population as a normal variant (Worth & Wollin, 1966).

A recessively inherited variety of endosteal hyperostosis (Van Buchem disease) is characterised by progressive mandibular enlargement from childhood, and in adult life signs and symptoms resulting from sclerotic encroachment on optic and acoustic foramina. Serum alkaline phosphatase is markedly elevated. Radiographically, there is marked thickening of the skull starting in the base and extending to the vault, and increased density of the mandible after puberty. There is increased density of the cortices of tubular bones with narrowing of the marrow cavity.

Sclereosteosis, also an autosomal recessive trait, is clinically and radiologically almost indistinguishable from Van Buchem disease. Sclereosteosis has been differentiated by a high frequency of hyperostosis in the nasal and facial bones, producing a broad, flat nasal bridge and ocular hypertelorism with minor hand malformations. The latter consist of cutaneous syndactyly, radial deviation of the second and third fingers and absent or hypoplastic nails (Beighton et al, 1976). Recent family studies from South Africa suggest that endosteal hyperostosis (Van Buchem disease) and sclereosteosis may be the same entity (Cremin, 1979).

Tubular stenosis (Caffey-Kenny)

This disorder is characterised by narrowing of the medullary cavity and myopia. In some patients, tetanic seizures due to hypocalcaemia in infancy occur (Kenny & Linarelli, 1966; Caffey, 1967).

Inheritance. Tubular stenosis is inherited as an autosomal dominant trait.

Natural history. Medullary stenosis maybe recognised at an incidental radiographic study or as part of the investigation of the infant with clinical manifestations of hypocalcaemia. Other clinical features include delayed closure of the anterior fontanelle and early onset myopia.

Radiographically there is widening of the diaphyseal cortex in the long bones and short tubular bones of the hands and feet, without overall widening of the diaphyses leading to reduction of the medullary cavity. Rarely, vertebrae, pelvis, carpals, tarsals and skull may show increased density.

Pachydermoperiostosis

This is an unusual condition characterised by progressive thickening of the skin and clubbing of the fingers with onset in adolescence. Radiographic findings are similar to those observed in hypertrophic (pulmonary) osteoarthropathy without evidence of primary pulmonary neoplastic lesions (Rimoin, 1965).

Inheritance. Pachydermoperiostosis is inherited as an autosomal dominant trait.

Natural history. Those affected develop a massive appearance of the limbs, which maybe disproportionately long, and thickening of the facial skin with seborrhoeic hyperplasia. Complaints of easy fatigability, joint pain and blepharitis are frequent.

The skeletal changes include cortical thickening and sclerosis of the tubular bones, thickening of the calvaria and base of the skull, which may lead to conductive and/or sensory hearing loss, and narrowing of other intervertebral foramina resulting in neurological symptoms.

Frontometaphyseal dysplasia

This produces a clinically striking facial appearance with a pronounced supraorbital ridge resulting from a torus-like bony overgrowth of the supraorbital ridges of the frontal bones (Fig. 52.7).

Inheritance. The disorder is inherited as an X–linked dominant trait (Gorlin & Winter, 1980).

Natural history. The prominent supraorbital ridge which extends across the entire frontal bone may be recognised at birth, although in some cases not till later. It is associated radiographically with poor development of the frontal and other paranasal sinuses and with mandibular hypoplasia. The pelvis shows an unusually abrupt flare. The metaphyses of all the long and short tubular bones are undermodelled. Hirsutism, scoliosis and conductive deafness with various alterations of the modelling of the tubular bones may be present.

Craniometaphyseal dysplasias

This may also be a genetically heterogeneous group of disorders. Both autosomal dominant (Fig. 52.8) and recessive inheritance have been described with overlap in the clinical and radiographic findings between both groups of patients (Gorlin et al, 1969). The recessive variety is very rare.

Natural history. There is wide variability in the onset of symptoms and signs in families showing a dominant mode of inheritance, but some cases have been recognised in infancy. Clinically, both dominant and recessively inherited varieties show progressive facial dysmorphology with broad osseous prominence of the nasal root extending across the zygoma (Fig. 52.8). Dif-

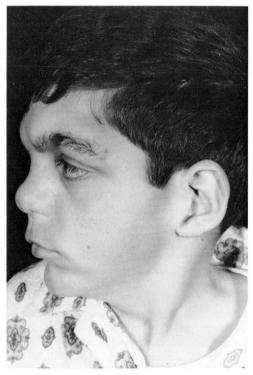

Fig. 52 .7 Frontometaphyseal dysplasia. Boy aged 12 years showing torus-like hyperostosis of frontal bone extending across the cranium (from Danks et al, by permission of the publishers, American Journal of Diseases in Children 123: 254–258).

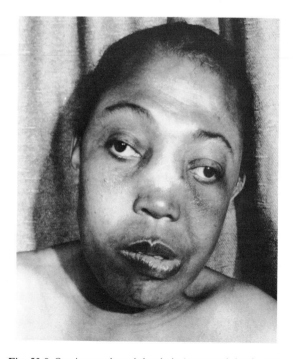

Fig. 52.8 Craniometaphyseal dysplasia (autosomal dominant) in woman aged 42 showing hyperostosis of nasal process of frontal bone and adjacent maxilla and mandible (from Rimoin, et al, 1969, by permission of the publishers, Birth Defects Original Article Series 5 (4): 96–104).

ficulty with breathing and encroachment on the nasal passages may be recognised in the first 6 months of life. Signs and symptoms of sclerotic encroachment on cranial foramina vary in severity from patient to patient but may be unusually severe.

The essential radiological features are hyperostosis of the skull, nasal and maxillary bones extending bilaterally across the zygoma with failure of pneumatisation of the paranasal sinuses and mastoids, and hyperostosis of the mandible. The long bones show flaring and decreased density of the metaphyses (Ehrlenmeyer flask deformity) due to a failure of remodelling of the metaphyses during growth. Hyperostosis and sclerosis of the mandible develops but is less severe than in craniodiaphyseal dysplasia.

Treatment. As in craniodiaphyseal dysplasia, the cosmetic and neurological problems in craniometaphyseal dysplasia maybe considerable. Plastic surgery for the facial hyperostosis has been successfully performed.

Osteodysplasty (Melnick-Needles)

This disorder or group of disorders is characterised by 'abnormally shaped' bones (Melnick & Needles, 1966).

Inheritance. Osteodysplasty is inherited as an autosomal dominant trait. Danks et al (1974) have described a severe 'precocious form' of osteodysplasty inherited as an autosomal recessive trait.

Natural history. The age at diagnosis is variable, and affected individuals usually present because of an abnormal gait with bowing of the extremities. Occasionally, dislocation of hips or delayed closure of the anterior fontanelle occurs. On the whole, these patients do not have short stature, and psychomotor development and adult height are normal. Facial appearance appears to be somewhat typical, with slight exophthalmus, protruding cheeks, a high, narrow forehead, prominent orbital rims, micrognathia and malaligned teeth. The lower thorax is narrow. There is incurving of the distal segments of the thumbs.

Radiographically, there is uneven thickening of the cortex of long bones, which have irregular contours and multiple constrictions producing a wavy border. The diaphyses are slightly curved and show metaphyseal modelling defects. Characteristically, there is coxa valga and dislocation of the hips is frequent. The ribs appear wavy, the pelvis is triangular and the iliac wings appear to be narrowed in the supra-acetabular portion.

DISORDERS OF MINERALISATION AND MINERAL METABOLISM

These disorders involve defective mineralisation, defective mineral metabolism or defective hormonal interactions with skeletal tissue during development.

Hyperphosphatasaemia with osteoectasia

In this disorder, progressive skeletal deformation is associated with marked elevation of alkaline phosphatase. As the clinical and radiological findings resemble Paget disease it has sometimes been known as juvenile Paget disease (Iancu et al, 1978).

Inheritance. The disorder is inherited as an autosomal recessive trait.

Natural history. The disease usually has its onset between 2 and 3 years, when painful deformity of the extremities develops and lead to gait abnormalities and sometimes fractures. The clinical findings are similar to those of Paget disease in adults but are more generalized and symmetric in distribution. Short stature ultimately results. The skull is large, and radiographically the diploe is widened and there is loss of normal calvarial structure. Bony texture is variable with dense areas (showing a teased cotton-wool appearance) interspersed with lucent areas. Demineralisation is seen throughout the remainder of the skeleton. The long bones appear cylindrical, even fusiform, and deformed with the loss of normal metaphyseal modelling. Pseudocysts with a dense bony halo maybe seen throughout the long bones.

Differential diagnosis.

1. Marked elevation of serum alkaline phosphatase may be observed in a wide variety of disorders of density of cortical bones or metaphyseal remodelling. It is commonly observed with osteopetrosis, craniodiaphyseal dysplasia, and Van Buchem disease. However, the clinical and radiographic findings in osteoectasia are distinctive and unlike those in the foregoing conditions.

2. Infantile cortical hyperostosis (Caffey disease). This disorder is usually recognised in the first 3 months of life and is characterised by a febrile course with marked swelling of soft tissues over the face and jaws and progressive cortical thickening of the long and flat bones (Maroteaux, 1979). The elevation of alkaline phosphatase is usually mild. Infantile cortical hyperostosis is characterised by repeated exacerbations with spontaneous regression after several years. Caffey disease is not familial. Corticosteroids have been demonstrated to be beneficial in relieving clinical symptoms during exacerbations.

Treatment: Clinical, radiographic and histopathologic amelioration of the skeletal lesions following treatment with human calcitonin, has been reported (Woodhouse et al 1972, Whalen et al 1977).

Hypophosphatasia

This includes a number of conditions with overlapping phenotype but differing modes of inheritance characterised by bowing deformities of the skeleton of varying severity and a reduced serum alkaline phosphatase due to total absence of the bone/liver isozyme. There is also elevation of serum and urine phosphorylethanolamine (Rasmussen & Bartter, 1978).

Congenital lethal hypophosphatasia

Neonates with this disorder show disproportionately short limbs with bowing or angulation deformity. The skull vault is thin and membraneous. Radiographic studies show extremely poor ossification throughout the skeleton with thin ribs, hypoplastic vertebrae, demineralised facial bones and markedly reduced ossification of the skull vault. The metaphyses of the long bones are frayed and splayed, sometimes with a moth-eaten appearance (Currarino, 1973).

Inheritance. The disorder is inherited as an autosomal recessive trait.

Pathogenesis. The alkaline phosphatase in chondro-osseous tissue is important in the hydrolysis of phosphate esters to release phosphate ion for normal calcification. In congenital hypophosphatasia a deficiency in the production or stability of bone alkaline phosphatase enzyme leads to a deficiency in the availability of free phosphate necessary for calcification.

Natural history. In the most severe cases death occurs prenatally or in the newborn period due to respiratory distress. The serum alkaline phosphatase is low and the bone/liver isozyme measured in cultured fibroblasts is extremely low (Mulivor et al, 1978).

Genetic counselling and prenatal diagnosis. There is a 25% recurrence risk for hypophosphatasia in sibs. Prenatal diagnosis by measurement of the bone/liver isozyme in cultured amniotic cells is feasible (Mulivor et al, 1978). Ultrasound studies in one instance failed to record abnormality in ossification of the fetal skull although in general, ultrasound examination of the fetal skull between 16 and 20 weeks gestation has been reported to show diminished ossification indicating an affected fetus (Garber et al, 1979).

Hypophosphatasia tarda

Into this group fall patients with clinical, laboratory and radiographic evidence of hypophosphatasia which is of a milder degree (Rassmussen & Bartter, 1978).

Inheritance. Both autosomal dominant and autosomal recessive modes of inheritance have been observed.

Natural history. Bowing of the legs may be recognised in early childhood. Premature craniosynostosis and premature loss of the teeth are also found. The serum alkaline phosphatase is reduced, and in both serum and urine there is elevation of phosphorylethanolamine.

Differential diagnosis. 1. Pseudohypophosphatasia. This term was used by Scriver and Cameron (1969) to describe patients with clinical and radiographic findings of hypophosphatasia in the presence of a normal serum alkaline phosphatase but elevated urinary phosphorylethanolamine.

X–linked hypophosphataemic rickets

X–linked hypophosphataemic rickets (XLH) is recognised in infancy with bowing of the legs and radiographic evidence of rickets resistant to vitamin D therapy.

Inheritance. XLH is inherited as an X–linked dominant trait.

Pathogenesis. The discovery and investigation of the Hyp mouse, a rachitic mouse with vitamin D-resistant hypophosphataemia has shed much light on the possible pathogenesis of human XLH rickets. Hyp is an X–linked trait in the mouse and therefore homology with human XLH follows (Ohno, 1967). In the Hyp mouse it has been demonstrated that there is an intrinsic partial defect in the transport of phosphate across the renal brush border and epithelium of the small intestine (Tenenhouse et al, 1978). Hypophosphataemia is the primary abnormality leading to the development of rickets. In human X–linked hypophosphataemic rickets, the renal phosphate handling is impaired, but opinions differ on whether there is impaired transport of phosphate at the intestinal level (Glorieux et al, 1972). Some heterogeneity in phosphate transport would not be surprising, as there are at least four alleles in the mouse for the copper transport defect leading to mottled mice (Danks, 1977).

Natural history. Abnormal vertical growth can be observed by 12 months and bow legs leading to abnormal gait recognised in hemizygous males soon after. In heterozygous females the findings are much more variable. Some heterozygous females have only low serum phosphate while others demonstrate the full manifestations of the disease. While growth rate is consistently disturbed, the growth of the children with XLH generally parallels the normal growth curves (Steendjik, 1976). In some mildly affected individuals growth may accelerate at puberty and cross the third percentile. In others, the growth spurt of puberty may aggravate bowing of the legs.

Dentition may be late, and abnormal development of the maxillofacial region has been reported. The poor dental development may be associated with spontaneous dental abscesses. Deformities of the limbs are not limited to varus deformity. Valgus and sitting deformities may also develop.

In adults bowing of the legs and short stature may persist. In some patient's, evidence of active osteomalacia may be present. Overgrowth of bone at the site of muscle attachments may lead to joint limitation and various neurological compressive syndromes (Rasmussen & Anast, 1978).

Differential diagnosis.

1. Autosomal dominant hypophosphataemic bone disease (HBD). This can be distinguished from XLH by the absence of frank rachitic changes on skeletal X–ray in the presence of short stature with leg bowing and a low serum phosphorus (Scriver et al, 1977). Clinical manifestations appear in late infancy. Leg bowing and short stature are less severe than in XLH, with comparable

reduction of serum phosphorus. There is a similar selective impairment in renal tubular reabsorption of phosphorus but no abnormality in red cell membrane phosphorus transport (Scriver et al, 1977).

2. Vitamin D-dependency rickets (VDD). This syndrome appears to be biochemically heterogeneous with two forms presently delineated.

a. Autosomal recessive VDD rickets. These patients have early infancy onset of hypocalcaemia, normal or low serum phosphorus, elevated serum alkaline phosphatase, generalised aminoaciduria and clinical and radiographic findings of severe rickets. Serum 25-hydroxy vitamin D is normal, but serum 1,25-dihydroxy vitamin D is below the limits of detection (Fraser et al, 1973). The disorder presumably results from defective 1-α hydroxylation of 25-hydroxy vitamin D.

b. Target organ resistance to 1,25-dihydroxy vitamin D. Brooke et al (1978) reported a 22-year old black patient with symptomatic osteomalacia, hypocalcaemia and hyperaminoaciduria from the age of 15 years. In this patient, plasma 25-hydroxy vitamin D was normal, but plasma 1,25-dihydroxy vitamin D was markedly increased. Osteomalacia in the face of elevated serum 1,25-dihydroxy vitamin D is thought to be due to impaired target organ responsiveness.

3. 'Steroid'-sensitive hypophosphataemic rickets. Dent (1976) has summarised the findings in a single patient with clinical and radiographic findings of hypophosphataemic rickets who appeared to respond to a small dose of cortisone and vitamin D.

4. Tumour rickets-delayed hypophosphataemic rickets of McCance. The onset of hypophosphataemia and rickets has been variable. McCance's (1947) patient had an unclassifiable tumour in the femur while Prader's case had a rib tumour identified as an osteoclastoma. Cure followed removal of the tumour. The cases have been reviewed by Salassa et al (1970).

Treatment. Oral supplementation with phosphate combined with vitamin D has demonstrated effectiveness in correcting hypophosphataemia, normalising growth and reducing bowing deformities of the lower limbs (Glorieux et al, 1972). Scriver et al (1976) recommended an acidic oral phosphate supplement, as this is better tolerated. To be effective, phosphate must be given in five divided doses at 3–4 hour intervals throughout the day. Phosphate therapy alone leads to the development of secondary hyperparathyroidism (Glorieux et al, 1972). Vitamin D_2 10–15 $\times$ 10^3 units can be used. However since 1,25-dihydroxy vitamin D_3 has been shown to be particularly effective in correcting the growth disorder in XLH (Chan & Bartter, 1979), this must be the vitamin D of choice in the management of XLH.

Genetic counselling. For XLH there is a 50% chance that a male child of an affected or carrier female will have hypophosphataemic rickets. Only a proportion of heterozygous females manifest the complete syndrome with short stature and leg deformities. All the daughters of affected males will be carriers or manifest the disorder.

Pseudohypoparathyroidism and related disorders

The clinical findings common to this group of disorders are disporportionate short stature with selective distal shortening of tubular bones, predominantly of metacarpals, but also of metatarsals and phalanges. There is also a high frequency of mental retardation and ectopic, usually subcutaneous calcification (Nagant de Deuxchaisnes & Krane, 1978).

In pseudohypoparathyroidism (PHP), the somatic abnormalities are associated with serum findings of hypoparathyroidism, i.e. low serum calcium and elevated serum phosphorus with resistance to the effects of circulating and exogeneous serum parathormone (PTH).

In pseudo-pseudohypoparathyroidism (Albright et al, 1952) (PPHP), the somatic features of PHP occur in the presence of normal serum chemistries and normal end organ responsiveness to exogeneous PTH.

As PHP and PPHP are often both found in the same family, it is likely that they represent variability within the same dominant genetic disorder. Furthermore, physiological studies of parathormone-induced urinary cyclic AMP response suggest that this group of disorders is genetically heterogeneous (Nagant de Deuxchaisnes & Krane, 1978).

Inheritance. While PHP appears to be genetically heterogeneous, the evidence suggests that in the majority the disorder is inherited as a dominant trait. In view of reported male-to-male transmission some forms of PHP and PPHP are likely to represent autosomal dominant inheritance, but many of these dominant cases may represent examples of type E brachydactyly (Mann et al, 1962). The elevated female/male sex ratio of 2.1:1 observed in some studies (Spranger & Rohwedder, 1965) must be explained by genetic heterogeneity with X–linked dominant inheritance, selection bias in favour of females or by the fact that the disease is more severe in females than males (Spranger & Rohwedder, 1965). Mann et al (1962) have observed that males are not more severely affected than females, a fact which can be reconciled with autosomal rather than X–linked inheritance.

Cederbaum and Lippe (1973) have reported a family in which two sibs (a brother and sister) had classic PHP while both parents and grandparents appeared to be completely normal. This raises the possibility that there is an autosomal recessive form of PHP.

Drezner et al (1973) have described a patient who had normal serum phosphate and a subnormal phosphaturic response to exogeneous parathyroid extract but normal cyclic AMP response, presumably representing a further disorder, pseudohypoparathyroidism type II.

Pathogenesis. The demonstrable defect in serum and urinary cyclic AMP (c-AMP) generation by endogeneous parathormone (PTH) suggest that a defect in hormone binding at the PTH receptor in the pathway of generation of c-AMP. Farfel et al (1980) have recently demonstrated, in 5 of 10 patients with PHP type I and in one patient with PHP type II, deficiency of a protein, the N protein which mediates between the PTH receptor and c-AMP generation. That 5 out of 10 patients representing one family did not show a defect in their assay system confirms the proposed genetic heterogeneity in pseudohypoparathyroidism.

Natural history. Symptomatic hypocalcaemia may be the presenting sign. Seizures, tetanic episodes and evidence of ectopic or intracranial calcification may also bring a child to attention. Mental retardation or a family history of short stature and mental retardation may be recorded. Affected individuals develop short stature with moderate obesity and dental anomalies. These consist of delayed eruption, enamel hypoplasia, dentin hypoplasia and teeth with short blunt roots.

Short digits arise from early closure of the epiphyses of the short tubular bones of the hands. The fourth and fifth digits are most often involved and the second least of all. The commonest phalanx affected is the distal first due to premature closure of its epiphysis. Cone-shaped epiphyses maybe seen at the base of both first metacarpals.

Other skeletal anomalies are seen but less frequently. Radius curvus, cubitus valgus, coxa valga and vara and genu valgum and varum have been reported. Ectopic calcification usually appears in infancy and may be located in any site, but most commonly in the extremities around large joints.

Mental retardation is present in some 75% of cases with pseudohypoparathyroidism (PHP). The mean IQ is in the order of 60 (Smith, 1976). Lenticular opacities have been reported in 44% of patients.

Complications.

1. Diabetes mellitus. There are a number of reports of the coexistence of diabetes mellitus and PHP and of diabetes mellitus in the families of patients with PHP (Nagant de Deuxchaisnes & Krane, 1978). Whether this is a true association or represents the segregation of a common trait (diabetes mellitus) in these cases is not established.

2. Hypothyroidism. This appears to have a real but rare association with PHP (Nagant de Deuxchaisnes & Krane, 1978). The majority of cases with both features have primary hypothyroidism although secondary hypothyroidism with diminished TSH response to TRH has also been reported.

Differential diagnosis.

1. Causes of hypoparathyroidism and hypocalcaemia. These include both primary and secondary hypoparathyroid states and are excellently reviewed by Nagant de Deuxchaisnes and Krane (1978).

2 Syndromes of mental retardation, obesity, short stature and brachydactyly. These include Turner syndrome (XO gonadal dysgenesis), basal cell naevus syndrome, Gardner syndrome and type E brachydactyly.

Treatment. The aim of treatment is to normalise serum calcium with supplementary dietary calcium and vitamin D. Treatment does not prevent the progression of lenticular opacities but may improve mental functioning.

Vitamin D_2 has been used conventionally in the treatment of pseudohypoparathyroidism in a dose of 50 000 to 100 000 units per day. Additional calcium as lactate or gluconate can be added to achieve a blood calcium level of 2.12–2.37 mmol/l (8.5 to 9.5 mg/100 ml). Where available, 1,25-dihydroxy vitamin D_3 which was shown to be effective in the treatment of PHP with ready control of serum calcium, is now probably the vitamin D of choice in management.

REFERENCES

Albright F, Forbes A P, Henneman P H 1952 Pseudopseudohypoparathyroidism. Trans. Ass. Amer. Phycns. 65: 337–350

Allen D I, Saunders A M, Northway W H, Williams G F, Schafer J A 1970 Corticosteroids in the treatment of Engelmann's disease: progressive diaphyseal dysplasia. Pediatrics 46: 523

Ballet J J, Griscelli C, Coutris C Milhaud G Maroteaux P 1977 Bone-marrow transplantation in osteopetrosis. Lancet 2: 1137

Beighton P, Durr L, Hamersma H 1976 The clinical features of sclerosteosis. A review of the manifestations in twenty-five affected individuals. Annals of Internal Medicine 84: 393–397

Biering A, Iverson T 1955 Osteogenesis imperfecta associated with Ehlers-Danlos syndrome. Acta Paediatrica 44: 279–286

Brenton D P, Dent c E 1976 Idiopathic juvenile osteoporosis. In: Bickel H, Stern J (eds) Inborn errors of calcium and bone metabolism. MTP Press, Lancaster, ch 15, p 222

Brooke M H, Bell N H, Love L et al 1978 Vitamin D-dependent rickets type II: resistance of target organs to 1,25 dihydroxy vitamin D. New England Journal of Medicine 298: 996–999

Buyse M, Bull M 1978 A syndrome of osteogenesis imperfecta and cataracts. Birth Defects Original Article Series 14 (6B): 95–98

Caffey J 1967 Congenital stenosis of medullary spaces in tubular bones and calvaria in two proportionate dwarfs, mother and son, coupled with transitory hypocalcemic tetany. American Journal of Roentgenology 100: 1–14

Carey M C, Fitzgerald O, McKieman E 1968 Osteogenesis imperfecta in twenty-three members of a kindred with heritable features contributed by a non-specific skeletal disorder. Quarterly Journal of Medicine 37: 437–439

Cederbaum S D, Lippe B M 1973 Probable autosomal recessive inheritance in a family with Albright's hereditary osteodystrophy and an evaluation of the genetics of this disorder. American Journal of Human Genetics 25: 638–645

Chan J C M, Bartter F C 1979 Hypophosphatemic rickets : effect of 1,25-dihydroxyvitamin D on growth and mineral metabolism. Pediatrics 64: 488–495

Coccia P F, Krivitt W, Cervenka J et al 1980 Successful bone-marrow transplantation for infantile malignant osteopetrosis. New England Journal of Medicine 302: 701–708

Cremin B J 1979 Sclerosteosis in children. Pediatric Radiology 8: 173–177

Currarino G 1973 Hypophosphatasia. In: Kaufman H J (ed) intrinsic diseases of bones. S Karger, Basel, p 469–494

Daentl D L et al 1978 Familial nephrosis, hydrocephalus, thin skin, blue sclerae syndrome: clinical, structural and biochemical studies. Birth Defects Original Article Series 14 (6B): 315–339

Danks D M, Mayne V, Koxlowski K 1974 A pricocious autosomal recessive type of osteodysplasty. Birth Defects Original Article Series 10 (12): 124–127

Danks D M 1977 Copper transport and utilisation in Menkes' syndrome and in mottled mice. Inorganic Perspective in Biology and Medicine 1: 73–100

Dent C 1976 Metabolic forms of rickets (and osteomalacia). In: Bickel H, Stern J. inborn errors of calcium and bone metabolism. MTP Press, St Leonardgate

Drezner M, Neelon F A, Lebovitz H E Pseudohypoparathyroidism type II: a possible defect in the reception of the cyclic AMP signal. New England Journal of Medicine 289: 1056–1060

Farfel Z, Brickman A S, Kaslow H R, Brothers V M, Bourne H R 1980 Defect of receptor-cyclase coupling protein in pseudohypoparathyroidism. New England Vournal of Medicine 303: 237–242

Fraser D, Kooh S W, Kind H P, Holick M F, Tanaka Y, De Luca H F 1973 Pathogenesis of hereditary vitamin D-dependent rickets. An inborn error of vitamin D metabolism involving defective conversion of 25-hydroxy vitamin to 1α,25-dihydroxy vitamin D. New England Journal of Medicine 289: 817–822

Garber A P, Sillence D O, Lachman R S et al 1979 Discordance between ultrasound and radiographic/biochemical findings in the prenatal diagnosis of congenital lethal hypophosphatasia. Proc. Birth Defects Conference 61A

Glorieux F H, Scriver C R, Reade T M, Goldman H, Roseborough A 1972 Use of phosphate and vitamin D to prevent dwarfism and rickers in X–linked hypophosphatemia. New England Journal of Medicine 287: 481–487

Gorlin R J, Winter R B 1980 Fronto metaphyseal dysplasia – evidence for X–linked inheritance. American Journal of Medical Genetics 5: 81–84

Gorlin, R J, Spranger J, Koszalka M F 1969 Genetic cranio-tubular bone dysplasias and hyperostosis, a critical analysis. Birth Defects Original Article Series 5: 79–95

Graham C B, Rudhe, U, Eklof O 1973 Osteopetrosis. In: Kaufman H J (ed) intrinsic diseases of bones. Progress in Pediatric Radiology, vol 4.S. Karger, Basel, p 375–402

Greenfield G, Romano A, Stein R, Goodman R M 1973 Blue sclerae and keratoconus: key features of a distinct heritable disorder of connective tissue. Clinical Genetics 4: 8–16

Houston C S, Gerrard J W, Ives E J 1978 Dysosteosclerosis. American Journal of Roentgenology 130: 988–991

Iancu T C, Almagor G, Friedman E, Hardoff R, Front D 1978 Chronic familial hyperphosphatasemia. Radiology 129: 669–676

Kenny F M, Linarelli L 1966 Dwarfism and cortical thickening of tubular bones. Transient hypocalcemia in a mother and a son. American Journal of Diseases of Children 3: 201–207

Lachman R, Hall J G 1979 The radiographic prenatal diagnosis of the generalised bone dysplasias and other skeletal abnormalities. Birth Defects Original Article Series 15 (5A): 3–24

Levin L S, Brady J M, Melnick M 1980 Scanning electron microscopy of teeth in dominant osteogenesis imperfecta. Support for genetic heterogeneity. American Journal of Medical Genetics 5: 189–199

Macpherson R I 1974 Craniodiaphyseal dysplasia, a disease or group of diseases? Journal of the Canadian Association of Radiology 25: 22–23

Mann J B, Alterman S, Hill A G 1962 Albright's hereditary osteodystrophy comprising pseudohypoparathyroidism and pseudo-pseudohypoparathyroidism, with a report of two cases representing the complete syndrome occurring in successive generations. Annals of Internal Medicine 56: 315–342

Marks S S, Walker D G 1976 Mammalian osteopetrosis – a model for studying cellular and humoral factors in bone resorption. In: Bourne G H (ed) the biochemistry and physiology of bone, 2nd edn, vol 4. Academic Press, New York

Maroteaux P 1979 Bone diseases of children. J B Lippincott, Philadelphia

McCance R A 1947 Osteomalacia with Looser's nodes (milkman's syndrome) due to a raised resistance to vitamin D acquired about the age of 15 years. Quaterly Journal of Medicine 16: 33–46

Melnick J C, Needles C F 1966 An undiagnosed bone dysplasia: a 2 family study of 4 generations and 3 generations. American Journal of Roentgenology 97: 39–48

Milhaud G, Labat M L 1978 Thymus and osteopetrosis. Clinical Orthopedics 135: 260–271

Mulivor R A, Mennuti M, Zackai E H, Harris H 1978 Prenatal diagnosis of hypophosphatasia: genetic, biochemical and clinical studies. American Journal of Human Genetics 30: 271–282

Murray R O, McCredie J 1979 Melorheostosis and the sclerotomes: a radiological correlation. Skelet. Radiol. 4: 57–71

Nagant de Deuxchaisnes C, Krane S M. In: Avioli L V, Krane S M (eds) Metabolic bone disease, vol 2. Academic Press, New York

Neuhauser G, Kaveggia E G, Opitz U M 1976 Autosomal recessive syndrome of pseudogliomatous blindness, osteoporosis and mild mental retardation. Clinical Genetics 9: 324–332

Ohno S 1967 Sex chromosomes and sex linked genes. Springer, New York

Rasmussen H, Anast C 1978 Familial hypophosphatemic (vitamin D-resistant) rickets and vitamin D-dependent rickets. In: Stanbury J B, Wyngaarlen J B, Frederickson D S (eds) The metabolic basis of inherited disease. McGraw-Hill, New York, p 1537

Rasmussen H, Bartter F C 1978 Hypophosphatasia. In: Stanbury J B, Wyngaarden J B, Fredrickson K S (eds) The metabolic basis of inherited disease, 4th edn. McGraw Hill, New York, p 1340

Reeves J D, August C S, Humbert J R, Weston W L Host defences in infantile osteopetrosis. Pediatrics 64: 202–205

Riedner E D, Levin L S, Holliday M J 1980 Hearing patterns in dominant osteogenesis imperfecta. Archives of Otolaryngology 106: 737–40

Rimoin D L 1965 Pachydermoperiostosis (idiopathic clubbing and periostosis). Genetic and physiologic considerations.

New England Journal of Medicine 272: 923–931

Saint-Martin J, Peborde J, Dupont H, Béguère A, Labes A 1979 Malformations osseuses complexes d'évolution léthale. Archives Français de Pédiatrie 36: 188–193

Salassa R M, Jowsey J, Arnaud C D 1970 Hypophosphatemic osteomalacia associated with 'non-endocrine' tumors. New England Journal of Medicine 283: 65–70

Saraux H, Frezal J, Roy C, Avon J J, Hyat B, Lamy M 1967 Pseudo-gliome et fragilité osseuse héréditaire à transmission autosomale recessive. Ann. Ocul. (Paris) 200: 1241–1252

Scriver C R, Cameron P 1969 Pseudohypophosphatasia. New England Journal of Medicine 281: 604

Scriver C R, Glorieux F H, Reade T M, Tenenhouse H S 1976 X–linked hypophosphatemia and autosomal recessive vitamin D dependency: models for the resolution of vitamin D refractory rickets. In: Bickel H, Stern J (eds) Inborn errors of calcium and bone metabolism MTP Press, St Leonardsgate

Scriver C R, MacDonald W, Reade I, Glorieux F H, Nogrady B 1977 Hypophosphatemic non-rachitic bone disease: an entity distinct from X–linked hypophosphatemia in the renal defect, bone involvement and inheritance. American Journal of Medical Genetics 1: 101–117

Shapiro J E, Phillips J A, Byers P H et al Prenatal diagnosis of lethal perinatal osteogenesis imperfecta (01 type II). Journal of Pediatrics 100: 127–134, 1982

Sillence D O, Senn A S, Dank D M 1979 a Genetic heterogeneity in osteogenesis imperfecta. Journal of Medical Genetics 16: 101–116

Sillence D O, Rimoin D L, Danks D M 1979 b Clinical variability in osteogenesis imperfecta – variable expressivity or genetic heterogeneity. Birth Defects Original Article Series OAS 15 (5B): 113–129

Smith D 1982 Recognizable patterns of human malformation 3rd edn. W B Saunders, Philadelphia

Sparkes R S, Graham C B 1972 Camurati-Engllmann disease. Journal of Medical Genetics 9,73–85

Spranger J W, Rohwedder J 1965 Zur Genetik der Osteodystrophia Hereditaria Albright. Medizinische Welt 41: 2308–2312

Steendijk R 1976 Aspects of growth and bone structure in hypophosphatemic rickets. In: Bickel H, Stern J (eds) Inborn errors of calcium and bone metabolism LMTP Press, St Leonardgate

Sugiura Y, Yamada Y, Koh J 1974 Pyknodysostosis in Japan: report of six cases and a review of Japanese literature. Birth Defects Original Article Series 10 (12): 78–98

Sykes, B, Francis M J O, Smith R 1977 Altered relation of two collagen types in osteogenesis imperfecta. New England Journal of Medicine 296: 1200–1203

Tenenhouse H S, Scriver C R, McInnes R R, Glorieux F H 1978 Renal handling of phosphate in vivo and in vitro by the X–linked ph–pophosphatemic male mouse (Hyp/X). Evidence for a defect in the brush border membrane. Kidney International 14: 236–244

Whalen J P, Horwith M, Krook L et al 1977 Calcitonin treatment in hereditary bone dysplasia with hyperphosphatasemia: a radiographic and histologic study of bone. American Journal of Roentgenology 129: 29–35

Woodhouse N J Y, Fisher M T, Sigurdsson et al 1972 Paget's disease in a five year old: acute response to human calcitonin. British Medical Journal 4: 267–269

Worth H M, Wollin D G 1966 Hyperostosis corticalis generalisata congenita. Journal of the Canadian Association of Radiology 17: 67–74

Yu J S, Oates K, Walsh K H, Stuckey S J 1971 Osteopetrosis. Archives of Diseases in Childhood 46: 257–263

53

Abnormalities of bone structure

W. A. Horton

In the past few decades many disorders have been delineated which are characterized by abnormal skeletal development, collectively termed the skeletal dysplasias. A large number of these, designated the osteochondrodysplasias, are thought to result from disturbances in the normal ossification process. The osteochondrodysplasias have been subdivided into three categories: defects of growth of tubular bones and/or spine, disorganized development of cartilage and fibrous components of the skeleton, and abnormalities of density of cortical diaphyseal structure and/or metaphyseal modelling (Rimoin, 1979).The disorders comprising the second category are the subject of this chapter. They can best be understood in the context of the normal ossification process.

The skeleton normally develops and grows through a combination of two distinct forms of ossification: endochondral and membranous (Rimoin & Horton, 1978). In the latter bone develops directly from fibrous tissue. The calvarium, clavicles, body of the mandible, spinous processes of the vertebrae and part of the pelvis arise in this fashion. In addition, diaphyseal widening of individual bones occurs in this manner. The remainder of the skeleton develops through endochondral ossification, a more complex process in which a cartilage precursor for each bone is formed and is subsequently transformed into true bone. The cartilage anlagen arise early in embryonic development, and by mid pregnancy, ossification has spread throughout each bone leaving only the epiphyses as cartilageous structures. Continued proliferation of this epiphyseal cartilage, predominantly that portion that borders the ossification front (the endochondral growth plate) is responsible for linear growth of the bone. Highly organized zones of proliferative, hypertrophic and degenerative cartilage can be identified within the growth plate. As the slowly progressing ossification front penetrates the growing cartilage (chondrosseus junction), true bone is laid down. Initially, it is immature or woven bone, but with modelling, this is replaced by mature or lamellar bone. [The maturation process occurs in membraneous ossification as well.] Secondary centers of ossification which exhibit a similar sequence of events also develop in the epiphyses during late fetal life and throughout childhood. With the completion of puberty, cartilage growth ceases and the entire structure is transformed into bone.

Certain generalizations can be made about the disorders discussed in this chapter. Several of them, such as hereditary multiple exostoses or enchondromatosis, are characterized by aberrant growth plate activity. The lesions in these disorders are restricted to bones which arise by endochondral ossification. The activity of these lesions tends to parallel that of the normal growth plate, i.e. growth during childhood, quiescence after puberty. In contrast, bone maturation is disturbed in other of the disorders, such as fibrous dysplasia of bone. Puberty seems to have little effect on these lesions which may affect all bones. Thus, the clinical features in these disorders are often determined by the relationship of the specific abnormality to the normal ossification process.

DYSPLASIA EPIPHYSEALIS HEMIMELICA

Dysplasia epiphysealis hemimelica (DEH) is a developmental disorder of childhood characterized by asymmetrical growth of epiphyseal cartilage. Originally described as tarsomegalie in 1926, several designations have been used: tarso-epiphyseal aclasis, chondrodystrophy epiphysairi, benign epiphyseal osteochondroma, carpal osteochondroma, osteochondroma of the distal femoral epiphysis, epiphysealis hyperplasia, and intra-articular osteochondroma of the astragalus (Kettlecamp et al, 1966; Barta et al 1973). The term DEH was introduced by Fairbank (1956) to distinguish this condition from multiple epiphyseal dysplasia and chondrodystrophica punctata. DEH has been extensively reviewed by several authors (Fairbank, 1956, Kettlecamp et al, 1966, Theodorou & Lantis, 1968, and Barta et al, 1973).

Males are affected approximately three times as often as females. Symptoms usually arise between the ages of two and fourteen years but have been described as early as 18 months (Fasting & Bjerkreim, 1976). In a few cases the diagnosis has been established during adulthood. Joint deformity especially at the knee and ankle, restricted motion, and occasionally pain, call attention to the condition. Bony hard swelling is found at the sites of the lesions which are usually confined to one side of a limb. The medial side is mainly affected in the leg, whereas, in the arm, which is involved infrequently, the radial side predominates. The most common sites in order of decreasing frequency are: talus, distal femoral epiphysis, distal tibial epiphysis, proximal tibial epiphysis, tarsal navicular, median cuneiform and distal fibular epiphysis. The axial skeleton is rarely involved, but lesions of the pubis (Kettlecamp et al, 1966) and scapula (Bigliani et al, 1980) have been reported. Multiple lesions occur in about two thirds of the patients.

Skeletal radiographs reveal irregular enlargement of the affected epiphyses and tarsal and carpal bones. There is usually a lobulated multicentric mass adjacent to one side of the epiphysis or bone. In young children multiple ossification centres may be seen within this mass, but with time these fuse to form a single ossified mass which eventually becomes part of the adjacent bone. Mild widening of the metaphysis of affected bones may also be seen. When the talus is affected, the ossification centres may appear prematurely.

The histological examination of the lesions show nests of proliferating and hypertrophic chondrocytes surrounding ossification centres. The process resembles the normal pattern of endochondral ossification associated with secondary ossification centres; it is also indistinguishable from the pattern seen in osteocartilagenous exostoses.

The lesions and their secondary deformities tend to increase during the first few years of life, afterwhich they become somewhat quiescent and enlarge only slightly as the child continues to grow. Both shortening and lengthening of the affected limbs compared to unaffected limbs has been described. New ossification centres may appear radiographically; however, as described earlier, these fuse with each other and the normal portion of the bone. Following puberty there is little change. Treatment must be individualized and usually involves excision of the lesions that contribute to deformities and interfere with normal function. Malignant degeneration of the lesions has not been described.

All cases of DEH reported to date have been sporadic. Moreover, in one instance, one of a pair of monozygotic twins was affected (Donaldson et al, 1953). Hensinger et al (1974), however, reported the autosomal dominant transmission of DEH together with intracapsular chondromas, extraskeletal chondromas, and osteochondromas.

HEREDITARY MULTIPLE EXOSTOSES

The formation of numerous cartilage capped exostoses which give rise to deformities of the growing skeleton characterizes hereditary multiple exostoses. The syndrome has been recognized as a familial entity for well over a century. Many terms including diaphyseal aclasis, multiple osteochondromas, multiple osteocartilagenous exostoses, hereditary deforming osteochondrodysplasia and multiple exostoses have also been applied to it.

The clinical and radiographic features have been delineated by Solomon (1963, 1964). The vast majority of patients are discovered during the first decade of life. Bony lumps of the scapula and tibia are usually noted first, probably because of the conspicuous nature of these areas. Skeletal radiographs at this time, however, usually show lesions in other bones. Palpable masses have been detected soon after birth in affected infants in instances in which the child was known to be at risk for the condition. The lesions characteristically appear and increase in size during childhood. After completion of puberty, no new lesions form and the activity of those lesions present ceases. Asymptomatic ones may be detected by X–ray at any age however. In addition, some lesions may actually disappear with time. The lesions are juxtaepiphyseal in origin and most frequently are found at the ends of tubular bones, vertebral borders of the scapula, iliac crest and ribs. Involvement of vertebral bodies, patella, carpal and tarsal bones is rare; however, the lesions can arise in any bone which develops by endochondral ossification. The radiographic appearance of the individual lesions varies considerably. In general, they appear as projections of the bone from which they come; the overlying cortex and inner marrow cavity are continuous with those of the parent bone.

The earliest lesion viewed radiographically is an asymmetric overgrowth of the metaphyseal cortical bone which lies immediately adjacent to the growth plate. As the parent bone lengthens two patterns may evolve. Normal growth of the juxtaepiphyseal metaphyseal bone may resume, so that as the bone elongates, the exostosis appears to migrate toward the disphysis (Fig. 53.1). Alternatively, the exostosis may continue to expand at the metaphysis producing an irregular club or sometimes cauliflower shaped end of the bone (Fig. 53.2). Pedunculated lesions which point away from the joint may also be seen near the metaphysis. The behaviour of the lesions is unpredictable, varying from one bone to another within the same individual and even within the same bone (Solomon, 1963).

In two thirds of patients the clinical picture is dominated by skeletal deformities distinct from the actual exostoses. They result from reduced linear growth of the affected long bones. In a study of 76 patients, Solomon (1961) found that forearm deformities, including bowed radius, conical ulna and radiohumeral dislocations, were present in 50% of patients, while genu valgum, valgus deformities of the ankles, and deformities of the hands were present in 21, 45 and 17%, respectively. Except for

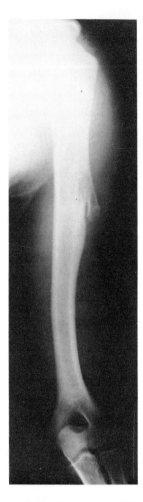

Fig. 53.1 Radiograph showing exostosis of the diaphysis of the humerus in a 16 year old boy with hereditary multiple exostoses.

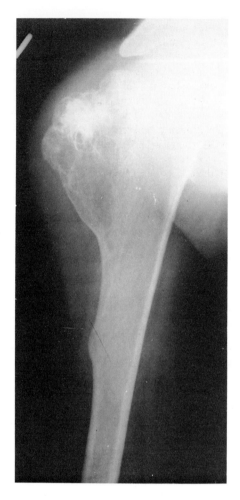

Fig. 53.2 Radiograph showing exostosis of the proximal humerus in 18 year old female with hereditary multiple exostoses.

the valgus deformities of the ankles, these deformities were asymmetrical. Scoliosis and pelvic and thoracic deformities were occasionally found as well. Short stature due to shortened extremities was common (41%) but was rarely severe. Shapiro et al (1979) noted frequent limb length discrepancies.

The most serious complication of this syndrome is malignant degeneration of the exostoses. Although development of chondrosarcoma has been reported in as high as 25% of patients (Jaffe, 1943), it is probably much lower, in the range of five to ten per cent of patients (Solomon, 1974; Ochsner, 1978). The tumors tend to occur in the pelvic girdle most commonly arising from the ilium or proximal femur and less often in the shoulder girdle. The diagnosis is most frequently made in the early thirties, and the first signs are usually swelling and rarely pain or neurologic symptoms (Ochsner, 1978).

The tumours generally grow slowly and metastasize late. Since the exostoses do not normally enlarge after completion of puberty, any swelling or pain associated with the lesion especially in the pelvic or shoulder region, should suggest malignant change. Other rare complications include large pelvic exostoses which cause urinary obstruction and renal failure, malposition of a pregnant uterus, intestinal obstruction and spinal cord compression (Solomon, 1963; Vinstein & Franken, 1971). Treatment depends upon the particular deformities and complications that occur. Most patients do require surgery, however. The most common procedures include removal of exostoses which interfere with function, contribute to deformity, produce compression or are suspected of undergoing malignant degeneration; epiphysiodeses to compensate for reduced growth of affected bones; excision of the radial head in cases of humero-radial dislocation; and correctional osteotomies for specific deformities (Shapiro et al, 1979).

Examination of an exostosis histologically shows a projection of trabecular bone covered by a cartilage cap. In children and adolescents columns of normally appearing proliferating and hypertrophic chondrocytes are found along the bony margin. The appearance is very similar to a normal growth plate except that the chondroosseous junction is irregular and collections of hypertrophic chondrocytes are incorporated into the bone (Spjut et al, 1971). In the adult, the cartilage is reduced to a thin rim or is absent altogether.

Hereditary multiple exostoses is inherited as an autosomal dominant trait. When studied radiographically, there is essentially complete penetrance. Males and females are equally affected, but there is little tendency toward similarity in the distribution and type of lesions and deformities within families (Solomon, 1964).

Several theories have been proposed to explain the pathogenesis of the cartilagenous tumours. Virchow originally postulated that a fragment of the growth plate becomes separated, rotated 90 degrees and proceeds to grow in the new direction (Spjut et al, 1971). Others have suggested that collections of chondrocytes arising from the proliferative layer of the metaphyseal perichondriun give rise to the tumour or that a defect in that perichondrial ring which normally surrounds the hypertrophic and degenerate zones of the growth plate permits the aberrant cartilage growth (Solomon, 1963). Langenskiold (1967) speculated that a layer of undifferentiated cells at the chondroosseous junction fails to differentiate into osteoblasts, as normally occurs and instead retains its chondrogenic potential producing the abnormal cartilage growth. Ogden (1976) has recently proposed that a biochemical defect exists which prevents synchronous cartilage division at the growth plate. Cells at the periphery, which may be under less physical constraint, are permitted to expand multidirectionally producing the exostosis. Increased excretion of mucopolysaccharides in the urine was reported in 1960 by Lorincz. However, Solomon (1964), who performed more extensive studies, found that mucopolysaccharide excretion was normal in adults and only slightly increased in affected children; he felt that the abnormalities simply reflected the increased bulk cartilage in these children.

Despite the lack of understanding regarding the origin of the exostoses, certain aspects of the disorder have been defined. The distribution of lesions is related to the growth rate of the individual bones; sites contributing the greatest to the overall skeletal growth show the highest frequency of exostoses. In addition, the normal process of bone remodeling affects the evolution of the individual lesions, explaining the phenomena of migration and disapparance of exostoses (Solomon, 1963).

Table 53.1 Clinical features in 13 reported cases of the Langer-Giedion syndrome

Feature	Occurrence
Typical facies	13/13
Microcephaly	11/12
Sparse scalp hair	13/13
Prominent ears	13/13
Micrognathia	6/11
Mental retardation	12/13
Delayed speech	10/12
Hearing loss	4/8
Short stature of post-natal onset	13/13
Multiple exostoses	13/13
Cone-shaped epiphyses	13/13
Winged scapula	8/11
Perthes-like bone changes	5/10
Loose skin	6/7
Skin nevi	7/11
Lax joints	6/12
Multiple fractures	3/13
Frequent respiratory infections	4/8
Delayed puberty	1/4
Male	9/13
Normal karyotype	3/3

LANGER-GIEDION SYNDROME

In the Langer-Giedion syndrome, multiple exostoses occur as a component of a multisystem disorder. Also known as the tricho-rhinophalangeal syndrome type II and acrodysplasia with exostoses, this syndrome is very rare. The first two cases were described independently by Langer (1968) and Giedion (1969). Hall, together with Langer, Giedion and others reported 5 additional patients and delineated the syndrome in 1974. Seven more cases have been added to the literature (Kozlowki et al, 1977; Stoltzfus et al, 1977; Murachi et al, 1979; Ourthys & Beemer, 1979; Wilson et al, 1979; Buhler et at, 1980). Of the fourteen total cases, thirteen are quite similar. An analysis of the clinical features based on these patients is tabulated in Table 53.1. Heavy eyebrows, large bulbous nose with thickened alae and septum, prominent elongated philtrum, thin upper lip together with mild microcephaly, large poorly developed protruding ears, and sparse scalp hair comprise the characteristic craniofacial appearance. Other consistent features have included mental retardation, delay in the onset of speech, short stature, multiple exostoses, cone-shaped epiphyses and loose skin. The mental retardation is generally mild to moderate in degree. In one patient who was initially considered to be mentally retarded, intelligence was eventually determined to be normal after a profound hearing deficit was found (Ourthys & Beemer, 1979). A hearing loss has been detected in half the patients tested. The delay of speech development has been observed in at least two patients with normal audiograms, however, and it appears to be out of proportion to the degree of mental retardation.

The multiple exostoses are similar in clinical behaviour and radiographic appearance to those seen in hereditary multiple exostoses. Diminished linear growth of affected bones and secondary deformities occur as well. No cases of malignant degeneration have been reported but the oldest patient yet described is only 22 years old (Wilson et al, 1979).

Several types of cone-shaped epiphyses have been described by Giedion (1969). All patients with this syndrome have had the type 12 in which the distal epiphyses of the metacarpal and proximal epiphyses of the phalanges of the hand are affected. Small conical shaped epiphyses appear to invaginate into the adjacent metaphyses often with fusion and widening of the metaphyses (Hall et al, 1974). These abnormalities are not visible radiographically before age 3 to 4 years, however, because ossification of the epiphyses in the hand bones is insufficient before this age. Epiphyseal irregularities have been found in other parts of the skeleton. In particular, Perthes-like changes in the capital femoral epiphyses have been seen in half the patients. This generalized epiphyseal disturbance is probably responsible for the short stature exhibited in all the cases.

The occurrence of multiple fractures has been mentioned as a component of the syndrome; however, it has been demonstrated in only three of the thirteen patients. Moreover, one patient had only a single traumatic fracture of the humerus (Gorlin et al, 1969), and the two others were identical twins who showed generalized skeletal demineralization. In fact, Hall et al (1974) questioned whether this feature was a part of the syndrome or simply a second abnormality restricted to the twins.

Although most of the children have cutaneous involvement, it has varied with age. The loose skin seems to be most striking during early childhood and regresses or even disappears between the ages of 6 and 14 years. Small brown to black maculopapular nevi are found on the face, scalp, neck and upper trunk of the older children, but have not been seen prior to age 4 years.

All cases reported to date have been sporadic and 9 of the 13 typical cases have been male. Two of the males were monozygotic twins. The additional patient reported by Buhler et al (1980) was a 13-year-old girl who had many manifestations of the syndrome including similar facial appearance, mental retardation, short stature, exostoses, and cone-shaped epiphyses. She lacked several features, however, such as sparse scalp hair and bulbous nose and had suffered severe birth asphyxia which could have explained the microcephaly and mental retardation. Moreover, she exhibited evidence of precocious puberty during the second year of life. In contrast, one of the typical cases had delayed puberty (Wilson et al, 1979) and three others underwent pubertal development at the normal age. This patient's most atypical feature was an abnormal karyotype 46 XX del (8)(q24). Unbanded karyotypes done at 1 and 10 years of age were reported to be normal, but banded studies done at age 13 years revealed the deletion. Chromosome studies on the parents were normal.

The aetiology of the Langer-Giedion syndrome is unclear. The abnormal karyotype in the atypical patient suggests the possibility that a small deletion in the long arm of chromosome 8 may be responsible. Normal karyotypes have been reported in 3 of the typical cases, however (Kozlowski et al, 1977; Wilson et al, 1979; Murachi et al, 1979). Further chromosome studies with high resolution banding techniques (Yunis, 1980) may resolve this issue. A new mutation of a dominant gene has also been suggested by Murachi et al (1979). They observed that the mean paternal age in six cases which they reviewed was 33.3 years, substantially higher than the average paternal age in the general population. The mean maternal age was normal.

ENCHONDROMATOSIS

Enchondromatosis is another rare disorder of the developing skeleton. It was originally described by Ollier who called it dyschondroplasia but it has been variably referred to an Ollier's disease, multiple enchondromatosis, multiple enchondromas, internal enchondromatosis (Fairbank, 1948). It must be distinguished from a similar but yet distinct disorder, Maffucci syndrome, in which the combination of multiple enchondromas and cutaneous hemangiomas and other tumours is found.

The manifestations of the disorder result from the occurrence of cartilaginous tumours in the metaphyses of bones that are formed in cartilage. They have been best described by Fairbank (1948). Both long and short tubular bones are preferentially involved and the more rapidly growing ends of these bones are the most frequently affected sites. For example, lesions in the region of the knee joint and at the lower ends of the radius and ulna are particularly common sites, while the phalanges and the pelvis are somewhat less common. The scalpula, ulna, ribs, sternum, base of the skull, and facial bones are rarely affected, and the cuboid bones, such as the vertebrae, carpal and tarsal bones, usually escape. Tumours do not occur in the calvarium. By definition, more than one lesion must be present; however, the involvement may vary considerably from enchondromas affecting a single limb to tumours throughout the skeleton. In the latter instance, the lesions are asymmetric and bilateral in the majority of cases (Mainzer et al, 1971).

The characteristic deformities result from direct expansion of the tumours and from reduced linear growth of the affected bones. The most common deformities include phalangeal enlargement, asymmetric shortening of the limbs, bowing of the long bones, ulnar deviation of the wrist, dislocation of the radial head and genu valgum. In rare instances when the base of the skull is involved, facial asymmetry and cranial nerve compression may occur. Fractures of the affected bones are uncommon. Considerable variability has been noted regarding the severity of the deformities ranging from asymptomatic lesions detected only by X–ray to extensive disfigurement and disability, e.g. massive swelling of fingers and toes.

The disorder is usually detected during childhood but has been identified at birth in an infant who exhibited asymmetrical limb shortening (Mainzer et al, 1971). The appearance of new lesions as well as tumour growth and progression of deformities tends to occur in an unpredictable fashion during childhood. The lesions often regress and deformities stabilize after puberty. Renewed growth during adulthood should suggest sarcomatous degeneration. The occurrence of this complication is probably less than in the Maffucci syndrome (below), but actual figures are not known.

Radiographically the lesions vary from a minute foci of incompletely calcified epiphyseal cartilage extending linearly from the growth plate into the metaphysis of the bone to large tumourous masses of cartilage which produce massive metaphyseal enlargement (Fig. 53.3). Irregular calcifications are often found within the tumour. Thinning and disruption of the cortex of the overlying bone may occur, and there may be abnormal metaphyseal modelling. As well, radiolucent defects often extend into the shaft of the bone (Lachman & Horton, 1977). The radiographic changes of enchondromatosis may be influenced by age (Mainzer et al, 1971). For example, despite shortening of a bone, typical lesions may not be seen during infancy. Furthermore, there may be a gradual 'filling in' of the lesions with normal appearing bone after puberty.

The tumour pathologically consists of lobulated masses of irregularly dispersed chondrocytes encased within bone. Proliferative and hypertrophic cells are found, and some areas resemble the normal endochondral growth plate. In tissue from older patients intracartilaginous ossification may be seen (Spjut et al, 1971).

Enchondromatosis has occurred in a sporadic fashion in almost all cases reported to date. Both sexes are affected, but it is more common in males (Fairbank, 1948). The source of the metaphyseal enchondromas is not known. They may represent unresorbed portions of growth plate tissue that become incorporated into the metaphysis as the bone lengthens or may arise *de novo* within the metaphysis.

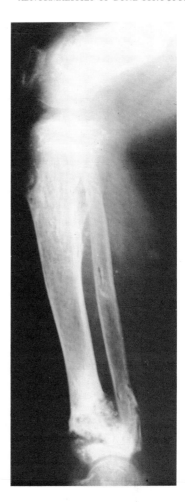

Fig. 53.3 Radiograph showing enchondromas in distal femur and proximal and distal tibia and fibula in a 12 year old boy with enchondromatosis.

MAFFUCCI SYNDROME

In 1891 an Italian, Maffucci, described a patient with enchondromas and superficial hemangiomas. Today the syndrome in which this combination occurs bears his name; however, it is recognized that the manifestations are much more extensive. The skeletal manifestations are similar to those seen in isolated enchondromatosis. Expanding cartilaginous tumours in the metaphyses of tubular bones, primarily, develop during childhood. The metacarpals and phalanges of the hand are the most common sites, although lesions are frequently observed in the tibia, fibula, femur, radius, ulna and humerus as well (Lewis & Ketchum, 1973). The tumours tend to be asymmetric and bilateral and cannot be distinguished radiographically or histologically from those found in patients with enchondromatosis. Likewise, tumor expansion and shortening of involved bones leads to a similar array of deformities. Spontaneous fractures through areas of advanced rarefication have been reported in 26% of patients in one series (Anderson, 1965). Cranial nerve palsies due to involvement of the base of the skull have also been described (Loewinger et al, 1977).

The major nonskeletal manifestation of the disorder is the occurrence of simple or cavernous cutaneous hemangiomas (Anderson, 1965). Usually located on the limbs, they lie in the deep layers of the skin and subcutaneous tissues. Their size varies from a few millimeters in diameter to many centimeters. They are not limited to the skin however, but may also be found throughout the viscera. There is a slight tendency for the hemangiomas and enchondromas to show a similar distribution with regard to laterality, but no direct relationship exists between the two. Phlebectasia is commonly observed, and thrombosis and subsequent calcification often occur within the vascular spaces. In fact, phleboliths seen on X–ray are found in nearly half the patients with this condition (Anderson, 1965). In reporting a patient with enchondromas and fibromuscular dysplasia of cerebral arteries, Slagsvold et al (1977) speculated that this arterial lesion might represent another vascular manifestation of the disorder. Lymphangiomatosis has been described in a number of cases (Lewis & Ketchum, 1973, Loewinger et al, 1977). Other nonskeletal manifestations seen in the Maffucci syndrome include vitiligo, hyperpigmentation and nevi (Loewinger et al, 1977). The majority of the soft tissue lesions are painless, although mild discomfort as well as increased skin temperature may accompany the hemangiomas (Lewis & Ketchum, 1973).

The skeletal abnormalities usually do not present until early or mid childhood, but the hemangiomas are often detected at or shortly after birth. The clinical picture through puberty is dominated predominately by the skeletal lesions; as with enchondromatosis, it is unpredictable. After the completion of puberty, however, the enchondromas usually do not progress, although this is not invariable (Anderson, 1965). The predisposition to neoplasia during adulthood is well established. The greatest risk is for sarcomatous degeneration of the enchondromas which has been estimated to occur in 15 to 19% of patients (Anderson, 1965; Lewis & Ketchum, 1973). The risk does not correlate with the severity of involvement. Malignant degeneration of hemangiomas and lymphangiomas also occurs, and patients may develop multiple primary tumours. There are also reports of many other malignant and benign tumours occurring in patients with the Maffucci syndrome. These include osteosarcoma, fibrosarcoma, glioma, mesenchymal ovarian carcinoma, carcinoma of the pancreas, uterine polyps and fibroids, adrenal cortical adenomas, thecoma of the ovary and multiple fibromas (Braddock

& Hadlow, 1966; Lewis & Ketchum, 1973). Chromophobe adenoma of the pituitary has been noted in 7 of 114 reported cases (Schnell & Genuth, 1976). The author has observed a parathyroid adenoma in one patient as well. Because of the isolated nature of most of these reports, it is not clear if these associations are significant or simply coincidental. Sudden enlargement of either skeletal or non-skeletal tumours during adulthood, however, should make one suspicious of malignant degeneration.

The treatment consists of orthopedic and surgical intervention to minimize deformities and for cosmetic purposes. Careful surveillance for malignant degeneration of both skeletal and nonskeletal tumours is essential.

The Maffucci syndrome occurs in all races with equal sex distribution. All cases have been sporadic and affected women have produced unaffected offspring (Lewis & Ketchum, 1973). Normal karyotypes have been obtained in several instances (Lewis & Ketchum, 1973). To explain the numerous mesenchymal tumours, it is generally thought that the syndrome results from a generalized defect in the mesodermal tissues (Anderson, 1965; Lewis & Ketchum, 1973; Loewinger, 1977), however, the nature of this defect is unknown.

METACHONDROMATOSIS

Metachondromatosis is a distinct syndrome in which both exostoses and enchondromas are found. Only 10 cases have been reported. Nine were members of two families in which the trait showed autosomal dominant transmission (Maroteaux, 1971; Giedion et al, 1975). The other was a sporadic case described by Lachman et al (1974). In addition, Cameron (1957) reported a patient (case no.2) who may have had this syndrome. The patient exhibited multiple exostoses, enchondromas involving the metatarsal and tarsal bone of the left foot and a single hemangioma of the left big toe.

Clinically, the patients may be short and usually present with exostoses, preferentially affecting the tubular bones of the hands and feet. In contrast to the lesions seen in hereditary multiple exostoses which point away from the epiphyses, the exostoses in this syndrome point toward the joint. In addition to the exostoses, irregularly calcified lesions which are sometimes separated from bone have been observed near the epiphyses (Giedion et al, 1975). An unusual feature of the syndrome is the tendency for the tumours to regress and actually disappear in adulthood (Maroteaux, 1971; 1971; Giedion et al, 1975).

The enchondromata are found in the metaphyses of long bones and in the iliac crest which is an unusual location for the tumours in enchondromatosis and the Maffucci syndrome (Fig. 53.4). Irregularity of the end

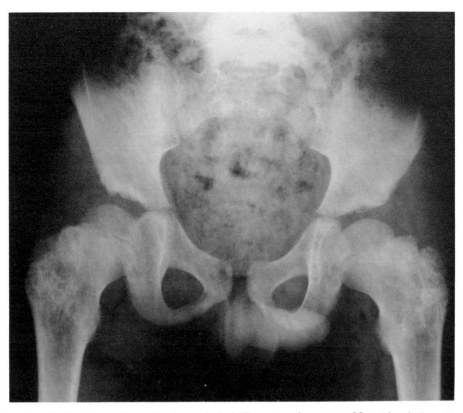

Fig. 53.4 AP radiograph of pelvis showing enchondromas in both iliac crest and exostoses of femoral necks in an 8 year old boy with metachondromatosis. (Courtesy of R S Lachman, Los Angeles, C A).

plates of the vertebral bodies has also been seen. Presumably this defect together with the metaphyseal involvement by enchondromata is responsible for the short stature. Treatment consists of surgery when indicated. The risk of malignant degeneration of the cartilaginous tumours is not known.

FIBROUS DYSPLASIA OF BONE

Fibrous dysplasia of bone is characterized by the replacement of bone by dysplastic fibrous tissue. Although initially confused with osteitis fibrosa cystica of hyperparathyroidism, it was recognized as a separate entity in 1937 by Albright et al who described the skeletal lesions in association with increased skin pigmentation and endocrine disturbances. Five years later, Lichtenstein and Jaffe (1942) delineated the pathologic features of the skeletal lesions which they termed fibrous dysplasia of bone and observed that the extraskeletal abnormalities did not occur when only a single bone was involved. The disorder has since been defined further by several reviews in which the features of nearly 300 patients have been examined (Fries, 1957; Stewart et al, 1962; Harris et al,

1962; Leeds & Seaman, 1962; Reed, 1963; Firat & Stutzman, 1968; Henry, 1969). Although there has been a tendency to classify fibrous dysplasia on the basis of whether or not extraskeletal features are found, it appears more appropriate to divide it on the basis of whether the lesions involve one or more than one bone since the extraskeletal features occur only in the latter instance.

Monostotic fibrous dysplasia
Patients with monostotic disease are thought to be much more common than those with the polyostotic form. The most frequently affected sites in monostotic fibrous dysplasia are the craniofacial bones, including the skull, maxilla, and mandible; ribs; femur; tibia; and humerus. The pelvis, other long bones, vertebrae, and tarsal bones are occasionally involved (Harris et al, 1962; Firat & Stutzman, 1968; Henry, 1969). The lesions in the extremities usually present during adolescence with pain, swelling, and pathologic fractures. The craniofacial lesions are often heralded by swelling, asymmetric growth of the skull or face and occasionally unilateral proptosis; they tend to occur in the second and third decade. Rib lesions are often asymptomatic and may be

discovered at any age, often as an incidental finding on a chest X–ray (Henry, 1969).

The earliest radiographic change consists of a loss of density at the site of the lesion. Later there is expansion of the bone with erosion and thinning of the cortex from within. The shaft may exhibit a 'ground glass' appearance, upon which prominent trabeculae are superimposed. In long bones the lesions appear to begin in the metaphysis and extend into the diaphysis (Stewart et al, 1962). Sclerosis may be associated with .involvement of the facial bones.

The lesions tend to grow slowly prior to adolescence, however, their activity is variable (Smith, 1965; Gross & Montgomery, 1967). After puberty, they usually become inactive; but, Henry (1969) observed that several patients developed symptoms, often pathologic fractures of long bones, beyond this age. He also noted that fibrous dysplasia may become activated or reactivated during pregnancy. Malignant degeneration does occur, but rarely. Schwartz and Alpert (1964) calculated the incidence to be approximately 0.4% of patients. Osteogenetic sarcoma was the predominant tumour and occurred at an average age of 32 years following a mean lag time of 13.5 years after the initial presentation. Several of the patients in whom malignant degeneration has occurred have received previous radiation therapy (Harris et al, 1962; Schwartz & Alpert, 1969).

Although the radiographic appearance of fibrous dysplasia is characteristic, it is not pathognomonic. Therefore, in the monostotic form, a biopsy is necessary to confirm the diagnosis. Histologically, the lesions consist of poorly defined partially calcified trabeculae of bone embedded within dense, cellular fibrous tissue. The bone is immature (woven) in type; no lamellar (mature) bone is found. The trabeculae are rimmed by only a few osteoblasts, and there is a paucity of osteoclasts (Fries, 1957; Harris et al, 1962; Reed, 1963; Spjut et al, 1971). These changes seem to vary little with age. Cysts, dense fibrosis, islands of cartilage and lamellar transformation of woven bone, have also been described. Reed (1963) feels that these changes are nonspecific and reflect previous surgery, trauma, fractures and hemorrhage.

All cases of monostotic fibrous dysplasia have occurred on a sporadic basis. Males and females are equally affected. The pathogenesis of the condition is poorly understood. In 1942 Lichenstein and Jaffe proposed that a defect in the bone forming mesenchyme results in the replacement of normal bone by dense fibrous tissue. This tissue then gives rise through metaplasia to woven bone which fails to mature into lamellar bone. Although the latter portion of this hypothysis, i.e. arrest of bone maturation, is still widely held (Fries, 1957; Reed, 1963; Spjut et al, 1971), the nature of the primary defect remains unknown.

The treatment of monostotic fibrous dysplasia involves surgery to remove abnormal tissue. If this is not possible curettage of the lesion and packing it with bone chips is indicated. Treatment is successful when the lesion is completely removed. However, if not, recurrence is common.

Polyostotic fibrous dysplasia

In polyostotic fibrous dysplasia, the McCune-Albright or Albright syndrome, bone lesions which are identical to those found in the monostotic form of the disease occur in multiple bones in association with abnormal skin pigmentation and a variety of endocrine disturbances. The bone lesions are the only invariable component of the syndrome. They are found throughout the skeleton, although the most frequent sites are the femur, tibia, pelvis, phalanges, ribs, humerus, and base of the skull (Harris et al, 1962). The radiographic appearance of the extracranial lesions is essentially the same as seen in monostotic fibrous dysplasia. (Fig 53.5) Cranial involvement is usually characterized by diffuse sclerosis of the base of the skull often involving the sphenoid, sella turcica and roof of the orbit, together with thickening of the occiput and obliteraton of the paranasal sinuses. Radiolucent areas may be scattered through these areas of increased density.

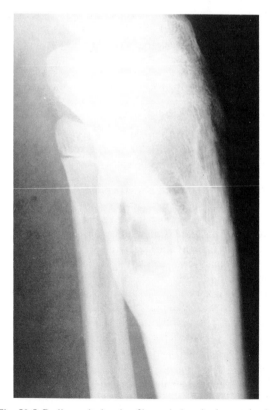

Fig. 53.5 Radiograph showing fibrous lesions in the proximal tibia via 14 year old female with polyostotic fibrous dysplasia.

The bone lesions are usually evident by age 10 years, and patients most often present with a limp, leg pain, or fracture (Harris et al, 1962). Deformities are common; they include leg length discrepancy, coxa vara, shepherd's-crook deformity of the femur, bowing of the tibia, Harrison's groove's and protrusio acetabuli. Most patients have at least one fracture and many have repeated ones. Extensive craniofacial involvement may produce facial deformities as well as cranial nerve compression, hearing loss, sinusitis, and lacrimal duct obstruction (Leeds & Seaman, 1962). Spinal cord compression has been associated with vertebral involvement (Montoya et al, 1968). The progression of the deformities is often associated with the extension of existing lesions. Puberty seems to have no effect on such extension or on the incidence of fractures. New lesions may appear usually after puberty, and spontaneous improvement rarely occurs (Harris et al, 1962). An elevation of serum alkaline phosphatase may be found.

Malignant degeneration has been reported more often in polyostotic than in monostotic fibrous dysplasia (Schwartz & Montgomery, 1964). It is thought that the higher incidence in the former is due to the greater number of lesions; the risk per lesion is the same in both (Gross & Montgomery, 1967). The risk is relatively low, 0.4% of patients, and the complication occurs less often in the craniofacial region than in other parts of the skeleton (Leeds & Seaman, 1962). Several of the patients with this complication have received prior radiation therapy (Gross & Montgomery, 1967).

The extraskeletal manifestations of polyostotic fibrous dysplasia involve the skin and endocrine glands. The cutaneous lesions consist of brown flat patches of pigmentation. They follow an irregular contour and are frequently evident at birth. They may be extensive and may, but not necessarily, overlie the bone lesions (Rimoin & Hollister, 1979).

Sexual precocity occurs in about one-third of patients, mostly females. In contrast to the sequence of events seen in normal girls undergoing puberty, and in most types of sexual precocity, vaginal bleeding usually occurs first and may precede breast development and the appearance of axillary and pubic hair by many years (Benedict, 1962). It may appear as early as three months of age. The early bleeding is usually scant and irregular and normal menstrual periods begin at the time of expected puberty. Moreover, fertility appears to be unaffected (Rimoin & Hollister, 1979). Accelerated skeletal maturation accompanies the sexual precocity. Laboratory findings in patients exhibiting this feature have been difficult to interpret. Gonadal and adrenal steroids have been found to be elevated in the plasma (Danon et al, 1975), however, both low (Benedict, 1962 and Danon et al, 1975) and high (Lightner et al, 1975) levels of circulating gonadotropins have been observed. Benedict (1962)

noted that in three such cases in which ovarian tissue had been examined, no evidence of ovulation was found. However, active spermatogenesis was seen in a testicular biopsy from a six year old boy with this condition (Hall & Warrick, 1972).

Hyperthyroidism is a common feature, occurring in 30% of patients in one series (Benedict, 1962). It may also contribute to the accelerated skeletal maturation. The thyroid abnormality is mild and distinct from Graves disease in that occular changes are lacking and histologically there is no lymphocytic infiltration in the thyroid tissue. Instead, diffuse hyperplasia is found (Hall & Warrick, 1972). Thyroid stimulating hormone levels have been determined to be low on three occasions (DiGeorge, 1975). Features of acromegaly and pituitary gigantism have been described several times, and an elevation of growth hormone has been detected at least once (Hall & Warrick, 1972; Lightner et al, 1975). Cushing's syndrome due to bilateral adrenal hyperplasia has been documented at least three times (Danon et al, 1975; Aarskog et al, 1968).

Two theories have evolved to explain the endocrine manifestations of the syndrome. The first states that hypersecretion of hypothalamic hormones leads to overactivity of various target endocrine glands (Hall & Warrick, 1972; Lighter et al, 1975). The other proposes autonomous hyperplasia of multiple endocrine glands (Danon et al, 1975; Giovanelli et al, 1978). The evidence to date gives the greatest support to the latter hypothesis (DiGeorge, 1975; Giovanelli et al, 1978), however, the relationship between the endocrine disturbances and fibrous dysplasia of bone is unknown.

Other abnormalities have rarely been observed in patients with polyostotic fibrous dysplasia and may be components of this syndrome. Multiple intramuscular myxomas have been noted in 11 patients (Wirth et al, 1971). They tend to develop in clusters, especially in the thigh region, and usually present during adulthood. Hyperplasia of reticuloendothelial tissue and both lymphoid and myeloid metaplasia have also been described (DiGeorge, 1975).

Except in two instances, the reported cases of polyostotic fibrous dysplasia have all been sporadic. Hibbs and Rush (1952) reported a mother with skin pigmentation, possible precocious puberty and fibrous lesions of several bones. A biopsy of a bone lesion was consistent with fibrous dysplasia. Her daughter had cystic bone lesions of multiple bones but no skin or endocrine abnormalities. A biopsy was also consistent with fibrous dysplasia. Firat and Stutzman (1968) described a mother and daughter both with documented hyperparathyroidism and cystic bone lesions (maxilla and mandible in the mother and mandible only in the daughter). Neither had skin or other endocrine manifestations. A bone biopsy in the mother showed dysplastic fibrous tissue consistent with fibrous dysplasia of bone although osteitis fibrosa cystica was also considered. With the reservation that the bone lesions might have resulted from the hyperparathyroidism, the authors raised the possibility that hyperparathyroidism might be another endocrine feature of the disorder.

CHERUBISM

In 1933 Jones reported four sibs with an unusual facial appearance; they appeared to be looking toward the heavens. He coined the term 'cherubism.' Despite the introduction of numerous more descriptive designations, including familial multilocular cystic disease of the jaws, familial fibrous dysplasia of the jaws, familial fibrous swelling of the jaws, familial bilateral giant cell tumour of the jaw, familial intraosseus fibrous swelling of the jaws, disseminated juvenile fibrous dysplasia of the jaws and familial osseus dysplasia of the jaws, the term cherubism seems to be firmly established (Thompson, 1959). By 1970 over 70 cases had been described. The clinical features of cherubism vary considerably (Thompson, 1959; Burland, 1962; Khosla & Korobkin, 1970). In general, the affected children present with painless symmetrical swelling of the jaws between the ages of 18 months and 7 years. The swelling progresses rapidly over the next two to three years after which it slows until puberty. Depending on the severity, the swelling can range from little more than broadening of the lower jaw to marked fullness of the lower face associated with thickening of the maxilla. In the most severe cases, maxillary expansion pushes the floor of the orbit upward. The cherubic look results from the combination of the displaced orbit and poorly supported lower eyelid; the altered facial contour permits the rim of sclerae to be exposed above the lower eyelid (Burland, 1962). It is uncommon.

Maxillary involvement occurs only when mandibular involvement is severe. When present, it may be viewed intraorally. The aveolar processes may become thickened and the vault of the palate obliterated to the extent that speech is impaired. Dental abnormalities including delayed eruption, missing or displaced teeth, premature loss of deciduous teeth and absence of permanent molars has been observed. Enlargement of submandibular lymph nodes has also been described frequently. After puberty there is a gradual normalization of the facial appearance, although in most cases there is some degree of residual enlargement (Burland, 1962). Treatment varies with the degree of involvement and may often not be needed because of the tendency toward spontaneous improvement.

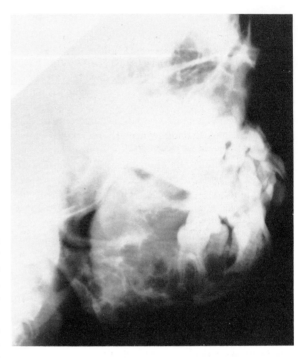

Fig. 53.6 Lateral radiograph of the jaw showing the multilocular lesions mandible in 8 year old girl with cherubism.

Radiographs of the mandible taken during childhood reveal bilateral symmetrical well-defined multilocular radiolucent areas associated with expansion of bone and cortical thinning (Fig. 53.6) (Cornelius & McClendon, 1969). The mandibular rami are always involved. The entire mandible may become involved except for the chondyles which are always spared (Khosla & Korobkin, 1970). Similar changes are seen in the maxilla when it is affected. The maxillary sinuses may be obliterated. In adults the radiolucent areas fill in with granular bone and become dense and sclerotic. The radiographic changes of the young are pathognomonic but those seen in adults are not.

Histologically, the bone is replaced by cellular fibrous tissue containing scattered trabeculae of woven bone and numerous collections of giant cells which resemble osteoclasts. Interestingly, the bone affected by the pathologic process is derived from the first branchial arch. The basic abnormality is unknown.

Cherubism is an autosomal dominant trait. A review of 21 families showed that the penetrance is 100% in males and 50 to 70% in females (Anderson & McClendon, 1962). There is considerable variability however, and X–rays may be needed to detect mildly affected individuals especially during adulthood.

REFERENCES

Albright F, Bulter A M: Hampton A O, Smith P 1937 Syndrome characterized by osteitis fibrosa disseminata, areas of pigmentation and endocrine dysfunction with precocious puberty in females. New England Journal of Medicine 216: 727–746

Anderson D E: McClendon J L, 1962 Cherubism – hereditary fibrous dysplasia of the jaws. OS, OM and OP 15 (Suppl 2): 5–16

Anderson I F, 1965 Maffucci's syndrome, report of a case with a review of the literature. South African Medical Journal 39: 1066–1070

Aarskog D, Tveterras E 1968 McCune-Albright's syndrome following adrenalectomy for Cushing's syndrome in infancy. Journal of Pediatrics 73: 89–96

Barta O, Schanzl A, Szepesi J 1973 Dysplasia epiphysealis hemimelica. Acta Orthopaedica Scandinavica 44: 702–709

Benedict P H 1962 Endocrine features in Albright's syndrome (fibrous dysplasia of bone). Metabolism 11: 30–45

Bigliani L U, Neer C S, Parisien N, Johnson A D 1980 Dysplasia epiphysealis hemimelica of the scapula, a case report. Journal of Bone and Joint Surgery 62 A: 292–294

Braddock G T F, Hadlow V D 1966 Osteochondroma in endochondromatosis (Ollier's disease). Journal of Bone and Joint Surgery 48 B: 145–149

Bühler U K, Bühler E M, Stolder G R, Jani L, Jurik L P 1980 Chromosome deletion and multiple cartilagenous exostoses. European Journal of Pediatrics 133: 163–166

Burland J G 1962 Cherubism, familial bilateral osseous dysplasia of the jaws. OS, OM and OP 15(Suppl 2): 43–68

Cameron J M 1957 Maffucci syndrome. British Journal of Surgery 44: 596–598

Cornelius E A, McClendon J L 1969 Cherubism – hereditary fibrous dysplasia of the jaws. American Journal of Radiology 106: 136–143

Danon M, Robboy S J, Kim S, Scully R, Crawford J D 1975 Cushing syndrome, sexual precocity, and polyostotic fibrous dysplasia (Albright syndrome) in infancy. Journal of Pediatrics 87: 917–921

DiGeorge A M 1975 Albright syndrome, is it coming of age? Journal of Pediatrics 87: 1018–1020

Donaldson J S, Sankey H H, Girdany B R, Donaldson W F 1953 Osteochondroma of distal femoral epiphysis. Journal of Pediatrics 43: 212–216

Fairbank H A T 1948 Dyschondroplasia, synonyms Ollier's disease, multiple enchondromata. Journal of Bone and Joint Surgery 30 B: 689–708

Fairbank T J 1956 Dysplasia epiphysealis hemimelica (tarso-epiphyseal aclasis). Journal of Bone and Joint Surgery 38 B: 237–257

Fasting O J, Bjerkreim I 1976 Dysplasia epiphysealis hemimelica. Acta Orthopaedica Scandinavica 47: 217–225

Firat D, Stutzman L 1968 Fibrous dysplasia of the bone, review of twenty-four cases. American Journal of Medicine 44: 421–429

Fries J W 1957 The roentgen features of fibrous dysplasia of the skull and facial bones, a critical analysis of thirty-nine pathologically proved cases. American Journal of Roentgenology 77: 71–88

Giedion Von A 1969 Die periphcre dysostose (PD)-ein sammelhegriff. Fortschr Roentgenstr 110: 507–524

Giedion A, Kesztler R, Muggiasca F 1975 The widened spectrum of multiple cartilagenous exostosis (MCE). Pediatric Radiology 3: 93–100

Giovannelli G, Bernasconi S, Banchini G 1978 McCune-Albright syndrome in a male child, a clinical and endocrinologic enigma. Journal of Pediatrics 92: 220–226

Gorlin R J, Cohen M M, Wolfson J 1969 Tricho-rhino-phalangeal syndrome. American Journal of Diseases of Children 118: 595–599

Gross C W, Montgomery W W 1967 Fibrous dysplasia and malignant degeneration. Archives of Otolaryngology 85: 97–101

Hall B D, Langer L O, Giedion A, Smith D W, Cohen M M, Beals R K, Brandner M 1974 Langer-Giedion syndrome. Birth Defects, Original Article Series 10: 147–164

Hall R, Warrick C 1972 Hypersecretion of hypothalamic releasing hormones, a possible explanation of the endocrine manifestations of polyostotic fibrous dysplasia (Albright's syndrome). Lancet 1: 1313–1316

Harris W H, Dudley H R, Barry R J 1962 The natural history of fiberous dysplasia, an orthopedic, pathologic, and roentgenographic study. Journal of Bone and Joint Surgery 44 A: 207–233

Henry A 1969 Monostatic fibrous dysplasia. Journal of Bone and Joint Surgery 51 B: 300–306

Hensinger R N, Cowell H R, Ramsey P L, Leopold R G 1974 Familial dysplasia epiphysealis hemimelica associated with chondromas and osteochondromas, a report of a kindred with variable expression. Journal of Bone and Joint Surgery 56 A: 1513–1516

Hibbs R E, Rush H P 1952 Albright's syndrome. Annals of Internal Medicine 37: 587–593

Jaffee H L 1943 Hereditary multiple exostoses. Archives of Pathology 36: 335–357

Jones W A 1933 Familial multilocular cystic disease of the jaws. American Journal of Cancer 17: 946–950

Kettlekamp D B, Campbell G J, Bonfiglio M 1966 Dysplasia epiphysealis hemimelica, a report of fifteen cases and a review of the literature. Journal of Bone and Joint Surgery 48 A: 746–766

Khosla V M, Korobkin M 1970 Cherubism. American Journal of Diseases of Children 120: 458–461

Kozlowski K, Harrington G, Barylak A, Bartoszewica B 1977 Multiple exostoses mental retardation syndrome (ale-calo or MEMR syndrome), description of two childhood cases. Clinical Pediatrics 16: 219–224

Lachman R S, Cohen A, Hollister D, Rimoin D L 1974 Metachondromatosis. Birth Defects, Original Article Series 10: 171–178

Lachman R S, Horton W A 1979 Endochondromatosis. In: Bergsma D (ed) Birth Defects Compendium, 2nd edn., Alan Liss Inc, New York, p 392–393

Langenskiöld A 1967 The development of multiple cartilaginous exostoses. Acta Orthopaedica Scandinavica 38: 259–266

Langer L O 1968 The thoracic-pelvic-phalangeal dystrophy. Birth Defects, Original Article Series 4: 55–64

Leeds N, Seaman W B 1962 Fibrous dysplasia of the skull and its differential diagnosis, a clinical and roentgenographic study of 46 cases. Radiology 78: 570–582

Lewis R J, Ketcham A S 1973 Maffucci's syndrome, functional and neoplastic significance, case report and review of the literature. Journal of Bone and Joint Surgery 55 A: 1465–1479

Lichtenstein L, Jaffe H L 1942 fibrous dysplasia of bone, a condition affecting one, several or many bones, the graver cases of which may present abnormal pigmentation of the skin, premature sexual development, hyperparathyroidism or still other extraskeletal abnormalities. Archives of Pathology 33: 777–816

Lightner E S, Penny R, Frasier S D 1975 Growth hormone excess and sexual precocity in polyostotic fibrous dysplasia (McCune-Albright syndrome), evidence for abnormal hypothalamic function. Journal of Pediatrics 87: 922–927

Loewinger R J, Lichtenstein J R, Dodson W E, Eisen A Z 1977 Maffucci's syndrome, a mesenchymal dysplasia and multiple tumour syndrome. British Journal of Dermatology 96: 317–322

Lorincz A E 1960 Urinary acid mucopolysaccharides in hereditary deforming chondrodysplasia (diaphyseal aclasia) Federation Proceedings 19:148

Mainzer F, Minagi H, Steinbach H L 1971 The variable manifestations of multiple enchondromatsis. Radiology 99: 377–388

Maroteaux P 1971 Metachondromatose Z Kinderheilk 109: 246–261

Montoya G, Evarts C M, Dohn D F 1968 Polyostotic fibrous dysplasia and spinal cord compression. Journal of Neurosurgery 29: 102–105

Murachi S, Itoh H, Sugiura Y 1979 Tricho-rhino-phalangeal syndrome type II, the Langer-Gieldion syndrome. Japanese Journal of Human Genetics 24: 27–36

Ochsner P E 1978 Zum problem der neoplastischen entarung bei multiplen kartilagnáren exostosen. Zeitschrift für Orthopädie 116–369–378

Ogden J A 1976 Multiple hereditary osteochondromata, report of an early case. Clinical Orthop Rel. Res 116: 48–60

Oorthuys J W E, Beemer F A 1979 The Langer-Giedion-syndrome (tricho-rhino-phalangeal syndrome type II). European Journal of Pediatrics 132: 55–59

Reed R J 1963 Fibrous dsyplasia of bone, a review of 25 cases. Archives of Pathology 75: 480–495

Rimoin D L 1979 International nomenclature of constitutional diseases of bone with bibliography. Birth Defects, Original Article Series 15: 1–29

Rimoin D L, Horton W A 1978 Short stature, Part I. Journal of Pediatrics 92: 523–528

Rimon D L, Hollister D W 1979 Fibrous dysplasia, polyostotic. In Birth defects compendium. Bergsma D (ed), Alan Liss Inc, New York, p 444–445

Schall A M, Genuth S M 1976 Multiple endocrine adenomas in a patient with the Maffucci syndrome. American Journal of Medicine. 61: 952–956

Schwartz D T, Alpert M 1964 The malignant transformation of fibrous dysplasia. American Journal of Medical Science 247: 1–20

Shapiro F, Simon S, Glimcher M J 1979 Hereditary multiple exostoses; anthropometric, roentgenographic, and clinical aspects. Journal of Bone and Joint Surgery 61 A: 815–824

Slagsvold J E, Bergsholm P, Larsen J L 1977 Fibromuscular dysplasia of intracranial arteries in a patient with multiple enchondromas (Ollier's disease). Neurology 27: 1168–1171

Smith J F 1965 Fibrous dysplasia of the jaws. Archives of Otolaryngology 81: 592–603

Solomon L 1961 Bone growth in diaphyseal aclasia. Journal of Bone and Joint Surgery 43 B: 700–716

Solomon L 1963 Hereditary multiple exostosis. Journal of Bone and Joint Surgery 45 B: 292–304

Solomon L 1964 Hereditary multiple exostoses. American Journal of Human Genetics 16: 351–363

Solomon L 1974 Chondrosarcoma in hereditary multiple exostosis. South African Medical Journal 48: 671–676

Spjut H J, Dorfman H D, Fechner R E, Ackerman L V 1971 Tumors of bone and cartilage, Fasicle 5, Atlas of Tumor Pathology. Armed Forces Institute of Pathology, Washington DC

Stewart M J, Gilmer W S, Edmonson A S 1962 Fibrous dysplasia of bone. Journal of Bone and Joint Surgery 44 B: 302–318

Stoltzfus E, Ladda R L, Lloyd-Still J 1977 Langer-Giedion syndrome, type II tricho-rhino-phalangeal dysplasia. Journal of Pediatrics 91: 277–280

Theodorou S, Lantis G 1968 Dysplasia epiphysialis hemimelica (epiphyseal osteochondromata), report of two cases and review of the literature. Helvetica paediatrica Acta 2: 195–204

Thompson N 1959 Cherubism, familial fibrous dyslasia of the jaws. British Journal of Plastic Surgery 12: 89–103

Vinstein A L, Franken E A 1971 Hereditary multiple exostoses, a report of a case with spinal cord compression. Radiology 112: 405–407

Wilson W G, Herrington R T, Aylsworth A S 1979 Pediatrics 64: 542–545

Wirth W A, Leovitt D, Enzinger E M 1971 Multiple intramuscular myxoma, another extraskeletal manifestation of fibrous dysplasia. Cancer 27: 1167–1173

Yunis J J 1980 Nomenclature for high resolution human chromosomes. Cancer Genetics and Cytogenetics 2: 221–229

54

Dysostoses

J. G. Hall

INTRODUCTION

The dysostoses are that group of disorders in which the skeletal involvement is predominantly manifested in malformations of individual bones, which can occur singly or in combinations. By comparison, the dysplasias have a generalised abnormality in cartilage or bone growth and development, or both. A discussion of the dysostoses becomes a discussion of specific conditions in which malformations of individual bones are observed. In some ways it becomes only a listing of specific conditions, since at this time very little is known about the pathogenesis of the dysostoses or what the specific patterns of their involvement may reflect about developmental processes. The revised International Nomenclature of Constitutional Diseases of Bones (Rimoin et al, 1979), will be followed in this discussion. In the International Nomenclature, the dysostoses are broken down into those primarily concerned with craniofacial involvement, those with predominantly axial involvement and those with predominant involvement of the extremities. These designations are arbitrary for the convenience of organization and categorization on clinical grounds, and in no way reflect basic mechanisms. In most cases, the other systems which may be involved will probably be the best clue to the basic mechanism of disease.

The dysostoses with craniofacial involvement are discussed in the chapter on craniofacial syndromes. Many of the dysostoses with predominantly axial involvement and with predominant involvement of the extremities will be included here. Only conditions which have been relatively well defined will be discussed. With the burgeoning of clinical genetics and dysmorphology, numerous syndromes have been and are being described. In many cases, malformations in individual bones are part of these newly defined syndromes. However, it is impossible to cover the variability and spectrum of many of the newly described or, as yet, poorly defined disorders in the scope of this chapter. Numerous excellent books on syndromes include extensive discussion of the dysostoses (Beighton, 1978; Bergsma, 1979; Gorlin et al, 1976;

Maroleaux, 1979; poznanski, 1974; Smith, 1976; Taybi, 1975; Temtamy & McKusick, 1978).

The dysostoses include a number of conditions in which there is absence or partial absence of a bone or set of bones. Limb and skeletal development occur before the eighth week of gestation; consequently the predominant features of the dysostoses may occur early in development. Many of these major malformations would be readily apparent prenatally with ultrasonography; therefore, genetic counselling and prenatal diagnosis are considerations for many of the conditions. Where a malformation would not be detected by ultrasound, prognoses are generally good.

DYSOSTOSES WITH PREDOMINANTLY AXIAL INVOLVEMENT

Vertebral segmentation defects including the Klippel-Feil anomaly (Klippel-Feil sequence)

Abnormal segmentation can involve any of the vertebral bodies (Fig. 54.1) but is most frequently seen in the cervical area. (Fig 54.2) Cervical vertebral segmentation anomalies are referred to as the Klippel-Feil anomaly or syndrome (Klippel-Feil sequence) in spite of the fact that there are actually several distinct subcategories, as defined by Gunderson et al (1967). The mechanism which leads to the malformations seen in the Klippel-Feil anomaly appears to be a failure of the normal segmentation and fusion processes of the mesodermal somites, which would occur between the third and seventh weeks of gestation.

Clinically, the head of patients with cervical involvement seems to sit directly on the thorax, often with the presence of pterygium colli. The hairline usually seems low, the neck is short and there is almost always limitation of head movement. The scapula is frequently high. If true neurological compromise is present, it may imply that the spinal cord has been compressed or even that there is a congenital structural anomaly of the spinal cord. The most severe form of cervical segmentation defects are discussed under spondylocostal dysplasia.

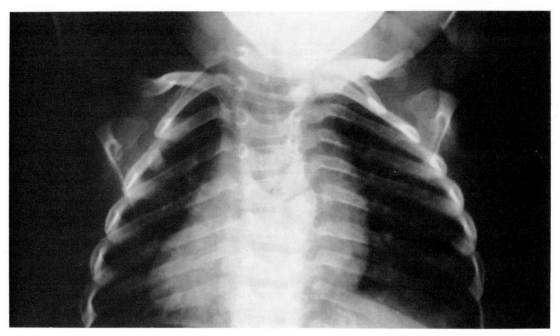

Fig. 54.1 Klippel-Feil anomaly. Radiograph of thoracolumbar spine. Note right sixth thoracic, hemivertebrate and associated changes in T5.

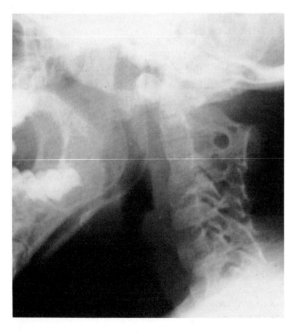

Fig. 54.2 Klippel-Feil anomaly, Radiograph of cervical spine. Note fusion of posterior elements of C1 to occiput and fusion and partial rotation of C2–C5.

Segmentation abnormalities in the C2–C3 area may lead to subluxation and secondary cord compression; thus, careful flexion and extension films of the neck should always be taken of patients with the Klippel-Feil anomaly. Abnormal segmentation in the thoracic and lumbar area can lead to scoliosis, either congenital, or developing during early childhood. Subluxation of the vertebrae can also occur in the thoracic or lumbar region leading to spinal nerve compression.

Multiple system congenital anomalies are seen frequently with multiple vertebral fusion defects, but no specific patterns have been repeatedly described. Congenital heart disease is occasionally present. Cleft palate or submucous cleft may be present in as many as 20% of the cases. Hearing loss, unilateral renal agenesis, limb anomalies, partial facial paralysis and ptosis are among the anomalies frequently reported (Gunderson et al, 1967).

Maroteaux (1979) has separated vertebral segmentation defects into anomalies of the cervical occipital region including vertebral blocks, malformations of the baso-occipital bone, abnormalities of the dens and abnormalities of the lumbosacral region. This distinction is useful, both in identifying which areas are involved and in considering the potential neurological complications.

In 1967, Gunderson distinguished three types of cervical vertebral fusion defects which also help to sort out familial types of vertebral fusion and the presence or absence of other system involvement. These are: type I – vertebral fusions containing massive fusion of many cervical and upper thoracic vertebrae (Fig. 54.1 and 2); type II – those containing fusions of only one or two interspaces, usually C2–C3 or C5–C6; but there can be intrafamilial variability, and hemivertebrae and occipitocervical fusion may be present; type III – patients in whom both cervical fusion and lower thoracic or lumbar fusion occur.

In type I (massive fusion of many cervical and upper thoracic vertebrae) most cases are sporadic and many have multiple anomalies of other organ systems. There are case reports of a second affected sib or a sib with multiple congenital anomalies, raising the possibility of a rare recessive gene being responsible for the anomalies. Family members may also have a small increased risk of neural tube defects or multiple vertebral anomalies (Wynne–Davies, 1975).

In type II (fusion of only one or two interspaces, most commonly C2–C3 or C5–C6) there are usually no other anomalies. When the fusion is in the cervical area, genetic forms are relatively frequent. An autosomal dominant disorder is known in which there is C2–C3 fusion. Occipitocervical fusion may also be seen in some affected members of these families. Fusion of C5–C6 with narrowing of C5–C6 has been reported to occur in an autosomal recessive pattern in several families. Variable cervical fusion with kyphoscoliosis was seen in other families in an apparent dominant pattern.

Type III (multiple vertebral segmentation anomaly including both cervical fusion and lower thoracic or lumbar fusion) is often associated with multiple organ anomalies and neurological compromise. Usually, it is a sporadic occurrence. However, Wynne-Davies (1975) has recognised families with an apparent autosomal dominant inheritance with marked variability within the family as to which and how many vertebrae are affected. It is not clear whether this type is distinguishable or distinct from various spondylocostal dysplasias.

Differential diagnosis of Klippel-Feil anomaly includes Turner syndrome, Noonan syndrome, Morquio syndrome, spondylothoracic dysostosis, spondylocostal dysostosis and Goldenhar syndrome.

A subdivision of vertebral segmentation anomalies has been designated the Wildervanck or cervical-oculo-acoustic syndrome, which may well be an X–linked dominant, since it appears to affect exclusively females. It is characterised by congenital perceptive deafness, paralysis with retraction of the bulb of one or both eyes (Duane syndrome), facial hypoplasia and asymmetry, fusion of cervical vertebrae and elbow hypoplasia. Radiological studies have shown that the deafness is due to a bony malformation of the middle ear (Start & Borton, 1973).

Sprengel deformity (Sprengel sequence)

Sprengel deformity is characterised by a high, medially rotated scapula. It occurs as an isolated event unilaterally or bilaterally or in association with a variety of abnormalities. Sprengel deformity presumably results from a failure of the normal embryological descent of the scapula from the neck to the normal thoracic position during the second month of gestation. The scapula is usually hypoplastic, having the fetal shape of an equilateral triangle. Because it lies higher and closer to the midline, it may produce a lump in the upper back and lead to restricted movement of the shoulder. In 20–50% of cases, there is accumulation of connective tissue or even bony fusion between the scapula and ribs or vertebrae. Even though 90% of cases are unilateral, associated anomalies occur in more than half of the cases. Scoliosis, hemivertebrae, fused vertebrae, spina bifida occulta, cervical ribs, missing ribs, fused ribs, clavicular anomalies and hypoplasia of the muscles of the shoulder girdle are seen. Association with situs inversus has been described, as have chest deformities (Offer, 1970).

Surgery may be needed, both to improve function of the shoulder and back, and to improve cosmetic appearance. Surgery usually involves removal of the scapulovertebral communication. Without surgery, exercise and stretching seem to be of little value. Most cases of Sprengel deformity are sporadic; however, a few families have been described with autosomal dominant transmission (Zadek, 1934). Marked variability occurred in those families.

Spondylocostal dysostoses

There are a number of spondylocostal dysostoses in which abnormal spinal segmentation and malformations of the ribs occur. Clinically, these patients have a short neck and/or trunk. Other visceral malformations are not generally seen. This group of dysostoses falls into two major groups: (1) mild varieties, which may be inherited as a dominant condition, and (2) a more severe variety, which may be inherited as an autosomal recessive trait.

Dominantly inherited multiple segmentation anomalies of vertebrae have been reported. There may be hemivertebrae, fused vertebrae, butterfly vertebrae and various rib anomalies. A family with mild ptosis has also been described by Faulk et al (1970). Because of marked variability within these families, X–ray studies are needed to establish the possibility of hemivertebrae or fusion (Poznanski et al, 1970a). The families with dominantly inherited Klippel-Feil anomaly (Gunderson et al, 1967) may represent the same condition as the families with dominantly inherited spondylocostal dysostosis. The report of Wynne-Davies (1975) suggests that these families may be at a slightly increased risk for neural tube defects.

The families with the recessively inherited types of multiple segmentation anomalies of vertebrae have all had marked shortening of the thorax. The diagnosis is readily apparent because the disproportion of the short trunk is dramatic when compared to the relatively long limbs; however, there appear to be several forms. In the Jarcho-Levin spondylothoracic dysostosis, the severe disproportion of the trunk and limbs gives a crab-like appearance on X–ray because of the marked platyspondyly of the fused vertebrae. Many children with the Jarcho-Levin spondylothoracic dysostosis syndrome die during infancy, probably from respiratory complications. Jarcho-Levin syndrome has an excess of affected females and is primarily seen in Puerto Ricans. Cantu et al (1971) have reported a family with less severe vertebral fusion, inherited as an autosomal recessive trait in which survival is better, probably because the chest is larger. This may be the same condition as that reported by Norum and McKusick (1969). A Mennonite family with spondylocostal dysplasia was also reported to have renal anomalies (Lasamassima et al, 1979).

Differential diagnoses of the spondylocostal dysostoses include the Klippel-Feil syndrome, mesomelic dysplasias, Poland syndrome and the short rib polydactyly syndromes.

Osteo-onychodysostosis (nail-patella syndrome)

Osteo-onychodysostosis is a dominantly inherited condition with the three major clinical features of dysplasia of the nails, absence or hypoplasia of the patella (Fig. 54.3), and the presence of iliac horns (pyramidal spurs just outside of the sacroiliac line (Fig. 54.4). AB blood group is known to be linked with this disorder. The tendency to develop renal abnormalities can be a serious complication which seems to have a familial aggregation (Maroteaux, 1979).

The disorder is recognised at different ages, depending on the degree of involvement. Some patients have difficulty walking because of instability of the knee. Others are basically asymptomatic and only recognised as a part of family studies. Height is usually normal.

The nails are small and concave, may be striated or rough and dysplastic, and sometimes are greyish or fragile and brittle. The patellae are small, laterally dislocated and may be bipartate or absent (Fig. 54.3). Prominence of the medial femoral condyle, hypoplasia of the lateral femoral condyle and proximal tibial distortion is seen. Hypoplasia of knee tendons may contribute to instability of the knee. At the elbow, hypertrophy of the medial condyle with hypoplasia of the radial head and lateral subluxation results in decreased pronation/supination. Hypoplasia of the lateral humeral condyle may also be seen. These elbow and knee changes are usually bilateral. Iliac horns arising from the central area of the outer surface of the iliac wing are usually pyramidal in shape and

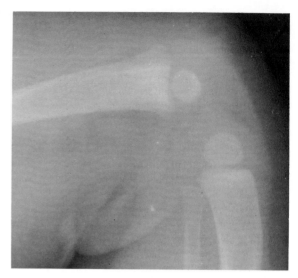

Fig. 54.3 Nail-patella syndrome (osteo-onychodysostosis). Radiograph knee. Note absence of the patella, and proximal tibial distortion.

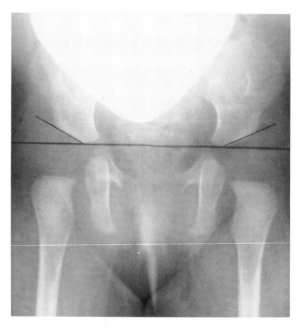

Fig. 54.4 Nail-patella syndrome (osteo-onychodysostosis). Radiograph of pelvis. Note flaring of iliac wings with definitive iliac horns.

are diagnostic (Fig. 54.4). The iliac horns may be asymmetric but always occur bilaterally. They are palpable in 70% of patients but are usually of no medical significance. Flaring of the iliac wing and a small iliac angle are often seen, as well as concavity or even a notch in the anterior border of the iliac wing (Taybi, 1975). Other skeletal anomalies include clubfoot (equinovarus, calcaneovalgus or, most frequently, pes planus), dislocated hips and contractures of other major joints (Lucas, 1967).

The renal lesion in the nail-patella syndrome resembles chronic glomerulonephritis or chronic pyelonephritis. Clinically, there is proteinuria and uraemia in 30% of patients. Accumulation of abnormal collagen fibers and thickening of the basement membrane can be found in the glomeruli on autopsy. These changes may represent a basic structural defect present as part of the disease rather than a phenomenon which is secondary to glomerular sclerosis (Morita et al, 1973).

Therapy is limited to surgical correction, especially of the knee, in order to achieve greater stability. All patients should be screened for renal problems, especially those in families with a history of renal involvement.

Differential diagnoses include distal arthrogryposis, Turner syndrome and trisomy 8 mosaicism. Incontinentia pigmenti and ectodermal dysplasias have similar nail abnormalities but have skin changes which are not seen in the nail-patella syndrome. Thus, an important distinguishing feature of the nail-patella syndrome is ectodermal involvement (nails) without changes in skin and hair.

Cerebro-costo-mandibular syndrome (Rib-Gap syndrome)

A specific syndrome exists in which there are rib gaps (consisting of uncalcified fibrous or cartilagenous tissues), Pierre-Robin anomaly (micrognathia, cleft palate, glossoptosis) and vertebral dysplasia. Abnormalities of the brain, neck or trachea and heart, mental retardation and polycystic kidneys are also seen (McNicholl et al, 1970).

X–rays show gaps in the dorsal portions of the ribs with fragmented ossification and absence of normal costovertebral articulations. Lesions are bilateral but not necessarily symmetrical. Subluxation of the elbows is also occasionally seen. Most infants die in the newborn period of respiratory insufficiency due to a 'flail chest'. Mental retardation and microcephaly may be secondary to anoxia because of respiratory compromise (Langer & Hermann, 1974).

The condition appears to be an autosomal recessive trait but with marked variability within families, such that one child may be mentally retarded while another may not. In addition, LeRoy (personal communication) recently reported an affected mother with two affected children, suggesting genetic heterogeneity and autosomal dominant inheritance in that family.

Rib gaps are seen in a number of conditions and are thus not pathognomonic for the diagnosis of cerebro-costo-mandibular syndrome. Differential diagnoses should include Goldenhar syndrome, Covesdem syndrome (Wadia et al, 1978) and oculovertebral syndrome. Cases with the Pierre-Robin anomaly and vertebral anomalies should have X–ray studies for rib gaps (Weyers & Thier, 1978).

PREDOMINANTLY LIMB INVOLVEMENT

Acheiropodia

Acheiropodia is an autosomal recessively inherited condition with absence deformities of both upper and lower limbs usually with symmetrical involvement. The limb malformation involves a terminal transverse hemimelia (below the elbow) in the upper limbs and a terminal transverse hemimelia of the distal third of the lower limbs. This inherited condition can be differentiated from other terminal transverse hemimelia conditions in that the latter usually have unilateral involvement of the upper limbs and the lower limbs are rarely involved, whereas the defects in acheiropodia are usually uniform and bilateral, and involve both upper and lower limbs. In addition, there are no other associated abnormalities in acheiropodia.

Acheiropodia (absence of the hands and feet) has only been seen in inbred Brazilian kindreds of Portuguese origin (Freire-Maia, 1970). Prenatal diagnosis would be possible using serial real-time ultrasound.

Differential diagnoses include the thalidomide syndrome, amniotic bands and Hanhart syndrome (characterised by bird-like face, micrognathia, peromelia and opisthodontia) (Garner & Bixler, 1969).

Radioulnar and humeroradial synostoses

Radioulnar or humeroradial synostosis (bony fusion at the elbow joint) can occur as an isolated phenomenon or in association with several specific syndromes.

In *radioulnar* synostosis, a bony dysplasia of the elbow joint is seen on X–ray and there is impaired pronation/supination of the arm. A number of families have been reported in which there is not true synostosis. Consequent limitation of function is usually minimal. Isolated congenital radioulnar synostosis was reported by Hansen and Anderson (1970) in 37 cases. Familial cases were bilateral and sporadic cases were both unilateral and bilateral.

Radioulnar synostosis is seen in a number of chromosomal syndromes, specifically the XXXY syndrome. In addition, radioulnar synostosis can be seen in the Poland syndrome, SC or pseudothalidomide syndrome, the Pfeiffer syndrome, Nievergelt-Perlman syndrome or in association with the Kleeblatschadel deformity of the skull.

Clinically, patients with *humeroradial* synostosis have an immobile elbow joint, and bony fusion is seen on X–ray examination. Surgical manipulation may be necessary to improve function. Isolated humeroradial synostosis can be inherited as an autosomal recessive trait

(Frostad, 1940) or can be a sporadic occurrence (Stranak & von Oberender, 1971).

Humeroradial synostosis is often a component of multiple synostosis syndromes, such as the brachymeso-symphalangism syndrome, an autosomal dominantly inherited condition with coalition of the carpal and tarsal bones, brachydactyly and occasional vertebral anomalies. Hunter et al (1976) have reported an apparent case of the SC phocomelia syndrome or pseudothalidomide syndrome in which there was dwarfism with humeroradial synostosis.

Brachydactyly

Brachydactyly, or shortening of the digits due to abnormal development of either the phalanges or metacarpals, is seen as either an isolated malformation (in a variety of different forms) or in conjunction with anomalies of one or more other systems. Bell (1951) classified the isolated brachydactylies into seven definitive groups (A1–3, B, C, D and E)on the basis of his review of 124 pedigrees with 1336 individuals affected with brachydactyly. Bass (1968) later described brachydactyly type A4. Familial reports of each type of isolated brachydactyly have shown an autosomal dominant pattern of inheritance.

In brachydactyly type A1, all middle phalanges are short or hypoplastic, and the proximal phalanges of the thumbs and halluces are shortened. In the most severe cases, fingers are approximately one half their normal length. In milder cases, hypoplasia of the middle phalanges is less severe, and the index and little fingers are the most severely affected. Severe cases have both cosmetic and functional problems. In brachydactyly type A2, shortening is predominantly seen in the second digits. The middle phalanx has a characteristic triangular shape as a result of a continuous epiphysis from proximal to distal ends on the shortened side. Consequently, growth of the phalanx is outward and results in angulation. Affected individuals may appear clinically normal. Type A3 is characterised by shortening of the middle phalanx of the fifth finger. Epiphyses may be cone-shaped. And finally, type A4 has shortening of all middle phalanges but is also associated with nail dysplasia and bifid distal phalanges of the thumb and hallux. Brachydactyly A4 can be confused with brachydactyly B; however, the latter is distinguished by hypoplasia of the distal phalanges (Temtamy & McKusick, 1978).

Differential diagnosis of brachydactyly type A includes a number of the chondrodysplasias. Specifically, brachydactyly A2 is seen in Rubinstein-Taybi syndrome, Pfeiffer syndrome and Apert syndrome. Brachydactyly A3 is seen in Down syndrome, several conditions with X chromosomal aberrations, Russell-Silver syndrome, Coffin-Siris syndrome, oral-facial-digital (OFD) syndrome types I and II, oto-palato-digital syndrome (OPD), focal dermal hypolasia, oculo-dental-digital syn-

drome (ODD), Holt-Oram syndrome, thrombocyto-poenia–absent radius syndrome (TAR), Noonan syndrome, Bloom syndrome, Seckel syndrome and Fanconi anaemia.

In type B brachydactyly, in addition to shortening of middle phalanges, there is shortening or complete absence of the terminal phalanges. Digits on the radial side of the hand are usually less severely affected than digits on the ulnar side of the hand (Temtamy & McKusick, 1978). Deformities are consistently symmetric and the feet are less severely affected. Soft tissue syndactyly, symphalangism, carpal and tarsal fusions, and shortening of metacarpals and metatarsals may be additional features. Deformities can be severely debilitating.

Differential diagnosis of brachydactyly B should include brachydactyly A4 and the Sorsby syndrome, which is distinguished by macular coloboma, occasional renal anomalies and includes brachydactyly B.

Brachydactyly type C has marked variability. However, characteristically, the middle and proximal phalanges of digits two and three, and the middle phalanges of digit five are shortened. It is striking that the fourth digit is basically normal and extends beyond the other digits. There is marked ulnar deviation of the proximal phalanx of the index finger. Short metacarpals and symphalangism are occasionally seen, and there is only minimal involvement of the feet. Short stature may be an associated feature. X–ray studies show delayed maturation of ossification centres and hypoplasia, aplasia or early fusion of the epiphyses (Temtamy & McKusick, 1978).

Brachydactyly type D is characterised by a shortened broad terminal phalanx of the thumbs and great toes. The deformity is attributed to an early closure of the epiphysis at the base of the distal phalanx of the thumb (Temtamy & McKusick, 1978).

Differential diagnoses of brachydactyly D should include heart–hand syndrome II (Tabatznik), Rubinstein-Taybi syndrome and Robinow syndrome.

Finally, brachydactyly type E is characterised by shortening of one or all of the metacarpals or metatarsals. Terminal phalanges are often short, and hyperextensibility of the hands is common. There may be mild short stature (Temtamy & McKusick, 1978).

Families with brachydactyly E associated with one of the following features have been reported: microcornea, keratoconus and hypertension. Differential diagnosis of brachydactyly E includes Turner syndrome, Albright syndrome, naevoid basal cell carcinoma syndrome, cryptodontic brachymetacarpalia, Ruvalcaba syndrome, Biemond syndrome type I, 5p-syndrome and Tuomaala syndrome and acrodysostosis.

Symphalangism

Symphalangism, or fusion of the phalanges, can be

inherited as an autosomal dominant trait with synostoses of various other joints. Both proximal (McKusick et al, 1964) and distal (Steinberg & Reynolds, 1948) forms have been described. Families with distal symphalangism are rare whereas proximal symphalangism is a much more common phenomenon. In addition, distal symphalangism tends to be an isolated anomaly and proximal symphalangism can have other associated abnormalities. Synostosis of the metacarpophalangeal joint has also been described, but only in one family (McKusick, 1978).

In the dominantly inherited proximal symphalangism, more than one joint or finger are involved (Fig. 54.5 and 6), but variability in age of onset and severity is seen within families. Involvement of other bones can be seen, such as coalition or fusion of the tarsal and carpal bones, scoliosis, craniosynostosis and deafness in affected family members. Therefore, careful evaluation of all joints, spine and skull should be done in family members of a patient affected with symphalangism. By contrast with other types of contractures and dysostotic processes, individuals with symphalangism may actually be made worse (i.e. have more rapid fusion) by vigorous physical therapy.

A difficult and as yet unanswered question is whether proximal dominantly inherited symphalangism is a different entity from dominantly inherited multiple synostosis or simply represents variability of expression of a dominant gene. A number of kindreds with autosomal dominantly inherited symphalangism and multiple synostosis syndrome have shown a conductive deafness with onset usually at the age of 2 or 3 years with progression throughout childhood (or at adolescence in multiple synostosis syndrome). A bony fusion of the stapes and petrous part of the temporal bone has been demonstrated at surgery in a number of patients. Excision of this fused area has frequently been successful in partial or complete restoration of hearing loss (Strasburger et al, 1965).

Several theories have been proposed for the mechanism causing symphalangism. Most probably, symphalangism is caused by a developmental defect at the interzone of the phalanges prior to the time of joint cavity formation (Duken, 1921). This absence of differentiation at the interzone allows cartilages to rest upon one another and ultimately fuse to form a single cartilage rather than a joint space. Symphalangism may be present at birth; however, X–ray examination at birth may not show complete bony fusion but simply a narrowing of the interzone.

Differential diagnoses include multiple synostosis, diastrophic dysplasia, fibrodysplasia ossificans, Pillay

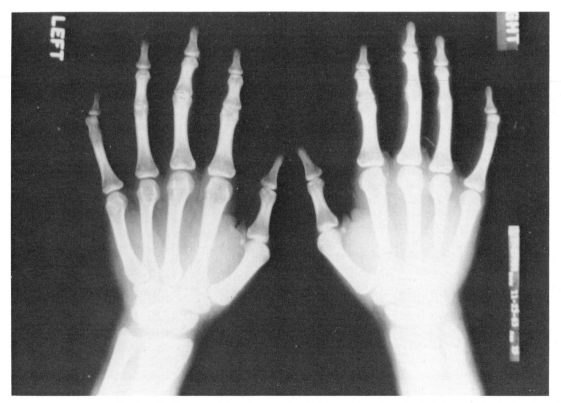

Fig. 54.5 Proximal symphalangism. Radiograph of dorsal view of hands. Note fusion of proximal phalanges on digits 4 and 5 and partial fusion of the proximal phalanges on digits 2 and 3.

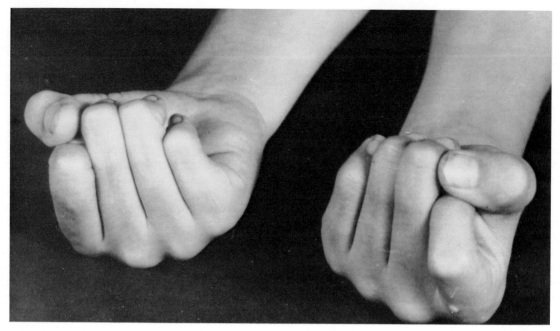

Fig. 54.6 Proximal symphalangism. Hands held in fist. Note absence of flexion creases over the proximal phalanges on digits 3, 4 and 5, and partial function of the proximal joint of digit 1 bilaterally.

syndrome, Apert syndrome, Pfeiffer syndrome and brachydactyly types A, B and C with or without short stature.

Polydactyly

Polydactyly, or the presence of a supernumerary digit or a portion of an extra digit, can be classified into two major groups: those with a preaxial addition or those with a postaxial addition.

Isolated postaxial polydactyly has long been recognised as a specific entity and is very common in black children. Autosomal dominant inheritance with reduced penetrance or multifactorial inheritance among black families has been suggested because of the skipping of the trait in one or more generations. In the same family with apparent dominant inheritance, variability of expression is so marked that the gene is clinically manifested as fully developed extra digits (type A) in some black family members and simply as rudimentary supernumerary digits or postminimi (type B) in others (Temtamy & McKusick, 1978).

Postminimi can be removed at birth by occluding the skin tag with a tight thread or string; the tag subsequently drops off. An adult so treated may often be unaware that he even had polydactyly, and a careful family history should therefore be taken from parents. By contrast, extra digits involving bone or cartilage must be excised surgically to avoid osteomyelitis.

Preaxial polydactyly, on the other hand, is much less common than postaxial polydactyly and has been subdivided into four different categories by Temtamy and McKusick (1978): type 1 – preaxial thumb polydactyly; type 2 – polydactyly of a triphalangeal thumb; type 3 – polydactyly of an index finger and type 4 – preaxial polydactyly and syndactyly. All types are inherited as autosomal dominant traits, but variability and reduced penetrance have been reported.

Polydactyly is associated with a number of specific syndromes, the most notable of which are the chondrodysplasias, such as Ellis-van Creveld (chondroectodermal dysplasia), Jeune syndrome (asphyxiating thoracic dysplasia), the short rib/polydactyly syndromes, the acrocephalosyndactylies, hypothalamic hamartoblastoma syndrome (Hall et al, 1980), Meckel syndrome, trisomy 13 and 18, Laurence-Moon-Biedl syndrome, Biemond syndrome type II, oral-facial-digital syndrome II and III and Kaufman syndrome. For the specific dysostotic changes found in other bones in these syndromes consult Taybi (1975).

Camptodactyly

Camptodactyly is clinically manifested by soft tissue flexion contractures of the fingers at one or several joints. Contractures may be present at birth or develop in childhood; they may be stationary or progressive. Camptodactyly may be seen as an isolated malformation, be inherited as an autosomal dominant trait or occur as a feature of many syndromes. There can be extreme variability within families. Camptodactyly does not usually interfere with function unless it is very severe at birth or vigorous physical therapy is not begun early enough.

There are probably a number of different aetiologies of camptodactyly, one of which is misplaced, hypoplastic or absent tendons (Stevenson et al, 1975; Zadek, 1934).The types of contractures seen in camptodactyly do benefit from surgical repair by reattaching the tendon, soft tissue release, and physical therapy with stretching exercises. Both fingers and toes can be affected. Other forms may represent early aging, inflammatory response or deterioration of connective tissue which would lead to fibrosis and contracture of tendons.

Camptodactyly is seen as a feature of many other conditions. Differential diagnosis of isolated camptodactyly includes Dupuytren (late onset) and distal arthrogryposes (congenital). Conditions with autosomal dominant patterns of inheritance and distal contractures include Freeman-Sheldon or 'whistling face' syndrome, trismus pseudocamptodactyly, Hanley syndrome of camptodactyly, dwarfism, hypogonadism, pectus carinatum and ptosis, camptodactyly with sensorineural hearing loss, Emery-Nelson syndrome, congenital contractural arachnodactyly and the distal arthrogryposes (Hall et al, 1981). Recessively inherited conditions with camptodactyly include the multiple pterygium syndrome, Pena-Shokeir, Neu-Laxova, Zellweger syndrome, Kuskokwim syndrome, adducted thumb syndrome (Christian syndrome) and others. Camptodactyly is frequently associated with chromosomal anomalies.

Syndrome of multiple synostoses

The syndrome of multiple synostoses has been described as a highly variable dominant condition in which there can be synostoses of all the joints. Various combinations of synostoses can be seen within the family, with some affected individuals having nothing more than symphalangism while others may have fusion of elbows, wrists, fingers, metacarpals, metatarsals and coalition of the ankle bones. Deafness may also be a feature, but characteristically fusions in the middle ear do not occur until adolescence. Growth is normally not affected. A typical facies has been described with a narrow nose and hypoplasia of the alae nasae (Maroteaux, 1979). As stated earlier, it is not yet clear whether this condition is distinct from autosomal dominant proximal symphalangism; however, the severity of involvement of distal phalanges (i.e. absence and hypoplasia of middle phalanges as well as consistency of carpal and tarsal coalitions) suggests it may be a distinct entity.

X–ray findings may show bony fusion of the joint, or early joint changes may be present simply as a narrowing of the joint space. The aetiological mechanism behind multiple synostoses is probably the same as for symphalangism. What determines which joints are affected is unknown. Differential diagnosis includes diastrophic dysplasia, fibrodysplasia ossificans, Pillay syndrome, Apert syndrome, Pfeiffer syndrome, brachydactylies A, B and C, and Emery-Nelson syndrome.

Ectrodactyly

The term ectrodactyly ('ektromo' denoting abortion and 'daktylos' finger) should be reserved for a specific hand deformity characterised by transverse terminal aphalangia or partial to total absence of distal segments of fingers. However, the term has been used for the split-hand or lobster claw deformity and in the EEC syndrome (ectrodactyly, meaning split-hand, ectodermal dysplasia, clefting), and so has come to be misleadingly associated with split-hand.

The true ectrodactyly malformation may involve one or more phalanges (aphalangia), one or more digits (adactylia) or the full hand (acheiria – see earlier) and even part of the upper arm. More severe manifestations are hemimelia or amelia. All of these malformations are considered to represent various degrees of severity of the same malformation and may be due to an intrauterine vascular occlusion or insufficiency. True ectrodactyly is usually sporadic and unilateral. Reports of familial ectrodactyly probably represent brachydactyly B. In a study by Birch – Jensen (1949), 19 individuals affected with true ectrodactyly had 51 normal children. However, a higher incidence of associated malformations in patients and their families has been reported (Grebe, 1964). Associated malformations which have been reported are spina bifida, hydrocephalus and meningomyelocoele. A report by Kohler (1962) of a family in which there was ectrodactyly in two individuals and a terminal transverse hemimelia in a third, suggests that there is a genetic basis for the terminal transverse defects in this family.

Differential diagnosis includes amniotic band syndrome, (Jones et al, 1974).

PREDOMINANT LIMB INVOLVEMENT WITH OTHER ASSOCIATED ABNORMALITIES

The Poland syndrome

The two major components of the Poland syndrome are unilateral symbrachydactyly and ipsilateral aplasia of the sternal head of the pectoralis major muscle. Clinically, there is unilateral absence of the normal anterior axillary fold and shortening or reduction of the digits associated with tissue webbing or syndactyly. There can be marked variability in the degree of reduction of the limb. Most reports of the Poland syndrome indicate that cases have apparently been sporadic; aetiological heterogeneity is probable; however, intrauterine vascular compromise is suspected in many cases. Fuhrmann described a family with apparent autosomal dominant inheritance, but mild clinical manifestations. (Temtamy & McKusick, 1978)

The isolated malformations of either symbrachydactyly or unilateral aplasia of the sternal head of the pectoralis major muscle are also sporadic. Poland syndrome has been found to be more common in males (3:1). The right side is more commonly involved than the left (2:1) (Goldberg & Mazzei, 1977). Analogous malformations have been seen in the lower limb. Several reported cases have been associated with the use of vascular constricting agents by the mother in early pregnancy (David, 1972). The question of an increased risk for leukemia in Poland syndrome has been raised (Goldberg & Mazzei, 1977).

The Poland syndrome has also been seen in association with other upper limb and trunk anomalies, such as radioulnar synostosis, Sprengel deformity, coalition of the carpal bones, camptodactyly, polydactyly, skin dimples, deficiencies of the rib cage, scoliosis and kyphosis. Other skeletal anomalies include cervical ribs, club foot, metatarsus adductus and syndactyly of the toes. Visceral anomalies reported include dextrocardia, herniation of the lungs, inguinal and umbilical hernias, cryptorchidism, ipsilateral hypoplasia of the kidney, encephalocoele and microcephaly (Goldberg & Mazzei, 1977).

Roentgenograms show syndactyly, polydactyly, hypoplasia of the long bones of the arm and hand, absence of the metacarpals and phalanges and relative hyperlucency of the ipsilateral hemithorax. Rib deformities and lung herniation can also be seen (Taybi, 1975).

Because some patients have features similar to the Moebius syndromè, an overlap between these conditions is possible. If both conditions are secondary to intrauterine vascular compromise, it is not surprising that there would be overlap with regard to the amount and degree of involvement. Symbrachydactyly conditions and the acrocephalosyndactylies should be considered in the differential diagnosis.

Rubinstein-Taybi syndrome

Individuals affected with the Rubinstein-Taybi syndrome typically have broad toes and thumbs and a very specific facies with beaked nose. The facies is unusual even in infancy, and in addition to the prominent nose there is an antimongoloid slant to the eyes and a highly arched palate. The broad thumbs and toes are very characteristic and appear spatulate, short, stubby, flattened and wide. The broad-toed appearance is the result of both soft tissue and bony tissue changes which can be seen on X–ray of the terminal phalanx. Duplication of the proximal or distal phalanx of the thumb has been reported (DerKaloustian, 1972). All reported patients have been mentally retarded (with IQ estimates below 50); microcephaly is seen in over half the cases. EEG abnormalities have been reported, as has absence of the corpus callosum. Short stature is a common feature. In a study of 105 patients, approximately 80% were below the third percentile for height (Rubinstein, 1969). Other

features that have been noted are cardiac malformations, cryptorchidism, duplicated kidneys or ureters, absence of the kidney and hydronephrosis or hydroureter (Smith, 1976).

X–ray changes include short and wide terminal phalanges of the thumbs and great toes, short, wide and tufted terminal phalanges in most fingers, flaring of ilia and retardation of skeletal maturation (Taybi, 1975).

Aetiology of the Rubinstein-Taybi syndrome is unknown. Most cases of Rubinstein-Taybi syndrome are sporadic; however, there are a few reports of familial cases. Temtamy and McKusick (1978) favour a small chromosomal aberration. Familial recurrence, on the whole, is very rare. Thus, autosomal recessive inheritance seems unlikely. A new dominant mutation has been suggested, but paternal ages have not been significantly advanced. There may be aetiological heterogeneity.

Differential diagnoses include brachydactyly D, Robinow syndrome and chromosomal aberrations.

Fanconi anaemia

Fanconi anaemia is characterised clinically by pancytopoenia, hyperpigmentation, short stature and radial and renal defects. In some cases, not all of these clinical features are present and severity of the features present can be extremely variable.

The pancytopoenia is usually progressive. Average age of onset has been estimated as 8 years and all marrow elements are involved. However, anaemia may precede decrease in white blood cells or platelets or viceversa. Reports of haematological symptoms have varied from 17 months to 22 years. Fetal haemaglobin has been recorded as elevated, and in some cases there have been reduced numbers of erythrocytes and leucocytes, and decreased levels of platelet hexokinase (Schroeder et al, 1976).

Hyperpigmentation of the skin is probably the most consistent clinical feature and appears as fine generalised hypermelanosis often presenting prior to haematological manifestations. Café-au-lait spots are also seen.

The most common bony defects are radial abnormalities with a hypoplastic, absent, digitalised or supernumerary thumb, hypoplasia of the first metacarpal, hypoplasia or absence of the radius and greater multangular and navicular bones. Bifid thumbs, retarded skeletal maturation, osteoporosis, microcephaly with thick calvarium, syndactyly and hip dislocation have been reported (Dosik et at, 1970; Esparza & Thomson, 1966).

Patients should be evaluated for renal abnormalities, and those with external ear anomalies for associated deafness. Other abnormalities that should be looked for on examination are spina bifida, Klippel-Feil anomalies, scoliosis, rib abnormalities, Sprengel deformity and flat or clubbed feet.

Complications usually result from pancytopoenia with

bleeding, pallor and recurrent infections. Therapy with testosterone and hydrocortisone has been helpful, although life expectancy is reduced. Patients have a predisposition to leukaemia and other tumours. Cancer deaths are increased threefold compared to the general population (Swift & Hirschhorn, 1971). Bone marrow transplantation may offer an alternative therapy in the future.

Fanconi anaemia appears to be inherited as an autosomal recessive trait; however, genetic heterogeneity has been postulated. A high incidence of consanguinity and occurrence in sibs and cousins has been noted (Schroeder et al, 1976). Intrafamilial variability of clinical features and age of onset does occur. There is an apparent excess of affected males. Chromosomal aberrations are seen, and include an increased number of chromatid breaks, gaps, exchange figures and endoreduplication. Prenatal diagnosis has been reported on several cases looking at chemically induced chromatid breaks and has thus far been successful (Auerbach et al, 1981).

Differential diagnosis should include TAR and the Holt-Oram syndrome.

Thrombocytopoenia–absent radius syndrome (TAR)

Thrombocytopoenia–absent radius is inherited as an autosomal recessive trait. The cardinal clinical features are thrombocytopoenia (usually with symptoms in the newborn period) and bilateral absence of the radius with the presence of both thumbs (i.e. each hand has five digits).

The thrombocytopoenia is congenital and on a hypomegakaryocytic basis. It is usually present at birth (90% are symptomatic during the first 4 months). Thrombocytopoenia gradually improves over the first 2 years, and platelets may even be in a normal range in adulthood. Viral illnesses, particularly gastrointestinal viral illness, will often aggravate the thrombocytopoenia. Leukaemoid reactions are seen in 60 to 70% of patients during the first year. Eosinophilia has been reported in 50% of the patients. Anaemia is thought to be the result of blood loss but may be due to hypoplasia of red blood cells during the first year (Bergsma, 1979).

The radius is absent bilaterally in all cases (Figs. 54.7 and 8). The ulna is absent bilaterally in about 20% of the cases and is usually hypoplasic in other cases. Occasionally, the ulna is absent unilaterally (Bergsma, 1979). The humerus may be short and dysplastic. The thumbs are always present.

Deformities of legs and hips are occasionally seen, e.g. dislocated hips, tibial torsion, abnormal tibiofibular joints, stiff knees, dislocation of the patella and camptodactyly of the toes with occasional club foot (Hall, 1969). Congenital cardiac abnormalities are seen in one third of the cases, the most frequent being tetralogy of Fallot and septal defects.

Complications are related to thrombocytopoenia and symptomatic bleeding. Death before 1 year of age occurred in 35–40% of patients in the past, mostly because of intracranial bleeding. This should be preventable by proper platelet transfusion (preferably from one donor). There may be delayed motor function because of hand malformation; however, eventual good function can be expected. Other complications of skeletal anomalies include nerve compression of the wrist and arthritis. TAR patients seem to have an increased incidence of allergy to cow's milk which precipitates episodes of low platelets.

Differential diagnosis should include Holt-Oram syndrome, pseudothalidomide syndrome and Fanconi anaemia. Prenatal diagnosis by demonstration of the absence of the radius using ultrasound has been successful (Luthy et al, 1979).

Oral-facial-digital syndrome

The oral-facial-digital (OFD) syndrome has been subdivided into two types, somewhat similar clinically but with different patterns of inheritance: OFD type I (Papillon-Leage) and OFD type II (Mohr). In both types, the clinical manifestation of the face are striking, with hypertelorism, epicanthal folds, micrognathia, epidermoid cysts, hypotrichosis and hypertrophic frenulae with clefts of the alveolar margin, lips and tongue. There is dystropia canthorum, a broad nasal root, and hypoplasia of the alar cartilage and malar bone (Maroteaux, 1979).

OFD type I is clinically distinguished by cleft palate, ventral clefts and hamartomas of the tongue, dental anomalies, alopecia and evanescent milia in infancy. Mental retardation is seen in approximately 50% of the cases and is apparently associated with CNS malformations in conjunction with the polycystic anomalies that have been seen in the kidneys of a number of autopsied cases. In contrast, OFD type II is clinically distinguished by normal intelligence, normal hair, normal teeth, no lateral oral frenulae, conductive hearing loss, and short stature (Gorlin et al, 1976).

On X–ray, OFD type I is characterised by brachydactyly (due to short metacarpals, metatarsals and phalanges and usually showing an irregular distribution), clinodactyly, syndactyly, camptodactyly, cone-shaped epiphyses and an increased nasion-sella basion angle. Preaxial polydactyly has been seen in a few cases. In OFD type II, or Mohr syndrome, there is polysyndactyly of the toes, usually symmetric with partial reduplication of the hallux, and postaxial polydactyly primarily of the hand. Clinodactyly, brachydactyly, metaphyseal irregularity and flaring, and supernumerary sutures of the skull are also seen (Taybi, 1975).

OFD type I is inherited as an X–linked dominant trait with lethality in the male. All cases have been females with the exception of a phenotypic male who turned out

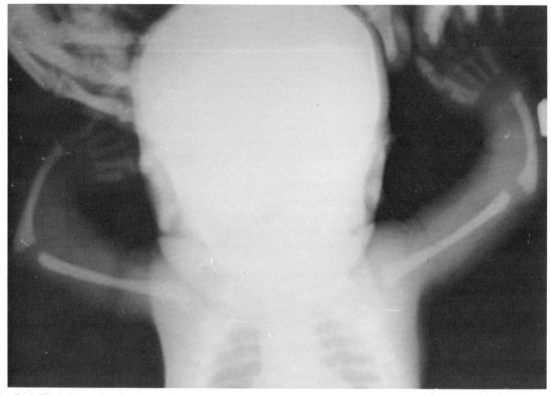

Fig. 54.7 Thrombocytopoenia–absent radius syndrome (TAR). Radiograph of chest and upper limbs. Note absence of radius bilaterally, presence of thumb and shortening of ulna.

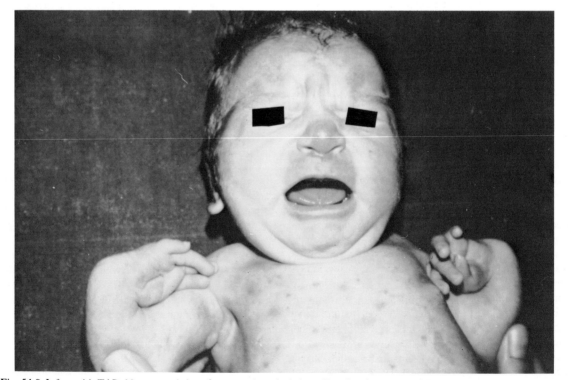

Fig. 54.8 Infant with TAR. Note curved short forearm, ulnar deviation of hand and presence of thumb bilaterally.

to have an XXY karyotype. OFD type II is inherited as an autosomal recessive trait.

Differential diagnoses include Ellis-van Creveld syndrome, holoprosencephaly and frontonasal dysplasia.

Holt-Oram syndrome

The Holt-Oram syndrome is characterised by autosomal dominant inheritance (with penetrance of at least 90%), congenital heart disease and radial ray defects. The characteristic hand malformation is digitilisation of a triphalangeal thumb so that the thumb is attached in the same plane as the other fingers. However, in some cases the thumb is absent or rudimentary. In addition, the more severe cases show absence or hypoplasia of the radius, or even the ulna and humerus. The most common cardiac defect is an atrial septal defect of the ostium secundum type. Cardiovascular abnormalities are also extremely variable. Other defects that have been described are patent ductus arteriosus, pulmonary hypertension, ventricular septal defect and transposition of the great vessels with a prolonged PR interval. Marked variability of limb and heart malformations may occur within the same family. Complications are usually related to heart disease, and severe cases die within the first year of life (Kaufman et al, 1974).

The bony changes which may be seen on X–ray are triphalangeal, hypoplastic, proximally placed or absent thumb, an abnormally shaped scaphoid bone, additional carpal bones or lack of ossification of the carpals, particularly the os centrale, a long ulnar styloid, carpal fusions, an apparent increase in length of the first metacarpal and shortening of the fifth middle phalanx with clinodactyly, a prominent or posterior projection of the medial epicondyle, clavicular hypoplasia, deformed humeral head and small rotated scapulae (Poznanski, 1970a).

The Holt-Oram syndrome is distinct from other radial ray defect syndromes in that there are no abnormalities of the kidneys or gastrointestinal tract, no deafness, no ear malformations, no mental retardation and no specific haematological disorder. Differential diagnoses include Poland syndrome, heart-hand syndrome II (Tabatznik), Fanconi anaemia, TAR, the VACTERL association and the thalidomide syndrome.

Femoral hypoplasia–unusual facies syndrome

A distinct pattern of malformation was characterised by Daentl et al in 1975 and was designated femoral hypoplasia–unusual facies syndrome (Fig. 54.9). Clinical features include femoral hypoplasia, or absence of the femur, and the unusual facial features of upslanting palpebral fissures, short nose with broad nasal tip, long philtrum, thin upper lip, micrognathia and cleft palate. In addition, renal anomalies, lower vertebral anomalies and deformed pelvis have been reported. With multiple surgery and the use of prosthetic devices, most patients are

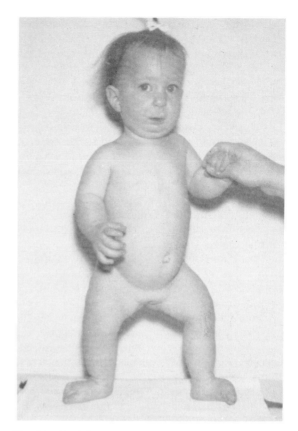

Fig. 54.9 Focal femoral hypoplasia with unusual facies syndrome. Note the short upper leg, short nose with broad nasal tip, long philtrum, thin upper lip, micrognathia and left equinovarus deformity of the foot.

ambulatory and quite functional socially. Intelligence is completely normal.

Some infants have been born to diabetic mothers, and the clinical similarities with the caudal regression syndrome might suggest a common aetiology (Assemany, 1972). Shortening of the humerus and restricted motion at the elbows and Sprengel deformities found in some infants would suggest that this syndrome is not confined to the lower limbs and that a similar mechanism could be acting upon both upper and lower limbs. Thus far, all reports have been of sporadic cases, but prenatal diagnosis could be offered for reassurance, using real-time ultrasound in an attempt to demonstrate presence of the femur.

Differential diagnosis includes proximal focal femoral hypoplasia *without* unusual facies, which is a relatively frequent sporadic orthopaedic anomaly.

Hand-foot-genital syndrome (hand-foot-uterus syndrome)

The hand-foot-uterus syndrome is an autosomal dominantly inherited condition with variable expressivity.

Clinical features include small feet with unusually short halluxes and short abnormal thumbs. Females with the disorder have duplication anomalies of the genital tract and decreased fertility. Males have been reported with cryptorchidism and hypospadius; however, these seem to be distinct embryologically from the female genital duplication anomalies.

Radiographic findings include short first metacarpals and metatarsals, short fifth fingers with clinodactyly, trapezium-scaphoid fusion in the wrist, cuneiform-navicular fusion in the foot, an os centrale and a long ulnar styloid (Poznanski, 1970b).

Genital tract anomalies are variable but are felt to represent different degrees of expression of the same underlying developmental problem. Duplication of the uterus varies in severity from a full double uterus to a uterus duplex unicornis. In addition, some patients have duplication of the cervix with septate vagina. These structural anomalies result in fertility complications; however, normal pregnancies are possible.

Abnormalities are present at birth and can be detected by hysterosalpingogram, ultrasound or laparotomy. Congenital heart disease has been reported in some patients; therefore, a careful cardiovascular examination is warranted.

Differential diagnosis includes Holt-Oram syndrome, trisomy 18, Ellis-van Creveld syndrome, and Cornelia de Lange syndrome.

Focal dermal hypoplasia (Goltz syndrome)

Focal dermal hypoplasia has been observed almost exclusively in females. It appears to be an X – linked dominant condition with lethality in males. Clinical features include cutaneous changes, skeletal defects, digital malformations, ocular anomalies and oral-dental anomalies.

The most striking clinical features in all of the cases of this syndrome are the widespread foci of dermal hypoplasia with herniation of fat (appearing as yellow-brown nodules) and red streaking of the skin, forming frequent papillomas of the lips, gums, vulva and anus. The areas of dermal hypoplasia appear as atrophy or absence of skin; however, the epidermis is intact. Telangiectasia and hypo- and hyperpigmentation are seen. Surgery is indicated for removal of lesions (e.g. angiofibromas) which are in areas prone to trauma. The hair is sparse, sometimes blonde or almost white in colour with patchy areas of alopecia. Nails may be absent, hypoplastic, dystrophic, spoon-shaped or grooved. Teeth are congenitally absent or malformed.

Digital anomalies include syndactyly, polydactyly, camptodactyly and absence deformities. Most individuals are short in stature and have vertebral anomalies, kyphosis and scoliosis. The skull is described as rounded, and there is asymmetry of the face, trunk and limbs. A number of different ocular changes have been described. They include microphthalmia, colobomas, strabismus and nystagmus. The ears may be large and prominent. There is occasional mental retardation.

The degree of clinical severity varies widely. Some patients may have only skin changes or simply syndactyly, whereas others may show full manifestations of the syndrome with microphthalmus, bilateral coloboma, iris ectopia lentis, hypoplasia of the teeth and severe cutaneous, skeletal and digital malformations (Goltz et al, 1970; Wodnianski, 1957).

Increased spontaneous breakage of chromosomes has been reported (Ferrara et al, 1967), a characteristic of conditions predisposing to cancer. The possibility of using fetoscopy for prenatal diagnosis exists but has not been reported.

Differential diagnoses should include incontinentia pigmenti, congenital poikiloderma (Thomsen's type) and naevus lipomatosus cutaneous superficialis.

REFERENCES

Assemany s, Muzzo S, Gardner L 1972 Syndrome of phocomelic diabetic embryopathy. American Journal of Diseases of Childhood 123: 489–491

Auerbach A, Adler, Chaganti R S K 1981 Prenatal and postnatal diagnosis and carrier detection of Fanconi anemia by a cytogenetic method. Pediatrics 67: 128–135

Bass H N 1968 Familial absence of middle phalanges with nail dysplasia – a new syndrome. Pediatrics 42: 318

Beighton P 1978 Inherited disorders of the skeleton. In: Emery E (ed) Genetics in medicine and surgery. Churchill Livingstone, New York

Bell J 1951 On brachydactyly and symphalangism. In: penrose L S (ed) Treasury of human inheritance. Cambridge University Press, London, vol 5, p 1–31

Bergsma D 1979 Birth defects compendium, 2nd edn. National Foundation March of Dimes. Alan R Liss, New York

Birch-Jensen A 1949 Congenital deformities of the upper extremities. Ejnar Munksgaard, Copenhagen

Cantu J M, Urrusti J, Rosales G, Rojas A 1971 Evidence for autosomal recessive inheritance of costovertebral dysplasia. Clinical Genetics 2: 149–154

Casamassima A C, et al 1979 Spondylocostal dysostosis associated with anal urogenital anomalies in a Mennonite sibship (personal communication)

Daentl D L, Smith D W, Scott C I, Hall B D, Gooding C A 1975 Femoral hypoplasia – unusual facies syndrome. Journal of Pediatrics 87: 107–111

David T J 1972 Nature and etiology of the Poland anomaly. New England Journal of Medicine 287: 487–489

DerKaloustian V M 1972 The Rubinstein-Taybi syndrome – clinical and muscle electron microscopy study. American Journal of Diseases of Childhood 123: 897

Dosik H et al 1970 Leukemia in Fanconi anemia: cytogenetic

and tumor virus susceptibility studies. Blood 3: 341–352

Duken J 1921 Ueber die Beziehunger zwischen Assimilation Shypophalangie und Aplasie der Interphalangealgelenke. Virchows Arceriv für Pathologische Anatomie 233: 204

Esparza A, Thompson W R 1966 Familial hypoplastic anemia with multiple congenital anomalies (Fanconi syndrome) – report of three cases. Rhode Island Medical Journal 49: 103–110

Faulk W P, Epstein C J, Jones 1970 Familial posterior lumbosacral vertebral fusion and eyelid ptosis. American Journal of Diseases of Childhood 119: 510–512

Ferrara A, Fontana V, Numsen G 1967 Bloom syndrome in an oriental male. New York Journal of Medicine 67: 3258–3262

Freire-Maia N 1970 The handless and footless families of Brazil. Lancet i: 519–520

Frostad H 1940 Congenital ankylosis of the elbow joint. Acta Orthopaedica XI (3–4): 296–306

Garner L G, Bixler D 1969 Micrognathia, an associated defect of Hanhart syndrome, types II and III. Oral Surgery 27: 601–606

Goldberg M J, Mazzei R J 1977 Poland syndrome: a concept of pathogenesis based on limb bud embryology. Birth Defects 13 (3D): 103–115

Goltz R W, Henderson R R, Hitch J M, Ott J E 1970 Focal dermal hypoplasia syndrome. A review of the literature and report of two cases. Archives of Dermatology 101: 1–11

Gorlin R J, Pindborg J J, Cohen M M 1976 Syndromes of the head and neck, 2nd edn. McGraw-Hill, New York

Grebe H 1964 Missbildungen der Gliedmassen. In: Becker P E (ed) Humangenetik II. Georg Thieme, Stuttgart

Gunderson C H, Greenspan R H, Glaser G H, Lubs H A 1967 The Klippel-Feil syndrome: genetic and clinical reevaluation of cervical fusion. Medicine 46 (6): 491–511

Hall J G 1969 Thrombocytopenia with absent radius. Medicine 48: 411

Hall J G et al 1980 Congenital hypothalamic hamartoblastoma, hypopituitarism, imperforate anus, and postaxial polydactyly – a new syndromce Part I: clinical, causal, and pathogenetic considerations. American Journal of Medical Genetics 7: 47–74

Hall J G, Reed S D, Greene G 1982. Distal arthrogryposis: a newly recognized condition with distal congenital contractures and its variants. American Journal of Medical Genetics 11: 185–239

Hansen O H, Andersen N O 1970 Congenital radio-ulnar synostosis. Acta Orthopaedica Scandinavica 41: 225–230

Hunter A G, Cox D, Rudd N 1976 The genetics of and associated clinical findings in humero-radial synostosis. Clinical Genetics 9: 470–478

Jones K L, Hall B D, Hall J G, Ebbins A J, Massaud H, Smith D W 1974 A pattern of cranio-facial and limb defects secondary to aberrant tissue bands. Journal of Pediatrics 84: 90–95

Kaufman R, Rimoin D, McAlister W, Hartman A 1974 variable expression of the Holt-Oram syndrome. American Journal of Diseases of Childhood 127: 21–25

Kohler H G 1962 Congenital transverse defects of limbs and digits. Archives of Diseases of Children 37: 263

Langer L O, Hermann J 1974 The cerebrocostomandibular syndrome. Birth Defects 10 (7): 167–170

Lucas G L 1967 Hereditary onycho-osteodysplasia (nail-patella syndrome) masquerading as arthrogryposis. Southern Medical Journal 60: 751–755

Luthy D, Hall J G, Graham B 1979 The use of fetal radiography in the prenatal diagnosis of thrombocytopenia with absent radius. Clinical Genetics 15 (6): 495–499

Majewski F, Lenz W, Pfeiffer R A, Tunte W 1972 Das oro-facio-digitale Syndrome. Zeitschrift Für Kinderheilkunde 112: 89–112

Maroteaux P 1979 Bone diseases of children. J P Lippencott Philadelphia

McKusick V A 1978 Mendelian inheritance in man. Johns Hopkins University Press, Baltimore

McKusick C A, Eldridge R, Hostetler J A, Egeland J A 1964 The distribution of certain genes in the older order Amish. Cold Spring Harbor Symposia on Quantitative Biology 29: 101

McNicholl B, Egan-Mitchell B, Murray J P, Doyle J F, Kennedy J D, Crone L 1970 Cerebro-costo-mandibular syndrome. Archives of Diseases of Children 45: 421–424

Morita T, Laughlin L, Kawrano K, Kimmelstiel P, Suzuki Y, Churg J 1973 Nail patella syndrome. Archives of Internal Medicine 131: 271–277

Norum R A, McKusick V A 1969 Costovertebral anomalies with apparent recessive inheritance. Birth Defects 5: 326–329

Otter G D 1970 Bilateral Sprengel's syndrome with situs inversus totalis. Acta Orthopaedica Scandinavica 41: 402–410

Poznanski A 1974 The hand in radiologic diagnosis. W B Saunders, Philadelphia

Poznanski A, Gall J, Stern A 1970a Skeletal manifestations of the Holt-Oram syndrome. Radiology 94: 45–53

Poznanski A K, Stern A M, Gall J C 1970b Radiographic findings in the hand-foot-uterus syndrome (HFUS). Radiology 95: 129–134

Rimoin D L, Fletcher B D, McKusick V A 1968 Spondylocostal dysplasia. American Journal of Medicine 45: 948–953

Rimoin D L, Hall J G, Maroteaux P 1979 International Nomenclature of Constitutional Diseases of Bone with Bibliography. Birth Defects Original Article Series XV (10)

Rubinstein J H 1969 The broad thumbs syndrome – progress report 1968. Birth Defects 5 (2): 25

Schroeder T M, Tilgen D Kruger J, Vogel F 1976 Formal genetics of Fanconi anemia. Human Genetics 32: 257–288

Smith D W 1976 Recognizeable patterns of malformation, 2nd edn. W B Saunders, Philadelphia

Stark E W, Borton T E 1973 Klippel-Feil syndrome and associated hearing loss. Archives of Orolaryngology 97: 415

Steinberg A G, Reynolds E L 1948 Further data on symphalangism. Journal of Heredity 39: 23

Stevenson R E, Scott C I, Epstein M 1975 Dominantly inherited ulnar drift. Birth Defects 11 (5): 75

Stranak V, von Oberender 1971 Über einen Fall von angeborener Synostosis humero-radialis bilateralis. Beitrage zur Orthopädie 18: 460–464

Strasburger A K, Hawkins M R, Eldridge R, Hargrave R L, McKusick V A 1965 Symphalangism: genetic and clinical aspects. Bulletin of Johns Hopkins 117 (2): 108–127

Swift M R, Hirschhorn K 1971 Fanconi anemia. Annals of Internal Medicine 65 (3): 496–503

Taybi H 1975 Radiology of syndromes. Year book Medical Publishers, Chicago

Temtamy S A, McKusick V A 1978 The genetics of hand malformations. Birth Defects XIV (3)

Wadia R S, Shirole D, Dikshit M 1978 Recessively inherited costovertebral segmentation defect with mesomelia and peculiar facies. Journal of Medical Genetics 15: 123–127

Weyers H, Thier C V 1958 Malformations mandibulofaciales et délimitation d'un syndrome oculo-vertébral. Journal Génétique Humaine 7: 143

Wilson M G, Mikity V G, Shinno N W 1971 Dominant inheritance of Sprengel's deformity. Journal of Pediatrics 79 (5): 818–821

Wodniansky P 1957 Ueber die Formen der congenitalen Poikilodermie Archiv Feur Klinische und experimentelle Dermatologie 205: 331–342

Wynne-Davies R 1975 Congenital vertebral anomalies: aetiology and relationship to spina bifida cystica. Journal of Medical Genetics 12 (3): 280

Zadek 1934 Congenital absence of the extensor pollicus longus of both thumbs. Operation and cure. Journal of Bone and Joint Surgery 16: 432–434

55

Arthrogryposes (congenital contractures)

J. G. Hall

INTRODUCTION

Arthrogryposis multiplex congenita (AMC) is a term which has been used for almost a century to describe conditions with non-progressive multiple congenital joint contractures. The conditions which have been called arthrogryposis range from well-known syndromes, to non-specific combinations of joint contractures. The term has become descriptive rather than diagnostic, and now is used in connection with a very heterogeneous group of patients, all of whom have multiple congenital joint contractures in common.

Although arthrogryposis is said to be a rare condition with an incidence of 1 in 5–10 000 liveborn, many kinds of congenital contractures, such as club feet and dislocated hips, are relatively common. The term arthrogryposis implies a more generalized involvement of multiple joints with congenital contractures, and is most often reserved for non-progressive conditions which involve more than one body area.

The medical literature on arthrogryposis or congenital contractures of the joints is very confusing. Over the last 50 years, more than 150 articles have been published describing what is said to be arthrogryposis, but the term has been used very loosely, first as a diagnostic term, but more recently as a clinical sign or as a general category of disorders. In addition to the imprecise use of the term, the medical literature on arthrogryposis is confusing because many authors fail to describe clinical features of their cases. They have often lumped a number of patients with congenital contractures together who in actuality represent many different specific entities, and then have made generalizations about recurrence, management, prognosis and treatment. This chapter will attempt to sort out some of the major known clinical entities with congenital contractures, to describe a clinical approach to distinguishing heterogeneity, to discuss the differential diagnosis of congenital contractures, and to make some comments about genetics and recurrence risk.

It has become increasingly apparent, both in animal studies such as those by Drachman and Coulombre (1962), and from human work particularly well-defined by David Smith (1977, 1978), that anything which leads to decreased movement in utero may also lead to congenital contractures or fixation of joints.

The studies of Drachman and Coulombre (1972) demonstrated temporary paralysis by curarization of chick embryos at various times in development resulted in multiple congenital contractures. The immobilized chick developed fixation of various joints, depending on what time in morphogenesis the immobilization occurred. DeMyer and Baird (1969) have shown that intrauterine removal of amniotic fluid in rats could lead to limitation of movement of joints and congenital contractures. The work of Doctors Smith and Graham has demonstrated that uterine compression in humans can lead to a variety of deformities, and in particular, fixation of joints.

It appears that any process which limits movement during development of a fetus or embryo may lead to congenital contractures. The in utero process may well be similar to the postnatal process of wearing a cast for a broken bone. When the cast is taken off, there is usually residual limitation of movement in joints which were immobilized. The growing embryo or fetus which has superimposed limitation of movement may develop even more marked contractures because the process of growth appears to accentuate contractures in joints with limited range of motion. In this regard, most congenital contractures may be considered deformities rather than primary malformations. The timing during development plays a critical role in the severity of contractures, in the position of joints, and in the secondary changes which occur with growth of the individual.

The potential causes of limitation of movement in utero fall most easily into four categories: 1) myopathic processes including myopathies and abnormal muscle structure and function, such as absence of muscles and congenital myopathies; 2) neuropathic processes including abnormalities in nerve structure or function such as meningomyelocele, failure of nerves to form, migrate or myelinate, and congenital neuropathies; 3) abnormal connective tissue including joint and tendon abnormalities, such as diastrophic dysplasia or abnormal tendon attachments; and 4) limitation of space or restriction of

Table 55.1 Musculoskeletal abnormalities and congenital contractures

Entity	Type AMC	Primary features	Contractures Body area	Position
Absence of dermal ridges	I	1. absent dermal ridges 2. bilateral flexn. contractures 3. bilateral webbing of toes 4. congenital milia	fingers toes	flexed
Absence of DIP creases	I	1. absent DIP creases 2. flexion limitation 3. palmar contracture	hands	flexed
Amniotic bands (Streeter)	I	1. ring-like constrictions 2. +/– other visceral anomalies	limbs	variable
Amyoplasia	I	1. loss of muscle tissue and replacement with fat 2. contractures 3. round face, midline hemangioma 4. increased frequency deformation anomalies (smashed digits, etc.)	hands elbows shoulders hips knees feet	flexion extension IR flexn, CDH +/– extnsn or flexion equino varus
Antecubital Webbing	I	1. elbow dysplasia 2. antecubital web 3. +/– carpal wrist abnormalities	elbow +/– wrist	flexion carpal fusion
Camptodactyly	I	1. camptodactyly	fingers only	fixed flexn
Clasped thumbs, congenital	I	1. extensor muscles and tendons of thumb weak or absent	thumb (bilateral)	flexed at MP and DIP joints, radial deviation (adducted)
Coalition	I	1. calcaneus-navicular 2. scaphoid – astragalus 3. talus-navicular 4. calcaneus – scaphoid	feet toes	fusion +/– contractures
Contractures, continuous muscle discharge and titubation	I	1. contractures 2. myokymia 3. ataxia and titubation	hand feet all extremities	fixed flexn stiffened
Distal arthrogryposis		1. clenched hand with overlapping fingers at birth – opens to ulnar deviation (90%) 2. usually calcaneo valgus but all combinations (80%) 3. other major joint contractures 4. +/– trismus, short stature, cleft lip, cleft palate, scoliosis	fingers hands elbows hips knees feet toes	clenched, overlap, then open and ulnar deviate +/– flexn or extnsn calcaneo valgus or equino varus overlap, camptodactyly
Humero-radial synostosis (HRS)	I	Familial 1. AD 100%; are bilateral AR 91% Sporadic 2. 62% have hypoplasia of hand and 77% have involvement of ulna	hand wrist elbow shoulder hips knees feet	46% of sporadic humeroradial synostosis 38% of sporadic 25% of AR 50% of AD
Impaired pronation, supination of forearm (familial)	I	no synostoses	forearm	reduction of supination-pronation

Progression	Lab test, X–rays, Autopsy findings	Inheritance	Incidence	References
milia-transient (disappear 1st 6 months)	chromosomes normal; skin biopsy normal, dermometer normal	AD	13 affected out of 24 individuals, 3 generations	Baird (1964)
progressive	X–rays: no bone fusion; chromosomes normal	AD	4 generations with 8 affected affected daughter and mother	Fried, K. (1976) Lambert, D. (1977)
		sporadic		Smith, D. (1976)
improves with therapy	CNS: ↓ # anterior horn cells in some cases; Muscle: variation in fibre diameter, small fibres, replacement muscle tissue with fat and C.T.; EMG: normal and abnormal	apparently sporadic	1/100,000	Price (1932) Drachman (1961) Hall (1982)
worse with time	X–ray; +/– fusion humerus and ulnae, +/– dysplastic condyle, +/– trochlea dysplasia	AD	4 families reported	Shin Shun (1954) Mead (1963)
	shortness of deep flexor tendons	AD		Welch (1966)
surgical treatment, tendon transplant		AD	≈ 50 reported by 1952	White (1952) Weckesser (1968)
	X–rays: synostosis; Differential diagnosis: peroneal spastic foot	AD		Bersani (1957) Wray (1963)
	abnormal muscle fibres (small)	AD	3 affected/2 generations	Hanson (1977)
good therapy response, improves with time	X–ray: hip dislocation, mild scoliosis	AD (variable)		Fisk, J. (1974) Lacassie, Y. (1977) Sack, G. (1978) Hall (1982)
	X–rays: humeroradial synostosis	sporadic, AR and AD	26 sporadic, 4 AD, 5 AR	Fuhrman (1966) Keutel (1970) Stranack (1971) Say (1973) Hunter (1976)
	X–rays: flattening of radial head, but no displacement, no abnormal curvature of radial shaft or synostosis	AD	4 affected/3 generations	Thompson, J. (1968)

Table 55.1 (cont'd)

Entity	Type AMC	Primary features	Contractures Body area	Position
Liebenberg syndrome	I	1. prominence of radial head 2. unusual slope of olecranon process 3. brachydactyly 4. streblomicrodactyly	elbows fingers wrists	limited ROM flexion, clinodactyly 5 flexion
Nievergelt-Pearlman	I	1. synostoses of feet and hands 2. elbow dysplasia	hand elbows foot	clinocamptodactyly radioulnar synostoses talipes, tarsal synostoses
Poland anomaly	I	1. dysplasia of upper limb 2. absent pectoral major (costal head) 3. +/– occult polysyndactyly and radioulnar synostoses (Peterson)	elbow	radioulnar synostosis (occasional)
Radioulnar synostosis	I	1. radioulnar synostosis	hand elbow (1/3 of cases) forearm	pronation fixed 10–30° extension limitation reduced pronation
Symphalangism		1. symphalangism – hands, feet 2. deafness variable	fingers foot	clinodactyly, ankylosis of 1st and 2nd phalanges, absent PIP creases inability to invert and evert 'double ankle'
Symphalangism/brachydactyly	I	1. brachydactyly 2. symphalangism – (proximal and distal) 3. +/– club feet 4. +/– craniosynostosis 5. +/– scoliosis just before menarche	hands } hips } feet	flexed 'clubbed'
Tel Hashomir camptodactyly	I	1. camptodactyly 2. distinct facial features 3. multiple musculoskeletal defects, short stature	fingers feet toes	camptodactyly clubbed, pes planus deformed
Trismus pseudocamptodactyly	I	1. inability to open mouth fully 2. camptodactyly with wrist dorsiflexed but straightening with wrist flexion	fingers } toes } +/– feet jaw	flexed when hand is dorsiflexed pes cavus, equino varus trismus

movement within the uterus, such as in the case of twins (Schinzel et al, 1979), structural anomalies of the uterus, amniotic bands or chronic leakage of amniotic fluid. The earlier any one of these processes occurs, the more severe the contractures are predicted to be. In a given individual or specific entity, several processes can be at work which may accentuate deformities.

An approach to sorting out various types of congenital contractures includes careful definition and documentation of what areas of the body are involved in the process, a natural history of complications and response to therapy, laboratory data such as muscle biopsies, autopsies

including CNS histopathology and chromosome studies, photographs at various ages and careful family, delivery and pregnancy histories.

The differential diagnosis of congenital contractures is extensive. Tables 55.1, 55.2 and 55.3 outline most of the more common conditions which must be considered. Many of them can be recognized by specific clinical features and/or by laboratory tests. The clinical approach we have found most useful has been to first distinguish 3 categories of congenital contractures on a clinical basis: 1) primarily limb involvement; 2) limb involvement plus other malformations or anomalies; 3) limb involvement

Progression	Lab test, X–rays, Autopsy findings	Inheritance	Incidence	References
	X–ray: fusion triquetrum and pisiform	AD	10 affected/5 generations	Liebenberg (1973)
	chromosomes normal; X–ray: radio ulnar synostoses, talipes, tarsal synostoses	AD	only one affected 3 children and father (Nievergelt) daughter and mother (Pearlman)	Dubois (1970) Spranger (1976)
	X–ray: hypoplasia of middle phalanges, rib deficiencies, radioulnar synostosis	sporadic	over 100 reports (1977)	Goldberg (1977) Peterson (1977)
	X–rays: synostosis	AD	rare 220 cases reported plus 27 cases (Hansen)	Hansen, O. (1970)
	X–ray: PIP fusion +/– DIP fusion, +/– talus and naviculus fusion	AD	351 affected/10 generation	Strasburger (1965) Hermman (1974)
	lab data normal; X–rays: carpal fusion, +/– flat vertebrae	AR	2 patients	Walbaum, R. (1976)
		AD	5 affected/3 generation 5 affected/2 generation	Ventruto, V. (1976) Sillence, D. (1978)
	Lab: WNL; Path: bilateral absence of peronei and extensor hallucis longus	AR	2 families	Goodman (1976)
	pathology: short finger, leg and foot flexor tendons	AD	7 families	Ter Haar (1971) Mabry (1974)

plus central nervous system dysfunction and mental retardation. Tables 55.1, 55.2 and 55.3 are organized on the basis of this clinical approach. There is obvious overlap because some individuals with a condition may have only involvement of limbs, and others in the same family or with the same condition may have more widespread involvement. Similarly, in some conditions with congenital joint contractures, a characteristic feature is mental retardation, but there may be affected individuals who do not have mental retardation. Nevertheless, we have found this approach to be the most useful for the clinician.

The second aspect of the clinical approach is outlined in Table 55.4, with documentation of the various important differential features of the pregnancy, delivery and family histories, physical examination, course or natural history, and laboratory tests. These have proved to be most important in distinguishing different types of arthrogryposis. Thus, in the course of a work-up of a patient with congenital contractures, definition of these areas may be helpful in arriving at a specific diagnosis.

It is impossible to describe in detail all the conditions with congenital contractures, but it seems appropriate to emphasize several of the frequently observed conditions under the three categories.

Table 55.2 Multiple system abnormalities and congenital contractures

Entity	Type AMC	Primary features	Contractures Body area	Position
Camptomelic dysplasia	II	1. curvature of long bones, particularly femur and tibia 2. pretibial dimpling over curves 3. cleft palate 4. hypoplasia of facial bones, scapulas and fibula 5. +/– ambiguous genitalia 6. +/– craniosynostosis	hips elbows feet	CDH synostosis calcaneo valgus
Conradi-Hünermann (chondrodysplasia punctata)	II	1. hypertelorism, prominent forehead 2. cataracts (17%) 3. limb contractures (27%) 4. atrophodenna follicularis/alopecia	large joints +/– feet	flexion clubbed
Contractural arachnodactyly	II	1. contractural arachnodactyly 2. kyphoscoliosis 3. crumpled ear helix 4. club foot +/– 5. +/– CHD	fingers elbows knees ankles feet +/–	flexion PIP limitation supination & pronation flexed calcaneous w/dorsiflxn adduction of forepart
Craniocarpotarsal dystrophy (Whistling face, Freeman-Sheldon)	II	1. flat stiff immobile face, cheeks bulge, antimongoloid eyes, microstomia, high arch palate, 'H' shaped tissue band chin 2. hand contractures 3. +/– talipes equinovarus or calcaneo valgus 4. +/– deafness	fingers hands thumbs feet +/– hallux	ulnar shift limited PIP movement absence DIP crease (95%) adducted calcaneo valgus or equino varus (80%) camptodactyly
Diastrophic dysplasia	II	1. dwarfism 2. joint contractures/'hitch-hiker thumb' 3. scoliosis/vertebral instability 4. abnormal ears 5. cleft lip, +/– abnormal tracheal ring	thumb fingers hip +/– feet	adducted ankylosis PIP joint dislocated equino varus
Focal femoral dysplasia	II	1. cleft palate, long philtrum, short nose with hypoplastic alae nasae, micrognathia 2. shortened limbs 3. joint contractures	elbow hips feet toes	fixed in flexion dislocated equino varus clinodactyly
Hand muscle wasting and sensori-neural deafness	II	1. flexion contracture of hands 2. hearing loss/deafness 3. absence of PIP & DIP flexion creases 4. proximally placed thumbs	fingers wrist elbow toes	camptodactyly, ulnar deviation limitation of pronation and supination limited extension ulnar deviation, camptodactyly
Holt-Oram	II	1. abnormalities of shoulders, hands and wrists 2. cardiac defects (structural) 3. abnormal joint structure (rare)	hands wrists shoulders knee foot	usually hypoplasia, +/– synostosis hypoplasia genu valgus talocalcaneal synostosis (rare)
Kneist syndrome	II	1. short trunk dwarfism, S/S 2. kyphoscoliosis 3. joint enlargement with limitation 4. myopia, deafness, cleft palate 5. +/– mucopolysacchariduria	hands fingers hips ankles	flexed

Progression	Lab test, X–rays, autopsy findings	Inheritance	Incidence	References
Lethal, perinatal or death in infancy observed	X–rays: bowing of long bones; pathology: abnormal enchondral ossification; chromosomes: ambiguous genitalia	AR		Thurman (1973) Khajavi (1976) Hall, B (1980)
	X–ray: punctate calcifications, tubular bones-mildly short, scoliosis-abnormal vertebrae; pathology: epiphyses abnormal	AD	65 patients reviewed by Spranger 27% had contractures	Smith (1976) Spranger (1972)
improves with age (knees the worst)	EMG: no response to galvanism in quadriceps; X–ray: bones gracile, kyphoscoliosis	AD	at least 14 kindreds by 1971	Bass (1978) Temtamy (1978) Beals (1971) Reeve (1960)
contractures may progress with age	pathology: fibrous bands around mouth, shortening of flexor tendons	AD AR (2 families) (Alves 1977)	at least 10 kindreds, 20 sporadic reports	Pfeiffer (1972) Cox (1974) Sauk (1974)
progressive (probably due to weight bearing)	X–ray: precocious calcification of cartilage, pathology: abnormal epiphyses, hypertrophied auricular cartilage and calcifications	AR	rare	Lamy (1960) Temtamy (1978)
	vertebral anomalies	(associated with maternal diabetes) sporadic	at least 6 cases	Smith (1976) Gleiser (1978)
	pathology: muscle mass distally: audiogram: sensori-neural loss; EMG, ECG: normal; X–ray: wide diaphysis in phalanges, metatarsals, metacarpals	AD (variable expression)	12 affected/5 generation	Stewart (1971)
	pathology: CHD	AD	over 108 cases reported between 1960 and 1972	Poznanski (1971) Brans (1972) Kuafman (1974)
	lab: some with high keratin sulphate excretion; X–ray: irregular ossification of epiphyses	AD heterogeneous		Spranger (1974) Kim, H. (1975)

Table 55.2 (cont'd)

Entity	Type AMC	Primary features	Contractures	
			Body area	Position
Kuskokwim	II	1. multiple joint contractures 2. +/− pigmented nevi and ↓ corneal reflexes	elbows ⎫ knees ⎬ ankles ⎭ feet	flexed +/− web equino valgus or varus
Larsen dysplasia	II	1. hypertelorism, low nasal bridge, flat round face 2. multiple joint dislocations 3. hand anomalies – long fingers 4. vertebrae anomalies +/− short stature	hands ⎫ fingers ⎬ elbow ⎫ hips ⎬ knees ⎭ feet	↑ # creases camptodactyly anterior dislocations equino varus or valgus
Leprechaunism	II	1. IUGR 2. specific facies 3. hirsutism 4. loose skin, dry 5. contractures	hands feet	flexion talipes varus
Megalocornea with multiple skeletal anomalies	II	1. megalocornea 2. IUGR 3. saddle nose, hypertelorism, frontal bassing, large low set ears 4. mild micrognathia 5. finger flexion, club feet, kyphoscoliosis	fingers feet	flexion equino varus
Metaphyseal dysostosis (Jansen)	II	1. small thorax 2. characteristic facies 3. flexion joint deformities 4. wide irregular metaphyses	knee ⎫ hip ⎬	flexion deformities
Metatropic dysplasia	II	1. short stature/kyphoscoliosis 2. prominent joints with restricted mobility, but ↑ finger extensibility 3. pelvic hypoplasia	knee ⎫ hip ⎬	flexed
Moebius	II	1. facial diplegia (VI and nerve) 2. joint contractures 3. difficulty swallowing	hand knees foot	camptodactyly ≈ 1/6 flexed, genu valgum clubbed ≈ 1/3
Multiple Pterygium syndrome	II	1. multiple webs 2. joint contractures, camptodactyly 3. vertebral anomalies +/− S/S 4. +/− cleft lip and palate, antimongoloid slant, ptosis	fingers hands ⎫ elbows ⎪ hips ⎬ knees ⎪ ankles ⎭ feet	camptodactyly flexion deformities equino varus or calcaneo valgus
Nail Patella (Hereditary Onycho Osteodysplasia)	II	1. nail dysplasia 2. absent or hypoplastic patella 3. joint contractures 4. +/− kidney disease	fingers elbow ⎫ knee ⎬ foot	ulnar deviation (5th finger clino-camptodactyly) flexed pes planus, talipes, equinovarus
Nemaline Myopathy	II	1. hypotonic, respiratory problems 2. congenital heart disease 3. short 1st metacarpal, clinodactyly 4. bilateral talipes varus	fingers feet	clinodactyly talipes varus

Progression	Lab test, X–rays, autopsy findings	Inheritance	Incidence	References
	pathology: muscle atrophy; X–ray: +/– patella migration, normal muscle and nerve function	AR	17 cases (7 families Eskimos)	Petajan (1969) Wright (1969)
diminished cartilage rigidity at birth, improved with time	X–ray: poor ossification of phalanges, CDH, juxtacalcaneal accessory bone, hypoplasia of humerus distally	AR and AD	rare, Larsen reported 6 cases/5yrs.	Latta, R. (1971) Silverman (1972) Spranger (1974)
lethal	autopsy: renal hyperplasia, focal changes in liver, calcified deposits in kidneys, abberation of endocrine system, brain-normal	AR		Donohue (1954) derKaloustian (1971)
	lab: WNL; chromosomes: normal; X–ray: kyphoscoliosis, thin cortical bone of skull	consanguinity	1 case	Frank (1973)
progressive	X–ray: hypercalcemia, hyperostosis of calvarium, lack of metaphyseal ossification gives gross irregular cyst like areas	AD	very rare	Sutcliffe (1966) Spranger (1977)
progressive	X–ray: platyspondyly/kyphoscoliosis, pelvic hypoplasia, short limbs-metaphyseal flaring, epiphyseal irregularity, hyperplastic trochanters	AD and AR?	17 cases reported by 1966	Rimoin (1976) Smith, D. (1976)
	EMG: frontalis, abicularis oculi, facial and external rectusno response; pathology: muscle hypoplasia	AD		Sprofkin (1956) Smith (1976)
non-progressive	pathology: skin, spinal cord and brain normal, muscle hypoplasia, fatty replacement	AR	(AR)	Srivastava (1968) Chen (1980)
	X–ray: pathognomonic iliac horns, absent patella, subluxation of radial heads	AD		Lucas, G. (1967) Spranger (1976)
lethal	autopsy: papillary muscle anomaly, myocardial scarring, hepatic fibrosis; pathology muscle: rods in muscle fibres	AD, (AR?)	at least 20 cases	Neustein (1973) McComb (1979)

Table 55.2 (cont'd)

Entity	Type AMC	Primary features	Contractures Body area	Position
Neurofibromatosis	II	1. neurofibromas 2. cafe au lait spots (multiple) 3. contractures +/− congenital	hands elbows hips knees feet	flexion
Oculo-dental-digital S.	II	1. small sunken eyes, thin nose 2. severe hypoplasia of enamel, microdontia 3. phalangeal hypoplasia, camptodactyly of 4th and 5th	fingers hallux	camptodactyly abduction
Ophthalmo-mandibulo melic dysplasia	II	1. fusion of temporomandibular joint 2. eyes-blindness from corneal opacities 3. joint contractures, mild limb shortening	fingers hands elbows	camptodactyly ulnar deviation radiohumero dislocation, limited extension
Oral cranial digital syndrome	II	1. cleft lip and palate 2. hypoplastic inflexible distally placed thumbs 3. bilateral elbow deformities 4. microcephalus, mild MR	thumb elbow toes	IP inflexibility limited extension camptodactyly
Osteogenesis imperfecta, congenital lethal 'Crumpled Bone Type' (Type II)	II	1. short limbs 2. fractures-poor mineralization, wormian bones 3. blue sclerae, shallow orbits, small nose 4. +/− contractures, hydrocephalus	wrists elbows knees feet	flexed flexed webbing
Oto-palato-digital	II	1. deafness-conductive 2. dwarfism/bone dysplasia 3. adontia, soft cleft palate 4. characteristic facies: hypertelorism, frontal bossing 5. mild MR	fingers wrists elbows toes	broad distal phalanges limited supination limited extension clinodactyly, broad distal phalanges
Pfeiffer	II	1. craniosynostoses, brachycephaly 2. syndactyly 3. +/− contractures	elbow +/− feet +/−	radioulnar synostoses mild calcaneo varus
Popliteal pterygium	II	1. popliteal web 2. cleft palate, cleft lip, lip pits, frenulae 3. syndactyly 4. nail anomalies, absence deformities of digits 5. equino varus 6. +/− ankyloblepharon filiforme adnatum	knee +/− foot	flexion with web equino varus
Prader-Willi habitus, osteoporosis, hand contractures	II	1. MR 2. short stature 3. obesity 4. genital abnormalities 5. hand and feet contractures	hands feet	flexed
Pseudothalidomide syndrome (Roberts syndrome)	II	1. microbrachycephaly, +/− craniosynostosis 2. limb reduction 3. +/− cleft lip and palate 4. characteristic facies 5. moderate to severe MR 6. +/− IUGR	elbows knees feet	radiohumeral synostosis femorotibial fusion talipes, calcaneo valgus

Progression	Lab test, X–rays, autopsy findings	Inheritance	Incidence	References
can be progressive	histopathology: neurofibromas	AD	1/3000 have NFT but contractures rare	Relkin (1965) Kibbe (1968)
	chromosomes: normal X–rays: absence of middle phalanges of toes, widening long and short tubular bones and ribs and clavicles	AD	7 patients total	Gorlin (1963) Spranger (1976)
	chromosomes: normal; X–rays: fusion temporomandibular joint	AD	father and 2 children	Pillay (1964)
	X–rays: 1st metacarpals-small, radius dislocated; chromosomes: normal	AR	5 out of sibship of 6 affected	Juberg (1969)
lethal, often stillborn	X–ray: wormian bones, fractures, cystic changes – long bones, flattened vertebrae, poor mineralization, crumpled bones	AR	few cases	Sharma (1964) Guha (1969)
	X–ray: facial bones hypoplastic; 2° ossification center at base of metacarpals and tarsals, short metacarpals, broad distal phalanges, pectus	X–linked recessive	rare	Taybi (1962) Gorlin (1970)
	X–ray: broad distal phalanges	AD	rare	Spranger (1974) Smith (1976)
	pathology: free edge of web (cord-like) contains nerve and blood vessel	AD	at least 48 cases, 26 familial, 22 isolated	Gorlin (1968) Escobar (1978) Hall (1982)
	X–ray: wormian bones, osteoporosis; chromosomes: normal; thyroid: normal	AR?	2 brothers	Urban (1979)
can be lethal	chromosomes: can have 'puffing' pnenomena; pathology: CHD, renal anomalies	AR	over 30 reports	Hermann (1969) Freeman (1974) Grosse (1975) Ladda (1978)

Table 55.2 (cont'd)

Entity	Type AMC	Primary features	Contractures	
			Body area	Position
Puretic	II	1. joint contractures 2. face/skull deformities 3. large subcutaneous nodes 4. skin lesions 5. infections: skin, eyes, nose, ears	5th finger arms legs	camptodactyly fixed flexn contractures
Sacral agenesis	II	1. lower limb hypoplasia with contractures 2. +/– others	shoulders hips feet	Sprengel's flexion equino varus
Schwartz-Jampel	II	1. small stature, IUGR 2. myotonia 3. fixed facies 4. contractures; pectus 5. blepharophimosis; myopia	fingers wrists hips toes +/– feet	limitation equino varus
SED congenita	II	1. short trunk 2. myopia 3. lag in epiphyseal mineralization	elbows knees hips	joint limitation, flexion
Sturge-Weber	II	1. flat facial hemangiomata 2. meningeal hemangiomata with calcifications 3. MR +/– seizures 4. Buphthalmos, glaucoma	large joints	paresis ≈ 30% of cases, flexion
Tuberous Sclerosis	II	1. glioma-angioma lesions, phakomata, seizures 2. adenoma sebaceum, shagreen patch ↓ pigment patches 3. +/– joint contractures	fingers 1–3 feet toes	flexed equino varus flexed
VATER Association	II	1. vertebral/vascular defects 2. anal atresia 3. tracheoesophageal fistula 4. esophageal atresia 5. radial/renal defects	hand and arm	'clubbed'
Weaver Syndrome	II	1. macrosomia 2. accelerated skeletal maturation 3. camptodactyly 4. unusual facies	fingers +/– feet	camptodactyly talipes equino- varus
Winchester Syndrome	II	1. craniofacial asymmetry, brachydactyly 2. faint corneal opacities 3. malar flush, thick facial skin	fingers elbows knees toes	flexed
X-Trapezoidocephaly, Midfacial Hypoplasia, Cartilage Abnormalities	II	1. unusual facies/craniosynostosis 2. contractures 3. radiohumeral synostosis 4. congenital contractures of femur	fingers wrist elbows ankles toes 3, 4, 5	flexed flexion at 190°, carpal synostoses radiohumeral synostosis tarsal synostosis flexed

Progression	Lab test, X−rays, autopsy findings	Inheritance	Incidence	References
progressive contractures from early infancy	histopathology: skin ↓ collagen, ↑ soluble protein, tumours, ↓ fat content, altered connective tissue	AR	rare	Puretic, S. (1962)
	X−rays: absence sacrum	maternal uterine teratogen?	Bony abnormalities in ≈ 1% of diabetic mother Pederson (1964)	Blumel (1959) Assemany (1972)
progressive	X−ray: fragmentation and flattening of femoral epiphysis, pectus	AR	at least 7 cases reported	Aberfeld (1965) Smith (1976)
progressive	lab: urine keratosulfate; X−rays: flat epiphyses, ↓ mineralization os pubis, talus, calcaneus, knee centers	AD	20 cases − 1966	Spranger (1974) Smith, D. (1976)
	pathology: cerebral cortical atrophy, sclerosis, double contour convolutional calcifications seen on X−ray	sporadic		Smith (1976)
can be progressive	autopsy: brain-tuberous sclerosis lesions; X−rays: no bone changes	AD variable		Sandbank (1964)
	chromosomes: normal; pathology: CHD, anal atresia, TE fistula, renal anomaly	sporadic		Temtamy (1974) Smith (1976)
	X−ray: broad distal femurs and ulnae	sporadic	2 cases (1974)	Weaver, D. (1974) Smith, D. (1976)
	lab: not MPS; pathology: swelling and degeneration of mitochondria, dilation of endoplasmic reticulum (fibroblastic function disorder?)	AR	4 cases in 2 families	Hollister (1974) Goodman (1977)
	ECG, EMG, lab: WNL; X−ray: radiohumeral synostoses, tarsal synostoses		1 case	Antley (1975)

Table 55.3 Abnormal CNS and congenital contractures

Entity	Type AMC	Primary features	Contractures	
			Body area	Position
Adducted thumbs	III	1. thumbs flexed 2. micrognathia, cleft palate 3. craniostenosis 4. microcephaly, dysmyelination 5. swallowing difficulties	thumbs elbows, wrists, knees } feet	flexed, adducted limited extension clubbed
Cerebro-oculo-facio-skeletal (COFS)	III	1. microcephaly, IUGR 2. cataracts, microphthalmia, micrognathia, abnormal ears 3. overlapping flexed fingers 4. calcaneo valgus 5. hypotonia	fingers elbows } hips } knees } feet	flexed, medially deviated flexion calcaneo vagus
Cloudy corneae, diaphragmatic defects, distal limb deformities	III	1. coarse face, cloudy corneae 2. cleft palate 3. hypoplasia/aplasia lung 4. digitalization thumbs 5. distal limb deformities 6. IUGR 7. +/– absent diaphragm	fingers thumbs	flexion PIP digitalization
Craniofacial/brain anomalies/IUGR	III	1. IUGR/psychomotor delay 2. craniofacial dysostosis 3. joint contractures 4. progeroid appearance	toes } fingers } elbows hips knees feet	camptodactyly flexed limited extension clubbed
Cryptorchidism, chest deformity, contractures	III	1. cryptorchidismno testes 2. chest deformity, pulmonary disorders 3. hypoplasia of muscle and absence of subcutaneous fat 4. MR severe, dolicocephaly 5. flexed knees, arachnodactyly 6. IUGR	knees	flexed
Faciocardiomelic	III	1. IUGR 2. microretrognathia, microstomia, epicanthal folds, abnormal ears, microglossia, glossoptosis 3. short/webbed neck 4. short limbs 5. CHD, complex 6. talipes varus	hands feet	radial deviation talipes varus
Fetal alcohol syndrome	III	1. microcephaly/IUGR 2. characteristic facial features 3. joint contractures palmar creases (73%) 4. +/– CHD (50%) 5. genital anomalies (50%)	fingers elbow hips	limitation dislocation flexion
FG syndrome	III	1. MR, large head 2. hypotonia +/– joint contractures 3. imperforate anus and other GI abnormalities 4. +/– CHD 5. seizures; CNS anomalies 6. +/– contractures	fingers wrists knees ankles } feet }	ulnar deviation radial deviation limited extension lateral displacement

Table 55.3 Abnormal CNS and congenital contractures (cont.)

Progression	Lab test, X–rays, autopsy findings	Inheritance	Incidence	References
	chromosomes: normal; EMG: abnormal; cine esophagoscopy: abnormal; lab: proteinuria, pathology: displaced tendons, dysmelination, long, slender bones	AR	4 children, 3 of similar Amish ancestry 1	Christian (1971) Fitch (1975)
lethal progressive	chromosomes: normal radiographs: platyspondyly, membranous cranial bones decreased ossification, osteoporosis; pathology: dysmyelination	AR	at least 20 cases	Preus (1977) Pena (1978)
lethal	chromosomes: normal; X–rays: hands and feet-rudimentary digit development; pathology: hypoplasia lungs and diaphragm			Fryns (1979)
lethal	EEG abnormal; EMG normal; lab: CMV in saliva of 1 sib, chromosomes: normal	AR	2 sibs	VanBiervielt (1977)
lethal (8 months, 4½ years, 11 years)	chromosomes, lab: normal; pathology: ↓ subcutaneous fat, atrophic musculature	AR or X–linked recessive	3 sibs	VanBenthem (1970)
lethal	lab, chromosomes: normal; pathology: complex CHD; X–ray: delayed bone age, shortened limbs, thumb hypoplasia, short metacarpals	AR consanguinity	3 male sibs	Cantú (1975)
	pathology: CNS abnormal; CHD	teratogen	11 cases 30 cases 127 cases from France	Jones/Smith (1973) Hanson, J. (1976) Mulvihill (1976)
	chromosomes: normal; pathology: CNS abnormal	X–linked		Opitz (1974) Riccardi (1977)

Table 55.3 (cont'd)

Entity	Type AMC	Primary features	Contractures Body area	Position
Marden-Walker	III	1. blepharophimosis 2. joint contractures, pectus 3. +/– hypotonia congenital 4. characteristic facies: immobile depressed nasal bridge	wrists elbows hips knees ankles feet	flexion equinovarus
Meningomyelocele	III	1. spinal lesion 2. paralysis → joint contractures 3. others +/–	usually lower limbs depending on lesion position	flexed
Mietens	III	1. corneal opacity, strabismus, nystagmus 2. flexion elbows 3. growth failure 4. MR	elbows knees	flexed limited extension (70°–150° limit)
Miller-Dieker (Lissencephaly)	III	1. lissencephaly – brain with smooth surface and large ventricles, seizures 2. IUGR 3. CHD 4. hypotonia 5. camptodactyly	hands	camptodactyly
Multiple Pterygium Lethal	III	1. multiple pterygium 2. IUGR 3. contractures 4. facies 5. lung hypoplasia	hands elbows hips knees feet	flexion calcaneo valgus
Myotonic Dystrophy-Severe Congenital (SCMD)	III	1. poor suck, difficulty swallowing 2. generalized hypotonia 3. facial diplegia 4. talipes equinovarus 5. cataracts, ptosis, MR	legs knees phalanges feet	frog position hyperextension talipes equinovarus
Neu Laxova	III	1. lissencephaly, microcephaly, absence of corpus callosum 2. flexion deformities 3. short neck, hypertelorism, micrognathia, exophthalmos 4. syndactyly, edema 5. IUGR	fingers wrists elbows hips knees ankles feet	overlapping flexed rocker bottom
Neuromuscular disease of larynx	III	1. IUGR 2. abnormal CNS 3. Pierre Robin facies 4. respiratory distress, absent arytenoid cartilage 5. no visceral malformations	hands feet 3rd finger	clubbed flexion
Nezelof syndrome	III	1. joint contractures 2. liver disease (pigment overload and biliary stasis) 3. renal dysfunction	hand foot	'clubbed' R talipes calcaneas L talipes equinus
Pena-Shokeir (ankylosis, facial anomalies and pulmonary hypoplasia)	III	1. CNS abnormalities IUGR 2. ankylosis 3. pulmonary hypoplasia 4. polyhydramnios, small placenta 5. hypertelorism, micrognathia	hands elbow hip knee feet	camptodactyly flexed ankylosis clubbed

Table 55.3 (cont'd)

Progression	Lab test, X–rays, autopsy findings	Inheritance	Incidence	References
lethal	pathology: atrophic muscles, CHD, microcysts in kidneys, ↓ muscle fibre size; hematology and urine: normal	sporadic	2 cases Fitch and Marden 3	Fitch (1971)
can be lethal		multifactorial		Smith, D. (1976)
	X–rays: metacarpal bone age ↑, head of radius dislocated bilaterally, epiphyses absent, shortened ulna and radius, clinodactyly; chromosomes: normal	AR	4 sibs	Mietens (1966)
lethal	autopsy: lissencephaly, PDA, L renal agenesis, duodenal atresion	AR	2 siblings	Miller, J. (1962) Fontaine (1977)
lethal	pathology: lung hypoplasia, cerebellar hypoplasia-1 case; chromosomes: normal	AR	3 families	Gillin (1976) Hall (1981)
progressive changes from normal muscle histology and EMG, life expectancy limited	biopsy: muscular dystrophy, pathology: abnormal CNS	AD		Harper (1975) Zellweger (1967) (1973) Bell (1972) Swift (1975)
lethal	chromosomes: normal; pathology: lissencephaly, absence corpus callosum, cerebellar hypoplasia, lung hypoplasia, small placenta, short umbilical cord	AR		Neu (1971) Laxova (1972) Lazjuk (1979)
lethal	autopsy: absent L arytenoid cartilage, brain abnormal neuromyopathic changes in limb and laryngeal intrinsic muscles, normal chromosomes			Schmitt (1978)
lethal	autopsy: rarefaction of anterior horn cells	AR	4 affected sibs/North African descent	Nezelof, C. (1979)
lethal	pathology: lung hypoplasia; chromosomes: normal	AR	at least 8 cases	Punnett (1974) Pena (1976) Hunter (1979)

Table 55.3 (cont'd)

Entity	Type AMC	Primary features	Contractures	
			Body area	Position
Popliteal pterygium with facial clefts	III	1. popliteal web 2. cleft lip and palate, facial clefts, hypoplastic nasal tip, frenulae, ankyloblepharon filiforme adnatum, corneal aplasia 3. microcephaly, IUGR 4. absent digits, nail anomalies, syndactyly	knee	flexion, web
Potter Syndrome	III	1. renal agenesis 2. flattened face, large floppy ears, micrognathia, chin skin crease 3. joint contractures 4. oligohydramnios, lung absent	hands wrists elbows hips knees ankles feet	'spade like' fixed flexion clubbed
Pseudotrisomy 18	III	1. micrognathia, abnormal ears 2. +/− CHD; genito-urinary anomalies 3. flexion deformities; clubfoot 4. MR	fingers knees feet	overlapping flexed flexed clubbed
Zellweger syndrome (Cerebrohepatorenal)	III	1. CNS impairment, IUGR 2. joint contractures 3. congenital glaucoma 4. hypertrophy of clitoris 5. visceral anomalies	hands fingers knees feet	ulnar deviation, flexed flexion clubbed
46XXY/48XXXY		1. bilateral aniridia/exophthalmos/glaucoma 2. severe MR 3. webbing 4. cryptorchidism 5. pes equino varus	elbows knees	flexion, cubital webbing flexion, popliteal webbing
49XXXXX and 49XXXXY		1. MR 2. scoliosis 3. hypertelorism 4. contractures, clinodactyly of 5th finger	hands elbows knees +/− feet	clinodactyly radioulnar synostosis flexed equino varus, pes planus
4p trisomy		1. MR, IUGR 2. small spherical nose, nasal aplasia 3. scoliosis 4. S/S	fingers hand feet hallux	flexion clubbed varus, calcaneo valgus valgus
trisomy 8/trisomy 8 mosaicism		1. moderate MR 2. high prominent forehead, long face, thick everted lower lip, large ears 3. skeletal malformations 4. +/− cryptorchidism testicular hypoplasia 5. deep palmar-plantar creases	hands elbows hips knees feet	camptodactyly ankylosed articulations, absent patellae clubbed, hallux valgus
trisomy 9		1. MR, brachycephaly 2. CHD 3. bulbous nose 4. abnormal genitalia	fingers hands feet	overlapping clubbed

Table 55.3 (cont'd)

Progression	Lab test, X–rays, autopsy findings	Inheritance	Incidence	References
lethal		AR	2 families	Bartsocas (1978) Hall (1981)
lethal	chromosomes: normal autopsy: +/– absent uterus and vagina, pulmonary hypoplasia, kidneys and ureters absent or rudimentary	sporadic		Passarge (1965) Gellis, S. (1969)
lethal	chromosomes: normal	AR	at least 6 reported cases	Burks (1964) Hook (1965) Hongre (1972)
lethal	chromosomes: normal; X–ray: calcification density over ischium and hip joints, stippling of patella and hands; pathology: agenesis corpus callosum, lissencephally, renal cysts; ECG, EEG: abnormal	AR	at least 15 reports	Bowen (1964) Poznanski (1970)
progressive ↓ blindness		chromosome abnormality	1 case	Pashayan (1973)
	X–ray: thick sternum, scoliosis, radioulnar synostosis	chromosome abnormality	4 cases	Holmes (1972)
1/3 die in childhood	X–ray: scoliosis; abnormal vertebrae, hips, iliac alae, sacrum, costal hypoplasia, decreased ossification	chromosome abnormality	23 cases	DeGrouchy (1977)
normal lifespan	pathology: +/– cardiopathy, +/– renal anomaly	chromosome abnormality	2/3-mosaic at least 30 cases	DeGrouchy (1977) Yunis (1977)
lethal	pathology: PDA, VSD +/– cerebral abnormalities; X–ray: dislocation knees, elbows, hips	chromosome abnormality	at least 10 cases	DeGrouchy (1977) Yunis (1977)

Table 55.3 (cont'd)

Entity	Type AMC	Primary features	Contractures	
			Body area	Position
trisomy 9q		1. MR 2. small face, beaked nose, micrognathia 3. amyotrophy	fingers hips ⎫ knees ⎬ hallux	long, tapering index overlaps at right angle flexion hammertoe
10q trisomy		1. MR/microcephaly 2. hypotonia 3. CHD	fingers lg. joint toes	taper dislocations hammer
trisomy 10p		1. IUGR, dolicocephaly 2. skeletal anomalies 3. lips inverted 4. hypotonia	finger hands ⎫ elbows ⎬	camptodactyly flexion
11q trisomy		1. MR 2. +/– renal anomalies, cardiopathy 3. +/– agenesis corpus callosum 4. contractures	elbows hips +/– feet	synostosis, fixed flexion ABD clubbed
trisomy 13		1. MR, microcephaly, holoprosencephaly 2. multiple visceral anomalies 3. bilateral cleft lip 4. microphthalmia 5. hexadactyly	fingers feet	overlapping calcaneo valgus
partial trisomy 14 (proximal)		1. severe MR 2. prominent nose, MR, cupid bow mouth 3. severe MR	fingers hips feet	flexion CDH
15 trisomy (proximal)		1. MR – IQ ≈ 20 2. seizures, hypotonia	fingers ⎫ toes ⎬ +/– feet	malpositioned clubbed
trisomy 18		1. corneal opacities/cataracts 2. abnormal ears 3. short neck, webbed 4. cryptorchidism 5. limb anomalies 6. visceral anomalies	fingers hands ⎫ elbows ⎮ hips ⎬ knees ⎭ feet	overlapping flexion calcaneo valgus

FREQUENTLY OBSERVED CONDITIONS

Primary limb involvement (see Table 55.1)

Amyoplasia

Amyoplasia is probably the most common condition with severe multiple congenital contractures and is referred to as 'classical arthrogryposis' by most orthopedists. One third of all patients in our large study of congenital contractures had amyoplasia (Hall et al 1982a). Amyoplasia is characterized by very specific positioning and symmetrical limb involvement, and usually involves all four limbs; however, occasionally only the arms or only the legs are affected. Affected individuals have fibrous bands and fatty tissue where muscles would normally be, suggesting that the muscle or muscle anlage was formed embryologically but failed to develop in a normal way. These patients usually have firmly fixed joints (Fig. 55.1). The feet are almost always in equinovarus position, the wrists are almost always flexed, the shoulders are internally rotated, the elbows are usually straight at birth but may be flexed and almost always develop some flexion with growth. There may be slight webbing of skin across the hips which may be flexed or extended in abduction or adduction. The knees may be extended or flexed.

Table 55.3 (cont'd)

Progression	Lab test, X–rays, autopsy findings	Inheritance	Incidence	References
retarded	pathology: amyotrophy	chromosome abnormality	3 cases	DeGrouchy (1977)
one half die in 1st year	pathology: cardiac, renal malformations; X–ray: scoliosis	chromosome abnormality	9 cases	DeGrouchy (1977)
usually lethal	pathology: cardiac – 1/3, renal, ocular abnormalities; X–ray: diaphyses, metaphyses are slender and narrow	chromosome abnormality	9 cases	DeGrouchy (1977)
one half die within one year	X–ray: acetabulum dysplasia, radioulnar synostosis; pathology: visceral malformations +/–	chromosome abnormality	14 cases	Yunis (1977) DeGrouchy (1977)
mean life expectancy – 130 days	pathology: oculocerebral malformations, cardiac, renal abnormalities	chromosome abnormality	1/4000– 1/10,000 L.B.	Yunis (1977) DeGrouchy (1977)
staturoponderal retardation	pathology: cardiopathy	chromosome abnormality	at least 8 cases	Yunis (1977) DeGrouchy (1977)
			15 cases	DeGrouchy (1977)
lethal	pathology: cerebral, ocular, cardiac, renal malformations; X–ray: +/– vertebral anomalies, CDH	chromosome abnormality	1/8000 births	Yunis (1977) DeGrouchy (1977)

Early physical therapy is extremely important to loosen contractures that are present at birth and thereby give whatever muscle is present a chance to strengthen rather than atrophy. Surgery is important to align the limbs in positions of function.

Most individuals have no other system involvement; however, there are a variety of other structural deformities that can be seen in amyoplasia. There is a very high frequency of hemangiomas or birthmarks over the midface. The face is usually somewhat round and flat with mild micrognathia. About 5% of the cases have had amniotic bands on one or more limbs. A small number of children have decrease in size of the distal digit with mild syndactyly or webbing. Often at birth, but definitely with time, there is undergrowth of an affected limb, much like the disuse atrophy seen in polio. Intelligence is within normal limits, unless there was trauma or anoxia at birth.

There appears to be an increased incidence of amyoplasia in identical twins with one normal twin and one affected twin; often the affected twin has only arms or only legs involved (Hall et al, 1982c). All cases have been sporadic, and many have reproduced having all normal children. Prenatal diagnosis in subsequent pregnancies can be offered for reassurance using serial real time ultrasound to detect normal limb movement. Most prob-

Table 55.4 Approach to congenital contractures

I History

1. *Pregnancy* (anything decreasing in utero movement leads to congenital contractures)
   a. Infectious (rubella, rubeola, coxsackie, enterovirus)
   b. Fever (above 102° – relation to time in gestation)
   c. Nausea (viral encephalitis)
   d. Drugs (curare, robaxin, alcohol)
   e. Fetal movement (polyhydramnois, one place, rolling decreased)
   f. Oligohydramnios, chronic leakage
   g. Trauma
2. *Delivery history*
   a. Presentation (breech, transverse)
   b. Length of gestation
   c. Initiation of labour
   d. Length of labour
   e. Traumatic delivery (limb, CNS)
   f. Intrauterine mass, twin
   g. Abnormal placenta +/– membranes
   h. Unusual cord position, length
   i. Time of year, geographic location
3. *Family history*
   a. Marked variability within family
   b. Change with time – degenerate vs. improve
   c Increased incidence of congenital contractures in second and third degree relatives
   d. Hyperextensibility present in some families
   e. R/O myotonic dystrophy, myasthenia gravis in parents (particularly mother)
   f. Consanguinity
   g. Advanced paternal age
   h. Increased stillbirths or miscarriages

II Newborn evaluation

1. *Description of contractures*
   a. Which limbs and joints
   b. Proximal vs. distal
   c. Flexion vs. extension
   d. Amount of limitation (fixed vs. passive vs. active movement)
   e. Characteristic position of rest
   f. Severity (firm vs. some give)
               PHOTOGRAPHS!!
   g. Complete fusion or ankylosis vs. soft tissue contracture
2. *Other anomalies*
   a. Deformities
      (i) Genitalia (cryptorchid, lack of labia, microphallus)
      (ii) Limbs (pyterygium, amniotic bands, cord wrapping, absent patella, dislocated radial heads, dimples)
      (iii) Jaw (micrognathia, trismus)
      (iv) Facies (asymmetry, flat bridge of nose, hemangioma)
      (v) Scoliosis
   b. Malformations
      (i) Eyes (small, corneal opacities, malformed, ptosis, strabismus)
      (ii) CNS (structural malformation, seizures, MR)
      (iii) Palate (high, cleft, submucous)
      (iv) Limb (deletion, radioulnar synostosis)
      (v) Dermatoglyphics (asbent, distorted, crease abnormalities)

(vi) Skull (craniosynostosis, asymmetry, microcephaly)
      (vii) Heart (congenital anomalies vs. cardiomyopathy)
      (viii) Lungs (hypoplasia vs. weak muscles)
      (ix) Other visceral anomalies
3. *Other features*
   a. Neurologic examination
      (i) Vigorous vs. lethargic
      (ii) Deep tendon reflexes (present vs. absent, slow vs. fast)
   b. Muscle
      (i) Mass (normal vs. decreased)
      (ii) Fixtures (soft vs. firm)
      (iii) Fibrous bands
      (iv) Normal Attachments
      (v) Change in time
   c. Connective tissue
      (i) Skin (soft, doughy, thick, extensible)
      (ii) Hernias (inguinal, umbilical, diaphragmatic)
      (iii) Joints (thickness, symphalangism)

III Course

1. *Changes with time*
   a. Developmental landmarks (motor vs. social and language)
   b. Growth of affected limbs
   c. Progression of contractures
   d. Lethal vs. CNS damage vs. stable vs. improvement
   e. Asymmetry (develops or progresses)
   f. Trunk vs. limb changes
   g. Intellectual abilities
   h. Socialization
2. *Response to therapy*
   a. Spontaneous improvement
   b. Response to physical therapy
   c. Response to casting
   d. Which surgery at which time
   e. Development of motor strength proportionate to limb size

IV Laboratory

1. *Tests*
   a. Documentation of range of motion and position with photographs
   b. X-rays if:
      (i) bony anomalies
      (ii) disproportionate
      (iii) scoliosis
      (iv) ankyolosis
   c. Chromosomes if:
      (i) multiple system involvement
      (ii) CNS abnormality (eye, microcephaly, MR, lethargic, degenerative)
      (iii) consider fibroblasts if lymphocytes were normal.
   d. Viral Cultures +/– specific antibodies in newborn
   e. EMG +/– muscle biopsy +/– nerve conduction
      (i) ↑ CPK
      (ii) abnormal tone, muscle mass, slow reflexes
   f. CPK if:
      (i) generalized weakness
      (ii) doughy or decreased muscle mass
      (iii) progressively worse
   g. Eye examination (opacities, retinal degeneration)

Table 55.4 (cont'd)

2. *Autopsy*
   a. Visceral anomalies
   b. CNS – brain neuropathology
   c. Spinal cord (number and size of anterior horn cells, limbs vs. trunk)
   d. Ganglion, peripheral nerve
   e. Eye (neuropathology)
   f. Muscle tissue from different muscle groups (EM & special stains)
   h. Fibrous bands replacing muscle
   i. Other malformations
3. *Documentation*
   a. Photographs
   b. X-rays
   c. Range of motion
   d. Chromosomes

Diagnosis
1. *R/O known syndromes*
2. *R/O environmental cause*
3. *Familial vs. sporadic*
4. *R/O chromosomal*

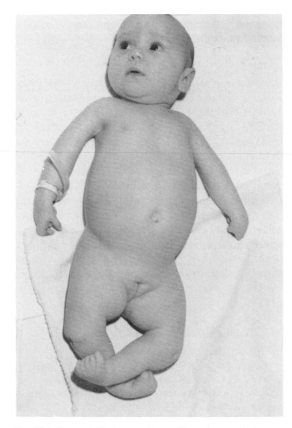

Fig. 55.1 Amyoplasia in a newborn. Note characteristic internally rotated shoulders with decreased muscle mass, extended elbows, hand contractures, equino varus deformities of the feet, dimples and flexion contractures at the knees. The face is round, the nose short and upturned, there is a midline hemangioma.

ably, the condition is secondary to some type of environmental agent. Recurrence has not been reported within families.

Distal arthrogryposis
Distal arthrogryposis is characterized by a very specific positioning of hands in the newborn period, and primarily distal contractures of the limbs (Hall et al, 1982b) (Fig. 55.2). The condition appears to have autosomal dominant inheritance, and is quite responsive to physical therapy. The hand positioning in the newborn is similar to that seen in trisomy 18, with a clenched fist and overlapping fingers (Fig. 55.3). With physical therapy, the hand usually opens up but there is often some residual ulnar drift of the fingers. Foot positioning is variable. Both equino varus and calcaneovalgus feet have been seen within the same family as well as in a single individual. Both the hand and foot abnormalities appear to be due to misplaced tendons. There are a number of cases in which this has been documented at surgery. Occasionally, affected family members have contractures of the hips, knees, and elbows. There can be marked variability in involvement within a family.

Some families with this disorder have been reported as familial camptodactyly, contractural arachnodactyly, and Freeman-Sheldon syndrome (autosomal dominantly inherited conditions which may have very similar abnormalities in the hands and feet). We have seen a number of sporadic cases but there is evidence of advanced paternal age among those cases, suggestive of new dominant mutations.

Most affected individuals have no non-orthopedic malformations; however, there are several subcategories of

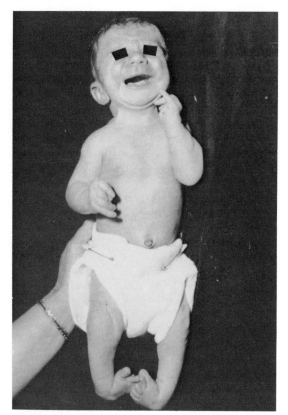

Fig. 55.2 Distal arthrogryposis in a newborn. Note predominant distal contractures, with overlapping finger contractures, ulnar deviation and clubfeet.

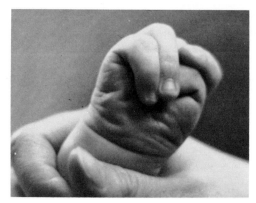

Fig. 55.3 Distal arthrogryposis newborn hand. Note clenched fist and overlapping fingers similar to hand position in Trisomy 18.

distal arthrogryposis which may have additional physical abnormalities. One of these, often referred to as the Gordon syndrome, (designated Distal IIA in our review of distal contractures) has the additional features of cleft palate and short stature in some affected family members (approximately 30–50%). The presence of short stature and clefting in an affected individual seems to be related to the severity of involvement of joints.

We have recognized a second subcategory of distal arthrogryposis in which there is limitation of jaw movement, +/– micrognathia in association with more generalized congenital contractures. The hand contractures are in an unusual position with hyperextension of the metacarpal phalangeal joint, and flexion of the other finger joints. Individuals with this condition may, in addition, have horizontal grooves on their chins. Approximately one third have had mild mental retardation. All of our cases appear to be sporadic. There is a higher-than-expected incidence of other joint anomalies within the family, and it is not entirely clear whether or not this is a polygenic or extremely variable dominant disorder. We call it distal arthrogryposis with trismus (or Distal IIE) for want of a better term (Hall et al, 1982b).

Distal arthrogryposis seems relatively responsive to physical therapy and surgical procedures. Some individuals and families are so mildly affected that one is not able to recognize any residual deformity, and only by talking to the grandparents is it found there were mild contractures at birth.

Symphalangism
Symphalangism is a well-known autosomal dominant condition. Some affected individuals and families are born with congenital contractures and develop fusion of various bones. Affected individuals may also have dislocated hips, short stature and conductive deafness due to fusion of the stapes and the petrous bone (Strasburger et al, 1965). There is a great deal of intra-familial variability, but the diagnosis is made by the recognition of characteristic fusion of phalanges which may not be present or obvious in early childhood. Individuals in affected families should be carefully examined for subtle signs of physical involvement that might ordinarily be overlooked. Surgery may be different than in other types of congenital contractures because of the expected fusion of bones. Physical therapy may exacerbate and hasten early fusion.

Limb involvement with other malformations (see Table 55.2)
The second major category of conditions with congenital contractures is that in which there are congenital contractures of the limbs in association with anomalies or malformations of other areas of the body.

Freeman-Sheldon
Perhaps the most common of these is Freeman-Sheldon, or Whistling Face syndrome, in which there are congenital contractures, primarily of the hands and feet with overlapping fingers and ulnar deviation, in associ-

ation with limitation in mouth movement secondary to constriction of muscles around the mouth. There is a characteristic 'H' shaped connective tissue band on the chin (Fig. 55.4). Individuals with Freeman-Sheldon syndrome may also have scoliosis, mid-face hypoplasia, coloboma of the alae nasae, ptosis and an antimongoloid slant of the eyes. Freeman-Sheldon syndrome appears to be more resistant to therapy than distal arthrogryposis.

It is clear that there is interfamilial and intrafamilial variability, but that autosomal dominant inheritance is the most common mode of inheritance. On the other hand, there appears to be a recessive form which is more severe (Alves & Azevedo, 1977) and is even lethal in some affected individuals. We are aware of a Mexican family in which physical findings were relatively severe in 3 affected siblings. The parents were entirely normal (Amendares, 1980).

Contractural arachnodactyly
Contractural arachnodactyly is a well-defined condition with autosomal dominant inheritance characterized by congenital contractures, long, thin extremities, a crumpling of the helix of the ear and kyphoscoliosis. Various chest deformities are seen as well, with pectus excavatum or carinatum. More recently there has been a suggestion of some overlap with the Marfan syndrome, in that some individuals with contractural arachnodactyly may have structural abnormalities of the heart with mitral valve prolapse and/or aortic aneurisms (Bass et al, 1980).

A variety of chondrodystrophies, such as diastrophic dysplasia and osteogenesis imperfecta also fall into this second category of congenital contractures associated with other malformations. In addition, Potter syndrome is a frequently observed condition in which the congenital contractures appear to be secondary to oligohydramnios.

Congenital contractures with CNS dysfunction (see Table 55.3 and Fig. 55.5)
The third category of conditions with congenital contractures is that in which there are congenital contrac-

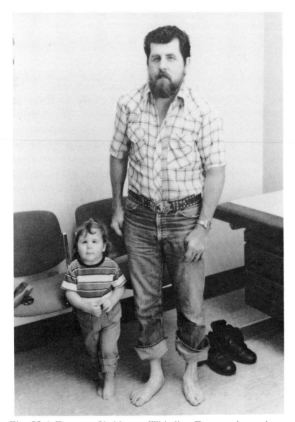

Fig. 55.4 Freeman Sheldon or Whistling Face syndrome in father and daughter. Note hand and foot contractures, more severe in father who has a very small left foot. The eyes are deeply set with an antimongoloid slant, the mouth is small and there is a mild groove in the chin. Both have short stature and short necks.

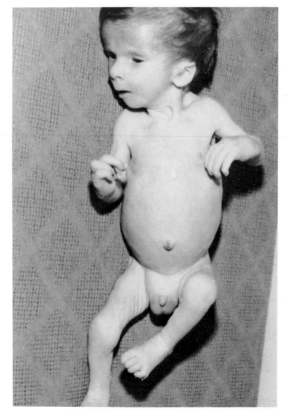

Fig. 55.5 Congenital contractures associated with central nervous system dysfunction. Note all limbs have flexion contractures, there is microcephaly with an abnormally shaped head and an unusual facies. The infant has microophthalmia, abnormally shaped ears, a thin upper lip, long philtrum, and micrognathia and a large inguinal hernia.

tures of the limbs associated with CNS malformations or dysfunction.

Trisomy 18

Probably the most frequent condition in this category is trisomy 18, which is characterized by intrauterine growth retardation, visceral anomalies with extremely high incidence of heart disease, radial limb anomalies, short sternum, small pelvis, facial paralysis and a typical positioning of fingers with overlapping fingers, clenched fists and rocker bottom feet.

Trisomy 8 mosaicism

Trisomy 8 mosaicism also frequently presents with congenital contractures and is often characterized by absence of patella and deep furrows in the palms or soles. Individuals with trisomy 8 mosaicism may only be identified with fibroblast karyotype.

There have been a number of our patients who have a variety of other chromosomal anomalies, which may only be recognized because of fibroblast karyotypes. Thus, the first step in arriving at a diagnosis in this CNS group is to eliminate those individuals with chromosomal abnormalities by doing fibroblast karyotypes.

Cerebro-oculo-facial-skeletal syndrome

Cerebro-oculo-facial-skeletal syndrome (COFS) seems to be one of the more common lethal conditions with contractures, characterized by structural abnormalities of the brain, demyelinization, and underdevelopment of the eye. The natural history of this degenerative condition has shown that in some families, some affected individuals are born with contractures, and others are not but develop contractures later in life (Scott-Emnakpor et al, 1977). However, in our experience it appears to be one of the more common causes of congenital contractures with CNS involvement, resulting in neonatal death.

In addition to chromosomal anomalies and specific syndromes (see Table 55.3) within this third category of arthrogryposis with CNS disorders, there is a very high incidence of lethality and death within the first two years of life. Autopsies are helpful in making a diagnosis.

GENETICS

There are some generalizations which can be made about the genetic aspects of arthrogryposis. In the past, when a child with arthrogryposis or congenital contractures was born to normal parents with an unremarkable family history, the parents were given an empiric polygenic multifactorial 5% recurrence risk that they might have another affected child. However, with careful documen-

tation, a specific diagnosis can be reached in probably half of the patients seen with congenital contractures. For instance, amyoplasia appears to have no recurrence risk at all. Distal forms of arthrogryposis may have as much as a 50% recurrence risk. In the category of individuals with CNS involvement, the recurrence risk may be as high as 25% with an average risk of 10–15%. (This implies, of course, that there is a high incidence of autosomal recessive disorders within this category.)

Prenatal diagnosis may be possible in some conditions, utilizing real time serial ultrasound studies trying to define fetal movement (Miskin et al, 1979). There is at least one reported case of failure to make the diagnosis in an infant with multiple joint contractures utilizing real time ultrasound during the second trimester (Benzie et al, 1976). However, if a family is at risk, prenatal diagnosis should be offered.

APPROACH (for the approach to patients with congenital contractures see Table 55.4)

Histories

Pregnancy history, delivery history, and family history are all extremely important, and several points should be kept in mind in their analysis.

Pregnancy history

The question of intrauterine infections should always be considered in the evaluation of infants with congenital contractures, particularly with neurological impairment. Not infrequently, the mother has had an infection that can lead to secondary CNS damage and was not aware of it. It is appropriate to do IgM studies in the newborn with congenital contractures looking for increased levels which would indicate intrauterine infection and in addition, specific titers can be pursued (rubella, coxsackie, enterovirus). Seasonal and geographical variables may be indicators of a viral infection and should be investigated. Maternal fever above 102° for an extended period may lead to CNS damage. Secondary contractures may result in the fetus because of abnormal nerve growth or migration associated with hyperthermia (Smith et al, 1978). A history of nausea in the mother is of importance as a high frequency of pregnancies which result in congenital contractures have been noted to be associated with nausea at various times in pregnancy. It is not known whether the nausea is due to a maternal viral infection or to discomfort or irritation because of an abnormal positioning of the fetus. Both need to be considered. Use of drugs during the pregnancy by the mother which would lead to decreased movement such as robaxin and curare (muscle relaxants) or drugs which may lead to potential CNS damage and secondarily affect fetal movement such as alcohol should be specifically asked about when taking a pregnancy history. A carefully reviewed pregnancy history frequently shows abnormal fetal movement (decreased movement, movement in only one area, or a 'swimming motion'). Polyhydramnios during the pregnancy may lead to fetal compromise or placental insufficiency. Oligohydramnios or chronic leakage of fluid may cause fetal constraint and secondary deformational contractures.

Delivery history

Delivery history is usually abnormal either because of an abnormal presentation or difficulty in delivery due to abnormal and fixed joints. It is not unusual that a fracture occurs during delivery; it certainly does not imply fragile bones. Babies with congenital contractures have been erroneously diagnosed as osteogenesis imperfecta by untrained individuals simply on the basis of fractures. The length of gestation is usually normal, although certain conditions such as trisomy 18 may go post-delivery date, and other factors such as congenital infections may lead to early delivery. The length of labour is often prolonged because of difficulty in delivering due to the unusual position of the joints. Breech and transverse positioning are relatively common. Both CNS and limb trauma not infrequently occur during delivery.

Careful examination of the uterus for structural uterine anomalies or abnormal uterine size is important. The placental membranes and cord insertion need to be examined looking for amniotic bands or vascular compromise. The umbilical cord may be shortened or may be wrapped around a limb and actually lead to compression of that limb.

Family history

A careful family history is important. We have certainly observed marked variability within families as to severity of contractures; congenital contractures may actually have worked themselves out by the time parents of an affected child reach adulthood. A large number of family members have other kinds of tissue abnormalities such as hyperextensibility, dislocated joints, club feet and dislocated hips (Hall et al, 1982d). A surprising number of children with arthrogryposis are secondary to known complications of a genetic disorder. Tuberous sclerosis and neurofibromatosis are occasionally seen in association with congenital contractures of the joints. Infants with congenital contractures are known to be born to mothers affected with myotonic dystrophy and myasthenia gravis. Thus, careful family histories with special attention to these four disorders should be pursued. Consanguinity, multiple stillbirths or miscarriages and advanced paternal age should be asked about.

Physical examination

Careful newborn examination and documentation is extremely important. Photographs are extremely helpful. Position of contractures with active and passive range of motion should be carefully measured and described. The definition of whether the contractures are proximal or distal, in flexion or extension, the amount of limitation and characteristic position at rest is important to document. A variety of secondary anomalies, including deformities and malformations, have been seen in children with congenital contractures. These anomalies may well give some clue to the underlying basic process, and to differential diagnosis. Careful documentation of the neurologic status and of muscles, as to muscle tissue presence and texture are important. Other connective tissue findings should be documented.

Laboratory tests

On the whole, laboratory tests have not been extremely useful in making a diagnosis in cases of congenital contractures. EMG, muscle biopsies, nerve conduction studies, and muscle enzyme studies are quite often interpreted to have nonspecific results. Muscle biopsies often show fatty tissue and connective tissue replacements, variation in fiber size or decreased fiber diameter, all nonspecific signs of muscle atrophy. Roentgenograms are useful in ruling out specific bone dysplasias, and in documenting scoliosis.

SUMMARY

Multiple congenital contractures are relatively frequent and often part of recognizable syndromes. Marked heterogeneity does exist as seen in Tables 55.1, 55.2 and 55.3. Careful work-up should lead to a specific diagnosis in over half the cases allowing more specific prognostication, counselling and therapy.

REFERENCES

Alves A F, Azevedo E S 1977 Recessive form of Freeman-Sheldon's syndrome or 'whistling face'. Journal of Medical Genetics 14(2): 139–141

Amendares S 1980 personal communication

Bass H N, Marcy S M, Sparkes R S, Crandall B F 1980 Congenital contractural arachnodactyly and aortic aneurysm in the same family. Abstract Birth Defects Conference New York

Benzie R J, Malone R, Miskin M, Rudd N, Schofield P 1976 Prenatal diagnosis by fetoscopy with subsequent normal delivery: report of a case. Journal of Pediatrics 126(2): 287–288

DeMyer W, Baird I 1969 Mortality and skeletal malformations from amniocentesis and oligohydramnios in rats: cleft palate, clubfoot, microstomia and adactyly. Teratology 2: 33–38

Drachman D B, Coulombre A J 1962 Experimental clubfoot and AMC. Lancet ii: 523

Hall J G, Reed S D 1982 Teratogens associated with congenital contractures in humans and in animals. Teratology 25: 173–191

Hall J G, Reed S D, Driscoll E P 1982a Part I Amyoplasia: a frequently seen sporadic condition with congenital contractures. American Journal of Medical Genetics (in press)

Hall J G, Reed S D, Greene G 1982b Distal arthrogryposis: Delination of new entities – review and norologica discussion. American Journal of Medical Genetics 11: 185–239

Hall J G, Hermann J, McGillivray B, Partington M, Schinzel A, Shapiro J, Reed S D 1982c Part II Amyoplasia: twinning in amyoplasia – a specific type of arthrogryposis with an apparent excess of discordant identical twins. American Journal of Medical Genetics. In Press

Hall J G, Reed S D, Scott C I, Rodgers J G, Jones K L, Carnneau A 1982d Three distinct types of X–linked arthrogryposis seen in 6 families. Clinical Genetics 21: 81–97

Miskin M, Rothberg R, Rudd N, Benzie R J, Shine J 1979 Arthrogryposis multiplex congenita prenatal assessment with diagnostic ultrasound and fetoscopy. Journal of Pediatrics 95(3): 463–464

Schinzel A, Smith D W, Miller J R 1979 Monozygotic twinning and structural defects. Journal of Pediatrics 95(6): 921–930

Scott-Emuakpor, Heffelfinger J, Higgins J V 1977 A syndrome of microcephaly and cataracts in 4 siblings. American Journal of Diseases of Children 131: 167

Smith D W 1977 An approach to clinical dysmorphology. Journal of Pediatrics 91(4): 690–692

Smith D W, Clarren S K, Harvey M A 1978 Hyperthermia as a possible teratogenic agent. Journal of Pediatrics 92(6): 878–883

Strasburger A K, Hawkins M R, Eldridge R, Hardgrave R L, McKusick V A 1965 Symphalangism: genetic and clinical aspects. Bulletin of the Johns Hopkins Hospital 117: 108–127

REFERENCES TO TABLES

Aberfeld D C, Hinterbuchner, Schneider M 1965 Myotonia, dwarfism diffuse bone disease and unusual ocular and facial abnormalities (a new syndrome). Brain 88: 313

Antley R, Bixler D 1975 X-trapezoidocephaly, midfacial hypoplasia and cartilage abnormalities with multiple synostoses and skeletal fractures. BDOAS 11(2): 397–401

Assemany S, Muzzo S, Gardner L 1972 Syndrome of phocomelic diabetic embryopathy. American Journal of Diseases of Children 123: 489–491

Baird H W III 1964 Kindred showing congenital absence of dermal ridges and associated anomalies. Journal of Pediatrics 64: 621–631

Baird H W III 1968 Absence of fingerprints in four generations. Lancet II: 1250

Bartsocas C S, Papas C V 1972 Popliteal pterygium syndrome. Journal of Medical Genetics 9: 222–226

Beals R K, Hecht F 1971 Congenital contractural arachnodactyly. Journal of Bone & Joint Surgery 53A(5): 987–993

Bell D B, Smith D W 1972 Myotonic dystrophy in the neonate. Journal of Pediatrics 81(1): 83–86

Bersani F A, Samilson R L 1957 Massive familial tarsal synostosis. Journal of Bone & Joint Surgery 39A(5): 1187–1189

Blumer J, Evans B C, Eggers G 1959 Partial and complete agenesis or malformation of the sacrum with associated anomalies. Journal of Bone & Joint Surgery 41A(3): 497–518

Bowen P, Lee C S N, Zellweger H, Lindenberg R 1964 A familial syndrome of multiple congenital defects. Bulletin of the Johns Hopkins Hospital 114: 402–414

Bowen P, Conradi G J 1976 Syndrome of skeletal and genitourinary anomalies with unusual facies and failure to thrive in Hutterite sibs. BDOAS 12(6): 101–108

Brans Y W, Lintermans J P 1972 The upper limb cardiovascular syndrome. American Journal of Diseases in Children 124: 779–783

Burks J, Sinkford S 1964 Clinical tris E syndrome (16–18): a cytogenetic enigma. Clinical Pediatrics 3(4): 233–235

Cantu J M, Hernandex A, Ramirez J, Bernal M, Rubio G, Urrusti J, Franco-Vazquez S 1975 Lethal faciocardiomelic dysplasia – a new autosomal recessive disorder. BDOAS XI(5): 91–98

Chen H, Chang C, Misra R, Peters H, Grijalva N, Opitz J 1980 Multiple pterygium syndrome. American Journal of Medical Genetics 17(2): 92–102

Christian J C, Andrews P A, Conneally P M, Muller J 1971 The adducted thumbs syndrome (an autosomal recessive disease with arthrogryposis, dysmyelination, craniostenosis and cleft palate). Clinical Genetics 2: 95–103

Clarren S, Ellsworth C, Sumi M, Streissguth A, Smith D W 1978 Brain malformations related to prenatal exposure to ethanol. Journal of Pediatrics 92(1): 64–67

Cox D, Pearce W G 1974 Variable expressivity in craniocarpotarsal dysplasia. BDOAS X(5): 243–248

Cox D J, Simmons F B 1974 Midline vocal cord fixation in the newborn. Archives of Otolaryngology 100: 219

deGrouchey J, Turleau C 1977 Clinical atlas of human chromosomes. John Wiley and Sons, New York

Der Kaloustian V. Kronfol N, Takla R, Habash A, Khazin A, Najjar S 1971 Leprechaunism. American Journal of Diseases in Children 122: 442–445

Donner M, Rapola J, Somer H 1975 Congenital muscular dystrophy: a clinico-pathological and follow-up study of 15 patients. Neuropaediatrie 6, 239–258

Donohue W L 1954 Dysendocrinism. Journal of Pediatrics 45: 739–748

Drachman D 1961 Arthrogryposis multiplex congenita. Archives of Neurology 5: 89–93

Drachman D B, Coulombre A J 1962 Experimental clubfoot and arthrogryposis multiplex congenita. Lancet II: 523–526

Dubois H J: Nievergelt Pearlman syndrome 1970 Synostosis in feet and hands with dysplasia of elbows. Journal of Bone & Joint Surgery 52B(2): 325–329

Escobar V, Weaver D D 1978 Facio-genito-popliteal syndrome. BDOAS XIV(6B): 185–192

Fisk J 1974 Congenital ulnar deviation of the fingers with clubfoot deformities. Clinical Orthopedics and Related Research 104: 200–205

Fitch N, Karpati G, Pinsky L 1971 Congenital blepharophimosis, joint contractures and muscular hypotonia. Neurology 21: 1214–1220

Fitch N, Levy E P 1975 Adducted thumb syndromes. Clinical Genetics 8: 190–198

Fontaine G, Farriaux J P, Blanckaert D, Lefebvre C 1977 Un nouveau syndrome polymalformatif complexe. Journal de Génétique Humaine 25(2): 109–119

Frank Y, Ziprowski M, Romano A, Stein R, Katznelson M, Cohen B, Goodman R M 1973 Megalocornea associated with multiple skeletal anomalies: A new genetic syndrome? Journal de Génétique Humaine 21: 67–72

Fried K, Mundel G 1976 Absence of distal interphalangeal creases of fingers with flexion limitation. Journal of Medical Genetics 13: 127–130

Fryns J P, Moerman F, Goddeeris P, Bossuyt C, Van den Berghe H 1979 A new lethal syndrome with cloudy corneae, diaphragmatic defects and distal limb deformities. Human Genetics 50: 65–70

Fuhrmann W, Steffens C, Rompe G 1966 Dominant erbliche doppelseitige dysplasie und synostose de Ellenbogengelenks. Humangenetik 3: 64–77

Gillin M E, Pryse-Davis J 1976 Case report – pterygium syndrome. Journal of Medical Genetics 13(3): 249–251

Gleiser S, Weaver D D, Escobar V, Nicholas G, Escobedo M 1978 Femoral hypoplasia-unusual facies syndrome from another viewpoint. European Journal of Paediatrics 128: 1–5

Goldberg J H, Mazzei R J 1977 Poland syndrome: A concept of pathogenesis based on limb bud embryology. BDOAS 13(3D): 103–115

Goodman R M, Katznelson M, Hertz M, Katznelson A 1976 Camptodactyly with muscular hypoplasia, skeletal dysplasia and abnormal palmar creases: Tel Hashomer camptodactyly syndrome. Journal of Medical Genetics 13: 136–141

Goodman R M, Gorlin R J 1977 Atlas of the face in genetic disorders (2nd ed). Saint Louis: Mosby

Gorlin R, Sedano H, Cervenka J 1968 Popliteal pterygium syndrome. Pediatrics 41(2): 503–509

Gorlin R J 1970 Inheritance of the oto-palato-digital syndrome. Americal Journal of Diseases in Children 119: 377

Gorlin R J, Pindborg J J, Cohen M M 1976 Syndromes of the head and neck. McGraw Hill, New York (2nd ed)

Goutieres F, Aicardi J, Farkas E 1977 Anterior horn cell disease associated with pontocerebellar hypoplasia in infants. Journal of Neurology, Neurosurgery & Psychiatry 40: 370–378

Grosse F R, Pandel C, Wiedemann H 1975 The tetraphocomelia-cleft palate syndrome. Humangenetik 28: 353–356

Guha D K, Rashmi A, Khanduja P C, Kochhar M 1969 Intrauterine osteogenesis imperfecta with arthrogryposis multiplex and regional achondroplasia. Indian Pediatrics 6(12): 804–807

Hall J G, Reed S D, Greene G 1982 Distal arthrogryposis: A newly recognized condition with distal congenital contractures and its variants. American Journal of Medical Genetics (in press)

Hall J G, Reed S D, Rosenbaum K, Guershanik J, Chen H, Wilson K 1982 Distinguishing specific entities with limb ptergia: A report of eleven patients. American Journal of Medical Genetics (in press)

Hall J G, Reed S D, Driscoll E P 1982 Amyoplasia: A frequently seen sporadic condition with congenital contractures. American Journal of Medical Genetics (in press)

Hall J G, Hermann J, McGillivray B, Partington M, Schinzel A, Shapiro J, Reed S D 1982 Part II. Aymoplasia: Twinning in amyoplasia – a specific type of arthrogryposis with an apparent excess of discordant identical twins. American Journal of Medical Genetics (in press)

Hansen O H, Andersen O 1970 Congenital radio-ulnar synostosis. Acta Orthopaedica Scandinavica 41: 225–230

Hanson J, Jones K L, Smith D W 1976 Fetal alcohol syndrome: Experience with 41 patients. Journal of the American Medical Association 235: 1458–1460

Hanson P A, Martinez L B, Cassidy R 1977 Contractures, continuous muscle discharges and titubation. Annals of Neurology 1: 120–124

Harper P 1975 Congenital myotonic dystrophy in Britain. Archives of Disease in Childhood 50: 514

Hecht F 1969 Inability to open mouth fully: An autosomal dominant phenotype with facultative camptodactyly and short stature. BDOAS V(3): 96–102

Herrmann J 1974 Symphalangism and brachydactyly syndrome: Report of the WL symphalangism-brachydactyly syndrome: Review of literature and classification. BDOAS X(5): 23–53

Hollister D W, Rimoin D L, Lachman R, Cohen A, Reed W, Westin G 1974 The Winchester syndrome: A nonlysosomal connective tissue disease. Journal of Pediatrics 84(5): 701–709

Hook E B, Yunis J J 1965 Tris 18 syndrome in a patient with normal karyotype. Journal of the American Medical Association 193(10): 840–843

Hunter A G, Cox D W, Rudd N L 1976 The genetics of and associated clinical findings in humeroradial synostosis. Clinical Genetics 9: 470–478

Hunter A G W, Woerner S J, Montalvo-Hicks L D, Fowlow S B, Haslam R H, Metcalf P J, Lowry R B 1979 The Bowen-Conradi syndrome – a highly lethal autosomal recessive syndrome of microcephaly, micrognathia, low birth weight and joint deformities. American Journal of Medical Genetics 3: 269–279

Jones K L, Smith D W 1973 Recognition of the fetal alcohol syndrome in early infancy. Lancet II: 999–1001

Juberg R C 1969 A new familial syndrome of oral, cranial and digital anomalies. Journal of Pediatrics 74(5): 755–762

Kaufman R L, Rimoin D L, McAlister W H, Hartman A F 1974 Variable expression of Holt-Oram syndrome. American Journal of Diseases in Children 127: 21–25

Keutel J, Kindermann I, Möckell H: Eine wahrscheinlich autosomal recessiv verebte Skeletmissbildung mit Humeroradialsynostose. Humangenetik 9: 43–53

Khajavi A, Lachman R S, Rimoin D L, Schimke R N, Dorst J P, Ebbin A J, Handmaker S, Perrault G 1976 Heterogeneity in the campomelic syndromes: Long and short bone varieties. BDOAS 12(6): 93–100

Kibbe M H, Kaufman B, Funk R L 1965 Arthrogryposis multiplex congenita associated with Von Recklinghausen's disease. Virginian Medical Monthly 95: 344–350

Kim H J, Beratis N G, Brill P, Raab E, Hisrchorn K, Matalon R 1975 Kniest syndrome with dominant inheritance and mucopolysacchariduria. American Journal of Human Genetics 27: 755–764

Ladda R L, Stoltzfus E, Gordon S, Graham W 1978 Craniosynostosis associated with limb reduction malformations and cleft lip/palate: A distinct syndrome. Pediatrics 61(1): 12–15

Lambert D, Nivelon-Chevallier A, Chapuis J L 1977 Absence of DIP fold causing difficulty in extending fingers. Journal of Medical Genetics 14(6): 466–467

Lamy M, Maroteaux P 1960 Le nanisme diastrophique. Presse Médicale 68: 1977–1980

Latta R J, Graham C B, Aase J, Scham S M, Smith D W 1971 Larsen's syndrome: A skeletal dysplasia with multiple joint dislocations and unusual facies. Journal of Pediatrics 78: 291–298

Laxova R, Ohara P T, Timothy A D 1972 A further example of a lethal autosomal recessive condition in sibs. Journal of Mental Deficiency Research 16: 139–143

Lazjuk G I, Cherstvoy E D, Lurie I W, Nedzved M K 1978 Pulmonary hypoplasia, multiple ankyloses and camptodactyly: One syndrome or some related forms. Helvetica Paediatrica Acta 33: 73–79

Lazjuk G I, Lurie I W, Ostrowskaja T I, Cherstvoy E D, Kirillova I A, Nedzved M K, Usoev S S 1979 Brief clinical observation: The Neu-Laxova syndrome – a distinct entity. American Journal of Medical Genetics 3: 261–267

Liebenberg F 1973 A pedigree with unusual anomalies of the elbows, wrist and hands in five generations. South African Medical Journal 47: 745–748

Lowry R B, MacLean R, MacLean D M, Tischler B 1971 Cataracts, microcephaly, kyphosis and limited joint movement in two siblings: a new syndrome. Journal of Pediatrics 79: 282–284

Lucas G L 1967 Hereditary onycho osteodysplasia (nail-patella syndrome) masquerading as arthrogryposis. Southern Medical Journal 60: 751–755

Lurie I W, Cherstvoy E D, Lazjuk G I, Nedzved M K, Usoev S S 1976 Further evidence for AR inheritance of COFS syndrome. Clinical Genetics 10: 343–346

Mabry C, Barnett I, Hutcheson W, Sorenson H 1974 Trismus pseudocamptodactyly syndrome. Journal of Pediatrics 85(4): 503–508

MacLeod P, Patriquin H 1974 The whistling face syndrome – cranio-carpo-tarsal dysplasia. Clinical Pediatrics 13(2): 184–189

Maroteaux P, Bouvet J P, Briard M L 1972 La maladie des synostoses multiples. La Nouvelle Presse Medicale 45: 3041–3048

McComb R D, Markesbery W R, O'Connor W N 1979 Fatal neonatal nemaline myopathy with multiple anomalies. Journal of Pediatrics 94(1): 47–51

Mead C, Martin M 1963 Aplasia of the trochlea – an original mutation. Journal of Bone & Joint Surgery 45A(2): 379–382

Mietens C, Weber H 1966 A syndrome characterized by corneal opacity, nystagmus, flexion of elbows, growth failure and mental retardation. Journal of Pediatrics 69: 624–629

Miller J Q 1962 Lissencephaly in siblings. Neurology 12: 298

Mulvihill J J, Yeager A M 1976 Fetal alcohol syndrome. Teratology 13: 345–348

Mulvihill J J, Mulvihill C G, Priester W N 1980 Cleft palate in domestic animals: Epidemiologic features. Teratology 21: 109–112

Neu R 1971 A lethal syndrome of microcephaly with multiple congenital anomalies in three siblings. Pediatrics 47(3): 610–612

Neustein H S 1973 Neamline myopathy. Archives of Pathology 96: 192–195

Nezelof C, Dupart M, Jaubert F, Eliacha E 1979 A lethal familial syndrome associating arthrogryposis multiplex congenita, renal dysfunction and a cholestatic and pigmentary liver disease. Journal of Pediatrics: 258–260

Norman R M, Kay J M 1965 Cerebello-thalamo-spinal degeneration in infancy: An unusual variant of Werdnig-Hoffman disease. Archives of Disease in Childhood 40: 302–308

Norman R M 1961 Cerebellar hypoplasia in Werdnig-Hoffman disease. Archives of Disease in Childhood 36: 96–101

Opitz J M, Zurhein G, Vitale L, Shahidi N T, Howe J J, Chou S M, Shanklin D R, et al 1969 The Zellweger syndrome. BDOAS V(2): 144–160

Opitz J M, Kareggia E G 1974 Studies of malformation syndromes of man XXXIII: The FG syndrome. Z Kinderheilk 117: 1–18

Parker N 1963 Dystrophia myotonica presenting as congenital facial diplegia. Medical Journal of Australia 2: 939–944

Pashayan H, Dallaire L, McLeod P 1973 Bilateral aniridia, multiple webs and severe mental retardation in a 47,XXY/48,XXXY mosaic. Clinical Genetics 4: 125–129

Passarge E, Sutherland J M 1965 Potter's syndrome. American Journal of Diseases in Children 109: 80–84

Passarge E 1965 Congenital malformations and maternal diabetes. Lancet I: 324–325

Pena S D, Shokeir M 1970 Syndrome of camptodactyly, multiple ankyloses, facial anomalies and pulmonary hypoplasia – further delineation and evidence for autosomal recessive inheritance. BDOAS XII(5): 201–208

Pena S D J, Shokeir M H K 1974 Autosomal recessive cerebro-oculo-facio-skeletal syndrome. Clinical Genetics 5: 285–293

Pena S D, Shokeir M H 1976 Syndrome of camptodactyly, multiple ankyloses, facial anomalies and pulmonary hypoplasia – Further delineation and evidence for autosomal recessive inheritance. BDOAS XII(5): 201–208

Pena S D, Evans J, Hunter A G 1978 COFS syndrome revisited. BDOAS XIV(6B): 205–213

Petajan J H, Momberger G, Aase J 1969 Arthrogryposis syndrome. Kuskokwim disease in the eskimo. Journal of the American Medical Association 209(10): 1481

Pfeiffer R A, Ammerman M 1972 Das syndrom von Freeman and Sheldon. Zeitschrift für Kinderheilkunde 112: 43–53

Pillay V K 1964 Ophthalmo-mandibulo-melic dysplasia – a hereditary syndrome. Journal of Bone & Joint Surgery 46A: 858–862

Povysilová V, Macek M, Salichová J, Seemanova E 1976 Letál ni syndrom mnohocetnych malformaci u tři sourozencu. Ceskoslovenská Pediatrie 31: 190–194

Poznanski A K, Nosanchuk J S, Baublis J, Holt J F 1970 The cerebro-hepato-renal syndrome (CHRS) American Journal of Roentgenology, Radiotherapy & Nuclear Medicine 109(2): 313–322

Poznanski A K, Gall J C, Stern A M 1970 Skeletal manifestations of the Holt-Oram syndrome. Radiology 94: 45–53

Punnett H, Kistenmacher M L, Valdes-Dapena M, Ellison R T 1974 Syndrome of ankylosis, facial anomalies and pulmonary hypoplasia. Journal of Pediatrics 85: 375–377

Reeve R, Silver H, Ferrier P 1960 Marfan's syndrome (arachnodactyly) with arthrogryposis (amyoplasia congenita). American Journal of Diseases in Children 99: 101–106

Relkin R 1965 Arthrogryposis multiplex congenita Report of 2 cases, review of literature. American Journal of Medicine 39: 871–876

Riccardi V M 1977 The FG syndrome: Further characterization, report of a third family, and of a sporadic case. American Journal of Medical Genetics 1: 47–58

Rimoin D, Siggers D, Lachman R, Silberberg R 1976 Metatropic dwarfism, the Kneist syndrome and the pseudoachondroplastic dysplasias. Clinical Orthopedics 114: 70–82

Sack G 1978 A dominantly inherited form of arthrogryposis multiplex congenita with unusual dermatoglyphics. Clinical Genetics 14: 317–323

Sandbank U, Cohen L 1964 Arthrogryposis multiplex congenita associated with tuberous sclerosis. Journal of Pediatrics 64(4): 571–574

Sauk J J, Delaney J R, Reaume C, Brandjord R, Witkop C F 1974 Electromyography of oral-facial musculature in craniocarpaltarsal dysplasia (Freeman-Sheldon syndrome). Clinical Genetics 6: 132–137

Say B, Balci S, Atasu M 1973 Humeroradial synostosis. Humangenetik 19: 341–343

Schmitt H P 1978 Involvement of the larynx in a congenital 'myopathy' unilateral aplasia of the arytenoid, micrognathia and malformation of the brain – A new syndrome. Virchows Archiv für pathologische Anatomie und Physiologie und für Klinische Medizin 381: 85–96

Scott C I, Louro J M, Laurence K M, Tolarova M, Hall J G, Reed S D, Curry J R 1981 Comments on the New Laxova syndrome and CAD complex. American Journal of Medical Genetics 9: 165–175

Sharma N L, Anand J S 1964 Osteogenesis imperfecta with arthrogryposis multiplex congenita. Journal of the Indian Medical Association 43: 124–126

Shun-Shin M 1954 Congenital web formation. Journal Bone & Joing Surgery 36B(2): 268–271

Sillence D 1978 Brachydactyly, distal symphalangism, scoliosis, tall stature and club feet: A new syndrome. Journal of Medical Genetics 15: 208–211

Smith D W 1974 The VATER Association. American Journal of Diseases in Children 128: 767

Smith D W 1976 Recognizable patterns of human malformations. W B Saunders, Philadelphia

Smith R, Kaplan E 1968 Camptodactyly and similar atraumatic flexion deformities of the proximal interphalangeal joints of the fingers. Journal of Bone & Joint Surgery 50A(6): 1187–1203

Spranger J W, Schinzel A, Myers T, Ryan J, Giedion A, Opitz J 1980 Cerebro-arthro-digital syndrome. American Journal of Medical Genetics 5: 13–24

Spranger J W, Langer L O, Wiedemann H K 1974 Bone dysplasias. W B Saunders, Philadelphia

Sprofkin B E, Hillman J W 1956 Moebius syndrome: Congenital oculo-facial paralysis. Neurology 6: 50–54

Srivastava R 1968 Arthrogryposis multiplex congenita – case report of two siblings. Clinical Pediatrics 7(11): 691–694

Stewart J M, Bergstrom L 1971 Familial hand abnormality and sensorineural deafness – a new syndrome. Journal of Pediatrics 78: 102–110

Strňák V, Obereender H 1971 Über einen fall von agerborener synostosis humero-radialis bilateralis. Beiträge zur Orthopädie und Traumatologie 18(8): 460–464

Strasburger A K, Hawkins M R, Eldridge R, Hardgrave R L, McKusick V A 1965 Symphalangism: Genetic and clinical aspects. Bulletin of the Johns Hopkins Hospital 117: 108–127

Sugarman G I 1973 Syndrome of microcephaly, cataracts, kyphosis and joint contractures versus Cockayne's syndrome. Journal of Pediatrics 82: 351–352

Sutcliffe J 1966 Metaphyseal dyostosis. Annals of Radiology 9: 215–223

Taybi H 1962 Generalized skeletal dysplasia with multiple anomalies. American Journal of Roentgenology 88: 450–457

Taybi H 1975 Radiology of syndromes. Year Book Medical Publishers, Chicago

Temtamy S A, McKusick V A 1978 The genetics of hand malformations. BDOAS XIV(3)

Ter Haar B G A, Van Hoof R F 1974 The trismus-pseudocamptodactyly syndrome. Journal of Medical Genetics 11: 41–49

Thompson J S, McLaughlin P R, Heslin D J 1968 Impaired pronation-supination of the forearm: An inherited condition. Journal of Medical Genetics 5: 48–75

Thurmon T, Kityakara A 1973 Camptomelic Dwarfism. Journal of Pediatrics 83: 841–843

Urban M D, Rogers J G, Meyer W J 1979 Familial syndrome of mental retardation, short stature, contractures of the hands, and genital anomalies. Journal of Pediatrics 94(1): 52–55

Van Benthem L H, Driessen O, Haneveld G, Rietema H 1970 Cryptorchidism, chest deformities and other congenital anomalies in three brothers. Archives of Disease in Childhood 45: 590–592

Van Biervelt J P, Hendrickx G, van Ertbruggen I 1977 Intrauterine growth retardation with craniofacial and brain anomalies and arthrogryposis. Acta Paediatrica Belgica 30: 97–103

Ventruto V, Girolano R, Festa A, Romano A, Sebastio G, Sebastio L 1976 Family study of inherited syndrome with multiple congenital deformities: Symphalangism, carpal and tarsal fusion, brachydactyly, cranio-synostosis, strabismus, hip osteochondritis. Journal of Medical Genetics 13: 394–398

Walbaum R, LeJeune M, Poupard B, Lacheretz M, Fontaine G 1973 Le syndrome de Freeman-Sheldon (syndrome du Siffleur). Annals of Pediatrics 20: 357–364

Weaver D D, Graham C B, Thomas I T, Smith D W 1974 A new overgrowth syndrome with accelerated skeletal maturation, unusual facies and camptodactyly. Journal of Pediatrics 84: 547–552

Weckesser E, Reed J, Heiple K 1968 Congenital clasped thumb (congenital flexion adduction deformity of the thumb). Journal of Bone & Joint Surgery 50A(7): 1417–1428

Weinberg A G, Kirkpatrick J B 1975 Cerebellar hypoplasia in Werdnig-Hoffman disease. Developmental Medicine & Child Neurology 17: 511–516

White J W, Jenson W E 1952 The infant's persistent thumb – clutched hand. Journal of Bone & Joint Surgery 34A(3): 680–688

Williams R S, Holmes L B 1980 The syndrome of multiple ankyloses and facial anomalies. Acta Neuropathologica 50: 175–179

Winchester P, Grossman H, Lim W, Dounes B S 1969 A new acid mucopolysaccaridosis with skeletal deformities simulating rheumatoid arthritis. American Journal of Roentgenology 106: 121–128

Winter R M, Donna D, Crawford M D 1981 Syndromes of microcephaly, microphthalmia, cataracts, and joint contractures. Journal of Medical Genetics 18(2): 129–133

Wray J B, Herndon C N 1963 Hereditary transmission of congenital coalition of the calcaneus to the navicular. Journal of Bone & Joint Surgery 45A(2): 365–372

Wright D G, Aase J 1967 The Kuskokwim syndrome. Birth Defects V(3): 91–95

Yunis J J (ed) 1979 New Chromosomal Syndromes. Academic Press, New York

Zellweger H, Afifi A, McCormick W F, Mergner W 1967 Severe congenital muscular dystrophy. American Journal of Diseases in Children 114: 591–602

Zellweger H 1973 Early onset of myotonic dystrophy in infants. American Journal of Diseases in Children 125: 601–604

Zergollern L, Hitrec V 1976 Three siblings with Robert's syndrome. Clinical Genetics 9: 433–436

56

Common skeletal deformities

W.A. Horton

Familial aggregation of common skeletal deformities is well known. Often this is because the deformity is a component of a simply inherited syndrome, such as the scoliosis that usually occurs in diastrophic dysplasia, or the club foot that may be found in spondyloepiphyseal dysplasia congenita. Frequently, however, even after these syndromes have been excluded and only the idiopathic variety of the deformities is being considered, familial aggregation still exists. Much interest has been generated in attempting to define the role of genetic and nongenetic factors in these instances. Twin studies, family surveys, and analysis of individual pedigrees have been employed, and numerous potential environmental causes have been investigated. These various approaches have indicated that genetic factors play an important role in the aetiology of certain of the deformities, and in several instances, specific modes of inheritance have been identified. Genetic heterogeneity has frequently been uncovered. In certain cases, environmental factors have been incriminated and often their relationship to genetic predisposition defined. For some of them, however, the contribution of genetic factors remains undefined and in virtually all cases the precise mechanisms by which these factors predispose to the deformities are poorly understood. The goal of this chapter is to examine the current body of information concerning the inheritance of these common skeletal deformities.

IDIOPATHIC SCOLIOSIS

Scoliosis, curvature of the spine, results from a multitude of causes. Some of the more common ones include poliomyelitis with trunk paralysis, myelomeningocele, neurofibromatosis, and radiation therapy to one side of the trunk (Harrington, 1977). Scoliosis is also frequently associated with congenital anomalies, such as hemivertebrae, or abnormally segmented vertebral bodies and with certain of the skeletal dysplasias in which the spine is involved, such as the spondyloepiphyseal dysplasias and spondylometaphyseal dysplasias (Winter et al, 1968; Rimoin, 1975). In the vast majority of cases,

however, the aetiology is obscure, and the term idiopathic scoliosis is used.

The incidence of idiopathic scoliosis in the population varies considerably, ranging from 0.2 to 2–8% (Riseborough & Wynne-Davies, 1973; Harrington, 1977). It usually appears and shows the greatest progression during periods of rapid growth, infancy and adolescence. The process may begin during the juvenile period as well, but worsens during adolescence. In so-called infantile scoliosis, the curve usually appears during the first year of life, is typically to the left side, often resolves without treatment, and occurs most frequently in boys. It is common in Great Britain, comprising almost half of all cases of idiopathic scoliosis, but is uncommon in North America. Idiopathic scoliosis of the adolescent variety usually appears during the pubertal growth spurt, is to the right side and occurs predominantly in girls. Curves developing after the age of six years show the characteristics of adolescent scoliosis (Wynne-Davies, 1968).

Familial aggregation of idiopathic scoliosis has long been recognized. Many forms of inheritance have been postulated including autosomal dominant, X–linked dominant and multifactorial inheritance (Wynne-Davies, 1968; Filho & Thompson, 1971; Cowel et al, 1972; Riseborough & Wynne-Davies, 1973; Bonaiti et al, 1976; and Czeizel et al, 1978). Environmental factors also have been proposed to explain this phenomenon (DeGeorge & Fisher, 1967).

There have been many reports of twins with at least one member of the pair having scoliosis. Fisher and DeGeorge (1967) questioned the validity of those reported prior to 1967 because of insufficient radiographic studies. Those described after that time are listed in Table 56.1. Seventeen of the pairs exhibited adolescent scoliosis, while in one case (#18) it was the infantile variety. Seven of the pairs were monozygotic; all were concordant and all were female. Of the ten pairs of dizygotic twins with adolescent scoliosis, five were concordant, and five were discordant. In the latter group four were of unlike sex, and in three cases, it was the female who was affected. Thus, the concordance rate of 100% for monozygotic twins and 50% for dizygotic twins

Table 56.1 Twin studies in scoliosis*

Authors	Zygosity	Twin 1	Twin 2
1. Fisher & DeGeorge (1967)	MZ	F-A	F-A
2. Fisher & DeGeorge (1967)	MZ	F-A	F-A
3. Fisher & DeGeorge (1967)	MZ	F-A	F-A
4. Fisher & DeGeorge (1967)	MZ	F-A	F-A
5. Fisher & DeGeorge (1967)	MZ	F-A	F-A
6. Fisher & DeGeorge (1967)	MZ	F-A	F-A
7. Wynn-Davies (1968)	MZ	F-A	F-A
8. Fisher & DeGeorge (1967)	DZ	F-A	F-A
9. Fisher & DeGeorge (1967)	DZ	F-A	F-A
10. Fisher & DeGeorge (1967)	DZ	F-A	F-A
11. Fisher & DeGeorge (1967)	DZ	M-A	M-A
12. Wynne-Davies (1968)	DZ	M-A	M-U
13. Fisher & DeGeorge (1967)	DZ	F-A	M-A
14. Fisher & DeGeorge (1967)	DZ	F-A	M-U[†]
15. Fisher & DeGeorge (1967)	DZ	F-A	M-U
16. Fisher & DeGeorge (1967)	DZ	M-A	M-U[†]
17. Wynne & Davies (1968)	DZ	F-A	M-U
18. Wynne & Davies (1968)	DZ	M-A	F-U

* All cases were adolescent scoliosis except for # 18 in which
the affected boy had infantile scoliosis
† Curve of less than 10°
Abbreviations: MZ = monozygotic; DZ = dizygotic;
        F   = Female; M = Male; A = Affected;
        U   = Unaffected

with adolescent scoliosis illustrates the importance of genetic factors in the aetiology of the deformity. However, the marked preference for females indicates that the sex is a strong determinant as well. Similarly, the usual sex predilection for boys was observed in the one pair of infants with scoliosis.

A number of surveys have examined the incidence of scoliosis in family members (Table 55.2). They are difficult to compare because different methods and criteria for diagnosis were employed. For example, the diagnosis

was made by a questionnaire in the survey of DeGeorge and Fisher (1967), while X–rays were used by Cowel et al (1972) and photofluorography by Czeizel et al (1978). Moreover, although most of the surveys focused on adolescent scoliosis, some did not, such as the one of Wynne-Davies (1968) in which approximately half of the patients had infantile scoliosis. Despite these differences, the surveys showed similar trends. The parents and sibs of patients with scoliosis were affected much more frequently than the general population, the incidence ranging from 3 to 35% for parents and from 5 to 36% for sibs. Wynne-Davies (1968) noted that the percentage of relatives affected was lower in infantile scoliosis: 2.6% of first degree relatives of infantile scoliosis patients versus 12% in adolescent scoliosis. When the incidence of scoliosis among second and third degree relatives was examined, all the surveys showed a dramatic drop-off. Furthermore, females were consistently affected more often than males in all categories of relatives, and the frequency of affected relatives was the same for male and female probands (Riseborough & Wynne-Davies, 1973; Czeizel et al, 1978).

Several other observations were made in these surveys. For instance, plagiocephaly (molding of the head) was frequently present in patients with infantile scoliosis. It was on the same side as the curve and was transient in almost all cases (Wynne-Davies, 1968). 0ther abnormalities including mental retardation, epilepsy, club foot, inguinal hernia, upper limb deformities, cleft palate and a variety of congenital heart defects were observed in two surveys (Wynne-Davies, 1968; Riseborough & Wynne-Davies, 1973). However, except for the high incidence of scoliosis already mentioned, the frequency of the additional anomalies in relatives was the same as in the general population. A substantial elevation of maternal

Table 56.2 Scoliosis surveys in families

Author	DeGeorge & Fisher	Wynne-Davies	Filho & Thompson	Cowell et al	Riseborough & Wynne-Davies	Bonaiti et al	Czeizel et al
Year	1967	1968	1971	1972	1973	1976	1978
Location	New York	Edinburgh	Toronto	Wilmington	Boston	Paris	Budapest
No. probands	446	114	201	110	208	241	116
Method	Questionnaire	Exam	X–ray	X–ray	X–ray	Interview	Photofluoro-graphy,
Criteria		"rib hump"		10° curve	20° curve		10° curve
Incidence (%)							
Parents	19	3	6	35	11	7	3.4
(male/female)	(6/13)			(29/42)	(3/18)	(5/9)	(3/4)
Sibs	9	5	7	36	12	8	8
(male/female)					(4/17)	(5/12)	(7/10)
All relatives							
first degree			6.9	6.8	11.1	7.4	5.8
second degree			3.7	1.6	2.4	1.9	1.4
third degree			1.6	1.0	1.4	0.9	0.8

age was found for adolescent scoliosis in three of the surveys (DeGeorge & Fisher, 1967; Wynne-Davies, 1968; Riseborough & Wynne-Davies, 1973), but it was noted to be normal by Filho and Thompson (1971). Finally, Wynne-Davies (1968) observed several instances in which typical infantile and adolescent scoliosis occurred within the same family.

These surveys confirm that genetic factors are important in the aetiology of idiopathic scoliosis, especially in the adolescent variety (onset beyond 6 years). Moreover, the incidence figures in first degree relatives and rapid drop-off in second and third degree relatives indicate multifactorial inheritance. According to this model, the highest frequency of scoliosis should be found in the relatives of males, the least affected sex (Carter, 1965). However, the incidence of affected relatives was found to be approximately the same for affected males and females. The model also predicts that the frequency of affected relatives is related to the severity of the condition in the proband. This was not assessed in most of the surveys because of the numerous variables that influence the degree of scoliosis, such as age and treatment, although Czeizel et al (1978) showed a trend in this direction. In a small number of patients they also observed that the scoliotic curve was slightly greater in offspring of affected fathers compared to affected mothers and greater yet when both parents were affected.

There have also been many families reported in which members in several generations exhibited adolescent scoliosis (Garland, 1934; Gilly et al, 1963; Cowel et al, 1972; Robin & Cohen, 1975). Because no instance of male to male transmission was seen in seventeen families studied in depth, Cowel et al (1972) proposed X–linked dominant inheritance. Riseborough and Wynne-Davies (1973), however, challenged this interpretation because father to son transmission has been observed in the families described by the other authors, and it was also noted in one of their cases. Thus, families exhibiting autosomal dominant inheritance of scoliosis do exist.

In summary genetic factors appear to play a definite role in the causation of idiopathic scoliosis. The observation that infantile and adolescent scoliosis appear within the same families suggests that common genetic factors are involved in both, although they seem to be more important in the latter. Genetic heterogeneity exists with regard to adolescent scoliosis. In some families it appears to be transmitted as an autosomal dominant trait. In the majority, however, it seems to be inherited in a multifactorial manner. The female sex is a strong determinant in converting the genetic predisposition into clinical disease.

The mechanism through which genetic factors operate is unknown. An association between HLA-AW19 and scoliosis was reported by Bradford et al (1977a). Several investigators have observed abnormalities in collagen and proteoglycan (Ponseti et al, 1976; Bradford et al, 1977b; Francis et al, 1977; Bushell et al, 1978, 1979; Uden et al, 1980). In most of the studies, the biochemical alterations were most marked at the region of greatest spinal curvature making it difficult to determine if they were primary or secondary in nature. In one study, however, increased susceptibility of collagen to pepsin digestion was noted throughout the spine in patients with scoliosis compared to non-scoliotic individuals (Buschell et al, 1978, 1979). The authors proposed that the observation reflected a subtle collagen defect which predisposes to scoliosis. Such a defect might be inherited.

SPONDYLOLISTHESIS

The slippage of a vertebral body forward over the one below it is called spondylolisthesis. It most commonly involves the fifth lumbar vertebrae, although the fourth lumbar and occasionally other vertebrae may be affected. Patients usually are asymptomatic but may exhibit low back pain, stiffness or even neurologic symptoms (Haukipuro et al, 1978). In most instances the displacement is associated with and thought to be due to a defect in the pars interarticulars (posterior inferior process) of the vertebral arch (Wiltse, 1962). This defect is designated spondylolysis, and five types have been defined: dysplastic (congenital), isthmic, degenerative, traumatic, and pathologic, the most common being the isthmic type (Wiltse et al, 1976). Spina bifida occulta often accompanies the dysplastic type (Blackburne & Velikas, 1977).

Spondylolysis occurs in 4 to 8% of the general population over six years of age, whereas, spondylolisthesis is found approximately half as often (Haukipuro et al, 1978; Wynne-Davies & Scott, 1979). Familial aggregation of spondylolysis with and without displacement has been observed on several occasions. The dysplastic and isthmic forms of spondylolysis are found in these families. In reviewing the subject, spondylolysis Wynne-Davies and Scott (1979) noted that in most radiographic surveys of family members, about 27% of near relatives were affected. In their study, which was restricted to spondylolisthesis of the fifth lumbar vertebrae, 19% of relatives had spondylolysis. However, when subdivided according to the type of spondylolysis in the proband, 33 and 15% of relatives of patients with the dysplastic and isthmic forms respectively were affected. They also noted that the relatives sometimes had the opposite type of spondylolysis found in the index case.

Several individual families have been reported containing multiple affected members (Wiltse, 1962; Amuso & Mankin, 1967; Haukipuro et al, 1978; Shahriaree et al, 1979). Wiltse (1962) postulated autosomal recessive inheritance with incomplete penetrance, but most authors have concluded that autosomal dominant inheritance is more likely. In one study the penetrance was 75% for spondylolysis and approximately 30% of those patients showed some degree of slippage (Haukipuro et al, 1978).

The inherited abnormality appears to be a defect in the pars interarticularis of the vertebral arch. It can be either the dysplastic or isthmic type although the latter is more common (Wynne-Davies & Scott, 1979). Similarly, different vertebral bodies can be affected as evidenced by monozygotic twins who exhibited defects at different levels (Wiltse, 1962). Radiographically, the defects become evident between the ages of five and seven years (Wiltse, 1962). The process of fatigue fracture due to repeated stress and trauma, rather than an acute traumatic event, is thought to be responsible (Wiltse et al, 1975). The slippage, if it occurs, usually appears during adolescence concomitantly with the pubertal growth spurt. The displacement is greater if spina bifida occulta or other vertebral anomalies are present (Blackburn & Velikas, 1977). The occurrence of spina bifida seems to be aetiologically independent, however, since the incidence of spina bifida and other neutral tube defects is no greater in the patients' relatives than in the general population (Wynne-Davies & Scott, 1979).

CONGENITAL DISLOCATION OF THE HIP

Congenital dislocation of the hip (CDH) is characterized by the displacement of the femoral head outside the acetabulum prior to or slightly after birth. When lesser degrees of displacement occur so that the femoral head articulates with the outer margin of the acetabulum, the term congenital subluxation is used. Acetabular dysplasia refers to the development of an abnormally shallow acetabulum without actual displacement (Wedge & Wasylenko, 1978). CDH is a common birth defect but the incidence varies considerably throughout the world (Table 56.3), ranging from 0.6 per 1000 Caucasians living in Birmingham, England to 38 per 1000 North American Indians living in Arizona (Woolf et al, 1968). Although much of the discrepancy is due to different methods of ascertainment, criteria for diagnosis, etc, environmental and genetic factors are thought to be important as well. For example, CDH is more common in infants born in the winter months (Wynne-Davies, 1970; Bjerkreim & van der Hagen, 1974). Presumably, the wrapping of the child for warmth keeps the hips in the extended position in which dislocation is more likely. The practice of swaddling an infant to a cradle board with hips extended and adducted for the first few months of life is thought to account for the high incidence of CDH in certain American Indian groups (Carter & Wilkinson, 1964). Intrauterine posture is very important as well; both breech presentation and being the first infant

Table 56.3 Incidence of CDH

Location	Incidence (per 1000)
Birmingham, England	0.6
Oslo, Norway	1.0
Salford, England	1.6
New York City, USA	1.6
Malmo, Sweden	1.7
Salt Lake City, USA	9.1
Jerusalem, Israel	9.8
Budapest, Hungary	27.5
Arizona, USA (Navajo Indian)	38.0

born to a mother predispose to CDH (Wynne-Davies, 1970; Bjerkreim & van der Hagen, 1974). The female sex is perhaps the major determining factor. CDH occurs approximately six times as often in females as in males. It is though that the production of estrone by the fetal ovary and possibly relaxin by the fetal uterus, both of which increase ligamentous laxity, account for this sex predilection (Carter & Wilkinson, 1964; Woolf et al, 1968).

Familial aggregation of CDH has long been recognized. Twin studies have consistently shown a higher concordance rate for monzygotic than for dizygotic twins (Table 56.4). There have been several large surveys in which the incidence of CDH in relatives of probands with CDH has been determined (Table 56.5). In two of the recent studies the patients were divided into two groups: those having neonatal and those having late onset, depending upon whether the diagnosis was made before or after the age of four weeks. This was because prior to 1960 it was not appreciated that CDH could be diagnosed in the neonatal period; most cases were detected when the child began to walk. Thus the prior studies had dealt primarily with the late-onset type and it was not known if the patients diagnosed in the neonatal period represented the same or perhaps an aetiologically different group.

The incidence of CDH was found to be much higher in relatives of patients with CDH than in the general population in all of the surveys. For example, the incidence in sibs ranged from 2.2 to 14%, the highest being in Hungary, where the population incidence is high. In the two studies in which neonatal and late-onset CDH were separated, there were several instances in which both types were observed within the same family (Wynne-Davies, 1970; Bjerkreim & van der Hagen, 1974). Moreover, in one pair of dyzygotic twins, both types of CDH were found.

The sex preference for females was observed in affected sibs. For instance, the 5% of affected sibs reported by Record and Edwards (1958) was comprised of 1% brothers and 10% sisters. Similarly, the series of Carter and Wilkinson (1964) consisted of four per cent

Table 56.4 Twin studies in CDH

| Author (s) | Year | Concordance | |
		MZ	DZ
Idelberger	1951	10/29	3/109
Kanbara & Saskawa	1954	15/21*	3/6†
Wynne-Davies	1970	1/2	1/3
Czeizel et al	1975a	3/6	0/11

* Twins classified as monochorionic
† Twins classified as biovular
Abbreviations:
MZ = Monozygotic DZ = Dizygotic

Table 56.5 Family surveys of CDH

| Author (s) | Year | Type | Incidence (%) | | |
			Parents	Sibs	Children
Mueller & Seddon	1953	NS*	1.3	2.2	3.4
Record & Edwards	1958	NS		5.0	
Carter & Wilkinson	1964	NS		5.7	
Woolf et al	1968	NS	1.6	4.3	
Wynne-Davies	1970	neonatal	0.8	13.5	
		late onset	0.8	5.0	12.1
Bjerkreim & van der Hagen	1974	neonatal	1.8	6.0	
		late onset	2.7	8.5	
Czeizel et al†	1975a	NS	2.1	14.0	
		NS	2.3	14.0	

* NS = not specified
† Surveys at two locations reported

brothers and seven per cent affected sisters. In general the incidence of affected sibs was slightly greater when the proband was male (Woolf et al, 1968; Bjerkreim & van der Hagen, 1974; Cziezel et al, 1975a) as would be expected in polygenic inheritance. However, in the two surveys in which the data was subjected to statistical analysis, no significant difference was found (Wynne-Davies, 1970; Bjerkeim & van der Hagen, 1974). A dramatic dropoff in the incidence of CDH in second and third degree relatives compared to first degree relatives was observed by Wynne-Davies (1970), Bjerkreim and van der Hagen (1974), and Czietzel et al (1975a).

The genetic contribution to CDH appears to have two separate components. Based on the observation that the configuration of the acetabulum is determined by a multiple gene system (Record & Edwards, 1968), Carter and Wilkinson (1964) postulated that acetabular dysplasia inherited in this fashion interacted with ligamentous laxity, possibly transmitted as an autosomal dominant trait, to predispose an infant to CDH. Subsequent studies by Wynne-Davies (1970) and Cziezel et al (1975b) confirmed that 'normal' parents of children with CDH have acetabulae that measure radiographically to be more shallow than normal. In the first study the association was

noted only for late-onset type of CDH, however, it was observed in both types in the latter investigation.

Several studies have demonstrated the occurrence of generalized joint laxity in infants with CDH (Carter & Wilkinson, 1964a,b; Wynne-Davies, 1970; Cziezel et al, 1975b). This was observed especially for boys and, particularly, in the neonatal form. Furthermore, these studies showed that it was more common in family members than in the general population; but the mode of inheritance was difficult to determine, i.e. joint laxity is difficult to assess and quantitate and tends to decrease with age. Carter and Wilkinson (1963) postulated that this common form of joint laxity was an autosomal dominant trait. The basis for this speculation appears to have been a few families exhibiting autosomal dominant transmission of generalized joint laxity frequently associated with CDH (Carter & Sweetnam, 1958, 1960). Horton et al (1980), however, recently demonstrated that these particular families probably had a separate autosomal dominant trait which they termed familial joint instability syndrome. This syndrome can be distinguished from simple joint laxity as seen in CDH by its tendency to present at birth and its association with dislocation of several major joints in addition to the hip. Moreover, the incidence of CDH is approximately equal in males and females with this syndrome. Thus it is not clear if the joint laxity seen in typical CDH is truly an autosomal dominant trait as postulated or may be simply the extreme of normal joint mobility, possibly inherited in a polygenic fashion. In either case, simple familial joint laxity is very common. It occurs in five per cent of the normal population and conveys a small but definite risk for CDH (Carter & Wilkinson, 1964b; Wynne-Davies, 1970; Jessee et al, 1980).

Thus, CDH appears to be inherited as a multifactorial trait. Acetabular dysplasia transmitted in a polygenic manner and ligamentous laxity inherited in a polygenic or autosomal dominant fashion interact with a number of factors to bring about CDH. The other factors include female sex, which probably indicates it has a hormone basis, and others, as yet undefined, that influence the position of the hip before birth and during infancy. Although increased joint laxity may be associated with an early diagnosis and a shallow acetabulum with a later one, the two seem to act additively.

CLUB FOOT

Club foot is a relatively common congenital anomaly occurring at a rate of approximately one to three per 1000 live births (Cowel & Wein, 1980). It occurs as a component of a number of syndromes, especially those involving the nervous and connective tissue systems, but also as an isolated developmental anomaly, idiopathic congenital club foot. The idiopathic variety shows familial aggregation, but its inheritance is confusing. Many types of transmission including autosomal recessive, X–linked recessive, autosomal dominant, and multifactorial, have been proposed (Ching et al, 1969). Part of the confusion is due to the inclusion of patients with unrecognized syndromes in surveys of idiopathic congenital club foot. In addition, many investigators have considered club foot as a single entity, when in fact, it is comprised of three distinct anomalies: talipes equinovarus, talipes calcaneovalgus, and metatarsus varus. The limited number of genetic studies in which this heterogeneity has been appreciated have indicated that the three forms are separate entities (Palmer, 1964; Wynne-Davies, 1964; Ching et al, 1969; Palmer et al, 1974).

Talipes equinovarus

Talpies equinovarus is characterized by adduction of the forefoot, inversion of the heel and plantar flexion of the forefoot and ankle. It is seen in males approximately twice as often as in females and about 18% of patients exhibit additional minor abnormalities of connective tissues such as joint laxity, hernias, etc. (Wynne-Davies, 1964). In a study of 174 twin pairs, Idelberger (1939) reported the concordance to be 32% in monozygotic twins and 3% in dizygotic twins. In a survey of 110 families, Palmer (1964) described 43 families in which at least two members had the deformity. Noting instances in which multiple members and three generations of a family were affected, together with the occurrence of male to male transmission and an equal ratio of affected males to females, he suggested that autosomal dominant transmission with reduced penetrance was responsible for the deformity at least in certain families. A segregation analysis of data from many of these families and others ten years later (Palmer et al, 1974), however, suggested that multifactorial inheritance was more likely. The incidence in second and third degree relatives was higher than expected though. This mode of transmission was supported by studies done by Carter (1965) in which he found that the incidence of talipes equinovarus was 2.1, 0.61 and 0.20% in first, second and third degree relatives, respectively. In addition, a survey of relatives of 340 patients revealed that 2.9% of relatives had talipes equinovarus, while talipes calcaneovalgus and metatarsus varus were very infrequent (Wynne-Davis, 1964). Male relatives of affected females showed the highest rate. Thus, it appears that in most cases, talipes equinovarus is inherited in the multifactorial manner. The risk of recurrence to sibs is approximately 3% (Wynne-Davies, 1964; Palmer et al, 1974). Autosomal dominant inheritance cannot be excluded in some families.

Talipes calcaneovalgus

In this anomaly there is dorsal flexion of the forefoot and the plantar surface of the foot faces laterally. It is mild, often correcting spontaneously, and it occurs more often in girls, male: female ratio 0.61:1. It is frequently seen in first born children suggesting that uterine constraint might be an aetiologic factor. Like talipes equinovarus, other minor connective tissue abnormalities occur in approximately 18% of patients, especially congenital dislocation of the hip which was present in nearly 5% of patients. The incidence of affected sibs is 4.5% suggesting multifactorial inheritance (Wynne-Davies, 1964).

Metatarsus varus

Inversion and adduction of the forefoot are found alone in this anomaly. It resembles talipes calcaneovalgus in many respects. Often mild, it may go unnoticed. Girls are affected slightly more frequently than boys, and it is observed in approximately 4.5% of sibs. Again multifactorial inheritance is suggested. It differs, however, in that patients do not exhibit additional minor connective tissue abnormalities nor does there appear to be any excess of first born infants (Wynne-Davies, 1964).

JUVENILE OSTEOCHONDROSES

The juvenile osteochondroses are a group of disorders in which localized noninflammatory arthropathies result from regional disturbances of skeletal growth (Table 56.6). There is ischemic necrosis of either primary or secondary endochondral ossification centers (Pappas, 1967). Most of the abnormalities occur sporadically, but

Table 56.6 Juvenile osteochondroses

Region affected	Eponym	Inheritance
Capital femoral epiphysis	Legg-Perthes disease	–
Tibial tubercle	Osgood-Schlatter disease	–
Os calcis	Sever disease	–
Tarsal of navicular bone	Kohler disease	–
Head of second metatarsal	Freiberg disease	–
Vertebral bodies	Scheuerman disease	–
Medial aspect of proximal tibial epiphysis	Blount disease, tibia vara	AD
Subchondral areas of diarthroidal joints (particularly knee, hip, elbow and ankle)	Osteochondritis dissecans	AD
Capitellum of humerus	Panner disease	–
Patella	Larsen-Johansson disease	–

AD = Autosomal dominant

familial forms have been described. Legg-Perthes disease, osteonecrosis of the capital femoral epiphysis, has received the greatest attention. It has been reported as an autosomal dominant trait (Wamosher & Farhi, 1963),a sex influenced autosomal dominant trait with reduced penetrance (Wansbrough et al, 1959) and as a multifactorial trait (Gray et al, 1972). However, these studies were done, or in the case of Gray et al, data recorded, prior to the delineation of a number of simply inherited skeletal dysplasias which exhibit abnormal development of the capital femoral epiphyses. It seems likely that patients with these conditions may have been included in the studies, especially patients with the mild form of multiple epiphyseal dysplasia (Ribbing), an autosomal dominant trait in which involvement may be restricted to the capital femoral epiphyses (Rimoin, 1975). In the recent surveys in which attempts were made to exclude such patients (Fisher, 1972; Harper et al, 1976, and Wynne-Davies, 1978)the frequency in relatives was found to be very low; approximately one per cent of first degree relatives were affected and the incidence in second and third degree relatives approached that of the general population. Moreover, in the three pairs of unselected monozygotic twins reported, all were discordant for Legg-Perthes disease (Wynne-Davies, 1980). Thus in the vast majority of cases, this condition is not inherited.

Blount's diesease, a growth disturbance of the medial aspect of the proximal tibial growth plate, occurs in both infancy and adolescence. Pedigrees consistent with autosomal dominant transmission have been reported in the infantile form (Sibert & Bray, 1977). However, Bathfield and Beighton (1978) in a survey of 231 sibs of 110 patients with the infantile form found only 10 to be affected. They concluded that common environmental factors were largely responsible for the familial aggregation.

Osteochondritis dissecans involving multiple sites, especially the knees, hips, elbows and ankles has been reported as an autosomal dominant trait in several families (Stougaard, 1961; Hanley et al, 1967; Mubarak & Carroll, 1979).The condition is characterized by the separation of a small piece of articular cartilage and underlying bone to form a loose body within the joint. Overlap with other of the osteochondroses has been observed. For example, osteochondritis dissecans has been seen in patients with involvement of the tibial tubercle (Osgood-Schlatter disease), spine (Scheuermann's disease),the medial aspect of the proximal tibial epiphyses (adolescent Blount's disease), patella (Larsen-Johansson syndrome), and the capital femoral epiphyses (Legg-Perthe's disease) (Tobin, 1957; Hanley et al, 1967). Thus it appears to be a generalized disorder affecting growing epiphyses and may be inherited in some families.

REFERENCES

Amuso S J, Mankin H J 1967 Hereditary spondylolisthesis and spina bifida, report of a family in which the lesion is transmitted as an autosomal dominant through three generations. Journal of Bone and Joint Surgery 49A: 507–513

Bathfield C A, Beighton P H 1978 Blount disease, a review of etiological factors in 110 patients. Clinical Orthopedics and Related Research 135: 29–33

Bjerkreim I, van der Hagen C B 1974 Congenital dislocation of the hip joint in Norway. V. Evaluation of genetic and environmental factors. Clinical Genetics 5: 433–448

Blackburne J S, Velikas E P 1977 Spondylolisthesis in children and adolescents. Journal of Bone and Joint Surgery 59B: 490–494

Bonaiti C, Feingold J, Briard M L, Lapeyre F, Rigault P, Guivarch J 1976 Helv Paediatica Acta 31: 229–240

Bradford D S, Noreen H, Hallgren H M, Yunis E J 1977a Histocompatibility determinants in idiopathic scoliosis. Clinical Orthopaedics and Related Research 123: 261–265

Bradford D S, Oegema T R, Brown D M 1977b Studies on skin fibroblasts of patients with idiopathic scoliosis. Clinical Orthopaedics and Related Research 126: 111–118

Bushell G R, Ghosh P, Taylor T K F 1978 Collagen defect in idiopathic scoliosis. Lancet 2: 94–95

Bushell G R, Ghosh P, Taylor T K F, Sutherland J M 1979 The collagen of the intervertebral disc in adolescent idiopathic scoliosis. Journal of Bone and Joint Surgery 61B: 501–508

Carter C O 1965 The inheritance of common congenital

malformations. Progress in Medical Genetics 4: 59–84

Carter C, Sweetnam R 1958 Familial joint laxity and recurrent dislocation of the patella. Journal of Bone and Joint Surgery 40B: 664–667

Carter C, Sweetnam R 1960 Recurrent dislocation of the patella and of the shoulder, their association with familial joint laxity. Journal of Bone and Joint Surgery 42B: 721–727

Carter C O, Wilkinson J A 1964a Genetic and environmental factors in the etiology of congenital dislocation of the hip. Clinical Orthopedics and Related Research 33: 119–128

Carter C, Wilkinson J 1964b Persistent joint laxity and congenital dislocation of the hip. Journal of Bone and Joint Surgery 46B: 40–45

Ching G H S, Chung C S, Nemechek R W 1969 Genetic and epidemiological studies of clubfoot in Hawaii, ascertainment and incidence. American Journal of Human Genetics 21: 566–580

Cowell H R, Hall J N, Mac Ewen G D 1972 Genetic aspects of idiopathic scoliosis. Clinical Orthopedics and Related Research 86: 123–131

Cowell H R, Wein B K 1980 Genetic aspects of club foot. Journal of Bone and Joint Surgery 62A: 1381–1384

Czeizel A, Szentpetery J, Tusnady G, Vizkelety T 1975a Two family studies on congenital dislocation of the hip after early orthopedic screening in Hungary. Journal of Medical Genetics 12: 125–130

Czeizel A, Tusnady G, Vaczo G, Vizkelety T 1975b The

mechanism of genetic predisposition in congenital dislocation of the hip. Journal of Medical Genetics 12: 121–124

Czeizel A, Bellyei A, Barta O, Magda T, Molnar L 1978 Genetics of adolescent idiopathic scoliosis. Journal of Medical Genetics 15: 424–427

De George F V, Fisher R L 1967 Idiopathic scoliosis, genetic and environmental aspects. Journal of Medical Genetics 4: 251–257

Filho N A Thompson M W 1971 Genetic studies in scoliosis. Journal of Bone and Joint Surgery 53A: 199

Fisher R L 1972 An epidemiologic study of Legg-Perthes disease. Journal of Bone and Joint Surgery 54A: 769–778

Fisher R L, De George F V 1967 A twin study of idiopathic scoliosis. Clinical Orthopedics and Related Research 55: 117–126

Francis M J O, Smith R, Sanderson M C 1977 Collagen abnormalities in idiopathic adolescent scoliosis. Calc Tiss Res, 22: 381–384

Garland H G 1934 Hereditary scoliosis. British Medical Journal 1: 328

Gilly R, Stagnara P, Fredrich A, Dalloz C, Robert J M, Goldblatt B 1963 Les aspects medicaux de la scoliose structurale essentielle chez l'enfant. Lyon Med 95: 79–95

Gray I M, Lowrey R B, Renwick D H G 1972 Incidence and genetics of Legg-Perthes disease (osteochondritis deformans) in British Columbia, evidence of polygenic determination. Journal of Medical Genetics 9: 197–202

Hanley W B, McKusick V A, Barranco F T 1967 Osteochondritis dissecans with associated malformations in two brothers. Journal of Bone and Joint Surgery 49A: 925–937

Harrington P R 1977 The etiology of idiopathic scoliosis. Clinical Orthopedics and Related Research 126: 17–25

Harper P S, Brotherton B J, Cochlin D 1976 Genetic risks in Perthes disease. Clinical Genetics 10: 178–182

Hankipuro K, Keränen N, Koivisto E, Lindholm R, Norio R, Punto L 1978 Familial occurrence of lumbar spondylysis and spondylolisthesis. Clinical Genetics 13: 471–476

Horton W A, Collins D L, De Smet A A, Kennedy J A, Schimke R N 1980 Familial joint instability syndrome. American Journal of Medical Genetics 6: 221–228

Idelberger K 1939 Die Ergebnisse der zwillingeforschung beim angeborenen klumpfuss. Verh Deutsh-Orthop'ad Ges 33: 272–276

Idelberger K 1951 Die erbpathologic der sogenannten angeborenen H'uftverrenkung, M'unchen und Berlin. Urban & Schwarzenberg

Jessee E F, Owen D S, Sagar K B 1980 The benign hypermobile joint syndrome. Arth Rheum 23: 1053–1056

Kambara H, Sasakawa Y 1954 On twins with congenital dislocation of the hip. Journal of Bone and Joint Surgery 36A: 186–187

Mubarak S J, Carroll N C 1979 Familial osteochondritis dissecans of the knee. Clinics in Orthopedics and Related Research 140: 131–136

Muller G M, Seddon H J 1953 Late results of treatment of congenital dislocation of the hip. Journal of Bone and Joint Surgery 35B: 342–362

Palmer R M 1964 Hereditary club foot. Clinical Orthopedics 33: 138–146

Palmer R N, Conneally P M, Yu P L 1974 Studies of the inheritance of idiopathic talipes equinovarus. Orthopedic Clinics of North America 5: 99–108

Pappas A M 1967 The osteochondroses. Pediatric Clinics of North America 14: 549–570

Ponseti I V, Pedrini V, Wynne-Davies R, Duval-Beaupere G

1976 Pathogenesis of scoliosis. Clinical Orthopedics and Related Research 120: 268–280

Record R G, Edwards J H 1958 Environmental influences related to the aetiology of congenital dislocation of the hip. Brit J Prev Soc Med 12: 8–22

Rimoin D L 1975 The chondrodystrophies. Advances in Human Genetics 5: 1–118

Riseborough E J, Wynne-Davies R 1973 A genetic survey of idiopathic scoliosis in Boston, Massachusetts. Journal of Bone and Joint Surgery 55A: 974–982, 1973

Robin G C, Cohen T 1975 Familial scoliosis, a clinical report. Journal of Bone and Joint Surgery 57B: 146–147

Shahriaree H, Sajadi K, Rooholamini S A 1979 A family with spondylolisthesis. Journal of Bone and Joint Surgery 61A: 1256–1258

Sibert J R, Bray P T 1977 Probable dominant inheritance in Blount's disease. Clinical Genetics 11: 394–396

Stougaard J 1961 The hereditary factor in osteochondritis dissecans. Journal of Bone and Joint Surgery 43B: 256–258

Tobin W J 1975 Familial osteochondritis dissecans with associated tibia vara. Journal of Bone and Joint Surgery 39A: 1091–1105

Uden A, Nilsson I M, Willner S 1980 Collagen changes in congenital and idiopathic scoliosis. Acta Orthopedica Scandinavica 51: 271–274

Wamoscher Z, Farhi A 1963 Hereditary Legg-Calve-Perthes disease. American Journal of Diseases of Children 106: 131–134

Wansbrough R M, Carrie A W, Walker N F, Ruckerbauer G 1959 Coxa plana, its genetic aspects and results of treatment with the long Taylor walking caliper. Journal of Bone and Joint Surgery 41A: 135–146

Wedge J H, Wasylenko M J 1978 The natural history of congenital dislocation of the hip. Clinics in Orthopedics and Related Research 137: 154–162

Wiltse L L 1962 The etiology of spondylolisthesis. Journal of Bone and Joint Surgery 44A: 539–560

Wiltse L L, Widell E H, Jackson D W 1975 Fatigue fracture, the basic lesion in isthmic spondylolisthesis. Journal of Bone and Joint Surgery 57A: 17–22

Wiltse L L, Newman P H, Machab I 1976 Classification of spondylolisis and spondylolisthesis. Clinical Orthopedics and Related Research 117: 23–29

Winter R B, Moe J H, Eilers V E 1968 Congenitial scoliosis, a study of 234 patients treated and untreated. Journal of Bone and Joint Surgery 50A: 1–47

Woolf C M, Koehn J H, Coleman S S 1968 Congenital hip disease in Utah, the influence of genetic and nongenetic factors. American Journal of Human Genetics 20: 430–439

Wynne-Davies R 1964 Family studies and the cause of congenital club foot, talipes equinovarus, calcanovalgus and metatarsus varus. Journal of Bone and Joint Surgery 46B: 445–463

Wynne-Davies R 1968 Familial (idiopathic)scoliosis, a family survey. Journal of Bone and Joint Surgery 50B: 24–30

Wynne-Davies R 1970 A family study of neonatal and late-diagnosis congenital dislocation of the hip. Journal of Medical Genetics 7: 315–333

Wynne-Davies R 1980 Some etiologic factors in Perthes' disease. Clinical Orthopedics Related Research 150: 12–15

Wynne-Davies R, Gormley J 1978 The aetiology of Perthes' disease, genetic, epidemiological and growth factors in 310 Edinburg and Glasgow patients. Journal of Bone and Joint Surgery 60B: 6–14

Wynne-Davies R, Scott J H S 1979 Inheritance and spondylolisthesis, a radiographic family survey. Journal of Bone and Joint Surgery 61B: 301–305

Marfan syndrome

R. E. Pyeritz

HISTORICAL PERSPECTIVE

In 1896 the French pediatrician AB-J Marfan described a nearly six-year-old girl with long, thin limbs and fingers which he termed dolichostenomelia (Marfan, 1896); this girl also had multiple joint contractures and developed scoliosis. Several years later Achard (1902) described a patient who had losse-jointedness of the hands, hypognathism and dolichostenomelia and called the condition arachnodactyly. In retrospect, neither of these patients likely were affected by what now is called the classic Marfan syndrome. Over the next 40 years, the other features of the syndrome were coupled with the skeletal. In 1914, subluxation of the ocular lenses was associated with the dolichostenomelic habitus (Boerger, 1914), though two tall, loose-jointed sibs were noted to have ectopia lentis many years before (Williams, 1876). The heritable nature of the condition and primary involvement of tissue derived from embryonic mesoderm were first noted by Weve (1932) who also associated Marfan's name with the phenotype for the first time, calling the syndrome dystrophia mesodermalis congenita, typus Marfanis. The aortic complications of dissection and dilatation were clearly associated with the skeletal findings by Baer, Taussig and Oppenheimer (1943) and by Etter and Glover (1943), though reports of congenital heart disease and arachnodactyly had appeared previously (Salle, 1912; Piper & Irvine-Jones, 1926). McKusick (1955) drew wider attention to the spectrum of the cardiovascular problems encountered in living patients and postmortem specimens; of more fundamental importance was his labelling of the Marfan syndrome as a heritable disorder of connective tissue, the first of a long line of conditions to be so designated.

The clinical features, natural history and prognosis, and management of patients affected by the Marfan syndrome have been studied extensively in the past quarter-century, most notably by McKusick and colleagues (McKusick, 1972; Halpern et al, 1971; Murdoch et al, 1972A; Ose & McKusick, 1977; Pyeritz & McKusick, 1979; McDonald et al, 1981).

Marked clinical variability of skeletal manifestations led Murdoch and colleagues (1969) to separate a group of particularly loose-jointed patients into the marfanoid hypermobility syndrome. Beals and Hecht (1971) described the contractural arachnodactyly syndrome which they believe was the condition that affected Marfan's original patient.

Fair evidence exists that Abraham Lincoln, who was dolichostenomelic and loose-jointed, was affected by the Marfan syndrome (Gordon, 1962; Schwartz, 1964). A presently living direct descendant of Lincoln's uncle clearly has the condition. Some argue that Lincoln was in congestive heart failure, presumably secondary to aortic regurgitation, in the weeks before his assassination. The violinist Paganini was tall, asthenic, and loose-jointed and is said by some (Schoenfeld, 1978) to have been affected by the Marfan syndrome, though a type of Ehlers-Danlos syndrome is also a reasonable conjecture.

THE MARFAN PHENOTYPE

The Marfan syndrome is defined solely by clinical features and mode of inheritance at the present time. The most common clinical features comprising the phenotype appear in three systems: the skeletal; the ocular; and the cardiovascular. A summary of the most prevalent manifestations observed in 50 consecutive patients is shown in Table 57.1

Skeletal features: Mean height in the Marfan syndrome is greater than that of either unaffected sibs or the population average for similar sex, age, race and cultural background (Fig. 57.1). The limbs are disproportionately long compared with the trunk (dolichostenomelia). The increased length of the limbs may be estimated if the lower segment length (top of the pubic ramus to floor) is divided into the upper segment length (height minus lower segment). This US/LS ratio varies with age during normal growth but, in the person affected by the Marfan syndrome, is usually at least 2 standard deviations below the mean for age, race and sex (Fig. 57.2). The US/ LS ratio may be exaggerated by scoliosis or abnormal kyphosis. Arachnodactyly appears in numer-

Table 57.1 Features of the Marfan syndrome in 50 consecutive clinic patients. From Pyeritz and McKusick (1979)

Clinical feature	No. demonstrating feature
Ocular	35/50
ectopia lentis	30/50
myopia	17/50
Cardiovascular	49/50
mid-systolic click only	15/50
mid-systolic click & late systolic	
murmur	9/50
aortic regurgitant murmur	5/50
mitral regurgitant murmur only	3/50
prosthetic aortic valve	5/50
abnormal echocardiogram	48/50
aortic enlargement	42/50
mitral valve prolapse	29/50
prosthetic aortic valve	5/50
Musculoskeletal	50/50
arachnodactyly	44/50
arachnodactyly	44/50
US/LS 2SD below mean for age	36/47
pectus deformity	34/50
high, narrow palate	30/50
height >95 percentile for age	29/50
hyperextensible joints	28/50
vertebral column deformity	22/50
pes planus	22/50
Family history	40/47
additional documented cases of	
syndrome	40/47
sporadic cases (presumed new	
mutations)	7/47
unclear or unknown pedigree	3/50

ous other syndromes and remains in large part a subjective feature. Attempts to provide a radiographic criterion by means of the length-to-width ratio of hand bones (metacarpal index) have not demonstrated enough improvement in diagnostic power to justify the time, cost and radiation exposure (Eldridge, 1964; Emanuel et al, 1977). Simple manoeuvres such as the thumb sign (Steinberg, 1966) (positive if the thumb, when maximally opposed within the clenched hand, projects beyond the ulnar border, Fig. 57.3A) and the wrist sign (Walker & Murdoch, 1970) (positive if the distal phalanges of the first and fifth digits of one hand overlap when wrapped around the opposite wrist, Fig. 57.3B), are helpful when positive but are subject to observer interpretation and may reflect the longitudinal laxity of the hand rather than arachnodactyly.

Longitudinal overgrowth of the ribs produces anterior chest deformity, either depression (pectus excavatum or funnel chest, Fig. 57.4A) or protrusion (pectus carinatum or pigeon breast, Fig. 57.4B) of the sternum. Both defects may be present in the same patient. The chest is often asymmetric, with one set of costochondral junctions protruding more than the contralateral set. The

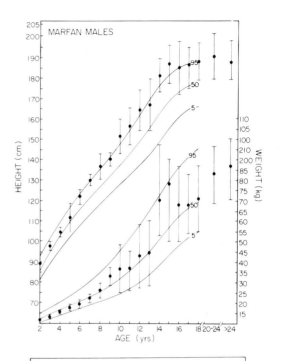

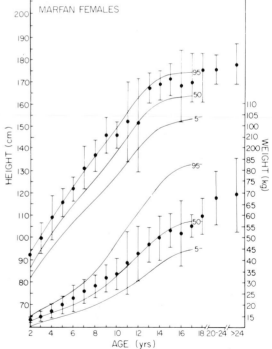

Fig 57.1 Growth in the Marfan syndrome. Plots of height and weight *vs* age for males (A) and females (B) who were not treated with hormones. Both cross-sectional and longitudinal data of about 200 caucasian patients were used in constructing these preliminary curves. The points show the means for persons grouped in one-year intervals and the bars show +/- one standard deviation. The curved lines show the 5, 50 and 95 percentiles of the unaffected population (adapted from National Center for Health Statistics Growth Charts, 1976).

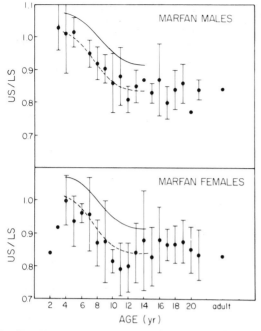

Fig. 57.2 Upper-to-lower segment ratios in the Marfan syndrome. The US/LS falls with increasing age through early puberty. The points show the means for caucasian patients grouped in one-year intervals and the bars show +/− one standard deviation. The solid curve is the mean and the dashed curve two standard deviations below the mean for unaffected caucasians (adapted from McKusick, 1972).

deformity is subject to considerable alteration during the time of rib growth.

Joint laxity is frequently present but has little diagnostic specificity. The fingers, wrists, elbows and knees (genu recurvatum) are commonly hyperextensible. Laxity of the carpal ligaments produces flat feet (pes planus, Fig. 57.5). Some patients have limited extension of fingers or elbows.

Scoliosis may occur at one or multiple sites along the vertebral column and generally worsens during periods of rapid growth, such as early adolescence (Robins et al, 1975). Mild degrees of curvature can best be appreciated clinically by observation of erect patients from behind as they bend forward at the hips with arms at full length and palms in contact; either the curve of the vertebral column will be more evident or one shoulder will be higher than the other. Thoracic scoliosis is usually obvious on the routine chest radiograph. Kyphosis of the thoracic or thoraco-lumbar region often accompanies scoliosis, but in many patients, even in the absence of scoliosis, a straightening of the usual mild thoracic kyphosis (straight-back syndrome) or even a thoracic lor-

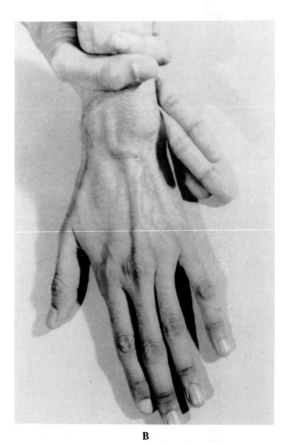

| A | B |

Fig. 57.3 Positive thumb (A) and wrist (B) signs in a 30-year-old man affected by the Marfan syndrome. Arachnodactyly is evident in 3B.

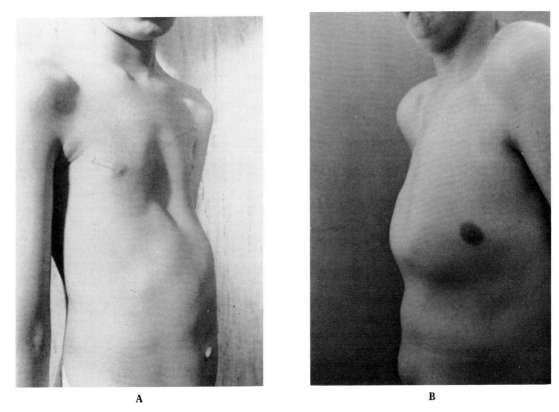

Fig. 57.4 Pectus excavatum (A) and carinatum (B) in the two young adolescent boys affected by the Marfan syndrome.

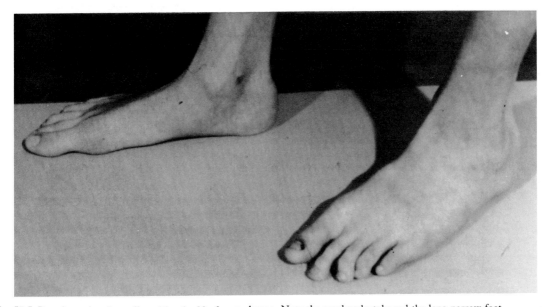

Fig. 57.5 Pes planus in a boy affected by the Marfan syndrome. Note the arachnodactyly and the long narrow foot.

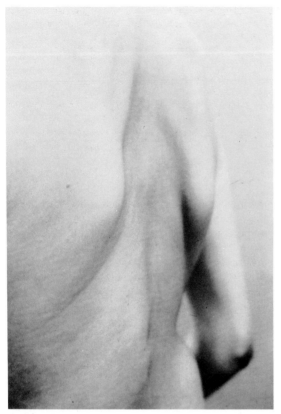

Fig. 57.6 Thoracic lordosis in the Marfan syndrome. The adolescent boy has a reversal of the usual thoracic kyphotic curve, resulting in a reduction of the antero-posterior diameter of the thorax. This type deformity is present in the 'straight back syndrome.'

dosis occurs, resulting in a reduced anteroposterior diameter of the chest (Fig. 57.6).

The hard palate is often narrow and highly-arched, being described as 'gothic,' resulting in crowding of the teeth and malocclusion.

Ocular manifestations: Subluxation of the lens (ectopia lentis) occurs in a proportion of cases variously estimated between 50 and 80%, is usually bilateral, and rarely progresses (McKusick, 1972; Cross & Jensen, 1975; Pyeritz & McKusick, 1979; Maumanee IH, personal communication). The lens is most commonly displaced upward, and the zonules remain intact, permitting normal accomodation (Fig. 57.7). Subluxation is usually present at the time of the first detailed ophthalmologic examination (Cross & Jensen, 1975) suggesting that the displacement frequently occurs in utero. Occasionally, the lens in the Marfan syndrome will dislocate into the anterior chamber (commonly as a result of trauma) and produce acute glaucoma. Most cases of glaucoma follow surgical extirpation of the lens (Cross & Jensen, 1975). A subluxed ocular lens is often not visible with the direct ophthalmoscope, but iridodenesis usually provides a clue to lens displacement. Any patient suspected of the Marfan syndrome must undergo a slit lamp examination with the pupils fully dilated.

The axial length of the globe is increased, contributing to myopia, an increased risk of retinal detachment, and lens subluxation (Table 57.2). As with glaucoma, the prevalence of retinal detachment increases following lens extraction (Maumanee IH, personal communication).

Studies of corneal shape (keratometry) show that

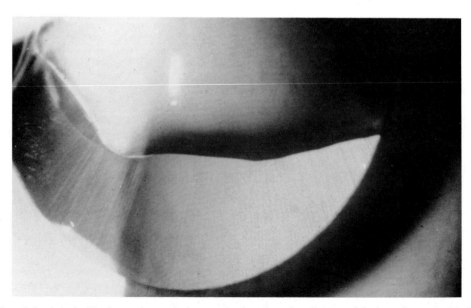

Fig. 57.7 Ectopia lentis in the Marfan syndrome. A photograph taken through a slit lamp of the lens of a young girl. The lens is dislocated superotemporally. Note the zonules which are stretched but intact.

Table 57.2 Axial length of the ocular globe in the Marfan syndrome (Adapted from I. H. Maumanee, Thesis, American Ophthalmological Society, 1981)

Age (yrs)	No. eyes measured	Mean length (mm ± S.D)
1–8	20	23.5 ± 0.8
9–14	23	24.5
15+	43	25.3 ± 2.50
All ages		
Without lens subluxation		23.4
With lens subluxation		26.0 (p<0.01)

Normal eyes have a mean axial length of 23 mm at age 3 yrs and between 23.5–24.7 mm at ages over 15 yrs.

Table 57.3 Corneal shape in the Marfan syndrome (Adapted from I. H. Maumanee, Thesis, American Ophthalmological Society, 1981)

Age (yr)	No. eyes measured	Mean keratometer reading (diopter ± S.D)
1–8	37	40.9 ± 2.4
9–14	28	40.8 ± 2.3
15+	72	41.9 ± 1.7

Normal, adult eyes have mean keratometer readings of 43.7 ± 0.2.

nearly all patients with the Marfan syndrome have relatively flat corneas (Table 57.3).

Myopia is frequent and may appear early and be severe. While abnormalities of the globe, retina, lens and cornea all may impair vision, a flat cornea tends to correct myopia.

Cardiovascular manifestations: The two most common cardiovascular features of the Marfan syndrome are mitral valve prolapse and dilatation of the ascending aorta. The former may result in mitral regurgitation while the latter may result in aortic regurgitation and predispose to aortic rupture or dissection. The mean age of death is reduced by 30-40% in persons affected by the Marfan syndrome and nearly all of the precocious deaths result from a cardiovascular complication (Murdoch et al, 1972a).

About 60% of patients have auscultatory signs of mitral or aortic valve pathology, but the rest have normal cardiovascular physical findings (Table 57.1; Brown et al, 1975; Pyeritz; et al, 1979).

Echocardiography has greatly enhanced the detection of the cardiovascular abnormalities, with a concomitant improvement in the ability to diagnose the Marfan syndrome. For example, whereas about one-third of the patients have single or multiple systolic clicks or systolic murmurs of presumed mitral origin, echocardiography shows that over 80% of all Marfan patients, irrespective of age or sex, have prolapse of at least the posterior mitral leaflet (Brown et al, 1975; Pyeritz et al, 1979; Pyeritz & McKusick, 1979). The prolapse is often pansystolic, with exaggerated leaflet excursion suggesting redundancy of valvular tissue.

The one-dimensional echocardiographic picture of the Marfan aorta is characteristic (Fig. 57.8). First, in both

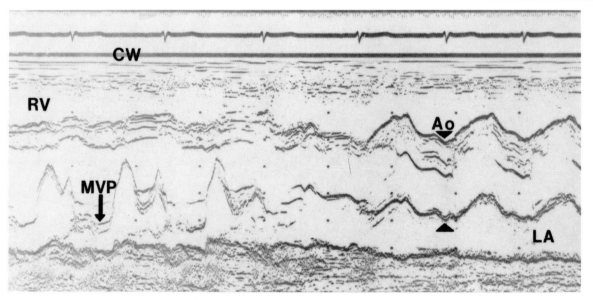

Fig. 57.8 Echocardiogram showing mitral valve prolapse and aortic dilatation. This 8-year-old boy had a normal clinical examination – no clicks or murmurs. Both leaflets of the mitral valve prolapse in mid-systole (M V P). The aortic root (Ao) has a diameter of 2.8 cm, greater than the upper limit of normal for either age or body surface. The right ventricle (R V, left atrium (L A) and chest wall (C W) are indicated.

children and adults, the diameter of the aortic root measured at the level of the aortic valve cusps is nearly always greater than the upper limit of the normal range, based on body-surface area. Second, the diameter of the aorta often increases in the region of the aortic valve and above. Third, if the root is moderately dilated, during mechanical systole the posterior aortic wall may paradoxically move posteriorly and the aortic cusps partially close. Rarely will a person in whom the diagnosis of the Marfan syndrome is strongly suspected on other grounds (skeletal, ocular, and auscultatory) have none of these echocardiographic abnormalities. In 5% of patients with the Marfan syndrome, a technically satisfactory echocardiogram is unobtainable, usually because of a severe pectus deformity or emphysema.

Cross-sectional echocardiography often displays the ascending aorta for a distance of 4-6 cm above the aortic valve (Pyeritz et al, 1980A). Computerized tomography or digital subtraction angiography may prove to be accurate methods for diagnosing and following aortic root size, but have not yet been adequately evaluated.

The chest radiograph is an insensitive technique for detecting early aortic root enlargement. Dilatation of the proximal ascending aorta is visible on the frontal radiograph only when substantial; mild to moderate enlargement is frequently hidden by the vertebral column and cardiac silhouette (Fig. 57.9).

No typical electrocardiographic abnormalities occur. Changes result from the chronic valvular regurgitation, usually after these lesions are clinically recognizable.

Axis deviations occur because of rotation of the heart by severe pectus excavatum or thoracic lordosis.

On aortography, the dilated Marfan aorta is characteristic (Fig. 57.10). The enlargement is symmetric and begins in the sinuses of Valsalva. Rarely does the dilatation extend as far as the innominate artery, and the ascending aorta has a gourd-like appearance when contrast material is injected.

Other clinical features: The predominant abnormality of the skin is the stria distensa, most commonly found over the shoulders and buttocks (Fig. 57:11A & B). Striae gravidarum can be marked in women affected by the Marfan syndrome. The skin is otherwise not unusually fragile or susceptible to bruising or poor healing. Frequently hernias occur, especially in the inguinal region. They may appear in early childhood, and a history of multiple repairs is not uncommon.

A number of case reports document the occurence of spontaneous pneumothorax and congenital lung abnormalities in Marfan patients (Bolande & Tucker, 1964; Lipton et al, 1971; Turner & Stanley, 1976). The prevalence of pneumothorax, bullous emphysema or other pulmonary problems in the Marfan syndrome is unknown.

Some patients have markedly reduced total lung capacity and residual volume ascribable to deforming kyphoscoliosis or pectus excavatum. Even in patients without thoracic distortion, forced vital capacity is consistently less than predicted (Pyeritz et al, unpublished).

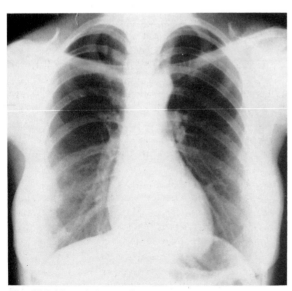

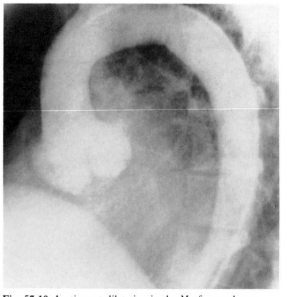

Fig. 57.9 Normal chest radiograph in the presence of aortic root dilatation. The proximal aorta of this 28-year-old woman affected by the Marfan syndrome measured 4:8 cm, nearly 50% greater than normal. This enlargement is hidden by the cardiac silhouette.

Fig. 57.10 Aortic root dilatation in the Marfan syndrome. The sinuses of Valsalva are symmetrically dilated to a moderate degree in this 37-year-old woman. While no aortic regurgitation is present, severe mitral regurgitation necessitated valve replacement in this patient.

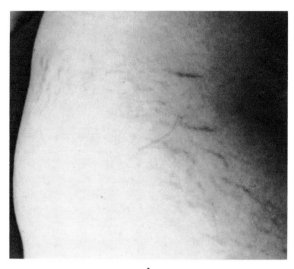

A

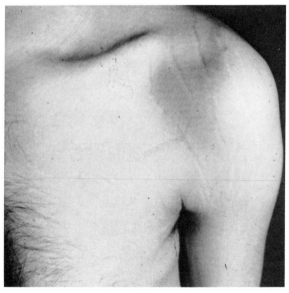

B

Fig. 57.11 Striae distensae in the Marfan syndrome. These characteristic skin lesions appear and expand with age. Striae usually first appear over the hips (A, an eight-year-old girl) and often occur over the shoulders (B, a 30-year-old man).

DIAGNOSIS

Each of the clinical features of the Marfan syndrome occurs with variable frequency in the general population. It is to be expected that several will occur together occasionally by chance alone. In determining which of such individuals are affected by a systemic connective tissue disorder, more diagnostic reliance is placed on the pres-

ence of hard manifestations (subluxed lenses, aortic dilatation, severe kyphoscoliosis and asymmetric deformity of the anterior chest) then on soft features (myopia, mitral prolapse, tall stature, joint laxity and arachnodactyly). Exceptional cases, such as an individual with ectopia lentis and an aneurysm of the ascending aorta with a normal habitus and a negative family history may rate the diagnosis of the Marfan syndrome, even though only two criteria are present. On the other hand, the familial occurrence of scoliosis, pectus excavatum, and mitral valve prolapse merits consideration of the Marfan syndrome because three of the criteria are present, but may well represent the mitral valve prolapse syndrome (Bon Tempo et al, 1975; Pyeritz et al, 1979 B; Pyeritz & McKusick, 1979).

Two laboratory test are required of any person in whom the Marfan diagnosis is suspected: slit lamp examination and one-dimensional echocardiography. The former is to establish whether ectopia lentis is present. Echocardiography is needed to determine if mitral valve prolapse and aortic root dilatation are present.

No single laboratory test can establish the diagnosis of the Marfan syndrome. No biochemical tests have proven to be either sensitive or specific for the Marfan syndrome.

Conditions which must be excluded routinely when considering the diagnosis of the Marfan syndrome include: homocystinuria; contractural arachnodactyly; marfanoid hypermobility syndrome; a number of the Ehlers-Danlos variants; and familial mitral valve prolapse. A variety of other conditions include one or more of the clinical features of the Marfan syndrome, but rarely would be confused; these are listed in Table 57:4.

Homocystinuria must be excluded in any patient thought to have the Marfan syndrome because the pleiotropic manifestations of the two conditions include the same organ systems. Homocystinuria is ruled-out by a negative cyanide-nitroprusside test of the urine, an easy screening test for disulfide accumulation; positive reactions necessitate further evaluation by quantitative amino acid analysis of urine and plasma (Mudd & Levy, 1978).

Contractural arachnodactyly and marfanoid hypermobility syndromes pose the same diagnostic problems as the Marfan syndrome, because of similar pleiotropic manifestations and extensive clinical variability. Some patients who clearly have the Marfan syndrome also have congenital contractures and abnormal ears (Pyeritz RE & Rosenbaum KN, unpublished).

Patients with Ehlers-Danlos Types I, II, or III may be asthenic and (rarely) have ectopia lentis(McKusick, 1972; Byers et al). Aortic dilatation and mitral valve prolapse occur frequently but the actual prevalence is unknown. Generally, the body proportions are not disturbed as in the Marfan syndrome. Severe joint laxity and skin elasticity argued against the Marfan syndrome.

Table 57.4 Clinical features common to both the Marfan syndrome and other syndromes (Adapted from Pyeritz et al, 1979B)

Skeletal
homocystinuria
congenital contractural arachnodactyly
marfanoid hypermobility syndrome
osteogenesis imperfecta
mitral valve prolapse syndrome
pseudoxanthoma elasticum
eunuchoidism or delayed puberty
Klinefelter syndrome (47,XXY)
trisomy 8 (47,XX or XY, +8)
Goodman camptodactyly syndrome B
Stickler syndrome
syndrome of nerve deafness, eye anomalies, and marfanoid habitus
nemaline myopathy
syndrome of pigmentary degeneration, cataract, microcephaly and arachnodactyly
myotonic dystrophy
multiple endocrine adenomatosis, type III
fragilitas oculi
Archard syndrome

Ocular
homocystinuria
familial ectopia lentis
Weill-Marchesani syndrome
Ehlers-Danlos syndrome, type VI
congenital contractural arachnodactyly
Marfanoid hypermobility syndrome
Stickler syndrome

Cardiovascular
syphilitic aortitis
Ehlers-Danlos syndromes, types I-IV and other variants
congenital contractural arachnodactyly
marfanoid hypermobility syndrome
familial bicuspid aortic valve
mitral valve prolapse syndrome
osteogenesis imperfecta
Erdheim cystic medial necrosis
relapsing polychondritis
ankylosing spondylitis
Reiter syndrome

Persons with the mitral valve prolapse syndrome lack ocular or aortic involvement but often have scoliosis, thoracic lordosis, asthenia, and pectus excavatum; these features are heritable as an autosomal dominant trait.

Genetic heterogeneity undoubtedly exists in the Marfan syndrome (McKusick, 1972; Pyeritz et al, 1979B). Discovery of a biochemical abnormality in one patient will enable definitive diagnosis in relatives; the same abnormality may not occur in another affected family and thus be of limited diagnostic utility.

The potential for diagnosing autosomal dominant conditions by linkage with restriction fragment length polymorphisms (RFLP) is exciting but untested (Botstein et al, 1980). With this method, the basic abnormality need not be known, so long as the phenotype is linked with a RFLP. Since only small amounts of DNA are needed to map RFLP, prenatal diagnosis by analysis of aminocyte DNA will be possible. At the present time, no method for prenatal diagnosis exists.

NATURAL HISTORY AND PROGNOSIS

Skeletal At birth affected children tend to be longer than normal, a discrepancy which persists, though the growth rate is no greater than their unaffected peers. The reduced upper to lower segment ratio compared with the normal population persists with increasing age (Fig. 57.3). The anterior chest deformity can change markedly during the course of growth of the ribs. A mild pectus excavatum in an infant can worsen in a matter of a few years, become asymmetric, and partially convert to a carinatum defect.

Joint laxity can lead to recurrent dislocation, most commonly of the first metacarpal-phalangeal joint and the patella. Laxity of the ankle and foot produces instability and various foot deformities in addition to pes planus. If they are untreated at an early age, severe lifelong gait disturbances can result. Pes cavus may occasionally develop. Joint laxity of the fingers, elbows and knees often lessens with age. Degenerative arthritic changes are commonplace in later life in joints that were once particularly lax. Protrusio acetabuli may be more frequent in the Marfan syndrome (Wenger et al, 1980) but the natural history and functional disability of this hip abnormality are undefined.

Scoliosis develops gradually, but progresses most rapidly during the adolescent growth spurt (Robins et al, 1975; Tolo VT, personal communication).

Ocular Sublaxation of the lens usually does not progress. Because the zonules remain intact, there is little tendency for the lens to migrate into either the anterior or posterior humors (Cross & Jensen, 1975). When the lens is present retinal detachments rarely occur; however, once the lens is extirpated, retinal detachment becomes much more common (Maumanee IH, personal communication). The degree of myopia may change substantially during the time of growth as various ocular structures change shape.

Cardiovascular Mitral valve prolapse may not be clinically or echocardiographically present during infancy but be noted several years later. The degree of prolapse, though difficult to evaluate noninvasively, may worsen with age. Mitral regurgitation does appear and progress hemodynamically in some patients who initially had only prolapse. Even in children the mitral regurgitation can become severe enough to warrant valve replacement (Phornphutkul et al, 1973; Soman et al, 1974; Friedman et al, 1978).

The size of the aortic root relative to body surface area

is generally larger than normal even in infancy and increases with age at a rate greater than normal. Moreover, aortic root dilatation does not cease at skeletal maturity. The aortic root enlarges symmetrically in the sinus of Valsalva region and for a short distance above the sinotubular ridge. The so-called annulus of the aortic valve may also dilate; however, it is the dilatation in the region of the sinotubular ridge that results in eventual failure of the cusps of the aortic valve to appose (Pyeritz et al, 1980B). As the aorta continues to dilate, the regurgitant flow increases. The left ventricular response to aortic regurgitation in the Marfan syndrome is qualitatively similar to that with other causes of chronic aortic regurgitation, but the following sequence of events may evolve more rapidly in the Marfan syndorme. The left ventricle dilates to compensate for the increased stroke volume required. Eventually the myocardium begins to fail and irreversible myopathic changes follow. The end-stage, if dissection or rupture of the aorta does not supervene, is death from congestive heart failure (McKusick, 1955).

The dilated ascending aorta is more susceptible than the undilated aorta to traumatic dissection or rupture (McDonald et al, 1981). Numerous cases of dissection or rupture, often associated with sudden death, have occurred in persons affected by the Marfan syndrome while they were playing contact sports such as basketball (Maron et al, 1980) or when they were involved in relatively minor deceleration injuries in automobile accidents.

Numerous case reports describe the rupture or dissection of the aorta and other large arteries in pregnant women affected by the Marfan syndrome. Because of the increase in cardiac output which occurs during the midtrimester, the dilated ascending aorta is under more strain than in the nonpregnant condition. The largest retrospective survey examined 105 pregnancies in 26 Marfan women. Only one death occurred, that due to endocarditis in a women with severe mitral valve disease which predated the pregnancy (McKusick, 1972; Pyeritz, 1981).

The records of 257 Marfan patients in the Johns Hopkins Hospital files were examined for life expectancy and causes of death (Murdoch et al, 1972). The study was performed at a time when medical and surgical therapy had virtually no beneficial impact on patient survival. Survival had fallen to 50% for men at age 40 years and for women at age 48 years, a reduction in expected life span of about 30-40% for both sexes.

The mean age of death of the 72 deceased patients was 32 years. The immediate cause of death was a cardiovascular complication in over 90%. Dissection or rupture of the aorta and chronic aortic regurgitation with congestive heart failure accounted for the vast majority of the deaths.

PATHOGENESIS

Numerous investigations of the biochemistry of tissues obtained from Marfan patients have failed to elucidate the underlying basic defects(s) or even establish reproducibly associated changes. It long has been supposed that the clinical features will be explicable by some abnormality in connective tissue, and research has focused on the proteins that occur in connective tissue, particularly collagen and elastin.

The fraction of collagen solubilized by standard extraction procedures is increased in biopsy specimens or fibroblast cultures obtained from Marfan patients (Macek et al, 1966; Laitinen et al, 1968; Priest et al, 1973). The resistance to denaturation of collagen types extracted from skin is not significantly different between Marfan samples and controls (Francis et al, 1974).

Marfan patients have long been known to excrete excess hydroxyproline (Prockop & Sjoerdsma, 1961). Excretion is increased in other abnormalities as well and during periods of rapid growth in normal people, while most adult Marfan patients have normal levels of urinary hydroxproline.

Cultured fibroblasts from the Marfan patients accumulate hyaluronic acid (Matalon & Dorfman, 1968). This accumulation is due to an increased rate of synthesis rather than defective degradation (Lamberg & Dorfman, 1973: Horwitz et al, 1979). A number of enzymes that are important in carbohydrate metabolism and which might be involved in post-translational modification of connective-tissue proteins have normal activity in Marfan fibroblasts (Matalon & Dorfman, 1968).

Marfan patients excrete less peptides containing desmosine in the urine (King & Starcher, 1979). Since desmosine arises only during the formation of lysyl-derived cross-links in elastin, these data provide indirect evidence for elastin involvement.

One patient had an abnormality of the alpha-2 chain of type I collagen detected by electrophoresis (Scheck et al, 1979). Analysis of cyanogen bromide-cleaved peptides showed an amino acid insertion in the helical portion of the chain; the triple helix of the collagen molecule was not destabilized, however (Byers et al, 1981). Eleven other patients were studied and did not have this defect. This insertion may represent one of the biochemical defects which produces the Marfan phenotype.

No consistent abnormalities of karyotype have appeared in Marfan patients.

Several animal models may have pertinence to the pathogenesis of the Marfan syndrome in humans. Feeding rats the lathyritic agent beta-aminoproprionitrile (BAPN) produces a phenotype resembling the Marfan syndrome with kyphoscoliosis, hernias, and aneurysms of the aorta. Dissection of the aorta in turkeys can be produced by adding BAPN to the feed (Barnett et al, 1957).

Copper deficiency in swine or fowl leads to aortic rupture (O'Dell et al, 1961). The histopathology and ultrastructure of the aortic wall in the Marfan syndrome, copper-deficient chicks, and BAPN-treated turkeys are similar (Simpson et al, 1980).

The primary defect in the Marfan syndrome is likely not to be an enzymopathy which (by gross phenotype) are nearly always mendelian recessive traits. A defect in the primary, secondary, or tertiary structure of a protein which results in the phenotype when the effective number of functional molecules is reduced seems more likely at this time.

GENETICS

A great many families in which multiple individuals affected by the Marfan syndrome occur have been studied (McKusick, 1972). The phenotype is equally prevalent and severe in males and females. Multiple generations are affected in some families; in some the phenotype can be traced through six generations. Male-to-male transmission occurs. All of these characteristics are consistent with autosomal dominant inheritance.

Reports of multiple affected sibs with ostensibly normal parents are rare and in no cases have both the parents been examined with sufficient detail to exclude their being mildly affected. Consanguinity has not been reported in these families.

No formal studies of the frequency of sporadic cases or of the evolutionary (or genetic) fitness of the Marfan syndrome have been published. McKusick (1972) estimated that 15% of patients had unaffected parents and most likely developed the Marfan syndrome form *de novo* mutation in a parental germ cell. Recently in our medical genetics clinic, of 138 consecutive Marfan patients, 41 had neither parent affected. While various biases may be reflected in which patients attend a clinic, these figures suggest that sporadic cases account for 15–30% of all patients. The average age of the fathers of such sporadic cases exceeds by some 7 years that of fathers in the general population (Murdoch et al, 1972B); the average age of the mothers of sporadic cases is not as advanced. This paternal age effect has been described in other autosomal dominant disorders such as achondroplasia. The progenitor cells of spermatozoa in the testes of older fathers have a longer time during which to mutate, through either exposure to mutagens or DNA replication errors, and for mutations to accumulate, since each mitosis of a mutated spermatogonia returns a replicated cell to the progenitor pool.

The marked degree of variability of expression of the Marfan gene undoubtedly explains the claims of 'nonpenetrance' which appear in the older literature. When presumed cases of 'nonpenetrance' or 'formes fruste' occurring in families in which other, well-documented cases of the Marfan syndrome occur are examined by sensitive methods (such as echocardiography), the assignment of the Marfan gene can be made with confidence (Pyeritz et al, 1979B).

The chromosomal location of a genetic locus determining the Marfan phenotype is unknown. The only attempts to determine a map position have been by means of linkage analysis.

Several studies examined linkage between the Marfan phenotype and a variety of blood group antigens and serum protein markers. Two earlier studies found no suspicions of linkage (Lynas & Merritt, 1958; Schleuterman et al, 1976). A recent study of a different population found a suggestion of linkage between the Marfan phenotype and Rh. The lod score was $+1.17$ at a recombination fraction of 0.30 (Mace, 1979).

The technique of linkage-analysis using restriction fragment length polymorphisms (Boststein et al, 1980) may provide evidence for the chromosomal location of genes capable of producing the Marfan phenotype before the biochemical defects are discovered.

PREVALENCE

Based on what was thought to be complete ascertainment of the phenotype in Northern Ireland, the mutation rate of the 'Marfan locus' was calculated (Lynas & Merritt, 1958). From this figure a minimal prevalence of 1-2 cases per 100 000 population was derived. The majority of cases of the Marfan syndrome followed at the Johns Hopkins Hospital live in the surrounding geographic area. Based on crude calculations of the size of this catchment area and the number of Marfan patients in the files, the prevalence was estimated as 4-6/100 000 (Pyeritz & Mckusick, 1979).

Since the manifestations of the Marfan syndrome may extend from the limits of the normal to the floridly 'classic' case in which the diagnosis is unquestionable, the actual prevalence of the Marfan syndrome may exceed the above estimate.

The Marfan syndrome probably occurs in all races and in all major ethnic groups that reside in the United States. Relative prevalences in ethnic groups elsewhere are unknown. Nothing is known about the geographic distribution of the Marfan syndrome, but no predilection is obvious in the United States.

PATHOLOGY

Gross pathology

Numerous reports of autopsies of patients affected by the Marfan syndrome appear in the literature (see McKusick (1972) for review). The aorta dilates in its most proximal region, the sinuses of Valsalva. The dilatation is symmetric and may extend above the sinotubular junction. The diameter of the ascending aorta usually returns to normal before the innominate artery, unless a DeBakey Type I dissection is present. The region of the upper aortic valve attachments is often the most widely dilated, resulting in failure of the cusps to coapt.

When dissection of the aorta occurs, the entry tear in the intima is frequently several centimetres above the aortic valve, in the area of greatest dilatation. Usually, when the aorta is not greatly dilated, dissections begin in the proximal ascending aorta. The dissection can either progress antegrade no further than the arch (DeBakey Type II) progress through the arch into the descending aorta (DeBakey Type I), or extend retrograde. In the latter case, attachments of the coronary arteries may be torn and the dissection may rupture into the pericardial sac producing tamponade. Any of these dissections can undergo rapid or gradual, stuttering evolution. Intimal tears in the absence of dissection are common in the dilated proximal ascending aorta.

The valve cusps are usually diaphanous and redundant. Fenestrations occur in a minority of aortic and mitral valve cusps. The aortic and mitral valves are prone to the development of bacterial endocarditis.

The pulmonary artery occasionally dilates in the proximal region.

Aneurysmal dilatation of coronary arteries has been reported but is uncommon. The coronary ostia may be abnormally positioned, either high in the aortic root or low because of the root dilatation.

No specific changes occur in the atria, ventricles or myocardium that are not attributable to the effects of chronic valvular regurgitation. Several patients have had clinical congestive heart failure out of proportion to their valvular disease and the existence of a cardiopathy associated with the Marfan syndrome has been suggested. Histopathologic studies of such patients are lacking.

Reports of gross ocular pathology are few and little can be said other than that the lenses tend to dislocate superiorly, the globes tend to be elongated in the antero-posterior direction, and the corneas are flatter than normal.

Published reports of gross pathology of bone, ligaments, and tendons show no particular abnormalities.

Histology and ultrastructure

The aortic wall characteristically shows most changes in the medial layer. The elastic fibers become progressively swollen, fragmented and reduced in number as the aortic diameter increases (Fig. 57.12). Lacunae appear in the media which are filled with a basophilic material, most likely proteoglycan. The term 'cystic medial necrosis' has been applied to these histologic changes, but is a misnomer and its use to be discouraged. Neither cysts nor necrosis are present. These histopathologic features are also seen in aortas from non-Marfan patients who had hypertension or aortic valve disease. The most reasonable

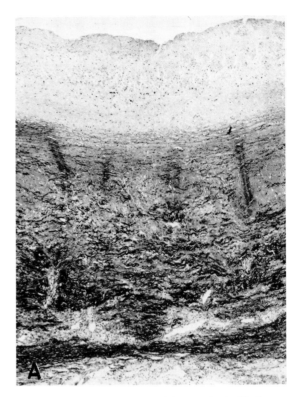

Fig. 57.12 Medial degeneration of the aorta in the Marfan syndrome.

explanation is that the histopathology indicates injury and repair regardless of the cause of the injury (Schlatmann & Becker, 1977). Electron microscopic examination confirms focal elastin fibre degeneration and associated abnormalities of collagen fibers (Scheck et al, 1979). The medial smooth muscle fibers appear shrunken and their basement membrane is greatly thickened. Other studies describe evidence of increased metabolic activity of smooth muscle cells (Scheck et al 1979).

Arteries elsewhere in the body may show evidence of medial disorganization but less than that present in the ascending aorta.

The aortic and mitral valve usually show myxomatous degenerative changes.

Cartilage biopsies from the iliac crest in three adolescent patients were examined by transmission electron microscopy. The chondrocytes had dilated endoplasmic recticulum, cytoplasmic vacuoles and increased glycogen stores (Nogami et al, 1979). Few reports of histologic changes in other tissues exist.

MANAGEMENT

No specific therapy exists for the underlying defect in the Marfan syndrome. Therapeutic efforts are directed at first establishing an accurate diagnosis, determining which problems are present at the time of diagnosis, anticipating the problems which will likely arise in the future, and pursuing certain prophylactic measures for specific problems. The patients should have one physician, knowledgeable about the syndrome, who serves as the primary physician, referring to subspecialists as need arises. The multidisciplinary approach is often best conducted in the setting of the academic medical institution.

Skeletal

All children with any evidence of abnormal spinal curvature and all adults with a progressive deformity should be evaluated by an orthopaedist semi-annually. Scoliosis greater than 20 degrees in children should be pursued aggressively with mechanical bracing and physical therapy. Spinal surgery is necessary when bracing fails to halt progression and in curves of greater than 45 degrees (Tolo VT, personal communication).

Scoliosis tends to progress most during rapid growth, especially in early adolescence. If this adolescent growth spurt can be shortened the scoliosis may not progress so far. A second benefit of decreasing the length of time that the bones have to elongate is a reduction in adult body height. Girls can be treated before menarche with oestrogen on a daily basis to induce puberty and epiphyseal closure. Progestogen is added five days each cycle to prevent dysfunctional bleeding. No conclusive data are yet available to show whether scoliosis is abated by this approach. Adult height has clearly been reduced in women who begin therapy before the menarche (Fig. 57.13).

Other orthopaedic problems associated with joint instability should be managed by an orthopaedic surgeon familiar with connective tissue disorders. The major indication for repair of anterior chest deformity is cardiopulmonary compromise. The proper age at which to perform repair of pectus excavatum and the long-term results have not been established. Repairs early in life provide many years for rib growth to depress the sternum and re-establish the deformity (Fig. 57.14).

Ocular

The patient should be evaluated annually by an ophthalmologist experienced in connective tissue disorders. Emphasis should fall on the correction of amblyopia, the direction and degree of lens subluxation, anterior chamber abnormalities, and detection of retinal detachment. The earliest symptoms of retinal detachment and the necessity of immediately seeking consultation should be explained to patients and their families. The subluxed lens rarely requires extirpation, except when adequate correction of visual acuity is impossible or in the rare instance of displacement into the anterior chamber.

Cardiovascular

The frequency of cardiologic evaluation depends on the

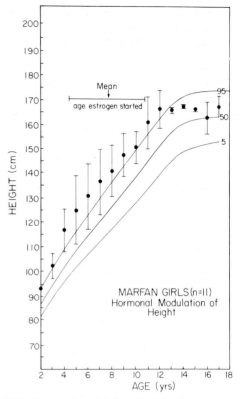

Fig. 57.13 Hormonal modulation of height in girls affected by the Marfan syndrome. In all cases treatment with ethinyl estradiol (0.05 mg/10 kg daily) and conjugated estrogen (Premarin^R, 10 mg on days 25–28 each menstrual cycle) was begun before menarche. Therapy was continued until the time menarche was likely to have occurred naturally or until bone maturation was well-advanced, whichever occurred first. Comparison with Figure 57: 1B shows early cessation of growth and reduction in height of the treated girls.

severity of the manifestation. If the patient has only mitral valve prolapse and a mildly dilated aorta without any valvular regurgitation, then an annual examination including an echocardiogram and EKG is sufficient. As the aorta dilates and as valvular regurgitiation appears and progresses, more frequent examinations are indicated.

The dilated aorta is susceptible to rupture or dissection, either spontaneously or following modest trauma. The shearing forces of ventricular ejection may be the driving forces behind dissection and dilatation. For these reasons, some restriction of patient activity seems warranted. Patients should not engage in contact sports, activities requiring maximal exertion or isometric exercise.

The use of propranolol to delay or prevent severe aortic complications rests on several premises, as yet unproven (Halpern et al, 1971; Pyeritz & McKusick, 1979; Pyeritz, 1980A). The first premise is that the risk of an aortic complication is proportionate to the diameter of the aorta. In most cases, aortic regurgitation results from streching of the upper valve cusp attachments at the sino-tubular junction. Likewise, since rupture and dissection depend on the tension or stress on the aortic wall, Laplace's relationship (wall tension is directly proportional to blood pressure and aortic radius and inversely proportional to wall thickness) applies (Pyeritz, 1980A). The second premise is that the ascending aortic dilatation is due to the repeated impulse of left ventricular ejection buffeting the intrinsically weak aortic wall. The final premise is that aortic enlargement can be prevented by reducing the static and dynamic forces acting on the proximal aorta. These premises led to the proposition that reducing stress on the proximal aorta over a long period of time would reduce the morbidity and mortality of the Marfan syndrome (Halpern et al, 1971). Propranolol reduces the rate of systolic aortic pressure rise through blockage of the beta-1 adrenergic receptors. Aortic dissection in turkeys, either spontaneous or induced by lathyritic agents, is preventable by oral administration of propranolol, independent of any effect on heart rate or blood pressure (Simpson et al, 1968). Early results of propranolol therapy in a small group of Marfan patients, most of whom had aortic regurgitation, were not encouraging (Ose & McKusick, 1977). Most of the subjects went on to die suddenly or require surgery. In retrospect the tension on the aortic wall, because of pre-existing dilatation, was already great, and propranolol likely had little effect. A prospective randomized trial of propranolol in patients of all ages is underway (Pyeritz, 1980A).

Surgical correction of the aorta and aortic valve is required in an acute emergency due to rupture, dissection, and severe left ventricular decompensation, when early signs of left ventricular strain appear in the presence of aortic regurgitation, and for substantial enlargement of the aorta even if the aortic regurgitation is mild (Pyeritz, 1980A; McDonald et al, 1981). Some patients require mitral valve replacement alone or in addition to aortic surgery. Use of a composite graft of prosthetic aortic valve sutured into one end of a prosphetic conduit has resulted in a dramatic decrease in perioperative mortality of aortic surgery in the Marfan syndrome (McDonald et al, 1981; Miller et al, 1980).

All patients are at risk of endocarditis regardless of whether demonstrable valvular abnormalities exist. They should be instructed in routine antibiotic prophylaxis with dental and genitourinary procedures.

Counselling

The major issue in genetic counselling is straight-forward, each affected person having a 50 % probability of passing the gene to any offspring irrespective of sex. When the Marfan syndrome is diagnosed in a young child and the family history is negative, the parents must be counseled about the risk of having subsequent affected children. Both parents must be carefully examined to insure that neither has signs of the Marfan gene before assurances are given that the risk that future offspring will be affected is slight.

Women affected by the Marfan syndrome must deal with two concerns. The first is the 50% risk that any offspring will inherit the syndrome. The second concerns the risk of cardiovascular problems during pregnancy. As described above, women without pre-existing murmurs do well during pregnancy (Pyeritz, 1981). Nonetheless, any woman who has echocardiographic evidence of moderate aortic dilatation should be counselled against pregnancy. Women who do decide to become pregnant are treated as high-risk pregnancies. Hospitalization during the final trimester and cesarean section are not routinely necessary.

Parents should be counseled about the range of intrafamilial variability possible in the Marfan syndrome. Affected offspring may be more or less severely involved than their parents.

Prevention

The only method of preventing the Marfan syndrome is through reproductive abstinence by affected parents. Even then, many new cases will appear through spontaneous mutation.

Prenatal diagnosis

No method now exists for prenatal diagnosis of the Marfan syndrome. The potential exists for prenatal diagnosis based either on a biochemical defect expressed in amniocytes or on linkage with restriction fragment length polymorphisms (Botstein et al, 1980).

REFERENCES

Achard C 1902 Arachnodactylie. Bullitens et Mémoires de la Societe Médicales Hôpital (Paris) 19: 834

Baer R W, Taussig H B, Oppenheimer E H 1943 Congenital aneurysmal dilatation of the aorta associated with arachnodactyly. Bulletin of the Hopkins Hospital 72: 309–331

Barnett B D, Bird R H, Lalich J J 1957 Toxicity of beta-aminoproprinoitrile for turkey poults. Proceedings of the Society for Experimental Biology and Medicine 94: 67–70

Beals R K, Hecht F 1971 Congenital contractural arachnodactyly: a heritable disorder of connective tissue. Journal of Bone and Joint Surgery 53A: 987–993

Boerger F 1914 Uber zwei von Arachnodaktyllie. Zeitschrift für Kinderheilk 12: 171

Bolande R P, Tucker A S 1964 Pulmonary emphysema and other cardiorespiratory lesions as part of the Marfan abiotrophy. Pediatrics 33: 356–366

Botstein D, White R L, Skolnick M, Davis R W 1980 Construction of a genetic linkage map in man using restriction fragment length polymorphism. American Journal of Human Genetics 32: 314–331

Brown O R, DeMots H, Kloster F E, Roberts A, Menashe V D, Beals R K 1975 Aortic root dilatation and mitral valve prolapse in Marfan's syndrome: an echocardiographic study. Circulation 47: 587–596

Cross H E, Jensen A D 1975 Ocular manifestations in the Marfan syndrome and homocystinuria. American Journal of Ophthalmology 75: 405–420

Eldridge R 1964 The metacarpal index: a useful aid in the diagnosis of the Marfan syndrome. Archives of Internal Medicine 113: 248–254

Emanuel R, Ng R A L, Marcomichekalis J et al 1977 Formes frustes of Marfan's syndrome presenting with severe aortic regurgitation: clinicogenetic study of 18 families. British Heart Journal 39: 190–197

Etter L E, Glover L P 1943 Arachnodactyly complicated by dislocated lens and death from rupture of dissecting aneurysm of the aorta. Journal of the American Medical Association 123: 88

Francis M J O, Sanderson M C, Smith R 1974 Skin collagen in idiopathic adolescent scoliosis and Marfan's syndrome. Clinical Science and Molecular Medicine 51: 467–474

Friedman S, Edmunds H L, Cuasco C C 1978 Long-term valve replacement in young children. Circulation 57: 981–986

Gordon A M 1962 Abraham Lincoln – a medical appraisal. Journal of the Kentucky Medical Association 60: 249

Halpern B L, Char F, Murdoch J L et al 1971 A prospectus on the prevention of aortic rupture in the Marfan syndrome with data on survivorship without treatment. Johns Hopkins Medical Journal 129: 123-129

Horwitz A, Appel A, Arcilla R A 1979 Hyaluronic acid production by cultured fibroblasts in Marfan syndrome (abst). Circulation 252: 59–60

King G S, Starcher B C 1979 Elastin catabolism: measurement of urine desmosine by radioimmunoassay. Clinical Research 27: 705A

Laitinen O, Uitto J, Iivananinen M et al 1968 Collagen metabolism of the skin in Marfan's syndrome. Clinical Chimica Acta 21: 321

Lamberg S I, Dorfman A 1973 Synthesis and degradation of hyaluronic acid in the cultured fibroblasts of Marfan's disease. Journal of Clinical Investigation 52: 2428–2433

Leier C V, Call T D, Fulkerson P K, Wooley C F 1980 The spectrum of cardiac defects in the Ehlers-Danlos syndrome. Annals of Intern Medicine 92: 171–178

Lipton R A, Greenwold R A, Seriff N S 1971 Pneumothorax and bilateral honeycombed lung in Marfan syndrome: report of a case and review of the pulmonary abnormalities in this disorder. American Review of Respiratory Disease 104: 924–928

Lynas N A, Merritt A D 1958 Marfan's syndrome in Northern Ireland. Annals of Human Genetics 22: 310

Mace M: (1979) A suggestion of linkage between the Marfan syndrome and the rhesus blood group. Clinical Genetics 16: 96–102

Marfan A B 1896 Un cas de déformation congénitale des quatre membres plus prononcée aux extrémitiés charactérisée par l'allongement des os avec un certain degré d' amonassement. Bullitens et Mémoires de la Societe Médicales Hôpital (Paris) 13: 220

Maron B J, Roberts W C, McAllister H A, et al 1980 Sudden death in young athletes. Circulation 62: 218–229

Matalon R, Dorfman A 1968 The accumulation of hyaluronic acid in cultured fibroblasts of the Marfan syndrome. Biochemistry and Biophysics Research Communications 32: 150–154

Maumanee I H 1981 The eye in the Marfan syndrome (thesis) American Ophthalmologic Society

McDonald G, Schaff H V, Pyeritz R E, McKusick V A, Gott V L 1981 Surgical management of patients with the Marfan syndrome and dilation of the ascending aorta. Journal of Thoracic and Cardiovascular Surgery 81: 180-186

McKusick V A 1955 The cardiovascular aspects of Marfan's syndrome: a heritable disorder of connective tissue. Circulation 11: 321–341

McKusick V A 1972 The Marfan syndrome. In: Heritable Disorders of Connective Tissue. 4th ed St. Louis Mosby pp 61–223

Mecek M, Hurych J, Chuapil M et al 1966 Study on fibroblasts on Marfan's syndrome. Humangenetik 3: 87

Miller C D, Stinson E B, Oyer P E, Moreno-Cabral R J, Reitz B A, Rossiter S J, Shumway N E (1980) Concomitant resection of ascending aorta aneruysm and replacement of the aortic valve. Journal of Thoracic and Cardiovascular Surgery 79: 388–401

Mudd S H, Levy H L 1978 Disorders of transulfuration. In: Stanbury J et al (eds) Metabolic Basis of Inherited Disease. New York McGraw-Hill pp 458–503

Murdoch J L, Walker B A, Halpern B L et al 1972 A Life expectancy and causes of death in the Marfan syndrome. New England Journal of Medicine 286: 804–808

Murdoch J L, Walker B A, McKusick V A 1972B Parental age effects on the occurrence of new mutations for the Marfan syndrome. Annals of Human Genetics 35: 331–336

Nogami H, Oohira A, Ozeki K, Oki T, Ogino T, Murachi S 1979 Ultrastructure of cartilage in heritable disorders of connective tissue. Clinical Orthopaedics 143: 251–259

O'Dell B L, Harfwick B L, Reynolds G, et al 1961 Connective tissue defect in the chick resulting from copper deficiency. Proceedings for the Society of Experimental Biology and Medicine 108: 402–405

Ose L, McKusick V A 1977 Prophyláctic use of propranolol in the Marfan syndrome to prevent aortic dissection. Birth Defects 13(3C): 163–169

Phornphutkol C, Rosenthal A, Nadas A C 1973 Cardiac manifestations of Marfan syndrome in infancy and childhood. Circulation 47: 587–596

Piper R K, Irvine-Jones E 1926 Arachnodactylia and its association with congenital heart disease. American Journal of Diseases of Childhood 31: 832–839

Priest R E, Moinuddin J F, Priest J H 1973 Collegen of Marfan syndrome is abnormally soluble. Nature (London) 245: 264–266

Prockop D J, Sjoerdsma A 1961 Significance of urinary hydroxyproline in man. Journal of Clinical Investigation 40: 843

Pyeritz R E, McKusick V A 1979 The Marfan syndrome: Diagnosis and management. New England Journal of Medicine 300: 772–777

Pyeritz R E, Brinker J A, Varghese P J 1979A Clinical and echocardiographic correlates in 127 Marfan patients (abst). Clinical Research 26: 196A

Pyeritz R E 1980A Cardiovascular diagnosis and management in the Marfan syndrome. Journal of Cardiovascular Medicine 5: 759–769

Pyeritz R E, Brinker J A, Fortuin N J et al 1980A Validation of M-mode echocardiographic diameter of the dilated ascending aorta. Clinical Research 28: 204A

Pyeritz R E, Murphy E A, McKusick V A 1979B Clinical variability in the Marfan syndromes. Birth Defects 15(5B): 155–178

Pyeritz R E, Brinker J A, Fortuin N J et al 1980B Annular dilatation does not cause aortic regurgitation in the Marfan syndrome. Clinical Research 78: 203A

Pyeritz R E 1981 Maternal and fetal complications of pregnancy in the Marfan syndrome. American Journal of Medicine 71: 784–790

Robins P R, Moe J H, Winter R B 1975 Scoliosis in Marfan's syndrome: its characteristics and results of treatment in thirty-five patients. Journal of Bone and Joint Surgery 57A: 358–368

Salle V 1912 Über einen Fall von angeborener abnormer Grosse der Extremitäten mit einem an Akromegalie erinnernden Symptomenkopmplex Jahrbuch Kinderheilk 75: 540–550

Scheck M, Siegel R C, Parker J et al 1979 Aortic aneurysm in Marfan's syndrome: changes in the ultrastructure and composition of collagen. Journal of Anatomy 129: 645–657

Scheutermann D A, Murdoch J L, Walker B A et al 1976 A linkage study of the Marfan syndrome. Clinical Genetics 10: 51–53

Schlatmann T J M, Becker A E 1977 Pathogenesis of dissecting aneurysm of the aorta: Comparative histopathologic study of significance of medial changes. American Journal of Cardiology 29: 21–26

Schoenfeld M R 1978 Nicolo Paganini – musical magician and Marfan mutant. Journal of the American Medical Association 239: 40-42

Schwartz H 1964 Abraham Lincoln and the Marfan syndrome. Journal of the American Medical Association 187: 473

Simpson C F, Boucek R J, Nobel N L 1980 Similarity of aortic pathology in Marfan's syndrome, copper deficiency in chicks and beta-aminoproprionitrile toxicity. Experimental and Molecular Pathology 32: 31–90

Simpson C F, Kling J M, Palmer R F The use of propranolol for the protection of turkeys from the development of beta-aminoproprinoitrile-induced aortic ruptures. Angiology 19: 414–418

Soman V R, Breton G, Hershkowitz M et al 1974 Bacterial endocarditis of the mitral valve in Marfan syndrome. British Heart Journal 36: 1247–1250

Steinberg I 1966 A simple screening test for the Marfan syndrome. American Journal of Roentgenology Radium Therapy and Nuclear Medicine 97: 118–124

Turner J A M, Stanley N N 1976 Fragile lung in the Marfan syndrome. Thorax 31: 771–775

Walker B A, Beighton P H, Murdoch J L 1969 The marfanoid hypermobility syndrome. Annals of Internal Medicine 71: 349–352

Walker B A, Murdoch J L 1970 The wrist sign: a useful physical finding in the Marfan syndrome. Archives of Internal Medicine 126: 276-277

Wenger D R, Ditkoff T J, Herring J A et al 1980 Protrusio acetabuli in Marfan's syndrome. Clinical Orthopaedics 147: 134–138

Weve H 1931 Uber arachnodakylie. Archiv Augenheilk 104: 1

58

Ehlers-Danlos syndrome

P. H. Byers, K. A. Holbrook, G. S. Barsh

INTRODUCTION

The Ehlers-Danlos syndrome (EDS) is a group of disorders characterized by abnormalities of skin, joints and other connective tissues (Beighton, 1970; McKusick, 1972; Hollister, 1978). In early descriptions of these disorders joint laxity and skin hyperextensibility were emphasized (Ehlers, 1901; Danlos, 1908), but as more patients were identified, skin fragility, easy bruising and the occasional complications of bowel and arterial rupture were recognized (Sack, 1936; Gottron, 1942; Barabas, 1967). During the last ten years the clinical and genetic heterogeneity has been explained, in part, by biochemical and ultrastructural studies which distinguish at least eight distinct varieties of the syndrome (Table 58.1) (Hollister, 1978; Pinnell, 1978; Bornstein and Byers, 1980).

This chapter provides a detailed clinical, genetic and biochemical summary of the eight recognized Ehlers-Danlos types and the information about collagen structure, biosynthesis, heterogeneity and tissue distribution which serves as the basis for understanding the pathophysiology of these disorders.

COLLAGEN TYPES

The collagens are a family of evolutionarily related, structurally similar proteins (see Bornstein & Sage, 1980 for review) which have distinguishing sequences, tissue distributions and cells of origin (Table 58.2).

Each collagen molecule contains three α chains arranged in a triple helical conformation that extends most of the length of the molecule. In most collagens one third of all amino acids is glycine distributed such that the sequence of the triple helical domains can be written $(Gly-X-Y)_n$, where X and Y can be most amino acids but are often proline (X) and hydroxyproline (Y). In tissues these molecules are arranged in fibrils or other higher order aggregates which are visible with the electron microscope.

Collagens can be divided into three groups on the basis of tissue distribution, and molecular and supramolecular structures: interstitial collagens (Types I, II and III), the basement membrane collagens (Type IV), and the cell-associated collagens (Type V). Type I, the most abundant collagen, is ubiquitous in distribution, and is the major connective tissue component of skin, bone, tendon, dentin, ligament and fascia. Most type I collagen molecules are heteropolymers which consist of two $\alpha 1(I)$ chains and one very similar chain $\alpha 2, [\alpha 1(I)]_2 \alpha 2$. The same $\alpha 1(I)$ chain, appears to be able to form a homopolymer, $[\alpha 1(I)]_3$ that is found in small amounts in normal tissues and in some pathological tissues. Type I collagen forms the large fibrils seen in most connective tissues, provides the tensile strength of skin and tendon, and forms the organic matrix of bone, the transparent matrix of the cornea and the opaque tissue of the sclera. Other major matrix macromolecules such as proteoglycans and glycoproteins interact with collagen to impart the unique structural and mechanical features to each tissue. Type II collagen, a homopolymer of the $\alpha 1(II)$ chain, $[\alpha 1(II)]_3$, is confined to cartilage and the nucleus pulposus of the intervertebral disc; an identical or closely related molecule is the collagenous constituent of the vitreous humor of the eye. Type III collagen is a homopolymer of $\alpha 1(III)$ chains, $[\alpha 1(III)]_3$. Its distribution parallels that of type I except that it is absent from bone. While it is a relatively minor component of skin in the adult, it constitutes more than 50% of dermal collagen in the fetus (Epstein, 1974), and may be important for the initial structuring of the tissue. Type III collagen is a major component of the walls of hollow organs of the gastrointestinal tract, the uterus and blood vessels. The molecular constitution of the type IV collagen molecules is uncertain although there appear to be three different collagen chains. These molecules are found in basement membranes and probably have different molecular configuration from the interstitial collagens since the helical domain is interrupted by short non-helical segments. The molecular configuration of the type V collagen molecules and their precise distribution in tissues are also uncertain.

Table 58.1 Ehlers-Danlos syndromes

Type	Clinical features	Inheritance	Biochemical disorder	Ultrastructural findings
I Gravis	Soft, velvety skin; marked skin hyperextensibility, fragility, and easy bruisability; 'cigarette paper' scars; large- and small-joint hypermobility; frequent venous varicosities; hernia. Prematurity due to ruptured fetal membranes is common.	AD	Not known	Large collagen fibrils, many irregular in shape.
II Mitis	Soft skin, moderate skin hyperextensibility, and easy bruisability; moderate joint hypermobility; varicose veins and hernia do occur but are less common than in type I. Prematurity is rare.	AD	Not known	Large collagen fibrils, many irregular in shape.
III Benign familial hypermobility	Skin is soft but otherwise minimally affected; joint mobility is markedly increased and affects large and small joints; dislocation is common.	AD	Not known	Large collagen fibrils, many irregular in shape.
IV Ecchymotic or arterial	Skin is thin or translucent or both; veins are readily visible over the trunk, arms, legs, and abdomen. Repeated ecchymosis with minimal trauma. Skin is not hyperextensible, and joints (except the small joints in the hands) are usually of normal mobility. Bowel rupture (usually affecting the colon) and arterial rupture are frequent and often lead to death.	AD AR	Decreased or absent synthesis of type III collagen. Altered secretion of type III collagen.	Thin dermis, small fibres, often engorged cells in dermis, fibrils of variable size.
V X-linked	Similar to EDS II; muscle haemorrhage may be more extensive	XR	Not known	Not known
VI Ocular	Soft, velvety, hyperextensible skin; hypermobile joints; scoliosis, scarring less severe than in EDS I; some patients have ocular fragility and keratoconus.	AR	Lysyl hydroxylase deficiency	Small collagen bundles fibrils normal or similar to those in EDS I
VII Arthrochalasis multiplex congenita	Soft skin; scars near normal. Marked joint hyperextensibility, congenital hip dislocation.	AD	Amino acid substitution at the NH$_2$ terminal cleavage site of proα2	Not known
		AR	NH$_2$ terminal protease deficiency	
VIII Periodontal form	Marked skin fragility with abnormal, atrophic pigmented scars, minimal skin extensibility and moderate joint laxity. Aesthenic habitus, generalized periodontitis.	AD	Not known	Not known

AD: Autosomal dominant
AR: Autosomal recessive
XR: X-linked recessive

BIOSYNTHESIS OF COLLAGENS

The biosynthesis of collagens is complex (Table 58.3) and involves many steps beyond the transcription of the genes (Pinnell, 1978; Prockop et al, 1979; Bornstein and Byers, 1980). The collagen genes appear to be almost ten times the size of the functional mRNA (Frischauf et al, 1978; Boyd et al, 1980; Vogeli et al, 1980). In the α2 gene of type I collagen there are about 50 coding sequences (exons), all of a relatively small size (54–108 bases), which are separated by larger intervening sequences (introns) of 100 to 3000 bases. The entire gene is transcribed and then spliced to yield a mature mRNA that contains about 5000 bases. The mRNA is trans-

Table 58.2 Structurally distinct collagen types

Type	Chain composition	Tissue distribution	Distinctive features
I	$[\alpha1(I)]_2\alpha2$	Almost ubiquitous.	Heteropolymer. Low hydroxylysine and carbohydrate content; forms large banded fibrils.
Type I Trimer	$[\alpha1(I)]_3$	Fetal tissues, inflammatory and neoplastic states.	Increased content of 3- and 4-hydroxyproline and hydroxylysine as compared to the heteropolymer.
II	$[\alpha1(II)]_3$	Cartilage, nucleus pulposus, vitreous.	Intermediate hydroxylysine and carbohydrate content.
III	$[\alpha1(III)]_3$	Same as type I except absent in bone and very low in tendon. Prominent in distensible tissues such as blood vessels, GI tract, fetal skin.	Helix terminates in cysteine-cysteine. More than 33% glycine. High 4-hydroxyproline, low hydroxylysine and carbohydrate content. Present in reticulin.
IV	$\alpha1(IV)$ $\alpha2(IV)$ composition uncertain	Lens capsule, parietal yolk sac, glomerular and other basement membranes.	Variable, but generally high 3-hydroxyproline, low alanine and arginine content. Enriched in hydrophobic amino acids, hydroxylysine, and carbohydrate. Contains cysteine.
	$[\alpha1(V)]_3$ $[\alpha1(V)]_2\alpha2(V)$	Fetal membranes, vascular tissue; minor component in bone and cartilage.	Low alanine, high hydroxylysyl and carbohydrate content. Intermediate content of hydrophobic amino acids.

Table 58.3 Pathway of collagen biosynthesis

Process	Cellular location
Gene transcription, processing to mature mRNA	Nucleus
Translation of mRNA, synthesis of prepro α chain	Ribosomes of rough endoplasmic reticulum
Cleavage of preproα chain to proα chain	RER membrane
Lysyl and prolyl hydroxylation, hydroxylysyl glycosylation, 'high' mannose addition	Cotranslational, RER membrane
Molecular assembly, disulphide bond formation, helix formation	Cisternae of RER
Processing of heterosaccharide	Golgi
Packaging of procollagen into secretory vesicles	Golgi
Secretion	Cell surface
Cleavage of amino terminal and carboxy-terminal propeptide extensions	Cell surface, extracellular space
Fibril formation	Extracellular space
Crosslink formation	Extracellular space

ported to the cytoplasm and translated on membrane-bound polysomes. A preproα chain, which contains an initial hydrophobic 'leader' sequence that facilitates transfer of the chain into the lumen of the rough endoplasmic reticulum, is synthesized and as the chain crosses the membrane, the 'leader' sequence is cleaved by an intramembrane endopeptidase to yield proα chains. The proα chains of most collagens are larger than the functional α chains in tissue by virtue of both aminoterminal

(160 amino acids) and carboxyterminal (300 amino acids) peptide extensions.

As cotranslational events certain lysyl and prolyl residues are hydroxylated by the enzymes lysyl and prolyl hydroxylase, respectively. These enzymes are distinct proteins which share cofactors (ferrous iron, ascorbate and α-ketoglutarate), and are located in the membranes of the rough endoplasmic reticulum. The degree of prolyl hydroxylation is dependent on collagen type and differs from tissue to tissue even for the same type of collagen. Lysyl hydroxylation and subsequent glycosylation also vary with collagen type. During translation some hydroxylysyl residues are glycosylated to form glucosyl-galactosylhydroxylysyl or galactosylhydroxylysyl and additional carbohydrate is added in the precursor-specific peptides.

After the synthesis of the proα chains is completed, the procollagen molecule is assembled (Table. 58.3). The three constituent chains first interact at sites within the COOH-terminal non-helical domain, the association is stabilized by interchain disulphide bond formation, and a triple helix is formed. The procollagen molecule is transported to the Golgi where the heterosaccharide moiety of the COOH-terminal nonhelical domain is modified. The intact procollagen molecule is transported to the cell surface in Golgi vesicles which fuse with the cell membranes to release their contents. Once secreted from the cell, procollagen is processed, by proteolytic cleavage, to collagen by specific endopeptidases which cleave the NH_2-terminal and COOH-terminal precursor specific peptides. The extent of cleavage varies with collagen type and may also depend on tissue specific factors. Type I procollagen is, for the most part, processed completely to collagen while type IV collagen may be processed little or not at all. However, the degree of processing may vary, even for type I collagen, since considerable NH_2-terminal precursor specific peptide is found in the papillary dermis, co-distributed with the helical domain of type I collagen, while virtually none is found in the reticular dermis.

The extracellular molecules assemble into fibrils or other higher order structures where they become covalently cross-linked to form highly stable structures. The cross-link precursors are lysyl or hydroxylysyl residues which are oxidatively deaminated by lysyl oxidase (Siegel, 1978). The resultant aldehydes then condense with adjacent lysyl or hydroxylysyl residues, or their respective aldehydes, to form covalent bifunctional cross-links; subsequently, polyfunctional cross-links involving additional lysyl or histidinyl residues can form (Eyre, 1980). The extent of fibril formation and of cross-link formation differs with collagen type, location, and age. The structure of the collagen fibril, its aggregation into bundles, and the mechanial properties of tissues depend not only on cross-linking but also on interactions with several other macromolecules, most notably proteoglycans and glycoproteins (Lindahl & Höök, 1978; Bornstein & Sage, 1980).

The complexity of collagen biosynthesis, involving substantial post-transcriptional mRNA processing and cotranslational and posttranslational protein processing provide many opportunities for error. In the Ehlers-Danlos syndrome, abnormalities in collagen gene expression and gene structure, and in intracellular and extracellular protein processing have all been implicated in pathogenesis of the different types. These are described in some detail in the following sections.

EHLERS-DANLOS, TYPE I (GRAVIS)

The gravis variety, or type I EDS, is the classic, severe disorder characterized by marked skin hyperextensibility and joint hypermobility (Fig. 58.1). Typically, the skin is soft, velvety in texture, and can be extended several centimetres away from attachment sites. The skin has increased compliance but returns to its original shape promptly and is not lax. It is fragile and there is easy bruising. Trauma results in gaping wounds which may bleed less than expected, but which heal with characteristic atrophic 'cigarette paper' scars. Areas of repeated trauma, such as elbows, knees, and shins often have marked pigment deposition in addition to the characteristic scarring. 'Molluscoid pseudotumors', small (0.5–1.5 cm) accumulations of connective tissue may form in the skin and some individuals develop palpable subcutaneous calcified nodules.

As many as 50% of infants with EDS I are born 4–8 weeks premature. The cause of prematurity is uncertain, but may be related to early rupture of the fetal membranes, as a result of mechanical alterations secondary to the primary connective tissue defect. The diagnosis of EDS I can be made in the perinatal period and family members are often proficient in distinguishing affected from unaffected newborns. The affected infants have softer skin than normal, increased skin extensibility and small joint hypermobility. Bruising in the newborn period is unusual, but begins as children start to crawl and stand. At this time, skin fragility is also evident and characteristic scars may appear on the forehead, under the chin, and on knees and elbows. Motor development may be somewhat slower than usual because the joint hypermobility often limits stability until muscle development is sufficient to overcome the ligamentous laxity. Intellectual development is normal.

Individuals with EDS I may have a variety of complications as a result of connective tissue involvement. Many people with the disorder have cardiovascular anomalies, the most common of which is the 'floppy' mitral valve. This common disorder may affect more than half of patients with EDS I. Other cardiac structural abnormalities are also seen and should be considered in all patients with the syndrome (Leier et al, 1980). Vascular rupture is a rare event among patients with EDS I in contrast to those with EDS IV (see below), but is encountered occasionally. Pes planus is common and mild to moderate scoliosis, especially in the lumbar region, is seen in some patients. It is our impression that the ligamentous laxity is associated with earlier than

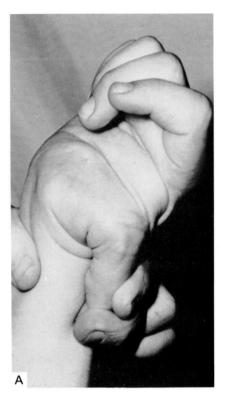
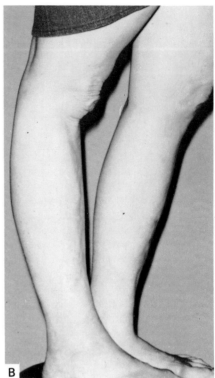
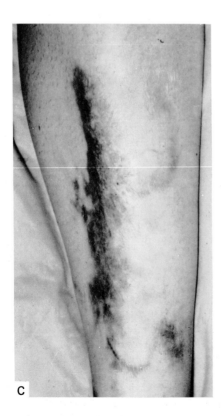
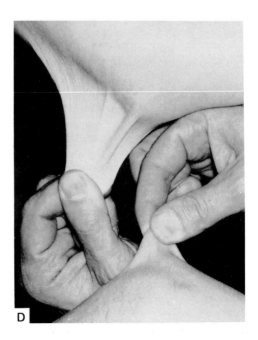

Fig. 58.1 The clinical features of type I EDS include (A) joint hypermobility, (B) and (C) abnormal 'cigarette paper' scars, and (D) skin hyperextensibility.

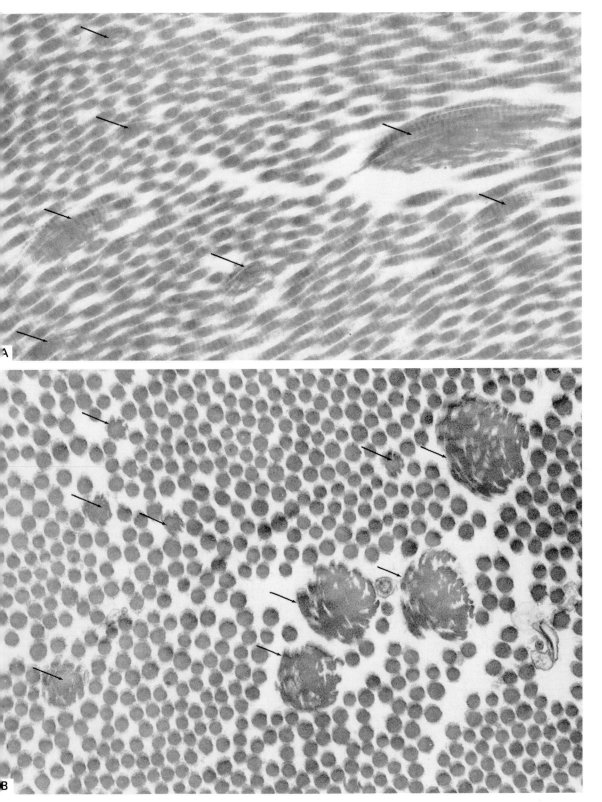

Fig. 58.2 Normal and abnormal appearing collagen fibrils are characteristics of the reticular dermis of individuals with dominant forms of the Ehlers-Danlos syndrome. The irregular, lobulated fibrils seen in cross section (A, arrows) correspond with the loosely aggregated conglomerate fibrils observed in longitudinal section — (B, arrows). X 30 000 (A), X 14,500 (B).

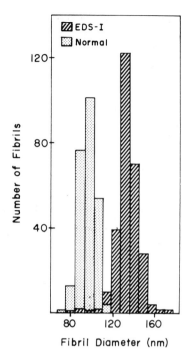

Fig. 58.2 (C) Histogram of collagen fibril diameters of normal individuals and of patients with type I Ehlers-Danlos syndrome.

usual degenerative arthritis. Pregnancy may be complicated by premature rupture of membranes of affected infants and by early labour for unknown reasons among some affected women carrying normal or affected children. Surgery in individuals with EDS I is generally uncomplicated, although tissues are more friable than usual and care must be taken to assure complete haemostasis. Sutures should be left in place two to three times longer than usual.

EDS I is inherited in an autosomal dominant manner with relatively little variation in expression. Although there are no distinctive biochemical tests, the diagnosis is generally not ambiguous in families. In the sporadic case the diagnosis of EDS V (in males) or EDS VI must be considered.

The biochemical basis of EDS I is unknown. Histologically, the dermal structure is altered so that the usual orthogonal weave of collagen bundles is defective. The collagen bundles are small, but the constituent fibrils are 10 to 40% larger than normal (110–140 nm compared to 90–100nm for control) (Vogel et al, 1979). Many fibrils are irregular in outline and some appear as poorly integrated structures (see Fig. 58.2). The mechanism by which the formation of collagen fibrils and of higher order structures is changed is not clear, although alterations in regions of the collagen molecule which direct intermolecular interaction, or abnormalities in other

macromolecules of the connective tissue matrix (e.g., proteoglycans or glycoproteins) might both produce disturbances of collagen fibril morphogenesis.

Recently, Shinkai et al, (1976) studied one patient with EDS I and found abnormalities in the biosynthesis of proteoglycans. Arneson et al (1980) described a family with features of EDS I and EDS II in which affected members appeared to have qualitative abnormalities in the fibronectin molecule (cold insoluble globulin or CIG). This glycoprotein is found circulating in plasma and the same or very closely related protein is present in most connective tissue matrices. In these patients, circulating fibronectin levels were normal and platelet aggregation in response to collagen (thought to be mediated, in part, by fibronectin) was abnormal but could be corrected by addition of fibronectin to their plasma. These patients, too, had abnormal collagen fibrils in skin. It is likely, then, that EDS I may be a biochemically heterogeneous disorder, the phenotypic manifestation of a number of molecular abnormalities which alter fibril formation and stability.

In the absence of definitive biochemical diagnostic tests, genetic counselling in the sporadic case can be difficult. Although there are no data available on the frequency of new dominant mutations in this disorder, if the clinical features are consistent with EDS I, and if EDS VI can be excluded, then it is likely that the patient has a disorder that is inherited in an autosomal dominant fashion.

EHLERS-DANLOS, TYPE II (MITIS)

The clinical features of EDS II, the mitis form, are similar to those of EDS I, but are milder. Skin is soft and velvety, but scarring and bruising are less than in EDS I, and joint hypermobility is less marked. Prematurity is rare and motor development is not as delayed as in EDS I. Like EDS I, EDS II is inherited in an autosomal dominant fashion and there is only modest variability in expression. The clinical course and natural history of the disorder are generally uncomplicated although many patients have the 'floppy' mitral valve syndrome and some develop early onset of degenerative arthritis. The ultrastructural features of the disease are similar to those of EDS I and the biochemical aetiology remains unknown. Evaluation and counselling should parallel those in EDS I.

EHLERS-DANLOS, TYPE III (BENIGN FAMILIAL HYPERMOBILITY)

EDS III, benign familial hypermobility is an autosomal dominant disorder with variable expression in which the major clinical features are large and small joint hypermobility. This disorder has considerable variability both within and among families. Joint hypermobility is generally accompanied by soft skin, but skin hyperextensibility is absent and scars are normal. The joint hypermobility may be dramatic in some individuals (see Beighton, 1970, for illustrations). The major problems associated with the disorder are recurrent joint dislocations. While surgical repair is generally satisfactory, recurrence is more common than in unaffected individuals.

The ultrastructural findings are similar to those in EDS I and EDS II, (Sevenich et al., 1980) but there are no distinctive biochemical findings. Counselling may present problems in sporadic cases. Because there is a wide range of normal in joint mobility (which can be augmented by training), establishing the diagnosis of EDS III may be difficult without a family history. Without a clear family history of EDS III, an individual with only modest joint laxity may represent normal variation.

EHLERS-DANLOS, TYPE IV (VASCULAR, ECCHYMOTIC, SACK-BARABAS)

EDS IV, the vascular or ecchymotic variety, was recognized as a distinct entity by Barabas in 1967, although Sack in 1936, and Gottron in 1942, probably described the same diseases. It is in this group of disorders, all due to abnormalities in metabolism of type III collagen, that some of the most extensive biochemical investigations have been done and in which heterogeneity is best recognized (Pope et al, 1975, 1977, 1980; Byers et al, 1979, 1981 a, b; Holbrook and Byers, 1981). Individuals with

EDS IV have fragile, thin or translucent skin, through which the venous pattern is readily visible (Fig. 58.3), marked bruising, and a characteristic facies (Pope et al, 1977). Some patients have soft skin which is mildly hyperextensible, but the majority have skin with normal texture and normal extensibility. Joint mobility is generally normal or hypermobility is limited to the small joints of the hands. In some patients with the 'acrogeric' form of the disorder, the skin over the distal extremities has an aged, atrophic appearance, and in others the skin on the hands has a fine, parchment quality. Venous varicosities are common and may be severe.

The major clinical complications are bowel, arterial and uterine rupture. Because of these dramatic complications, life expectancy is shortened. Both autosomal dominant and autosomal recessive forms of EDS IV have been described; in general, the autosomal dominant varieties appear to have better overall prognoses. The most frequent complication is bowel rupture of the colon, which usually occurs near or distal to the splenic flexure along the antimesenteric border. The small intestine is rarely, if ever, involved. Treatment is the same as for any acute bowel rupture, but because tissues of affected individuals are exceedingly friable, surgical repair of any lesion is often difficult. Since only the colon appears to be susceptible to spontaneous rupture, consideration should be given to removal if rupture recurs.

Major vessel rupture is another life-threatening complication. The clinical presentation depends on the location of the ruptured artery so that haemorrhagic stroke, haemothorax, haemoperitoneum, and compartmental syndromes may all result. Uterine rupture near term in pregnancy is an occasional complication.

The clinical features of the disorder are variable. In

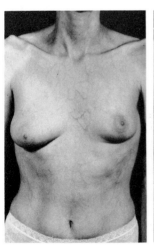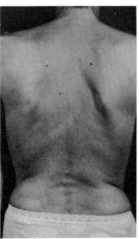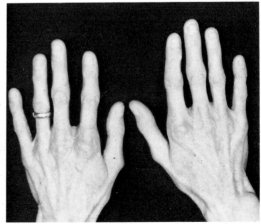

Fig. 58.3 This 26 year old woman has type IV EDS. Her skin is extremely thin and the venous vasculature can be seen over the chest, abdomen and back. She has elastosis perforans serpiginosa over both antecubital regions, and skin over her hands appears markedly aged. (From Byers et al, 1979).

some patients the diagnosis can be made early in infancy because of marked bruising· and thin skin. In other patients with a family history of the disorder the diagnosis may be suspected in infancy because of other complications such as cerebral hemorrhage. However, in many patients the diagnosis is not suspected unless there is a positive family history and even then the signs of the disease may be limited to mild bruising during childhood. Vessel and bowel rupture may be seen in children, although they occur most commonly in the third to fifth decades. Uterine rupture is more likely to occur during pregnancies in the 30's than earlier.

A summary of our experience with 23 affected individuals from nine families helps to evaluate the natural history of the disorder. Nineteen of these people are found in five families in which EDS IV is inherited in an autosomal dominant manner; the remaining four are the only affected member in their respective families in which there is no history of consanguinity. Of the 23 affected individuals, seven are now dead, three as a result of arterial rupture (ages 46, 23, and 12 years), two as a consequence of ruptured bowel (both at 39 years) and two from uterine rupture at term in pregnancy (ages 32 and 22). Nine of the sixteen survivors are well and have had no major complications of their disease, the oldest of whom is in her mid-40's. Of the remaining seven, one has had a spontaneous pneumothorax, one has severe periodontal disease, one had a spontaneous bowel rupture at 33, one patient has had a bowel rupture at 6, epiphyseal bleed at 12, stroke at 23 and a compartmental bleed at 26; two patients had intracranial hemorrhage in the neonatal period but have done well since, and one patient had a pneumothorax at 20, a femoral artery compartmental bleed at 21, and three episodes of bowel rupture in his early 20's. It should be recognized that EDS IV is an underdiagnosed disorder and those patients having difficulties are most likely to be referred to genetics centers or for diagnostic evaluation. This serves to emphasize the heterogeneity of the disorder and to demonstrate the difficulty in providing unambiguous genetic counselling.

The clinical diagnosis of EDS IV can be confirmed biochemically by the demonstration of decreased or absent type III collagen in affected tissues. Pathologically, dermis is thin and may be only 25% of normal thickness. There appears to be an increased amount of elastic fibres, but this is probably a relative increase since the total skin thickness is decreased. Collagen bundles are smaller than normal and, at the ultrastructural level, collagen fibrils are small in some patients and varied in size with a major component of small fibrils in others. Many patients have marked dilatation of the rough endoplasmic reticulum of dermal fibroblast in situ, evidence of decreased secretion of synthesized proteins (Fig. 58.4).

Studies of dermal fibroblasts in culture from patients with EDS IV have demonstrated several alterations in type III collagen metabolism. The first studies of such cells were consistent with absent synthesis since no type III procollagen was secreted by the cells in culture and the cultured cells did not stain with antibodies to type III procollagen (Pope et al, 1975; Gay et al, 1976). Subsequent studies of cells from other patients have demonstrated decreased, but not absent type III procollagen, or alterations in its secretion with intracellular storage (Byers et al, 1981a, b; Holbrook and Byers, 1981). In our families with autosomal dominant inheritance, four of five have evidence of intracellular storage of type III procollagen, as do three of four of the 'sporadic' cases. We have identified no patients in whom we can be sure of recessive inheritance on either genetic or biochemical grounds. It is clear from our studies and those of others that many individuals with EDS IV have a dominantly inherited disorder and in those families counselling with regard to inheritance is straightforward although prognosis may be variable. In those families, prenatal diagnosis is a consideration, since certain amniotic fluid cells synthesize and secret type III procollagen. Genetic counselling for the sporadic patient is a problem. Pope, et al, (1977) has suggested that some patients have a recessively inherited disorder on the basis of decreased levels of type III collagen in skin of some first degree relatives of an affected patient. It is important to realize, however, that since there is a decrease in genetic fitness some affected individuals would be expected to result from new mutations. Thus an affected individual in a nonaffected family might have a recessively inherited disorder or represent a new dominant mutation. Thus, genetic counselling for the sporadically affected individual is difficult and careful evaluation of the specific biochemical lesion may be the only effective means for providing accurate genetic information.

There is, at present, no demonstrated effective treatment for EDS IV. The catastrophic complications of artery and organ rupture are treated surgically. Vitamin C (ascorbic acid), which increases collagen synthesis, secretion, and molecular stability in vitro, has the potential for being effective in some patients (we have treated one patient with 1–3 gm/day for a year during which time there was an increase in type III collagen in skin and decrease in bruising), but requires a careful clinical trial before its general use can be advocated.

EHLERS-DANLOS, TYPE V (X–LINKED VARIETY)

Type V EDS is an X–linked variety of the disorder, first described by Beighton, (1970). Skin hyperextensibility is similar to that in EDS II, but joint mobility and bruis-

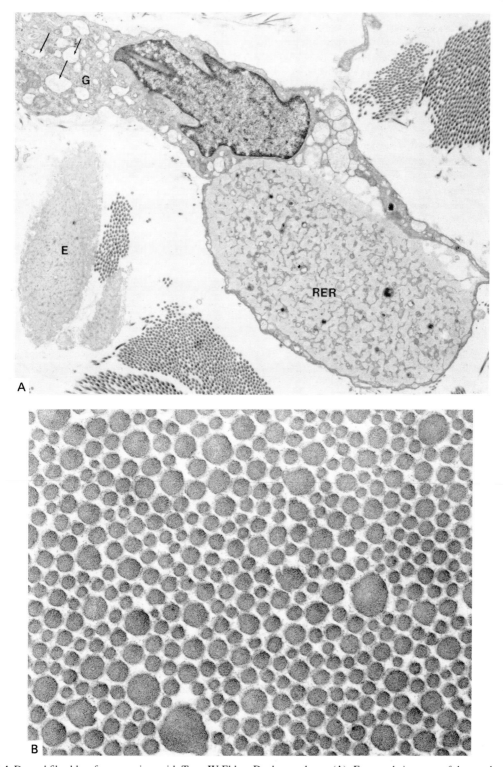

Fig. 58.4 Dermal fibroblast from a patient with Type IV Ehlers-Danlos syndrome (A). Engorged cirsternae of the rough endoplastic reticulum (RER) occupies a major portion of the cell. Other cisternae are not as dilated (arrows) and the Golgi [G] appears normal. Note the frayed margins of an elastic [E] fibre. X 5600.
(B) Collagen fibrils of irregular diameter are found in the reticular dermis of certain patients with type IV Ehlers-Danlos syndrome. X 45,600.

ing are less marked. The other typical features of EDS II, scars and pseudotumours, may be present and, in addition, intramuscular haemorrhage may occur. There has been considerable uncertainty and confusion as to the biochemical aetiology of this disorder. DiFerrante et al, (1975) described a family with an X–linked connective tissue disorder with some features of the Ehlers-Danlos syndrome, but clinically different from Beighton's patients. They measured lysyl oxidase activity in the medium of cultured dermal fibroblasts from these patients and found it to be decreased although the methods used for enzyme determination may not have been reliable (Siegel et al, 1979). Subsequently, Byers et al, (1976, 1980) described a second X–linked disorder which they considered to be a variety of cutis laxa. In addition to skin laxity, these males had skeletal anomalies and genitourinary tract diverticula. Both affected boys had low levels of lysyl oxidase in skin and low levels in medium of cells in culture. Their cells failed to cross–link collagen normally and did not synthesize normal amounts of cross–link precursors. Furthermore, both boys had low serum copper levels. MacFarlane and colleagues (1980) have identified two similar families. Finally, Siegel et al, (1979) recently examined Beighton's original X–linked families and could find no evidence of abnormalities in lysyl oxidase function or in cross–link generation. Thus, the biochemical basis of the X–linked form of EDS remains unknown.

Genetic counselling for the sporadic, moderately affected male with EDS may be difficult. Such individuals should be studied carefully for lysyl hydroxylase deficiency (EDS VI, an autosomal recessive disorder) by assay of skin collagen for hydroxylysine and of dermal fibroblasts for the enzyme. If these studies are negative, then, given a compatible clinical picture, the most likely diagnosis is EDS II, since it appears to be far more frequent than EDS V.

EHLERS-DANLOS, TYPE VI (OCULAR)

Type VI EDS was the first of the true molecular disorders of collagen metabolism to be recognized when Pinnell et al, (1972) described two sisters with lysyl hydroxylase deficiency that resulted in hydroxylysine deficient collagen. The two sisters described in the initial report had smooth, hyperextensible, velvety skin, moderate scarring and bruising, large and small joint laxity, a Marfan habitus with moderately severe thoracic kyphoscoliosis, and keratoconus with ocular globe fragility (Fig. 58.5). Since the initial description, several other patients have been identified who share many of these features, and as expected, there is some clinical heterogeneity (Sussman et al, 1974; Steinmann et al,

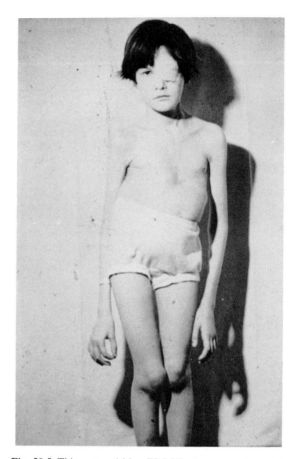

Fig. 58.5 This young girl has EDS VI, an autosomal recessive disorder characterized by reduced lysyl hydroxylation. She has a Marfanoid habitus, scoliosis, and lost her eye as a result of minor trauma. (Photograph courtesy of Dr Sheldon Pinnell, Duke University).

1975; Elsas et al, 1978; Krieg et al, 1979). With only a small number of these patients identified, the natural history of the disorder is not known. One of the early patients described died as a result of an aortic rupture in her early 50's; an affected brother had died earlier from a gastrointestinal hemmorhage (Sussman et al, 1974). Both had had intraocular haemorrhages previous to their fatal systemic hemorrhages. The other known patients are all less than 30 years old at this time.

The histopathology in this disorder is not well described. In two patients collagen fibril morphology is said to be normal, although in one fibre organization may be disrupted (Pinnell et al, 1972; Steinmann et al, 1975). We have examined skin from one patient with the disorder; she has normal fibril diameters but small fibres; there are many bizarre fibrils, such as seen in EDS I.

In most affected patients, there is virtually no hydroxylysine found in skin collagen: normally there are

Table 58.4 Lysyl hydroxylase activity in cultured cells from a patient with EDS VI. Data from Sussman et al (1974)

| | Lysyl hydroxylase | | Prolyl hydroxylase | |
	^{3}H cpm released	% control	^{3}H cpm released	% control
Control	850		11 100	88
EDS VI	100	12	9800	

Table 58.5 Partial amino acid composition of skin from control and EDS VI. Data from Sussman et al (1974)

	Control	EDS VI
4-OHpro	81	76
Pro	118	114
Gly	316	300
Ala	122	134
Hylys	4.2	0.24
Lys	28	31

approximately 5 residues of hydroxylysine per 1000 amino acids but in most affected individuals there is less than 0.5 residue (Tables 58.4 and 58.5; Steinmann et al, 1975) described a sib pair in whom hydroxylysine in skin was only modestly decreased, but who had virtually no measurably lysyl hydroxylase in cultured cells. All patients in whom it has been measured have very low lysyl hydroxylase levels in cultured cells (Tables 58.4 and 58.5). Parents of affected individuals generally have about half normal levels of the enzyme, consistent with autosomal recessive inheritance.

The major pathophysiologic effect of decreased lysyl hydroxylation in collagen is a decrease in the production of stable intermolecular cross–links which alters the physical properties of tissues. It is not certain whether the enzymatic deficiency affected all tissue, since collagen in skin (types I and III) is markedly deficient, collagen in ligament (type I) is underhydroxylated, but cartilage (type II) has normal levels of hydroxylysine. Lysyl hydroxylase requires ascorbic acids, ferrous iron and α-ketoglutarate as cofactors. Studies by Quinn and Krane (1976) indicated that the interaction of the abnormal enzyme with ascorbate was altered. Subsequently, Elsas et al (1978) suggested that treatment of patients with ascorbate could increase urinary excretion of hydroxylysyl glycosides and produce subjective decrease in bruising, although no change in skin hydroxylysine content was demonstrable.

As is the case for most enzymatic defects, EDS VI is an autosomal recessive disorder. Thus, the risk of recurrence in a family with one affected child is 25% for each pregnancy. The risk for each affected person to have

affected children is negligible unless he or she mates with a relative or other known carrier. As indicated above, counselling concerning the natural history of the disorder remains uncertain because of the paucity of information. The clinical disorder may be additionally heterogeneous since two children with a similar presentation, including ocular globe fragility, have been described who appear to have normal lysyl hydroxylation (Judisch et al, 1976). Prenatal diagnosis of lysyl hydroxylase deficiency is probably feasible using amniotic fluid cells in culture to assay for the enzyme.

EHLERS-DANLOS, TYPE VII (ARTHROCHALASIS MULTIPLEX CONGENITA)

Type VII EDS, arthrochalasis multiplex congenita, is characterized by extreme joint laxity, soft but non-fragile skin, minimal bruising and mild skin hyperextensibility (Lichtenstein et al, 1973; 1974). Several of the affected individuals had bilateral congenital hip dislocation, which was difficult to stabilize, and at older ages, had multiple dislocations of other joints.

When first described, all patients were thought to have abnormalities in the conversion of procollagen to collagen as a result of a defective amino terminal procollagen protease (Lichtenstein et al, 1973). While this apparently is true of the majority of affected patients, one was restudied recently and shown to have a structural abnormality in about half of the α2 chains of type I collagen that interferes with the enzymatic conversion of procollagen to collagen (Steinmann et al, 1980). Ultrastructural studies of skin from patients with EDS VII have been surprisingly normal, given the marked disturbances in fibril structure seen in the skin of animals with dermatosparaxis, a disorder in the enzymatic cleavage of the amino-terminal propeptide from procollagen (Lenaers et al, 1971; Holbrook et al, 1980). Because of the biochemical heterogeneity in this disorder, genetic counselling is dependent on determining the precise abnormality. If a deficiency of the amino terminal procollagen protease can be demonstrated, then the patient most likely has an autosomal recessive disorder, whereas the presence of a structural defect on either the α2 or α1(I) chain that interferes with conversion is likely to be inherited in an autosomal dominant manner.

EHELRS-DANLOS, TYPE VIII (PERIODONTAL FORM)

Stewart and his colleagues (1977) recently described two families in which periodontal disease was accompanied by marked bruising, joint hypermobility and skin hyperextensibility and all were inherited in an autosomal dominant manner. Remarkably, affected individuals had lost most of their teeth to periodontal disease by their early twenties. There have been no published biochemical or ultrastructural studies of these patients. Interestingly, periodontal disease may be a feature of EDS VI. Thus, careful biochemical studies will be needed to distinguish these two disorders.

DIFFERENTIAL DIAGNOSIS AND PRENATAL DIAGNOSIS

The Ehlers-Danlos syndrome is a heterogeneous group of disorders of connective tissue manifest primarily as abnormalities of skin, joints, vessels and hollow organs. Disorders in type I and type III collagen have been identified, and the clinical disorders due to alterations in these two different molecules can be readily distinguished. Some of the clinical manifestations of the EDS are seen in certain other inherited connective tissue disorders so that careful medical history and physical examination are necessary to confirm the diagnosis. In the Marfan syndrome, for example, joint hypermobility is common but the associated features of arachnodactyly, lens subluxation and skeletal abnormalities help to distinguish the two syndromes (Pyeritiz & McKusick, 1979). The Marfanoid hypermobility syndrome, because of the marked joint hypermobility may be difficult to distinguish from EDS III unless the clinician is aware of both syndromes (Walker et al, 1969). Some of the cutaneous manifestations of osteogenesis imperfecta (Sillence et al, 1979), thin skin and easy bruising, are similar to those in some of the Ehlers-Danlos syndrome but the presence of marked bone fragility help to distinguish the disorders. The differentiation between the true cutis laxa disorders and some varieties of the Ehlers-Danlos syndrome occasionally is confusing (see the discussion of EDS V, above). In cutis laxa, the elastic components of the skin are generally altered and the skin is lax and, in contrast to skin in the EDS, does not return to its original position rapidly.

Increased joint laxity and slow motor development are often seen in neuromuscular disorders and children with EDS I or EDS II are sometimes thought to have those conditions. Conversely, in the evaluation of joint laxity and slow motor development in children, the connective tissue disorders should be considered. Occasionally, individuals with EDS I, EDS II and EDS IV are thought to have bleeding disorders. In most instances careful hematological evaluations have yielded no identifiable abnormalities in hemostasis (but see discussion of EDS I above). Nonetheless, some individuals with EDS are considered to have unidentified disorders of haemostasis and it is not until the connective tissue problems are recognized that the correct diagnosis is made.

Amniotic fluid cells in culture make both type I and type III collagens, and process and secrete them in the same manner as dermal fibroblasts. As a result, prenatal diagnosis of those forms of the Ehlers-Danlos syndrome in which specific biochemical abnormalities are known is feasible. It must be emphasized, however, that such attempts must be preceded by the accurate diagnosis of the defect in each family and, because different amniotic fluid cells synthesize and secrete different collagens (Crouch and Bornstein, 1979), must be accompanied by careful studies of the appropriate type of normal amniotic fluid cells. Other potential problems in the prenatal diagnosis of disorders of collagen metabolism include the uncertainty about whether the collagen types synthesized and secreted by the developing fetal cells are the products of the same genes as expressed by adult cells, and similar questions about the relation of the developmentally active enzyme modifying systems to those of the adult.

The clinical descriptions and classification system for the Ehlers-Danlos syndrome that we have presented here do not include all the families that have been described with the disorder. It is sometimes difficult to classify new families with respect to this system, underlining the yet undescribed heterogeneity that still exists. We anticipate that as more families are studied by biochemical techniques, that many different disorders in metabolism of collagen (and other macromolecules) will be identified that will provide specific diagnostic criteria, more rational genetic counseling, and facilitate prenatal diagnosis of some of the very severe disorders.

Already, the study of these unusual connective tissue disorders has provided considerable insight into a number of facets of collagen metabolism: the importance of certain collagen cross–links, the regulation of collagen synthesis, and the manner in which development of some tissues is modulated. The application of many of the techniques of molecular biology promises insight into the structure of some of these abnormal genes and may provide even more detailed understanding of the disease mechanisms that will be useful in the clinical sphere.

REFERENCES

Arneson M A, Hammerschmidt D E, Furcht L T, King R A 1980 A new form of Ehlers-Danlos Syndrome: fibronectin corrects defective platelet function. Journal of the American Medical Association 244: 144–147.

Barabas A P 1967 Heterogeneity of the Ehlers-Danlos syndrome: description of three clinical types and a hypothesis to explain the basic defect. British Medical Journal 2: 612–614.

Barabas A P 1966 Ehlers-Danlos syndrome associated with prematurity and premature rupture of foetal membranes; possible increase in incidence. British Medical Journal 2: 682–684.

Beighton P 1970 The Ehlers-Danlos syndrome. William Heinemann Medical Books, London.

Bornstein P 1974 The biosynthesis of collagen. Annual Review of Biochemistry 43: 576–603.

Bornstein P, Byers P H 1980 Disorders of collagen metabolism. In: Bondy P K and Rosenberg L E (eds). Metabolic Control and Disease, 8th ed. W B Saunders Co, Philadelphia.

Bornstein P, Sage H 1980 Structurally distinct collagen types. Annual Review of Biochemistry 49: 957–1004.

Boyd C D, Tolstoshev P, Schafer M P, Trapnell B C, Coon H C, Kretschmer P J, Nienhuis A W, Crystal R G 1980 Isolation and characterization of a 15-kilobase genomic sequence coding for part of the α2 chain of sheep type I collagen. Journal of Biological Chemistry 255: 3212–3220.

Byers P H, Holbrook K A, Barsh G S 1981a Type IV Ehlers-Danlos syndrome. In: Proceedings of the Workshop on Heritable Disorders of Connective Tissue, W Akeson, P Bornstein, M J Glimcher (eds). C V Mosby, St. Louis

Byers P H, Holbrook K A, Barsh G S, Smith L T, Bornstein P 1981b Altered secretion of type III procollagen in a form of type IV Ehlers-Danlos syndrome: biochemical studies in cultured fibroblasts. Laboratory Investigation 44: 336–341

Byers P H, Holbrook K A, McGillivray B, MacLeod P M , Lowry R B 1979 Clinical and ultrastructural heterogeneity of type IV Ehlers-Danlos syndrome. Human Genetics 47: 141–150.

Byers P H, Narayanan A S, Bornstein P, Hall J G 1976. An X–linked form of cutis laxa due to deficiency of lysyl oxidase. Birth Defects: Original Article Series 12(5): 293–298.

Byers P H, Siegel R C, Holbrook K A, Narayanan A S, Bornstein P, Hall J G 1980 X–linked cutis laxa: defective collagen crosslink formation due to decreased lysyl oxidase activity. New England Journal of Medicine 303: 61–65.

Crouch E, Bornstein P 1978 Collagen synthesis by human amniotic fluid cells in culture: characterization of a procollagen with three identical α1(I) chains. Biochemistry 17: 5499–5509.

Danlos M 1908 Un cas de cutis laxa avec tumeurs par contusion chronique des coudes et des Mace de Lepinay. Bulletin of the Societé Francais Dermatologie 19–70.

DiFerrante N, Leachman R D, Angelini D, Donnelly P W, Francis G, Almazan A 1975 Lysyl oxidase deficiency in Ehlers-Danlos syndrome type V. Connective Tissue Research 3: 48–53.

DiFerrante N, Leachmann R D, Angelini P, Donnelly P W, Francis G, Almazen A, Segni G, Franzblau C, Jordan R D 1975 Ehlers-Danlos type V (X–linked form), lysyl

oxidase deficiency. Birth Defects Original Article Series II: (6) 31–37.

Ehlers E 1901 Cutis laxa, Neigung zu hemorrhagien in der Haut, Loekerung mehrerer artikulationen. Dermatalogische Zeitschrift 8: 173.

Elsas L J, Miller R L, Pinnell S R 1978 Inherited human collagen lysyl hydroxylase deficiency: ascorbic acid response. Journal of Pediatrics 92: 378–384.

Epstein E H Jr 1974 α1(III)$_3$ human skin collagen: release by pepsin digestion and preponderance in fetal life. Journal of Biological Chemistry 249: 3225–3231.

Eyre D R, Glimcher M J 1972 Reducible cross-links in hydroxylysine-deficient collagens of a heritable disorder of connective tissue. Proceedings of the National Academy of Science USA 69: 2594–2595

Eyre D R 1980 Collagen: Molecular diversity in the body's protein scaffold. Science 207: 1315–1322.

Fessler J H, Fessler L I 1978 Biosynthesis of procollagen. Annual Review of Biochemistry 47: 129–162.

Frischauf A M, Lerach H, Rosner C, Boedtker H 1978 Procollagen complementary DNA, a probe for messenger RNA purification and the number of type I collagen genes. Biochemistry 17: 3243–3249.

Gay S, Martin G R, Müller P K, Timpl R and Kühn K 1976 Simultaneous synthesis of types I and III collagen by fibrolasts in culture. Proceedings of the National Academy of Sciences USA 73: 4037–4040.

Gottron H 1940 Familiare acrogeria. Archives of Dermatology Berlin 181: 571–576.

Judisch G F, Waziri M, Krachmer J H 1976 Ocular Ehlers-Danlos syndrome with normal lysyl hydroxylase activity. Archives of Ophthalmology 94: 1489–1491.

Holbrook K A, Byers P H 1981 Ultrastructural characteristics of the skin in a form of Ehlers-Danlos syndrome type IV: storage in the rough endoplasmic reticulum. Laboratory Investigation 44: 342–350

Holbrook K A, Byers P H, Counts, D F, Hegreberg G A 1980 Dermatosparaxis in a himalayan cat: ultrastructural studies of dermis. Journal of Investigative Dermatology 74: 100–104.

Hollister D W 1978 Heritable disorders of connective tissue: Ehlers-Danlos syndrome. Pediatric Clinics of North America 25: 575–591.

Krieg T, Feldmann U, Kessler W, Müller P K 1979 Biochemical characteristics of Ehlers-Danlos syndrome type VI in a family with one affected infant. Human Genetics 46: 41–49.

Leier C V, Call T D, Fulkerson P K, Wooley C F 1980 The spectrum of cardiac defects in the Ehlers-Danlos syndrome, types I and III. Annals of Internal of Medicine 92: 171–178.

Lichtenstein J R, Kohn L D, Martin G R, Byers P H, McKusick V A 1974 Procollagen peptidase deficiency in a form of the Ehlers-Danlos syndrome. Transactions of the American Association of Physicians 86: 333–339.

Lichtenstein J R, Martin G R, Kohn L, Byers P H, McKusick V A 1973 Defects in conversion of procollagen to collagen in a form of Ehlers-Danlos syndrome. Science 182: 298–300.

Lindahl V, Höök M 1978 Glycosaminoglycans and their binding to biological macro-molecules. Annual Review of Biochemistry 47: 385.

MacFarlane J D, Hollister D W, Weaver D D, Brandt K D, Luzzati L L, Biegel A A 1980 A new Ehlers-Danlos syndrome with skeletal dysplasia. American Journal of Human Genetics 32: 118A.

McKusick V A 1972 Heritable disorders of connective tissue. C V Mosby Co, St. Louis.

Paglia L, Wilczek J, Diaz de Leon L, Martin G R, Hörlein D, Müller P 1979 Inhibition of procollagen cell-free synthesis by amino-terminal extension peptides. Biochemistry 19: 5030–5034.

Pinnell S R 1978 Disorders of collagen. In: Stanbury J B, Wyngaarden J B, Frederickson D S (eds). The Metabolic Basis of Inherited Disease. McGraw Hill Book Co, New York.

Pinnell S R, Krane S M, Kenzora J E, Glimcher M J 1972 A heritable disorder of connective tissue: Hydroxylysine-deficient collagen disease. New England Journal of Medicine 866: 1013–1020.

Pope F M, Martin G R, Lichtenstein J R, Penttinen R P, Gerson G, Rowe D W, McKusick V A 1975 Patients with Ehlers-Danlos syndrome type IV lack type III collagen. Proceedings of the National Academy of Sciences USA 72: 1314–1316.

Pope F M, Martin G R, McKusick V A 1977 Inheritance of Ehlers-Danlos type IV syndrome. Journal of Medical Genetics 14: 200–204.

Prockop D J, Kivirikko K I, Tuderman L, Guzman N A 1979 The biosynthesis of collagen and its disorders. New England Journal of Medicine 301: 13–23, 77–85.

Pyeritz R E, McKusick V A 1979 The Marfan syndrome: diagnosis and management. New England Journal of Medicine 300: 772–775.

Quinn R S, Krane S M 1976 Abnormal properties of collagen lysylhydroxylase from skin fibroblasts of siblings with hydroxylysine-deficient collagen. Journal of Clinical Investigation 57: 83–93.

Sack G 1936 Status dysvascularis; ein Fall von besonderer Zerreisslichkeit der Blutgefasse. Deutsches Archivfür Klinische Medizin 178: 663–669.

Schachter H, Roseman S 1980 Mammalian glycosyltransferases: their role in the synthesis and function of complex carbohydrates and glycolipids. In: The Biochemistry of glycoproteins and proteoglycans, W J Lennarz ed. Plenum Press, New York.

Siegel R C 1979 Lysyl oxidase. International Review of Connective Tissue Research 8: 73–118.

Siegel R C, Black C M, Bailey A J 1979 Cross-linking of collagen in the X–linked Ehlers-Danlos type V. Biochemical and Biophysical Research Communications 88: 281–287.

Sillence D O, Senn A, Danks D M 1979 Genetic heterogeneity in osteogenesis imperfecta. Journal of Medical Genetics 16: 101–116.

Stewart R E, Hollister D W, Rimoin D L 1977 A new variant of the Ehlers-Danlos syndrome: an autosomal dominant disorder of fragile skin, abnormal scarring and generalized periodontitis. Birth Defects 13(3B)85–93.

Steinmann B, Gitzelmann R, Vogel A, Grant M E, Harwood R, Sear C H J 1975 Ehlers-Danlos syndrome in two siblings with deficient lysyl hydroxylase activity in cultured skin fibroblasts but only mild hydroxylysine deficit in skin. Helvetica Pediatrica Acta 30: 255–274.

Steinmann B, Tuderman L., Peltonen L, Martin G R, McKusick V A, Prockop D J 1980 Evidence for a stuctural mutation of procollagen type I in a patient with the Ehlers-Danlos syndrome type VII. Journal of Biological Chemistry 255: 8887–8893.

Sussman M, Lichtenstein J R, Nigra T P, Martin G R, McKusick V A 1974 Hydroxylysine-deficient collagen in a patient with a form of the Ehlers-Danlos syndrome. Journal Bone and Joint Surgery 56A: 1228–1234.

Vogel A, Holbrook K A, Steinmann B, Gitzelmann R, Byers P H 1979 Abnormal collagen fibril structure in the gravis form (type I) of the Ehlers-Danlos syndrome. Laboratory Investigation 40: 201–206.

Vogeli G, Avvedimento E V, Sullivan M, Maizel J V, Lozang G, Adams S L, Pastan I, deCrombrugghe B 1980 Isolation and characterization of genomic DNA coding for α 2 chain of type I collagen. Nucleic Acids Research 8: 1823–1837.

Walker B A, Beighton P, Murdoch J L 1969 The Marfanoid hypermobility syndrome. Annals of Internal Medicine 71: 349–352.

59

Pseudoxanthoma elasticum and related disorders

R. M. Goodman

PSEUDOXANTHOMA ELASTICUM

Introduction

Pseudoxanthoma elasticum (PXE) is a genetically determined heterogeneous disorder with clinical manifestations that may involve many organ systems. Although this condition has been referred to by many names (Table 59.1), it was first described as an atypical xanthoma by Rigal (1881) and the first autopsy report was given by Balzer (1884). Subsequent clinicians have recognized that the skin involvement is the least serious of its clinical features. In addition to the xanthoma-like appearance of part of the skin, the most frequently encountered manifestations include angioid streaks and other chorioretinal changes which frequently impair vision, and degenerative vascular changes which account for upper gastrointestinal haemorrhage, cardiovascular symptoms and a variety of neurological complications.

Attempts to relate the diverse clinical findings to a single pathological change led to the belief that PXE represents a genetic defect involving elastic or collagen fibres (McKusick, 1972). Although the elastic fibre hypothesis is the oldest and currently the most widely held, much remains to be learned concerning the basic defect in this disorder (Goodman et al, 1963).

Clinical features

Skin and mucosa

It has been commonly thought that recognizable skin changes do not appear before the second decade of life or later, however, Goodman and coworkers (1963) noted that on careful questioning the majority of their patients were aware of skin changes between the ages of 3 and 12 years. One patient was told that lesions were present about the neck from birth. All areas of normal body folds are prone to involvement, especially the neck. The yellowish appearing skin becomes thickened, pebbled and grooved resembling coarse-grained Moroccan leather. With progression of the disease the skin develops lax, redundant and inelastic features. About the face, exaggeration of the nasolabial folds and chin creases is often striking, producing a distinct, sagging facial appearance

Table 59.1 Terms used for pseudoxanthoma elasticum.

Date	Author	Term
1881	Rigal	Diffuse xanthelasma
1884	Balzer	Atypical xanthoma
1896	Darier	Pseudoxanthoma elasticum (PXE)
1929	Grönblad and Strandberg	Grönblad-Strandberg syndrome = angioid streaks plus skin lesions of PXE
1933	Lewis and Clayton	Elastosis atrophicans
1938	Böck	Elastosis dystrophica
1940	Témine	Elastorrhexie systématisée
1952	Tunbridge et al	Pseudo-xanthoma pseudo-elasticum

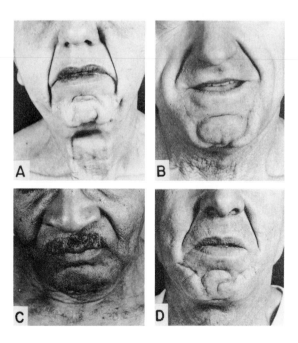

Fig. 59.1 Patients with PXE from three different families showing the prominent nasolabial folds as the skin about the face becomes lax. Altered skin changes about the neck can also be noted.

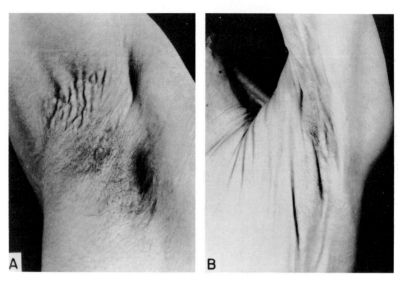

Fig. 59.2 Moderate (A) and marked (B) skin changes in the axilla.

(Fig. 59.1). Extreme laxity of the skin in the neck, axillary folds (Fig. 59.2) and abdominal wall has caused some patients to seek surgical intervention.

In some individuals the skin changes are exceedingly mild despite pronounced pathological changes in the eye and cardiovascular system. In addition to the characteristic skin changes described, some patients may have a different skin lesion which consists of ring-shaped plaques of closely grouped hyperkeratotic papules, 1-2 mm in size. Frequently a hyperkeratotic cap becomes dislodged to leave a small haemorrhagic depression which has been termed reactive perforating elastoma or Miescher's elastoma (Smith et al, 1962).

Calcinosis cutis has been observed in some patients, and calcification in the middle and deeper layers of the dermis may be noted readily by radiographic techniques.

Mucosal lesions similar to the characteristic skin findings have been observed on the inner aspect of the lower lip, buccal mucosa and in the rectum and vagina. Endoscopic examinations have also shown like lesions in the stomach and bladder.

Eye

The best described and most characteristic ocular lesion of PXE consists of peripapillary or radial 'angioid streaks'. Although angioid streaks are not pathognomonic of PXE, they are recognized in approximately 85% of cases, and a comparably large portion of all individuals with these streaks have PXE.

Depending upon the depth of retinal pigmentation these streaks appear grey, red or maroon. Lack of pigmentation of the streaks may be demonstrated by applying sufficient pressure upon the eye to occlude the retinal artery. Pallor of the vascular retina produced by this manoeuvre decreases visual contrasts and may lead to a virtual disappearance of the streaks (Goodman et al, 1963). In later stages, the streaks are bordered by proliferating scar tissue and retinal pigmentary epithelium. That angioid streaks are true cracks in Bruch's membrane beneath the retina is clinically substantiated by the observation of their tapering and their complimentary zigzag borders. They always underlie the retinal vessels.

Although probably not present at birth, these streaks usually develop in the second decade or later. They may persist for many years as the only ocular sign of PXE; however, chorioretinal changes usually appear. The development of haemorrhage or the appearance of chorioretinal scarring is an ominous sign.

Complete blindness usually does not occur but macular involvement frequently results in a diminution of visual acuity to 20/200, 20/400 or only the ability to see fingers at a few feet. When chorioretinal scarring and accompanying retinal pigment proliferation are extensive, angioid streaks may be obscured, although indistinct remnants of streaks usually persist at the periphery of such scars.

Some patients show only pigmentary mottling of the fundus and this is thought to be the earliest finding of an alteration in Bruch's membrane.

Berlyne and coworkers (1961) reported that persons presumed to be heterozygous for the PXE gene had an abnormally prominent choroidal vascular pattern but other studies (Goodman et al, 1963) have not been able to confirm this finding.

Gastrointestinal

The frequency of gastrointestinal haemorrhage in PXE is difficult to ascertain, but bleeding appears to be common and may be fatal. It may result from a peptic ulcer or hiatus hernia, but in most instances the source is not evident. Superficial ulceration and a friable oozing mucosal surface with diffusely scattered erosions have been seen by gastroscopy. Gastroscopy done in the absence of bleeding may show a yellowish papular gastric mucosa with lesions similar to those found in the oral and rectal mucosa. Redundancy of mucosal tissue of the lesser curvature of the stomach has been seen (Goodman et al, 1963).

Upper gastrointestinal tract bleeding in PXE has been known to occur in children as early as age 3 years but in most instances onset is in adulthood. Massive gastrointestinal haemorrhage has been observed during pregnancy suggesting that this state may be an influencing factor. In patients with upper gastrointestinal haemorrhage of unknown cause one should always look for the skin lesions noted in PXE.

The nature of the complex vascular anatomy of the stomach and its regulatory mechanism are fundamental to the understanding of the mucosal abnormalities and to the occurrence of gastrointestinal bleeding in PXE. As described by Bentley and Barlow (1952) the submucosal arterial plexus gives off spiraling branches which anastomose to form the mucosal plexus. These then arborize into a rich capillary bed. Arteriovenous shunts are present which can dilate to 140μm in calibre and can, when open, direct blood away from the mucosa and lead to pallor of the surface. Although the mechanism for the control of flow in this system is not well understood, it seems reasonable that alteration in the elastic tissue of the vessels might impair the normal regulation of gastric blood flow. This alteration could account for poor constriction of vessels and inadequate shunting of blood away from the mucosa with persistence of vascular dilation and resultant diffuse oozing from the mucosal surface. This hypothesis (Goodman et al, 1963) suggests that upper gastrointestinal haemorrhage in PXE occurs as the result of an alteration in vascular elastic tissue and impairment of the normal mechanism for the regulation of gastric blood flow.

Another possible mechanism for haemorrhage is entirely speculative: proliferation and calcification of nodular lesions in the stomach may be followed by perforation and ulceration, such as occurs in the skin in lesions of elastoma perforans of PXE.

Abdominal angina has been reported in several patients with PXE due to stenosis of the coeliac artery. The symptoms are usually of pain coming on 40–50 minutes after a meal.

Cardiovascular

It has long been known that the peripheral arteries are involved in the pathological process underlying PXE. Intermittent claudication has been described as early as

the age of nine and in other cases before the age of 36 years.

Radial and/or ulnar pulses are frequently absent in this disorder, but ischaemic symptoms are rather unusual in the upper extremities despite the severe angiographic changes that can be observed (Fig. 59.3). The lack of upper extremity symptoms may be due to the fact that collateral circulation from the interosseous artery provides adequate filling of the arterial system in the hand.

Calcification of peripheral arteries is frequently observed in PXE. The most common site is the femoral artery. Although calcification of vessels tends to increase with age, as does that of the skin, it has been reported to occur as early as the age of nine years. The media is the predominant site of calcium deposition within the artery.

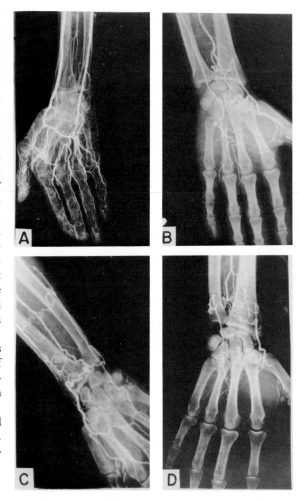

Fig. 59.3 (A) normal upper extremity arteriogram, (B-D) arteriograms in patients with PXE showing varying degrees of occlusive changes involving the radial, ulnar and digital arteries.

PXE patients are prone to premature atherosclerosis, and coronary arterial involvement can be demonstrated by the presence of angina pectoris, e.c.g. changes demonstrating myocardial infarction and radiographic evidence of occlusive coronary artery disease. McKusick (1972) mentions an 11 year-old girl with angina pectoris who at the age of 18 years showed disease in three vessels and the following year had a triple graft replacement.

The disease process in PXE may also involve the endocardium, heart valves and cardiac conduction system. Clinical manifestations may include cardiac enlargement, heart failure, arrhythmias and murmurs with valve deformity which result from the endocardial thickening (McKusick, 1972).

Hypertension is not uncommon in such patients and this has been shown to be due to renal vascular disease of the PXE type (McKusick, 1972). The presence of hypertension can be an influencing factor in the tendency to haemorrhage. Excessive uterine bleeding and intra-articular haemorrhage with formation of haemarthroses have been reported in a few patients (Altman et al, 1974).

Neurological

Various neurological signs and symptoms can be manifested in patients with PXE depending upon the location and severity of the vascular lesion (Iqbal et al, 1978). Patients may complain of paraesthesia and numbness. Aneurysms often involve the cerebral arteries with secondary complications. Subarachnoid haemorrhage has been a cause of death in some patients.

Frequent associations of prominent mental or psychiatric disturbances, such as forgetfulness or impaired memory, dull mentality, depression, psychoneurosis and mental deterioration, have been noted in association with PXE. The incidence of seizures is increased in this disorder but no specific e.e.g. abnormality has been observed.

Diagnosis

At present the diagnosis of PXE is based on distinct clinical and histological changes as no precise biochemical alteration has been found. The combination of the characteristic skin changes along with the presence of angioid streaks (Grönblad-Strandberg syndrome) is pathognomonic for the disorder. The involved skin shows characteristic histological changes involving masses of abnormal elastic-staining material within the mid-dermis and, less frequently, within the upper or lower dermis (Goodman et al, 1963). For the most part, this material is granular but in places rodlike structures are observed (Fig. 59.4). Tuberculoid areas with giant cells are found in the area of degeneration. Calcification of the degenerated material occurs, and it has now been documented that calcium deposition in elastic fibres is the earliest demonstrable histopathological change in PXE (Good-

man et al, 1963). Elastic fibres surrounding the sweat glands (Fig. 59.4) are thought to be among the first to show this early change (Goodman et al, 1963).

Further clinical documentation of PXE may be obtained by visual examination of the mucosal surface of the oral cavity, stomach, rectum and vagina, or by noting the characteristic occlusive changes in the upper extremities using the technique of brachial artery angiography.

Differential diagnosis

Actinic or senile elastosis may outwardly resemble the skin lesions of PXE but such changes are limited to the exposed surfaces of the body and histologically are distinguishable from PXE.

Angioid streaks occur in 8–15% of patients with Paget disease of bone. This disease shares with PXE a predisposition to calcification of the media of arteries, and the angioid streaks in the two disorders are clinically and histologically indistinguishable (Schmorl, 1931). However, the streaks in Paget disease are observed late in life when the bone changes are far advanced. A few cases with both Paget disease and PXE have been reported in detail as well as several less well documented cases (Woodcock, 1952; Shaffer et al, 1957).

It is estimated that 5% of all individuals homozygous for sickle cell disease have angioid streaks (Goodman et al, 1963). The pathology has not been defined, but description of abnormal elastic tissue in Bruch's membrane and the internal elastic lamella of ocular vessels may suggest involvement of the elastic tissue in this disorder – probably of the secondary type. Patients with both sickle cell disease and PXE have been reported (Geereats & Guerry, 1960; Goodman et al, 1963).

Angioid streaks have been observed in one person with familial hyperphosphataemia and metastatic calcification (McPhaul & Engel, 1961), in a patient with idiopathic thrombocytopenic purpura (Yatzkan, 1957) and in several instances of lead poisoning (De Simone & De Concilliis, 1958). The mechanism of streak production in these disorders is not known.

Genetics

Incidence and prevalence

Several hundred cases of PXE have been reported in the literature since the first case was described in 1881 by Rigal. Although this genetically determined disorder should be thought of as being rare, no racial or ethnic group appears to have a predilection and no distinct geographic distribution has been noted.

The frequency of PXE is not known. Berlyne and his group (1961) in England suggested that one case may occur among every 160 000 to 1 million persons. It is the impression of many (Goodman et al, 1963; McKusick, 1972) that it occurs more frequently than 1 in 160 000. (See section under inheritance).

PXE   HYPERCALCAEMIA

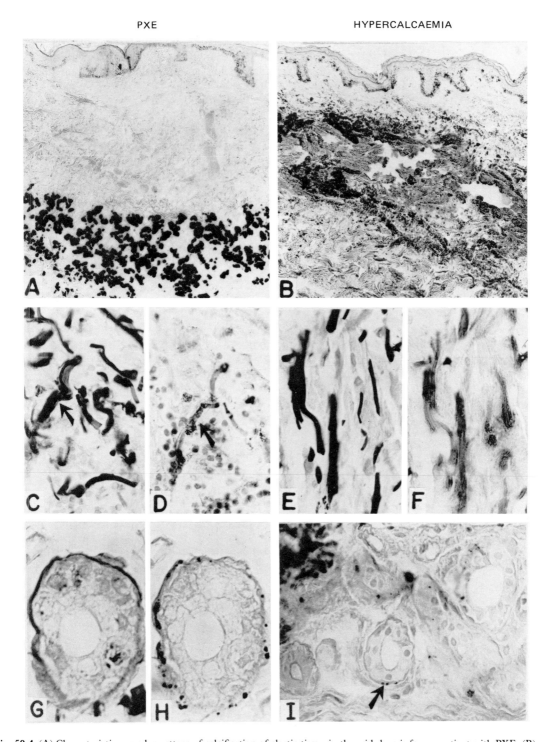

Fig. 59.4 (A) Characteristic granular pattern of calcification of elastic tissue in the mid-dermis from a patient with PXE. (B) Massive and nonspecific calcification in the skin of a patient with secondary hypercalcaemia due to leukaemia. (C) Elastic stain showing normal appearing elastic fibres in the skin of a patient with PXE. (D) Same fibres restained for calcium illustrating that some fibres are calcified despite the fact that they appear normal with the elastic stain. (E and F) The same as C and D in a patient with secondary hypercalcaemia due to leukaemia. (G) Elastic fibres surrounding a sweat gland from a patient with PXE. (H) Same sweat gland showing small foci of calcification in the elastic tissue. (I) Arrow points to small foci of calcification of elastic tissue about the sweat gland in a patient with transient idiopathic hypercalcaemia.

Sex ratio

Various observers have concluded, by tabulation of cases in the literature, that there is a preponderance of affected females (McKusick, 1972). A review of 106 cases of PXE from the Mayo Clinic (Connor et al, 1961) showed a 1:1.2 ratio of affected males to females. But within this group there were 32 cases with angioid streaks alone, the ratio then being 2.2:1 males to females. A major problem in ascertaining the sex distribution in PXE from reports in the literature is that females are more likely to seek medical advice when there is a cosmetic problem.

Inheritance

Extensive studies in the United Kingdom by Pope (1974a, 1974b, 1975) have firmly established that there is genetic heterogeneity in PXE. At present there appear to be two autosomal dominant and two recessive forms (Table 59.2).

Recessive type I is the most common (the classic type) and resembles dominant type I, although the vascular and retinal degenerative changes are milder. Upper gastrointestinal haemorrhage tends to be more common in affected females.

Recessive type II is an extremely rare variant which exhibits generalized cutaneous laxity and infiltration without systemic complications. Pope (1975) found only 3 affected families out of some 140 examined in Britain and none were found in the previous literature.

Dominant type I is the most severe form exhibiting the characteristic skin changes with cardiovascular complications and degenerative retinopathy leading to a marked loss in vision.

Dominant type II is about four times more common than dominant type I. This form is characterized by a canary-yellow macular skin lesion, minimal vascular symptoms and mild retinal changes with prominent choroidal vessels. Increased extensibility of the skin, blue sclerae, high-arched palate and myopia are also observed in this type.

Consanguinity has been found in at least 20% of cases with the classic recessive type I. Altman and co-workers (1974) estimated the prevalence of all forms of PXE in the Seattle area to be greater than 1 in 70 000.

Genetic counselling and prenatal diagnosis

Every effort must be made to establish the precise type of PXE afflicting the patient before proper genetic counselling is undertaken. Recurrence risks can then be given depending upon whether one is dealing with an autosomal dominant or recessive form or perhaps a new mutation.

Table 59.2 Clinical findings in autosomal dominant and recessive types of PXE (based on data presented by Pope, 1974a and b).

Characteristics	Genetic types			
	Autosomal dominant		Autosomal recessive	
	Dominant I (percent)	Dominant II (percent)	Recessive I (percent)	Recessive II (percent)
Cutaneous changes				
Classic peau d'orange and flexural rash	100	25	75	
Macular rash		70	15	
General increase of extensibility	10	65	10	
General cutaneous PXE				100
Vascular disease				
Angina	55			
Claudication	55			
Hypertension	75	10	20	
Haematemesis	10	5	15	
Ophthalmic abnormalities				
Severe choroiditis	75	10	35	
Angioid streaks	35	50	50	
Washed-out pattern		15	2	
Prominent choroidal-vessels		20		
Myopia	25	50	5	
Blue sclerae	10	40	10	
Other findings				
High arched palate		55	15	
Joint hypermobility		35	5	

Despite the fact that some investigators (Berlyne et al, 1961; Altman et al, 1974) have claimed that it is possible in some families to detect clinically those heterozygous for the type I recessive form of PXE, most do not believe that this is possible at present.

Prenatal diagnosis has not been done in this disorder but theoretically in the more severe forms it might be possible to use a skin biopsy from a commonly involved site to demonstrate early predisposition to calcification of the elastic tissue.

Basic defect

The basic defect in PXE is not known, although it is thought that the elastic fibre is primarily involved. It has been shown quite clearly that calcification of elastic fibres is not only frequent in PXE, but that it is always present in the various lesions which can be detected by light microscopy. Furthermore, it has been demonstrated that calcification is the earliest recognizable change, occurring in elastic fibres which appear normal under light microscopy (Goodman et al, 1963; Reeve et al, 1979). Such observations suggest that calcification represents a far more basic aspect of PXE than has been suspected previously (Akhtar & Brody, 1975). More recently, electron microscopy of elastic fibres from patients with PXE has shown that the principal alterations are in the elastin moiety of the elastic fibres (Ross et al, 1978). In contrast to the elastin moiety, the microfibrillar component of the elastic fibre appears to be normal. Further studies are needed to understand better the relationship between calcium deposition and the elastin moiety.

Prognosis and treatment

In considering the prognosis in patients with PXE it is important to know the genetic type. In general, the earlier the onset in PXE the more severe are the manifestations and thus the worse the prognosis. For the more severe forms of the disease life span is shortened by the various vascular complications involving the cardiovascular, gastrointestinal and central nervous systems.

Unfortunately no curative form of therapy is known. There have been a few isolated reports claiming that X–ray therapy (Carlborg, 1944) and tocopherol have produced improvement in the skin lesions (Stout, 1951). Ocular lesions have been treated with vitamin C in conjunction with calcium, and iodine and bismuth treatment has occasionally been used for resolving haemorrhages in the fundi (Carlborg, 1944). Although none of these treatments has been successful, there are certain supportive measures that are worth bearing in mind. Since the most disabling feature of this disease is progressive loss of vision, the use of visual aids is important. Redundant and unsightly skin folds about the neck can be improved by plastic surgery. Gastrointestinal haemorrhage usually should be treated conservatively, though surgical intervention may be life saving.

CUTIS LAXA

Introduction

The genetic form of cutis laxa is a very rare disorder of connective tissue often confused with the Ehlers-Danlos syndrome and the severe type of PXE. Kopp (1888) described the disorder in a father and son and Weber (1923) was the first to discuss the clinical differences between this disorder and the Ehlers-Danlos syndrome. Many designations have been used to describe cutis laxa and they include such terms as: chalazoderma, cutis pendula, dermatomegaly, dermatochalasia and systemic elastolysis when there are internal manifestations. Beighton (1972) recognized the presence of genetic heterogeneity in cutis laxa and commented on the clinical differences between the dominant and recessive forms.

Clinical features

Skin

Characteristically the skin has the appearance of being too large for the rest of the body and thus tends to sag extensively in those areas where it is normally loose, e.g. around the face and eyes (Goodman & Gorlin, 1977). Frequently the skin is wrinkled and appears prematurely aged so that an affected pubertal child will look older than his or her unaffected parents (Fig. 59.5). At birth, the skin may be soft and loose and nurses may comment on noticing a different 'feel' to the skin when compared to other infants. Even from birth the pendulous skin over the abdomen may cover the genitalia.

Unlike the skin in the Ehlers-Danlos syndrome, the skin in cutis laxa shows no fragility, bruisability or hyperextensibility. Some observers have noted that as affected individuals grow they tend to fill out their loose skin.

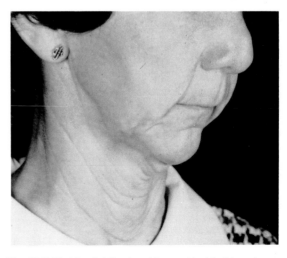

Fig. 59.5 Facial wrinkling in a 16 year-old girl with cutis laxa. (Courtesy of Professor P. Beighton).

Facial

A number of facial features are common to this disorder and they include the following: an unusually long upper lip, hooking of the nose with shortening of the columella and unusually long ear lobes (Beighton, 1970). Frequently the voice from birth may be deep and resonant in tone due to laxity of the vocal cords. Micrognathia, delayed or bizzare tooth eruption and thickening of the oral and pharyngeal mucosa have also been observed. A variety of eye findings have been noted and these include ectropion of the lids, ocular hypertelorism, iris hypoplasia, blue sclerae and microcornea.

Internal manifestations

A variety of internal organ findings have been reported, but lung involvement with emphysematous changes is one of the more common and severe manifestations of the recessive form of the disorder (McKusick, 1972). This may cause right ventricular enlargement, cor pulmonale and death at any early age. Pulmonary artery stenosis and extremely tortuous blood vessels along with dilation of the aorta have also been observed in the recessive form.

Inguinal, diaphragmatic, and unbilical hernias have been described as well as diverticulae of the oesophagus, stomach, intestine and bladder. Prolapse of the rectum and uterus has been reported.

Musculoskeletal changes include such findings as delayed somatic growth, hypotonia, late closure of the anterior fontanelle, hip dislocation and joint hyperextensibility.

Diagnosis

The clinical features are usually present at birth or in infancy with the skin changes giving a prematurely aged appearance to the affected individual. A skin biopsy shows a reduced number of elastic fibres which are fragmented and granular (Goltz et al, 1965). Byers and coworkers (1976) have shown that the skin fibroblasts from a patient with the X–linked type of cutis laxa synthesized diminished levels of lysyl oxidase when compared to control fibroblasts.

X–ray studies may show various types of herniations, prolapses and diverticula, while arteriographic studies may reveal pulmonary artery stenosis, dilation of the aorta and kinking of peripheral vessels (Meine et al, 1974).

Differential diagnosis

Cutis laxa may develop as a secondary manifestation in the later stages of certain infectious diseases affecting the dermis, or secondary to an allergic phenomenon such as a contact eczema or penicillin allergy (Rook et al, 1979). In the acquired forms of cutis laxa the skin changes are like those of the congenital or genetic form but they begin in adulthood.

More recently Linares et al (1979) reported an infant with generalized cutis laxa born to a cystinuric mother who took penicillamine throughout pregnancy. By the age of nine months the infant had normal skin. They postulated that the D-penicillamine treatment may have produced low blood copper levels accounting for the connective tissue changes present at birth. Walshe (1979) challenged the interpretation of the copper studies done by Linares et al (1979) and felt the skin changes could not be attributed to copper depletion.

Cutis laxa confined to the anterior abdominal wall and thorax and present from birth may occur in association with dysplasia of the abdominal musculature, deformity of the thorax and mediastinal hernia.

Loose skin folds may develop in certain areas of the body in patients with the Ehlers-Danlos syndrome, PXE, neurofibromatosis, blepharochalasis and leprechaunism, but these disorders usually can be differentiated from cutis laxa by their other clinical manifestations and/or skin histopathological findings.

Two other genetic syndromes having skin findings that should be considered in the differential diagnosis of cutis laxa are the wrinkly skin syndrome and geroderma osteodysplastica. These are discussed below.

Genetics

Incidence and prevalence

The genetic forms of cutis laxa are extremely rare and as of 1980 not more than 50 well documented cases have been reported in the medical literature. Almost all patients have been Caucasian.

Sex ratio

Except for the X–linked recessive form of cutis laxa no unusual sex ratio has been noted.

Inheritance

At present there are three known genetic forms of this disorder. The most common and severe type is transmitted as an autosomal recessive trait in which the parents are frequently consanguineous. A less commonly observed form is the relatively benign autosomal dominant type (Beighton, 1972). The reported mild sporadic cases are probably of this type. Byers and coworkers (1976) reported an X–linked recessive type in which the patients had mild joint hyperextensibility and bladder diverticula. It is this type that is associated with diminished levels of lysyl oxidase in skin fibroblasts.

Genetic counselling and prenatal diagnosis

As with any heritable disorder in which there is genetic heterogeneity, it is essential to know which form of the condition the patient is afflicted with before embarking on genetic counselling. Once this is established, recurrence risks can be given according to the mode of transmission be it autosomal dominant, recessive or X–linked recessive.

Theoretically it may be possible to offer prenatal diagnosis to those families at risk for the X–linked recessive type, based on a low level of lysyl oxidase in cultured skin fibroblasts from a male fetus at risk.

If a skin biopsy could be obtained using fetoscopy then a fetus at risk for the more severe autosomal recessive form of the disorder could possibly be diagnosed based on the histopathological features of cutis laxa.

Basic defect

The basic defect in cutis laxa is not known despite the observation of Byers and coworkers (1976) that in the X–linked form there is a diminished level of lysyl oxidase. Nevertheless, histopathologic studies using both light (Goltz et al, 1965) and electron microscopy (Hashimoto & Kanzaki, 1975) have shown that it is primarily the elastic fibre that undergoes change. Some investigators have postulated that there is increased susceptibility of elastin to the action of elastase, due to a deficiency of elastase inhibitor resulting from a disturbance of copper metabolism (Goltz & Hult, 1965). However, there is no evidence at present to support this hypothesis (Harris et al, 1978).

Prognosis and treatment

The autosomal recessive form often leads to death early in childhood due to cardiorespiratory complications. The dominant form is not a life-threatening condition in the early years of life but various complications, reflecting tissue weakness of internal organs, should be looked for as these patients age.

Plastic surgery should be considered to reduce the cosmetic disfigurement and to improve the psychosocial attitude of the patient. Periodic respiratory function studies should be done to ensure early diagnosis of associated emphysema. In children with heart failure, upper airway obstruction should be evaluated and tracheostomy considered.

WRINKLY SKIN SYNDROME

Clinical features

This genetic disorder of connective tissue was first described by Gazit and coworkers (1973) in three sibs of consanguineous parents.

At birth it was noted that all three affected sibs were hypotonic and small for dates although all were full-term. The most striking physical finding pertained to the skin. Over most of the body, except the face, the skin appeared dry and easily wrinkled, as noted about the abdomen in the sitting position (Fig. 59.6). Numerous skin wrinkles

were noted on the dorsal and ventral surfaces of the hands (Fig. 59.7) and feet. This wrinkled appearance of the skin about the hands and feet was present from birth. A reduction in the elasticity of skin about the hands was noted but there appeared to be no altered skin elasticity in other parts of the body. A prominent venous pattern

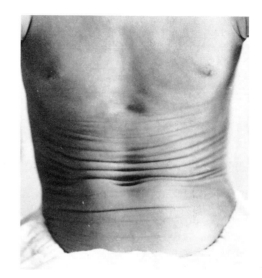

Fig. 59.6 Multiple abdominal skin wrinkles in a 9 year-old girl with the wrinkly skin syndrome.

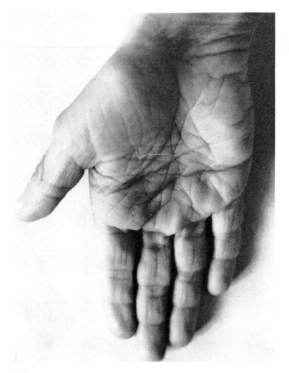

Fig. 59.7 Accentuated and multiple palmar creases in a 9 year-old girl with the wrinkly skin syndrome.

was observed on the anterior surface of the chest and the dorsal surface of the hands and feet. The skin did not sag, there was no evidence of abnormal scar tissue formation and no history of easy bruisability. The joints were not hyperextensible. The two affected sibs had kyphosis, 'winging' of the scapulae and poor muscle development. In addition one of them had microcephaly with moderate mental retardation along with myopic changes with old chorioretinitis and partial optic atrophy.

Diagnosis

At present the diagnosis of this syndrome is based on the clinical features described above. No distinct histopathological changes were observed from biopsied skin tissue studied under light microscopy. Both the collagen and elastic fibres appeared normal, however, electron microscopic examination of these fibres was not done.

Differential diagnosis

In cutis laxa the facial skin characteristically hangs loose giving a premature aged appearance to the patient. Furthermore, the elastic fibres in cutis laxa are reduced in number and are fragmented. These two distinct features of cutis laxa help in distinguishing it from the wrinkly skin syndrome. Hyperextensible skin and joints in the various forms of the Ehlers-Danlos syndrome, along with ease in bruisability and poor scar tissue formation, differentiate this disorder from the wrinkly skin syndrome.

Genetics

This condition is thought to be transmitted as an autosomal recessive trait. The parents of the three affected sibs reported by Gazit et al (1973) were unaffected first cousins of Jewish ancestry originating from Iraq. The author has recently observed this same disorder in two other sibs of Jewish Iranian background whose parents were also normal and first cousins.

The recurrence risk should be like that of any other autosomal recessive disorder. It is doubtful that fetoscopy would allow prenatal diagnosis of this disorder, especially since no characteristic histopathological findings have been observed in the skin.

Basic defect

The basic defect in this heritable disorder of connective tissue is not known.

Prognosis and treatment

Not enough is known about this syndrome to assess all its possible prognostic features. For example, there is no certainty that the microcephaly with mental retardation observed in one affected sib is part of the disorder. No special treatment other than symptomatic care is indicated.

GERODERMA OSTEODYSPLASTICA

Clinical features

This heritable disorder of connective tissue was first described by Bamatter and coworkers (1949) and is characterized by distinct facial and musculoskeletal findings.

The skin about the face gives the appearance of premature aging due to excessive wrinkling and atrophic changes (Fig. 59.8). Eye abnormalities may include microcornea, myopia and keratoconus. Frequently these patients have micrognathia and various dental anomalies. Premature wrinkling of the skin is also common about the abdomen and dorsal surface of the hands and feet.

Musculoskeletal findings include the following: short stature, excessive length of the upper extremities, stooped posture due to kyphoscoliosis, 'winging' of the scapulae, pes planus, hyperextensible joints with ease in dislocation, muscular hypotonia with a protuberant abdomen and hernias.

Diagnosis

The diagnosis of this syndrome is a clinical one and many of the above clinical features are present from early childhood. X–ray studies show generalized osteoporosis, platyspondyly and multiple incremental lines within bones

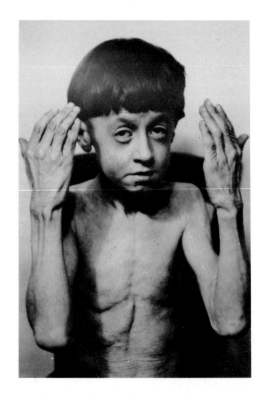

Fig. 59.8 A 10 year-old boy with geroderma osteodysplastica showing premature wrinkling of the skin. (Courtesy of Professor D. Klein).

like growth rings of a tree (Brocher, 1968). A skin biopsy shows atrophy of the epidermis and fragmentation of the elastic fibres.

Differential diagnosis

This syndrome must be differentiated from cutis laxa and the wrinkly skin syndrome. The laxity of the skin in geroderma osteodysplastica is not generally as severe as that observed in cutix laxa, and the extensive skeletal changes known to be present in the former are not found in either cutis laxa or the wrinkly skin syndrome. A skin biopsy from a patient with the wrinkly skin syndrome does not show specific changes, whereas characteristic findings have been observed in both cutis laxa and geroderma osteodysplastica.

Genetics

In the original Swiss family reported by Bamatter et al (1949), Boreux (1968) postulated that the disorder might be inherited as an X–linked recessive trait with mild manifestations in the female. Hunter and coworkers

(1978) reported two families with six affected children. Consanguinity and two fully affected females among the six children strongly support autosomal recessive transmission. Genetic heterogeneity in this rare syndrome is a possibility but actual verification must await reports of other families.

Genetic counselling must be based on the most likely mode of transmission for the family in question. Prenatal diagnosis has not been done in this disorder.

Basic defect

The basic defect in this syndrome is not known.

Prognosis and treatment

At present there is no evidence to suggest that affected individuals have a shortened life span. Because of their osteoporosis these patients are prone to fractures, especially of the vertebrae. Treatment for the osteoporosis is required. Possible orthopaedic intervention for correction of the kyphoscoliosis and plastic surgery for the facial skin involvement should be considered.

REFERENCES

Pseudoxanthoma elasticum

Akhtar M, Brody H 1975 Elastic tissue in pseudoxanthoma elasticum: ultrastructural study of endocardial lesions. Archives of Pathology 99: 667–671

Altman L K et al 1974 Pseudoxanthoma elasticum. Archives of Internal Medicine 134: 1048–1054

Balzer F 1884 Récherches sur les charactèrs anatomiques du xanthelasma. Archives of Physiology 4: 65–80

Bentley F H, Barlow T E 1952 The vascular anatomy of the stomach. Modern Trends in Gastroenterology. Butterworth and Co, London p 309

Berlyne G M et al 1961 The genetics of pseudoxanthoma elasticum. Quarterly Journal of Medicine 30: 201–212

Böck J 1938 Zur Klinik und Anatomie der Gefässählichen Streifen im Augenhintergrund. Zeitschuft für Augenheilkunde 95: 1

Carlborg U 1944 Study of circulatory disturbances, pulse wave velocity and pressure pulses in larger arteries in cases of pseudoxanthoma elasticum, and angioid streaks. A contribution to the knowledge of the function of the elastic tissue and the smooth muscles in larger arteries. Acta Medica Scandinavica 151: 1

Connor P J et al 1961 Pseudoxanthoma elasticum and angioid streaks, a review of 106 cases. American Journal of Medicine 30: 537–543

Darier J 1896 Pseudoxanthoma elasticum. Monatsh Prakt Dermatol 23: 609–617

De Simone S, De Concilliis U 1958 Strie angioidi della retina (considerazioni cliniche e patogenetiche). Archives of Otolaryngology 62: 161

Geereats W J, Guerry J 1960 Angioid streaks and sickle cell disease. American Journal of Ophthalmology 49: 450–470

Goodman R M et al 1963 Pseudoxanthoma elasticum: A clinical and histopathological study. Medicine (Baltimore) 42: 297–334

Gronblad E 1929 Angioid streak – pseudoxanthoma elasticum: Vorläufige Mitteilung. Acta Ophthalmologica (Kbh) 7: 329

Iqbal A et al 1978 Pseudoxanthoma elasticum: A review of neurological complications. Annals of Neurology 4: 18–20

Lewis G M, Clayton M D 1933 Pseudoxanthoma elasticum and angioid streaks. Archives of Dermatology and Syphilology 28: 546–556

McKusick V A 1972 Heritable disorders of connective tissue, 4 edn. C V Mosby, St Louis pp 475–520

McPhaul J J Jr, Engel F L 1961 Heterotopic calcification, hyperphosphatemia and angioid streaks of the retina. American Journal of Medicine 31: 488–492

Pope F M 1974a Autosomal dominant pseudoxanthoma elasticum. Journal of Medical Genetics 11: 152–157

Pope F M 1974b Two types of autosomal recessive pseudoxanthoma elasticum. Archives of Dermatology 110: 209–212

Pope F M 1975 Historical evidence for the genetic heterogeneity of pseudoxanthoma elasticum. British Journal of Dermatology 92: 493–510

Reeve E B et al 1979 Development and calcification of skin lesions in thirty-nine patients with pseudoxanthoma elasticum. Clinics in Experimental Dermatology 3: 291–301

Rigal D 1881 Observation pour servir á l'histoire de la chéloide diffuse xanthelasmique. Annals of Dermatology and Syphilology 2: 491–501

Ross R et al 1978 Fine structure alterations of elastic fibers in pseudoxanthoma elasticum. Clinical Genetics 13: 213–223

Schmorl G 1931 Anatomische Befunde bei einem Fall von Osteopoikilic. Fortschritte auf dem Gebiete der Roentgenstrahlen und der Nuklearmedizin 44: 1–8

Shaffer B et al 1957 Pseudoxanthoma elasticum. A case of Paget's disease and a case of calcinosis with arteriosclerosis as manifestations of the syndrome. Archives of Dermatology 76: 622–633

Smith E W et al 1962 Reactive perforating

feature of certain genetic disorders. Bulletin of the Johns Hopkins Hospital 11: 235–251

Stout O M 1951 Pseudoxanthoma elasticum with retinal angioid streaking, decidedly improved on tocopherol therapy. Archives of Dermatology and Syphilology 63: 510–511

Strandberg J 1929 Pseudoxanthoma elasticum. Zeitschrift für Haut – und Geschlechtskrankheiten 31: 689

Témine P 1940 Contribution à l'étude de l'elastorrhexie systématisée. Paris thesis et cie, Paris

Tunbridge R E et al 1952 The fibrous structure of normal and abnormal human skin. Clinical Science 11: 315

Woodcock C W 1952 Pseudoxanthoma elasticum, angioid streaks of retina and osteitis deformans. Archives of Dermatology and Syphilology 65: 623

Cutis laxa

Beighton P et al 1970 Plastic surgery in cutis laxa. British Journal of Plastic Surgery 23: 285–290

Beighton P 1972 The dominant and recessive forms of cutis laxa. Journal of Medical Genetics 9: 216–221

Byers P H et al 1976 An X–linked form of cutis laxa due to deficiency of lysyl oxidase; the collagen and elastin crosslinking enzyme. Birth Defects no 36: 293–298

Goltz R W et al 1965 Cutis laxa, a manifestation of generalized elastolysis. Archives of Dermatology 92: 373–387

Goltz R W, Hult A M 1965 Generalized elastolysis (cutis laxa) and Ehlers-Danlos syndrome (cutis hyperelastica); a comparative clinical and laboratory study. Southern Medical Journal 58: 848–854

Goodman R M, Gorlin R J 1977 Atlas of the face in genetic disorders. C V Mosby, St Louis. pp 106–107

Harris R B et al 1978 Generalized elastolysis (cutis laxa). American Journal of Medicine 65: 815–822

Hashimoto K, Kanazaki T 1975 Cutis laxa ultrastructural and biochemical studies. Archives of Dermatology 111: 861–873

Kopp W 1888 Demonstration zweier Fälle von 'Cutis laxa'. Münchener Medizinische Wochenschrift 35: 259–260

Linares A et al 1979 Reversible cutis laxa due to maternal D-penicillamine treatment. Lancet 2: 43

McKusick V A 1972 Heritable disorders of connective tissue, 4th edn. C V Mosby, St Louis pp 372–389

Meine F et al 1974 The radiographic findings in congenital cutis laxa. Radiology 113: 687–690

Rook A et al 1979 Textbook of dermatology, 3rd edn. Blackwell Scientific Publications, London. pp 1626–1627

Walshe J M 1979 Congenital cutis laxa and maternal D-penicillamine Lancet 2: 144–145

Weber F P 1923 Chalasodermia or "loose skin" and its relationship to subcutaneous fibroids or calcareous nodules. Urologic and Cutaneous Reviews 27: 407

Wrinkly skin syndrome

Gazit E et al 1973 Wrinkly skin syndrome: A new heritable disorder of connective tissuee. Clinical Genetics 4: 186-192

Geroderma osteodysplastica

Bamatter F 1949 Gérodermie ostéodysplastique héréditaire. Un nouveau biotype de la "progeria". Confinia Neurologica 9: 397

Boreux G 1969 A gérodermie ostéodysplastique à hérédite liéé au sexes, nouvelle entité clinique et génétique. Journal de Génétique Humaine 17: 137–178

Brocher J E W 1968 Roentgenologische Befunde bei Geroderma osteodysplastica hereditaria. Fortschritte anf dem Gebiete der Roentgenstrahlen und der Nuklearmedizin 109: 185–198

Hunter A G 1978 Geroderma osteodysplastica: a report of two affected families. Human Genetics 40: 311–325

Peptic ulcer

J. I. Rotter

INTRODUCTION

The familial aggregation of peptic ulcer disease and its association with such clear-cut genetic factors as blood group O and non-secretor status is well established. However, the genetics of this disorder or group of disorders has, until recently, been poorly delineated. Polygenic inheritance was the prevailing hypothesis proposed for peptic ulcer, based primarily on the finding of blood group associations and the exclusion of a simple mode of inheritance for all ulcer disease. Genetic heterogeneity was proposed as an alternative hypothesis that could explain both the familial aggregation of peptic ulcer disease and the lack of a simple Mendelian pattern of inheritance (Rotter & Rimoin, 1977). This concept states that peptic ulcer is not one disease, but a group of disorders with different genetic and environmental causes. Initially based on indirect evidence, genetic heterogeneity has now received direct support from genetic studies using subclinical markers such as serum pepsinogen I (Rotter, 1980a,b). The unravelling of the genetic heterogeneity of peptic ulcer has important clinical and aetiological implications, for if what is termed a 'disease' is in reality a number of disorders that are grouped together because of some common clinical feature, these distinct disorders may differ markedly in genetics, pathophysiology, interaction with environmental agents, natural history and response to therapeutic and preventative measures.

This chapter will discuss the current state of knowledge regarding the genetic basis of peptic ulcer. The concept of polygenic inheritance will be contrasted to that of genetic heterogeneity, and the methods for delineating genetic heterogeneity in a common disease such as ulcer will be described.

DISEASE DEFINITION AND DIFFICULTIES FOR GENETIC STUDIES

A peptic ulcer is a circumscribed loss of tissue occurring in those parts of the gastrointestinal tract exposed to acid and pepsin – in the main, the lower esophagus, stomach and upper intestine (duodenum) (Grossman et al, 1979; Grossman, 1981). Its typical symptom is epigastric abdominal pain, worse at night and relieved by meals. Such classical symptoms occur only in a portion of all ulcer patients, and many present with less classical abdominal pain or with an ulcer complication. Complications include bleeding into the gastrointestinal tract (which can range from chronic blood loss to a severe life threatening haemmorrhage), perforation (extension of the ulcer through the full thickness of the wall of the gastrointestinal tract), and obstruction of gastric emptying (from scarring and/or oedema and spasm). The diagnosis of a peptic ulcer is usually made by upper gastrointestinal radiography using a contrast material such as barium sulphate, or by direct visualization by endoscopy.

An ulcer is generally thought to occur when there is an imbalance between the 'aggressive' forces of acid and pepsin and the less defined 'defensive' forces of mucosal resistance and regeneration. The goal of ulcer therapy, both medical and surgical, is to hopefully correct this imbalance in order to promote ulcer healing, relieve symptoms, and prevent complications and recurrences. This is usually done by agents or methods that either buffer the acid produced (e.g. antacids) or reduce acid secretion (e.g. cimetidine, vagotomy), though protective agents such as prostaglandins and sulphated disacchar-ides are also being developed. A complete discussion of ulcer diagnosis and therapy is beyond the scope of this chapter and the reader is referred to more complete references of this area (Grossman et al, 1979; Grossman 1980a; 1981). Peptic ulcer tends to be an episodic, chronic disorder, characterised by symptomatic periods and pain free intervals. The natural history of ulcer is still being defined, and this may well differ as the different diseases leading to an ulcer are delineated by clinical, physiological and genetic studies.

Peptic ulcer is among the most common of chronic diseases, occurring in 5 to 10% of the population in their lifetime (depending on such factors as geography, population, level of health care) (Grossman, 1980b; 1981; Langman, 1979). This leads to a number of problems for genetic studies. Is a relative affected because he has the same genotype, shares the same environment, or has the chance occurrence of a common disorder? Even if peptic ulcer is a group of disorders, they are sufficiently common that different forms will occur in the same family by chance alone. The age of onset of peptic ulcer varies markedly. Therefore, it is impossible to say whether an individual who is clinically unaffected at any given time will become affected later in life. Like many common diseases, genetic studies of peptic ulcer have suffered from confusion engendered by the varying definitions of 'affected' used by different investigators. 'Affected' has ranged from a person who has abdominal pain to one with an endoscopically demonstrated crater. Probably the greatest obstacle limiting genetic studies has been ignorance of the basic defects in various kinds of peptic ulcer and correspondingly the lack of genetic markers that would disclose clinically unaffected individuals with the hereditary predisposition.

Despite these difficulties, we have known for many years that genetic factors play a role in the aetiology of peptic ulcer, based on three lines of evidence: family studies, twin studies, and blood group studies.

EARLY GENETIC EVIDENCE

Family studies

The first approach in looking for genetic factors in a common disease is to determine whether familial aggregation is present. One compares the incidence of the disease in relatives of patients with the incidence in the general population. If increased, this is often the first indication that genetic factors are important in a disease. Family aggregation was noted in the late 1800's, but as with many diseases, the majority of initial reports presented one or a few pedigrees with no control data. Subsequently individuals with peptic ulcer were shown to have an 'increased family history' of the disease (McConnell, 1966; 1980). Most reports indicated a positive family history in 20–50% of individuals with peptic ulcer, compared to the 5 to 15% in controls. While this information has been used to support the importance of genetic factors, it is of little value in testing genetic hypotheses, since the prevalence of a positive family history will vary greatly with the types of interview, family size, number of relatives included, and with the criteria used for defining an affected individual. A more accurate assessment of familial aggregation is obtained by comparing the prevalence of the disorder among specific relatives of an affected individual to that found among similar relatives of a control group. This was done in several excellent studies (see Table 60.1). The consistent observation was that the frequency of peptic ulcer was 2 to 3 times greater in the first degree relatives of peptic ulcer patients than

in similar relatives of controls or the general population. Because these differences persisted across generations and social classes, genetic factors were presumed to explain these findings.

Twin studies

Familial aggregation can conceivably be due to common environmental as well as common genetic factors. Twin studies represent an approach to resolving the question of the relative influence of genetics and environment. The frequency of concordance (both members of the twin pair affected) of monozygotic (identical) twins is compared with that of dizygotic (fraternal) twins. Monozygotic twins share all genes, and should be concordant for disorders with pure genetic aetiology. Dizygotic twins share on the average only half their genes and are no more alike genetically than any pair of siblings. If the characteristic being studied is genetically determined with no environmental influence, then one expects 100% concordance in monozygotic twins, and less in dizygotic twins. If the disorder is entirely environmental, one should see equal concordance between monozygotic and dizygotic twins. If an interaction between a genetic predisposition and an environmental agent is necessary for clinical expression, one would expect to find a higher concordance among monozygotic than dizygotic twins, but not 100%. For peptic ulcer the concordance in monozygotic twins is less than 100% but consistently exceeds that in dizygotic twins (Table 60.2). This difference persists when dizygotic twins are restricted to those pairs of like sex. We can conclude from the twin studies that a large part of the familial aggregation is due to genetic factors.

Blood group studies

The third line of evidence for genetic factors in ulcer came from studies of blood group associations. The goal of such disease association studies is to determine the prevalence of a disorder among individuals with well defined genetic traits, such as blood groups or serum enzyme polymorphisms (also known as qualitative gene markers). If there is a positive association between a given disease and a particular allele of a well defined genetic locus, then the genetically determined trait is usually considered to be of importance in the pathogenesis of the disorder under study. Soon after the original association between blood group A and gastric cancer was described, the same group of investigators demonstrated that peptic ulcer was associated with blood group O (Aird et al, 1954). Individuals with blood group O have a 30–40% greater incidence of peptic ulcer than those of the remaining blood groups (McConnell, 1966; 1980; Mourant el al, 1978). One might question whether this relatively small increased risk is real. Yet this observation has been repeated by many investigators in many

Table 60.1 Peptic ulcer in families

Author	Proband's diagnosis	Relatives studied	Criteria	Relatives of ulcer proband	Relatives of controls or population controls
Doll & Buch, 1950	Peptic ulcer	Brothers	Hospital	11.5%	4.6%
		Sisters	records (60%)	2.8%	0.9%
		Fathers	Patient's	16.4%	4.5%
		Mothers	account (40%)	4.3%	–
Wretmark, 1953	Peptic ulcer	Brothers	History	15.0%	6.6–8.1%
		Fathers	from	14.8%	3.6%
		Mothers	proband	7.4%	1.2%
Kuennsberg, 1962	Duodenal ulcer	Sons	History	7.9%	2.4%
		Daughers	from proband	5.1%	0.7%
Monson, 1970a	Peptic ulcer	Fathers	History	24.5%	14.4%
		Mothers	from	9.5%	4.5%
		Brothers	proband	14.3%	6.5%
		Sisters		3.7%	1.6%
Jirasek, 1971	Duodenal ulcer	Parents	History	14.7%	
		Sibs	from	9.9%	
	Duodenal Gastric	Parents	proband	10.0%	
	ulcer	Sibs		8.0%	1.5–4.8%
	Pyloric ulcer	Parents		8.0%	
		Sibs		7.1%	
	Gastric ulcer	Parents		12.1%	
		sibs		6.8%	
Kubickova &	Duodenal ulcer	First degree	History	9.5%	1.7%
Vesely, 1972		Second degree	from	2.9%	0.5%
		Third Degree	proband	1.4%	0.22%

Table 60.2 Peptic ulcer in twins

Author	Criteria	No. of pairs	Concordance MZ	DZ
Camerer (1936)	Often clinical	14	14%	14%
Huhn (1939)	Questionnaire, then X–ray	13	80%	0%
Doig (1957)	X–ray	10	50%	12.5%
Harvald & Hauge (1958)	Hospitalized	112	18%	7.2%
Marshall et al (1962)[*]	X-ray	58	14.3%	6.3%
Eberhard (1968)	X-ray	112	50.0%	14.1%
Pollin et al (1969)[+]	Medical records	837	11.3%	5.8%
Gotlieb–Jensen (1972)[‡]	X-ray of all twins	181	52.6%	35.7%

[*] Very young population.
[+] Duodenal ulcer only. Based on followup of US World War II veterans, whose care is still under the Veterans Administration.
[‡] An excellent detailed study using the Danish twin registry. Should be compared with Harvald and Hauge (1958), same twin source, to show what detailed investigation and an extra 10 years of followup reveals.

countries, and in different racial and ethnic groups throughout the world. The physiologic basis for the blood group O association remains unknown. Attempts have been made to relate it to the acid secretory capacity of the stomach as defined by serum pepsinogen or maximal acid output, but no consistent relationship has been delineated (McConnell, 1966; Langman, 1973; Lam and Sircus, 1975; Prescott et al, 1976). The next polymorphic genetic marker found to be associated with peptic ulcer was nonsecretor status (Clarke et al, 1956). Non-secretors are 40–50% more likely to have a duodenal ulcer than secretors (McConnell, 1966; Mourant et al,

1978). The effect of the two genes, O and nonsecretor, on the risk for ulcer seem to be multiplicative (Doll et al, 1961; Langman, 1973). The relative risk for a duodenal ulcer in a blood group O individual is 1.3 (30% increase over a non O individual), and the relative risk for duodenal ulcer in a nonsecretor is 1.5 (increased 50% over a secretor). Individuals who are both O and nonsecretor have a relative risk for duodenal ulcer of approximate 2.5 (hence the term multiplicative).

Many other gene marker associations have been reported with peptic ulcer (Table 60.3) (reviewed in Rotter, 1980b). As can be seen, some eight different genetic systems have been implicated at one time or another as predisposing to peptic ulcer, making peptic ulcer the most 'associated' disorder in man. Some of these associations, notably blood group O and blood group nonsecretor, are so well established that they are undeniably real. Others, such as Rh positivity, are of such small effect, relative risk 1.1 for duodenal ulcer, that they must remain of questionable importance. The remaining associations listed in Table 60.3 have only been examined in a few or even single studies, and so must be considered tentative. What can we conclude as regards the genetics of ulcer from this wealth of association data? There are two major possibilities. One is that each of these genes has a small effect in predisposing to peptic ulcer, a true polygenic system. The other is that each predisposes to a specific subgroup of peptic ulcer. If the latter hypothesis is true then as subgroups are delineated, one would expect stronger associations in certain group subgroups, and no association in others. In contrast, if these predispositions are truly polygenic in nature, then these associations should occur across ulcer groups. Our understanding of the nature of these various associations relation to peptic ulcer would be greatly enhanced if we

were able to delineate the physiologic basis of each of them. In the case of blood group O and nonsecretor status, the pathophysiologic relationships to ulcer remain unknown after more than 20 years of study. This is probably because the degree of the association is so small. It has been calculated that both O and nonsecretor combined contribute only 2.5 to 3% of the genetic variance to ulcer (Roberts, 1965; Edwards, 1965). In the case of α-1-antitrypsin deficiency, HLA antigens, and urinary pepsinogen phenotype, there are clinical or theoretical clues for the association. Thus even though the latter associations are still statistically tentative, the possibility of a pathophysiologic relationship makes them of interest.

GENETIC INTERPRETATIONS – POLYGENIC VS GENETIC HETEROGENEITY

It has thus been clear for a number of years that genetic factors predispose to peptic ulcer, but the mode of inheritance of this genetic predisposition had not been resolved. For over a decade, the hypothesis of polygenic or multifactorial inheritance was used to explain the genetics of peptic ulcer (Roberts, 1965; McConnell, 1966; Cowan, 1973). Peptic ulcer was placed in the polygenic category for two principal reasons. First, the inheritance of all ulcer disease could not be explained by any simple, single genetic defect – that is, the genetics of ulcer was not compatible with simple autosomal dominant, autosomal recessive, or X–linked modes of inheritance. Secondly, the demonstration of the gene marker associations, blood group O and blood group nonsecretor status, provided some direct support for the polygenic hypothesis, since more than one gene seemed to contrib-

Table 60.3 Gene marker associations with peptic ulcer[*]

Polymorphic allele with increased risk for ulcer	Genetic marker system	Number of reports	Relative risk	Comments
0	ABO	>200	1.3	well established
nonsecretor	ABH secretor	~ 40	1.5	well established
RH[+]	Rh	~ 30	1.1	very small relative risk
taster	PTC tasting	2	1.4–2.7	
decreased α–1–antitrypsin activity	α-1-antitrypsin	5	1.4–3.0	? a partial explanation of ulcer pulmonary disease association
Pg^A	urinary pepsinogen phenotyping	1	2.4	? related to quantitative pepsinogen I
B5, B12, Bw35[†]	HLA	4 (1 negative)	2.1–2.9	? an immunologic form of ulcer
G6PD deficiency	glucose-6-phosphate dehydrogenase	1	2.2	

For references see Rotter, 1980b

[*] Most associations are with duodenal ulcer, nonsecretor and alpha-1-antitrypsin are associated with duodenal and gastric ulcer.
[†] See also Ellis and Woodrow, 1979, and Gough and Giles, 1979.

ute a small but measureable tendency toward peptic ulcer and the presence of both genes had a multiplicative effect. However, while there may be a polygenic contribution to peptic ulcer, the alternative mechanism of genetic heterogeneity is probably much more important.

Genetic heterogeneity was proposed as an alternative hypothesis that could explain both the familial aggregation of peptic ulcer disease and the lack of a simple Mendelian pattern of inheritance (Rotter et al, 1976; Rotter & Rimoin, 1977). Furthermore, genetic heterogeneity would better account for the varying physiologic disturbances and diverse clinical manifestations that have been described in peptic ulcer patients. The concept of genetic heterogeneity states that a particular clinical disorder is, in reality, a group of distinct diseases with different aetiologies, both genetic and nongenetic, which by a variety of pathogenetic mechanisms, result in a similar clinical picture. In the absence of subclinical markers to help separate the different diseases, a number of distinct disorders may be lumped together in a common genetic

analysis, masking the existence of subsets of a variety of simply inherited disorders, in such a way that the familial aggregation observed would appear to conform with the polygenic model. There has an increasing realisation that peptic ulcer is not a single disorder, but a whole host of disorders with a common clinical manifestation, a hole in the lining of gastrointestinal tract in those areas exposed to acid and pepsin (Rotter et al, 1978; 1979d; 1980; Lam, 1979; Grossman, 1978).

Heterogeneity of a common disease can be demonstrated by the several methods listed in Table 60.4, and advances in all of these areas have contributed to our knowledge of ulcer heterogeneity. These methods are being increasingly utilized to define the heterogeneity of many common gastrointestinal diseases (see Rotter et al, 1980). The evidence for heterogeneity within peptic ulcer has accumulated rapidly over the last several years, and this concept has gained increasing widespread acceptance (Grossman, 1978; Rotter et al, 1979d; 1980; Lam, 1979). It should be noted that many of the lines of evi-

Table 60.4 Methods of demonstrating heterogeneity in a common disease, peptic ulcer

Method	Example
1. Rare genetic syndromes with peptic ulcer	MEA I and ZE, systemic mastocytosis, ulcer-tremor-nystagmus (see also Table 60.5).
2. Ethnic variability	*Ulcer incidence and site* DU more frequent in Europe, GU more frequent in Japan *Complications* Stenosis common in African and Indian DU, hemorrhage most common in Europe
3. Clinical genetic studies	*Ulcer site* Increased familial risk is site specific, i.e. GU or DU runs in families or twin pairs
4. Clinical evidence	*Age of onset* Childhood DU vs. adult DU Younger DU different complications than older DU
5. Heterogeneity of association with genetic polymorphisms	Blood group O associated with DU and not with GU of the body of the stomach
6. Physiological differences[+]	*GU vs Du* Acid secretion and serum pepsinogen I greater in DU than GU *Within Du* Acid hypersecretors and normosecretors Hyper PG I and normo PG I Increased and normal gastrin response Increased and normal rate of gastric emptying *Combined GU – DU* Positive gastrin-gastric acid correlation
7. Genetic studies utilizing physiologic abnormalities as subclinical markers	Hyperpepsinogenaemic I DU vs normopepsinogenaemic I DU Rapid emptying DU Antral G cell hyperfunction

DU – duodenal ulcer
GU – gastric ulcer
[†] – Includes biochemical, histologic, immunologic, etc.
    See text and Rotter et al, 1980; Rotter, 1980 a,b; 1981; Grossman et al, 1981.

dence for ulcer heterogeneity are genetic. This is not mere happenstance. As will become apparent in our discussion, genetic methods are powerful tools for dissecting out distinct disorders from among a broad phenotype. Because of limitations of space, we can discuss each of these only briefly, and the interested reader is referred to more extensive recent reviews (Rotter et al, 1980; Rotter, 1980b)

GENETIC SYNDROMES WITH PEPTIC ULCER

The existence of well defined genetic and rare clinical syndromes that feature peptic ulceration is an important demonstration of genetic and aetiologic heterogeneity. It also suggests that such heterogeneity may exist in common peptic ulcer. The existence of over 40 genetic syndromes with glucose intolerance and in some cases frank diabetes was an important early indicator of genetic heterogeneity within that group of disorders (Rimoin, 1967; Rimoin and Schimke, 1971; Rotter and Rimoin, 1981). Besides the demonstration of heterogeneity, the study of such disorders serves an even more important function – such rare disorders may elucidate different pathogenetic mechanisms that can lead to the ulcer diathesis, and in the process teach us much about normal physiology and common pathophysiology. This is precisely what has occurred in at least one such syndrome – the Zollinger-Ellison (ZE) syndrome.

Multiple endocrine adenoma syndrome, type I (MEA I)
MEA I is an autosomal dominant disorder characterized by pituitary, parathyroid and pancreatic adenomas (Ballard et al, 1964; Rimoin & Schimke, 1971; Schimke, 1976). Its familial nature was first described by Wermer (1954). Soon after, Zollinger and Ellison (1955) reported a triad of (1) fulminant peptic ulcer disease, with ulcers that could occur as far down the intestine as the jejunum and that would recur despite repeated operations, (2) gastric acid hypersecretion, with an elevated basal to maximal output ratio (greater than 0.6), and (3) non-beta islet cell tumours of the pancreas. This clinical syndrome was later shown to be due to secretion by the pancreatic tumours of the hormone gastrin, a major stimulant of acid secretion (Gregory et al, 1960; 1967). All the features of the syndrome, which include gastric hyperrugosity, hyperplasia, and hypersecretion, can be explained as consequences of the gastrin excess (Isenberg et al, 1973). Thus, this syndrome aided in the elucidation of normal and abnormal gastric physiology. Until the association of ulcer disease with the endocrine tumours was recognized, the pattern of inheritance for multiple endocrine adenomatosis elucidated, and the biochemical marker of increased plasma gastrin levels characterized, this specific entity was lost among the mass of peptic

ulcer patients. Gastrinoma of the pancreas and associated ulcer disease may also occur as a sporadic somatic mutation without familial aggregation and without endocrine tumours in other organs. The sporadic and familial forms seem equally common (Rimoin & Schimke 1971; Lamers et al, 1978; 1980). The diagnostic criteria of an elevated basal to maximal output ratio has essentially been replaced by the radioimmunoassay of gastrin in serum and the response of serum gastrin to a variety of stimuli, which included a protein meal, calcium and secretin (Lamers & van Tongeren, 1977; Deveney et al, 1977). With the distinctive marker of increased plasma gastrin as a tool, more and more patients are being diagnosed at a stage when they are clinically indistinguishable from 'common' peptic ulcer (Regan & Malagelada, 1978). Until recently, the recommended therapy for this severe form of ulcer disease was total gastrectomy, but many patients are being treated successfully with H2 blockers such as cimetidine, often in combination with other agents (Grossman, 1980a; Grossman, 1981).

Systemic mastocytosis
Another multisystem syndrome that includes peptic ulcer as one of its manifestations is systemic mastocytosis, a disorder characterized by flushing, maculopapular rash, pruritus, abdominal pain and diarrhea. Genetic factors would appear to be of major importance in this disorder, since six of eight reported monozygotic twin pairs have been concordant for the disorder (Selmanovitz et al, 1970). A number of familial cases of systemic mastocytosis have been reported and both dominant and recessive modes of inheritance have been suggested (Selmanovitz et al, 1970; Shaw, 1968). However, a careful review of the pedigrees reported by Shaw (1968) clearly demonstrate examples of incomplete penetrance and thus dominant susceptibility could be reasonably invoked to explain most pedigrees. This syndrome illuminates the role of another stimulant of acid secretion, histamine. These histamine excess syndromes can lead to gastric hypertrophy and gastric hypersecretion with high basal acid outputs, mimicking the Zollinger-Ellison syndrome, and to frank duodenal ulceration (Rotter, 1980b). Erosive gastroduodenitis and elevated acid secretion can occur without elevated blood levels of histamine, but with elevated gastric tissue stores of the secretatogue. This observation by Amman et al (1976) led them to conclude that it is the tissue, and not the serum, level of histamine that leads to gastrointestinal complications. This uncommon disorder demonstrates the important role of histamine in acid secretion, a role that has been confirmed by the discovery of the H-2 receptor (histamine receptor-2) blockers such as cimetidine, as potent inhibitors of gastric acid secretion (Grossman, 1980a; 1981; Grossman et al, 1981). Therapy now includes the use of H-1 and H-2 blockers, though even together these

are not always fully successful (Hirschowitz & Groarke, 1979; Achord and Langford, 1980).

Tremor-nystagmus-ulcer syndrome

Another distinct autosomal dominant syndrome associated with peptic ulcer consists of essential tremor, congenital nystagmus, duodenal ulcer, and a narcolepsy-like sleep disturbance. This was described in a family of Swedish-Finnish ancestry by Neuhauser et al (1976). Of 17 affected family members, 12 had essential tremor, 12 had nystagmus, and 8 had duodenal ulcer; the latter occurred almost exclusively in individuals with the neurologic syndrome and sometimes preceeding the onset of neurologic symptoms. Basal and maximal gastric acid outputs were unremarkable (range 1.9–4.0 meq/hr and 23.4–58.4 meq/hr, respectively). Both essential tremor and narcolepsy appear most often to be dominant disorders (Pratt, 1967; Baraitser and Parkes, 1978), and it might be useful to ascertain such a disorder through neurology clinics. However, this clinical entity was not identified in a series of 50 narcolepsy cases (Parkes, 1979).

Amyloidosis (Van Allen type)

Another dominant disorder accompanied by peptic ulcer is a distinct form of amyloidosis reported by Van Allen et al (1968). The term amyloidosis encompasses a variety of disorders which have in common the presence of infiltrates in various tissues of amyloid, a heterogeneous complex of insoluble proteins and/or protein polysaccharides. Amyloidosis can be secondary to chronic inflammation due to infections or autoimmune diseases, to deposition of immunoglobulin light chains in plasma cell cell dyscrasias, and in other cases can have a clear genetic basis. In fact, over a dozen hereditary disorders with amyloidosis as one of their cardinal features are recognized (McKusick, 1978; Glenner et al, 1978). In a large family of English-Scottish-Irish origin, Van Allen et al (1968) were able to identify 12 affected members in two generations, 8 of whom had confirmation of their amyloidosis by pathologic studies. Male to male transmission supported dominant inheritance. Duodenal ulcer occurred in 9 of the 12 affected individuals, with death due to perforation in one. The mechanism of the ulcer predisposition remains obscure but it appears not to be due to local amyloid infiltration. Other prominent features were chronic progressive sensorimotor neuropathy, involving the lower extremities most prominently and usually the means of presentation, and amyloid nephropathy leading to renal failure as the usual cause of death. Onset was on the average in the mid 30's and death in the late 40's. Other features included some individuals with deafness and cataracts. Gimeno et al (1974) appeared to have identified a similarly affected individual, with a prominent family history of ulcer, deafness and renal disease.

Other syndromes

The relationship of peptic ulcer to the above mentioned syndromes appears clear. There are several additional genetic disorders in which an increased incidence of peptic ulcer has been suggested. These include hyperparathyroidism (this association may be solely through MEA-I), cystic fibrosis, α-1-antitrypsin deficiency, carcinoid syndrome, a recently described disorder designated as 'stiff skin and multisystem disease', and pachydermoperiostosis (see Table 60.5) (Rotter, 1980b; Lam et al, 1981). Though less well established, each of these suggest the possibility of a different pathogenetic mechanism leading to peptic ulceration. In the case of hyperparathyroidism this may occur via increased acid secretion (Barreras, 1973). Grossman (1972) has argued that the increased incidence of duodenal ulcer and gastric hypersecretion in hyperparathyroid patients, if it occurs, could well be due to the coexistent occurrence of parathyroid with gastrin tumours as part of MEA-I. A systematic study of gastrin levels and their response to provocative agents in hyperparathyroid patients and their families is needed to answer this question. The association of duodenal ulcer and cystic fibrosis could occur through inadequate acid neutralization by deficient pancreatic secretions. The possible association of ulcer and α-1-antitrypsin deficiency is of interest because the association may be with both gastric and duodenal ulcer, and because it may serve as a model of deficient mucosal protection that could explain the more common association of chronic pulmonary disease with both gastric and duodenal ulcer (Rotter, 1980b; Rotter et al, 1982). The carcinoid ulcer association may be a manifestation of MEA-I, but there appears to be a specific risk for gastric ulcer, especially with bronchial carcinoids (Sandler et al, 1961). A newly described multisystem 'stiff skin syndrome' is of interest because of the coincident manifestation of calcium renal stones and peptic ulcer (Stevenson et al, 1979), which may have a common underlying mechanism in certain families (Rotter, 1980b). Lam et al (1981) have recently identified a Chinese family with four male members in two generations affected with pachydermoperiostosis and peptic ulcer. Duodenal ulcer was documented in the two male sibs, and the father and paternal uncle had typical ulcer pain. Acid and meal stimulated gastrin studies were normal, and the only physiological abnormality identified was hyperpepsinogenaemia I.

The recognition of these disorders is important not just for the implications for genetic heterogeneity, but because they illustrate that different pathogenetic mechanisms, e.g., excess gastrin or excess histamine, can result in peptic ulcer. Patients with these disorders should have specific genetic counselling and therapy. MEA I is an excellent example of how the alert physician, by making an accurate diagnosis, can then screen asymptomatic family members for the presence of subclinical

Table 60.5 Genetic syndromes with ulcer

Syndromes	Location of ulcer	Pathogenetic mechanism	Associated clinical findings	Pattern of inheritance
Genetic syndromes with peptic ulcer-relationship established				
Multiple endocrine adenoma, type I	DU	Excess gastrin	Pituitary-acromegaly (GH), infertility (prolactin) Parathyroid-renal stones, hypercalcaemia (PTH) Pancreas-hypoglycaemia (insulin), diabetes (glucagon)	Autosomal dominant
Sporadic gastrinoma	DU	Excess gastrin		Somatic mutation
Systemic mastocytosis	DU	Excess histamine	Skin lesions, urticaria	? (both dominant and recessive pedigrees reported)
Ulcer-tremor-nystagmus	DU	Unknown	Essential tremor, nystagmus, narcolepsy	Autosomal dominant
Amyloidosis, type IV	DU, ?GU	Unknown	Sensorimotor neuropathy, nephropathy, hearing loss, cataracts	Autosomal dominant
Genetic syndromes with peptic ulcer – relationship suggested, but not established				
Hyperparathyroidism	DU	? Calcium increasing gastric secretion	Hypercalcaemia, renal stones	Familial form-autosomal dominant
Cystic fibrosis	DU	? Deficient pancreatic secretion	Pulmonary disease, malabsorption	Autosomal recessive
α–1–antitrypsin deficiency	DU, GU	? Deficient mucosal protection	Pulmonary disease, cirrhosis	Autosomal recessive
Carcinoid syndrome	?GU	? Excess–5–hydroxy-tryptophan	Flushing, cyanosis, diarrhea. bronchoconstriction	?
Stiff skin syndrome	DU	Unknown	Stiff skin, joint enlargement, renal stones, diabetes	Autosomal dominant
Pachydermoperiostosis	DU	Unknown	Clubbing, thickened skin, increased periosteum of distal extremities	Autosomal dominant

disease, and, by detecting the endocrine tumors early, prevent or ameliorate many of their manifestations. The existence of these rare disorders also suggest that what we recognize as 'common' peptic ulcer may, in fact, comprise several disorders.

EPIDEMIOLOGICAL HETEROGENEITY – ETHNIC VARIABILITY

The marked ethnic variability in the prevalence, and especially in the clinical features, of peptic ulcer constitutes epidemiologic evidence for heterogeneity (Susser, 1967; Tovey & Tunstall, 1975; Tovey, 1979; Rotter, 1980b; Moshal, 1980). While duodenal ulcer is usually more common than gastric ulcer, this ratio varies widely over the globe; in a few cases, such as in Japan, gastric ulcer is more frequent. The absolute incidence also varies widely; e.g., the frequency of duodenal ulcer in Southwest American Indians is one-fourtieth that of United States whites. Male/female ratios also vary widely, from over 30 to 1 in rural Africa and India to about 2–3 to 1 in the United States. Most significantly, there is extensive ethnic and geographic variation in clinical characteristics, such as age of onset or complications. The incidence of young patients with duodenal ulcer is greatly increased in Hong Kong compared to Scotland (Lam & Sircus, 1975; Lam & Ong, 1976). A younger mean age of duodenal ulcer is also found in the high ulcer incidence areas of Africa and India compared to the mean age of the United Kingdom (Tovey & Tunstall, 1975; Tovey, 1979). The complications of pyloric stenosis as an indication for surgery is much more frequent in the high ulcer areas of south India and the Nile Congo watershed, whereas hemorrhage and perforation are more frequent complications in Europe. There are other unique features of rural African and Indian ulcer, including the occurrence of a fibrous tumour-like inflammatory mass around the duodenal bulb, and an increased frequency of postbulbar ulceration and choledochoduodenal fistula. While there is certainly extensive phenotypic heterogeneity on an ethnic basis, much of it could be due to environmental differences such as diet as well as due to genetic differences between the populations.

CLINICAL SUGGESTIONS OF HETEROGENEITY – GASTRIC ULCER VS DUODENAL ULCER

The demonstration of clinical, physiological, or genetic differences within a disorder that can be consistently related to other clinical features such as ulcer location or age of onset can also suggest genetic heterogeneity. In the case of gastric ulcer and duodenal ulcer, much of the evidence to indicate that these are separate and distinct disorders has been gathered in this fashion, using the ulcer location as the dividing criterion and then comparing other features – age of onset, complications, male/female ratio, acid secretion, etc (see Table 60.6). This separation was confirmed by the classic clinical genetic study of Doll and Kellock (1951). Starting with index cases with a radiographically defined ulcer site, Doll and Kellock painstakingly tracked down the actual radiographs of relatives who were reportedly also affected with peptic ulcer. They observed that the relatives of gastric ulcer probands had a 3 fold increased prevalence of gastric ulcer compared to the general population, however, duodenal ulcer occurred no more frequently among these relatives than in the general population. Likewise, the relatives of duodenal ulcer patients had 3 times as much duodenal ulcer compared to the control population, but no increased risk of gastric ulcer. Monson (1970a) confirmed these findings, observ-

ing twice as many duodenal ulcers as expected in the relatives of physicians with duodenal ulcer, yet no increase in gastric ulcer over that expected. This familial separation is termed independent segregation and is extremely strong evidence that gastric and duodenal ulcer are separate disorders.

Further genetic evidence validates this separation of gastric and duodenal ulcer. In the vast majority of like-sex twins concordant for peptic ulcer, the ulcer site has been observed to be identical (Gotlieb-Jensen, 1972). Blood group association studies also support this division, since heterogeneity of genetic polymorphism association is observed. In numerous studies, blood group O is consistently found to be associated with duodenal ulcer (with or without associated gastric ulcer) but not with primary gastric ulcer (McConnell, 1966; 1980; Langman, 1973; Mourant et al, 1978). Since blood groups are genetic polymorphisms that are inherited in a simple Mendelian fashion, these consistent differences in association are ascribed to genetic and hence aetiological differences between the disorders. Physiologic data also support this separation, as maximum gastric acid output and serum pepsinogen I are usually normal or even subnormal in gastric ulcer patients, while on the average both are increased in duodenal ulcer patients (Wormsley & Grossman, 1965; Samloff et al, 1975).

It might be appropriate here to deal with a common question. If gastric and duodenal ulcer are truly independent disorders, why do we observe the two together in the same patient more often than just the product of the two disorders in the populations at large (Bonnevie, 1975). The answer is probably further heterogeneity; that is, combined ulcer (gastric and duodenal) may well be a distinct form of ulcer disease separate from either primary gastric or primary duodenal ulcer. Support for this concept comes from the same study by Doll and Kellcok (1951) which suggested independent segregation of combined ulcer, that is the prevalence of combined ulcer was greater in the relatives with combined disease than in the relatives of probands who had either a solitary

Table 60.6 The evolution of the separation of gastric and duodenal ulcer

Method	Evidence
Clinical	Differences in age of onset, complications, male-female ratio
Clinical genetic	Independent segregation of gastric and duodenal ulcer
Heterogeneity of blood group associations	Blood group O associated with DU, pyloric and combined ulcer, but not with solitary gastric ulcer
Physiological	GU – Acid normosecretors, or subnormal (on the average)
	DU – Acid hypersecretors (on the average)
Ethnic variability	GU – more frequent in Japan
	DU – more frequent in Europe
Clinical genetic	Concordant twins – ulcer site concordant
Physiological	GU – normopepsinogenaemic I
	DU – hyperpepsinogenaemic I

gastric or solitary duodenal ulcer. Physiologic studies by Lam and Lai (1978) also support this separation. They found a positive correlation between gastric acid output and gastrin response to a protein meal in such patients, and a negative correlation in gastric ulcer patients and controls.

Heterogeneity within duodenal ulcer has also been claimed on clinical grounds, most actively by Lam and coworkers (Lam, 1979). Age of onset has been proposed as one dividing criterion. Childhood duodenal ulcer may well be distinct genetically from adult duodenal ulcer, analogous to the separation of juvenile from maturity onset diabetes (Rotter & Rimoin, 1981). Investigators have been impressed by the frequency of a 'positive' family history' (Cowan, 1973), and one study has reported that the first and second degree relatives of childhood duodenal ulcer patients are affected with a frequency twice that of relatives of adult probands (Sedlackova & Seemanova, 1973). In Hong Kong, Lam and Ong (1976) divided their duodenal ulcer patients on the basis of age of onset and found that their early-onset group (onset below age 20 years) had a significantly stronger family history, a frequency of blood group O similar to that of controls, more frequently presented with gastrointestinal bleeding as the first manifestation of the disease, and rarely had complications such as perforation, obstruction, intractable pain or secondary gastric ulcer, while, in contrast, their late-onset group (onset after age 30 years) had an infrequent family history of ulcer disease, an increased frequency of blood group O, presented less frequently with gastrointestinal bleeding, and had an increased frequency of complications such as perforation, pyloroduodenal stenosis, severe pain, virulent ulcer and secondary gastric ulcer.

Another means of looking for heterogeneity clinically is to examine the association of ulcer with other diseases within families. Based on preliminary observations in certain families, we have proposed that the association of ulcer with certain chronic diseases may occur because of the inheritance of a common defect that predisposes to both diseases (Rotter et al, 1979d). This may account for observations of the family aggregation of ulcer disease and renal stones (without hyperparathyroidism), ulcer and coronary artery disease, and ulcer and chronic obstructive pulmonary diseases. In the latter case, it has often been assumed that the ulcer is secondary to the pulmonary disease, yet the association is both with chronic pulmonary disease and lung cancer (Bonnevie, 1977), which have been shown to have a common familial component (Cohen et al, 1977). Although cigarette smoking is associated with both lung disease and ulcer, it does not fully account for the association of lung lesions and ulcer (Monson, 1970b). In addition, we have recently observed that, in many if not most cases, the ulcer disease precedes the pulmonary disease (Rotter et

al, 1982). α-1-antitrypsin deficiency may be a specific cause of this more general association (Rotter, 1980b).

PHYSIOLOGICAL HETEROGENEITY

There is extensive evidence for physiological heterogeneity in peptic ulcer. For example, in gastric ulcer patients mean levels of acid secretion and of serum pepsinogen I are decreased, whereas, in duodenal ulcer patients they are increased (Wormsley & Grossman, 1965; Samloff et al, 1975). It has been suggested that combined ulcer (gastric and duodenal ulcer) patients have a different pathophysiology, exhibiting a positive correlation of gastric acid output and gastrin response (Lam and Lai, 1978). Physiologic evidence for heterogeneity within duodenal ulcer includes: (1) the occurrence of duodenal ulcer in both acid hypersecretors and normosecretors, (2) the identification of hyperpepsinogenaemic I and normopepsinogenaemic I duodenal ulcer patients, (3) marked variability in the gastrin response to a protein meal, and (4) the observation that the rate of gastric emptying differs among duodenal ulcer patients (Rotter & Rimoin, 1977; Grossman, 1978; Lam, 1980; Rotter, 1980b). The recent suggestion of an association of certain HLA antigens with duodenal ulcer (Rotter et al, 1977a; Ellis & Woodrow, 1979; Gough & Giles, 1979), the report of antibodies to secretory IgA in certain duodenal ulcer patients (Kwitko & Shearman, 1978), and the observation of acid stimulating antibodies (Dobi et al, 1980), hint that there may be immunologic forms of peptic ulcer (Rotter, 1980b; Rotter & Heiner, 1982). Yet, each of these abnormalities is found in some, but not all, ulcer patients, Thus, rather than looking for a single defect in all ulcer patients, we should be emphasizing the differences between patients as clues to delineate different disorders.

GENETIC STUDIES UTILIZING SUBCLINICAL MARKERS

Possibly the most powerful method to demonstrate genetic heterogeneity is to utilize family studies to test whether the reported physiologic abnormalities have a genetic basis and if so, whether they serve as subclinical markers (Rotter, 1980a; b). Subclinical markers (predictors) are abnormalities proposed to have a role in the pathogenesis of the disease under study. They thus detect individuals with the abnormal genotype in addition to those with overt disease. They are important in genetic studies, because in many disorders not all individuals with the mutant genotype may manifest the disorder (reduced penetrance), the variability of the phenotype may be so great that the clinical features are too mild to be readily apparent (variable expressivity), or there may be a delayed age of onset of the disease, such that the younger genetically predisposed individuals are clinically normal. Thus subclinical markers maximize the number of affected individuals that can be detected. Until we identified subclinical markers in peptic ulcer we could not detect individuals genetically predisposed to ulcer until its clinical manifestations were full blown.

Subclinical markers can also be used to detect heterogeneity within a clinical syndrome. Simply because a given potential marker does not occur in all individuals with a clinically similar disorder, does not mean that it is unimportant in a subgroup of these individuals who may have a distinct, but previously unrecognized disease. For example, sickling of the red cells is an excellent subclinical marker in some patients with anaemia, whereas G6PD levels are a subclinical marker in another group of individuals. If anaemia was considered a single disease, then both sickling and G6PD levels would be rejected as good subclinical markers since they do not occur in all affected individuals. Similarly, in peptic ulcer numerous biochemical and physiologic abnormalities have been described in some, but not all, ulcer patients (Rotter, 1980a; 1980b). The proposition that distinct ulcer syndromes can be defined by the stratification of patients into groups according to different markers is being borne out by appropriate genetic-physiological studies. This has been done for several physiological traits including serum pepsinogen I, gastric emptying, and gastrin response to a protein meal.

The most extensive studies have utilized the radioimmunoassay of serum pepsinogen I (PGI) developed by Samloff (1979; 1980). Human serum pepsinogens, the precursors of pepsin, have been separated into two immunochemically distinct groups, one of fast electrophoretic mobility which is confined to the acid secreting part of the stomach (pepsinogen I, PG I), and the other of slower mobility which is found throughout the stomach and in the first part of the duodenum (pepsinogen II, PG II).

Studies of some 120 duodenal ulcer sibships, in collaboration with Drs McConnell and Ellis of Liverpool, have shown that about half of duodenal ulcer patients have hyperpepsinogenaemia I (hyper PG I) and the other half have normopepsinogenaemia I (normo PG I), both on a familial basis (Rotter et al, 1979a). That is, the hyper PG I duodenal ulcer and normo PG I duodenal ulcer, for the most part, segregate independently. Both forms of duodenal ulcer exhibit an increased risk for sibs for ulcer (some 20–25% of the sibs affected) compared to the population risk. Thus both forms demonstrate familial aggregation whose basis is presumably genetic. Other risk factors did not distinguish between the two groups, such as blood groups, or the male/female ratio which was 3 to 1 in both groups. A small series of twins

studied to date also support this separation of hyper and normo PG I duodenal ulcer (Rotter et al, 1977b). Also supporting this separation of hyper and normo PG I duodenal ulcer was the study of PG I levels in the clinically normal sibs of the duodenal ulcer sibships. The mean serum PG I of the normal sibs of the hyper PG I sibships was significantly greater than the clinically normal sibs of the normo PG I sibships. In fact the mean PG I level in the clinically normal sibs of the hyper PG I sibships was intermediate between the mean level in their sibs with duodenal ulcer and the mean level in healthy controls.

These sib studies and studies of extended families have also suggested that the familial aggregation of an elevated PG I is consistent with autosomal dominant inheritance (Rotter et al, 1979a; 1979b). In the sibships studied, 36 of 83 clinically normal sibs of hyper PG I sibships had an elevated PG I (Rotter et al, 1979a). Segregation analysis of the trait of an elevated PG I yielded segregation ratios bracketing the value of 0.5, supporting autosomal dominant inheritance of this trait. In the extended families studied, the vertical transmission of an elevated PG I was also characteristic of autosomal dominant inheritance. In each generation, approximately 50% of the offspring of members with an elevated PG I had an elevated PG I, all offspring of normo PG I members had a normal PG I, and there was male to male transmission of hyperpepsinogenaemia (Rotter et al, 1979b). Thus, these studies have delineated a major genetic factor, elevated serum pepsinogen I, that can identify individuals at risk and that may account for the major genetic predisposition of many, possibly even half, of duodenal ulcer patients. This does not mean that an elevated serum pepsinogen I itself predisposes to ulcer. More likely, it identifies those individuals with an increased mass of chief and parietal cells who are genetically predisposed on the basis of producing excess pepsin and acid. In family and sibling studies of hyperpepsinogenaemic I patients, some 40% of the relatives with an elevated pepsinogen I have clinical duodenal ulcer. Thus other factors, environmental and/or genetic, must also play a role in disease expression.

These accumulated studies suggest that there are at least two genetic subtypes of duodenal ulcer. In the hyper PG I type, the genetic predisposition to duodenal ulcer in apparently normal sibs can be identified by an elevated serum PG I level. The second type is characterised by normopepsinogenaemia I in both the ulcer proband and his sibs. This latter type of ulcer also appears to have a genetic basis as demonstrated by its familial aggregation, but other markers must be sought to identify the individuals at risk. One should not conclude from these studies that there are only two forms of duodenal ulcer. One might predict that the use of other subclinical markers might further subdivide these broad groups. Additional studies utilizing other physiological characteristics are just starting to further subdivide the hyperpepsinogenaemic I and normo-pepsinogenaemic I duodenal ulcer groups. Thus, there appears to be a subgroup of the normopepsinogenaemic I class in which rapid gastric emptying seems to be the inherited physiologic abnormality predisposing to ulcer (Rotter et al, 1979c). Familial hyperpepsinogenaemic I duodenal ulcer also seems to be separable into different groups. A group of patients with a markedly exaggerated gastrin response to a protein meal from an antral source (antral G cell hyperfunction) have also been shown to have hyperpepsinogenaemia I (Calam et al, 1979; Taylor et al, 1981). In addition, both the gastrin and pepsinogen I abnormalities were shown to have a familial basis. Both rapid emptying and postprandial hypergastrinaemia appeared to follow autosomal dominant inheritance patterns. Combining physiological studies and family history in a cross sectional study, Lam and Ong (1980) have presented evidence that there may be more than one form of early onset ulcer.

Thus pepsinogen I, gastric emptying, and gastrin response, have been demonstrated to be useful markers in genetic studies. There are a variety of additional potential subclinical markers for genetic studies of peptic ulcer (Rotter, 1980a; 1980b). The only other one examined in a family study has been maximum acid secretion. Fodor et al (1968) measured maximum acid output in 160 duodenal ulcer patients, 113 nonulcerated first degree relatives, and 155 healthy controls without a family history of ulcer. Acid secretion in the family members was found to be intermediate between the ulcer patients and controls, regardless of blood groups or secretor status. Since only the mean values were reported, we have no knowledge whether there was any segregation of elevated acid secretion, but the considerable overlap between normals and ulcer patients would complicate such analysis. It would be worthwhile, however, to re-examine Fodor's data with modern genetic analytic techniques.

It should be noted that the genetic-family method of studying potential markers is useful not only for demonstrating heterogeneity. Equally important, by showing cosegregation of the disease and the physiological marker in certain families, it can help demonstrate that a particular abnormality does in fact have a clear pathophysiological relationship to at least one type of peptic ulcer. Such studies can thus resolve any doubt about whether a give abnormality is a 'real' observation in peptic ulcer patients.

A GENETIC CLASSIFICATION

Thus, the accumulating evidence suggests that the genetic predisposition to peptic ulcer is not due principally to the cumulative effect of multiple, additive predisposing genes each with a small effect (the polygenic hypothesis), but rather that there are multiple forms of peptic ulcer, each with a different genetic basis. A classification of our evolving knowledge of peptic ulcer genetic and aetiological heterogeneity is shown in Table 60.7. It should be noted that polygenic inheritance and genetic heterogeneity are not necessarily mutually exclusive. There may well be a polygenic background upon which major predisposing genes act. While the studies mentioned above appear to be identifying major genes, such as hyperpepsinogenaemia I, which predispose to one form of peptic ulcer, this does not rule out the effect of genes such as blood group O, nonsecretor, and even male sex, as having an additional effects on the genetic predisposition. Such 'minor genes' may form the genetic background upon which the major disease predisposing genes exert their effects. In addition, some of the various heterogeneous forms may be polygenic in origin, as has been suggested for childhood duodenal ulcer. Cowan (1973) proposed that childhood duodenal ulcer may be an example of polygenic inheritance in that these children have 'more genes' (stronger family history) and therefore their disease is 'more severe' (younger age of onset). An alternative explanation is that 'adult' and 'childhood' duodenal ulcer are different disorders, with different average ages of onset, as is the case for adult and juvenile diabetes. The genetic physiological approaches enumerated here should be able to resolve this question.

Genetic counselling

At the present time, how do we counsel our ulcer patients and their families? We tell our ulcer patients that about 20% of their first degree relatives (parents, sibs, offspring) will also experience peptic ulcer disease in their lifetime.

Are the subclinical markers useful in genetic counselling? About 50% of patients with duodenal ulcer appear have hyperpepsinogenaemia I, and some half of their sibs and half of their offspring also have this trait and therefore have an increased risk (about 40%) of developing duodenal ulcer. Should efforts be made to identify these individuals so they will know they have this susceptibility? Should such individuals be told to avoid risk factors such as smoking cigarettes, and to seek medical care promptly if symptoms suggestive of ulcer occur? Studies need to be done to determine whether such an effort is worthwhile. If we should discover specific environmental factors which act in concert with a given genetic trait, such as hyperpepsinogenaemia I, to convert genetic predisposition into clinical disease, then it would obviously be desirable to identify those with the genetic trait so they could be warned to avoid the environmental factor.

In the case of the rare genetic syndromes that feature peptic ulceration, especially multiple endocrine aden-

Table 60.7 Classification of peptic ulcer genetic and etiologic heterogeneity

---

I. Peptic ulcer associated with rare genetic syndromes
   A. Relationship established
      1. Multiple endocrine adenomatosis, Type I (gastrinoma)
      2. Systemic mastocytosis
      3. Tremor-nystagmus-ulcer syndrome
      4. Amyloidosis, type IV
   B. Relationship suggested
      1. Hyperparathyroidism
      2. Cystic fibrosis
      3. α-1-antitrypsin deficiency
      4. Carcinoid syndrome
      5. Stiff skin syndrome
      6. Pachydermoperiostosis
II. Oesophageal ulcer
III. Gastric ulcer
   A. Accompanied by chronic gastritis
   B. Secondary to use of aspirin[†]
IV. Combined gastric and duodenal ulcer
V. Hyperpepsinogenaemic–I duodenal ulcer[††]
   A. Without postprandial hypergastrinaemia
   B. With postprandial hypergastrinaemia
   C. Secondary to retained antrum
VI. Normopepsinogenaemic–I duodenal ulcer
   A. Without rapid gastric emptying
   B. With rapid gastric emptying
VII. Childhood duodenal ulcer
   A. Normal acid secretion[*]
   B. Elevated acid secretion[*]
VIII. Immunologic form of duodenal ulcer[*]
   A. Antibody to secretory IgA
   B. Immunoglobulin stimulated acid secretion
IX. Peptic ulcer associated with other chronic diseases[*]
   A. Peptic ulcer and chronic lung disease
   B. Duodenal ulcer and renal stones (without hyperparathyroidism)
   C. Duodenal ulcer and coronary artery disease
X. Meckel's diverticulum

[†] Also occurs with other nonsteroidal antiinflammatory agents
[††] Also usually acid hypersecretors
[*] Tentative subdivisions
For further details, see Rotter 1980a; 1980b; 1981 and the text.

omatosis type I, a thorough search of all family members should be made for occult cases so the disease can be treated in its earliest stages before complications arise.

Future implications

The polygenic hypothesis suggests that all ulcer is a spectrum of one disease, and that pathophysiology and optimal therapy would be similar for all ulcer patients. In direct contrast, the implication of genetic heterogeneity is that the pathophysiology, and therefore optimal therapy, may well differ between different types of ulcer patients. Our goal as physicians and scientists is to recognize the full heterogeneity of this group of disorders, to develop specific methods for identifying individuals predisposed to each of the component disorders, and to define the specific environmental differences that lead to clinical expression in each kind of genetically predisposed individual. This may eventually lead to specific modes of therapy, prevention, and genetic counselling for each of the disorders that lead to the ulcer syndrome.

REFERENCES

Achord J L, Langford H 1980 The effect of cimetidine and propantheline on the symptoms of a patient with systemic mastocytosis. The American Journal of Medicine 69: 610–614

Aird I, Bentall H H, Mehigaro J A, Roberts J A F 1954 The blood groups in relation to peptic ulceration and carcinoma of the colon, rectum, breast and bronchus. British Medical Journal ii: 315–321

Ammann R W, Vetter D, Deyhle P, Tschen H, Sulser H, Schmid M 1976 Gastrointestinal involvement in systemic mastocytosis. Gut 17: 107–112

Ballard H S, Frame B, Hartsock R J 1964 Familial multiple

endocrine adenoma-peptic ulcer complex. Medicine 43: 481–516

Baraitser M, Parkes J D 1978 Genetic study of the narcoleptic syndrome. Journal of Medical Genetics 15: 254–259

Barreras R F 1973 Calcium and gastric secretion. Gastroenterology 64: 1168–1184

Bonnevie O 1975 The incidence in Copenhagen County of gastric and duodenal ulcers in the same patient. Scandinavian Journal of Gastroenterology 10: 529–536

Bonnevie O 1977 Causes of death in duodenal and gastric ulcer. Gastroenterology 73: 1000–1004

Calam J, Taylor I L, Dockray G J, Simkin E, Cooke A, Rotter J I, Samloff I M 1979 Subgroup of duodenal ulcer patients with familial G-cell hyperfunction and hyperpepsinogenemia I. Gut 20: A934

Camerer J W 1936 Z. Menschl. Vererb-U. Konstit. Lehre 19: 416, quoted in Gotlieb-Jensen, 1972

Clarke C A, Edwards J W, Haddock D R W, Howel Evans A W, McConnell R B, Sheppard P M 1956 ABO blood group and secretor character in duodenal ulcer. British Medical Journal 725–731

Cohen B H, Diamond E L, Graves C G, Kreiss P, Levy D A, Menkes H A, Permutt S, Quaskey S, Tockman M S 1977 A common familial component in lung cancer and chronic obstructive pulmonary disease. Lancet ii: 523–526

Cowan W K 1973 Genetics of duodenal and gastric ulcer. Clinics in Gastroenterology 2: 539–546

Deveney C W, Deveney K S, Jaffe B M, Jones R S, Way L W 1977 Use of calcium and secretin in the diagnosis of gastrinoma (Zollinger-Ellison syndrome). Annals of Internal Medicine 87: 680–686

Dobi S, Gasztonyi G, Lenkey B 1980 Immunoglobulin stimulated superacidity in duodenal ulcer. Acta Medica Academiae Scientarium Hungaricae 37: 51–59

Doig R K 1957 Illness in twins: duodenal ulcer. Medical Journal of Australia 2: 617–619

Doll R, Buch J 1950 Hereditary factors in peptic ulcer. Annals of Eugenics 15: 135–146

Doll R, Kellock T D 1951 The separate inheritance of gastric and duodenal ulcer. Annals of Eugenics 16: 231–240

Doll R, Drane H, Newell A C 1961 Secretion of blood group substances in duodenal, gastric and stomach ulcer, gastric carcinoma and diabetes mellitus. Gut 2: 352–359

Eberhard G 1968 Peptic ulcer in twins. A study in personality, heredity and environment. Acta Psychiatrica Scandinavica. Supplement 205

Edwards J H 1965 The meaning of the associations between blood groups and disease. Annals of Human Genetics 29: 77–83

Ellis A, Woodrow J C 1979 HLA and duodenal ulcer. Gut 20: 760–762

Fodor O, Vestea S, Urcan S, Popescu S, Sulica L, Ienicca R, Goia A, Ilea V 1968 Hydrochloric acid secretion capacity of the stomach as an inherited factor in the patheogenesis of duodenal ulcer. American Journal of Digestive Diseases 13: 260–265

Gimeno A, Garcia-Alix D, Segovia de Arana J M, Mateos F, Sotelo M T 1974 Amyloidotic polyneuritis of type III (Iowa-Van Allen). European Neurology 11: 46–57

Glenner G G, Ignaczak T F, Page D L 1978 The inherited systemic amyloidoses and localized amyloid deposits. In: Stanbury JB, Wyngaarden J B, Frederickson D S (eds) The Metabolic Basis of Inherited Disease, McGraw-Hill, New York p 1308–1339

Gotleib-Jensen K 1972 Peptic Ulcer: Genetic and Epidemiological Aspects Based on Twin Studies. Munksgaard, Copenhagen

Gough M J, Giles G R 1979 HLA antigens in duodenal ulceration. Gut 20: A919–20

Gregory R A, Tracy H J, French J M, Sircus W 1960 Extraction of a gastrin-like substance from a pancreatic tumor in a case of Zollinger-Ellison syndrome. Lancet i: 1045–1048

Gregory R A, Grossman M I, Tracy H J, Bentley P H 1967 Nature of the gastric secretagogue in Zollinger-Ellison tumors. Lancet ii: 543–544

Grossman M I 1972 Gastrointestinal hormones: some thoughts about clinical applications. Scandinavian Journal of Gastroenterology 7: 97–104

Grossman, M I 1978 Abnormalities of acid secretion in patients with duodenal ulcer. Gastroenterology 75: 524–526

Grossman M I 1980a New medical and surgical treatments of peptic ulcer disease. American Journal of Medicine 69: 647–649

Grossman M I 1980b Peptic ulcer, definition and epidemiology. In: Rotter J I, Samloff I M, Rimoin D L (eds) The Genetics and Heterogeneity of Common Gastrointestinal Disorders, San Francisco and New York, Academic Press, p 21–29

Grossman M I (ed) 1981 Peptic Ulcer, A Guide for the Practicing Physician, Year Book, Chicago

Grossman M I, Walsh J H, Isenberg J I, Meyer J H 1979 Peptic ulcer. In: Beeson P B, McDermott W, Wyngaarden J B (eds) Textbook of Medicine, W.B. Saunders, Philadelphia, p 1502–1520

Grossman M I, Kurata J H, Rotter J I, Robert A, Meyer J H, Richardson C T, Debas H T, Jensen D M 1981 Peptic ulcer – new therapies, new diseases. Annals of Internal Medicine 95: 609–627, 1981

Harvald B, Hauge M 1958 A catamnestic investigation of Danish twins. Acta Genetica 8: 287–294

Hirschowitz B I, Groarke J F 1979 Effect of cimetidine on gastric hypersecretion and diarrhea in systemic mastocytosis. Annals of Internal Medicine 90: 769–771

Huhn G 1939 Magenerkrankagen bei Zwillingen. Hamburg. Quoted in Gotlieb-Jensen, 1972

Isenberg J I, Walsh J H, Grossman M I 1973 Zollinger-Ellison syndrome. Gastroenterology 65: 140–65

Jirasek V 1971 Hereditary factors in the etiology of peptic ulcer. Acta Universitatis Carolinae Medicae 17: 383–456

Kubickova Z, Vesely K T 1972 The value of investigation of the incidence of peptic ulcer in families of patients with duodenal ulcer. Journal of Medical Genetics 9: 38–42

Kuenssberg E V 1962 Are duodenal ulcer and chronic bronchitis family diseases? Proceedings of the Royal Society of Medicine 55: 299–302

Kwitko A, Shearman D J C 1978 Antibodies to secretory IgA (SIgA) in duodenal ulcer disease. Gut 19: A437

Lam S K 1979 Duodenal-ulcer inheritance. Lancet i: 977–978

Lam S K 1980 Physiologic abnormalities and heterogenity in peptic ulcer. In: Rotter J I, Samloff I M, Rimoin D L (eds) Genetics and Heterogeneity of Common Gastrointestinal Disorders, New York, Academic Press, p 67–80

Lam S K, Sircus W 1975 Studies in duodenal ulcer, the clinical evidence for the existence of two populations. Quarterly Journal of Medicine 44: 369–387

Lam S K, Ong G B 1976 Duodenal ulcers, early and late onset. Gut 17: 169–179

Lam S K, Lai C L 1978 Gastric ulcers with and without associated duodenal ulcer have different pathophysiology. Clinical Science and Molecular Medicine 55: 97–102

Lam S K, Ong G B 1980 Identification of two subgroups of familial early onset duodenal ulcer. Annals of Internal Medicine 93: 540–544

Lam S K, Hui K K, Rotter J I, Samloff I M 1981 Pachydermoperiostosis and peptic ulcer. Gastroenterology, 80: 1202

Lamers C B H, Van Tongeren J H M 1977 Comparative study of the value of the calcium, secretin, and meal stimulated increase in serum gastrin in the diagnosis of the Zollinger-Ellison syndrome. Gut 18: 128–134

Lamers C B, Stadil F, Van Tongeren J H 1978 Prevalence of endocrine abnormalities in patients with the Zollinger-Ellison syndrome in their families. American Journal of Medicine 64: 607–612

Lamers C, Diemel C, Froeling P, Jansen J 1980 Hereditary of hypergastrinemic hyperchlorlydria syndromes. In: Rotter J I, Samloff I M, Rimoin D L (eds) The Genetics and Heterogeneity of Common Gastrointestinal Disorders, San Francisco and New York, Academic Press, p 81–89

Langman M J S 1973 Blood groups and alimentary disorders. Clinics in Gastroenterology 2: 497–506

Langman M J S 1979 The Epidemiology of Chronic Digestive Disease, Edward Arnold, London

Marshall A G, Hutchinson E O, Honisett J 1962 Hereditary in common diseases, a retrospective survey of twins in a hospital population. British Medical Journal i: 1–6

McConnell R B 1966 The Genetics of Gastrointestinal Disorders, Oxford University Press, London

McConnell R B 1980 Peptic ulcer, early genetic evidence--families, twins, and markers. In: Rotter J I, Samloff I M, Rimoin D L (eds) The Genetics and Heterogeneity of Common Gastrointestinal Disorders, New York, Academic Press, p 31–41

McKusick V A 1978 Mendelian Inheritance in Man, Catalogue of Autosomal Dominant, Autosomal Recessive, and X–linked Phenotypes, Johns Hopkins University Press, Baltimore

Monson R R 1970a Familial factors in peptic ulcer, the occurrence of ulcer in relatives. American Journal of Epidemiology 91: 453–466

Monson R R 1970b Duodenal ulcer as a second disease. Gastroenterology 59: 712–716

Moshal M G 1980 Ethnic differences in duodenal ulceration. In: Rotter J I, Samloff I M, Rimoin D L (eds) The Genetics and Heterogeneity of Common Gastrointestinal Disorders, San Francisco and New York, Academic Press, p 91–110

Mourant A E, Kopec A C, and Domaniewska-Sobczak K 1978 Blood Groups and Diseases: A Study of Associations of Diseases with Blood Groups and Other Polymorphisms. Oxford University Press, Oxford

Neuhauser G, Daly R F, Magnelli N C, Barreras R F, Donaldson R M, Opitz J M 1976 Essential tremor, nystagmus and duodenal ulceration. Clinical Genetics 9: 81–91

Parkes J D 1979 Personal communication

Pratt R T C 1967 The Genetics of Neurological Disorders. Oxford University Press, London

Pollin W, Allen M G, Hoffer A, Stabenau J R, and Hrubec Z 1969 Psychopathology in 15,909 pairs of veteran twins: evidence for a genetic factor in the pathogenesis of schizophrenia and its relative absence in psychoneurosis. American Journal of Psychiatry 126: 597–610

Prescott R J, Sircus W, Lai C L, and Lam S K 1976 Failure to confirm evidence for existence of two populations with duodenal ulcer. British Medical Journal ii: 677

Regan P T, Malagelada J R 1978 A reappraisal of clinical, roentgenographic and endoscopic features of the Zollinger-Ellison syndrome. Mayo Clinic Proceedings 53: 19–23

Rimoin D L 1967 Genetics of diabetes mellitus. Diabetes 16: 346–351

Rimoin D L, Schimke R N 1971 Endocrine pancreas. In: Genetic Disorders of the Endocrine Glands. Mosby, St. Louis, p 150–216

Roberts J A F 1965 ABO blood groups, secretor status, and susceptibility to chronic diseases: An example of genetic basis for family predispositions. In: Neel J V, Shaw M W, and Schull W J (eds) Genetics and the Epidemiology of Chronic Diseases. U.S. Government Printing Office, Public Health Service Publication No. 1163, p 77–86

Rotter J I 1980a Genetic approaches to ulcer heterogeneity. In: Rotter J I, Samloff I M, Rimoin D L, The Genetics and Heterogeneity of Common Gastrointestinal Disorders. Academic Press, San Francisco and New York, p 111–128

Rotter J I 1980b Peptic ulcer disease--more than one gene, more than one disease. In: Steinberg A G, Bearn A G, Motulsky A G, Childs B Progress in Medical Genetics, Volume 4 (new series), W.B. Saunders, Philadelphia p 1–58

Rotter J I 1981 Gastric and duodenal ulcer are each many different diseases. Digestive Diseases and Sciences 26: 154–160

Rotter J I, Gursky J M, Samloff I M, and Rimoin D L 1976 Peptic ulcer disease – further evidence for genetic heterogeneity. Excerpta Medica International Congress Series, No. 397: 96

Rotter J I, Rimoin D L 1977 Peptic ulcer disease – a heterogeneous group of disorders? Gastroenterology 73: 604–607

Rotter J I, Rimoin D L, Gursky J M, Teraski P I, and Sturdevant R A L 1977a HLA-B5 associated with duodenal ulcer. Gastroenterology 73: 435–437

Rotter J I, Rimoin D L, Samloff I M, McConnell R B, Gotlieb-Jensen K, Gadeburg O, and Hauge M 1977b The genetics of peptic ulcer disease – elevated serum group I pepsinogen concentrations in siblings and twins of ulcer probands. Gastroenterology 72: 1165

Rotter J I, Rimoin D L, Samloff I M 1978 Genetic heterogeneity in diabete mellitus and peptic ulcer. In: Morton N E, Chung C S (eds) Genetic Epidemiology, Academic Press, p 381–414

Rotter J I, Petersen G M, Samloff I M, McConnell R B, Ellis A, Spence M A and Rimoin D L 1979a Genetic heterogeneity of familial hyperpepsinogenemic I and normopepsinogenemic I duodenal ulcer disease. Annals of Internal Medicine 91: 372–377

Rotter J I, Sones J Q, Samloff I M, Richardson, C T, Gursky, J T Walsh J H and Rimoin D L 1979b Duodenal ulcer disease associated with elevated serum pepsinogen I, an inherited autosomal dominant disorder. New England Journal of Medicine 300: 63–66

Rotter J I, Rubin R, Meyer J H, Samloff I M, and Rimoin D L 1979c Rapid gastric emptying – an inherited pathophysiologic defect in duodenal ulcer? Gastroenterology 76: 1229

Rotter J I, Rimoin D L, and Samloff I M 1979d Genetic heterogeneity in peptic ulcer. Lancet i: 1088–1089

Rotter J I, Samloff I M, Rimoin D L (eds) 1980 The Genetics and Heterogeneity of Common Gastrointestinal Disorders, San Francisco and New York, Academic Press

Rotter J I, Rimoin D L 1981 Etiology of diabetes – genetics. In: Brownlee M (editor) Handbook of Diabetes Mellitus, Garland STPM Press, New York, p 3–93

Rotter J I, Monson R R, Grossman M I 1982 Duodenal ulcer and pulmonary disease, which comes first? Submitted for publication

Rotter J I, Heiner D C 1981 Are there immunological forms of duodenal ulcer, Journal of Clinical and Laboratory Immunology 7: 1–6

Samloff I M, Liebman W M, Panitch N M 1975 Serum group I pepsinogens by radioimmunoassay in control subjects and patients with peptic ulcer. Gastroenterology 69: 83–90

Samloff I M 1979 Serum pepsinogens I and II. In: Developments in Digestive Diseases, edited by Berk J E, Lea and Febiger, Philadelphia, p 1–12

Samloff I M 1980 Pepsinogens and their relationship to peptic ulcer. In: Rotter J I, Samloff I M, Rimoin D L (eds) The Genetics and Heterogeneity of Common Gastrointestinal Disorders, Academic Press, New York, p 43–49

Sandler M, Scheuler P J, and Watt P J 1961 5-Hydroxytryptophan secreting bronchial carcinoid tumor. Lancet ii: 1067–1069

Schimke R N 1976 Multiple endocrine adenomatosis syndromes. In: Advances in Internal Medicine, Volume 21, Gene H. Stollerman (ed), Year Book, Chicago, p 249–265

Sedlackova M, Seemanova E 1973 Genealogical investigation in a group of children with duodenal ulcer. Review of Czechoslovak Medicine 19: 81–88

Selmanowitz V J, Orentreich N, Tiango C C, Demis D J 1970 Uniovular twins discordance for cutaneous mastocytosis. Archives of Dermatology 102: 34–41

Shaw J M 1968 Genetic aspects of urticaria pigmentosa. Archives of Dermatology 97: 137–138

Stevenson R E, Lucas T, and Martin J R 1979 Stiff skin and multiple system disease in four generations. American Journal of Human Genetics 31: 84A

Susser M 1967 Causes of peptic ulcer: A selective epidemiological review. Journal of Chronic Diseases, 20: 435–456

Taylor I L, Calam J, Rotter J I, Vaillant C, Samloff I M, Cook A, Simkin E, Dockray G J 1981 Family studies of hypergastrinemic, hyperpepsinogenemic I duodenal ulcer. Annals of Internal Medicine, 95: 421–425, 1981

Tovey F I 1979 Progress report, peptic ulcer in India and Bangladesh. Gut, 29: 329–347

Tovey F I, Tunstall M 1975 Progress report, duodenal ulcer in black populations in Africa south of the Sahara. Gut, 16: 564–576

Van Allen M W, Frohlich J A, Davis J R 1969 Inherited predisposition to generalized amyloidosis, clinical and pathological study of a family with neuropathy, nephropathy, and peptic ulcer. Neurology 19: 10–25

Wermer P 1954 Genetic aspects of adenomatosis of endocrine glands. American Journal of Medicine 16: 363–371

Wormsley K G, and Grossman M I 1965 Maximal histalog test in control subjects and patients with peptic ulcer. Gut 6: 427–435

Wretmark G 1953 The peptic ulcer individual, a study in hereditary, physique and personality. Acta Psychiatrica Scandinavica and Neurologica (Supplement 84)

Zollinger R M, and Ellison E H 1955 Primary peptic ulcerations of the jejunum associated with islet cell tumors of the pancreas. Annals of Surgery 142: 709–728

61

Congenital pyloric stenosis

C. O. Carter

CLINICAL FEATURES

The first clear description of pyloric stenosis was by Hirschsprung in 1887. The onset of symptoms is usually from 2–6 weeks after birth with a mean of about 21 days, and is rare after 12 weeks. The presenting sign is abilious vomiting, which soon becomes projectile. This leads to failure to gain weight, dehydration, constipation and an alert and anxious facial expression. An experienced observer is able to feel an olive-shaped tumour at the outer edge of the right rectus muscle above the umbilicus. Abdominal peristalsis may become visible. On radiological examination by barium meal a characteristic thin and elongated lumen of the pylorus, the 'string sign', is apparent. The disease is self-limiting and, if the untreated child survives, the vomiting usually stops at about 16 weeks.

It appears that a period of postnatal feeding is required before symptoms develop. The condition has occasionally been found accidentally a few days after birth, for example at laparotomy on the second day for haematemesis (Kelsey et al, 1968) and at postmortem on the third day after death from meningitis (Laurence, 1963). There are reports of operation in the second half of the first week, for example on the fourth day (Meeker & Nicola, 1948), and one report back in 1927 of operation on the second day (MacHaffie, 1927). In premature infants the onset of symptoms is a little delayed but may develop well before the expected date of birth (Wilson, 1960). The condition rarely presents in adult life and may be associated with infantile pyloric stenosis in the children of these parents (Fenwick, 1953; Woo-ming, 1961). A further example is known to the author in which father and son were treated in infancy by Rammstedt's operation and grandfather by the same operation at the age of 40 years.

There are no strongly associated conditions. Conditions that cause vomiting in infancy, for example oesophageal hiatus hernia and phenylketonuria, are associated, perhaps by exacerbating minor degrees of pyloric stenosis. There is an association with oesophageal atresia, probably because this prevents prenatal swallowing of amniotic fluid. The association with indirect inguinal hernia is probably due to raised abdominal pressure from vomiting.

PATHOLOGY

On microscopic examination the pyloric muscle is enlarged, firm and pale. Histological examination of the tumour shows hypertrophy, mainly of the circular muscle, but also to lesser degree of the longitudinal muscle and elastic tissue of the pylorus. The mucosa of the pylorus is thickened and oedematous and it is the development of this which probably produces the partial obstruction of the pyloric canal. Wallgren (1946) observed that the radiological appearances were not present in newborn infants who later developed the disorder. The gastric mucosa is also inflamed, probably secondary to the obstruction.

No convincing explanation of the hypertrophy of the pyloric muscle has been found. There are sometimes degenerative changes in the neurons of the myenteric plexus, but these are probably secondary changes. Dodge (1970) was able to induce histologically similar pyloric tumours in puppies by injecting the mother bitch with pentagastrin, a synthetic analogue of the hormone gastrin, during pregnancy. The hypertrophy was increased when in addition the newborn puppies were given pentagastrin. The experiment has been successfully repeated by Karim et al (1974). However, serum gastrin is not raised either during fasting or after feeds in children with pyloric stenosis (Moazam et al, 1978).

DIFFERENTIAL DIAGNOSIS

The initial differential diagnosis is from the many other causes of vomiting of early onset at 2–6 weeks of postnatal life. In cases of early onset there is a more specific differential diagnosis from the rare cases of pyloric atresia or diaphragm and of high duodenal atresia and from functional pylorospasm. It is uncertain whether some cases of pylorospasm are mild examples of pyloric stenosis.

Experienced paediatricians usually make the diagnosis without difficulty and seldom need to seek radiological confirmation.

THERAPY

Complications of the condition are dehydration, loss of electrolytes, alkalosis and starvation. Sixty years ago the condition had a high mortality in Britain; death usually was from intercurrent infection. Higher survival rates were achieved in Scandinavia. Mortality changed rapidly after the introduction in 1912 of Rammstedt's operation of a linear cut through the pyloric musculature down to the mucosa. The changing pattern at The Hospital for Sick Children, London after the introduction of Rammstedt's operation is shown in Table 61.1 (Carter, 1961). In experienced centres mortality by operation after restoration of electrolyte balance is now less than 1%. Treatment with anti-spasmodic drugs (for example methyl atropine nitrate) in addition to gastric lavage has been tried. While such treatment is useful in tiding over a case of late onset into the age of natural recovery, most centres in Britain prefer the quick cure by operation for all but the most mild cases. In Scandinavia such medical treatment was more widely used, but now surgical treatment is usual.

SEQUELAE

There are no serious sequelae after operation. After medical treatment or after gastro-jejunostomy the pyloric hypertrophy may persist for several years. An apparent increase in the frequency of peptic ulcer in adult life has been claimed, but it is doubtful if there is really such an increase (Berglund & Rabo, 1973b). In a few cases treated medically, when the illness has been prolonged and there has been a marked weight loss, a moderate (3–4 cms) reduction in height, and a small, but not statistically significant, reduction in intelligence has been noted in patients at call-up for military service. These

patients did not differ from the remainder in mean birth weight. There is also a suggestion at later follow-up that in these patients there was a reduction in the percentage with children as compared with the general population (Berglund & Rabo, 1973a).

EPIDEMIOLOGY

Estimates of birth frequency are somewhat insecure since the diagnosis may be missed in severe cases with superadded infection and labelled gastroenteritis, and also missed in mild cases which are self-limiting. For North Europeans the birth frequency is probably 2 to 4 per thousand live births. Some typical figures per thousand live births from the UK are Newcastle 2.8 (Davison, 1946), Birmingham 3.1 (McMahon et al, 1951), Dundee 1.5 (Lawson, 1951), Aberdeen 4.5 (McLean, 1956), Edinburgh 3.6 (Smith, 1960), Belfast 2.6 (Dodge, 1975). For Gothenburg, Wallgren (1960) reported a figure of 2.0 and from Eastern Europe Czeizel (1972) reported a figure of 1.5. Both in Gothenburg and Belfast there was evidence of a decline in the incidence of the condition. There are indications that the conditon is less common in southern than in northern Europeans. For example Cachia and Fenech (1966) have reported a figure of 0.9 for Malta.

In non-Caucasian populations the condition is appreciably less common, for example Laron and Horne (1957) from Pittsburgh reported a rate in Whites of 1.3, but of only 0.5 per thousand in Negroes. In Hawaii (Shim et al, 1970) the rates were 1.9 in Caucasians and 0.5 in Japanese per thousand, and there were no cases in over 11 000 Chinese and only 2 in over 22 500 Philipinos. The male preponderance however appears similar in all races surveyed.

The sex ratio in Europeans is usually between 4 and 5 males to 1 female. Thus a 3 in 1000 birth frequency corresponds to about 1 in 200 males and 1 in 1000 female live births.

The condition is said to be more common in firstborn. The original observation by Still in 1927 was in part based on an unsuitable choice of controls. Since then the finding has been confirmed in some series but not in others. The effect is seen most clearly in the cases with a

Table 61.1 Treatment and number of survivors of children with pyloric stenosis from The Hospital for Sick Children, London, 1918–25.

Years	Rammstedt's operation		Medical treatment		Total	
	Survivors	Dead	Survivors	Dead	Survivors	Dead
1918–19	6	14	1	6	7	20
1920–21	25	26	4	14	29	40
1922–23	55	18	0	6	55	24
1924–25	72	15	0	1	72	16

later onset (McKeown et al, 1952; Nielsen, 1954). The effect may be due to less skilled handling of minor degrees of the condition by an inexperienced mother.

The maternal age distribution is similar to that in the general population.

No constant association of season of birth has been found (MacMahon et al, 1951; Campbell, 1969). Dodge (1975) found an excess born in the winter months; but the differences are doubtfully significant in the absence of any prior hypothesis.

Other observers have found an excess of parents in professional and managerial occupations (Dodge, 1975), but others (Czeizel, 1972) found no such difference.

The onset of illness has been found later in children fed four hourly than three hourly (Gerrard et al, 1955) and in children born in hospital than those born at home (McKeown et al, 1952).

In several series (Malmberg, 1949; Shim et al, 1970; Dean, 1970; Czeizel, 1972; Berglund & Rabo, 1973b) an increase in mean birth weight was found for patients as compared with controls. A reduced incidence has been found among children born prematurely (Wilson, 1960; Czeizel, 1972), but in these the diagnosis is less easily made since vomiting is less often projectile and gastric peristalsis less evident.

No consistent association with any particular maternal condition or prenatal history has been found. The proportion of patients fully breast fed did not differ appreciably from that of the controls (Dodge, 1975).

GENETICS

Twins

No large scale consecutive series of twins has been reported, but there is no doubt that the concordance of MZ twins is higher than that for DZ twins (Metrakos, 1953; Lamy et al, 1953), and that the concordance for MZ twins for clinical illness is well below 100% and probably below 50% (MacMahon & McKeown, 1955). There are reports both of a monozygotic twin pair (Lewis, 1944) and a dizygotic twin pair (Powell & Carter, 1951) in which the second twin on examination was found to have visible peristalsis and a tumour, but was asymptomatic.

First degree relatives

Because of the high mortality in earlier years of pyloric stenosis it is unlikely that parents will often be affected. In the author's London series (Carter & Evans, 1969) of 330 male patients treated between 1920 and 1939 and 233 female patients from 1920 to 1949 only one parent (a mother) was affected, but in the second series of 307 males treated from 1953 to 1962 and 119 females from 1950 to 1965, 8 of 426 fathers and 4 of 426 mothers had

Table 61.2 Pyloric stenosis: proportion of sibs affected.

| | London series | | Belfast series | |
	Brothers	Sisters	Brothers	Sisters
Male index patients	21/546 (3.8%)	15/565 (2.7%)	51/544 (9.4%)	13/428 (3.0%)
Female index patients	25/273 (9.2%)	10/263 (3.8%)	20/160 (12.5%)	6/159 (3.8%)

themselves been successfully treated by Rammstedt's operation, three of them being index patients in the earlier series.

An increased risk to sibs was however noted early (Cockayne & Penrose, 1943). The data in the two larger series from London (Carter & Evans, 1969) and Belfast (Dodge, 1973) are summarised in Table 61.2.

The findings are reasonably consistent except for the rather high figure for the proportion of brothers affected in the Belfast series. A noteworthy feature of both studies is the higher risk to the sibs of the female index patients. An early hypothesis (Cockayne & Penrose, 1943) for the mode of inheritance was that it was modified autosomal recessive. However in 1954 reports appeared both from Copenhagen (Nielsen, 1954), based on the medically treated series, and from London (Carter & Powell, 1954), based on a series in which the condition was confirmed at operation in both generations, that there was a substantial risk to the children of index patients. The later findings for the London series (Carter & Evans, 1969) are summarised in Table 61.3.

The findings suggest that the proportion of children affected is probably no different from the proportion of sibs affected. The higher proportion of relatives affected when the index patient is female is even more marked in the children than in the sibs.

The risks to first degree relatives appear, on the small numbers available, to be substantially increased where the index patient already has an affected relative. In the London series where the male index patient had already had an affected child 3 of 9 subsequent sons and 0 of 8 subsequent daughters were affected, for female index patients 3 of 9 subsequent sons and 2 of 4 subsequent daughters were affected. Similarly where the index patient had an older sib affected 0 of 9 subsequent brothers and 2 of 9 sisters were affected, for female index

Table 61.3 Pyloric stenosis: proportion of children affected.

	Sons	Daughters
Male index patients	19/347 (5.5%)	8/337 (2.4%)
Female index patients	20/106 (18.9%)	7/100 (7%)

patients 0 of 9 brothers and 0 of 2 sisters were affected. Combining the two groups the male index patients' proportions affected are 3 in 18 sons or brothers and 2 in 17 daughters or sisters, while for female index patients 3 in 18 sons or brothers and 2 in 6 daughters or sisters were affected.

Second degree relatives

In the earlier series information on aunts and uncles born at a time when diagnosis was unreliable would be far from complete. In a recent Hungarian series (Czeizel, personal communication) for male index patients 0 in 153 paternal, 1 in 180 maternal uncles, 0 in 146 paternal and 1 in 166 maternal aunts were affected; for female index patients 0 in 42 paternal, 0 in 42 maternal uncles, 0 in 33 paternal and 0 in 39 maternal aunts were affected. In the London series data were available for many nephews and nieces, a few half-sibs (Carter & Evans, 1969) and recently for a few grandchildren (Carter et al, 1980). These data are summarised in Table 61.4.

Within the limits of chance variation due to the small numbers affected the proportions affected of the different types of second degree relative are consistent and indicate risks of 2.2, 0.5, 4.3 and 1.7% for male and female relatives of male index patients and male and female relatives of female index patients respectively. The higher risk to relatives for female than male index patients, seen in first degree, is therefore also apparent in the second degree relatives.

Third degree relatives

While cousins are contemporary with the index patients and therefore in general diagnosis will be satisfactory, the parents of the index patient will not always have full knowledge of the health in infancy of their nephews and nieces. The findings in the London series (Carter & Evans, 1969) in first cousins are summarised in Table 61.5. It will be seen that for male index patients 0.9% of male and 0.2% of female cousins, and for female index patients 0.7% of male and 0.3% of female cousins were affected. The higher risk to the relatives of female patients is no longer present. The corresponding proportions in the smaller Hungarian series (Czeizel, personal communication) were 3 in 284, 1 in 280, 1 in 82 and 0 in 59, and therefore essentially similar to those in the London series.

MECHANISM OF INHERITANCE

Estimates of the 'K' value, that is the proportion of relatives affected divided by the birth frequency in the general population of the same sex, are given in Table 61.6.

A comparison of the values for children and sibs excludes any substantial element of recessive inheritance. In the case of female patients the K value is even higher for children than sibs. Any substantial element of X-linkage is excluded by the frequent instances of male to male transmission. Simple dominant inheritance with

Table 61.4 Second degree relatives of index patients.

| | Nephews and nieces | | | | Half-sibs | | | | Grandchildren | | | | Total | |
| | brothers' | | sisters' | | paternal | | maternal | | sons' | | daus.' | | | |
	sons	daus.	sons	daus.	bros.	sis.	bros.	sis.	sons	daus.	sons	daus.	male	female
Male index patients	1/125	0/123	5/137	1/157	0/18	0/20	1/11	0/23	0/27	1/17	1/41	0/35	8/359 (2.23%)	2/375 (0.53%)
Female index patients	3/36	0/38	1/51	0/53	1/12	0/11	0/7	0/6	0/5	1/3	0/5	1/5	5/116 (4.31%)	2/116 (1.72%)

Table 61.5 Pyloric stenosis: third degree relatives.

| | Children of | | | | | | | | Total cousins | |
| | fathers' brothers | | fathers' sisters | | mothers' brothers | | mothers' sisters | | | |
	male	female	male	female	male	female	male	female	male	female
Male index patients	6/697	1/634	7/624	1/600	5/603	1/579	7/759	3/767	25/2683 (0.93%)	6/2580 (0.23%)
Female index patients	3/389	2/344	1/393	1/407	4/411	0/404	3/445	1/413	11/1638 (0.67%)	4/1568 (0.26%)

Table 61.6 Approximate 'K' values for first, second and third degree relatives.

| | First degree | | | | Second degree | | Third degree | |
	bros.	sis.	sons	daus.	male	female	male	female
Male index patient	10	30	10	25	4	5	2	2½
Female index patient	20	40	40	70	10	15	1½	2½

penetrance determined by environmental factors is also improbable. On this hypothesis the higher K value for the sibs and children of female patients would have to be attributed to the need for a stronger environmental influence before a girl is affected, and that this environmental influence is common to families and shared, if anything, more strongly by parent and child than by sibs. Again on the simple modified dominant hypothesis the sharp fall off in the K value as one passes from first to second to third degree female relatives of female index patients (while the likelihood of carrying the gene involved declines only from 1/2 to 1/4 to 1/8) would have to be attributed to a rapid dilution of the environmental factor. Further it is difficult to visualise the mutant gene involved reaching such a high frequency in Caucasians when the condition had, until recently, such a high mortality. It would require a selective advantage of those who are heterozygous for the gene, but not clinically affected.

Both the effect of sex of patient and the sharp fall off with decreasing relationship to the index patient are expected if it is assumed that there is a substantial polygenic element in the genetic predisposition to develop the disorder, and that females are protected by their sex and require a stronger polygenic predisposition to develop the disorder than males. Fewer females reach the threshold beyond which they are at risk of developing the disorder, and those that do are more extreme deviants from

their population mean than are most males. The principle is illustrated in Figure 61.1. For example first degree male relatives of male patients will have a distribution for the polygenic predisposition about a mean halfway between the mean for the male population and that of male patients. First degree male relatives of female patients would be distributed about a mean half the greater distance between the mean for the female population and that of female patients. The increasing K value as one passes from male relatives of male patients, through female relatives of male and male relatives of female, to female relatives of female patients is explained by the model.

The sharp fall off in the K values for female index patients and their female relatives is also readily explained on the polygenic model, since the birth frequency is low. This is illustrated in Figure 61.2. The birth frequency in males is too high to give a fall off markedly different from the halving of the K value with each step away from the index patient expected on simple modified dominant inheritance.

In 1961 the author proposed a model with a major gene whose expression was modified by a polygenic background, sex and environment. Later, with more data available, it was apparent there was no need to postulate the major contribution of a single gene and that the polygenic model modified by sex and environment, the multifactorial threshold model, was sufficient with-

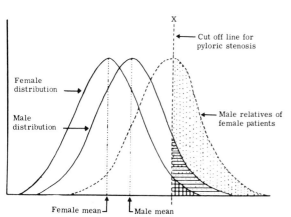

Fig. 61.1 Model for polygenic inheritance with sex modification, with a threshold beyond which patients are at risk for pyloric stenosis.

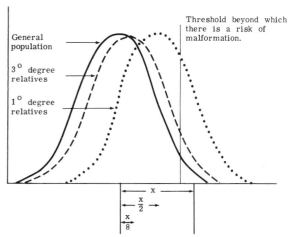

Fig. 61.2 Model for polygenic inheritance.

out involving a major gene (Carter & Evans 1969). Lalouel et al (1977) analysing the segregation ratios only in sibships, by parental mating types, in the series of Cockayne & Penrose (1943), McKeown et al (1951) and Carter & Evans (1969), concluded that the generalised single locus model gave a less satisfactory fit than either a mixed model or the multifactorial model. They noted that the two latter models gave an equally good fit, but that the multifactorial model was to be preferred as the more economical hypothesis. It is also easier to reconcile with the findings in second and third degree relatives for females. It is easier too to reconcile with the frequency

of the condition, since it is not unreasonable to suppose that there is stabilising selection, with selection against individuals at the other extreme of the polygenic predisposition.

The author and others have noted that the apparently higher risk to the children than sibs of female index patients suggests a direct maternal effect. However this could just be due to the size of the sample, and there is no indication yet that this influence is shared by the female index patients and their sisters and daughters, nor for maternal half-sibs to be more often affected than paternal (Carter et al, 1980).

REFERENCES

Bendix R M, Necheles H 1947 Hypertrophic pyloric stenosis. A follow-up study. Journal of the American Medical Association 135: 331–3

Berglund G, Rabo E 1973a A long-term follow-up investigation of patients with hypertrophic pyloric stenosis – with special reference to heredity and later morbidity. Acta Paediatrica Scandinavica 62: 130–2

Berglund G, Rabo E 1973b A long-term follow-up investigation of patients with hypertrophic pyloric stenosis – with special reference to the physical and mental development. Acta Paediatrica Scandinavica 62: 125–9

Cachia E A, Fenech F F 1966 Incidence of pyloric stenosis in Malta. Journal of Medical Genetics 3: 49–50

Campbell M A 1969 A question of seasonal variation of pyloric stenosis. Journal of Paediatrics 74: 1006–7

Carter C O 1961 Inheritance of congenital pyloric stenosis. British Medical Bulletin 17: 251–3

Carter C O, Powell B W 1954 Two-generation pyloric stenosis. Lancet 1: 746–8

Carter C O, Evans K A 1969 Inheritance of congenital pyloric stenosis. Journal of Medical Genetics 6: 233–9

Carter C O, Evans K, Warren J 1980 The grandchildren of patients with pyloric stenosis. Journal of Medical Genetics 17: 411–5

Cockayne E A, Penrose L S 1943 The genetics of congenital pyloric stenosis. Ohio Journal of Science 43: 1–16

Czeizel A 1972 Birth weight distribution in congenital pyloric stenosis. Archives of Disease in Childhood 47: 978–80

Davison G 1946 The incidence of congenital pyloric stenosis. Archives of Disease in Childhood 21: 113–4

Dean D 1970 Behandlungsergebnisse der hypertrophischen pylorusstenose bei 351 Sauglingen von 1945–1964. Archiv für Kinderheilkunde 181: 32–9

Dodge J A 1970 Production of duodenal ulcers and hypertrophic pyloric stenosis by administration of pentagastrin to pregnant and newborn dogs. Nature 225: 284–5

Dodge J A 1973 Genetics of hypertrophic pyloric stenosis. Clinics in Gastroenterology 2: 523–8

Dodge J A 1975 Infantile hypertrophic stenosis in Belfast 1957–69. Archives of Disease in Childhood 50: 171–8

Fenwick J 1953 Familial hypertrophic pyloric stenosis. British Medical Journal 2: 12–4

Gerrard J W, Waterhouse J A H, Maurice D G 1955 Infantile pyloric stenosis. Archives of Disease in Childhood 30: 493–6

Glasson M J, Bandrevics V, Cohen D H 1973 Hypertrophic

pyloric stenosis complicating oesophageal atresia. Surgery 74: 530–5

Hirschsprung H 1888 Falle von angeborenen Pylorusstenose, beobachtet bei sauglingen. Jahrbuch Kinderheilkunde 28: 61

Karim A A, Morrison J E, Parks T G 1974 The role of pentagastrin in the production of canine hypertrophic pyloric stenosis and pyloroduodenal ulceration. Abstract, British Journal of Surgery 61: 327

Kelsey D, Stayman J W, McLaughlin E D, Mebane W 1968 Massive bleeding in a newborn infant from a gastric ulcer associated with hypertrophic pyloric stenosis. Surgery 64: 979–89

Lalouel J M, Morton N E, MacLean C J, Jackson J 1977 Recurrence risks in complex inheritance with special regard to pyloric stenosis. Journal of Medical Genetics 14: 408–14

Lamy M, Poignan C, Maroteaux P 1953 The genetics of pyloric stenosis. Proceedings of the Royal Society of Medicine 46: 1062–3

Laron Z, Horne L M 1957 The incidence of infantile pyloric stenosis. American Journal of Diseases of Childhood 94: 151–4

Laurence K M 1963 Hypertrophic pyloric stenosis. Lancet 1: 224–5

Lawson D 1951 The incidence of pyloric stenosis in Dundee. Archives of Disease in Childhood 26: 616–7

Lewis F L K 1944 Pyloric stenosis in identical twins. British Medical Journal 1: 221

MacHaffie L P 1927 An early case of pyloric stenosis. Canadian Medical Association Journal 17: 946–7

McKeown T, MacMahon B, Record R G 1951 The familial incidence of congenital pyloric stenosis. Annals of Human Genetics 16: 260–81

McKeown T, MacMahon B, Record R G 1952 Evidence of postnatal environmental influence in the aetiology of infantile pyloric stenosis. Archives of Disease in Childhood 27: 386–90

McLean M M 1956 The incidence of infantile pyloric stenosis in the North-East of Scotland. Archives of Disease in Childhood 31: 481–2

MacMahon B, McKeown T 1955 Infantile hypertrophic pyloric stenosis: data on 81 pairs of twins. Acta Geneticae Medicae et Gemellologicae 4: 320–5

MacMahon B, Record R G, McKeown T 1951 Congenital pyloric stenosis. An investigation of 578 cases. British Journal of Social Medicine 5: 185–92

Malmberg N 1949 Hypertrophic pyloric stenosis – a survey of

136 successive cases – with special reference to treatment with Scopyl. Acta Paediatrica 38: 472–83

Meeker C S, DeNicola R R 1948 Hypertrophic pyloric stenosis in a newborn infant. Journal of Pediatrics 33: 94–7

Metrakos J D 1953 Congenital hypertrophic pyloric stenosis in twins. Archives of Disease in Childhood 28: 351–7

Moazam F, Rodgers B M, Talbert J L, McGuigan J E 1978 Fasting and postprandial serum gastrin levels in infants with congenital hypertrophic pyloric stenosis. Annals of Surgery 188: 623–5

Nielsen O S 1954 Familial predisposition to congenital pyloric stenosis. Acta Paediatrica 43: 522–8

Ovemin R I, Klein A 1968 Infantile pyloric stenosis: a 10 year survey. South African Medical Journal 42: 1056–60

Powell B W, Carter C O 1951 Pyloric stenosis in twins. Archives of Disease in Childhood 26: 45–9

Rammstedt W C 1912 Zur operation der angeborenen Pylorusstenose. Medizinische Klinik 8: 1702–5

Shim W K, Campbell A, Wright S W 1970. Pyloric stenosis in the racial groups of Hawaii. Journal of Pediatrics 76: 89–93

Smith I M 1960 Incidence of intussusception and congenital hypertrophic pyloric stenosis in Edinburgh children. British Medical Journal 1: 551–2

Still G F 1927 Place-in-family as a factor in disease. Lancet 2: 795–800 and 853–8

Wallgren A 1946 Preclinical stage of infantile hypertrophic pyloric stenosis. American Journal of Diseases of Childhood 72: 371–6

Wallgren A 1960 Is the rate of hypertrophic pyloric stenosis declining? Acta Paediatrica 49: 530–5

Wilson M G 1960 Pyloric stenosis in premature infants. Journal of Pediatrics 56: 490–7

Woo-ming M 1961 Familial relationship between adult and infantile hypertrophic pyloric stenosis. British Medical Journal 1: 476

62

Hirschsprung disease and other developmental defects of the gastrointestinal tract

E. Passarge

INTRODUCTION

Hirschsprung disease is an early childhood disease observed in about 1 per 5000 newborn. It has a remarkable sex ratio of 3.75 males to one female. The disease is characterized by chronic constipation leading to severe abdominal distension, megacolon, and possible secondary electrolyte disturbances. It may present in the neonatal period with ileus or sigmoid perforation. Although the first clinical description by Hirschsprung in 1887 was followed by good pathological studies in 1901 (Tittel, 1901) and 1924 (Dalla Valle, 1924), which demonstrated absence of intramural intestinal ganglion cells, it was not until 1948 that this was firmly established as the cause of the disease (Zuelzer & Wilson, 1948; Swenson & Bill, 1948). Since then, numerous studies have been devoted to the diagnosis, management, surgical procedures, and the genetic aspects (Ehrenpreis, 1970; Weinberg, 1974; Bolande, 1975). Genetic factors are implicated by the familial occurrence in 4% of cases. Genetic heterogeneity is suggested because congenital intestinal aganglionosis may occur as part of a variety of disorders, most notably trisomy 21, Waardenburg syndrome, cartilage hair dysplasia, phaeochromocytoma, and others.

Anatomical and embryological considerations

Intestinal mobility is controlled via three distinct enteric plexuses: the myenteric plexus of Auerbach, between the circular and longitudinal muscle layers of the muscularis propia, and two plexuses in the submucosal region. These are the superficial submucosal plexus of Meissner, just beneath the muscularis mucosa, and the deep submucosal plexus of Henle. The latter appears to be analogous to Auerbach's plexus (Baumgarten et al, 1973; Weinberg, 1974).

Ganglion cells of the normal myenteric plexuses are concentrated along the neural strands and the nodal points of a network of non-myelinated extrinsic nerve fibres. Nerve trunks are of vagal origin and largely acetylcholinesterase-positive. However, considerable morphological and histochemical heterogeneity appears to exist, and the complexities of the anatomical and physiological properties of enteric plexuses are not yet fully understood. As pointed out by Weinberg (1974), the enteric ganglion cells do not simply represent peripheral parasympathetic effector cells, but should be viewed as part of a complex neuroregulatory system (Baumgarten et al, 1973).

Apparently intramural intestinal ganglion cells reach the alimentary tract by migrating from the cephalic neural crest between the 6th and 12th week of embryogenesis (Hüther, 1954; Okamoto & Ueda, 1967; Andrew, 1971). This migration occurs in a defined time sequence with a cranial-caudal gradient. At 5 weeks gestation, paired vagal fibres extend to the upper oesophagus, and there are a few fine fibres from the periaortic and pelvic plexuses, but ganglion cells are still absent. At 6 weeks, neuroblasts are present in the oesophagus outside the circular layer and the stomach. At 8 weeks (18 mm embryo) ganglion cells are present in the small intestine and the rectum, but not the colon. At 12 weeks (70 mm) the entire plexus is innervated, presumably by further caudal ganglion cell migration. The most critical period seems to be between weeks 8 and 12, when most of the distal plexus develops.

The neuroblasts first reaching the alimentary tract form the myenteric plexus. The submucosal plexus is formed by neuroblasts migrating from the myenteric plexus across the circular muscle layer into the submucosa (Okamoto & Ueda, 1967). The submucosal plexus is also formed in the caudal direction, but later, during the third and fourth months of gestation. The outer longitudinal muscle layer develops from embryonic mesenchymal tissue after the myenteric plexus has been formed in the twelfth week (Okamoto & Ueda, 1967). In contrast to the apparently direct role of vagal nerve fibres, sympathetic and pelvic parasympathetic nerves are not involved in the development of the intramural plexus.

It should be noted that the intrinsic innervation of the anal canal differs from that of the intestines by a zone normally lacking ganglion cells (Weinberg, 1974). This zone may extend up to about 14–18 mm above the pectinate line, followed by another 4–5 mm with a reduced number of ganglion cells. This normal hypoganglionic zone may thus extend for up to 23 mm until the normal plexus is reached.

Thus, a diagnostic rectal biopsy must be taken 20–30 mm above the pectinate line. The orientation of the specimen must be clearly marked and it should be pinned to a flat surface prior to fixation to allow sectioning perpendicular to the plane of the plexus (Weinberg, 1974). A full-thickness biopsy of about 5 x 10 mm must be obtained to ensure that both layers of the muscle are present. Fragmented specimens pose considerable difficulties in interpretation. Different methods of biopsy including suction biopsy have been reviewed by Weinberg (1974).

Absence of intestinal ganglion cells
In classic Hirschsprung disease, ganglion cells of the mucosal and submucosal plexus are absent (*total aganglionosis*). The aganglionic segment extends from the supraanal region (see above) up to the sigmoid colon in 80–90% of patients. In others, the aganglionic segment may reach even up to the splenic flexure, and in some cases may involve the entire colon and small intestine. A reduced number of ganglion cells in the enteric plexus may be found in the distal colon, a condition called *hypoganglionosis* (Weinberg, 1974). It is not clear whether this constitutes a disease entity in terms of a defined aetiology. Usually, however, a hypoganglionic segment represents the transition between the aganglionic segment and the normal bowel. Another condition is *segmental aganglionosis*. Pathological findings and embryological considerations make it unlikely that this is a developmental defect. It is more likely to be the result of a localized vascular accident (Yntema & Hammond, 1954).

Genetic factors
Mainly three systematic genetic studies have been useful in estimating the recurrence risk of congenital intestinal aganglionosis in sibs (Bodian & Carter, 1963; Madsen, 1964; Passarge, 1967a, 1967b, 1973). The family data are summarized in Table 62.1 and indicate an overall recurrence risk between 2.3 and 13.6% depending on whether the index patient is male or female and the sex of the sib at risk. These data have been interpreted as possibly reflecting multifactorial inheritance (Passarge, 1967a, 1967b, 1973), though this is not entirely supported by the apparent higher risk among sisters of female index patients (or among sisters of male index patients in type II in Table 62.2).

The familial incidence is greater when the aganglionic segment is long. On the basis of different recurrence risks according to the length of the aganglionic segment in the index case, Passarge (1972, 1973) distinguished

Table 62.1 Congenital intestinal aganglionosis: frequency of affected sibs[a].

Index patients	Affected sibs	
	Brothers	Sisters
319 males	16/300 (5.3%)	7/305 (2.3%)
85 females	9/79 (11.4%)	11/81 (13.6%)

[a] Source of data: Bodian & Carter (1963), Madsen (1964), Passarge (1967). Cases with aganglionosis as part of systemic disorders not included.

Table 62.2 Congenital intestinal aganglionosis: frequency of affected sibs according to length of aganglionic segment[a].

Index patients		Affected Sibs	
		Brothers	Sisters
Type I:	182 males	4/73 (5.5%)	1/172 (0.6%)
	35 females	3/37 (8.1%)	1/35 (2.85%)
Type II:	28 males	10/148 (6.75%)	3/27 (11.1%)
	15 females	2/11 (18.2%)	1/11 (9.1%)

[a] Source of data as in Table 62.1. Length of aganglionic segment defined as type I for absence of intestinal ganglion cells caudal to the splenic flexure and as type II for absence anywhere further rostral to this point.

two types of congenital intestinal aganglionosis (CIA): type I and type II. Type I was defined as aganglionosis extending from the rectum up to the splenic flexure, thereby closely corresponding to classic Hirschsprung disease. Type II was defined as aganglionosis extending beyond this point into the transverse colon or even into the entire colon or small intestine. The data are summarized in Table 62.2. This distinction may be somewhat artificial, but it is supported by differences in the risk of recurrence (Table 62.2). The sex ratio also differs, being 5.2 in type I and 1.86 to 1 in type II.

Aganglionosis of the entire bowel has been reported in about 10 families including affected sibs (MacKinnon & Cohen, 1977; Talwalker, 1976). At present it is not clear whether this is a separate entity, possibly with autosomal recessive inheritance, or the result of over-reporting of a rare coincidence. In some cases nerve fibres were also absent, in contrast to the usual form where ganglion cells are lacking but nerve trunks are present.

Hirschsprung disease was not observed in 34 children of affected parents studied by Puri and Nixon (1977), but was in 2 and possibly 4 of 103 children reported by Carter et al (1981). Of these, 3 were born to parents with long segment disease. The authors considered there to be a genetic risk of about 2% for a parent with short segment disease and a high risk for a parent with long segment disease, bearing in mind that the length of the segment affected may differ in parent and child.

Evidence for genetic heterogeneity

Congenital intestinal aganglionosis may occur in a number of other disorders (Table 62.3). Earlier studies (Passarge, 1967) have shown that 2.5% of patients with Hirschsprung disease have trisomy 21 (Down syndrome). The reason for this rather frequent association, however, is not yet clear.

In view of the neural crest origin of intramural intestinal ganglion cells, melanocytes, and the sensory components of the spinal and cranial nerves, several recent observations reporting the association of intestinal aganglionosis and Waardenburg syndrome (Omenn & McKusick, 1979; Branski et al, 1979) are of particular interest. With an estimated incidence of Waardenburg syndrome with deafness of 2 per 100 000 and of Hirschsprung disease of 2 per 10 000, the chance association would be only 4 per one billion. Omenn & McKusick (1979) have rightly pointed out that this association must be significant.

A similar association of pigmentary anomalies and intestinal aganglionosis has been observed in several mouse mutants. These are the recessive alleles *piebald*, *piebald-lethal* and *lethal-spotting* (Lane, 1966). Homozygotes for *piebald-lethal* and *lethal-spotting* show a 100% incidence of aganglionosis. *Piebald* homozygotes and *piebald/piebald-lethal* compound heterozygotes have a 10% incidence for aganglionosis (Omenn & McKusick, 1979). These murine disorders represent genetically determined disturbances in cells derived from the neural crest, although the direct effects of the mutant alleles on the neural crest are not yet clear.

The occurrence of intestinal aganglionosis in such diverse disorders as trisomy 21 (chromosomal), Waardenburg syndrome and other forms of deafness (Mendelian), phaeochromocytoma (presumptive neural crest disorder), in addition to classic Hirschsprung disease (presumptive multifactorial) supports the contention that failure of the intramural intestinal ganglion cells to develop properly is aetiologically heterogeneous. It remains to be seen whether defects in migration from the neural crest account for all the observations. The complex development of the intramural intestinal neuroregulatory system leaves ample room for different genetic mechanisms leading to maldevelopment.

DEFECTS OF THE GROSS INTESTINAL ANATOMICAL STRUCTURE

Developmental defects of the gastrointestinal tract may occur alone, limited to one or several sites of the gastrointestinal tract, or they may be part of an overall developmental disorder. Clinically they usually lead to signs of obstruction, resulting from stenosis, atresia or impaired intestinal mobility, or to bleeding due to ulceration. Although occasionally familial occurrence has been observed in gastrointestinal malformations (see below), it may be noteworthy that Mendelian inheritance has not been established for any. In syndromes with gastrointestinal involvement, the overall disorder determines the aetiology of the gastrointestinal maldevelopment. Hence, it is important to recognize the presence of associated non-gastrointestinal defects, which may provide a clue to the recognition of genetic factors.

Intestinal atresia

About one third of congenital atresias involve the oesophagus, with or without concomitant tracheal fistula. However, familial occurrence is rare. The duodenum is the site of atresia in about 10%. In some series, up to one third of patients with duodenal atresia have been found to have an additional chromosome 21 (trisomy 21) (Warkany, 1971). Multiple intestinal atresias and jejunal atresia have been reported in sibs in the so-called 'apple peel syndrome' (Martin et al. 1976). Autosomal recessive inheritance has been assumed as an explanation, but has not been proven. Preferential reporting of coincidental findings could still explain the few observations. Intrauterine mesenteric artery accidents, perhaps as a consequence of the normal developmental rotation, appear just as likely a cause.

Malrotation

This is a common developmental failure, but little evidence for genetic factors is available. However, it is often part of a chromosomal or Mendelian disorder.

Duplication

Duplicated parts of the intestines are relatively common

Table 62.3 Congenital intestinal aganglionosis, frequently observed in association with other disorders.

Chromosomal disorders
Trisomy 21
Other chromosomal aberrations

Mendelian disorders
Deafness, different forms
Waardenburg syndrome
Cartilage hair dysplasia
Syndrome of congenital heart defect, broad halluces, and ulnar polydactyly in sibs (Laurence et al, 1975)
Aarskog syndrome (Hassinger et al, 1980)
Syndrome of microcephaly, hypertelorism, short stature and submucous cleft palate (Goldberg & Shprintzen, 1981).

Other disorders
Neuroblastoma
Phaeochromocytoma
Rubella embryopathy
Colon atresia
Other congenital defects

developmental defects, but genetic factors do not seem to be involved.

Anorectal malformations

Congenital malformations of the anus and rectum include anal stenosis, atresia or ectopy. They occur at a frequency of about 1 per 5000 births. About half of the patients also show other associated developmental defects. Pinsky (1978) has recently listed at least 26 different patterns of malformations involving anorectal anomalies. These include Mendelian, chromosomal, and non-genetic conditions.

One of the most frequent associations is the VATER/VACTERL complex, an acronym for vertebral, anal, tracheo-esophageal, renal and radial limb anomalies, including cardiovascular and nonradial limb anomalies which may also be present. Pinsky (1978) emphasized the aetiologic heterogeneity of these defects and warned of wrong estimates of the genetic recurrence risk unless the underlying phenotype is recognized.

REFERENCES

Andrew A 1971 The origin of intramural ganglia. Journal of Anatomy 108: 169

Baumgarten H G, Holstein A F, Stelzner F 1973 Nervous elements in the human colon of Hirschsprung's disease. Achives of Pathology and Anatomy 358: 113

Bodian M, Carter C O 1963 Family study of Hirschsprung's disease. Annals of Human Genetics 29: 261

Bolande R P 1975 Hirschsprung's disease, aganglionic or hypoganglionic megacolon. American Journal of Pathology 79: 189

Branski D, Neale J M, Brooks L J 1979 Hirschsprung's disease and Waardenburg's syndrome. Pediatrics 63: 803

Carter C O, Evans K, Hickman V 1981 Children of those treated surgically for Hirschsprung's disease. Journal of Medical Genetics 18: 87

Dalla Valle A 1924 Contributo alle conoscenza della forma famigliare del megacolon congenito. Pediatria 32: 569

Ehrenpreis T 1970 Hirschsprung's disease. Year Book Medical Publishers, Inc., Chicago

Goldberg R B, Shprintzen R J 1981 Hirschsprung megacolon and cleft palate in two sibs. Journal of Craniofacial Genetics and Developmental Biology 1: 185

Hassinger D D, Mulvihill J J, Chandler J B 1980 Aarskog's syndrome with Hirschsprung's disease, midgut malrotation, and dental anomalies. Journal of Medical Genetics 17: 235

Hirschsprung H 1887 Stuhlträgheit Neugeborener infolge von Dilatation und Hypertrophie des Colons. Jahrbuch Kinderheilkunde 27: 1

Hüther W 1954 Die Hirschsprung'sche Krankheit als Folge einer Entwicklungsstörung der intramuralen Ganglien. Beiträge zur pathologischen Anatomie und zur allgemeinen Pathologie 114: 161

Lane P W 1966 Association of megacolon with two recessive spotting genes in mouse. Journal of Heredity 57: 29

Laurence K M, Prosser R, Rocker I, Pearson J F, Richards C 1975 Hirschsprung's disease associated with congenital heart malformation, broad big toes, and ulnar polydactyly in sibs: a case for fetoscopy. Journal of Medical Genetics 12: 334

Lawrence A G, van Wormer D E 1961 Intussusception due to segmental aganglionosis. Journal of American Medical Association 175: 909

Mackinnon A E, Cohen S J 1977 Total intestinal aganglionosis. An autosomal recessive condition? Archives of Diseases in Childhood 52: 898

Madsen C M 1964 Hirschsprung's disease. Munksgaard, Copenhagen

Martin C E, Leonidas F C, Amoury R A 1976 Multiple gastrointestinal atresias, with intraluminal calcifications and cystic dilatation of bile ducts: A newly recognized entity resembling "a string of pearls". Pediatrics 57: 268

Okamoto E, Ueda T 1967 Embryogenesis of intramural ganglion of the gut and its relation to Hirschsprung's disease. Journal of Pediatric Surgery 2: 437

Omenn G S, McKusick V A 1979 The association of Waardenburg syndrome and Hirschsprung megacolon. American Journal of Genetics 3: 217

Passarge E 1967a The genetics of Hirschsprung's disease. Evidence for heterogeneous etiology and a study of sixty-three families. New England Journal of Medicine 276: 138

Passarge E 1967b Quelques considérations étiologiques et génétiques sur la maladie de Hirschsprung. Médecine et Hygiène 25: 240

Passarge E 1972 Genetic heterogeneity and recurrence risk of congenital intestinal aganglionosis. Birth Defects, Original Article Series (G.I Tract.) Vol. VIII, No 2: 63

Passarge E 1973 Genetics of Hirschsprung's disease. Clinics in Gastroenterology 2: 507

Pinsky L 1978 The syndromology of anorectal malformation (atresia, stenosis, ectopia). American Journal of Medical Genetics 1: 461

Puri P, Nixon H H 1977 Long-term results of Swenson's operation for Hirschsprung's disease. Progress in Pediatric Surgery 10: 87

Swenson O, Bill A H 1948 Resection of rectum and rectosigmoid with preservation of the sphincter for benign spastic lesions producing megacolon. Surgery 24: 212

Talwalker V C 1976 Aganglionosis of the entire bowel. Journal of Pediatric Surgery 2: 213

Tittel K 1901 Über eine angeborene Mißbildung des Dickdarms. Wiener Klinische Wochenschrift 14: 903

Warkany J 1971 Congenital malformations. Notes and comments. Year Book Medical Publishers, Chicago

Weinberg A G 1974 Hirschsprung's disease – A pathologist's view. In "Perspectives in pediatric pathology" II. Year Book Medical Publishers, Chicago, p 207

Yntema C C, Hammond W S 1954 Origin of intrinsic ganglia of trunk viscera from vagal neural crest in chick embryo. Journal of Comparative Neurology 101: 515

Zuelzer W W, Wilson J L 1948 Functional intestinal obstruction of congenital neurogenic basis in infancy. American Journal of Diseases in Childhood. 75: 40

63

The polyposes

A. M. O. Veale

Polypoid conditions of the gastrointestinal tract, particularly the colon and rectum, form an interesting group of diseases with familial polyposis coli, Peutz-Jeghers syndrome and Gardner syndrome showing simple Mendelian dominant inheritance. Other conditions appear to show familial aggregation of affected cases with the formal genetics remaining obscure. Of particular interest is the fact that adenomas of the colon and rectum in polyposis coli and Gardner syndrome are indistinguishable from isolated adenomas arising in the general population, and from those seen in association with cancer of the large bowel.

Just as the detailed study of inborn errors of metabolism yields a greater understanding of normal metabolic pathways, it may be that the polyposes contain clues concerning the pathogenesis of colorectal cancer. Collectively, the polyposes are not a common group of disorders when seen from the perspective of a general physician. To a geneticist, though, they are far from infrequent, and their study, apart from the intrinsic interest and its importance to the family members, may yield a greater understanding of carcinogenesis notwithstanding the considerable evidence implicating environmental factors in the causative chain. Genetic and environmental causes are not mutually exclusive, and individual differences in cancer susceptibility are now being increasingly recognised (Harris et al, 1980).

In this chapter we describe non-premalignant polyps, premalignant polyps and finally what evidence there is to suggest that genetic factors may play a role in the appearance of colorectal cancer.

A medical dictionary defines a polyp as: 'A morbid excrescence or protruding growth from a mucous membrane'. In considering polypoid conditions of the gastrointestinal tract, it is helpful to bear this definition in mind as it does not carry any implications with respect to the malignant potential that any given polyp may or may not have. This serves to remind us that in the investigation of a polyp the histology of the lesion is an essential piece of information required to arrive at a correct diagnosis.

Geneticists naturally tend to classify a group of diseases sharing some common feature (in this case, polyps) into those recognisable syndromes which are apparently not inherited, and those which are. There usually remains an indistinct group in which the inherited nature of its members is debatable. An alternative classification of polypoid lesions of the colon and rectum could be based on the malignant potential of the polyp based on histological criteria, followed by consideration of a further genetic subdivision.

Non-malignant or non-premalignant conditions would thus include:

1. Isolated hamartomas of childhood
2. Hyperplastic polyps
3. Juvenile polyposis
4. Peutz-Jeghers syndrome
5. Other benign forms of polyposis

Premalignant polypoid conditions are as follows:

1. Isolated adenomas of the rectum and/or colon
2. Multiple adenomas of the colon and rectum with or without associated lesions elsewhere
3. Other forms of multiple polyps which are not adenomas.

In this classification the term 'adenoma' is used in a generic sense as a grouped term to include neoplastic polyps in general such as an adenoma itself or tubular adenoma, the tubular-villous or papillary adenoma and the villous adenoma or villous papilloma.

NON-PREMALIGNANT POLYPS

Isolated hamartomas of childhood

These lesions are also known as juvenile, cystic or retention polyps, and are prone to torsion of their long pedicle and subsequent auto-amputation. The histological appearances are typical, with large amounts of loose connective tissue and cystic spaces containing mucus. Occasionally, a polyp of this kind may be found in association with multiple adenomas, but this is rare.

Hyperplastic polyps

These lesions are frequently seen on sigmoidoscopy and

colonoscopy, but are not regarded as having any malignant potential. They present as small raised areas a few millimetres across which macroscopically are indistinguishable from the early appearance of an adenoma with which they are often found in association. The microscopic appearances, however, are quite different with lengthening of the tubules which are dilated with mucus leading to flattening of the epithelial cells. There is also a diminution in the number of goblet cells. The potential of these lesions, also known as metaplastic polyps, is not known but they are at present regarded as benign even though they may be found in association with adenomas or carcinoma.

Juvenile polyposis

This condition, described by McColl et al (1964) and later by Veale et al (1966), is characterised by lesions more closely resembling the isolated hamartomas of childhood than those of an adenoma. The histological appearances show less connective tissue than commonly seen in the isolated lesions, with more irregularity of branching of the glands.

Sachatello (1972) divided the condition into 3 subgroups, the first corresponding to the isolated lesions described above, the second with multiple lesions confined to the large bowel, and a third with polypoid lesions throughout the gastrointestinal tract. Bussey et al (1978), however, emphasise the rarity of multiple juvenile polyposis, and attempt no subdivision of cases, apart from those with and without a history of other affected relatives. It is note-worthy that in their series of just over 50 cases in 36 families, three quarters of the families were of 'isolated' cases, and one quarter had from 2 to 5 affected family members. Other congenital anomalies such as congenital heart defects, malrotation of the gut, Meckel's diverticulum and hydrocephalus were found in nearly 20% of cases. At first it was thought that these abnormalities were confined to cases with no family history (Bussey, 1970), but this is no longer the case and the apparent distinction is blurred.

Even though the histological appearances in juvenile polyposis coli are not suggestive of any malignant potential, and the disease is in the meantime grouped with other non-malignant and non-premalignant conditions, there does seem to be some relationship with familial polyposis coli. In the first instance, although the majority of the lesions in juvenile polyposis coli show the typical histological appearances of the isolated cystic or retention polyp seen in childhood, a proportion show areas of epithelial atypia similar to that seen in adenomas. Secondly, in some families with juvenile polyposis coli there are relatives affected with multiple adenomatous polyposis and/or colonic or rectal carcinoma (Veale et al, 1966; Smilow et al, 1966; Bussey et al, 1978). In a family where a parent had adenomatous polyposis and two offspring had juvenile polyposis it was suggested by Veale et al (1966) that this variation between parent and offspring could be due to an allelic gene received from the unaffected parent and interacting with the gene for adenomatous polyposis received from the affected parent. This was purely speculative and families described since have given little support to the notion. The exact relationship between adenomatous and juvenile polyposis probably requires much more extensive data covering several generations in order to elucidate the problem. In the meantime, it seems logical to continue to include juvenile polyposis in the 'non-malignant' category. One should also remember that the term 'juvenile' does not necessarily mean that the condition is found only in children. The term refers more to the primitive nature of the connective tissue in the polyp rather than to the age of the patient.

Peutz-Jeghers syndrome

First described by Peutz (1921) and then by Jeghers et al (1949) the genetics of this condition is clear cut. Inherited as a Mendelian dominant, the characteristic findings are polyps of the gastrointestinal tract, and spots of skin pigmentation. The polyps may be present throughout the entire gastrointestinal tract, but in over 90% of cases the small bowel is involved, and in about one third of cases the colon and rectum as well (Louw, 1972). The skin pigmentation is shown as patches of melanin a few millimetres in diameter on the lips, oral mucosa and the hands and feet.

At first, it was thought that the polyps had considerable malignant potential, but Bartholomew and Dahlin (1958) and Bartholomew et al (1957) suggested that they were in fact local tissue malformations (hamartomas), and had little or no potential for undergoing malignant change. Bailey (1957) collected 67 cases from the literature and tabulated the distribution of the tumours together with details of their histology. In thirteen cases there was an adenocarcinoma of the small intestine, and in three cases a carcinoma of the large bowel. This emphasises an important difference between Peutz-Jeghers syndrome and familial polyposis coli (adenomatosis) where the risk of malignancy is high. The probability of malignant degeneration in Peutz-Jeghers syndrome has continued to be argued and it may be that the cases where malignancy does occur are the result of the concomitant occurrence of adenomas. Bussey (1975) reports knowledge of eighteen cases of definite cancer in patients with Peutz-Jeghers polyposis. Most of these cases occurred in the stomach and duodenum. Morson (1962) believes the risk of malignancy in Peutz-Jeghers polyps is low. The histological appearances of a Peutz-Jeghers polyp are in marked contrast to those seen in an adenoma. A tree-like proliferation of the muscularis mucosae is primarily involved in the formation of a Peutz-Jeghers polyp with the epithelium only secondarily involved. Furthermore, the epithelium is substantially normal with the same proportion of individual cells of different types in the same relationship to each other as in uninvolved epithelium. There is no increase in epithelial mitotic activity, or alteration in mucus secreting activity. For all these reasons the Peutz-Jeghers syndrome should be regarded as essentially a non-premalignant condition, especially as some of the few cases of malignancy reported were found to have associated adenomas (Dodds et al, 1972). The principle symptoms of Peutz-Jeghers polyposis are those arising from intussusception and/or intestinal obstruction.

Lipomatosis
Swain et al (1969) reported a condition resembling a generalised colorectal polyposis where there were deposits of fat in the submucosa. So far this condition has only been observed in children. Ordinary lipomas may also occur in the gastrointestinal tract, and are usually not multiple. Ling et al (1959) reported a case with multiple lipomas throughout the alimentary tract.

Cystic pneumatosis
Macroscopically this condition can be confused with adenomatosis because multiple gas filled cysts project into the lumen of the large bowel. The cause is unknown.

Inflammatory polyps
Any condition of the large bowel leading to patchy destruction of the mucosa may result in the formation of irregular tags of tissue projecting into the lumen, e.g. bacillary and amoebic dysentery, hyperplastic tuberculosis, bilharzia infection and ulcerative colitis. The latter carries a small risk of malignancy (1–2%), but it is probably the underlying cause of the ulcerative colitis rather than the mucosal tags themselves which leads to this.

Benign lymphoid polyposis
This condition arises as a result of non-neoplastic hypertrophy of lymphoid tissue normally present in the gastrointestinal tract. It must be distinguished from the conditions described by Cornes (1960; 1961) where the polyposis is secondary to some other pathological process. Benign lymphoid polyps are more frequently seen in children or young adults. Louw (1968) has described the condition appearing in three sibs.

PREMALIGNANT POLYPS

Isolated adenomas of the colon and rectum
The occurrence of single adenomas in the colon and rectum in adult patients over the age of 40 is commonplace, and not infrequently the number may be more than one.

Andren and Frieberg (1959) surveyed 3609 patients and found the incidence of adenomas increased steadily with age from 5% at 20 to nearly 15% at 70. Rider et al (1959) studied 9669 patients and found polyps in 537 (5.6%), a lower incidence than in other surveys. A most significant finding, however, was the re-examination of 372 of these patients with adenomas during a four to nine year follow up period. It was found that 41% of these patients had developed additional polyps. The authors concluded that new polyps were being formed faster in this group of patients than in the general population, and that they represented a group that were 'polyp prone'.

Woolf et al (1955) have described a large family in which isolated adenomas (1–4) occurred in nearly 50% of the adult members. They felt that there was good evidence in this family to suggest that the appearance of isolated adenomas may have been due to the segregation of a single gene predisposing to adenoma formation. Lynch et al (1979) have described two families in which there occurs the simultaneous appearance of patients with familial polyposis coli and others showing only isolated adenomas.

Bussey (1975) described the frequency of adenomas in a series of 1788 patients thought not to have familial intestinal polyposis. The vast majority had only a single lesion and only 15 patients had more than 6. Very rarely patients with 60 or 70 adenomas have been reported, but have not been thought to have familial polyposis coli, although any patient with more than 100 adenomas almost certainly has this condition. A possible genetic explanation for the occurrence of isolated adenomas will be discussed later. (See: 'A genetic model').

Familial polyposis coli
This condition was probably first described in the eighteenth century and several times in the nineteenth. Lockhart-Mummery (1925) first drew attention to the relationship between polyposis and cancer, and other reviews have been provided by Dukes (1952), Reed and Neel (1955), Veale (1965), Pierce (1968) and Bussey (1975). Multiple adenomas (>100) of the colon and rectum occurring in childhood or young adults is pathognomonic, although it must be remembered that the appearance of polyps may be delayed until middle or later life.

The average age at which patients with symptoms are first diagnosed is 35 years, and approximately 10% of such cases are not diagnosed until older than 50. Naturally, once an index case has been identified the investigation of relatives will yield positive cases who may be quite young. Polyposis affects both sexes equally and is inherited as an autosomal dominant trait. The risk of one or more of the adenomas undergoing malignant degeneration is virtually 100%. The condition should be treated surgically by total colectomy or sub-total colectomy with an ileorectal anastomosis and subsequent examination of the rectal stump at frequent intervals.

Until comparatively recently it was thought that the adenomatous lesions were confined to the colon and rectum, and that the occasional cases of polyposis of the entire gastrointestinal tract perhaps represented a distinct genetic entity (Yanemoto et al, 1969). Hoffman and Goligher (1971) reviewed the matter, and Ross and Mara (1974) reported two additional cases, one with adenocarcinoma of the jejunum with an associated adenoma 0.8 cms in diameter, and the other with adenocarcinoma of the ileum with a 25 cm length of the resected ileum showing multiple adenomatous polyps. It seems that the gastrointestinal lesions in familial polyposis coli are *not* confined to the colon and rectum, and that one should be alert to the possibility of adenomas in the small bowel as well. Even though this may not be a frequent complication, it should be borne in mind particularly in those patients who have had a successful surgical treatment of the large bowel for a number of years.

The Gardner syndrome (see below) characteristically shows a number of associated lesions, but quite apart from this, patients with familial polyposis coli sometimes show other manifestations of neoplastic activity. In his series of polyposis families Veale (1965) reported 11 unrelated cases of polyposis, all with affected relatives, all from different kindreds, none of which was thought to be affected with Gardner syndrome. The associated lesions found were fibroma of uterus, carcinoma of the uterus, sebaceous cyst and frontal bone osteomas, abdominal wall desmoid and frontal osteomas, mesenteric lymphangioma, thyroid adenoma and two abdominal desmoids, multiple lipomas, hepatoma, medulloblastoma, keloid in abdominal scar, and an abdominal desmoid. In addition to these cases, there were five isolated cases of polyposis (no affected relatives) showing similar lesions, and another isolated case with chronic lymphocytic leukaemia. There seems to be little doubt that patients with polyposis have some kind of predisposition to other forms of neoplastic activity, particularly the formation of desmoid tumours in the abdominal wall following surgery (McAdam & Goligher, 1970).

Gardner syndrome

The characteristic tetrad of gastrointestinal adenomas, fibromas, osteomas and epidermal cysts described by Gardner (1953) is much less frequent than the classical form of familial polyposis coli. In all respects, apart from the extra-colonic lesions, the two diseases are similar. In view of the fact that some patients with classical polyposis occasionally show some of the features of Gardner syndrome, and that in some kindreds assumed to have Gardner syndrome not all affected members show all the characteristic extra-colonic features, or when shown they

are not necessarily affected to the same degree, it is not surprising to find that there is some debate with respect to whether the two genes are distinct (Smith, 1968). Evidence in favour of Gardner syndrome being a separate disorder from familial polyposis coli is afforded by several large pedigrees with all affected members showing the characteristic lesions.

Utsunomiya and Nakamura (1975), however, were able to demonstrate occult osteomatous changes in the mandible not only in cases of Gardner syndrome, but also in the majority (19 out of 21 cases) of patients with polyposis coli. The authors now regard routine panoramic X-rays of the jaws as an essential part of their work-up of any polyposis family. They have been able to correctly predict the presence of colonic adenomatosis following such X-ray examination. As a result they have concluded that Gardner syndrome and classical familial polyposis coli should not be regarded as different aetiological categories, and that their findings are a further indication that familial polyposis coli can manifest other forms of neoplastic activity apart from that in the colon and rectum.

Cronkite-Canada syndrome

This is another form of polyposis of the colon and rectum with associated lesions. Originally described by Cronkite and Canada (1955) the characteristic lesions associated with general gastrointestinal polyposis were diffuse areas of skin pigmentation, alopecia and onychotrophia. All the cases described so far have been sporadic so it is difficult to know how to fit this syndrome in with the others. The condition is accompanied by intestinal malabsorption with disturbances of the plasma proteins and electrolytes. The prognosis is poor and a genetic causation remains to be proved.

Turcot syndrome

Turcot et al (1959) reported polyposis coli in association with malignant tumours of the central nervous system. Two sibs died at the ages of 17 and 21 from medulloblastoma and glioblastoma respectively. Previous polyposis had been diagnosed and treated surgically when the patients were aged 15 and 16. Two reports of isolated cases are cited by Bussey (1975) who also mentions another member of a polyposis family from the St Mark's Hospital series who died from a medulloblastoma. This patient was 'at risk' for developing polyposis, but at the time of death was not known to have been affected. This case from St Mark's is in addition to the one mentioned earlier (under 'familial polyposis coli') where the patient was known to have had polyposis. It has been suggested that Turcot syndrome may be an autosomal recessive trait if it does indeed represent a condition distinct from polyposis coli.

Other rare syndromes

Cornes (1960 and 1961) described cases with primary malignant lymphomas and carcinomas of the intestinal tract. These patients were found to have adenomas of the colon as well as malignant lymphomas, again demonstrating another facet in the relationship between adenoma formation and other neoplastic activity.

Von Recklinghausen disease (multiple neurofibromatosis) may occasionally produce multiple neurofibromas of the colon and rectum (Ghrist, 1963) and one case of polyposis coli has been found subsequently to have had neurofibromatosis (Bussey, 1975). A mixture of colonic neurofibromas and juvenile polyps has also been reported (Donnelly et al, 1969).

BOWEL CANCER IN THE POPULATION

The importance of adenomas as a predisposing factor to colorectal cancer in polyposis coli and Gardner syndrome is undisputed. Similarly, the occurrence of small adenomas (1–4) in the colon or rectum of a person not a member of a polyposis family is regarded as not without significance with respect to the development of a subsequent carcinoma. Adenomas are correctly regarded as premalignant lesions, even though the risk may be small. It should also be noted that so far there is nothing histologically which serves to distinguish an adenoma in a polyposis patient from an isolated adenoma arising spontaneously, independent of polyposis. Naturally, there has been speculation about whether or not there is a tendency towards familial aggregation in cases of colorectal cancer. We have already seen that Woolf et al (1955) suggested that in at least one family there was a tendency for isolated adenomas to appear as if determined by a single gene similar to the polyposis gene, but with a less powerful action.

Similarly, Lynch et al (1966, 1967 and 1973) have presented reports of families in which many members were affected with colorectal cancer, sometimes occurring in conjunction with cancer of the breast and endometrium. This has given rise to the notion of families which are 'cancer prone'. More generally, Macklin (1960) and Lovett (1976) have looked at the incidence of cancer in the relatives of unselected index cases with colorectal cancer and found that the incidence of colorectal cancer, particularly in first degree relatives, is much increased. Apart from the obvious 'cancer prone' families, polyposis coli and Gardner syndrome, the increased incidence of colorectal cancer in the relatives of index cases has hitherto been ascribed as probably due to environmental factors for which there is quite impressive evidence.

Numerous studies have reported that the incidence of colon cancer shows a striking positive correlation with dietary factors such as meat and fat intake, and a negative correlation with dietary fibre intake. Vitamin A and alcohol intake also seem to be involved. There are striking international differences in colorectal cancer indicating that it is probably a disease of 'life style', the incidence being highest in Western European-like countries. Native born Japanese have a very low incidence of large bowel cancer, but on migration to Hawaii or the USA the incidence soon approaches that of the host population, although there is some protection afforded if the immigrants seek to retain their national dietary habits. Similarly, McMichael (1980) has shown that European migrants from Italy, Yugoslavia and Greece have an increasing incidence of colorectal cancer depending on their length of stay in Australia. Seventh Day Adventists, who observe a strict dietary code, have also been much studied in the USA where it is found that their incidence of colorectal cancer is much lower than that of their non Seventh Day Adventist compatriots.

Considerable attention has been focussed on the role of intestinal bacteria in the causation of bowel cancer, particularly the ratio of anaerobes to aerobes in the faecal flora of individuals from groups with marked differences in colorectal cancer incidence. Similarly, concentrations of acid and neutral steroids in the faeces have also differed in patients on high and low protein diets. In this connection Watne and Core (1975) have reported differences in the faecal steroids found in polyposis patients from those in the general population. More importantly, Wilkins and Hackman (1974) have reported that normal patients are divisible into two distinct classes based upon the analysis of neutral sterols in faeces, which may be a reflection of an underlying genetic heterogeneity. Much animal experimental work has been done on the induction of colorectal cancer, and Hill (1975) has suggested that in humans the role of cocarcinogen and carcinogen is fulfilled by unsaturated and saturated bile acids interacting with colonic anaerobic bacteria. There is considerable evidence to invoke environmental factors in the causation of bowel cancer, but there are still areas of controversy such as disputes over the role (if any) of dietary cholesterol. Furthermore, the Mormons of Utah represent a group with a very high protein and meat intake, and yet have a low incidence of colorectal cancer (Enstrom, 1975). Dietary factors seem to have an 'immediate' effect in that immigrants assume the host population's incidence at a rate proportional to their exposure time but, surprisingly, there is no correlation in the host population between the incidence of colorectal cancer in spouses (Jensen et al, 1980).

A colorectal cancer hypothesis

Quite apart from the study of colorectal cancer itself, the epidemiology of adenoma formation in populations is informative. Hill (1978) reported the size of adenomas in different populations (high and low incidences of colorectal cancer), together with the frequency with which malignancy was found in adenomas of different sizes. Small adenomas (<1 cm) were relatively much more frequent in Japan than in England, but the percentage of large adenomas showing malignant changes was the same (approximately 50%) in each group. The distribution of small adenomas is fairly uniform throughout the large bowel, but the distribution of large adenomas is similar to that of carcinoma, showing an increased frequency as the site considered passes more distally. Hill et al (1978) interpreted these findings as indicating that the factors predisposing to small adenoma formation are different from those which conspire to induce small adenomas to become large. They propose that adenomas will only arise in persons of an appropriate genotype, and that an environmental factor (A) will induce the formation of small adenomas uniformly throughout the large bowel. Environmental factor (B) will cause small adenomas to become large, but with an effect showing an increasing gradient as we pass from proximal to distal. Finally, agent (C) induces malignancy in a high proportion of large adenomas, a small proportion of small adenomas and, rarely, in normal mucosa.

Hill et al then comment on the nature of the three factors postulated. They suggest that (A) must be ingested preformed and be of uniform concentration throughout the large bowel.

Factor (B) is probably a bacterial metabolite of the bile acids (already implicated in the causation of colorectal cancer) or something else related to dietary intake of fat or meat.

Factor (C) remains unknown.

A genetic model

Of particular interest to the writer is the genetic component of the model proposed by Hill et al (1978). The predisposing genotype is designated pp where p is an allele of the polyposis coli gene P first postulated by Veale (1965). The hypothesis was proposed to explain the absence of parent/child correlations in polyposis families in connection with various age related parameters, such as appearance of polyps, onset of malignancy, and age at death from cancer. Sib/sib correlations were statistically consistent with a value of $+0.5$, whereas parent/child values approached zero. There was also a suggestion of bimodality in the age distributions so that two polyposis genotypes were postulated: Pp with earlier onset and $P+$ with later onset, each distribution showing considerable overlap with the other. This theory is sufficient to explain the zero parent/child correlations and the values of $+0.5$ for sibs. It was further suggested that non-polyposis patients of genotype pp of frequency 9% in the general population represented those persons predisposed to adenoma formation.

Formal consequences of this are:

1. There should be an increased incidence of colorectal cancer among index cases with the condition. This is now well documented (Lovett, 1976).
2. There would be 'polyp prone' individuals in the population (Woolf et al, 1955, Rider et al, 1959, Brahme et al, 1974).
3. We would expect that families would occur from time to time in which there was a predominance of pp individuals. Such families would show a high incidence of colorectal cancer, and have been reported (Warthin, 1925; Macklin, 1960; Lynch & Krush, 1967; Lynch et al, 1973).
4. If there were a large bowel 'cancer proneness' bestowed upon an individual by virtue of his genotype it might be that this could manifest itself in other organs. Such an association in colon cancer families has been reported by Lynch et al (1966) and Lynch and Krush (1973) with respect to an increased frequency of endometrial cancer, breast cancer and multiple primary malignancies.
5. If 'cancer proneness' had a genetic basis there might be some manifestation of this in a tissue culture system.

Estimation of genetic parameters

If we assume the gene frequency of the p gene is u and $v = 1-u$, then the frequency of the pp genotype will be u^2. Given that the probability of developing cancer when of genotype pp is x, the frequency of cancer patients = u^2x which, for colorectal cancer, is approximately 0.03 in England and Wales. Among the parents of index cases with colorectal cancer the frequency of persons with genotype pp and cancer will be ux. An estimate of this quantity can be obtained from data based on that of Lovett (1976), but with 2 families now known to have polyposis coli omitted. The series now consists of 207 sets of parents nearly all of whom are dead, and for which there is reliable hospital and/or death certificate information concerning their bowel cancer status. A total of 36 out of 414 parents are known to have had colorectal cancer giving a value of $ux = 0.087$. Solving these two equations gives values for u and x of 0.34 and 0.25 respectively.

It is also possible to use sib data to obtain other equations involving u and x, but here the matter is complicated because of the nonexistence of a suitable body of data. Lovett's (1976) amended series of index cases includes 672 sibs of whom only 166 are at present dead. Among 104 of these who died in the period 1930-1970 there were 18 who died of colorectal cancer (17.31%) which is over 5 times the number of deaths expected. In view of the large number of sibs still alive, no formal segregation analysis is at present possible. Such an analysis is further complicated by the fact that the risk to sibs will vary between families due to the fact that the probabilities for parental genotypes will also vary with the incidence of cancer found among relatives. For example, the risk to a sib given no other family history of bowel cancer other than the index case is $(u+\frac{1}{2}v)^2x$, whereas if one parent is known to have had cancer the risk is $(u+\frac{1}{2}v)x$. More complicated expressions arise when there are other affected relatives such as uncles and aunts or additional affected sibs.

Additional complications in segregation analysis are introduced by the inherent biases in ascertaining families (truncate selection). In the meantime it would appear that in order to investigate familial aggregation of cancer, the families of index cases should be followed with the same persistence as that bestowed on undoubted genetic conditions such as polyposis coli. Notwithstanding the importance of environmental influences as demonstrated by the studies on immigrants, the lack of correlation in incidence between spouses seems to indicate that such factors might require the appropriate genetic predisposition to be effective.

Polyps, cancer and ABO blood groups

The possibility that familial aggregations of large bowel cancer might be the result of a combination of environmental factors and of relatives tending to share some common genetic factor such as a blood group, has been suggested. McConnell (1966) cites 11 investigations into an association between the ABO blood groups and colorectal cancer, and concludes that the overall impression is that the ABO blood groups do not seem to be involved. Fleming et al (1967) investigated the association with polyps of the colon or rectum (373 patients) and found a significant excess of blood group O (p <0.001) in patients with papillary adenomas. These represented 21 patients, of whom 16 were group O. The distribution of blood groups in patients with tubular adenomas did not differ from controls. Vogel and Krüger (1968) concluded, from their survey of the literature, that blood group A was over represented in colorectal cancer patients, but that this was weaker than the well known association with stomach cancer. More recent studies by

Bjelke (1973) reporting no consistent differences, are cited by Correa and Haenszel (1978).

Tissue culture systems

There has been considerable work done on the changes found in metabolic pathways within the cells which constitute the normal colonic and rectal mucosa. During differentiation of the cell types, various nucleic acid activities appear to be induced and others are repressed. Additional chemical changes are observed in tissue culture from cells derived from tubular and villous adenomas, but so far nothing has served to differentiate an adenoma from a polyposis coli or Gardner syndrome patient, and an isolated adenoma found in a non-polyposis patient. Danes (1975, 1976, 1979) has detected a major cytogenetic change in cultures of epithelial cells taken by skin biopsy in patients with Gardner syndrome. Such cultures have shown a greatly increased incidence of tetraploidy (30–40%) over the 2–3% found in normals. Similar findings were found in cell lines derived from colonic and rectal mucosa.

At first, the finding was thought to be confined to Gardner syndrome only and not polyposis coli. It appears, however, that some polyposis coli patients do show increased tetraploidy although Delhanty et al (1980) found the frequency similar in both polyposis coli and controls. Danes (1980) presented data showing results in controls, polyposis coli and Gardner syndrome. There does not seem to be any doubt that tetraploidy is much increased in Gardner syndrome, and only marginally so in polyposis coli. Of particular interest is the result in the controls where 7 out of 97 (7.2%) gave positive results. The importance of this type of approach is that not only might some in vitro manifestation of a major gene be apparent, but, more importantly, it may point the way to the early recognition of a 'cancer prone' genotype in the normal population. The subsequent genetic investigation of families, particularly those already recognised as having an increased risk, would enable a precise genetic analysis of a kind not at present possible.

REFERENCES

Andren L, Frieberg S 1959 Frequency of polyps of rectum and colon, according to age, and relation to cancer. Gastroenterology 36: 631
Bailey D 1957 Polyposis of the gastrointestinal tract: the Peutz Syndrome. British Medical Journal 2: 433
Bartholomew L G, Dahlin D C 1958 Intestinal polyposis and mucocutaneous pigmentation (Peutz-Jeghers syndrome). Minnesota Medicine 41: 848
Bartholomew L G, Dahlin D C, Waugh J M 1957 Intestinal pigmentation associated with mucocutaneous melanin

pigmentation (Peutz-Jeghers syndrome). Gastroenterology 32: 434
Bjelke E 1973 Epidemiological studies of cancer of the stomach, colon, and rectum: With special emphasis on the role of diet. 1-5, University Microfilms, Ann Arbor, Michigan. Cited by Correa P, Haenszel W. In: Klein G, Weinhouse S (eds) 1978 Advances in cancer research 26, Academic Press, New York, San Francisco, London.
Brahme F, Ekelund G R, Norden J G, Wenckert A 1974 Metachronous colorectal polyps: Comparison of

development of colorectal polyps and carcinomas in persons with and without histories of polyps. Diseases of the Colon and Rectum 17: 166 –171.

Bussey H J R 1970 Gastrointestinal polyposis. Gut 11: 970–978.

Bussey H J R 1975 Familial polyposis coli. The Johns Hopkins University Press, Baltimore, London.

Bussey H J R, Veale A M O, Morson B C 1978 Genetics of gastrointestinal polyposis. Gastroenterology 74: 1325–1330.

Cornes J S 1960 Multiple primary cancers: Primary malignant lymphomas and carcinomas of the intestinal tract in the same patient. Journal of Clinical Pathology 13: 483.

Cornes J S 1961 Multiple lymphomatous polyposis of the gastrointestinal tract. Cancer 14: 249

Correa P, Haenszel W 1978 The epidemiology of large bowel cancer. In: Klein G, Weinhouse S (eds) Advances in cancer research, Vol. 26, Academic Press, New York, San Francisco, London

Cronkite L W Jr, Canada W J 1955 Generalized intestinal polyposis: An unusual syndrome of polyposis, pigmentation, alopecia and onychotrophia. New England Journal of Medicine 252: 1011–1015

Danes B S 1975 The Gardner Syndrome: A study in cell culture. Cancer 36: 2337 (Supplement)

Danes B S 1976 Increased tetraploidy in cultured skin fibroblasts. Journal of Medical Genetics 13: 52

Danes B S 1979 In vitro evidence for adenoma-carcinoma sequence in large bowel. Lancet 2: 44–45

Danes B S 1980 In vitro tetraploidy in familial polyposis coli. Lancet 2: 200–201

Delhanty J D A, Pritchard M B, Bussey H J R, Morson B C 1980 Tetraploid fibroblasts and familial polyposis coli. Lancet 1: 1365

Dodds W J, Schulte W J, Hensley G T, Hogan W J 1972 Peutz-Jeghers syndrome and gastrointestinal malignancy. American Journal of Roentgenology 115: 374–377

Donnelly W H, Sieber W K, Yunis E J 1969 Polypoid ganglio-neurofibromatosis of the large bowel. Archives of Pathology 87: 537–541

Dukes C E 1952 Familial intestinal polyposis. Annals of Eugenics 17: 1

Enstrom J E 1975 Cancer mortality among Mormons. Cancer 36: 825 –841

Fleming T C, Caplan H W, Hyman G A, Kitchin F D 1967 ABO blood groups and polyps of the colon. British Medical Journal 2: 526–527

Gardner E J, Richards R C 1953 Multiple cutaneous and subcutaneous lesions occurring simultaneously with hereditary polyposis and osteomatosis. American Journal of Human Genetics 5: 139

Ghrist T D 1963 Gastrointestinal involvement in neurofibromatosis. Archives of Internal Medicine 112: 357–362

Harris C C, Mulvihill J J, Thorgierrson S S, Minna J D 1980 Individual differences in cancer susceptibility. Annals of Internal Medicine 92: 809–825

Hill M J 1975 The role of colon anaerobes in the metabolism of bile acids and steroids, and its relation to colon cancer. Cancer 36: 2387–2400

Hill M J 1978 Etiology of the adenoma-carcinoma sequence. In: Bennington J L (ed) The pathogenesis of colorectal cancer, W B Sanders Company, Philadelphia, London, Toronto. Ch 12, p 153–162

Hill M J, Morson B C, Bussey H J R 1978 Aetiology of adenoma-carcinoma sequence in large bowel. Lancet 1: 245–247

Hoffman D C, Goligher J C 1971 Polyposis of the stomach and small intestine in association with familial polyposis coli. British Journal of Surgery 58: 126–128

Jeghers H, McKusick V A, Katz K H 1949 Generalised intestinal polyposis and melanin spots of the oral mucosa, lips and digits. New England Journal of Medicine 241: 993–1005, 1031 –1036

Jensen O M, Bolander A M, Sigtryggsson P, Vercelli M, Nguyen-Dinh X, MacLennan R 1980 Large bowel cancer in married couples in Sweden. Lancet 1: 1161–1163

Ling C S, Leagus C, Stahlgren L H 1959 Intestinal lipomatosis. Surgery 46: 1054–1059

Lockhart-Mummery J P 1925 Cancer and heredity. Lancet 1: 427

Louw J H 1968 Polypoid lesions of the large bowel in children with particular reference to benign lymphoid polyposis. Pediatric Surgery 3: 195–209

Louw J H 1972 Polypoid lesions of the large bowel in children. South African Medical Journal 46: 1347–1352

Lovett E 1976 Family studies in cancer of the colon and rectum. British Journal of Surgery 63: 13–18

Lynch H T, Guirgis H, Swartz M, Lynch J, Krush A J, Kaplan A R 1973 Genetics and colon cancer. Archives of Surgery 106: 669–675

Lynch H T, Krush A J 1967 Heredity and adenocarcinoma of the colon. Gastroenterology 53: 517–527

Lynch H T, Krush A J 1973 Differential diagnosis of the cancer family syndrome. Surgery 136: 221

Lynch H T, Lynch Patricia M, Follett Karen L, Harris R E 1979 Familial polyposis coli: Heterogeneous polyp expression in two kindreds. Journal of Medical Genetics 16: 1–7

Lynch H T, Shaw M M, Magnuson C W, Larsen A L, Krush A J 1966 Hereditary factors in cancer: Study of two large mid Western kindreds. Archives of Internal Medicine 117: 206–212

McAdam W A F, Goligher J C 1970 The occurrence of desmoids in patients with familial polyposis coli. British Journal of Surgery 57: 618–631

McColl I, Bussey H J R, Veale A M O, Morson B C 1964 Juvenile polyposis coli. Proceedings of the Royal Society of Medicine 57: 896–897

McConnell R B 1966 The genetics of gastro-intestinal disorders. Oxford Monographs on Medical Genetics, Oxford University Press, London

McMichael A 1980 Personal communication

Macklin M T 1960 Inheritance of cancer of the stomach and large intestine in man. Journal of the National Cancer Institute 24: 551–571

Morson B C 1962 Precancerous lesions of upper gastrointestinal tract. Journal of the American Medical Association 179: 311

Peutz J L A 1921 Over een zeer merkwaardige, gecombineerde familiaire polyposis van de slijmoliezen van den tractus intestinalis met die van de neuskeelholte en gepaard met eigenaardge pigmentaties van huid-en slijmoliezen. Maandschrift Geneesk. 10: 134–146

Pierce E R 1968 Some genetic aspects of familial multiple polyposis of the colon in a kindred of 1422 members. Diseases of the Colon and Rectum 11: 321 –329

Reed T E, Neel J V 1955 A genetic study of multiple polyposis of the colon (with an appendix deriving a method of estimating relative fitness). American Journal of Human Genetics 7: 236

Rider J A, Kirsner J B, Moeller H C, Palmer W L 1959 Polyps of colon and rectum: Four year to nine year follow-up study of 537 patients. Journal of American Medical Association 170: 633

Ross Janice E, Mara J E 1974 Small bowel polyps and carcinoma in multiple intestinal polyposis. Archives of Surgery 108: 736–738

Sachatello C R 1972 Polypoid diseases of the gastrointestinal tract. Journal of Kentucky Medical Association 70: 540–544

Smilow P C, Pryor C A Jr, Swinton N W 1966 Juvenile polyposis coli: A report of three patients in three generations of one family. Diseases of the Colon and Rectum 9: 248–254

Smith W G 1968 Familial multiple polyposis: Research tool for investigating the etiology of carcinoma of the colon? Diseases of the Colon and Rectum 11: 17–31

Swain V A J, Young W F, Pringle E M 1969 Hypertrophy of the appendices epiploicae and lipomatous polyposis of the colon. Gut 10: 587–589

Turcot J, Despres J P, St Pierre F 1959 Malignant tumours of the central nervous system associated with familial polyposis of the colon. Diseases of the Colon and Rectum 2: 465–468

Utsunomiya J, Nakamura T 1975 The occult osteomatous changes in the mandible of patients with familial polyposis coli. British Journal of Surgery 62: 45–51

Veale A M O 1965 Intestinal polyposis. Eugenics Laboratory, Memoir Series (40): London

Veale A M O, McColl I, Bussey H J R, Morson B C 1966 Juvenile polyposis coli. Journal of Medical Genetics 3: 5–16

Vogel F, Krüger J 1968 Statistische Beziehungen zwischen den ABO-Bluntgruppen und Krankheiten mit Ausnahme der Infektionskrankheiten. Blut 16: 351–376

Warthin A S 1925 The further study of a cancer family. Journal of Cancer Research 9: 279–286

Watne A L, Core S S 1975 Fecal steroids in polyposis coli and ileorectostomy patients. Journal of Surgical Research 19: 157–161

Wilkins T, Hackman A 1974 Two patterns of neutral steroid conversion in the feces of normal North Americans. Cancer Research 34: 2250 –2254

Woolf C M, Richards R C, Gardner E J 1955 Occasional discrete polyps of the colon and rectum showing an inherited tendency. Cancer 8: 403

Yanemoto R M, Slayback J B, Byron R L Jr, Rosen R B 1969 Familial polyposis of the entire gastrointestinal tract. Archives of Surgery 99: 427–434

Cystic fibrosis

W. M. McCrae

INTRODUCTION

Cystic fibrosis is the most common inherited disease in Caucasian populations and one of the commonest causes of death in childhood. Although described in 1938 (Andersen) and now a very familiar problem to all paediatricians, the essential defect remains unknown and there is even some lingering doubt that it is in fact a single disease entity.

There seems to be abundant evidence that cystic fibrosis is inherited as an autosomal recessive trait. The expected occurrence of 1 in 4 among sibs has been demonstrated in a number of studies (e.g. Danksetal, 1965). It seems likely therefore that all the features of the disease should be attributable to a defect of a single protein. The defect in cystic fibrosis has not yet been identified at the molecular level and this leaves some room for conjecture that more than one mutant allele may be responsible for the disorder recognised as cystic fibrosis. This concept has some attraction for the clinician who is aware of the wide variation in the way in which the disease may present and the differences in the manner and speed with which the condition progresses to the fully developed phenotype. Some unconfirmed laboratory findings have been offered in support of genetic heterogeneity in this disease (Danes & Bearn, 1969). In studying cultured fibroblasts from patients with cystic fibrosis, Danes and Bearn (1969) reported at least two separate types of cell distinguishable by differences in metachromasia. These findings have not been confirmed and there is no substantial evidence to counter the general acceptance that the disease, although varying to some extent in the pattern of expression, is the result of a single mutant gene.

INCIDENCE

For many years standard textbooks have given the incidence of cystic fibrosis for Caucasian populations as approximately 1 in 2500 with an equal sex distribution. This implies a carrier rate of 1 in 20 to 25 and thus approximately 1 in 400 to 600 marriages would be 'at risk' of producing an affected child.

In part these estimates were based on autopsy records. Between 2 and 4% of autopsies in children's hospitals are performed on patients with cystic fibrosis. For the most part however, the estimates were computed from the number of cases which made themselves clinically manifest and were satisfactorily diagnosed.

It is now clear that these estimates are too low. In studies in which populations of newborns are universally screened for cystic fibrosis the incidence has been found to be at least 1 in 1800 (Stephan et al, 1975). It has been claimed in other Caucasian populations that the incidence may be even higher (Sweet, 1977). The difference from previous estimates is probably due to the inclusion of cases of cystic fibrosis where the expression of the disease is so mild that it would not have been recognised under normal circumstances.

Cystic fibrosis is principally a disease of Caucasian children although it has also been diagnosed in Negroes, Indians, American Indians and Japanese. The incidence in these races, although probably very low, is not known precisely. It is of interest that although previously unknown in Arabs, 17 cases were discovered in Baghdad by a single clinical team in a few months (Al-Hassani, 1976).

BASIC DEFECT

The clinical features of cystic fibrosis are the result of: (a) an abnormality of all exocrine glands; and (b) a susceptibility to respiratory infection, the site of the infection being the lower respiratory airways. The genetics of the condition suggests that these abnormalities should all result from a defect of a single abnormal enzyme or protein.

Cystic fibrosis is an epithelial disease. The organs of the epithelium develop in response to an interaction with mesenchymal cells, so that cystic fibrosis could perhaps be caused by a mesenchymal defect. The epithelial glands, however, are initially normal in structure, disruption of a gland occurring in the course of the disease as a result of a defect in secretion. Epithelial glands are acinar-ductal structures. As the disease progresses, alterations in the secretions which increase their viscosity lead to obstruction of the ducts and subsequent structural damage. The vas deferens and associated structures, however, represent a special case in that ductal blockage, injury and reabsorption occur during embryonic development resulting in sterility in males. In cystic fibrosis the embryonic development of all other organs is normal.

The cause of the abnormality in secretion is unknown but is being investigated at the various levels of (a) control of secretion, (b) intracellular events associated with secretion and (c) the biochemistry of exocrine gland products.

Spock et al (1967) reported that serum from cystic fibrosis patients disorganised the beat of cilia in explants of respiratory mucosa from rabbit trachea. This observation has since been confirmed using other animal tissues including oyster gills (Bowman et al, 1969) and fresh water mussels (Besley et al, 1969). Investigation suggests that the factor inhibiting ciliary movement is a heat labile protein with a molecular weight of between 2500 and 10 000, usually bound to IgG (Wilson & Fundenberg, 1978). Unfortunately the assay methods for this factor have given inconsistent results and the significance of the factor in relation to the pathology of the disease has not been established. However, this factor has attracted great research interest. Since it has been shown that a similar substance can be isolated from culture medium of long term lymphoid lines and peripheral blood leucocytes from those harbouring the C.F. gene (Wilson & Fundenberg, 1978) it may prove to be an effective genetic marker. It is also possible that its presence may be directly related to the basic enzyme or protein defect.

The main cause of death in cystic fibrosis is the severe chronic lower respiratory tract infection. This susceptibility to infection cannot be explained by any defect in immune function. Both B-cell and T-cell systems are normal. There is, however, some conjecture about the role of the alveolar macrophage. A defect in its function could explain both the occurrence and the site of infection since it has a major role in maintaining the sterility of the lower respiratory tract.

PATHOLOGY

Pancreas

In 15 to 20% of cases there is no defect of pancreatic function at the time of diagnosis; in the others the degree of impairment varies widely. The initial defect is a failure of production of water and bicarbonate. The pancreatic enzymes continue to be produced but the resulting secretion becomes increasingly viscous until ductules become blocked. The related acini undergo dilatation and rupture with escape of enzymes into the supporting structures where a fibrous reaction is provoked.

The absence of pancreatic secretions from the lumen of the upper intestine produces a form of malabsorption which has certain characteristics. Only those ingestants which require digestion before absorption are affected. Iron absorption is not impaired and indeed because of the abnormally low pH in the upper jejunum, iron absorption is enhanced. Anaemia is not a feature of the disease. Absence of pancreatic lipase results in particularly severe steatorrhoea. Fat globules can often be seen on examination of the stool. This is not the case in any of the other common causes of malabsorption in childhood.

Liver and bile ducts

The initial abnormality in the liver is the accumulation of excess mucus in the bile ducts which dilate and proliferate (Oppenheimer & Esterly, 1975). Increased fibrosis is provoked in the portal areas and these areas expand and become linked together. The cirrhosis then progresses until it becomes clinically significant by causing portal hypertension. Hepatocellular injury is not a prominent feature. Enzyme measurements and other liver function tests are not helpful in following the progress of the disease. Of those reaching adult life some 20% will have evidence of portal hypertension. Jaundice is unusual and presents only very late in the disease.

Intestine

Meconium ileus

Approximately 10% of cases of cystic fibrosis present in the neonatal period with meconium ileus. The intestinal obstruction is caused by inspissation of the meconium in the distal ileum. The plug of putty-like material produced has a high protein content as the result of absence of proteolytic enzymes, secretion of abnormally viscid mucus and reduced water secretion by the pancreas and biliary system. The obstruction may be complicated by volvulus or perforation. The presence of the plug during late stages of embryonic development may also result in a degree of atresia of the lower gut.

Mucus production

Throughout the gut goblet cells are distended and the crypts are often filled by eosinophilic material. These abnormalities can be demonstrated by rectal biopsy.

The distension of Brunner's glands can be demonstrated radiologically following a barium meal.

Rectal prolapse

Rectal prolapse is a common complication of untreated cystic fibrosis in the first two or three years of life. This is due to a number of factors, the chief of which are the near vertical course of the rectum at this age, diarrhoea, cough and diminution of ischiorectal fat resulting from poor nutrition. Cystic fibrosis should be suspected whenever rectal prolapse occurs in this age group (Shwachman, 1975).

Sweat glands

As is the case in other serous glands the sweat gland in cystic fibrosis is structurally normal. The sweating rate is also normal but variable. At very low sweating rates the sodium and chloride concentrations approach normal values. At high sweating rates produced by heat, exercise or stimulation by pilocarpine, the sodium and chloride concentrations become abnormally high (i.e. above 70 mmol/l) due to defective absorption of these ions from the fluid secreted at the base of the gland as it passes outwards through the duct (di Sant'Agnese et al, 1953).

In hot climates this defect may be a troublesome predisposing factor to heat exhaustion.

As this abnormality of sweating is characteristic of cystic fibrosis its chief importance is as diagnostic evidence of the disease.

Reproductive system

Approximately 97% of male cystic fibrosis patients are sterile. The anatomical basis is bilateral absence or atrophy of the epididymis, vas deferens and seminal vesicles (see above). Aspermia is accompanied by a reduced semen volume. The patients are not impotent (Landing et al, 1969).

In females delayed menarche is common. Fertility is reduced to about one fifth of normal probably due to abnormal viscosity of the cervical mucus. Maternal mortality is also increased (Cohen et al, 1980).

Pulmonary disease

In cystic fibrosis the lungs are peculiarly susceptible to infection both by common pathogenic bacteria and also by organisms which do not behave as pathogens in normal subjects. Along with the progress of the infection there is a concomitant alteration in the secretion of mucus which is both promoted by the presence of infection and at the same time increases the susceptibility to further infections by interference with lung drainage. It is the state of the lung pathology which determines the quality of the patient's life, and respiratory infection is the usual cause of death.

At birth the lungs are structurally normal. For reasons unknown but conceivably due to a defect of alveolar macrophage function, the peripheral airways become infected. At first the common pathogens are *Haemophilus influenzae* and *Staphylococcus aureus*. Later in the course of the illness, especially after there has been extensive use of antibiotics, the most troublesome organism is *Pseudomonas*. In most cases the *Pseudomonas* is present in its usual 'rough' form but in time the dominant organism becomes the mutant mucoid *Pseudomonas* which is almost never found as a pathogen except in the cystic fibrosis lung.

In response to the presence of infection there is hypertrophy in the mucus secreting tissues in the airway. Submucous glands hypertrophy. The proportion of globet cells in the respiratory mucosa increases and the goblet cells are found more peripherally in the small airways than in the normal lung. The presence of excess mucus predisposes to further infection.

The pathology which begins as bronchiolitis progresses to chronic bronchitis and bronchiectasis.

The respiratory dysfunction is the result of airway obstruction. Vital capacity is reduced while residual volume and functional residual capacity are increased (Wood et al, 1976).

Cardiovascular disease

With longer survival of the patients, cardiovascular complications are being encountered more frequently. These complications can be expected when the vital capacity has fallen below 60% of normal. The combination of low pO_2 and pulmonary hypertension leads to right ventricular hypertrophy and failure. It has been noted that the low pO_2 affects the contractility of both ventricles so that left ventricle function also deteriorates in the late stage of the disease (Goldring et al, 1964).

Diabetes mellitus

The incidence of diabetes mellitus increases with age, and results from increasing encroachment on the islet cells as the pancreatic lesion progresses. The prevalence in the total population of cystic fibrosis patients is approximately 1 in 100.

This diabetes is mild and easily controlled. It is not accompanied by ketosis, retinopathy, neuropathy or other complications. It does not adversely affect the prognosis of the cystic fibrosis patient (Kellman & Larsson, 1975).

DIAGNOSIS

Sweat test

Diagnosis of cystic fibrosis by demonstration of the basic molecular defect is not possible. Diagnosis therefore depends on recognising certain constant and characteristic features of the phenotype.

Of these the most reliable is the abnormality in sweat production. The significance and relationship of elevated sweat sodium and chloride to the disease was first described in 1953 (di Sant'Agnese et al, 1953). Elevated sweat electrolyte concentrations occur in a few other conditions - severe malnutrition, diabetes insipidus, adrenal insufficiency and glucose-6-phosphatase deficiency – but these are conditions which could not be confused clinically with cystic fibrosis. More troublesome is the elevation of sweat electrolytes which occurs with ageing. Normal adults (i.e. over 17 years) at high sweating rates may occasionally have values for sweat sodium and chloride which lie within the range usually associated with cystic fibrosis. In childhood however, the sweat test is a good diagnostic tool provided it is done with meticulous care and by a laboratory with frequent experience of the test and good quality control (Shwachman & Mohmoodian, 1979).

The method of testing now preferred is that of pilocarpine iontophoresis (Gibson & Cook 1969). Both sodium and chloride should be measured as a check. A difference of more than 30 mmol/l between the concentration of either of the two ions in repeat tests indicates technical error. It is also useful to measure potassium concentration. Since potassium concentration is not affected in cystic fibrosis, a report of a high potassium suggests that the specimen of sweat has been affected by evaporation and the result should be discarded.

Most clinicians would accept that a concentration of sodium over 70 mmol/l and chloride over 60 mmol/l (measured in a minimum collection of 100 mgs of sweat) are significantly abnormal and consistent with the diagnosis of cystic fibrosis. If the test has been correctly performed very similar results should be obtained if the test is repeated under similar conditions. Schwarz (1974) noted that in cystic fibrosis sodium loss resulting from diarrhoea, and the malnutrition due to malabsorption, may cause increased aldosterone production which may lower the sodium concentration in sweat and raise the potassium concentration. Thus when the disease is treated the sodium level may rise and the potassium fall. These changes are of interest but not sufficient to cause confusion in clinical practice.

The sweat test remains the corner-stone of the diagnosis of cystic fibrosis. Evaluation and standards have been the subject of a very full report by a committee of the National Research Council, Washington D. C. (Howell, 1976).

Pancreatic function tests

Pancreatic function tests are not usually required for the diagnosis of cystic fibrosis. The tests are unpleasant for the child. Pancreatic achylia may occur in other conditions such as familial chronic pancreatitis and Scwachman syndrome. Conversely pancreatic function may be normal in as many as 15 to 20% of cases at presentation.

Pancreatic function tests are therefore done only when additional evidence is required to support a series of equivocal sweat tests.

Meconium testing

As explained above, deficiency of pancreatic enzymes leads to defective digestion of protein and the resulting excess of protein contributes to the abnormal character of the meconium.

The Boehringer-Mannheim (B-M) test strip (with tetrabromophenolphthalein as an indicator) used as a dip-stick test on meconium produces a blue colour when the concentration of protein exceeds 20mg/gm dry weight. The test is therefore positive in cystic fibrosis except in the 15 to 20% of cases where pancreatic function is normal at birth. False positive results are also frequent especially in premature infants and twins. In one random series of 34 300 tests, even experienced laboratory staff produced a false positive rate of 0.5% (Stephan, 1975). With inexperienced staff 1% of the tests were falsely reported as abnormal.

The test is therefore of limited usefulness and insufficient on its own to establish a diagnosis of cystic fibrosis.

TREATMENT

There is no specific therapy. Treatment is supportive only but can significantly improve both the quality and duration of life.

The main burden of the disease results from the respiratory component. Infection has not been effectively prevented by the use of prophylactic antibiotics or by vaccines. It is not possible to maintain a sterile lower respiratory tract for any length of time. In the long term the best that can be achieved is to maintain a balance between the patient and the invading pathogens, so that the infection remains contained and the patient is able to grow and develop normally and lead a normal life.

Exercise promotes chest drainage and the patients should be encouraged to take an active part in some form of sport (e. g. swimming, trampolining, squash). Lung function is improved by regular postural drainage and physiotherapy. It is also possible that physiotherapy, by helping to clear the airways of excess secretions, also lessens the frequency of infection. To be effective physiotherapy must be carried out twice or three times daily. At first, in the young child, this is done by the parents, but it is helpful if friends or relatives are willing to learn the necessary techniques and give occasional relief to the parents in their prolonged burden of care. As the patient gets older the physiotherapy techniques can be altered so that the patient becomes progressively less dependent on the help of others. The teenager can carry out his treatment quite independently, except during exacerbation of infection. Continuing guidance to the family by an experienced physiotherapist is an essential part of management and it is important for the morale of both patient and family that independence, in relation to physiotherapy, should be achieved as soon as possible.

Exacerbation of infection should be treated as early as possible with appropriate antibiotics. To this end it is best if the patient is seen frequently by his paediatrician (e.g. every four weeks) and that the paediatrician should have the support of a bacteriologist with knowledge of the special problems of cystic fibrosis. When early in the disease the infecting organism is *Staphylococcus*, *Haemophilus* or *Pneumococcus* a wide range of antibiotics is available. In the later stages of the disease when the principal pathogen is a mucoid *Pseudomonas*, antibiotic treatment is less satisfactory. At present the best prospects seem to be offered by a combination of one of the newer aminoglycocides such as Tobramycin and one of the new penicillins, Ticarcillin or Azlocillin. Even with these drugs complete eradication of the organism is unusual, but with the energetic use of intravenous antibiotics and physiotherapy good clinical improvement can be achieved.

The cardiovascular complications of cystic fibrosis are now seen more frequently than before because of longer survival. They are difficult to prevent and the effectiveness of treatment has so far not been adequately studied.

The progress of liver disease likewise cannot be prevented. When portal hypertension results however, shunt operations can be carried out very successfully without the complication of encephalopathy which is met with in other forms of liver disease such as alcoholic cirrhosis.

The nutritional problems of cystic fibrosis are usually easily managed. Almost all patients can be maintained on a normal diet. It is helpful if the diet is rich in protein. Occasionally when the pancreatic deficiency is very severe it may be necessary to restrict the dietary fat. Pancreatic extracts are given in sufficient dosages to secure adequate digestion and absorption. The effectiveness of treatment may be judged by the patient's growth and weight gain as well as the character of the stools. When steatorrhoea is not adequately controlled the stools are foul smelling and persistence of this smell may cause social embarrassment to the patient. The dosage of pancreatic enzymes should be increased until this problem is removed. The effectiveness of enzyme treatment can be improved if an alkali is also given orally to secure a more normal pH in the upper jejunum.

PROGNOSIS

The prognosis in cystic fibrosis is very variable and difficult to forecast for the individual patient. Where two or more sibs are affected, experience with an older child gives no guidance as to the course of the illness and subsequent outcome in later children.

The course of the illness is influenced by social conditions, the aggressiveness of management and the standard of comprehensive care. However, the best guide to prognosis is the extent of irreversible pulmonary involvement at the time of diagnosis. Those who present with established pulmonary disease in the first month of life do badly. Those who present later but yet before pulmonary disease is obvious do relatively well. In one large series (Stern et al, 1976) the mean follow up time from diagnosis was over 14 years.

FAMILY EFFECTS OF CYSTIC FIBROSIS

When cystic fibrosis is diagnosed the whole family becomes involved. If the genetics of the disease is adequately explained and fully understood by the parents there should then be no recrimination between the parents, and in this sense the disease should have no disruptive effects on the family. The divorce rate in affected families is in fact no greater than in the general population.

Many parents have feelings of guilt which may remain troublesome even after the fullest discussion over several years.

Parents are anxious and often depressed. In the author's experience 70% of mothers of cystic fibrosis children are receiving antidepressant drugs at any one time. Some anxieties can be alleviated. Many mothers go in constant fear of further pregnancy. Advice from an expert in contraception can be helpful. Many parents have not been fully informed about the course of the disease and the manner in which death is likely to occur. They are often in constant fear of the child's sudden death. Reluctance of paediatricians to discuss the subject of the child's death before the event is unhelpful.

Financially the disease may be a burden to the family even where medical services are provided free of cost. Travel even to free clinics may be expensive, but more important is the impulse in parents to indulge their affected child in ways which lead to insupportable expense.

The child too suffers emotionally. In early childhood behaviour disorders are extremely common as a result of the parents' reluctance to discipline the affected child about whom they have disturbing feelings of guilt. At school, performance tends to be poor, not because of breaks in attendance caused by illness, but through low standards of expectation by parents and teachers because of the child's disability. The emotional pressures become cumulative as the patient matures. There is the increasing realisation of the threat of physical disorder as well as impending difficulties in employment resulting from a combination of poor physique and poor educational attainments. This distressing period is often made worse by increasing isolation. Retardation of growth and development as well as increase in symptoms may make it impossible to hide the condition and 'differences' from peers. At this stage of the illness rejection of treatment and support is common as a result of a feeling of hopelessness.

GENETIC COUNSELLING

Genetic counselling is an extremely important part of management when a family is affected by cystic fibrosis. Unfortunately it is subject to a number of pitfalls.

Timing is an essential consideration. When the parents are first given the diagnosis and some indication of the prognosis their reaction is one of shock, and during this period of reaction little of the information offered is absorbed. For the following several weeks a period of mourning is experienced and the parents will continue to reject further distressing information. Thereafter the parents emerge into a more receptive and positive state of mind and full discussion of the implications of the disease can reasonably be conducted and plans made for the future. At this stage parents will often deny that any previous instruction has been offered, but will readily accept explanations and seek advice.

Language may be a problem. Words such as 'gene' may be meaningless to parents with poor education and even a precise and accurate explanation may not be understood.

A considerable minority of people have difficulty with the concept of probability. In explaining that the chance of a further child being affected is 1 in 4 it should not be too readily assumed that it has been fully understood and it may be necessary to emphasise that this is the risk for *each* and *all* succeeding pregnancies.

In Scotland (McCrae et al, 1973) when genetic counselling has been carefully given, parents decide in almost equal numbers to take one of three courses of action: (i) to have no more children because they already have the number of children that they planned i.e. the diagnosis of cystic fibrosis does not influence family planning, (ii) to have no more children because of the risk of a further child being affected, (iii) to accept the risk and proceed to a further pregnancy. It is noticeable that in making the choice morbidity is of more concern than mortality. A death from meconium ileus may not be too discouraging an experience but long continued disability caused by the disease is more likely to deter the parents from a further pregnancy.

The counsellor should be aware that when parents have decided to have no further children they may need help to follow their intention. Family planning advice may be required.

Prenatal diagnosis

There is no reliable method for the diagnosis of cystic fibrosis in utero. Following Danes and Bearn's report (1968) of a genetic marker for cystic fibrosis it was thought that it might be possible to diagnose cystic fibrosis by the study of metachromasia in cells cultured from amniotic fluid. Subsequent investigation has shown the technique to be unreliable (Nadler et al, 1969). An alternative technique has not yet been described.

SCREENING

Limited screening including all sibs of known cases is obligatory. This is best carried out using the conventional sweat test. Universal screening of all newborns would certainly be desirable for three purposes.

1. Enumeration. Because of the wide variation in severity of the condition and the occurrence of cases so mild that they do not present until adulthood, the true incidence of cystic fibrosis in different populations and races is unknown. Only universal screening could produce the required information.

2. Life studies. If large series of subjects with cystic fibrosis could be followed from birth rather than from the onset of functional disorder the natural history of the disease would be better understood. As yet it has not been possible to study the possibility that environmental factors may influence or even initiate the series of pathological changes to which the cystic fibrosis homozygote is subject.

3. Family planning. Since cystic fibrosis may present late the parents may have embarked on further pregnancies before they are aware that subsequent pregnancies are at risk.

Whether universal screening would have a place in routine medical practice is more problematical. It seems likely that early diagnosis and treatment should improve the outcome, and there is some objective evidence that this is so (Warwick & Progue, 1969). At present however, universal screening seems impractical. No simple and reliable test is available which could be used in the neonatal period. It has been suggested that meconium could be tested routinely as described above and that infants giving a positive result could have the diagnosis confirmed or refuted by a sweat test performed perhaps at the age of 6 weeks when adequate sweat samples are relatively easy to obtain. Due to the failings of the meconium test and the technical finesse required by the sweat test such a programme would give unsatisfactory results. It would also be expensive. It has been estimated that detection of a single case by this method would cost £10 000 (McCrae, 1977).

Universal screening, although desirable must await the development of an acceptable screening test, which in its turn probably depends on knowing the basic biochemical defect.

FUTURE PROSPECTS

Patients with cystic fibrosis now survive longer than was the case a few years ago. The total amount of clinical care required is therefore increasing and new problems are achieving importance, especially in relation to education, employment and emotional stress.

Bronchopulmonary disease remains the chief hazard to the patient. Newly developed antibiotics are useful but perhaps other approaches may be tried such as the early immunisation of the patient against *Pseudomonas aeruginosa*. Such a preventive approach would be encouraged if sensible and practical methods could be developed for the early detection of disease before lung damage has occurred.

The basic defect in this disease remains unknown. Further study of the C.F. factor may lead to better understanding of the disease. Meanwhile the discovery of this factor may prove immediately useful. Promising preliminary results have been reported using an antiserum produced in mice by the injection of C.F. factor isolated from patients by iso-electric focusing. If such an antiserum can be shown to react with the serum of heterozygotes and with amniotic fluid from an affected fetus, this will allow much improved genetic counselling and also the prospect of prenatal diagnosis (Dunn, 1980; Gurwitz et al, 1980).

REFERENCES

Al-Hassani 1976 personal communication

Andersen D H 1938 Cystic fibrosis of the pancreas and its relation to coeliac disease: A clinical and pathological study. American Journal of Diseases of Children 56: 344–399

Besley G T N, Patrick A D, Norman A P 1969 Inhibition of motility of gill cilia of Dreissena by plasma of cystic fibrosis patients and parents. Journal of Medical Genetics 6: 278–280

Bowman B H, Lockart L H, McCombe M L 1969 Oyster ciliary inhibition by cystic fibrosis factor. Science 164: 325–326

Cohen L F, di Sant' Agnese P A, Freidlander J 1980 Cystic fibrosis and pregnancy. Lancet 2: 842–844

Committee for a study for evaluation of testing for cystic fibrosis. D A Howell Chairman 1976 Evaluation for testing for cystic fibrosis. Journal of Pediatrics 88: 711–750

Danes B S, Bearn A G 1968 A genetic marker in cystic fibrosis of the pancreas. Lancet 1: 1061–1063

Danes B S, Bearn A G 1969 Cystic fibrosis of the pancreas. A study in cell culture. Journal of Experimental Medicine 129: 793

Danks D M, Allan J, Anderson C M 1965 Genetic study of fibrocystic disease of the pancreas. Annals of Human Genetics 28: 323–356

Di Sant' Agnese P A, Darling R C, Perera G A, Shea E 1953 Abnormal electrolyte composition of sweat in cystic fibrosis of the pancreas. Clinical significance and relationship to disease. Pediatrics 12: 549–563

Dunn L 1980 Cystic fibrosis. Nature 286: 844

Gibson L E, Cook R E 1959 A test for the concentration of electrolytes in sweat in cystic fibrosis of the pancreas utilising pilocarpine by iontophoresis. Pediatrics 23: 545–549

Goldring R M, Fishman A P, Turino G M, Cohen H I, Denning C R, Anderson D H 1964 Portal hypertension and cor pulmonale in cystic fibrosis of the pancreas. Journal of Pediatrics 65: 501–524

Gurwitz D, Corey M, Francis P W J, Crozier D, Levison H 1980 Perspectives in cystic fibrosis. Pediatric Clinics of North America 26: 603–615

Kellman N I, Larsson Y 1975 Insulin release in cystic fibrosis. Archives of Disease in Childhood 50: 205–209

Landing B H, Wells T R, Wang G 1969 Abnormality of the epididymis and vas deferens in cystic fibrosis. Archives of Pathology 88: 569–580

McCrae W M 1977 in Philips G I, Wolfe J N. ed Clinical Practice and Economics. Pitman Medical London 31–45

McCrae W M, Cull A M, Burton L, Dodge J 1973 Cystic fibrosis. Parents' response to the genetic basis of the disease. Lancet 2: 141–143

Nadler H L, Wodnicki J M, O' Flynn N E 1969 Cultivated amniotic fluid cells and fibroblasts from families with cystic fibrosis. Lancet 2: 84–85

Oppenheimer E H, Esterly J R 1975 Hepatic changes: Young infants with cystic fibrosis. Journal of Pediatrics 86: 683–684

Schwarz V 1974 The development of the sweat glands and their function. Daves J, Dobbing J ed. Scientific foundations of paediatrics. Heinemann, London p 544–546 Heinemann, London p 544–546

Shwachman H 1975 Gastro-Intestinal manifestation of cystic fibrosis. Pediatric Clinics of North America 224: 787–805

Shwachman H, Mohmoodian A 1979 Quality of sweat test performance in the diagnosis of cystic fibrosis. Clinical Chemistry 25(1): 158–161

Spock A, Heick H M C, Cress H et al 1967 Abnormal serum factor in patients with cystic fibrosis of the pancreas. Pediatric Research 1: 173–177

Stephan V, Busch E W, Kollberg H, Hellsing K 1975 Cystic fibrosis detection by means of a test-strip. Pediatrics 55: 35–38

Stern R C, Boar T F, Doershuk C F, Tucker A S, Primiano F F, Matthews L W 1976 Course of cystic fibrosis in 95 cases. Journal of Pediatrics 89: 406–411

Sweet E M 1977 Causes of delayed respiratory distress in childhood. Proceedings of the Royal Society of Medicine 70: 863–866

Warwick W J, Progue R E 1969 Computer studies in cystic fibrosis. Lawson ed. Proceedings of 5th International Cystic Fibrosis Conference, London. C Nicholas and Co Ltd p 320–332

Wilson G B, Fundenberg H H 1978 Separation of ciliary dyskinesis substances found in serum and secreted by cystic fibrosis leucocytes and lymph cell lines, using protein A-Sepharose C.L-4B. Journal of Laboratory and Clinical Medicine 93: 463–482

Wood R E, Boat T F, Doeshuk C F 1976 Cystic fibrosis. State of the art. American Review of Respiratory Disease 113: 833–875

65

Asthma and other allergic conditions

J. A. Raeburn

INTRODUCTION

Allergy of the respiratory tract is a very common condition and causes a considerable morbidity and mortality. As many as 10% of the population may be affected in childhood (Williams & McNicol, 1975; Soothill, 1976) but, as the child grows, there is a reduction in the disproportionate narrowing of the airways; therefore asthma symptoms may moderate. There are many different causes of asthma, but a useful clinical classification is into an extrinsic type, provoked by a wide range of external allergens, and intrinsic asthma which develops later in life without allergic sensitivity and in the absence of a family history. In contrast, patients with extrinsic asthma frequently have a positive family history of allergic disorders. The clinical distinction between these two main types of asthma is often disputable and many genetic studies suffer from the consequent difficulty in classification. However the high prevalence of asthma and the strong familial tendency suggest that a genetic approach might lead to useful methods of prevention.

Allergic disorders of the respiratory tract and of other regions, particularly the skin, often coexist either in an individual patient or in one family (Reeves, 1977). This phenomenon suggests that the inherited feature is the immunological response to certain external allergens. However there are many enigmatic aspects. For example, in patients with both asthma and atopic eczema why do exacerbations of asthma often coincide with improvement in the eczema and vice versa? Another unsolved question is that the abnormal reactivity can be localised to one site in one affected family member and to another site in his affected relatives. In this chapter we will concentrate on respiratory allergy, principally allergic rhinitis and asthma, and on atopic dermatitis. All three conditions are very common and they are frequently associated.

INVESTIGATIONS IN ATOPIC DISEASES

Atopic disorders suffer from the lack of reliable markers of disease, whether clinical, immunological or biochem-

ical. Therefore there are no accurate figures for the population incidence, estimates varying widely between 2 and 20% (Seah & Wilkinson, 1974). Table 65.1 lists the main information required in the investigation of an atopic patient; the extent to which such investigations are completed will depend on the severity of the condition in the index patient or his family. The various investigations need not be described in detail here (see Reeves, 1977), but it is worth stressing that unless a personal and family history has been obtained that is accurate and detailed, the specialist investigations will provide little useful information.

Skin prick tests can be performed simultaneously on many members of the family and can give semi-quantitative information about the degree of atopy (Pepys, 1975). The solutions used in prick testing can be chosen on the basis of known precipitants of atopic attacks, but usually a wide range of allergens as well as a control solution will be tested in each patient, thus giving a profile of the skin reactivity. However, reactivity in the asthmatic's skin may differ from the bronchial reactivity. A further limitation is that children below three years of age have a reduced skin reactivity to histamine and allergens (Aas, 1975). Loeffler and colleagues (1973) showed that there is a good correlation between serum IgE levels and the skin test reactions; for example only 11% of subjects with negative skin tests had elev-

Table 65.1 Plan of investigation of the atopic family.

A Clinical information
   i) Allergic history of the proband
   ii) Allergic history of the first and second degree relatives
   iii) Distribution of allergy in affected family members
   iv) Other conditions eg susceptibility to infection in family members and index patient.
B Side room tests
   i) Skin prick tests
   ii) Eosinophil counts in blood (and sputum)
C Specialist investigations
   i) Total serum immunoglobulin E (IgE) level
   ii) Antigen-specific IgE levels
     (based on radioallergosorbent tests)
   iii) Provocation tests

---

ated serum levels of IgE (over 800 units/ml) whereas 83% of skin test positive subjects had elevated levels.

Immunoglobulin E and atopy

The great majority of patients who have elevated IgE levels suffer from the common atopic disorders but there is considerable overlap between atopic and non-atopic populations (see Table 65.2 based on Adkinson, 1976 and Barnetson et al, 1980).Of the atopic patients the highest serum IgE levels occur in atopic eczema; in patients with allergic asthma or hay fever levels are much lower (Barnetson et al, 1980). Barnetson and his colleagues also noted that the very high IgE concentrations occurred in atopic eczema patients who had food allergies and positive allergen-specific responses to foods. This observation, coupled with the considerable variance of IgE levels in each group, suggests that within atopy there are many disease subgroups within which IgE variation could be much smaller. It is likely that such subgroups could be the result of genetic heterogeneity. Additional markers of atopy are therefore required in order to subclassify the range of allergy.

MODE OF INHERITANCE IN ATOPY

Reports of a familial basis for asthma date back to the last century and the various authors have suggested either autosomal dominant or autosomal recessive inheritance as well as multifactorial transmission (Bias, 1973; Schwartz, 1952; Adkinson, 1920). There has been a similar dispute for all atopic disorders and for many years the prevalent view ranged from autosomal dominant (Spain & Cooke, 1924) to autosomal recessive inheritance (Tips, 1954). Recently the heterogeneity of atopy has been better appreciated and Kaufman and Frick (1976) suggested the multifactorial mode of inheritance, following a prospective study which attempted to classify different types of allergy as well as the varying environmental influences, particularly diet. Despite these contradictions about the mode of inheritance, all studies show firstly that allergy is very common and secondly that the recurrence risk is high if a parent or sib is affected.

The genetic heterogeneity of atopic disorders is almost certainly very marked and is reminiscent of the heterogeneity recognised in diabetes ten years ago. Some families undoubtedly show inheritance fully compatible with a single gene, autosomal dominant, disorder. In all atopic diseases, however, susceptible individuals may fail to express the condition if they do not encounter the appropriate antigen(s) at a specific phase of their immunological development. Figure 65.1 shows the pedigree of a family suffering from severe asthma which in most individuals is triggered by mild respiratory infections. At the age of 21 the monozygotic twins in the second generation (II) were thought to be discordant for asthma. The onset of that disease in one twin was at age 14 and in the other was at 24. In this family autosomal dominant inheritance is the likely cause of the susceptibility to asthma but the disease does not develop spontaneously, it requires an appropriate environmental trigger.

Sibbald and Turner-Warwick (1979) have emphasized the importance of distinguishing the two main clinical subtypes of asthma in any genetic studies of the disease. Their study of 416 probands showed that asthma occurred in 13.3% of first degree relatives of extrinsic (atopic) asthmatics and in 7.6% of first degree relatives of intrinsic (non-atopic) asthmatics, a highly significant reduction in the latter group (p < 0.001). However it is

FAMILY H.

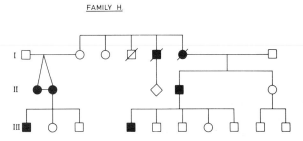

Fig. 65.1 The affected members of this family had asthma which was usually precipitated by an upper respiratory infection of viral type. Unless the consequent bronchoconstrictive symptoms were energetically treated, usually with short-term high doses of steroids, the subsequent exacerbations of asthma could persist for many months. Autosomal dominant inheritance of a susceptibility gene is the simplest model to explain this family.

Table 65.2 Total serum IgE levels in different adult populations.

Population	No. studied	Range of IgE levels (international units per ml)	Geometric mean
Non-atopic adults	102	1–3824	26.7
Unselected adults (allergy not excluded)	73	2.5–7896	43.8
Asthma/hay fever adults	28	10–1900	160
Atopic eczema adults	32	40–45 000	2800

frequently difficult to classify asthma as either extrinsic or intrinsic and the above authors recognised at least two intermediate groups. They were unable to determine the mode of inheritance but in a separate study, Sibbald (1980) showed that there is probably no genetic basis for differences between males and females as regards the prevalence of asthma.

Lubs (1972) carried out a postal survey of those twins recorded at the Swedish twin registry to ascertain the prevalence of allergic disorders and to determine the heritability. There were responses from both twins in 74.5% of the register population, providing data on almost 7000 twin pairs. Table 65.3 summarises the data for asthma, hay fever and eczema. The concordance rate for monozygotic twins in this study was lower (15.4–24.4%) than in previous, but much smaller, twin samples. Nevertheless the differences between these values and the concordance rates for dizygotic twins (4–16.2%) strongly suggest a hereditary component. These data can only apply to the populations from which the twins were derived and similar large studies of prevalence are needed for any population in which genetic approaches to prevention are anticipated. An interesting observation in Lubs' (1972) study is that migraine, classified as an allergic disorder, had a prevalence of 8% and also showed increased concordance in monozygotic twins. Oakshot (personal communication 1980) has found that the incidence of migraine is increased in families affected by the common atopic diseases.

GENETIC COUNSELLING IN ALLERGIC DISORDERS

In view of the genetic and clinical heterogeneity of all allergic disorders the estimation of recurrence risks is problematical. The author's approach is to take a careful family history, noting the occurrence of any type of allergy in the first and second degree relatives of the proband. In preparing pedigrees note is also taken of diseases which may be associated with atopy such as

Table 65.3 Allergic disorders in twins (based on Lubs, 1972).

Disease group	Prevalence (%)	Concordance (%)*	
		Monozygotic	Dizygotic
Asthma	3.8	19.0	4.8
Hay fever	14.8	21.4	13.6
Eczema	2.5	15.4	4.0
Asthma or hay fever or eczema	18.2	24.4	16.2

* The concordance for monozygotic twins in each disease group significantly exceeded that for dizygotic twins (p < 0.01 in all four comparisons)

immune deficiency syndromes or autoimmune disorders. Where there are affected family members it is useful to enquire about the age of onset and any known precipitating factors because this information gives an indication of possible methods of prevention.

Having examined the pedigree and all clinical data a Mendelian form of inheritance may be suggested which forms the basis of a risk estimate. For example the offspring of the asthmatic son of the identical twin in Figure 65.1 would have a 50% risk of inheriting the susceptibility. X–linked recessive atopic diseases have not yet been described but in the differential diagnosis of severe eczema in the young male, the X–linked Wiskott-Aldrich syndrome should be considered.

Autosomal recessive inheritance is a possibility if the atopic disorders occur only in one sibship, and two possible syndromes are 'asthma associated with aspirin intolerance' (occasionally with nasal polyposis) or 'asthma with short stature and elevation of serum levels of IgA,' (McKusick, 1978). One further condition which is probably autosomal recessive is bronchomalacia in which flaccidity of the bronchi can simulate many aspects of asthma without, however, any other evidence of atopy. Cystic fibrosis (C.F.) families show an increase of atopy in both homozygotes and obligate heterozygotes for the causative gene. This phenomenon has not yet been adequately explained but the genetic counsellor should perhaps consider the possibility of cystic fibrosis in the offspring of a couple, both of whom are atopic. A pilot study in Edinburgh (Jansen & Raeburn, 1977 – unpublished observations) showed that the presence of atopy in both parents was insufficient evidence on which to base prospective counselling for cystic fibrosis; however laboratory tests to identify carriers of the C.F. gene may in the future be useful here.

Having excluded those atopic families which show a Mendelian form of inheritance, empirical risk figures can be used to estimate the chances of further individuals being affected. Table 65.4, based on data from van Arsdel and Motulsky (1959), Leigh and Marley (1967), Lubs (1972) and Gerrard et al (1976), gives the risk of atopies in a child some of whose first-degree relatives are affected.

In assessing the risk of asthma two other aspects need consideration. Firstly, if a proband has asthma *plus* either allergic rhinitis or eczema, then the risk to first degree relatives is doubled (Lubs, 1972). Secondly, in the adult age groups the risk of asthma increases by a factor of two from age 45 to 65 years (Leigh & Marley, 1967). The empiric figures from Table 65.4 will give an approximate risk of atopic diseases in certain situations, which will help parents to make decisions about their future family. In addition the figures will help clinicians to identify high risk subjects *before* atopic diseases have developed, so that preventive management can be instituted. Genetic

Table 65.4 Empiric risk of atopic disease in children with affected first degree relatives.

Disease	Affected sib, normal parents (%)	One parent affected (%)	Both parents affected (%)
Asthma[†]	10	26	34
Hay fever*	6	12	insufficient data
Atopic dermatitis[†]	14	34	57
Any atopic disease	20	35	50

[†] The risk given is the risk of the same atopic disease.
* The risk given is the risk of asthma in the child whose first degree relatives have hay fever – the risk of hay fever is much higher but the clinical consequences are less severe.

counselling in the field of allergy will therefore involve an accurate diagnosis, careful pedigree analysis, calculation of appropriate Mendelian or empiric risk figures, discussion with the consultand(s) and an active approach to prevention.

THE PREVENTION OF ALLERGIC DISEASES

For most allergic diseases the susceptible individual is clinically and immunologically normal at birth and prenatally. However Taylor et al (1973) showed that about half of the infants at high risk of atopy on genetic grounds had low immunoglobulin A (IgA) levels at age 3 months and an 'overshoot' at one year. The infants with this 'transient IgA deficiency' were much more likely to develop infantile atopy than other 'high risk' babies who had normal IgA levels throughout. Since the transient IgA deficiency precedes the development of reaginic allergy (Soothill, 1976), IgA studies may therefore identify the atopic subjects at a stage at which intervention may be considered. For example Matthew et al (1977) have shown that a single allergen avoidance regimen, based on breast feeding, could significantly reduce the incidence of atopic dermatitis at 6 months and also at 1 year of age. Whether this initial allergen avoidance can permanently reduce the individual's risk of atopy remains to be seen, but there is evidence that reaginic allergy occurs at specific stages of immunological development and therefore this approach may not necessitate life-long avoidance of major allergens. In addition to dietary measures, avoidance of inhaled antigens from animal or plant dusts can also be instigated in addition to therapy, such as disodium cromoglycate, which may prevent histamine release into lung tissue following antigen exposure. Transient IgA deficiency is unlikely to detect all individuals with susceptibility to atopic diseases. An additional approach is based on a search for

either linkage to the HLA loci or association with specific HLA haplotypes. Ragweed pollinosis is always associated with intense skin reactivity to antigen E, the major antigen of ragweed pollen. Affected subjects all have severe hay fever following contact with ragweed pollen, and often concomitant asthma. Analysis of several studies of HLA haplotypes in this disease has recently shown that it is due to a gene or genes linked to the HLA-B locus (Braun, 1978). Thus HLA testing in families with this disease will often detect 'at risk' subjects at a presensitisation stage. Prospective studies in susceptible families will provide a further model for the prevention of allergic diseases.

HLA studies in asthma families have shown no association with a particular HLA antigen, such as occurs between HLA B27 and ankylosing spondylitis. Although early studies suggested a small increase in the A1–B8 haplotype, the results were no longer statistically significant when correction was made for the number of antigens studied (see Braun, 1978). Turton et al (1979) confirmed the lack of association with known antigens of the A, B and C loci in 40 extrinsic asthma patients as well as in 41 patients with intrinsic asthma and 41 with allergic bronchopulmonary aspergillosis. In addition the haplotype segregation in the sibs of probands with or without asthma did not differ from that predicted. These negative results are disappointing but they indicate the need for study of other immunological and genetic markers in asthma.

For many subjects who are at risk of respiratory allergy the best prospects for disease prevention lie in measures taken in early infancy or childhood. Some however will be free from any form of allergy until adult life when contact with new agents provokes specific sensitisation. An appropriate area for application of preventive management would be in the wide field of industrial health, for a wider knowledge of atopic disorders will indicate which individuals should avoid specific situations (eg some asthma subjects should not work in factories producing biological detergents). If genetic studies or immunological markers are used prospectively to identify high risk individuals then the possibilities for prevention are very great in many industries which range from coal mining to natural and synthetic chemical purification and manufacture. Although some allergic diseases may be mild, a careful study of allergy may suggest ways of preventing life-threatening asthma states or chronic handicapping atopic dermatitis.

ACKNOWLEDGEMENTS

It is a pleasure to acknowledge the help of several colleagues in the preparation of this chapter, particularly Dr I P Gormley and Professor A E H Emery.

REFERENCES

Aas K 1975 Diagnosis of immediate type respiratory allergy. Pediatric Clinics of North America 22: 1: 33–42

Adkinson J 1920 The behaviour of bronchial asthma as an inherited character. Genetics 5: 363–418

Adkinson N F 1976 Measurement of total serum immunoglobulin E and allergen-specific IgE antibody. In: Rose N R, Friedman H (eds) Manual of Clinical Immunology, Ch 79, p. 590–602

van Arsdel P P, Motulsky A G 1959 Frequency and heritability of asthma and allergic rhinitis in college students. Acta Genetica 9: p 101–114

Barnetson R StC, Merrett T G, Ferguson A 1980 Hyperimmunoglobulinaemia E in atopy (Abstract) In: Preud'homme J L, Hawken V A L (eds) 4th International Congress of Immunology. French Society of Immunology, Paris. Ch 13.1.02

Bias W B 1973 The genetic basis of asthma. In: Austen K F, Lichtenstein L M (eds) Asthma: Physiology Immunopharmacology and Treatment, Academic Press, New York. p 39–44

Braun W E 1978 Current status of HLA and disease associations. In: HLA and Disease, A comprehensive review, CRC Press Inc., Boca Raton. Ch 7, p 29–33

Gerrard J W, Vickers P, Gerrard C D 1976. The familial incidence of allergic disease. Annals of Allergy 36: 10–15

Kaufman H S, Frick O L 1976 The development of allergy in infants of allergic parents: a prospective study concerning the role of heredity. Annals of Allergy 37: 410–415

Leigh D, Marley E 1967 Bronchial Asthma. Pergamon Press, Oxford

Loeffler J A, Cawley L P, Moeder M 1973 Serum IgE levels - correlation with skin test reactivity. Annals of Allergy 31: 331–336

Lubs E M L 1972 Empiric risks for genetic counselling in families with allergy. Journal of Pediatrics 80: 26–31

Matthew D J, Taylor B, Norman A P, Turner M W, Soothill J F 1977 Prevention of eczema. Lancet 1: 321–324

McKusick V A 1978 Mendelian Inheritance in Man, 5th edn. The Johns Hopkins University Press, Baltimore. p 428

Pepys J 1975 Skin testing. British Journal of Hospital Medicine 14: 412–417

Reeves W G 1977 Atopic disorders. In: Holborow E J, Reeves W G (eds) Immunology in Medicine, Academic Press, London. Ch 22, p. 749–779

Schwartz M 1952 Heredity in Bronchial Asthma. Munksgaard, Copenhagen

Seah P P, Wilkinson D S 1974 Eczema. In Fry L, Seah P P (eds) Immunological aspects of skin diseases. MTP, Lancaster, England. Ch 6, p 234–284

Sibbald B 1980 Genetic basis of sex differences in the prevalence of asthma. British Journal of Diseases of the Chest 74: 93–94

Sibbald B, Turner-Warwick M 1979 Factors influencing the prevalence of asthma among first degree relatives of extrinsic and intrinsic asthmatics. Thorax 34: 332–337

Soothill J F 1976 Some intrinsic and extrinsic factors predisposing to allergy. Proceedings of the Royal Society of Medicine 69: 439–442

Spain W C, Cooke R A 1924 Studies in specific hypersensitiveness. Journal of Immunology 9: 521–569

Taylor B, Normal A P, Orgel H A, Stokes C R, Turner M W, Soothill J F 1973 Transient IgA deficiency and pathogenesis of infantile atopy. Lancet 2: 111–113

Tips R L 1954 A study of the inheritance of atopic hypersensitivity in man. American Journal of Human Genetics 6: 328–343

Turton C W G, Morris L, Buckingham J A, Lawler S D, Turner-Warwick M 1979 Histocompatibility antigens in asthma: population and family studies. Thorax 34: 670–676

Williams H E, McNicol K N 1975 The spectrum of asthma in children. Pediatric Clinics of North America 22: 43–52

66

Alpha₁-antitrypsin deficiency and related disorders

J. Lieberman

ALPHA₁-ANTITRYPSIN (α₁AT)

Introduction: α₁AT and pulmonary emphysema

The discovery of alpha₁-antitrypsin (α₁AT) deficiency (Laurell & Eriksson, 1963) has achieved much significance over the past 17 years:

1. It has emphasized the potential role of cellular proteases in the pathogenesis of disease;
2. It has clarified the role of α₁AT as one of the organism's defense mechanisms;
3. It has led to a better understanding of the pathogenesis of pulmonary emphysema;
4. It has provided a tool for geneticists to study inheritance and gene mapping.

Laurell and Eriksson (1963) had observed 5 patients who lacked an α₁AT globulin peak on their serum protein paper electrophoresis. It was well-known at that time that the α₁-globulin peak was formed primarily by the α₁AT glycoprotein, whereas other α₁-globulins (α₁-lipoprotein and the orosomucoid) contributed minimally to this electrophoretic peak. Subsequent measurement of the serum-trypsin-inhibitory-capacity (STIC) in these 5 patients, a measurement of α₁AT activity, revealed a marked deficiency. Three of the 5 patients had emphysema, as did 9 of 14 additional cases with pronounced α₁AT deficiency reported later by Eriksson (1964). Detailed family studies of these patients, measuring the STIC, clearly demonstrated that the defect was inherited through two codominant autosomal genes, with heterozygotes having intermediate levels (approximately 60% of normal) of α₁AT activity, and deficient homozygotes having approximately 15% of normal levels. Eriksson (1965) summarized and extended these studies in his classical monograph.

These preliminary observations were quickly confirmed worldwide. It was generally reported that the classical presentation for patients with severe α₁AT deficiency is that of a male or female, between 20 and 60 years of age (average 45 years) with insidious onset of shortness of breath progressing rapidly to a typical presentation of pulmonary, panacinar, emphysema. Essentially all are cigarette smokers. The clinical presentation of emphysema in these patients is somewhat unusual as compared to others with normal α₁AT in that the disease primarily involves the basilar portions, rather than the apical portions, of the lungs. Involvement of the lung bases is usually apparent on the chest roentgenograph, but is also demonstrable by perfusion and ventilation lung scans; the latter show a delay in ventilation of the bases as well as a delay in clearing of the radioactive material from the lung bases (Welch et al, 1969; Fallat et al, 1973). Otherwise, pulmonary physiologic studies typically show obstructive changes with increased residual volumes, increased compliance, reduced airflow from the lungs (FEV₁), and reduced diffusing capacity. Although the majority of patients present in this classical fashion, some present with symptoms of bronchial asthma (Makino et al, 1970), chronic bronchitis (Falk et al, 1971), or bronchiectasis (Longstreth et al, 1975). A positive family history for obstructive lung disease is frequently obtained from these subjects.

Initially, the lung disease associated with α₁AT deficiency did not appear to be an important clinical entity since early studies had suggested that only 1% of emphysema patients had severe α₁AT deficiency. Eriksson (1965) had emphasized that only those with severe α₁AT deficiency (perhaps 0.04% of the population) were prone to develop lung disease. Persons with intermediate deficiency were thought to be adequately protected. However, a renewed burst of clinical interest in α₁AT deficiency resulted in 1969 (Lieberman; Kueppers et al), when it was reported that both heterozygotes and homozygotes with α₁AT deficiency were present in increased numbers among patients with pulmonary emphysema. We reported a prevalence of 25.8% with α₁AT deficiency in 66 patients at Long Beach Veterans Administration Hospital, of which 10.6% had severe deficiency and 15.2% had intermediate deficiency. Kueppers et al (1969) obtained similar data. Since 5% of the population were estimated to have an intermediate deficiency of α₁AT, a screening and preventive programme seemed plausible and clinical interest in α₁AT deficiency became pertinent. A number of reviews of α₁AT have been written (Lieberman, 1973; Kueppers & Black, 1974; Talamo, 1975;

Carrell & Owen, 1976; Eriksson, 1978; Kueppers, 1978; Lieberman, 1980) and may be referred to for additional information.

α_1AT deficiency in pathogenesis of pulmonary emphysema

Functions of α_1AT

Alpha$_1$-antitrypsin is a broad spectrum protease inhibitor with a relatively low molecular-weight of approximately 50 000 daltons. Table 66.1 lists the proteases that are or are not inhibited by α_1AT. It is generally believed that the inhibition of granulocytic proteases by α_1AT is most important for protecting the human organism against autodigestion. Granulocytic elastase especially has destructive actions on mammalian lung; administration of this enzyme to animal models can produce emphysema, and concurrent administration of α_1AT can prevent this effect. Leucocytes, when present due to infectious or inflammatory stimuli in the lungs, release proteolytic enzymes either through cellular death or during the act of phagocytosis. Normally the α_1AT in the interstitial spaces binds and inhibits the leucocytic proteases. When levels of α_1AT are inadequate, the uninhibited proteolytic enzymes digest the alveolar septi and produce the pathologic picture we recognize as pulmonary emphysema. Experimental support of this concept was provided by demonstrating that leucocytic proteases are capable of digesting lung tissue and that α_1AT

Table 66.1 Enzymes inhibited or not inhibited by α_1AT.

Enzyme	Reference
Enzymes inhibited	
Trypsin	Eriksson (1965)
Chymotrypsin	Bloom & Hunter (1978)
Elastase	Turino et al (1969)
Granulocyte proteases (elastase, chymotrypsin-like enzyme, and	Lieberman & Gawad (1971)
collagenase)	Lieberman & Kaneshiro (1972)
Plasmin (in vitro)	Laurell (1975)
Human factor XI(PTA)	Heck & Kaplan (1974)
Renin	Scharpe et al (1976)
Urokinase	Clemmenson & Christensen (1976)
Bacterial subtilisin	Wisher & Dolovich (1971)
Acrosomal proteinase	Schumacher (1971)
Thrombin	Machovich et al (1977)
Enzymes not inhibited	
Kallikrein	Heck & Kaplan (1974)
Plasminogen activator	Heck & Kaplan (1974)
Papain	
Ficin } Plant proteases	Sasaki et al (1974)
Bromelain	
Plasmin (in vivo)	Laurell (1975)
Hyaluronidase	
Pepsin	Lieberman (1971)
Anhydrotrypsin	Moroi et al (1975)

strongly inhibits this activity (Lieberman & Gawad, 1971; Janoff et al, 1972, 1979). Tuttle and Jones (1975) studied the histologic distribution of α_1AT in frozen sections of human lung with fluorescent antibody and found specific fluorescence for α_1AT in the lining of the terminal airways and alveoli in some of their cases. This suggests that α_1AT may be distributed in lung in association with pulmonary surfactant, and that the increased concentration of α_1AT on the surface lining of such lungs may reflect a protective action at this site.

Other effects have been demonstrated for α_1AT which may contribute to tissue damage when α_1AT is deficient. For example, Arora et al (1978) showed that α_1AT is 'an effector of immunological stasis'. They demonstrated that α_1AT suppresses the immune response of mouse spleen cells against sheep red cells. If this mechanism can be interpreted to indicate a more widespread immunoregulatory role for α_1AT, then the immunologic response to an antigen might be enhanced when α_1AT is reduced or absent, so that more leucocytic cells would respond to an antigenic stimulus and more cellular proteases would be available for tissue destruction. Similar observations were made by Glasgow et al in 1971.

Another effect of trypsin inhibitors was demonstrated by Mirsky and Foley in 1945, but has not been discussed in the literature recently. Mirsky and Foley showed that trypsin inhibitors have an antibiotic action, and conversely, that certain antibiotics such as penicillin, have a weak but definite antiproteolytic action. These authors claim that the rise of antiprotease in blood during a variety of pathologic states may play an important role in resistance to infection.

The lung apparently is the organ most dependent upon the protective action of α_1AT. The lung preferentially incorporates α_1AT (Ishibashi, 1978; Moser, 1978), and tends to retain active antitrypsin for longer periods of time than other mammalian tissues. The presence of leucocytes in the lungs, on the other hand, must result from either: (1) infection, (2) inflammation and irritation, as by cigarette smoking, etc., or (3) the sequestration of leucocytes within the pulmonary capillaries in the basilar portions of the lungs. Sequestration of leucocytes has been described as a natural phenomenon within the lung bases (Bierman et al, 1955), but the process is strikingly enhanced during acute trauma to the lungs and may actually cause complete occlusion of pulmonary capillaries as in 'shock lung' (Ratliff, 1971; Wittels et al, 1974). The natural storage of leucocytes within the basilar pulmonary capillaries could be the reason for enhanced emphysematous damage to the lung bases in individuals with reduced serum concentrations of α_1AT. Alveolar macrophages also contain proteases, and greater emphasis is being accorded these cells in recent investigative studies (see below).

Inherited vs acquired α₁AT deficiency

An important concept regarding the role of α_1AT in the pathogenesis of emphysema is that the same mechanism for damage to lung parenchyma can account for the disease whether a genetic deficiency of α_1AT exists or not. In other words, a 'relative' deficiency of inhibitor may be acquired in individuals without the genetic predisposition. First of all, smokers have significantly higher mean serum levels of α_1AT than non-smokers (Ashley et al, 1980; Lellouch et al, 1979; Rees et al, 1975). α_1AT is an acute-phase-reactant-protein that responds to stresses, such as infection, inflammation, cancer, pregnancy, and oestrogenic hormones. The increased serum levels in the smokers suggest that this may be a protective mechanism against the proteolysis induced by cigarette smoke. However, recent evidence indicates that cigarette smoke can directly suppress protease inhibition in vitro (Carp & Janoff, 1978; Janoff & Carp, 1977; Gadek et al, 1978; Janoff et al, 1979) and actually induces a functional deficiency of antiprotease in the lower respiratory tract of humans (Gadek et al, 1979) and rats (Janoff et al, 1979). This effect on α_1AT may be due to an oxidant in cigarette smoke, since treatment with a reducing agent is capable of restoring the elastase-inhibitory capacity of rat serum (Janoff et al, 1979). Johnson (1980) showed that inhalation of ozone inactivates α_1-antiprotease on the air space side of the lung to create a localized deficiency that might contribute to the development of emphysema. The case against cigarette smoke was strengthened further when Blue and Janoff (1978) showed that human polymorphonuclear leucocytes released their content of elastase when incubated in vitro in the presence of cigarette smoke condensate. Similarly, Hinman et al (1980) and Kuhn and Senior (1978) showed that macrophages from cigarette smokers synthesized and secreted greater amounts of elastase than did macrophages from non-smokers. Cigarette smoking, therefore, increases the production and release of cellular proteases, and simultaneously, reduces elastase-inhibitory activity, thereby producing a functional or relative deficiency of α_1AT. Since cigarette smoking is the basis for the development of pulmonary emphysema in most subjects, whether genetically deficient in α_1AT or not, it seems quite likely that the same mechanism is involved in either case.

With this knowledge about the effect of cigarettes on the protease-antiprotease balance, it would appear that inheritance of an intermediate deficiency of α_1AT would predispose individuals to the development of pulmonary emphysema if they smoke cigarettes, since the level of α_1AT activity is reduced to begin with. In addition, the acute-phase-reactant property of α_1AT is less effective with an intermediate, heterozygous deficiency (Lieberman & Mittman, 1973), so that the protective rise in α_1AT concentration would be diminished. The effects of an intermediate deficiency of α_1AT are currently being debated (see below).

Other diseases associated with α₁AT deficiency

The preceding discussion suggests that organs and tissues other than the lungs may also be subject to damage by a genetic or relative deficiency of protease inhibition. However, only liver disease, especially juvenile hepatitis or cirrhosis, has been definitely linked with α_1AT deficiency.

Juvenile hepatitis or cirrhosis

The association of α_1AT deficiency and idiopathic juvenile cirrhosis was first reported by Sharp et al (1969), who reported 7 children with juvenile cirrhosis who were homozygous deficient for α_1AT. This association has since been confirmed by others. An intensive screening program of 200 000 infants by Sveger (1976) in Norway, revealed 120 infants with severe α_1AT deficiency of whom 14 had prolonged obstructive jaundice, 9 had severe clinical and laboratory evidence of liver disease, and 5 had only laboratory evidence of liver disease. Ninety-eight of the other infants with severe α_1AT deficiency did not have clinical liver disease, but approximately half had abnormal liver function tests.

The variability of occurrence of liver disease in patients with severe α_1AT deficiency suggests that an additional provocative factor may be required. This factor must be one that could induce hepatic inflammation, which ordinarily would be limited by normal levels of α_1AT. We suggested that the presence of Australia antigen (HAA) might be a factor in the development of liver disease in these individuals (Lieberman et al, 1972). Porter et al (1972) found that 3 of 5 infants with neonatal hepatitis and severe α_1AT deficiency had Australia antigen in their serum and that Australia antigen or antibody was present in one or both parents of these children and in the parents of even those children whose serum was negative. Confirmation of this association, however, has not appeared. Bradfield and Wells (1978) postulated that Kupffer cells and their intracellular proteolytic enzymes may be the link between α_1AT deficiency and liver damage. They stated that Kupffer cells tend to release proteolytic enzymes into the liver parenchyma during phagocytosis, and that increased Kupffer cell activity could cause damage if α_1AT is deficient.

The occurrence of liver disease in adults with α_1AT deficiency (severe and intermediate) has also been reported (Campra et al, 1973; Triger et al, 1976; Fisher et al, 1976; Chan et al, 1978; Morin et al, 1975; Kueppers et al, 1976), but the association remains controversial.

α₁AT in cancer

A possible association between cancer and α_1AT deficiency has been sought, since protease inhibitors have been shown to normalize the growth pattern of certain cancer cells (Goetz et al, 1972) and since unlimited nuclear division of neoplastic cells is dependent on protease activity (O'Neill, 1974). To date, only hepatocellular carcinoma has been detected with increased frequency in subjects with α_1AT deficiency. In these patients, α_1AT globules (see discussion below) are found in the hepatoma cells and, in some instances, in their metastases (Lieberman, 1974). Both PiZZ and PiMZ phenotypes have been found in patients with hepatomas. Another type of tumour, the yolk sac or endodermal sinus tumour, has also been found to contain α_1AT globules (Palmer et al, 1976). The human yolk sac was shown to be a site of synthesis of α_1AT as well as of serum albumin, prealbumin and transferrin (Gitlin & Perricelli, 1970).Thus, the presence of α_1AT in yolk sac tumours seems appropriate but unrelated to α_1AT deficiency. Tellerman et al (1977) found that the serum levels of α_1AT and alpha fetoprotein were elevated in patients with yolk sac tumours; the fetoprotein, however, was a better tumour marker than was α_1AT.

Care must be taken when evaluating cellular globules which have immunologic reactivity for α_1AT as being a marker for Pi^Z. Abramowsky et al (1980) detected such globules in an undifferentiated (embryonal) sarcoma of the liver in a 14 year old boy. The globules were shown to contain α_1AT protein by immunofluorescent techniques, but when studied under the EM, the globules consisted of phagolysosomal structures and were therefore distinct from those described in α_1AT deficiency. Abramowsky et al believe that the globules may represent trapping of serum proteins by the malignant cell.

Other diseases

In addition to emphysema, infantile hepatitis and hepatocellular carcinoma, the list of diseases reported in association with α_1AT deficiency has been growing over the years (see Table 66.2). In some instances only a single case was reported, whereas with others multiple conflicting reports have appeared. Glomerulonephritis and angiitis or vasculitis may be associated with α_1AT deficiency, but confirmatory reports are needed. A number of reports claim that rheumatoid arthritis is associated with α_1AT deficiency, but the number of negative reports in this regard is quite large. Fibrosing alveolitis, panniculitis, periodontal disease, anterior uveitis and psoriasis have all been reported in association with α_1AT deficiency, but confirmation is required. In most instances, the rationale behind an association between α_1AT deficiency and a specific tissue damage is thought to be the lack of protection against proteolysis during an inflammatory process.

Methods for detecting α_1AT deficiency

A laboratory manual has been prepared by Talamo et al (1980) that contains methodology and references for most of the current procedures used for testing α_1AT.

Table 66.2 Diseases reported in association with α_1AT deficiency.

Disease	Reference
Multiple cases studied (cumulative)	
Angiitis and glomerulonephritis	Brandrup (1978)
	Miller & Kuschner (1969)
	Lubec et al (1976)
	Moroz et al (1976)
Rheumatoid arthritis	*For an association:*
	Cox & Huber (1976, 1980)
	Buisseret et al (1977)
	Arnaud et al (1977, 1979)
	Against an association:
	Geddes et al (1977)
	Sjoblon & Wollheim (1977)
	Karsh et al (1979)
	Brackertz & Kueppers (1977)
	Walsh & McConkey (1977)
Fibrosing alveolitis	Geddes et al (1977)
Panniculitis	Rubinstein et al (1977)
Anterior uveitis	Brewerton et al (1978)
	Brown et al (1979) – negative report
Peptic ulcer	Andre et al (1975)
	Blenkinsopp (1977) – negative report
	Lieberman (1969) – negative report
Psoriasis	Beckman et al (1980)
Thrombocytopenia &/or platelet function defects	Miale et al (1977)
Reduced C4	LeProvost (1975)
Pre-albumin deficiency	Premachondra & Yu (1979)
IgA deficiency	Casterline et al (1978)
	Robert et al (1979)
Paraproteinaemias	Ananthakrishan et al (1979)
Autism	Walker-Smith & Andrews (1972)
Coeliac disease	Walker-Smith & Andrews (1972)
Glucose intolerance	Santiago (1974)
Chronic pancreatitis	Novis et al (1978)
	Lankisch et al (1978) – negative report
Periodontal disease	Peterson & Marsh (1979)
Hepatocellular carcinoma	Lieberman (1974)
	Palmer & Wolfe (1976)
Single case reports or a family study	
Multisystem fibrosis	Palmer et al (1978)
Extrahepatic bile duct hypoplasia	Christen et al (1975)
Pemphigus vulgaris	Benitz-Bribensca (1972)
Severe combined immuno-deficiency	Gelfand et al (1979)
Hypercholesterolaemia	Victorino et al (1978)
Multiple sclerosis	Samad & O'Connell (1972)
Growth hormone deficiency	Schydlow et al (1979)
Multiple endocrine adenomatosis	Alder et al (1979)
Cystathioninuria and renal iminoglycinuria	Halal et al (1979)
Pancreatic fibrosis	Freeman et al (1976)
Mannosidosis	Perelman et al (1975)
Intestinal mucosal atrophy	Greenwald et al (1975)
Cardiomyopathy	Torp (1975)

Serum protein electrophoresis

Serum protein electrophoresis is the most readily available procedure capable of giving a rough estimate of α_1AT concentration (Lieberman et al, 1969). The severe deficiency can be diagnosed directly by visual evaluation of the electrophoretic scan. A missing or plateau configuration to the α_1-globulin peak on cellulose-acetate-electrophoresis is usually diagnostic of severe α_1AT deficiency. An intermediate deficiency state can also be suggested if the observer is experienced in viewing these scans, but quantitation of the α_1-globulin peak is usually inaccurate, since accurate quantitation of the small α_1-globulin peak can be difficult (Lieberman et al, 1969).

Immunologic assays

Radial immunodiffusion is most commonly used in clinical laboratories for evaluating the α_1AT concentration. The procedure requires a specific antibody against human α_1AT plus accurate standards for quantitation. Electroimmunodiffusion is a more rapid method using the same concepts of antigen-antibody interaction.

Enzymatic assays

Specific enzymatic assays which evaluate α_1AT activity are more rapid than radial immunodiffusion and do not usually require standards with each run. Inhibitory capacity for either trypsin or elastase can be measured. To date, an inactive antitrypsin variant has not been discovered, so that the enzymatic assays and immunologic assays can be used interchangeably. Should an inactive variant of α_1AT be discovered, then both types of quantitative procedures will be required for its detection.

Problems arise with the quantitative measurements when one is particularly interested in detecting individuals with intermediate or heterozygous deficiency states, because the acute-phase-reactive properties of α_1AT cause its blood levels to fluctuate in response to acute illnesses. The α_1AT levels in individuals with a severe deficiency do not respond to these stresses, but the levels with an intermediate deficiency can rise into the low normal range. Some years ago we recommended use of a provocative test with diethylstilbestrol to determine whether the α_1AT was already maximally stimulated in a subject whose α_1AT concentration was in the low normal range; the STIC in a normal person rose above 1.2 units, but remained below 1.2 units in a person with intermediate α_1AT deficiency (Lieberman et al, 1971). However, provocative testing has not been required since the advent of Pi phenotyping.

Protease inhibitor (Pi) typing

α_1AT phenotyping was discovered by Fagerhol of Norway (1968). He determined that α_1AT was a polymorphic protein with molecular variants that had different mobilities on acid-starch gel electrophoresis. With this procedure, the α_1AT protein breaks up into at least 5 peaks

in the acid gradient; these include 3 major peaks and 2 minor peaks. The pattern of these peaks is similar for most variants of α_1AT, but the variants usually differ in their mobility towards the anode. The difference in mobility of these peaks may be due to differences in sialic acid content (Yoshida & Wessels, 1978), but each of the 5 α_1AT peaks retains antitrypsin activity (Langley & Talamo ,1975).

Fagerhol has named the polymorphism of α_1AT the 'Pi' (Protease inhibitor) system and has developed the following nomenclature: Pi^M is the most frequently described form of α_1AT which has medium mobility in an acid gradient. Variants with faster mobility have been assigned letters lower than M in the alphabet, and variants with slower mobility have been assigned letters higher than M in the alphabet. A meeting was held in Rouen, France in 1978 to standardize the nomenclature for the Pi system and for determining specific methods for assigning names to newly discovered variants (Cox et al, 1980). Figures 66.1a and b are taken from Cox et al's report of this meeting and show the most current summary of variants of α_1AT and the names applied to the variants. The standard for assigning a letter to a variant is basically dependent upon its mobility on isoelectric focusing in a pH range of 3–5. In spite of the apparent complexity of the Pi system and the rather large number of variants described to date (approximately 30), the system is really simple and practical for detecting deficient variants. Most disease states have been associated with the Z variant whose characteristics are summarized in Table 66.3. The homozygous Z phenotype causes a severe deficiency of α_1AT, whereas the heterozygous Z phenotype (MZ) causes intermediate deficiency. Heterozygous or homozygous phenotypes, which include the other slightly deficient variants (I, P, S), can occasionally cause intermediate deficiency states. Other severely deficient variants reported include only a 'null' gene, the Mduarte (Lieberman et al, 1976) and Mmalton (Cox, 1975) variants. The Mduarte variant resembles the Pi^Z form in its clinical effects but cannot be detected directly by Pi typing since it has normal mobility. Examples of 'Pi' typing patterns on isoelectric focusing are shown in

Table 66.3 Characteristics of the Pi^Z variant of α_1AT.

PiZZ phenotype – causes severe deficiency of α_1AT.
PiMZ phenotype – causes intermediate deficiency of α_1AT.
Hepatic globules – PiZZ and PiMZ associated with hepatocytic globules – PAS positive, diastase resistant, immunologically related to α_1AT, in RER under the electron microscope.
Acid gradient electrophoresis
  Slow mobility; low concentration.
Increased heat lability
Reduced content of sialic acid
  None in PiZ from liver
  Half normal in PiZ from serum
Serum levels do not rise in response to oestrogens or other 'acute-phase-reactant' stimuli

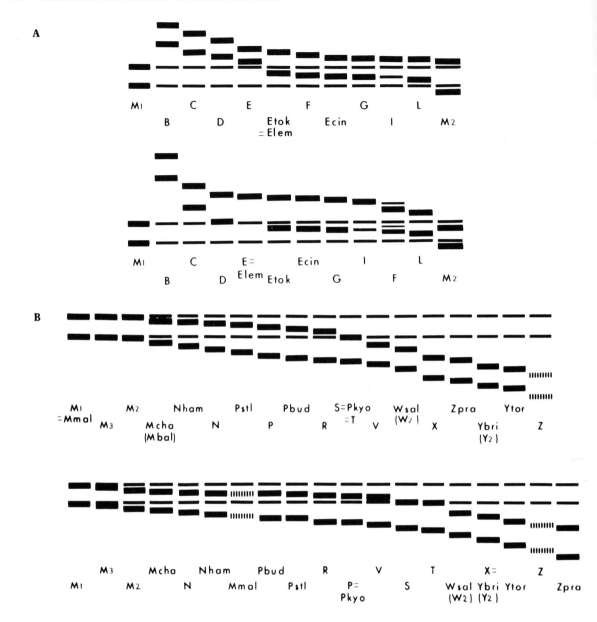

Fig. 66.1 Pi variants showing the two major bands of each variant. Top: acid starch gel electrophoresis. Bottom: isoelectric focusing in acrylamide. Narrow bands indicate position of M1. Dashed bands indicate deficiency alleles. (a) variants anodal to M; (b) variants cathodal to M. From Cox et al (1980), with permission of the author and publisher.

Figure 66.2 and some crossed immunoelectrophoresis patterns are shown in Figure 66.3.

$\alpha_1 AT$ globules in hepatocytes

Sharp (1971) was the first to detect the presence of globules in the hepatocytes of children with juvenile cirrhosis and homozygous (ZZ) $\alpha_1 AT$ deficiency. These globules stained with PAS, were immunoreactive for $\alpha_1 AT$, and were diastase resistant. We subsequently detected similar globules in the liver of adult patients without liver disease who were carriers of the Z variant (both homozygous and heterozygous) (Lieberman et al, 1972; Gordon et al, 1972). The presence of these globules has since been accepted as reflecting the Pi^Z variant, and the globules have been shown to contain inactive PiZ $\alpha_1 AT$ (Matsubara et al, 1974) within rough endoplasmic reticulum (RER) as seen under the electron-microscope (EM). These globules were found mainly periportally and var-

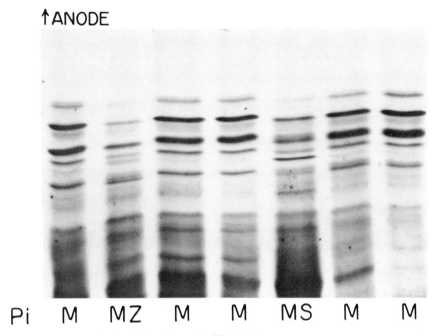

Fig. 66.2 Pi type patterns as seen on isoelectric focusing gels (pH 3.0–5.0).

ied considerably in size and concentration in different parts of a liver or in livers from different individuals. It is believed that the liver globules result from a block in release of incompletely synthesized $\alpha_1 AT$ of the Z variant. The Pi^{Mduarte} variant also was found to be associated with similar liver globules, resembling the Pi^Z variant in this respect (Lieberman et al, 1976).

Detection of the $\alpha_1 AT$ liver globules has been used in some post-mortem studies to link hepatoma, cirrhosis or emphysema with $\alpha_1 AT$ (Pi^Z) deficiency. Recently, some words of caution have been expressed regarding the specificity of the liver globules, since similar globules were seen in some individuals with normal PiMM phenotypes and normal levels of $\alpha_1 AT$ (Fisher et al, 1976; Bradfield & Blenkinsopp, 1977; Reintoft, 1979) and in a patient with a PiS phenotype (Kelly et al, 1979). Reintoft (1979) found that these 'non-$\alpha_1 AT$' globules were located primarily around central veins and were of almost uniform size in contrast to the $\alpha_1 AT$ globules which were found periportally and usually varied in size. The non-$\alpha_1 AT$ globules in some instances showed antigenicity for $\alpha_1 AT$, but more consistently showed antigenicity for IgG. Under the EM, the non-$\alpha_1 AT$ globules appeared to be composed of loose or compact granular material within lysosomal structures and thus to differ from $\alpha_1 AT$ globules which are found inside dilated RER (Reintoft, 1979). It would appear that EM studies of the liver are necessary to specifically identify the $\alpha_1 AT$ globules even though the globules may show antigenicity for $\alpha_1 AT$.

The non-$\alpha_1 AT$ globules seen in hepatocytes may result from hepatic congestion or may reflect hyaline necrosis of the liver (Kern et al, 1969).

Sites of synthesis for $\alpha_1 AT$

Although the liver is the primary site of synthesis for $\alpha_1 AT$, a number of other sites have been found where $\alpha_1 AT$ appears to localize. These sites include the pancreatic islet cells (McElrath et al, 1979; Rea & Desmet, 1978; Rea et al, 1977), mast cells (Rea & Desmet, 1978), polymorphonuclear leucocytes (Briebiesca & Horta, 1977), platelets (Bagdasarian & Colman, 1978), and the surface of mitogen-stimulated human lymphocytes (Lipsky et al, 1979). In the pancreatic islets, the immunoreactive $\alpha_1 AT$ is localized to the peripheral cells of the islets, but the immunostaining of these islet cells becomes less intense the longer the paraffin embedded tissues are stored. In platelets, the protease inhibitor resembles $\alpha_1 AT$ in its antigenic identity and molecular weight (Bagdasarian & Colman, 1978). $\alpha_1 AT$ was localized to the platelet granules, but a considerable amount was membrane bound.

The presence of $\alpha_1 AT$ antigenic material in the plasma of polymorphonuclear leucocytes and monocytes suggests that the intracytoplasmic proteases of these phagocytic cells may be held inactive by the inhibitor, but it is not known whether these cells synthesize their own $\alpha_1 AT$.

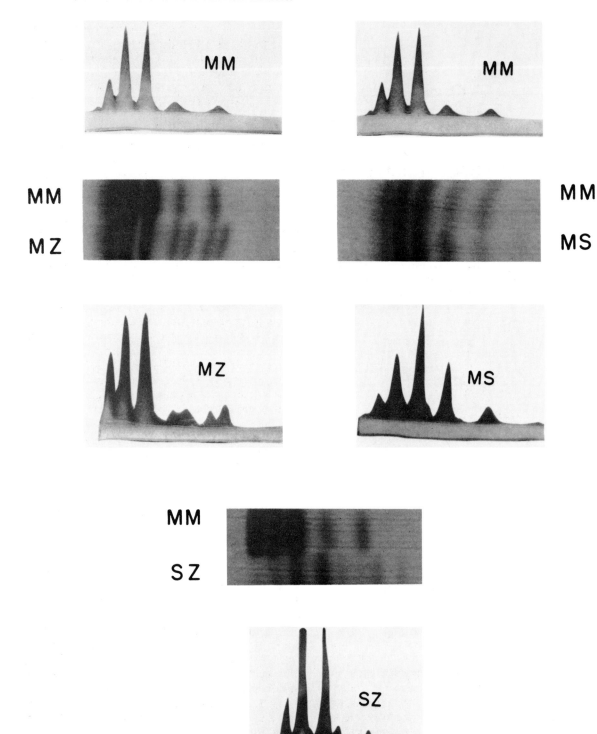

Fig. 66.3 Common Pi type patterns as seen by immunofixation of acid-starch gel electrophoresis and by crossed antigen-antibody electrophoresis.

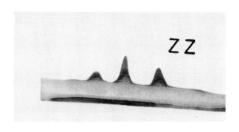

ZZ

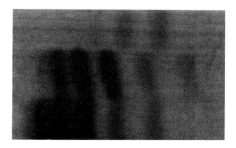

ZZ

SS

MM

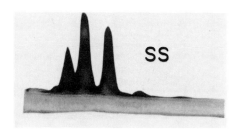

SS

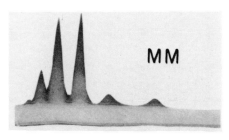

MM

Fig. 66.3 (cont'd)

Genetics of α_1AT

One of the few non-controversial aspects of α_1AT is the statement that α_1AT is inherited via two codominant autosomal alleles. The Pi^M allele is the major form of α_1AT detected in all populations studied. The prevalence of the other variants, especially the Pi^S, Pi^Z and Pi^F, varies within different populations and they provide an excellent tool for genetic studies of populations. Table 66.4 lists the allele frequencies for the M, S, Z and F forms of antitrypsin in the various populations and ethnic groups studied to date. A number of broad conclusions can be drawn from these data:

1. The Pi^S allele has its highest prevalence in Spain and Portugal. The next highest rates are seen in Frenchmen from the middle South of France and in French Canadians. This association tends to point out the origin of French Canadians, and also reflects the ethnic origin of the Southern French people to Spain and Portugal. Similarly, the Pi^S allele is more predominant in the southern part of the Netherlands (below the Rhine) than the northern part (Dijkman et al, 1980). Since prehistoric times, the Rhine has formed the ethnic border between Saxons and Franks; this may be the reason for differences in Pi types between populations on either bank of the river. Dijkman et al also observed clustering of α_1AT deficiency in small rural communities in which the populations move relatively little and consanguinity may have played a role. As one travels further north in Europe, the prevalence of Pi^S decreases considerably. The Pi^S gene is absent among orientals and African blacks.

2. The Pi^Z allele has a lower prevalence in the south of Europe, in Lapps from either Finland, Norway or Sweden, and among the Dutch from northeast Holland. The Pi^Z is essentially absent in African Blacks, Orientals and Indians. It has an unusually high frequency among the Maoris of New Zealand. Janus et al (1975) discussed the possible association of the high Pi^Z frequency in Maoris with the high incidence of chronic respiratory disease and liver disease in these people. The incidence of cirrhosis and hepatomas in male Maoris ranks third highest in the world after Polynesian Hawaiians and Hawaii Chinese. Janus and Carrell (1975) have published some clinical studies of the diseases found in Maoris with severe antitrypsin deficiency, and hopefully they will follow up with similar studies in the heterozygotes.

3. The Pi^F variant has an overall lower frequency than Pi^S or Pi^Z wherever it has been studied, but seems to be essentially missing from Spain and Portugal. Apparent Pi^F antitrypsin bands sometimes appear with old sera, so that the frequency of Pi^F may be overestimated in some studies.

4. The increased frequency of Pi^X in Malaysians is of interest (frequency of 0.007); it was not found among the Chinese or Indians of the same country.

It would appear that the Pi^Z variant, which is the variant most commonly associated with deficient serum levels of α_1AT, is primarily found in Caucasians of northern European extraction, as well as in the New Zealand Maoris. Studies performed in our laboratory a number of years ago suggested that Americans derived from northern and central European countries had an increased prevalence of intermediate antitrypsin deficiency as compared to others from the Mediterranean area, Blacks, Mexican-Americans, or those of American-Indian extraction. These studies were done on Americans

Table 66.4 Gene frequencies for Pi^M, Pi^S, Pi^Z and Pi^F for various populations.

Population	No.	Pi^M	Pi^S	Pi^Z	Pi^F	Reference
Spain	378	0.866	0.112	0.012	0.003	Fagerhol & Tenfjord (1968)
	576	0.881	0.114	0.005	0	Goedde et al (1973)
Portugal	36	0.859	0.141	0	0	Fagerhol & Tenfjord (1968)
	189	0.920	0.059	0.023	0	Geada et al (1976)
	330	0.865	0.115	0.018	0	Martin et al (1976)
Greece	504	0.960	0.028	0.002*	0.006	Fertakis et al (1974)
	400	0.959	0.003	0.016	0.013	Kellermann & Walter (1970)
Germany	262	0.967	0.023	0.019	0.010	Goedde et al (1970)
	517	0.879	0.021	0.009	0.090	Kellermann & Walter (1970)
	200	0.980	0.020	0.003	0.003	Kueppers (1971)
	229	0.961	0.024	0.011	0.004	Kuhn & Spielmann (1979)
Italy (North)	202	0.951	0.030	0.010	0.007	Klasen et al (1978)
Poland	3560	0.982	0.016	0.001	0.001	Szczeklik et al (1974)
France						
Normandy	394	0.901	0.066	0.022	0.009	Morin et al (1975)
Lyon	1653	0.902	0.071	0.014	0.004	Arnaud et al (1977)
Brittany	280	0.896	0.075	0.023	0.004	Sesboue et al (1978)
Other	1520	0.910	0.079	0.006*	0.001	Robinet-Levy & Rieunier (1972)
	934	0.983	0.019	0.001*	0.006	Vandeville et al (1972)
French-Canadians	390	0.892	0.092	0.006	0	Joly et al (1980)
United Kingdom	5237	0.930	0.050	0.014*	0	Cook (1975)
Southern England	926	0.924	0.048	0.022	0.002	Arnaud et al (1979)
Northern Ireland	1000	0.936	0.039	0.020	0.002	Blundell et al (1975)
Netherlands	708	0.956	0.030	0.005	0.006	Klasen et al (1977)
	1474	0.828	0.016	0.012	0.002	Hoffman & van den Broek (1976) Dijkman et al (1980)
Finland	548	0.966	0.017	0.014	0.002	Arnaud et al (1977)
	223	0.9955	0	0.005	0	Fagerhol et al (1969)
	300	0.972	0.015	0.013	0	Beckman et al (1980)
Norway	2830	0.946	0.023	0.016	0.013	Fagerhol (1967)
Sweden	1869	0.981	0.010	0.008	0.0003	Beckman et al (1980)
Lapps						
Finnish	468	0.996	0.003	0.001	0	Fagerhol et al (1969)
Norwegian	302	0.992	0	0.008	0	Fagerhol et al (1969)
Swedish	217	0.995	0.005	0	0	Beckman et al (1980)
Canada	426	0.928	0.048	0.016	0	Moroz et al (1976)
	360	0.960	0.036	0.004	0	Ostrow et al (1978)
USA (Whites)	1381	0.937	0.043	0.014	0.001	Lieberman et al (1976)
	1933	0.948	0.036	0.012	0	Pierce et al (1975)
Japan	100	1.000	0	0	0	Roberts et al (1977)
	1271	1.000	0	0	0	Miyake et al (1979)
Malaysia						
Malaysians[†]	908	0.979	0.015	0	0	Lie-Injo et al (1978)
Chinese	371	0.981	0.019	0	0	" " "
Indians	231	0.976	0.024	0	0	" " "
Blacks						
Mozambique	274	0.982	0.002	0	0.164	Kellerman & Walter (1970)
American	186	0.989	0.008	0	0	Lieberman et al (1976)
" "	204	0.980	0.010	0.005	0	Pierce et al (1975)
Bantu	132	1.000	0	0	0	Vandeville et al (1974)
The Gambia (West Africa)	701	1.000	0	0	0	Welch et al (1980)
New Zealand Maori	487	0.959	0.005	0.035	0.001	Janus et al (1975)
American Indians	230	0.939	0.039	0.004*	0.010	Vandeville et al (1972)
Thailand	852	0.963	0.018	0.011	0.006	Pongpaew & Schelp (1980)

* Pi^Z may be underestimated due to technical limitations.

[†] $Pi^X = 0.007$

by taking histories of ethnic and national background, and by measuring serum-trypsin-inhibitor-capacity (Mittman & Lieberman, 1973)

One important practical point related to these national studies is that all investigations to determine the prevalence of α_1AT deficiency-states in a specific disease must have adequate control studies for the specific population being investigated. It would be foolhardy to compare an experimental group from one area to a control population from another.

The recent discovery of subtypes of the Pi^M (M1, M2 and M3) has expanded the capabilities for utilizing α_1AT as a tool in genetics. Unfortunately, the terminology has not been standardized, and papers are being published with different names for the Pi^M subtypes. The terminology suggested by Frants and Eriksson (1978) will most likely become the standard. Frants and Eriksson found that the Pi^{M2} allele was rather high in Finns (0.12) but low in west African Bozo (0.04). The Pi^{M3} was found with a frequency of 0.3 in Dutch, 0.08 in Finns and 0.02 in Bozo. Frants and Eriksson discuss the validity of using this Pi^M polymorphism for population genetic studies, linkage analysis and parentage testing. Many laboratories are still having difficulty in detecting the three major subtypes of PiM; apparently the ability to detect these subtypes varies with different batches of polyacrilamide used in the gel (Kueppers, personal communication). I will not review in detail the literature that has already appeared in this area, since it would be premature; a discussion of the Pi^M subtypes is a topic for future review.

Genetic linkage studies with α_1AT

The α_1AT (Pi) and immunoglobulin-G (Gm) loci have been shown to be linked autosomally with a recombination fraction of 19% in males and 26% in females. (Gedde-Dahl et al, 1972, 1975). Attempts to link further the Pi system to chromosomal markers have not been successful; Schmidt et al (1975) showed no linkage to chromosomal markers or to four polymorphic red cell antigens, or to HLA antigens. They concluded that the Pi locus does not appear to be on chromosomes 2, 3, 13, 14, 21 or 22 within measurable distance of the markers used. Noades and Cook (1976) eliminated the possibility of linkage between Gm or Pi and the markers A-Hp, S-ec, ACP₁ or Gc, and Weitkamp et al (1976) found no indication for linkage between Pi and the red cell acid phosphatase gene. Weitkamp et al (1978) also confirmed the linkage established by Gedde-Dahl between Pi and Gm and found evidence for a difference in recombination frequency between males heterozygous for PiMZ vs PiMS. They postulated that the altered gene for Pi^Z may affect recombination of the two variant forms. Fagerhol (1976) further discussed the genetics of α_1AT and its implications.

Segregation distortion for the Pi^Z allele was reported simultaneously by two laboratories (Iammarino et al, 1979; Chapuis-Cellier & Arnaud, 1979). Both groups reported a significant increase in PiMZ offspring in families where the male parent was MZ. In contrast, when the mother carried the Z allele, the distribution of phenotypes in the children did not differ significantly from the expected frequency. These observations suggest that a selective advantage is associated with the expression of the Pi^Z allele in male gametes. Dr Diane Cox (1980) questions the interpretation of these data since she has found errors in the calculations due to failure to correct for ascertainment bias. In addition, data from Cox's laboratory failed to show the marked segregation difference between mothers and fathers carrying the Z variant. Mittman (1980) also could not demonstrate the occurrence of segregation distortion in 19 families studied. The question regarding segregation distortion for the Pi^Z variant remains an open question, and further studies are necessary.

α_1AT and chromosome aberrations

Aarskog and Fagerhol (1970) examined Pi phenotypes in 32 Norwegian families where chromosome aberrations had been found. Of 7 families with sex chromosome mosaics, 5 had Pi phenotypes other than the most common MM type; FM, MS and SS were found in unexpectedly high numbers in these families. Kueppers et al (1975) confirmed these findings in the families of 21 patients with sex chromosome mosaicism. The prevalence of heterozygotes among the parents of patients with sex chromosome mosaicism was significantly higher than in control populations and included MF, MS and MZ phenotypes. They could not discern whether the higher prevalence for heterozygosity was due to the contribution of the mother or the father to the total group. Fineman et al (1976) provided additional data to support these studies and suggested that decreased α_1AT activity may also be an aetiologic factor in trisomy 21. They suggested that a practical benefit of these observations may be the identification by α_1AT phenotyping of individuals with a significantly increased risk of producing children with chromosome abnormalities.

Effects of α_1AT deficiency on reproduction

α_1AT deficiency has been suspected of enhancing reproductive capacity since penetration of cervical mucus and fertilization of the ovum by spermatozoa involve the enzymatic action of both acrosomal hyaluronidase and proteases. Increased proteolytic activity by sperm or reduced inhibition could increase penetrability of the ovum and thereby increase fertility. The content of proteolytic enzyme inhibitors in cervical mucus also varies with the menstrual cycle so that the protease inhibitor level is lowest during the female's most fertile interval (Schumacher & Pearl, 1965). Thus, an inborn reduction in protease inhibitory activity could theoretically enhance the opportunity for sperm penetration and fertilization.

Fagerhol and Gedde-Dahl (1969) found a deficiency of the normal $MM \times MM$ genotype combinations in families selected for large family size, suggesting that individuals with α_1AT variants may have a high fertility. They found that heterozygosity for α_1AT occurred more frequently among mothers than fathers. An increased number of individuals with reduced α_1AT activity were also detected among twins and parents of twins (Lieberman et al, 1979); both monozygotic and dizygotic twins had the same prevalence of α_1AT deficiency. It is therefore possible that both increased fertility and twinning may be heterozygote advantages in α_1AT deficiency. Aarskog et al (1978) performed α_1AT Pi typing on 30 couples suffering recurrent miscarriages, and found only 2 couples with Pi heterozygosity in both partners, which was possibly entirely fortuitous. The observation is rather remarkable, however, and might imply a possible relationship to fetal wastage in such couples.

Molecular structure of α_1AT variants
Studies of the amino acid and carbohydrate content of human α_1AT from serum and liver show no gross variations between the normal M type and the Z type, except for the sialic acid content. (See Lieberman (1980) for a summary of these studies). Sialic is reduced from 7 residues per molecule in Pi^M to 3 residues per molecule in Pi^Z from serum, and is totally lacking in Pi^Z from liver. Hercz et al (1978) also studied the Z variant isolated from human liver and, contrary to previous findings, found an absence of both galactose and sialic acid, an appreciable decrease in N-acetyl glucosamine, and an almost twofold increase in mannose residues. Hercz et al, calculated that the Z protein from liver contains only three oligosaccharides with 2 N-acetyl glucosamines and 7 mannose residues per chain. They stated that the presence of only 3 oligosaccharides in this protein indicates an interference with glycosylation of a particular asparagine residue which could be the consequence of an amino acid substitution in the Z variant protein. Transfer of core carbohydrates from lipid bound to protein oligosaccharide can take place only in the rough endoplasmic reticulum (RER) so that glycoproteins may not be free to leave the RER until the process is completed. Thus, defective glycosylation may interfere with the passage of glycoproteins from the RER to the smooth endoplasmic reticulum (SER) and lead to stagnation of the liver Z variant in the RER. It is possible that the enzyme, which should remove excess mannose, resides in the SER, so that the extra mannose remains as long as the Z variant is confined to the RER. Hercz et al, further stated that some of the liver Z variant molecules may become fully glyco-

sylated and subsequently leave the RER thereby providing a small amount of Z variant in the serum with a carbohydrate composition similar to that of the M variant. Hercz et al's observations indicate that the microheterogeneity of α_1AT is not due to uneven sialylation, but rather due to variations in the content of charged amino acids in the isoproteins. A number of α_1AT variants have been purified and analyzed by peptide finger-printing and amino acid analysis. Table 66.5 lists these variants and the amino acid substitutions causing the microheterogeneity. In most instances, a glutamic acid is replaced by another amino acid; lysine in the Pi^Z, valine in the Pi^S, aspartic acid in $Pi^{Balhambra}$ and in Pi^{M2}.

Yoshida and Wessels (1980) have studied the sialic acid content of the multiple components of the human α_1AT pattern obtained in acid-starch gel electrophoresis. They found that the most acidic components contained more sialic acid per molecule than the basic components. The molecular sizes of these components were identical, excluding the possibility of polymerization of α_1AT during electrophoresis. Therefore, the multiple components of the inhibitor are primarily due to differences in the sialic acid content of each component so that the 3 major components contain 8, 7 and 6 sialic acid residues per molecule respectively.

Induction of α_1AT deficiency in animal models
A large body of literature has appeared regarding the experimental induction of pulmonary emphysema by protease administration to animals. The field was recently reviewed by Karlinsky and Snider (1978) in a State of the Art article. The two enzymes most capable of producing emphysema in animals are papain and elastase. The emphysema-producing effects of papain were actually shown by Snider et al (1974) to be related to the elastolytic content of the enzyme preparation rather than its esterolytic activity. Enzymes without elastolytic activity are not effective for producing experimental emphysema. The experiments suggest that destruction of lung

Table 66.5 Amino acid substitutions in variants of α_1AT.

α_1AT variant	Reference	Pi^M	Amino acid variant
Z	Yoshida et al (1976) Jeppson et al (1976)	Glutamic acid	Lysine
S	Yoshida et al (1977) Owen & Carrell (1976)	Glutamic acid	Valine
Balhambra	Yoshida et al (1979)	Glutamic acid Lysine	Aspartic acid Aspartic acid
		Pi^{M1}	
M2	Yoshida et al (1979)	Glutamic acid	Aspartic acid

elastin is basic to the development of pulmonary emphysema in both experimental animals and man.

Most animal models use papain or elastase alone to induce emphysema. A somewhat different approach was used by Blackwood et al (1979) in which D-galactosamine was administered to rats to produce a transient reduction in serum-elastase inhibitory capacity, and thereby to enhance the development of emphysema from intravenous injections of pancreatic elastase. The degree of severity of the emphysema correlated with the trypsin- and elastase-inhibitory capacities at the time of the elastase injection. D-galactosamine apparently causes a transient reduction in serum α_1AT concentration by impairing protein synthesis from the liver. This type of experiment resembles somewhat the transient effects that cigarette smoke might have on α_1AT function, thereby enhancing the tendency to damage the lungs and induce emphysema.

Proteolytic enzymes themselves can inactivate α_1AT when present in excess. Baumstark et al (1977) demonstrated a rapid inactivation of α_1AT by elastase, and similar effects were shown with bacterial proteinases (Lieberman et al, 1975; Moskowitz & Heinrich, 1971; Morihara et al, 1979) so that antitrypsin inactivation could play a role in the tissue destruction associated with severe infection and inflammation. Sandhaus and Janoff (1974) showed that hepatocyte acid cathepsins were also capable of degrading human α_1AT, however the significance of this phenomenon is questionable, since the acid pH required for demonstrating cathepsin activity can itself degrade the α_1AT (Carrico et al, 1976).

Role of intermediate α_1AT deficiency state in predisposing to pulmonary disease

An editorial by Mittman (1978) recently reviewed the significance of the PiMZ phenotype as a risk factor for chronic obstructive lung disease. The role has been hotly debated over the past 12 years, although the argument seems rather academic if we believe that an acquired or relative deficiency of α_1AT contributes to the pathogenesis of emphysema. A lower baseline level of α_1AT would certainly enhance the detrimental actions of cigarette smoke in altering the protease to protease-inhibitor balance.

Four methods have been used for evaluating the significance of intermediate α_1AT deficiency as a predisposing factor for lung disease. These are:

1. Determining the prevalence of intermediate α_1AT deficiency among patients with pulmonary emphysema

This was the first type of study that incriminated an intermediate deficiency of α_1AT as predisposing to emphysema. From 4 to 25% of patients with emphysema were found to have an intermediate deficiency in various studies. Most recently, Matzen et al (1977) reported 8

variants of α_1AT among 35 patients with COPD (23%) as compared to 13% with α_1AT variants among 426 patients without respiratory disease. More specifically, Lochon et al (1978) detected 25% of his emphysematous patients to have an MZ phenotype. Lebeau and Rochemure (1978) also claim to have confirmed the pathogenetic role of the MZ phenotype.

2. Detection of abnormal pulmonary function in subjects with intermediate α_1AT deficiency in general populations

The majority of such studies have failed to show significant abnormalities of pulmonary physiology among random individuals found to have an MZ or intermediate α_1AT deficiency state. The most recent studies showing either negative (Chan-Yeung et al, 1978; Ostrow et al, 1978; McDonagh et al, 1979; Buist et al, 1979; Pride et al, 1980; Horton et al, 1980) or positive (Kanner et al, 1979; Larson et al, 1977) findings are referenced. Larson et al (1977) studied a representative population of 50 year old men in Sweden. They found that non-smoking PiMZ subjects did not differ from non-smoking PiM controls, whereas smoking heterozygotes showed a significant loss of elastic recoil, enlarged residual volumes, and increased closing capacity, but no signs of obstructive ventilatory impairment. Most of these smoking PiMZ individuals reported mild exertional dyspnoea. This study is nearly ideal in that the subjects were old enough to have allowed the detrimental effects of cigarette smoking and deficient α_1AT to become discernible. In another recent study, Kozarevic et al (1978) found an apparent physiologic impairment associated with the Pi^Z heterozygosity that produced a shift in the relationships between the different lung volumes without overall hyperinflation, namely, an increase in residual volume at the expense of vital capacity. However, Kozarevic et al did not feel that the Pi^Z gene accounted for much of the COPD found in their population due to the low prevalence of the Pi^Z gene (less than 1%).

The difficulties in obtaining significant information in this type of study are discussed in detail by Mittman (1978). The important aspects of his discussion relate to the likelihood that patients with the MZ phenotype may already have become symptomatic and have removed themselves from the so-called 'healthy' population. In addition, Mittman argues that if the overall risk for developing emphysema is 5% in a general population, and if the MZ phenotype merely doubles the risk, then one would expect that 10% of subjects with the MZ phenotype will have emphysema and 90% will not. Such studies therefore would have trouble proving a significant association.

3. Longitudinal studies

Longitudinal studies should be effective in providing

meaningful data, especially if the population being followed is divided into smokers and non-smokers, since α_1AT deficiency should increase the rate of lung deterioration over a period of time. Ostrow and Cherniack (1972) have shown that changes in lung elasticity due to ageing may be accelerated in the heterozygous state. In a more recent study, Kanner et al (1979) observed that COPD patients with higher levels of α_1AT had more favourable rates of change of FVC and FEV_1 over a 2 to 6 year period of follow up. The actual phenotype was not determined in this study. In contrast, Horton et al (1980) followed 68 PiMZ subjects and a group of matched controls over a 6 year period but found no statistically significant differences between the mean spirometric parameters.

4. Detection of α_1AT deficiency at autopsy by the presence of α_1AT globules in hepatocytes

In this type of study, one assumes that the majority of individuals with α_1AT hepatocytic globules at autopsy are heterozygotes for the Z gene. Aagenaes et al (1972) state the homozygotes can be distinguished from heterozygotes by the percentage of hepatocytes containing globules. Homozygotes were found to have 20 to 70% positive hepatocytes, whereas the heterozygotes had a maximum of 5% hepatocytes with globules. Erkisson et al (1975) found macroscopic emphysema in 50% of 26 subjects having positive liver inclusions as compared to a prevalence of 18% with macroscopic emphysema among 100 PAS negative subjects. Reintoft (1977) in a similar study found that 10 of 15 subjects (67%) positive for the hepatic globules exhibited post-mortem signs of chronic pulmonary disease of varying severity.

It would appear from all that has been written regarding the role of intermediate antitrypsin deficiency in the pathogenesis of pulmonary emphysema that nothing definite can be decided by surveys of healthy populations. Logic plus the findings of an increased prevalence of intermediate antitrypsin deficiency among patients with pulmonary emphysema must dictate what our attitude should be in consulting with patients having this degree of deficiency. I consider those with intermediate α_1AT deficiency to have an increased predisposition to lung damage, and I give them stern warning that they must not smoke cigarettes nor expose themselves to unusual lung pollutants or irritations. It is certainly possible that other genetic or environmental factors may contribute to the development of lung disease in certain individuals with intermediate α_1AT deficiency as compared to others (Kueppers et al, 1977). One such variable may be the inherited level of leucocytic protease; this will be discussed below.

Treatment of α_1AT deficiency

There is no 'practical' method for treating a genetic deficiency of α_1AT at this time. However, a number of different approaches are being considered, and these are as follows:

Use of purified human α_1AT

The defect that produces a deficiency of circulating α_1AT seems clearly to be the result of defective biosynthesis and release of α_1AT from the liver. No differences in catabolic rates have been detected between the Z and the normal M protein (Laurell et al, 1977; Glaser et al, 1977; Kueppers & Fallat, 1969). Because of this, and since intravenously injected α_1AT is preferentially deposited within the lungs (Moser et al, 1978; Makino & Reed, 1970; Ishibashi et al, 1978), it would appear that use of purified human α_1AT therapeutically has rationale. However, the half-life of α_1AT is relatively short, from 3 to 6 days (Makino & Reed, 1970; Moser et al, 1978; Jones et al, 1978; Yu and Gan, 1978; Kueppers & Fallat 1969; Glaser et al, 1977; Laurell et al, 1977), and the material is relatively expensive, so that such therapy would seem to be impractical at this time.

Cohen (1979) calculated that an initial loading dose of 15 grams of α_1AT would be necessary to increase the blood concentration in severely deficient individuals to that found in normal persons. Additional injections of 7.4 grams every 5 days would then be necessary to maintain this normal concentration. If there were 100% efficiency in obtaining α_1AT, the regimen would require approximately 850 units of blood per year for fractionation. Dr Cohen was left with the feeling that the replacement of α_1AT was an impossible task. However, Cohen states that enough of α_1AT is discarded during commercial fractionation of albumin and gamma globulin in the United States each year, so it might not be as impossible a task as he had originally thought.

Use of synthetic elastase inhibitors

Synthetic elastase inhibitors would have the benefit of specifically inhibiting elastase, of having the capability of being produced in large amount and for a cheaper price, and of having a longer half-life than the natural α_1AT. Dr James C. Powers of Atlanta, Georgia, has been a leader in efforts to produce useful synthetic inhibitors for therapy (Powers et al, 1977), but such compounds have not been used therapeutically to the present time. The synthetic inhibitors primarily studied till now have been chloromethyl ketones. Kleinerman et al (1980) tested one of these compounds (alanyl-alanyl-prolyl-alanine) for its effect on the experimental induction of emphysema in hamsters with elastase, and found: (1) it had significant antielastase activity in vivo, (2) it markedly decreased the extent of elastase-induced emphysema, and (3) it did not produce any adverse toxic effects on the hamster. The chemical was administered intraperitoneally to the hamster prior to and immediately after the intratracheal instillation of elastase. Janoff and Dearing (1980) tested the effectiveness of another chloromethyl ketone (methyloxysuccinal-alanyl-alanyl-prolyl-valine-chloromethyl ketone) for prevention of experimental emphysema in mice and found that those mice receiving the chloromethyl ketone within 15 minutes before instillation of intratracheal elastase were protected from the development of emphysema. In contrast, however, no significant protection was afforded by treatment with chloromethyl ketone one hour or more before challenge with the elastase, or at any time after challenge.

This approach to the treatment of α_1AT deficiency most likely will be limited by the potential toxicity of these compounds when administered over prolonged intervals. The inhibitors must also be shown to be effective when administered after the pathologic lung changes have already begun.

Stimulation of α_1AT production by the liver

α_1AT is an acute-phase-reactant-protein whose synthesis and serum levels fluctuate in response to certain stresses placed upon the human organism. Shulman et al (1952) found that elevation of trypsin inhibition was a non-specific indicator of disease and tissue destruction. Abnormal elevation of trypsin inhibition had the same significance as an elevated fibrinogen concentration or an elevation of the sedimentation rate. With this knowledge in mind, our laboratory (Lieberman & Mittman, 1973) and Kueppers (1968) studied the ability of diethylstilbesterol and typhoid vaccine respectively, to stimulate α_1AT levels in individuals with antitrypsin deficiency (ZZ and MZ, etc.). We both found that PiMZ heterozygotes showed half the normal response to these stimuli, and that individuals with the homozygous PiZZ deficiency did not respond at all.

Brown and Pollack (1970) studied the direct effects anti-inflammatory drugs on elastase and collagenase and found variable effects induced by both non-steroidal and steroidal anti-inflammatory drugs. Only phenylbutazone inhibited elastase, steroids had no effect, and other drugs (ASA, indomethacin, etc.) induced activation of the proteases. These studies did not look at an effect on α_1AT. More recently, Pitt and Lewis (1979) found that low doses of hydrocortisone and prednisone caused an elevation of plasma α_1AT in the rat without any adverse effects on the liver. A similar effect in man has not been observed (Lieberman, personal observation).

Dickinson et al (1969) tested the effect of testosterone treatment on various plasma proteins and amino acids in man and found that testosterone decreased trypsin-inhibitor levels. However, Gadek et al (1980) used the synthetic androgen Danazol^R and found that it induced the hepatocyte to increase production of various proteins; α_1AT levels rose from an approximate mean of 30 mg/dl to approximately 45 mg/dl in individuals with homozygous Z or MduarteZ phenotypes. The α_1AT in one SZ individual rose from approximately 83 mg/ml to 160 mg/ml indicating that the S variant is more capable of

responding to Danazol^R and also to diethylstilbesterol (see Lieberman & Mittman, 1973). Gadek et al claim that Danazol^R may provide a means of improving the antiprotease balance in α_1AT deficient individuals and thereby impede the progression of their lung disease. However, I do not believe that the minimal increase in antitrypsin concentration reported in these patients is enough for a protective action.

Liver transplantation

Sharp et al (1971) were the first to show that α_1AT deficiency can be corrected completely by liver transplantation. Unfortunately, few of these patients survived for any length of time. Putnam et al (1977) replaced the liver in a 16 year old girl with advanced cirrhosis and severe α_1AT deficiency, converting the phenotype to that of the donor (PiMM), and raising the recipient's serum levels of α_1AT to normal. When the liver was rejected 16 months later, it was replaced with a homograft from a heterozygous MZ donor and the phenotype was again found to change to that of the new donor. Hood et al (1980) recently reported their accumulated experience of liver transplantation for advanced liver disease with α_1AT deficiency. Their 7 cases confirmed that the α_1AT phenotype became that of the donor without reversion back to the original phenotype after periods of up to 3 years. Terblanche et al (1979) and Macdougall et al (1980) have recently reviewed their total accumulated experience with liver transplantation in general.

Another potential method of providing donor liver cells to synthesize normal α_1AT could involve a transplant of fetal liver cells, without a total homotransplant of a liver. Touraine et al (1979) performed such a transplant of fetal liver cells in a patient with Fabry disease and found both objective and subjective clinical improvement in one patient.

A summary of the current status of treatment for α_1AT deficiency was presented at a meeting of the Pulmonary Disease Advisory Committee of the Division of Lung Disease of the National Heart, Lung and Blood Institute in October 1978 (see Cohen, 1979). They concluded that:

1. α_1AT replacement in persons with PiZZ phenotype and pulmonary emphysema has a strong likelihood of preventing the progression of emphysema.

2. If replacement of this enzyme inhibitor can stop the progression of the emphysema, it would be logical to try to replace the function of α_1AT in patients with the deficiency using safe, inexpensive, low-molecular weight synthetic inhibitors of elastase.

3. If either of the preceding two agents (plasma α_1AT or synthetic inhibitors) prevents the development of emphysema, then a trial of low-molecular weight elastase inhibitors in more common varieties of emphysema is a logical next step.

4. If safe elastase inhibitors can be developed, they should be tried in common forms of emphysema, regard-

less of the results in those patients with a PiZZ phenotype.

The problem involved in testing any drug or medication for correcting α_1AT deficiency and for testing its effect on pulmonary emphysema relates to the fact that emphysema is a long term disease. It would take many years to prove effectiveness; a type of study that both investigators and drug companies are loath to undertake.

Screening programmes for α_1AT deficiency

Neonatal screening

Initial interest in screening for α_1AT deficiency was aimed at detecting newborn infants who might be subject to respiratory distress syndrome. Evans et al (1972) had observed that such infants had low levels of α_1AT in their cord blood and believed initially that this might be related to the genetic defect. It was subsequently shown that these infants tended to lose serum proteins, including α_1AT, into the air spaces of their lungs because of increased pulmonary capillary permeability. The parents of such infants did not have α_1AT deficiency or any unusual preponderance of α_1AT variants in their phenotypes.

Subsequent screening programmes have been aimed specifically at detecting infants with the genetic form of α_1AT deficiency to associate the deficiency with neonatal cholestasis or cirrhosis, or to determine the occurrence of unusual respiratory problems in childhood with the deficiency. Laurell and Sveger (1975) performed the first such screening programme with a drop of blood on filter paper from 108 000 newborn Swedish infants by quantitatively measuring α_1AT concentration with an electroimmunoassay compared to a simultaneous measurement of transferrin. With this technique, primarily those infants with severe α_1AT deficiency were detected; the PiZ phenotype occurred at a rate of 1 per 1433 infants. The method was not capable of detecting all infants with an intermediate or heterozygous phenotype.

Sveger (1978) later undertook a screening programme utilizing a dried blood spot on filter paper that was originally submitted for the Guthrie test. Serum concentration of α_1AT was determined by electroimmunoassay and Pi typing by isoelectric focusing. Sveger found a variety of significant symptoms in about 30% of PiZ children.

O'Brien et al (1978) screened 107 038 infants with blood specimens also routinely collected on filter paper. The blood specimens were obtained by heel prick from infants upon the day of discharge from the hospital, and a second sample was obtained in most of the infants at 4 to 6 weeks of age. Twenty-one homozygous deficient (PiZ) infants were identified; an incidence of 1 in 5000. Of the 18 infants studied and followed, only 1 had neonatal hepatitis, although 5 had hepatomegaly or biochemical abnormalities indicating some hepatic damage.

After 3 to 6 years, all of these children were asymptomatic, although 4 of them continued to have hepatomegaly and biochemical evidence of liver damage. It is of interest that 9 of the 21 PiZ infants detected were missed on the initial sample, but were identified on the sample drawn 4 to 6 weeks later. The blood samples from these infants were screened initially by measuring the trypsin-inhibitory-capacity from the filter-paper sample, and Pi typing was performed on every infant with an abnormal screening test. The accuracy of the screening test was evaluated by comparing the screening method to a standard procedure performed with cord blood samples. The screening test using dry blood samples detected all specimens with trypsin-inhibitory-activity of less than 0.5 mg/ml. O'Brien et al (1978) state that 'since there is currently no specific therapy for α_1AT deficiency or for the liver disease associated with it, and since prognosis is uncertain, they do not recommend routine neonatal screening for α_1AT deficiency at the present time'.

Dijkman et al (1980) undertook a screening programme of newborns in the eastern part of the Netherlands utilizing electroimmunoassay for screening, followed by Pi-typing in suspected cases. In 95 033 newborn screened, the mean frequency of deficiency was 8 in 10 000 including PiZ, SZ, and S phenotypes. They found more Pi^Z north of the Rhine and Pi^S south of the Rhine in the Netherlands. The screening method employed drops of blood obtained by heel prick and collected on filter paper in a similar fashion to that employed by Sveger. The ratios between the heights of α_1AT and transferrin peaks was used as described by Laurell and Sveger (1972).

It would appear from reviewing these attempts at neonatal screening that the methods employed were not completely satisfactory, since some cases were missed on the initial screening attempt, and since only severe antitrypsin deficiency could be detected. The conclusions of O'Brien et al (1978) seem appropriate in that routine neonatal screening for α_1AT deficiency is not to be recommended at this time because of inability to provide specific therapy and because the number of cases found is quite small.

Childhood or adult screening programmes

The major purpose of screening older children or adults for α_1AT deficiency would be for a preventive medical approach to detect individuals with antitrypsin deficiency and warn them of their unusual predisposition to lung disease, especially the development of pulmonary emphysema should they smoke cigarettes. The value of this programme would be markedly enhanced if it were proven that the intermediate deficiency state indeed predisposed to lung disease. Many of us are convinced that it does, and that screening programmes would be of value for older children and young adults especially.

We undertook a screening programme in the junior high schools of Long Beach, California, and found the 7th grade students (13 years old) to be highly receptive as were their parents (Lieberman et al, 1977). Most of the deficient individuals had an MZ phenotype with intermediate antitrypsin deficiency. Of 1841 7th grade junior high school students, antitrypsin deficiency states were detected only in white subjects (3.04%) and not in 461 subjects of other races. The purpose for detecting these individuals was to warn them against taking up the cigarette smoking habit and also against accepting a type of employment where extreme environmental air pollution exists. It is of interest that a number of other surveys in hazardous environmental industries found very few with intermediate antitrypsin deficiency or abnormal phenotypes. It is as if these individuals screen themselves out from such employment either because they have already developed respiratory disease or they have experienced some respiratory symptoms that cause them to seek employment elsewhere.

GENETIC VARIATION IN PROTEASE CONTENT OF LEUCOCYTES

Studies with α_1AT indicate that an imbalance of the protease to protease-inhibitor levels can result in damage to lung tissue and the development of pulmonary emphysema. A logical extention of the α_1AT investigations, therefore, would be a study of leucocytic protease relationships to the pathogenesis of pulmonary emphysema. Galdston et al (1973) measured the leucocyte lysosomal elastase-like esterase in family members of two α_1AT deficient probands and in 12 control subjects with normal α_1AT and free of lung disease. Two levels of elastase activity were found among the family members; one level like that in the control group and the other, one-half this level. The investigators interpreted this to mean that the lower level of leucocytic elastase activity reflected a genetic variation that was protective for some members with reduced α_1AT. In other words, normal elastase-like esterase was associated with an unfavourable clinical course in the presence of intermediate or low α_1AT (Galdston et al, 1973, 1977). In a subsequent study, Galdston et al (1977) reported that individuals with chronic obstructive pulmonary disease, of either MM, MZ or ZZ phenotypes, differed from healthy controls of the same Pi types by having greater mean leucocyte-lysosomal elastase-like activity than controls of the same Pi types without lung disease. The individuals with lung disease also had a greater number of polymorphonuclear leucocytes and a history of having smoked a greater number of cigarettes within their lifetimes. However, in these individuals, the elastase-like activity was unrelated to the number of leucocytes, suggesting that the enzyme level

was an associated variable of COPD and not necessarily a result of the disease.

More recently, Galdston et al (1979) suggested that more elastase becomes bound to alpha$_2$-macroglobulin (α_2M) when antitrypsin is deficient, and that elastase bound to α_2M retains some of its elastolytic activity. Thus, in the presence of normal M serum, only about 6% of the neutrophilic elastase activity is retained toward elastin, whereas approximately 12% of the activity is retained in the presence of Z serum. The authors postulated that increased binding of elastase to α_2M when α_1AT is deficient may increase the turnover of soluble elastin and contribute to lung damage.

Lam et al (1979) also found greater neutrophil-elastase content in patients with abnormal lung function and a PiMZ phenotype than in those with normal lung function and the same Pi type. They concluded that the neutrophil elastase content was a significant risk factor in MZ deficient subjects, and that neutrophil elastase and smoking interact to produce abnormal lung function in PiMZ subjects.

A slightly different concept was suggested by Martin and Taylor (1979) who had examined 71 patients with COPD and 46 healthy controls. They found that leucocytic elastase activity from patients with lung disease interacted abnormally with α_1AT so that increased residual activity was present despite adequate amounts of α_1AT for total inhibition. This was seen in 33 of 71 patients with COPD as compared to 6 of 46 normal control subjects. This observation is somewhat similar to Galdston's findings of an increased reaction with α_2M and increased residual elastase activity when α_1AT is deficient.

Kramps et al (1980) found higher leucocyte elastase-like activity in 16 PiMM patients with emphysema than in healthy control subjects. These authors concluded that increased levels of leucocyte elastase may be a contributing factor in persons without α_1AT deficiency, but not in persons with α_1AT deficiency. In contrast, Abboud et al (1979) did not find significant differences in mean lysosomal elastase or protease activity between COPD patients and controls with normal α_1AT, although a few of their COPD patients did have higher concentrations of neutrophil-elastase. In patients with α_1AT deficiency, however, both the elastase and protease content per 10^8 neutrophils was significantly higher in homozygous and heterozygous Pi^Z COPD patients as compared to normal subjects and PiM COPD patients. Abboud et al conclude that the concentration of neutrophilic elastase and protease may be an important risk factor in patients with Z or MZ phenotypes and in a few patients with M phenotype.

Despite this number of supportive, though somewhat contradictory reports, a number of negative reports were also published. Klayton et al (1975) measured a series of leucocytic enzymes and found none of them to be associated with the development of COPD or with smoking history in heterozygotes, but they did find that cigarette smoking was a significant determinant of the development of COPD in heterozygotes. Similarly, Taylor and Kueppers (1976) found no differences in concentration of leucocytic elastase between patients with COPD and controls, but they found an almost fourfold increase in the prevalence of a slow electrophoretic type of elastase in the COPD patients. They concluded that there may be a qualitative rather than a quantitative difference in elastase which could play a role in the pathogenesis of COPD in patients with normal α_1AT phenotypes.

One can conclude from these studies that there is some significance to variation in leucocytic elastase activity that may play a role in the pathogenesis of pulmonary disease. Additional work in this area is indicated.

LEUCOCYTIC CHEMOTACTIC FACTOR INACTIVATOR

Normal human serum contains an inactivator of chemotactic factors for neutrophilic leucocytes (Berenberg & Ward, 1973). Ward and Talamo (1973) found that human serum deficient in α_1AT was also deficient in this naturally occurring chemotactic-factor-inactivator. The serum-donors with this combined deficiency all had severe pulmonary emphysema. The deficiency of chemotactic-factor-inactivator was not observed in patients with clinically similar pulmonary disease who had normal α_1AT.

Ward and Talamo (1973) do not believe that α_1AT and chemotactic-factor-inactivator are identical, since α_1AT

works by binding to the enzymes in stoichiometric fashion whereas the chemotactic-factor-inactivator appears to destroy the chemotactic factor in an enzymatic manner. Thus, according to Ward and Talamo, our concepts of how α_1AT deficiency works in predisposing to pulmonary emphysema should be modified to take into account a deficiency of the chemotactic-factor-inactivator.

Grady et al (1979) suggest that proteases themselves may have chemotactic activity. They found that a variety of inhibitors of serine-proteases and also protease substrates inhibit chemotaxis of human polymorphonuclear leucocytes in addition to inhibiting the esterase activity of these cells. They claim that serine-protease-activity may function during induction of chemotaxis, so that inhibition of enzyme activity also inhibits chemotaxis. This information could shed more light on the association of α_1AT with a deficiency of chemotactic-factor-inactivator, but implicates α_1AT as playing the role of a chemotactic-factor-inactivator contrary to the beliefs of Ward and Talamo.

Lam et al (1980) also measured the serum chemotactic-factor-inactivator in 22 subjects with chronic airflow obstruction and in 19 healthy subjects with PiM and PiMZ phenotypes. They observed that subjects with chronic airflow obstruction had significantly lower chemotactic-factor-inactivator activity than normal subjects, irrespective of the α_1AT phenotype. However, the lowest levels were found in those with chronic airflow obstruction and a PiZZ phenotype. Lam et al (1980) believe that the deficiency of serum chemotactic-factor-inactivator may be important in the pathogenesis of chronic airflow obstruction, particularly in those with severe α_1AT deficiency.

REFERENCES

Aagenaes O, Matlary A, Elgjo K, Munthe E, Fagerhol M 1972 Neonatal cholestasis in alpha$_1$-antitrypsin deficient children. Acta Paediatrica Scandinavica 61: 632–642

Aarskog D, Aarseth P, Fagerhol M K 1978 Alpha$_1$-antitrypsin (Pi) types in recurrent miscarriages. Clinical Genetics 13: 81–84

Aarskog D, Fagerhol M L 1970 Protease inhibitor (Pi) phenotypes in chromosome aberrations. Journal of Medical Genetics 7: 367–370

Abboud R T, Rushton J M, Grzybowski S 1979 Interrelationships between neutrophil elastase, serum alpha$_1$-antitrypsin, lung function and chest radiography in patients with chronic airflow obstruction. American Review of Respiratory Disease 120: 31–40

Abramowsky C R, Cebelin M, Choudury A, Izant R J 1980 Undifferentiated (embryonal) sarcoma of the liver with alpha$_1$-antitrypsin deposits: Immunohistochemical and ultrastructural studies. Cancer 45: 3108–3113

Ananthakrishnan R, Biegler B, Dennis P M 1979 Alpha$_1$-antitrypsin phenotypes in paraproteinaemias. Lancet 1: 561–562

Andre F, Andre C, Lambert R, Descos F 1974 Prevalence of alpha$_1$-antitrypsin deficiency in patients with gastric or duodenal ulcer. Biomedicine 21: 222–224

Arnaud P, Koistinen J, Wilson G B, Fudenberg H H 1977b Alpha$_1$-antitrypsin (Pi) phenotypes in a Finnish population. Scandinavian Journal of Clinical and Laboratory Investigation 37: 339–343

Arnaud P, Cellier C C, Vittoz P, Creyssel R 1977a Alpha$_1$-antitrypsin phenotypes in Lyon, France. Human Genetics 39: 63–68

Arnaud P, Galbraith R M, Faulk W P, Ansell B M 1977 Increased frequency of the MZ phenotype of alpha$_1$-protease inhibitor in juvenile chronic polyarthritis. Journal of Clinical Investigation 69: 1442–1444

Arnaud P, Galbraith R M, Faulk W P, Black C 1979a Pi phenotypes of alpha$_1$-antitrypsin in Southern England: Identification of M subtypes and implications for genetic studies. Clinical Genetics 15: 406–410

Arnaud P, Galbraith R M, Faulk W P, Black C, Hughes G V 1979b Alpha$_1$-antitrypsin in adult rheumatoid arthritis. Lancet 1: 1236–1237

Arora P K, Miller H C, Aronson L D 1978 α₁-antitrypsin is an effector of immunological stasis. Nature 274: 589–590

Ashley M J, Corey P, Chan-Yeung M 1980 Smoking, dust exposure, and serum alpha₁-antitrypsin. American Review of Respiratory Disease 121: 783–788

Bagdasarian A, Colman R W 1978 Subcellular localization and purification of platelet α₁-antitrypsin. Blood 51: 139–156

Baumstark J S, Lee C T, Luby R J 1977 Rapid inactivation of α₁-protease (α₁-antitrypsin) by elastase. Biochimica et Biophysica Acta 482: 400–411

Bechman G, Beckman L, Nordenson I 1980 Alpha₁-antitrypsin phenotypes in Northern Sweden. Human Heredity 30: 129–135

Beckman G, Beckman L, Liden S 1980 Association between psoriasis and the α₁-antitrypsin deficiency gene Z. Acta Dermatovenereologica 60: 163–164

Berenberg J L, Ward P A 1973 Chemotactic factor inactivator in normal human serum. Journal of Clinical Investigation 52: 1200–1206

Bierman H R, Kelly K H, Cordes F L 1955 The sequestration and visceral circulation of leucocytes in man. Annals of the New York Academy of Sciences 59: 850–862

Blackwood R A, Cerreta J M, Mandl I, Turino G M 1979 Alpha₁-antitrypsin deficiency and increased susceptibility to elastase-induced experimental emphysema in a rat model. American Review of Respiratory Disease 120: 1375–1379

Blenkinsopp W K, 1978 Alpha₁-antitrypsin bodies, Piᶻ phenotype, and peptic ulcer. Gut 19: 157–158

Bloom J W, Hunter M J 1978 Interactions of α₁-antitrypsin with trypsin and chymotrypsin. Journal of Biological Chemistry 253: 547–559

Blue M L, Janoff A 1978 Possible mechanisms of emphysema in cigarette smokers. Release of elastase from human polymorphonuclear leucocytes by cigarette smoke condensate in vitro. American Review of Respiratory Disease 117: 317–325

Blundell G, Frazer A, Cole R B, Nevin N C 1975 Alpha₁-antitrypsin phenotypes in Northern Ireland. Annals of Human Genetics 38: 289–294

Bradfield J W B, Wells M 1978 Liver disease caused by Lysosomal enzymes released from Kupffer cells. Lancet 1: 836

Brandrup F, Ostergaard P A 1978 α₁-antitrypsin deficiency associated with persistent cutaneous vasculitis. Archives of Dermatology 114: 921–924

Brewerton D A, Webley M, Murphy A H, Ward A M 1978 the α₁-antitrypsin phenotype MZ in acute anterior uveitis. Lancet 1: 1103

Bribiesca L B, Attias J L, de la Vega G 1972 Pemphigus vulgaris associated with alpha₁-antitrypsin deficiency. Sobretiro de Patologia X; 41–48

Bribiesca L B, Horta R F 1978 Immunofluorescent localization of alpha₁-antitrypsin in human polymorphonuclear leucocytes. Life Sciences 21: 99–104

Brown J H, Pollock S H 1970 Inhibition of elastase and collagenase by anti-inflammatory drugs. Proceedings of the Society for Experimental Biology and Medicine 135: 792–795

Brown W T, Mamelok A E, Bearn A G 1979 Anterior uveitis and alpha₁-antitrypsin. Lancet 2: 644

Buisseret P D, Penbrey M E, Lessof M H 1977 α₁-antitrypsin phenotypes in rheumatoid arthritis and ankylosing spondylitis. Lancet 2: 1358–1359

Buist A S, Sexton G J, Azzam A M H, Adams B–E 1979 Pulmonary function in heterozygotes for alpha₁-antitrypsin deficiency: A case control study. American Review of Respiratory Disease 120: 759–766

Campra J L, Craig J R, Peters R L, Reynolds T B 1973 Cirrhosis associated with partial deficiency of alpha₁-antitrypsin in an adult. Annals of Internal Medicine 78: 233–238

Carp H, Janoff A 1978 Possible mechanisms of emphysema in smokers. In vitro suppression of serum elastase-inhibitory capacity by fresh cigarette smoke and its prevention by antioxidants. American Review of Respiratory Disease 118: 617–621

Carrell R W, Owen M C 1976 α₁-antitrypsin: Structure, variation and disease. Essays in Medical Biochemistry 4: 83–119

Carrico R J, Lieberman J, Yeager F 1976 The source of a minor alpha₁-antitrypsin in variant serum. American Review of Respiratory Disease 114: 53–57

Casterline C L, Evans R, Battista V C, Talamo R C 1978 Selective IgA deficiency and Pi ZZ-antitrypsin deficiency. Chest 73: 885–886

Chan C H, Steer C J, Vergalla J, Jones E A 1978 Alpha₁-antitrypsin deficiency with cirrhosis associated with the protease inhibitor phenotype SZ. American Journal of Medicine 65: 978–986

Chan-Yeung M, Ashley M J, Corey P, Maledy H 1978 Pi phenotypes and the prevalence of chest symptoms and lung function abnormalities in workers employed in dusty industries. American Review of Respiratory Disease 117: 239–245

Chapuis-Cellier C, Arnaud P 1979 Preferential transmission of the Z deficient allele of α₁-antitrypsin. Science 205: 407–408

Christen H, Bau J, Halsband H 1975 Hereditary alpha₁-antitrypsin deficiency associated with congential extrahepatic bile duct hypoplasia. Klinische Wochenschrift 53: 90–91

Clemmensen I, Christensen F 1976 Inhibition of urokinase by complex formation with human α₁-antitrypsin. Biochimica et Biophysica Acta 429: 591–599

Cohen A B 1979 Opportunities for the development of specific therapeutic agents to treat emphysema. American Review of Respiratory Disease 120: 723–727

Cook P J L 1975 The genetics of α₁-antitrypsin: a family study in England and Scotland. Annals of Human Genetics 38: 275–287

Cox D W 1975 Deficiency allele of α₁-antitrypsin PiMmalton (abstract). American Journal of Human Genetics 27: 29A

Cox D W 1980 Transmission of Z allele from heterozygotes for α₁-antitrypsin deficiency. American Journal of Human Genetics 32: 455–457

Cox D W, Huber O 1976 Rheumatoid arthritis and alpha₁-antitrypsin. Lancet 1: 1216–1217

Cox D W, Huber O 1980 Association of severe rheumatoid arthritis with heterozygosity for α₁-antitrypsin deficiency. Clinical Genetics 17: 153–160

Cox D W, Johnson A M, Fagerhol M K 1980 Report of nomenclature meeting for α₁-antitrypsin. Human Genetics 53: 429–433

Doeglas H M G, Bleumink E 1975 Protease inhibitors in plasma of patients with chronic urticaria. Archives of Dermatology 111: 979–985

Dickinson P, Zinneman H H, Swaim W R, Doe R P, Seal US 1969 Effects of testosterone treatment on plasma proteins and amino acids in men. Journal of Clinical Endocrinology and Metabolism 29: 837–841

Dijkman J H, Penders T J, Kramps J A, Sonderkamp H J A, van den Broek W G M, ter Haar B G A 1980 Epidemiology of alpha₁- antitrypsin deficiency in the Netherlands. Human Genetics 53: 409–413

Eberle V F, Adler G, Kern H F, Martini G A 1979 Polypoid gastric heterotopy of the small intestine in a patient with primary hyperparathyroidism and alpha₁-antitrypsin deficiency belonging to a MEA-family. Zeitschrift fur Gastroenterologie 1: 354–365

Eriksson S 1964 Pulmonary emphysema and alpha₁-antitrypsin deficiency. Acta Medica Scandinavica 175: 197–205

Eriksson S 1965 Studies in α_1-antitrypsin deficiency. Acta Medica Scandinavica 177: Supplementum 432, 85pp

Eriksson S 1978 Proteases and protease inhibitors in chronic obstructive lung disease. Acta Medica Scandinavica 203: 449–455

Eriksson S, Moestrup T, Hagerstrand I 1975 Liver, lung and malignant disease in heterozygous (PiMZ) α_1-antitrypsin deficiency. Acta Medica Scandinavica 198: 243–247

Evans H E, Keller S, Mandl I 1972 Serum trypsin inhibitory capacity and the idiopathic respiratory distress syndrome. Journal of Pediatrics 81: 588–592

Fagerhol M K 1967 Serum Pi types in Norwegians. Acta Pathologica et Microbiologica Scandinavica 70: 421–428

Fagerhol M K 1968 The Pi system. Genetic variants of serum. Series Haematologica 1: 153–161

Fagerhol M K 1976 The genetics of alpha₁-antitrypsin and its implications. Postgraduate Medical Journal 52 Supplement 2: 73–83

Fagerhol M K, Eriksson A W, Monn E 1969 Serum Pi types in some Lappish and Finnish populations. Human Heredity 19: 360–364

Fagerhol M K, Gedde-Dahl T 1969 Genetics of the Pi serum types. Human Heredity 19: 354–359

Fagerhol M K, Tenfjord O W 1968 Serum Pi types in some European, American, Asian and African populations. Acta Pathologica et Microbiologica Scandinavica 72: 601–608

Falk G A, Smith J P 1971 Chronic bronchitis: A seldom noted manifestation of homozygous alpha₁-antitrypsin deficiency. Chest 60: 166–169

Fallat R J, Powell M R, Kueppers F, Lilker E 1973 ¹³³Xe ventilatory studies in α_1-antitrypsin deficiency. Journal of Nuclear Medicine 14: 5–13

Fertakis A, Tsourapas A, Douratsos D, Angelopoulos B 1974 Pi phenotypes in Greeks. Human Heredity 24: 313–316

Fineman R M, Kidd K K, Johnson A M, Breg W R 1976 Increased frequency of heterozygotes for α_1-antitrypsin variants in individuals with either sex chromosome mosaicism or trisomy 21. Nature 260: 320–321

Fisher R L, Taylor L, Sherlock S 1976 α_1-antitrypsin deficiency in liver disease: The extent of the problem. Gastroenterology 71: 646–651

Frants R R, Eriksson A W, 1978 Reliable classification of six PiM subtypes by separator isoelectric focusing. Human Heredity 28: 201–209

Freeman H J, Weinstein W M, Shnitka T K, Crockford P M, Herbert F A 1976 Alpha₁-antitrypsin deficiency and pancreatic fibrosis. Annals of Internal Medicine 85: 73–76

Gadek J E, Fells G A, Crystal R G 1979 Cigarette smoking induces functional antiprotease deficiency in the lower respiratory tract of humans. Science 206: 1315–1316

Gadek J E, Fulmer J D, Gelfand J A, Frant M M, Petty T L, Crystal R G 1980 Danazol-induced augmentation of serum α_1-antitrypsin levels in individuals with marked deficiency of this antiprotease. Journal of Clinical Investigation 66: 82–87

Galdston M, Janoff A, Davis A L 1973 Familial variation of leukocyte lysosomal protease and serum α_1-antitrypsin as determinants in chronic obstructive pulmonary disease. American Review of Respiratory Disease 107: 718–727

Galdston M, Melnick E L, Goldring R M, Levytska V, Curasi C A, Davis A L 1977 Interactions of neutrophil elastase, serum trypsin inhibitory activity, and smoking history as risk factors for chronic obstructive pulmonary disease in patients with MM, MZ, and ZZ phenotypes for alpha₁-antitrypsin. American Review of Respiratory Disease 116: 837–846

Galdston M, Levytska V, Leener I E, Twumasi D Y 1979 Degradation of tropelastin and elastin substrates by human neutrophil elastase, free and bound to alpha₂-macroglobulin in serum of the M and Z (Pi) phenotypes for alpha₁-antitrypsin. American Review of Respiratory Disease 119: 435–441

Geada H M, Albino J P, Manso C 1976 Polymorphism of α_1-antitrypsin in a Portuguese population. Human Genetics 32: 109–113

Gedde-Dahl T, Fagerhol M K, Cook P J L, Noades J 1972 Autosomal linkage between the Gm and Pi loci in man. Annals of Human Genetics 35: 393–399

Gedde-Dahl T, Cook P J L, Fagerhol M K, Pierce J A 1975 Improved estimate of the Gm-Pi linkage. Annals of Human Genetics 39: 43–50

Geddes D M, Webley M, Brewerton D A 1977 α_1-antitrypsin phenotypes in fibrosing alveolitis and rheumatoid arthritis. Lancet 2: 1049–1051

Gelfand E W, Cox D W, Lin M T, Dosch H M 1979 Severe combined immune-deficiency disease in patients with α_1-antitrypsin deficiency. Lancet 2: 202

Gitlin D, Perricelli A 1970 Synthesis of serum albumin, prealbumin, alpha fetoprotein, alpha₁-antitrypsin and transferrin by the human yolk sac. Nature 228: 995–997

Glaser C B, Karic L, Fallat R J, Stockert R 1977 Alpha₁-antitrypsin. Plasma survival studies in the rat of the normal and homozygote deficient forms. Biochimica et Biophysica Acta 495: 87–92

Glasgow A H, Cooperband S R, Schmid K, Parker J T, Occhino J C, Mannick J A 1971 Inhibition of secondary immune responses by immunoregulatory alphaglobulin. Transplantation Proceedings III: 835–837

Goedde H W, Benkmann H G, Christ I, Singh S, Hirth L 1970 Gene frequencies of red cell adenosine deaminase, adenylate kinase, phosphoglucomutase, acid phosphatase and serum α_1-antitrypsin (Pi) in a German population. Humangenetik 10: 235–243

Goetz I E, Weinstein C, Roberts E 1972 Effects of protease inhibitors on growth of hamster tumour cells in culture. Cancer Research 32: 2469–2474

Gordon H W, Dixon J, Rogers J C, Mittman C, Lieberman J 1972 Alpha₁-antitrypsin accumulation in livers of emphysematous patients with α_1AT deficiency. Human Pathology 3: 361–370

Grady P G, Davis A T, Shapira E 1979 The effect of some protease substrates and inhibitors on chemotaxis and protease activity of human polymorphonuclear leucocytes. Journal of Infectious Diseases 140: 999–1003

Greenwald A J, Johnson D S, Oskvig R M, Aschenbrener C A, Randa D C 1975 α_1-antitrypsin deficiency, emphysema, cirrhosis, and intestinal mucosal atrophy. Journal of the American Medical Association 231: 273–276

Halal F, Scriver C R, Cox D W, Jaber L, Varsano I 1979 Cystathioninuria, renal iminoglycinuria and α_1-antitrypsin deficiency in the same family: relevance in medical practice. CMA Journal 121: 64–67

Heck L W, Kaplan A P 1974 Substrates of Hageman factor. I. Isolation and characterization of human factor XI (PTA) and inhibition of the activated enzyme by α_1-antitrypsin. Journal of Experimental Medicine 140: 1615–1630

Hercz A, Katona E, Cutz E, Wilson J R, Barton M 1978 α_1-antitrypsin: The presence of excess mannose in the Z variant isolated from liver. Science 201: 1229–1232

Hinman L M, Stevens C A, Matthay R A, Gee J B L 1980 Elastase and lysozyme activities in human alveolar macrophages. Effects of cigarette smoking. American Review of Respiratory Disease 121: 263–271

Hoffman J J M L, van den Broek W G M 1976 Distribution of alpha₁-antitrypsin phenotypes in two Dutch population groups. Human Genetics 32: 43–48

Hood J M, Koep L J, Peters R L, Schroter G P J, Weil R, Redeker A G, Starzl T E 1980 Liver transplantation for advanced liver disease with alpha₁-antitrypsin deficiency. New England Journal of Medicine 302: 272–275

Horton F O, Mackenthun A V, Anderson P S, Patterson C D, Mannarsten J F 1980 Alpha₁-antitrypsin heterozygotes (Pi type MZ). A longitudinal study of the risk of development of chronic air flow limitation. Chest 77: 261–263

Iammarino R M, Wagener D K, Allen R C 1979 Segregation distortion of the α_1-antitrypsin Pi Z allele. American Journal of Human Genetics 31: 508–517

Ishibashi H, Shibata K, Okubo M, Tsuda-kawamura K, Yanase T 1978 Distribution of α_1-antitrypsin in normal granuloma, and tumor tissues in rats. Journal of Laboratory and Clinical Medicine 91: 575–583

Janoff A, Carp H 1977 Possible mechanisms of emphysema in smokers. Cigarette smoke condensate suppresses protease inhibition in vitro. American Review of Respiratory Disease 116: 65–72

Janoff A, Carp H, Lee D K, Drew R T 1979a Cigarette smoke inhalation decreases α_1-antitrypsin activity in rat lung. Science 206: 1313–1314

Janoff A, Dearing R 1980 Prevention of elastase-induced experimental emphysema by oral administration of a synthetic elastase inhibitor. American Review of Respiratory Disease 121: 1025–1029

Janoff A, Sandhaus R A, Hospelhorn V D, Rosenberg R 1972 Digestion of lung proteins by human leucocyte granules in vitro. Proceedings of the Society for Experimental Biology and Medicine 140: 516–519

Janoff A, White R, Carp H, Harel S, Dearing R, Lee D 1979b Lung injury induced by leucocytic proteases. American Journal of Pathology 97: 111–129

Janus E D, Carrell R W 1975 Alpha₁-antitrypsin deficiency in New Zealand. New Zealand Medical Journal 81: 461–467

Janus E D, Joyce P R, Sheat J M, Carrell R W 1975 Alpha₁-antitrypsin variants in New Zealand. New Zealand Medical Journal 12: 289–291

Jeppsson J O, 1976 Amino acid substitution in α_1-antitrypsin PiZ. FEBS Letters 65: 195–197

Joly J, Richer G, Boisvert F, Laverdiere M 1980 Alpha₁-antitrypsin phenotypes in French Canadian newborns. Human Heredity 30: 1–2

Jones E A, Vergalla J, Steer C F, Bradley-Moore P R, Vierling J M 1978 Metabolism of intact and desialylated α_1-antitrypsin. Clinical Science and Molecular Medicine 55: 139–148

Johnson D A 1980 Ozone inactivation of human α_1-proteinase inhibitor. American Review of Respiratory Disease 121: 1031–1038

Kanner R E, Renzetti A D, Klauber M R, Smith C B, Golden C A 1979 Variables associated with changes in spirometry in patients with obstructive lung diseases. American Journal of Medicine 67: 44–50

Karlinsky J B, Snider G L 1978 Animal models of emphysema. American Review of Respiratory Disease 117: 1109–1133

Karsh J, Vergalla J, Jones E A 1979 Alpha₁-antitrypsin phenotypes in rheumatoid arthritis and systemic lupus erythematosus. Arthritis and Rheumatism 22: 111–113

Kellermann G, Walter H 1970 Investigations on the population genetics of the α_1-antitrypsin polymorphism. Humangenetik 10: 145–150

Kelly J K, Taylor T V, Milford-Ward A 1979 Alpha₁-antitrypsin Pi S phenotype and liver cell inclusion bodies in alcoholic hepatitis. Journal of Clinical Pathology 32: 706–709

Kern W H, Mikkelsen W P, Turrill F L 1969 Significance of hyaline necrosis in liver biopsies. Surgery, Gynecology and Obstetrics 129: 749–754

Klasen E C, Franken C, Voleers W S, Bernini L F 1977 Population genetics of α_1-antitrypsin in the Netherlands. Human Genetics 37: 303–313

Klasen E C, D'Andrea F, Bernini L F 1978 Phenotype and gene distribution of alpha₁-antitrypsin in a North Italian population. Human Heredity 28: 474–478

Klayton R, Fallat R, Cohen A B 1975 Determinants of chronic obstructive pulmonary disease in patients with intermediate levels of alpha₁-antitrypsin. American Review of Respiratory Disease 112: 71–75

Kleinerman J, Ranga V, Rynbrandt D, Sorensen J, Powers J C 1980 The effect of the specific elastase inhibitor, alanyl alanyl prolyl alanine chloromethylketone, on elastase-induced emphysema. American Review of Respiratory Disease 121: 381–387

Kozarevic D, Laban M, Budimir M, Vojvodic N, Roberts A, Gordon T, McGee D L 1978 Intermediate alpha₁-antitrypsin deficiency and chronic obstructive pulmonary disease in Yugoslavia. American Review of Respiratory Disease 117: 1039–1043

Kramps J A, Bakker W, Dijkman J H 1980 A matched-pair study of the leucocyte elastase-like activity in normal persons and in emphysematous patients with and without alpha₁-antitrypsin deficiency. American Review of Respiratory Disease. 121: 253–261

Kueppers F 1968 Genetically determined differences in the response of alpha₁-antitrypsin levels in human serum to typhoid vaccine. Humangenetik 6: 207–214

Kueppers F 1971 Alpha₁-antitrypsin: Physiology, genetics and pathology. Humangenetik 11: 177–189

Kueppers F 1978 Inherited differences in alpha₁-antitrypsin. In: Litwin S D (ed) Lung Biopsy in Health and Disease; Genetic Determinants of Pulmonary Diseases, Marcel Dekker, Inc, Ch 2, p 23–74

Kueppers F, Black L F 1974 α_1-antitrypsin and its deficiency. American Review of Respiratory Disease 110: 176–194

Kueppers F, Dickson E R, Summerskill W H J 1976 Alpha₁-antitrypsin phenotypes in chronic active liver disease and primary biliary cirrhosis. Mayo Clinic Proceedings 51: 286–288

Kueppers F, Fallat R J 1969 α_1-antitrypsin deficiency: A defect in protein synthesis. Clinica Chimica Acta 24: 401–403

Kueppers F, Fallat R, Larson R K 1969 Obstructive lung disease and alpha₁-antitrypsin deficiency gene heterozygosity. Science 165: 899–901

Kueppers F, Miller R D, Gordon H, Hepper N G, Offord K 1977 Familial prevalence of chronic obstructive pulmonary disease in a matched pair study. American Journal of Medicine 63: 336–342

Kueppers F, O'Brien P, Passarge E, Rudiger H W 1975

Alpha$_1$-antitrypsin phenotypes in sex chromosome mosaicism. Journal of Medical Genetics 12: 263–264

Kuhn C, Senoir R M 1978 The role of elastases in the development of emphysema. Lung 155: 185–197

Kuhnl P, Spielmann W 1979 Investigations on the Pi polymorphism in a German population. Forensic Science International 14: 135

Lam S, Abboud R T, Chan-Yeung M, Rushton J M 1979 Neutrophil elastase and pulmonary function in subjects with intermediate alpha$_1$-antitrypsin deficiency (MZ phenotype). American Review of Respiratory Disease 119: 941–951

Lam S, Chan-Yeung M, Abboud R, Kreutzer D 1980 Interrelationships between serum chemotactic factor inactivator, alpha$_1$-antitrypsin deficiency, and chronic obstructive lung disease. American Review of Respiratory Disease 121: 507–512

Langley C E, Talamo R 1975 Antitryptic activity of alpha$_1$-antitrypsin Pi bands in starch gel. In: Peeters N (ed) Protides of the Biological Fluids, Pergamon Press, Elmsford, New York pp 497–500

Lankisch P G, Koop H, Winckler K, Kaboth U 1978 α_1-antitrypsin in pancreatic diseases. Digestion 18: 138–140

Larsson C, Eriksson S, Dirksen H 1977 Smoking and intermediate alpha$_1$-antitrypsin deficiency and lung function in middle-aged men. British Medical Journal 2: 922–926

Laurell C B 1975 Relation between structures and biologic function of the protease inhibitors in the extracellular fluid. In: Peeters N (ed) Protides of the Biological Fluids, Pergamon Press, Elmsford, New York, p 3–12

Laurell C B, Eriksson S 1965 The serum α_1-antitrypsin in families with hypo-α_1-antitrypsinemia. Clinica Chimica Acta 11: 395–398

Laurell C B, Eriksson S 1963 The electrophoretic α_1-globulin pattern of serum in α_1-antitrypsin deficiency. Scandinavian Journal of Clinical and Laboratory Investigation 15: 132–140

Laurell C B, Nossling B, Jeppsson J O 1977 Catabolic rate of α_1-antitrypsin of Pi type M and Z in man. Clinical Science and Molecular Medicine 52: 457–461

Laurell C B, Sveger T 1975 Mass screening of newborn Swedish infants for α_1-antitrypsin deficiency. American Journal of Human Genetics 27: 213–217

Lebeau B, Rochemaure J 1978 Variations du taux d'alpha$_1$-antitrypsine chez les sujets atteints de broncho-pneumopathies aigues. Roles du phenotype Pi et de la fonction hepatique. La Nouvelle Presse Medicale 7: 3521–3525

Lellouch J, Claude J R, Thevenin M 1979 α_1-antitrypsine et tabac, une etude de 1296 hommes sains. Clinica Chimica Acta 95: 337–345

Lieberman J 1969 Heterozygous and homozygous alpha$_1$-antitrypsin deficiency in patients with pulmonary emphysema. New England Journal of Medicine 281: 279–284

Lieberman J 1971 Alpha$_1$-antitrypsin and pepsin inhibition. New England Journal of Medicine 285: 524

Lieberman J 1973 Alpha$_1$-antitrypsin deficiency. Medical Clinics of North America 57: 691–706

Lieberman J 1974 Emphysema, cirrhosis, and hepatoma with alpha$_1$-antitrypsin deficiency. Annals of Internal Medicine 81: 850–851

Lieberman J 1980a Alpha$_1$-antitrypsin. In: Schmidt RM (ed) Handbook Series in Clinical Laboratory Science Section I: Hematology, Volume III, pp 195–204

Lieberman J 1980b Alpha$_1$-antitrypsin deficiency. In: Simmons D H (ed) Current Pulmonology, Volume 2, Houghton Mifflin Professional Publishers, ch 2, p 41–68

Lieberman J, Gawad M A 1971 Inhibitors and activators of leucocytic proteases in purulent sputum. Journal of Laboratory and Clinical Medicine 77: 713–727

Lieberman J, Kaneshiro W 1972 Inhibition of leucocytic elastase from purulent sputum by alpha$_1$-antitrypsin. Journal of Laboratory and Clinical Medicine 80: 88–101

Lieberman J, Borhani N O, Feinleib M 1979 α_1-antitrypsin deficiency in twins and parents-of-twins. Clinical Genetics 15: 29–36

Lieberman J, Gaidulis L, Klotz S D 1976a A new deficient variant of α_1-antitrypsin (Mduarte). Inability to detect the heterozygous state by antitrypsin in phenotyping. American Review of Respiratory Disease 113: 31–36

Lieberman J, Gaidulis L, Roberts L 1976b Racial distribution of α_1-antitrypsin variants among junior high school students. American Review of Respiratory Disease 114: 1194–1198

Lieberman J, Gaidulis L, Schleissner L A 1976c Intermediate alpha$_1$-antitrypsin deficiency resulting from a null gene (M-phenotype). Chest 70: 532–535

Lieberman J, Gawad M A 1971 Inhibitors and activators of leucocytic proteases in purulent sputum. Digestion of human lung and inhibition of alpha$_1$-antitrypsin. Journal of Laboratory and Clinical Medicine 77: 713–727

Lieberman J, Kaneshiro W, Gaidulis L 1975 Interference with alpha$_1$-antitrypsin studies in stored serum by presumed bacterial proteases. Journal of Laboratory and Clinical Medicine 86: 7–16

Lieberman J, Mittman C 1973 Dynamic response of α_1-antitrypsin variants to diethylstilbestrol. American Journal of Human Genetics 25: 610–617

Lieberman J, Mittman C, Gordon H W 1972 Alpha$_1$-antitrypsin in the livers of patients with emphysema. Science 175: 63–65

Lieberman J, Mittman C, Kent J R 1971 Screening for heterozygous α_1-antitrypsin deficiency. III. A provocative test with diethylstilbestrol and effect of oral contraceptives. Journal of the American Medical Association 217:1198–1206

Lieberman J, Mittman C, Schneider A S 1969 Screening for homozygous and heterozygous α_1-antitrypsin deficiency. Protein electrophoresis on cellulose acetate membranes. Journal of the American Medical Association 210: 2055–2060

Lieberman J, Silton R M, Agliozzo C M, McMahon J 1975 Hepatocellular carcinoma and intermediate α_1-antitrypsin deficiency (MZ phenotype). American Journal of Clinical Pathology 64: 304–310

Lie-Injo L E, Ganesan J, Herrera A, Lopez C G 1978 α_1-antitrypsin variants in different racial groups in Malaysia. Human Heredity 28: 37–40

Lipsky J J, Berninger R W, Hyman L R, Talamo R C 1979 Presence of alpha$_1$-antitrypsin on mitogen-stimulated human lymphocytes. Journal of Immunology 122: 24–26

Lochon B, Vercaigne D, Lochon C, Fournier M, Martin J P, Derenne J P, Pariente R 1978 Emphysema pan-lobulaire: relations avec le taux d'alpha$_1$-antitrypsin serique le phenotype Pi et le systeme H.L.A. La Nouvelle Presse Medicale 7: 1167–1170

Longstreth G F, Weitzman S A, Browning R J, Lieberman J 1975 Bronchiectasis and homozygous alpha$_1$-antitrypsin deficiency. Chest 67: 233–235

Lubec V G, Weissenbacher G, Balzar, Bugajer-Gleitmann H 1976 Alpha$_1$-antitrypsin bei Kindern mit glommerularen Nierenkrankheiten. Wiener Klinische Wochenschrift 88: 271–274

Macdougall, B R D, McMaster P, Calne R Y, Williams R 1980 Survival and rehabilitation after orthotopic liver transplantation. Lancet 1: 1326–1328

Machovich R, Borsodi A, Blasko G, Orakzai S A 1977 Inactivation of α and β-thrombin by antithrombin-III, α₂-macroglobulin and α₁-proteinase inhibitor. Biochemical Journal 167: 393–398

Makino S, Chosy L, Valdivia E, Reed C E 1970 Emphysema with hereditary alpha₁-antitrypsin deficiency masquerading as asthma. Journal of Allergy 46: 40–48

Makino S, Reed C E 1970 Distribution and elimination of exogenous alpha₁-antitrypsin. Journal of Laboratory and Clinical Medicine 75: 742–746

Martin J P, Sesboue R, Charlionet R, Ropartz C, Pereira M T 1976 Genetic variants of serum α₁-antitrypsin (Pi types)in Portuguese. Human Heredity 26: 310–314

Martin W J, Taylor J C 1979 Abnormal interaction of α₁-antitrypsin and leucocyte elastolytic activity in patients with chronic obstructive pulmonary disease. American Review of Respiratory Disease 120: 411–419

Matsubara S, Yoshida A, Lieberman J 1974 Material isolated from normal and variant human liver that immunologically crossreacts with alpha₁-antitrypsin. Proceedings of the National Academy of Sciences 71: 3334–3337

McDonagh D J, Nathan S P, Knudson R J, Lebowitz M D 1979 Assessment of alpha₁-antitrypsin deficiency heterozygosity as a risk factor in the etiology of emphysema. Journal of Clinical Investigation 63: 299–309

McElrath M J. Galbraith R M, Allen R C 1979 Demonstration of alpha₁-antitrypsin by immunofluorescence on paraffin-embedded hepatic and pancreatic tissue. Journal of Histochemistry and Cytochemistry 27: 794–796

Matzen R N, Bader P I, Block W D 1977 Alpha₁-antitrypsin deficiency in clinic patients. Annals of Clinical Research 9: 88–92

Miale T D, Lawson D L, Demian S, Teague P O, Wolfson S L 1977 Possible involvement of blood platelet/megakaryocyte system in alpha₁-antitrypsin deficiency. Lancet 2: 93–94

Mihas A A, Hirschowitz B I 1976 Alpha₁-antitrypsin and chronic pancreatitis. Lancet 2: 1032–1033

Miller F, Kuschner M 1969 Alpha₁-antitrypsin deficiency, emphysema, necrotizing angiitis and glomerulonephritis. American Journal of Medicine 46: 615–623

Mirsky I A, Foley G 1945 Antibiotic actions of trypsin inhibitors. Proceedings of the Society for Experimental Biology and Medicine 59: 34–35

Miyake K, Suzuki H, Oka H, Oda T, Harada S 1979 Distribution of α₁-antitrypsin phenotypes in Japanese: Description of Pi M subtypes by isoelectric focusing. Japanese Journal of Human Genetics 24: 55–62

Mittman C 1978 The PiMZ phenotype: Is it a significant risk factor for the development of chronic obstructive lung disease? American Review of Respiratory Disease 118: 649–652

Mittman C, 1980 Additional supporting data. American Journal of Human Genetics 32: 457–458

Mittman C, Lieberman J 1973 Screening for α₁-antitrypsin deficiency. Israel Journal of Medical Sciences 9: 1311–1318

Mittman C, Lieberman J, Marasso F, Miranda A 1971 Smoking and chronic obstructive lung disease in alpha₁-antitrypsin deficiency. Chest 60: 214–221

Morihara K, Tsuzuki H, Oda K 1979 Protease and elastase of Pseudomonas aeruginosa: inactivation of human plasma α₁-proteinase inhibitor. Infection and Immunity 24: 188–193

Morin T, Feldmann G, Benhamou J P, Martin J P, Rueff B, Ropartz C 1975 Heterozygous alpha-antitrypsin deficiency and cirrhosis in adults, a fortuitous association. Lancet 1: 250–251

Moroi M, Yamasaki M, Aoki N 1975 Association of human α₁-antitrypsin with anhydrotrypsin. Journal of Biochemistry (Tokyo), 78: 925–928

Moroz S P, Cutz E, Cox D W, Sass-Kortsak A 1976a Liver disease associated with alpha₁-antitrypsin deficiency in childhood. Journal of Pediatrics 88: 19–25

Moroz S P, Cutz E, Balfe J W, Sass-Kortsak A 1976b Membranoproliferative glomerulonephritis in childhood cirrhosis associated with alpha₁-antitrypsin deficiency. Pediatrics 57: 232–238

Moser K M, Kidikoro Y, Marsh J, Sgroi V 1978 Biologic half-life and organ distribution of radiolabeled human PiM and PiZ alpha₁-antitrypsin in the dog. Journal of Laboratory and Clinical Medicine 91: 214–222

Moskowitz R W, Heinrich G 1971 Bacterial inactivation of human serum alpha₁-antitrypsin. Journal of Laboratory and Clinical Medicine 77: 777–785

Noades J E, Cook P J L 1976 Family studies with the Gm:Pi linkage group. Cytogenetics Cell Genetics 16: 341–344

Novis B H, Banks S, Young G O, Marks I N 1975 Chronic pancreatitis and alpha₁-antitrypsin. Lancet 2: 748

O'Brien M L, Buist N R M, Murphey W H 1978 Neonatal screening for alpha₁-antitrypsin deficiency. Journal of Pediatrics 92: 1006–1010

O'Neill F J 1974 Limitation of nuclear division by protease inhibitors in cytochalasin-B-treated tumor cells. Journal of the National Cancer Institute 52: 653–657

Ostrow D N, Cherniack R M 1972 The mechanical properties of the lungs in intermediate deficiency of α₁-antitrypsin. American Review of Respiratory Disease 106: 377–383

Ostrow D N, Manfreda J, Tse K S, Dorman T, Cherniack R M 1978 Alpha₁-antitrypsin phenotypes and lung function in a moderately polluted northern Ontario community. Canadian Medical Association Journal 118: 669–672

Owen M C, Carrell R W 1976 Alpha₁-antitrypsin: molecular abnormality of S variant. British Medical Journal 1: 130–131

Palmer P E, Wolfe H J 1976 α₁-antitrypsin deposition in primary hepatic carcinoma. Archives of Pathology and Laboratory Medicine 100: 232–236

Palmer P E, Safaii H, Wolfe H J 1976 Alpha₁-antitrypsin and alpha-fetoprotein. Protein markers in endodermal sinus (yolk sac) tumors. American Journal of Clinical Pathology 65: 575–582

Palmer P E, Wolfe H J, Kostas C I 1978 Multisystem fibrosis in alpha₁-antitrypsin deficiency. Lancet 1: 221–222

Perelman R, Nathanson M, Lepastier G, Lesavre Ph, Plainfosse B, Chirazi S, Seringe Ph 1975 Mannosidose associee a l'absence d'alpha-1-antitrypsine. Annales Pediate 22: 385–396

Peterson R J, Marsh C L 1979 The relationship of alpha₁-antitrypsin to inflammatory periodontal disease. Journal of Periodontology 50: 31–35

Pierce J A, Eradio B, Dew T A 1975 Antitrypsin phenotypes in St. Louis. Journal of the American Medical Association 231: 609–612

Pitt E, Lewis D A 1979 Stimulatory action of steroidal anti-inflammatory drugs on plasma alpha₁-antitrypsin levels in the rat. British Journal of Pharmacology 66: 454–455

Pongpaew P, Schelp F P 1980 Alpha₁-protease inhibitor phenotypes and serum concentrations in Thailand. Human Genetics 54: 119–124

Porter C A, Mowat A P, Cook P J L, Haynes D W G, Shilken R W 1972 α₁-antitrypsin deficiency and neonatal hepatitis. British Medical Journal 2: 435–439

Powers J C, Gupton B F, Harley A D, Nishino N, Whitley R J 1977 Specificity of porcine pancreatic elastase, human leucocyte elastase and cathepsin G. Inhibition with peptide chloromethyl ketones. Biochimica et Biophysica Acta 485: 156–166

Premachandra B N, Yu S Y 1979 Association of prealbumin deficiency with alpha$_1$-antitrypsin deficiency. Metabolism 28: 890–894

Prevost C L, Frommel D, Dupuy J M 1975 Complement studies in alpha$_1$-antitrypsin deficiency in children. Journal of Pediatrics 87: 571–573

Pride N B, Tattersall S F, Pereira R P, Hunter D, Blundell G 1980 Lung distensibility and airway function in intermediate alpha$_1$-antitrypsin deficiency (PiMZ). Chest 77: 253–255

Putnam C W, Porter K A, Peters R L, Ashcavai M, Redeker A–G, Starzl T–E 1977 Liver replacement for alpha$_1$-antitrypsin deficiency. Surgery 81: 258–261

Ratliff N B, Wilson J W, Mikat E, Hackel D B, Graham T C 1971 The lung in hemorrhagic shock. IV. The role of neutrophilic polymorphonuclear leukocytes. American Journal of Pathology 65: 325–332

Ray M B, Desmet V J 1978 Immunohistochemical demonstration of alpha-1-antitrypsin in the islet cells of human pancreas. Cell and Tissue Research 187: 69–77

Ray M B, Desmet V J 1978 Immunohistochemical immunoreactivity in islet cells of adult human pancreas. Cell and Tissue Research 185: 63–68

Rees E D, Hollingsworth J W, Hoffman T R, Black H, Hearn T L 1975 Smoking and disease. Effect on serum antitrypsin in hospitalized patients. Archives of Environmental Health 30: 402–408

Reintoft I 1977 Alpha-1-antitrypsin deficiency. Experience from an autopsy material. Acta Pathologica et Microbiologica Scandinavica 85: 649–655

Reintoft I 1979 Alpha-1-antitrypsin globules in livers from a medicolegal autopsy material. Acta Pathologica et Microbiologica Scandinavica 87: 447–450

Roberts A, Kagan A, Rhoads G C, Pierce J A, Bruce R M 1977 Antitrypsin and chronic obstructive pulmonary disease among Japanese-American men. Chest 72: 489–491

Robert J, Souillet G, Chapuis-Cellier C, Ghipponi J, Bienvenu J, Frobert Y, Carron R 1979 Immunite non specifique et role aggravant d'un phenotype abnormal de l'alpha-1-antitrypsine chez les enfants atteints de deficit selectif en IgA. La Nouvelle Press Medicale 8: 2659–2662

Rodriquez J R, Seals J E, Radin A, Lin J S, Mandl I, Turino G M 1975 The role of leukocyte elastase in the pathogenesis of obstructive lung disease. American Review of Respiratory Disease 111: 929

Rubenstein H M, Jaffer A M, Kudrna J C, Lertratanakul Y, Chandrasekhar A J, Slater D, Schmid F R 1977 Alpha$_1$-antitrypsin deficiency with severe panniculitis. Report of two cases. Annals of Internal Medicine 86: 742–744

Samad I A, O'Connell C J 1972 Serum alpha$_1$-antitrypsin deficiency. Chest 61: 307–308

Sandhaus R A, Janoff A 1974 Degradation of human α_1-antitrypsin by hepatocyte acid cathepsins. American Review of Respiratory Disease 110: 263–272

Santiago J V, Dew T A, Haymond M, Williamson J R, Kilo C, Kipnis M, Pierce J A 1974 Glucose intolerance in α_1-antitrypsin deficiency. Journal of Clinical Investigation 53: 70A

Sasaki M, Yamamoto H, Iida S 1974 Interaction of human serum proteinase inhibitors with proteolytic enzyme of animal, plant and bacterial origin. Journal of Biochemistry (Tokyo), 75: 171–177

Scharpe S, Eid M, Cooreman W, Lauwers A 1978 α_1-antitrypsin, an inhibitor of renin. Biochemical Journal 153: 505–507

Schmitt M G, Phillips R B, Matzen R N, Rodey G 1975 α_1-antitrypsin deficiency: A study of the relationship between the Pi system and genetic markers. American Journal of Human Genetics 27: 315–321

Schumacher G F B 1971 Inhibition of rabbit sperm acrosomal protease by human alpha$_1$-antitrypsin and other protease inhibitors. Contraception 4: 67–78

Schumacher G F B, Pearl M J 1965 Alpha$_1$-antitrypsin in cervical mucus. Fertility and Sterility 19: 91–99

Schydlower M, Waxman S H, Patterson P H 1979 Coexistence of deficiency in alpha$_1$-antitrypsin and in growth hormone. New England Journal of Medicine 300: 364–365

Sesbout R, Charlionet R, Vercaigne D, Guimbretiere J, Martin J P 1978 Genetic variants of serum alpha$_1$-antitrypsin (Pi types) in Bretons. Human Heredity 28; 280–284

Sharp H L 1971 Alpha$_1$-antitrypsin deficiency. Hospital Practice, May: 83–96

Sharp H L, Bridges R A, Krivit W, Freier E F 1969 Cirrhosis associated with alpha$_1$-antitrypsin deficiency: A previously unrecognized inherited disorder. Journal of Laboratory and Clinical Medicine 73: 934–939

Shulman N R 1952 Studies on the inhibition of proteolytic enzymes by serum. Journal of Experimental Medicine 95: 605–618

Sjoblom K G, Wollheim F A 1977 Alpha$_1$-antitrypsin phenotypes and rheumatic diseases. Lancet 2: 41

Snider G L, Hayes J A, Franzblau C, Kagan H M, Stone P J, Korthy A 1974 Relationship between elastolytic activity and experimental emphysema inducing properties of papain preparations. American Review of Respiratory Disease 110: 254–262

Sveger T 1978 α_1-antitrypsin deficiency in early childhood. Pediatrics 62: 22–25

Sveger T 1976 Liver disease in alpha$_1$-antitrypsin deficiency detected by screening of 200,000 infants. New England Journal of Medicine 294: 1316–1321

Szceklik A, Turowska B, Mysik G C, Opolska B, Nizankowska E 1974 Serum alpha$_1$-antitrypsin in bronchial asthma. American Review of Respiratory Disease 109: 487–490

Talamo R C 1975 Basic and Clinical Aspects of the alpha$_1$-antitrypsin. Pediatrics 56: 91–99

Talamo R C, et al 1978 Alpha$_1$-antitrypsin laboratory manual. U.S. Department of Health, Education and Welfare. DHEW Publication No. (NIH) 78–1420

Talerman A, Haije W G, Baggerman L 1977 Alpha$_1$-antitrypsin (AAT) and alphafoetoprotein (AFP) in sera of patients with germ-cell neoplasms: Value as tumour markers in patients with endodermal sinus tumour (yolk sac tumour).International Journal of Cancer 19: 741–746

Taylor J C, Kueppers F 1977 Electrophoretic mobility of leucocyte elastase of normal subjects and patients with chronic obstructive pulmonary disease. American Review of Respiratory Disease 116: 531–536

Terblanche J, Koep L J, Starzl T E 1979 Liver transplantation. Medical Clinics of North America 63: 507–521

Torp A 1975 Myocardial biopsy in a case of cardiomyopathy and partial α_1-antitrypsin deficiency with liver engagement. Acta Medica Scandinavica 197: 137–140

Touraine J L, Malik M C, Perrot H, Maire I, Revillard U P, Grosshans E, Traeger J 1979 Maladie de Fabry: deux malades amellores par la greffe de cellules de foie foetal. La Nouvelle Presse Medicale 8: 1499–1503

Triger D R, Millward-Sadler G H, Czaykowski A A, Trowell

J, Wright R 1976 Alpha₁-antitrypsin deficiency and liver disease in adults. Quarterly Journal of Medicine 45: 351–372

Turino G M, Senior R M, Garg B D, Keller S, Levi M M, Mandl I 1969 Serum elastase inhibitor deficiency and α_1-antitrypsin deficiency in patients with obstructive emphysema. Science 165: 709–711

Tuttle W C, Jones R K 1975 Fluorescent antibody studies of alpha₁-antitrypsin in adult human lung. American Journal of Clinical Pathology 64: 477–482

Vandeville D, Martin J P, Ropartz C 1974 α_1-antitrypsin in polymorphism of a Bantu population: Description of a new allele PiL. Humangentik 21: 33–38

Victorino R, Silveira J C B, Geada H, Moura M C 1978 Familial hypercholesterolaemia with alpha₁-antitrypsin deficiency. British Medical Journal 1: 413–414

Walker-Smith J, Andrews J 1972 Alpha₁-antitrypsin, autism, and coeliac disease. Lancet 2: 883–884

Walsh L, McConkey B 1977 Alpha₁-antitrypsin and rheumatoid arthritis. Lancet 2: 564–565

Ward P A, Ralamo R C 1973 Deficiency of the chemotactic factor inactivator in human sera with α_1-antitrypsin deficiency. Journal of Clinical Investigation 52: 516–519

Weitkamp L R, Cox D W, Johnston E, Guttormsen S A, Schwartz R H, Bias W B, Hsu S H 1976 Data on the genetic linkage relationships between red cell acid phosphatase and alpha₁-antitrypsin variants Z, S, I, and F. Cytogenetics and Cell Genetics 16: 359–363

Weikkamp L R, Cox D, Guttormsen S, Johnston E, Hempgling S 1978 Allelic specific heterogeneity in the Pi:Gm linkage group. Cytogenetics and Cell Genetics 22: 647–650

Welch M H, Richardson R H, Whitcomb W H, Hammarsten J F, Guenter C A 1969 The lung scan in α_1-antitrypsin deficiency. Journal of Nuclear Medicine 10: 687–690

Welch S G, McGregor I A, Williams K 1980 α_1-antitrypsin (Pi) phenotypes in a village population from the Gambia, West Africa. Human Genetics 53: 223–235

Wicher V, Dolovich J 1971 Interactions of Bacillus subtilis alkaline proteinases with α_2-macroglobulin and α_1-antitrypsin. International Archives of Allergy and Applied Immunology 40: 779–788

Wittels E H, Coalson J J, Welch M H, Guenter C A 1974 Pulmonary intravascular leucocyte sequestration. A potential mechanism of lung injury. American Review of Respiratory Disease 109: 502–509

Yoshida A, Wessels M 1978 Origin of the multiple components of human α_1-antitrypsin. Biochemical Genetics 16: 641–649

Yoshida A, Chillar R, Taylor J C 1979a An α_1-antitrypsin variant, Pi B Alhambra with rapid anodal electrophoretic mobility. American Journal of Human Genetics 31: 555–563

Yoshida A, Ewing C, Wessels M, Lieberman J, Gaidulis L 1977 Molecular abnormality of Pi S variant of human alpha₁-antitrypsin. American Journal of Human Genetics 29: 233–239

Yoshida A, Lieberman J, Gaidulis L, Ewing C 1976 Molecular abnormality of human alpha₁-antitrypsin variant (Pi-ZZ) associated with plasma activity deficiency. Proceeding of the National Academy of Sciences 73: 1324–1328

Yoshida A, Taylor J C, van den Brock W G M 1979b Structural difference between the normal PiM₁ and the common PiM₂ variant of human α_1-antitrypsin. American Journal of Human Genetics 31: 564–568

Yu S D, Gan J C 1978 Effects of progressive desialylation on the survival of human plasma α_1-antitrypsin in rat circulation. International Journal of Biochemistry 9: 107–115

67

Kartagener syndrome and its variants

P. S. Gerald and E. S. Schneeberger

INTRODUCTION

Kartagener syndrome is clinically characterized by the presence of situs inversus, bronchiectasis and recurrent sinusitis. The recent discovery in these patients of various electron microscopic defects in the axial (axonemal) structure of their cilia and sperm tails, associated with immotility or dysfunction of these structures, has permitted the recognition of a number of variants of this syndrome. In addition, it is now evident that only a proportion, perhaps half, of individuals with abnormal cilia have recurrent respiratory disease without cardiac malrotation. For this reason, the phrases immotile-cilia syndrome and ciliary-dyskinesia syndrome are becoming the preferred designations. The syndrome is probably recessively inherited. No consistent abnormality has been detected in presumed heterozygotes.

HISTORY

The combination of situs inversus with respiratory disease received particular attention following Kartagener's publication in 1933 (Kartagener, 1933). Its familial nature was recognized in several subsequent papers (Rott, 1979). The unusual association of a congenital malformation with recurrent respiratory disease aroused considerable, but generally futile, speculation as to the pathogenesis of the disorder. The first notable insight in this direction resulted from the publication in 1975 of studies of three infertile males from two unrelated sibships (Afzelius et al, 1975; Pedersen & Rebbe, 1975). All three males exhibited both immotility of their sperm and an ultrastructural defect of the axonemal structure of the sperm tail. Since the axonemal structures of cilia and sperm were known to be comparable, it was expected and subsequently proven that cilia, like sperm, were immotile and had a similar structural defect. With the recognition that the ciliary abnormality was the probable underlying basis for the respiratory manifestations of this syndrome, it was possible to show that many, perhaps half, of individuals with the ciliary defect lacked the car-

diac malrotation. This led to the suggestion that this syndrome should be renamed the immotile-cilia syndrome (Eliasson et al, 1977). Although most of the patients initially studied had apparently identical axonemal defects (described below), variant patterns were occasionally encountered. In a few of these variants, some degree of ciliary movement was observed, but was believed to be disorganized and ineffective. Since the characteristic clinical features can exist in the absence of total ciliary immotility, it has been suggested that ciliary dyskinesia is the more appropriate designation for this syndrome (Sturgess et al, 1980).

NORMAL AXONEMAL STRUCTURE

Cilia and sperm have similar axonemal structures (Fig. 67.1) and consist of 9 outer microtubular doublets and two central microtubules. The latter are partially surrounded by the central sheath, which is connected to the outer doublets by radial spokes. The microtubules designated as the outer doublets in Fig. 67.1 have three types of structure attached to them. These are the dynein arms, the nexin links and the radial spokes. The dynein arms, which are firmly attached to one doublet, form intermittent connections to the adjacent doublet. One or more of the proteins in the dynein arms have ATPase activity (Gibbons, 1965; Satir, 1965). It is currently believed that the dynein arms function through this ATPase activity to make and break connections with the adjacent doublet. The motion of cilia and sperm tails depends upon the sliding of the microtubules relative to one another (Satir, 1965), while the nexin links are thought to be responsible for maintaining the axonemal structure and for limiting the extent of sliding. The intermittent attachments provided by the dynein arms are vital to this process and hence to ciliary motility. In addition to their morphologic distinctiveness, the outer and inner arms differ in their protein components (Huang et al, 1979).

The normal role of the radial spokes is less clearly delineated. There is evidence that they interact with the

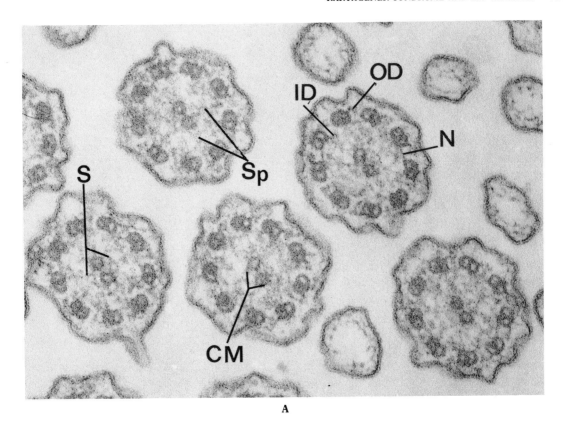

A

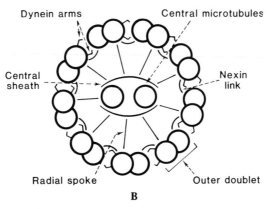

B

Fig. 67.1 (A) Nasal brush biopsy from a normal individual showing five similarly oriented cilia as judged by the alignment of the two central microtubules (CM). The outer (OD) and inner (ID) dynein arms are attached to one of the tubules of the outer doublets. The central sheath (S), spokes (SP) and nexin links (N) are indicated. Mag. x147,000. (B) Schematic diagram of axonemal structure of a cilium.

central sheath at the start of bending and in some way serve to convert the sliding into bending motion (Warner & Satir, 1974). From their location in the axoneme, it would be expected that they would serve, as is implicit in their name, to maintain the orientation of the central pair of microtubules relative to the outer doublets. This is consistent with the altered arrangements of microtubules seen in patients with radial spoke defects (Sturgess et al, 1979).

It should be appreciated that the schematic diagram of Fig. 67.1 dramatically oversimplifies the axonemal structure. The remarkable constancy of the axonemal structure, from plants to humans, should not be interpreted as indicating a simple molecular composition. The latest biochemical studies indicate that approximately 100 different proteins are present in the axonemal structure (Piperno et al, 1977). A comparable multiplicity of genetic determinants may reasonably be expected.

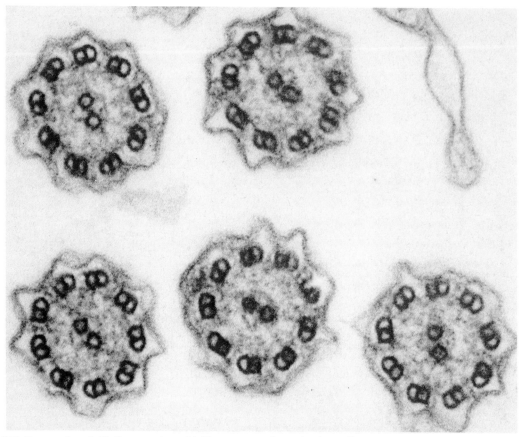

Fig. 67.2 Cross section of cilia from a patient with Kartagener syndrome in whose cilia both inner and outer dynein arms are absent. Note that the central microtubules are randomly oriented. Mag. x167,000.

The foregoing emphasis upon the details of the axonemal structure reflects the greater amount of information available in this area. It should not be forgotten, however, that a typical ciliated epithelial cell has many cilia upon its surface and that their motion must be coordinated if it is to be effective. Further, each of the epithelial cells of a given organ must be properly oriented if the direction of mucociliary transport is to be effective and physiologically appropriate. Little or nothing is known about the factors responsible for interorganelle and intercellular communication and for cellular orientation that are necessary to meet these requirements.

AXONEMAL DEFECTS IN MAN

The first Kartagener syndrome patients examined were found to have an at least superficially similar axonemal defect (Afzelius et al, 1975; Pedersen & Rebbe, 1975; Eliasson et al, 1977). In these patients, the dynein arms, both inner and outer, were either totally absent or pres-

ent only as shortened projections (Fig. 67.2). These features were evident in both spcrm tails and respiratory cilia. Similar findings were observed in cilia from bronchial and nasal epithelium, and even from ciliated cells of the middle ear (Fischer, 1978). The dynein arms were also shown to be absent in the cilia of epithelial cells lining the fallopian tubes (Jean et al, 1979).

A common accompaniment of the dynein defect is a somewhat randomized orientation for adjacent cilia, as judged by the orientation of the central pair of microtubules (Fig. 67.2). Normally, a line drawn through the two central microtubules of one cilium is remarkably parallel to comparably drawn lines for adjacent cilia. The non-parallel nature of these lines in patients with Kartagener syndrome (and the various variants to be described subsequently) is highly characteristic of this disease. The non-uniform orientation of the cilia is even more readily discerned by examining the basal body located at the base of each cilium. In human ciliated epithelium, the basal body has a lateral spur projecting from it parallel to the cell surface. In normal individuals, the spurs of adjacent

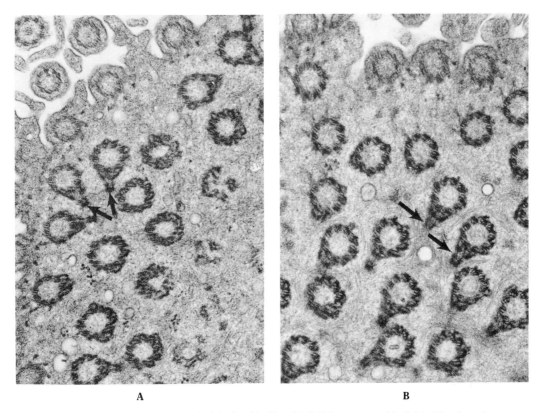

A   B

Fig. 67.3 Section of ciliated cells cut at the level of the basal bodies. (A) Cell from a normal individual in whom the spurs attached to the basal bodies are all oriented in the same direction (arrows). (B) Cell from patient in whose cilia there was a lack of both inner and outer dynein arms. The lateral spurs show a random orientation (arrows). Mag. x42,000.

cilia have a strikingly similar orientation, which contrasts markedly with the findings in the various forms of Kartagener syndrome (Fig. 67.3A and B).

Sturgess et al (1979) have described a patient with clinically classical Kartagener syndrome, two of whose sibs were affected with recurrent respiratory disease without situs inversus. In all three individuals, the outer dynein arms were present, while the inner arms and radial spokes were missing. (Absence of the inner arms was noted subsequent to publication, according to a personal communication from Dr Sturgess.) Associated with the lack of radial spokes, and perhaps as a consequence of this absence, was an eccentric displacement of the central pair of microtubules and, in some cilia, a movement of an outer doublet towards the centre. Since these features were common to all three patients, and not noted in any of the previously described Kartagener syndrome patients with absence of both dynein arms, it can be assumed that the absence of radial spokes in this family represents a distinct genetic entity. The one male in this sibship also had a moderately reduced sperm count, which contrasts with the normal sperm counts usually present in the Kartagener syndrome patients with absence of both dynein arms.

These and other patients with different types of axonemal defects emphasize the need to develop a terminology that takes these differences into account. In accord with the suggestion of Sturgess et al (1980), we will refer to these different morphologic and functional axonemal defects as various types of ciliary dyskinesia. The usual form of ciliary dyskinesia, with absence of both inner and outer dynein arms, will be designated type 1 and the absent radial spoke category will be called type 2 (Table 67.1).

A clinically classical Kartagener syndrome patient examined by the present authors may also be of type 2 (Schneeberger et al, 1980). This male was severely oligospermic, had unusually prominent outer dynein arms while inner arms and nexin links were undetectable (Fig. 67.4A and B). Only 46% of cilia, however, lacked radial spokes and exhibited eccentric inner microtubules and centrally displaced outer doublets. A sibling of this patient was said to have died in infancy of cyanotic congenital heart disease, but it was not possible to obtain further details.

Sturgess et al (1980) have described two sibs affected with what they have tentatively labelled as type 3 ciliary dyskinesia (Table 67.1). In ciliary cross sections from

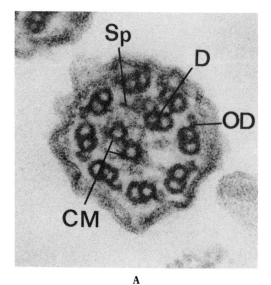

A

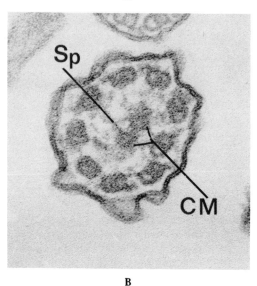

B

Fig. 67.4 Cilia from a patient whose cilia have prominent outer (OD) but no inner dynein arms. No nexin links were seen in any of the cilia examined. (A) One of the cilia in which the two central microtubules (CM) are eccentrically placed and an outer doublet (D) is displaced centrally. The spokes (SP) appear disorganized. (B) One of the cilia in which the central microtubules (CM) are eccentrically placed and the spokes (SP) are disorganized. However, the 9 outer doublets form the usual outer ring. Mag. x210,000.

both of these patients, the central pair of microtubules was missing and one outer doublet (identified in sperm tails as the doublet in the number one position in the ring) was displaced to the central area for at least part of the length of the cilium. Both of these patients had chronic respiratory disease but no cardiac malrotation.

Table 67.1 Varieties of ciliary dyskinesia.

Type	Axonemal defect	Sperm exam.	Relative frequency
1	Complete or partial absence of inner and outer dynein arms. Randomized orientation of adjacent cilia.	Immotile, normal count	Common
2	Absence of radial spokes, inner dynein arms and nexin links. Outer dynein arms present and may be unusually prominent. Randomized orientation of adjacent cilia.	Immotile, moderately to markedly reduced in number	Rare
3	Displacement of (number 1) doublet to the interior with absence of central microtubules. Dynein arms and radial spokes are normal.	Reduced motility (10% of normal), normal count	Very rare
4	Supernumerary single microtubules both inside and outside the ring of doublets. Occasional absence of one or both central microtubules. Partial or complete absence of inner and outer dynein arms. Randomized orientation of adjacent cilia.	No information	Rare

In the one male patient, there was a normal sperm count but only 10% motility.

Still other variant axonemal patterns have been described, but generally not as familial disorders. While it is likely that many of these represent distinct genetic disorders, the evidence is accordingly less certain. In this category is the patient of Neustein et al (1979) with chronic respiratory disease but without cardiac malrotation. The ciliary cross sections from this patient were characterized by the presence of supernumerary single-

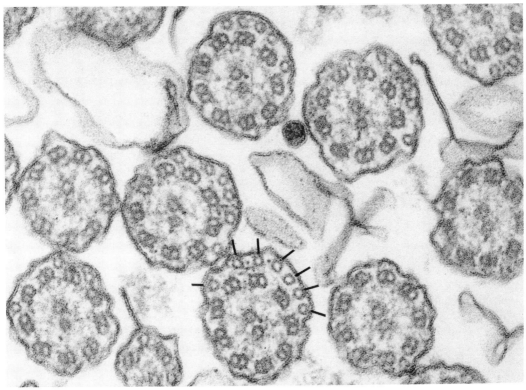

Fig. 67.5 Cilia from patient with supernumerary singleton microtubules. In this field five of eight cilia have three to seven supernumerary outer single microtubules (small lines). Dynein arms are absent. Mag. x131,000.
Figures 67.1A, 67.2, 67.3A & B, 67.4A & B and 67.5 reproduced with permission of the authors and publisher from Schneeberger et al (1980).

ton microtubules. The supernumerary microtubules were present in the central area (the typical central pair was either absent or replaced by supernumerary microtubules) or between the ring of outer doublets and the ciliary membrane. Dynein arms were said to be present but were difficult to identify. Sperm could not be examined since the patient was preadolescent. We have tentatively classified this patient as type 4 ciliary dyskinesia (see Table 67.1).

A patient with some of the features of this type 4 disease has been examined by the present authors (Schneeberger et al, 1980). This patient has situs inversus, recurrent respiratory disease and pectus excavatum (severe enough to justify elective surgical correction). In all cilia examined, there was complete or partial absence of both inner and outer dynein arms, although the remaining axonemal structures were normal. In 38% of his ciliary cross sections, from 1 to 9 supernumerary singleton microtubules could be identified in the space between the ring of outer doublets and the ciliary membrane (Fig. 67.5). In an additional 5% of cilia there was either absence of the central pair, or 1 to 2 single microtubules were within the ring of outer doublets. Sperm

analysis was precluded by this patient's preadolescent status.

Still other varieties of defects have been recognized (Afzelius & Eliasson, 1979) and undoubtedly many more will be found in the future. At the moment, it is not clear whether these additional, and often subtler, differences represent entities that are genetically distinct from those listed in Table 67.1. For this reason we have not included them as defined types in the Table.

PATHOPHYSIOLOGY

The serendipitous discovery of sperm immotility in Kartagener syndrome led to the identification of the axonemal defect that is now believed to be the primary abnormality in this disorder. It is of historical interest that several reports (Arge, 1960; Grewal et al, 1965) prior to the discovery of the axonemal defect noted the presence of infertility and relative or absolute immotility of the sperm in Kartagener syndrome patients. The association of sperm immotility and dynein arm defects was clinical confirmation of the explanation for sperm motility independently deduced from experimental studies (Gibbons, 1965; Satir, 1965). It is assumed that the infertility is a direct consequence of sperm immotility.

Although the motility of cilia has been much less studied than that of sperm tails, the remarkable similarity of the axonemal structures of these two organelles suggested that the information available on sperm motility could be applied in toto to ciliary motility. Studies in vivo of mucociliary transport have confirmed that the lack of motility in cilia matches that in sperm (Mossberg et al, 1978).

It is reasonable to expect that this defect in mucociliary transport would cause ineffective removal of bacteria and their toxic products, with consequent increase in severity and chronicity of infection of organs exposed to the external environment. Since some patients have partial motility of sperm and cilia, it might be that they would be less affected by respiratory disease. Unfortunately, there are not yet enough data to attempt this correlation.

It is also possible that components of the axoneme responsible for generating motility of the cilium might additionally have a role in movement of non-axonemal structures. This possibility led to the investigation and consequent demonstration, by Caleb et al (1977), of a defect in cell migration in one patient with Kartagener syndrome. No other published studies of this sort are available. (Dr Harvey Cohen examined the present authors' patient with type 2 ciliary dyskinesia but was unable to detect any similar abnormalities.) Nonetheless, the results of Caleb et al (1977) suggest that the susceptibility to respiratory infections might be influenced by factors other than ciliary motility.

Organs lined with ciliated epithelium that are not exposed to the external environment do not show an increased frequency of infection. Nonetheless, some functions of these organs might be altered by ciliary dyskinesia. This might possibly account for the severe, chronic headaches experienced by some patients with ciliary dyskinesia, even when no active sinusitis is present (Afzelius, 1979). Since ependymal cells are ciliated, ciliary dyskinesia might also result in impaired circulation of the cerebrospinal fluid. The slight enlargement of the ventricular system noted (Afzelius, 1979) in patients with Kartagener syndrome might be attributable to this mechanism.

None of the currently available studies of ciliary dyskinesia provide any real evidence for the pathogenesis of the cardiac malrotation. It has been speculated (Afzelius, 1976) that the movement of embryonic cells might be guided by ciliary activity. If so, the presence of ciliary dyskinesis might cause cell movement to be undirected, so that situs inversus and situs solitus would be equally likely to occur. This speculation is consistent with the findings in mice homozygous for a gene for situs inversus (*iv/iv*). These mice have an equal frequency of situs

solitus and situs inversus (Layton, 1976). This murine defect is not the result of ciliary dyskinesis, however, since the sperm of *iv/iv* males are normally motile (personal communication from Dr Roy Stevens).

The presence of sperm motility in the *iv/iv* mouse, as well as the lack of respiratory disease, implies that the mechanism producing situs inversus in these animals differs from that operative in the human ciliary dyskinesia syndromes. This leads to the prediction that humans might also have a genetically determined form of situs inversus without ciliary dyskinesia and respiratory disease. This is consistent with the clinical impression that only a small proportion of patients with situs inversus have significant respiratory disease (Rott, 1979). A more definitive statement on this point must await a detailed study of situs inversus patients without respiratory disease.

In patients with clinically typical Kartagener syndrome, the situs inversus is total and cardiac function is normal. Since the connection between axonemal defects and cardiac malrotation is not clearly delineated, it is possible that some forms of axonemal defect might produce partial malrotation, with its associated abnormal cardiac function. In an effort to assess this possibility, the authors have examined cilia from several patients with congenital heart disease due to malrotation. None of these patients had significant respiratory disease. Although several had a higher than normal frequency of microtubular defects (such as absence of one or both central microtubules), none had defects as dramatic as those already described. It is uncertain whether these findings constitute genuine axonemal defects.

In many reports of Kartagener syndrome patients, one or both parents are described as having an increase in respiratory infections. This raises the question of the manifestions of this disorder in heterozygotes. Since the disease is probably autosomal recessive, the fathers of patients with Kartagener syndrome are both presumptive heterozygotes and obviously fertile. The present authors have examined electron microscopically the cilia of the parents of one patient (with probable type 2 disease). Except for a slight increase in the frequency of microtubular defects, no abnormalities were found. The sperm from the father of this patient were normal in number, but had approximately 50% of normal movement (Schneeberger et al, 1980). Additional studies of obligate heterozygotes are required before it will be possible to determine if heterozygotes have either gross axonemal defects or symptoms.

KARTAGENER SYNDROME IN OTHER SPECIES

Situs inversus and recurrent respiratory infections (Carrig et al, 1974) have been reported in the dog. Unfortunately, no studies of axonemal structures were conducted.

A recessive disorder in mice (*hpy/hpy*), with hydrocephaly and polydactyly accompanied by male infertility and defective sperm tail formation, has been described (Bryan, 1977). Cilia from these mice were said to be abnormal in cross section and only the outer dynein arms were recognizable. Homozygous *hpy* mice do not have situs inversus or respiratory disease, however, so this animal is not a suitable model for studies of ciliary dyskinesia.

A more satisfactory model for the analysis of the genetic factors determining axonemal structure and function is offered by the alga Chlamydomonas. This single celled organism has four flagellae whose axonemal structure is remarkably similar to that of human cilia and sperm tails. The flagellae provide motive power to the organism and enable it to move toward light. Mutants with immotile (paralyzed) flagellae may be identified with ease as individuals unable to swim toward a light source. Genetic analysis of a series of paralyzed flagellar mutants demonstrates that many different loci determine flagellar activity (Randall & Starling, 1976). Current research on paralyzed flagellar mutants is emphasizing the correlation between ultrastructural changes and the concomitant alterations in flagellar proteins (Luck et al, 1977; Huang et al, 1979). These studies have shown, for example, that more than a dozen different proteins participate in the formation of the radial spokes (Luck et al, 1977).

Although Chlamydomonas serves as an ideal system for correlating genetic, ultrastructural and protein analytic information, there is as yet no direct means of comparing human and Chlamydomonas mutants, nor do any of the available Chlamydomonas mutants seem to duplicate exactly the known human defects. It is hoped that transformation of paralyzed flagellar mutants to normal activity by isolated human DNA fragments will become possible and permit direct comparison of the genetic defects in these two species.

GENETICS

Although the familial nature of Kartagener syndrome was noted even before Kartagener's original publication (Rott, 1979), there have been relatively few attempts to analyze this syndrome genetically. Cockayne's review in 1938 of 'transposition of the viscera' (Cockayne, 1938) included but did not distinguish instances of clinically typical Kartagener syndrome from individuals with situs inversus without respiratory disease. (Only a minority of individuals with situs inversus have respiratory disease (Rott, 1979). The majority, therefore, presumably do not have Kartagener syndrome.) Cockayne's evidence for recessive inheritance of situs inversus has been rather

non-critically applied to Kartagener syndrome by some subsequent writers. Rott (1979) has reviewed published cases that meet the criteria for Kartagener syndrome and believes that the occurrence of the syndrome in sibs and of consanguinity in the parents renders recessive inheritance beyond doubt.

Afzelius (1979) was able to collect family information for 15 patients with the immotile cilia syndrome, both with and without situs inversus. These patients had a total of 23 sibs, only 4 of whom were also affected. While this fraction is consistent with recessive inheritance Afzelius (1979) cites a personal communication from Dr Anne Child stating that the proportion of affected sibs in her experience is less than the predicted 25%.

Several papers on the immotile cilia syndrome state the belief that only half of such patients will have situs inversus (Rott, 1979). Since most original publications do not state the means of ascertainment with precision, it is difficult to estimate this fraction with confidence. It can only be stated that a significant number of patients with ciliary dyskinesia and without situs inversus have been identified and that the proportion of ciliary dyskinesia patients that have situs solitus may be as high as 50%. Much of the confidence in this last figure is derived from the similar figure obtained in the studies of the *iv/iv* mouse (Layton, 1976).

MEDICAL MANAGEMENT

The recurrent pulmonary, sinus and otic disease produce significant morbidity in these patients. (As was previously noted, the cardiac status in situs inversus totalis is functionally normal.) Antibiotic therapy and avoidance of infection, combined with centesis of sinus and otic cavities are the only approaches possible at present. Control of pulmonary infections, augmented with physiotherapy, hopefully will lessen the likelihood of bronchiectasis developing. These conventional approaches have only a mildly to moderately ameliorating effect in the average patient.

If the presumptively missing protein(s) in the various ciliary dyskinesias could be identified and introduced into respiratory epithelial cells, replacement therapy might actually be accomplished, since ciliary regeneration is a well recognized property of these cells. In vitro attempts along these lines have produced modest but, at least, initial success (Forrest, 1979).

DIAGNOSIS AND GENETIC COUNSELLING

Diagnosis presently depends upon the demonstration of an axonemal defect in cilia (and/or sperm). This diagnostic approach can be supplemented by direct examination of ciliary movement (Rutland & Cole, 1980) or by demonstration of delayed pulmonary clearance (Mossberg et al, 1978).

All presently known forms of ciliary dyskinesia are probably recessively inherited. The risk of recurrence among descendants of affected males is nil, in view of their expected infertility. Females with the disease are fertile. In the absence of consanguineous matings, their progeny will all be heterozygotes and generally asymptomatic.

No means of prenatal diagnosis are known.

REFERENCES

Afzelius B A 1976 A human syndrome caused by immotile cilia. Science 193: 317–319

Afzelius B A 1979 The immotile-cilia syndrome and other ciliary disease. International Review of Experimental Pathology 19: 1–43

Afzelius B A, Eliasson R 1979 Flagellar mutants in man: On the heterogeneity of the immotile-cilia syndrome. Journal of Ultrastructure Research 69: 43–52.

Afzelius B A, Eliasson R, Johnsen O, Lindholmer C 1975 Lack of dynein arms in immotile human spermatozoa. Journal of Cell Biology 66: 225–232

Arge E 1960 Transposition of the vicera and sterility in men. Lancet 1: 412–414

Bryan J H D 1977 Spermatogenesis revisited. IV. Abnormal spermiogenesis in mice homozygous for another male-sterility-inducing mutation, hyp (hydocephalic-polydactyl). Cell and Tissue Research 180: 187–201

Caleb M, Lecks H, South M A, Norman M E 1977 Kartagener's syndrome and abnormal cilia. New England Journal of Medicine 297: 1012–1013

Carrig C B, Suter P F, Ewing C O, Dunggworth D L 1974 Primary dextrocardia with situs inversus associated with sinusitis and bronchitis in a dog. Journal of the American Veterinary Medical Association 164: 1127–34

Cockayne E A 1938 The genetics of transposition of the viscera. Quarterly Journal of Medicine 7: 479–493

Eliasson R, Mossberg B, Camner P, Afzelius B A 1977 The immotile-cilia syndrome. New England Journal of Medicine 297: 1–6

Fischer T J, McAdams J A, Entis G N, Colton R, Ghory J E, Ausenmoore R W 1978 Middle ear ciliary defect in Kartagener's syndrome. Pediatrics 62: 443–445.

Forrest J B, Rossman C M, Newhouse M T, Ruffin R 1979 Activation of nasal cilia in immotile cilia syndrome. American Review of Respiratory Disease 120: 511–15

Gibbons I R 1965 Chemical dissection of cilia. Archives de Biologie (Liege) 76: 317–352

Grewal K S, Dixit R P, Dutta B 1965 Kartagener's syndrome associated with arrested spermatogenesis and sterility. Journal of the Indian Medical Association 45: 608–612

Huang B, Piperno G, Luck D J L 1979 Paralyzed flagella mutants of Chlamydomonas reinhardtii. Journal of Biological Chemistry 254: 3091-3099

Jean Y, Langlais J, Roberts K D, Chapdelaine A, Bleau G 1979 Fertility of a woman with nonfunctional ciliated cells in the fallopian tubes. Fertility and Sterility 31: 349–350

Layton W M, Jr 1976 Random determination of a developmental process. Journal of Heredity 67: 336–338

Luck D, Piperno G, Ramanis Z, Huang B 1977 Flagellar mutants of Chlamydomonas: Studies of radial spoke-defective strains by dikaryon and revertant analysis. Proceedings of the National Academy of Sciences USA 74: 3456–3460

Mossberg B, Afzelius B A, Eliasson R, Camner P 1978 On the pathogenesis of obstructive lung disease. A study on the immotile-cilia syndrome. Scandinavian Journal of Respiratory Disease 59: 55–65

Neustein H B, Church J, Cohen S 1979 Dysmorphology of cilia. Journal of the American Medical Association 241: 2423

Pedersen H, Rebbe H 1975 Absence of arms in the axoneme of immobile human spermatozoa. Biology of Reproduction 12: 541–544

Piperno G, Huang B, Luck D J L 1977 Two-dimensional analysis of flagellar proteins from wild-type and paralyzed mutants of Chlamydomonas reinhardtii. Proceedings of the National Academy of Sciences USA 74: 1600–1604

Randall J, Starling D 1976 Genetic determinants of flagellum phenotype in Chlamydomonas reinhardtii. In: Lewin R (ed) The genetics of algae. Blackwell Scientific Publishing and University of California Press, Botanical Monographs, Vol 12

Rott H D 1979 Kartagener's syndrome and the syndrome of immotile cilia. Human Genetics 46: 24–261

Rutland J, Cole P J 1980 Non-invasive sampling of nasal cilia for measurement of beat frequency and study of ultrastructure. Lancet 2: 564–565

Satir P 1965 Studies of cilia II. Examination of the distal region of the ciliary shaft and the role of the filaments in motility. Journal of Cell Biology 26: 875–834

Schneeberger E E, McCormack J, Issenberg H J, Schuster S R, Gerald P S 1980 Heterogeneity of ciliary morphology in the immotile-cilia syndrome in man. Journal of Ultrastructure Research 73: 34–43

Sturgess J M, Chao J, Turner J A P 1980 Transposition of ciliary microtubules. New England Journal of Medicine 303: 317–322

Sturgess J M, Chao J, Wong J, Aspin N, Turner J A P 1979 Cilia with defective radial spokes. New England Journal of Medicine 300: 53–56

Warner D, Satir P 1974 The structural basis of ciliary bend formation. Journal of Cell Biology 63: 35–63

Congenital heart defects

V. V. Michels and V. M. Riccardi

INTRODUCTION

Congenital heart defects include all primary structural malformations of the heart and intrathoracic great vessels resulting from an error in morphogenesis. The term congenital heart defect (CHD) does not include morbid processes (diseases) that occur after the embryologic heart has formed, whether or not they are congenital and/or heritable. This chapter will include discussions of cardiac defects per se, but except for endocardial fibroelastosis, will exclude diseases such as the Marfan syndrome in which abnormal supporting and connective tissue may result in secondary gross structural abnormalities.

A CHD may occur as an isolated defect in an otherwise normal infant as a result of a localized error of morphogenesis. Alternatively, CHDs may occur in conjuction with other abnormalities as part of a syndrome, a complex or association. A 'syndrome' is defined as a recognized pattern of malformations presumably having the same aetiology and currently not interpreted as the consequence of a single *localized* error in morphogenesis. A 'complex' refers to a malformation together with its subsequently derived structural changes, and an 'association' is a recognized pattern of malformations that occur together more frequently than by chance alone but which currently are not considered to constitute a syndrome or complex (Smith, 1976). The occurrence of a CHD as an isolated abnormality, or as part of a syndrome, complex or association, does not necessarily imply a common aetiology for the defects. The aetiology of CHDs is heterogeneous, and the exact nature of the defect, such as ventricular septal defect (VSD) or tetralogy of Fallot, is generally not specific for a particular aetiology. Aetiology may be single gene Mendelian, polygenic/multifactorial, teratogenic, chromosomal, or unknown. The evaluation of an individual with a CHD must take into account these various aetiologies in addition to whether the defect is isolated or associated with other abnormalities.

As with any medical problem, a thorough present history, past history including details of maternal health, pregnancy and developmental milestones, and family history must be obtained. During the physical examination, in addition to the cardiac findings, specific attention should be directed to evidence for other congenital defects. Other defects could be major and interfere significantly with the patient's health or function of a body part, for example cleft palate; or defects may be minor; such as rudimentary extra digits, low-set ears, mild micrognathia, or syndactyly. The individual findings may be inconsequential to the overall health of the individual, but they may provide valuable clues about the correct diagnosis or aetiology. In some instances, examination of other family members may be necessary to establish a correct diagnosis. Laboratory tests and specialized procedures necessary for diagnosis of the specific cardiac lesion are obviously indicated. Depending on the results of the medical and family history and physical examination, the patient may require chromosome analysis, viral cultures and serum antibody titres, slit lamp examination of the eyes, skeletal X–rays, intravenous pyelography, computerized axial tomography of the brain, audiometric evaluation, or formal psychometric testing. Clearly, the evaluation and care of a patient with CHD is not limited to concerns about the cardiac status, but must take into account any potential or actual associated abnormalities, and must be viewed in the context of aetiologic heterogeneity.

ISOLATED CONGENITAL HEART DEFECTS

The overall incidence of CHDs among all births (stillbirths and live births) is 8.14 per 1000 as determined by the Collaborative Study of Cerebral Palsy, Mental Retardation, and Other Neurologic and Sensory Disorders of Infancy and Childhood in a prospective evaluation of 56 109 births (Mitchell et al, 1971). This overall incidence is similar for all ethnic groups that have been studied (Anderson, 1977). Thirty percent of patients had an associated extra-cardiac malformation or mental retardation; however, these included relatively minor malformations such as inguinal herniae. On the other hand, the average follow-up time for surviving children was $3\frac{1}{2}$

years, and in some cases problems such as mild mental retardation may not have been detected. Estimates of the frequencies of associated malformations in other studies range from 9 to 42 %; a 25% incidence of major malformations was found in a comprehensive study group that included autopsy and clinic patients with significant CHD (Greenwood et al, 1975).

In spite of the variability in estimates derived from different studies, it is apparent that in most patients CHDs are isolated lesions. It is also apparent that additional defects are approximately ten times more frequent than in the general population (in which the overall incidence of major birth defects is 3 to 5%). One must therefore have a high index of suspicion about other anomalies in infants who present with a cardiac defect, and it is imperative that the physician consider the possibility that the heart defect is only the most obvious element of a multisystem disorder. In general, the most common malformations associated with a CHD are those of the musculoskeletal system (8.8%). Central nervous system disorders are present in 8.5%, renal-urinary tract malformations in 5.3%, and gastrointestinal anomalies in 4.2% (Greenwood, 1975). Knowledge about particular syndromes or associations can be helpful in directing one's attention to a given organ. For example, preductal coarctation of the aorta has a higher association with renal lesions than do other cardiac defects (Mitchell et al, 1971) and this fact might prompt performance of intravenous pyelography in these patients. Approximately 1.8% of patients with CHD have a cleft palate; although this is a relatively low rate of association, it is a ten fold increase in the incidence of cleft palate over that in the general population (Warkany, 1971).

Alternatively, patients with congenital defects of other organ systems may have a statistically increased risk for a cardiac defect. For example, approximately 15% of patients with oesophageal malformations have an associated heart defect (Greenwood & Rosenthal, 1976).

When additional congenital malformations are found, it is important to determine the nature of the multisystem involvement. Abnormalities in two or more systems may result from two primary abnormalities or may constitute a field defect. A 'field defect' is defined as a constellation of two or more malformations that result from a developmental error in a single embryologic field. The DiGeorge complex is an example of a field defect in which a primary abnormality in the fourth branchial arch and third and fourth pharyngeal pouches results in hypoplasia of the thymus and parathyroid glands in addition to aortic arch or conotruncal anomalies. Similarly, secondary consequences must be considered in any case of multisystem involvement. Secondary defects are generally deformations, alterations in shape and/or structure of a previously normally formed part; they are the results of primary malformations. For example, some cases of

patent ductus arteriosus (PDA) may be due to damage or enlargement resulting from increased volume flow related to preductal coarctation of the aorta.

Finally, one must consider coincidence when two types of disorder or birth defect are present in the same individual. For example, autosomal dominant neurofibromatosis is not usually associated with CHDs, but case reports of this association have appeared in the literature (Neiman et al, 1974). The incidence of CHD is 0.8% and the incidence of neurofibromatosis is 1 per 3300 live births (Bergsma, 1979). Therefore one could expect a chance association of these two conditions in approximately 1 per 400 000 live births.

Whether other defects associated with CHDs are due to coincidence, secondary consequences, or field defects may be readily apparent in some cases and unclear in others. Repeated evaluations and long term follow-up may be required before these confounding factors can be sorted out. Patients with apparently isolated CHDs must be re-evaluated to ensure that the defect is not part of an unsuspected multisystem disorder.

Aetiology

The aetiology of isolated CHDs includes single gene mutations, polygenic/multifactorial influences, teratogens, and other unknown factors. The great majority of isolated defects are due to polygenic and/or multifactorial causes. Although the terms 'polygenic' and 'multifactorial' are often used interchangeably, strictly speaking 'polygenic' refers to the influence of two or more genes that act together to account for a given phenotype. 'Multifactorial' is a more general term that may include the effects of one or more genes, environmental agents or other unknown factors that act together to influence the presence and nature of a given phenotype. In practice, one can rarely distinguish between the two possible sets of factors.

Single gene mutations are well known causes of isolated CHDs. Any one type of heart defect does not specify a cause, and only occasionally gives a clue about the underlying gene abnormality. A positive family history is usually, but not always, the clue that leads one to suspect Mendelian inheritance. For example, families with atrial septal defects (ASDs) in multiple generations suggest autosomal dominant inheritance (McKusick, 1978; #10880). In other instances, the nature of the heart defect raises suspicion that the defect is heritable. For example, secundum type ASD with prolonged atrioventricular conduction should lead one to consider a single gene aetiology even if a positive family history is not obtained (McKusick, 1978; #10890).

Moreover, a positive family history for a given defect does not in itself prove that the condition is inherited. For example, a family with four sibs having primum type ASD has been reported (Yao et al, 1968); the parents were normal. This family situation suggests but does not prove autosomal recessive inheritance. Multifactorial/polygenic inheritance or a common environmental factor or teratogen cannot be excluded. Similarly, there are reports of many other types of heart defect affecting two or more family members. These reports include families with Ebstein anomaly (McKusick, 1978; #22470), hypoplastic left heart (McKusick, 1978; #24155), coarctation of the aorta (McKusick, 1978; #12000), and patent ductus arteriosus (McKusick, 1978; #16910), to name a few. Single gene inheritance cannot be excluded and may in fact be the aetiology in some of these families. Studies of large series of patients with these defects give empiric recurrence risks compatible with multifactorial inheritance. The studies on tetralogy of Fallot serve as an example of this phenomenon in which most cases of a particular heart defect are probably of multifactorial aetiology though there are a few families with multiple family members suggesting a single gene aetiology. One six-generation pedigree (Pitt, 1962) was reported in which eleven of 275 members had a CHD, and six of these patients had tetralogy of Fallot or a variant thereof. The author interpreted these findings as an instance of autosomal dominant inheritance with reduced penetrance. However in another large study of 100 index patients with classical tetralogy of Fallot and their families, a tendency to familial aggregation of the condition and of other CHDs compatible with multifactorial inheritance was discerned (Boon et al, 1972). Whether a single gene is responsible for the heart defect in some families or whether multiple occurrences are due to multifactorial inheritance cannot always be established.

Teratogens must also be considered as a cause of isolated CHDs. The teratogenic rubella virus usually causes multiple defects; however 21% of infants with congenital rubella had single defects, many of which were accounted for by patent ductus arteriosus (PDA). Ventricular septal defect (VSD), ASD, tetralogy of Fallot, pulmonic stenosis (PS) and pulmonary branch stenosis (PBS) can also result from intrauterine rubella infection (Dudgeon, 1967).Other viral agents including Coxsackie Group B virus and those responsible for cytomegalic inclusion disease, influenza and mumps have been implicated but not proven to cause CHDs (Jackson, 1968). At the present time rubella can be considered as the only well documented viral teratogen, but it is possible that other viral agents will some day be shown to cause CHDs.

Similarly, drugs are often implicated as teratogenic agents, but relatively few are well documented to have this effect. It is sometimes more difficult to prove that an isolated CHD in a human is due to a specific drug than when the heart defect is part of a characteristic syndrome. Lithium as a cause of the Ebstein anomaly is an exception. This relatively rare heart defect was noted to occur frequently in offspring of women being treated with lithium for depression. Another way to identify drugs that can induce isolated CHDs is through large survey studies of the effects of drugs taken by mothers during pregnancy. Data from the Collaborative Perinatal Project (Heinonen et al, 1977) did not provide conclusive evidence that any of the drugs studied result in isolated CHDs, although it did strengthen previous suggestions that exogenous female sex hormones taken early in pregnancy may cause CHDs. It must be remembered that these types of study do not conclusively rule out the possibility that these agents could cause isolated CHDs at very low rates in the population or could cause CHDs in certain susceptible individuals. These types of concern lead to the mandate that pregnant women should be given medications only if necessary for their own health or the health of their fetus.

Evidence for teratogenicity of drugs in laboratory animals is more extensive. The fact that dextroamphetamine induced CHDs in genetically predisposed mouse strains (Nora et al, 1968) supports the possibility that drugs can induce defects in certain susceptible humans. Other agents that induce CHDs in animals include trypan blue, hypervitaminosis A, and aspirin; the defects induced are variable, even for a given agent. Other conditions besides drug administration that induce malformation include vitamin A and folic acid deficiencies, X–irradiation, and hypoxia. Frequently littermates of inbred animal strains were not concordant for specific defects, indicating as yet unexplained variable susceptibility of genetically identical animals (Warkany, 1971). Although X–irradiation and hypoxia have documented teratogenic potential in rats, neither has been shown to be a definite cause for isolated CHDs in humans under usual conditions.

Other factors to consider in the pathogenesis of CHDs include maternal health. Maternal cyanotic CHD with accompanying hypoxia does not appear to result in a higher incidence of offspring with CHD than expected when the recurrence risk associated with multifactorial disorders is taken into account (Jackson, 1968). However, maternal diabetes mellitus (Heinonen et al, 1977) systemic lupus erythematosus (Chameides et al, 1977) and phenylketonuria (Fisch et al, 1969) are examples of disease states that can adversely affect the development of the heart.

In addition to viral and drug teratogens, nutritional deficiency states, environmental agents and maternal health, there are probably other currently unknown agents or conditions that result in isolated CHDs.

Types of defect

Atrial septal defect (ASD)

ASDs account for approximately 15% of CHDs (Cascos, 1972), with an overall incidence of 0.6 to 0.7 per 1000 births (Heinonen, 1976). In approximately 84% of cases,

ASD is the only cardiac defect (Cascos, 1972). Of the two types of ASD, ostium secundum defects are more common, with an incidence of 0.56 per 1000 births (Heinonen, 1976). This type of defect seems to result from an abnormality in the degenerative process in the septum primum that normally forms the ostium secundum, such that the opening which forms is too large; or the defect may result from malposition of the ostium secundum in relation to the septum secundum that ordinarily covers it. A third possibility is that the septum secundum forms improperly so that the ostium is unguarded. The secundum type of defect is separated from the atrioventricular valves by septal tissue while the ostium primum defects have no septal tissue separating them from the atrioventricular valves; this latter results from failure of the septum primum to fuse with the atrioventricular canal cushion tissue. The defect is often accompanied by clefts of the mitral and/or tricuspid valve(s), suggesting that the defect may result from deficient development of the atrioventricular canal cushions rather than from the septum itself. Ostium primum defects are closely related to atrioventricular canal defects in which there is a common channel between both atria and ventricles in addition to cleft mitral and tricuspid valves. This defect clearly arises from abnormal development of the atrioventricular canal cushions (Jackson, 1968). Most cases of isolated ASD are inherited as a multifactorial condition, and empiric recurrence risk figures are compatible with this type of inheritance. The risk for sibs being affected with a similar CHD is 3.6% when no other relatives are affected (Nora et al, 1967). There is a female preponderance with a male:female ratio of 0.64; in keeping with predictions based on multifactorial inheritance, the risk for sibs of male patients is 5% and of female patients is 2.5% (Cascos, 1972). Autosomal dominant transmission of isolated ASD in some families is well documented (McKusick, 1978; #10880). In addition, there is an autosomal dominant syndrome of secundum type ASD with atrioventricular conduction defects (McKusick, 1978; #10890). In patients with nonfamilial secundum type ASDs the incidence of first degree atrioventricular block is only in the range of 6 to 19% (Kahler et al, 1966).

Other aetiologies of ASD include intrauterine rubella infections (Dudgeon, 1967), maternal systemic lupus erythematosus in which case congenital heart block is also present (Chameides et al, 1977), and maternal phenylketonuria (Fisch et al, 1969). Exposure of the embryo to excessive female hormones in the form of oral contraceptives has also been implicated as a cause of isolated primum type ASD (Heinonen, 1977). There are many other aetiologies for ASD as a part of syndromes and malformation complexes, and in one series 15% of patients had extracardiac abnormalities (Cascos, 1972).

Ventricular septal defect (VSD)
The incidence of isolated VSD is 2.19 per 1000 births,

and this lesion accounts for approximately 25% of CHDs (Nora et al, 1966). The defect can result from failure of normal ingrowth of tissue from the muscular septum, atrioventricular cushions, and/or conal ridges. Most cases of isolated VSD are multifactorial in origin. The risk of a sib being affected with VSD or a similar form of heart defect is 4.5% and for affected offspring is 3.7% when there is only one case of CHD in the family. It must be remembered when taking the family history that 10 to 25% of VSDs may close spontaneously. If two first degrees relatives have CHDs the recurrence risk figures double. There are no documented instances of isolated VSD being due to a single abnormal gene. However, congenital rubella (Dudgeon, 1967), maternal phenylketonuria (Fisch et al, 1969), and possibly embryonic exposure to oral contraceptives (Heinonen et al, 1977) can cause VSDs.

Conotruncal abnormalities
Abnormalities related to faulty conotruncal septation include tetralogy of Fallot, as well as some instances of isolated VSD and isolated PS (Patterson et al, 1974), transposition of the great artries (TGA) and double outlet right ventricle. The overall incidence of this group of defects is 0.87 per 1000 births (Heinonen, 1976). Conotruncal septation refers to the division of the single primitive heart tube into two distinct outflow tracts from two swellings that arise in the truncal region at 30 days gestation and grow towards each other in a spiral fashion and fuse to form the septum that divides the truncus arteriosus into the pulmonary artery and aorta. At the same time, two additional swellings in the conus region grow towards each other and fuse to form the division between the outflow tracts just below the aortic and pulmonary valves (Miller, 1979). Evidence that conotruncal septation is under genetic control arises from studies of the Keeshond dog model (Van Mierop et al, 1977; Patterson et al, 1974). These data and those from human pedigrees (Pitt, 1962) are consistent with multifactorial inheritance of conotruncal septation defects. However, it has been suggested that in some cases with strongly positive family histories, a single gene defect with incomplete penetrance may be responsible and that recurrence risk may then be higher than the usually quoted risk figures derived from large series of patients (Miller & Smith, 1979).

Transposition of the great vessels seems to be due to complete lack of rotation of the truncoconal septum. The conotruncal wall itself is presumed to be involved in this failure of rotation since the coronary ostia remain associated with the aorta (Jackson, 1968). The recurrence risk for first degree relatives is approximately 2.0% (Nora et al, 1970). This defect is particularly common in infants of diabetic mothers, the overall empiric risk for a CHD in offspring of diabetics being 5% (Nora & Nora, 1978). Transposition of the great vessels and other truncoconal anomalies also seem to be particularly common among the heart defects present in infants exposed in utero to oral contraceptive agents (Heinonen, 1977). The tetralogy of Fallot is a more common abnormality of conotruncal septation that seems to result from unequal partitioning of the conus at the expense of the right ventricular outflow tract and pulmonary trunk (Van Mierop et al, 1977). Recurrence risk for first degree relatives is approximately 2.7% (Nora et al, 1970). It has been observed in infants with congenital rubella infection (Dudgeon, 1967) and may be particularly common in infants born to mothers with phenylketonuria (Lenke & Levy, 1980).

Coarctation of the aorta

The incidence of coarctation of the aorta is 0.37 to 0.44 per 1000 births (Miller, 1971). The coarctation usually occurs either immediately proximal or immediately distal to the ductus arteriosus. There are two theories regarding the development of this defect. The more popular theory is that the aorta may fail to grow at a localised point; the second possibility is that a localised segment of the aorta may contain ductus-like tissue that undergoes constriction at birth on the same basis as the normal ductus (Jackson, 1968). Recurrence risk figures are compatible with multifactorial inheritance and range from 1.0 to 1.8% for first degree relatives.

Patent ductus arteriosus (PDA)

The incidence of PDA as an isolated CHD is 0.6 per 1000 births (Mitchell et al, 1971).Perinatal factors related to prematurity or to high altitude-induced hypoxia may delay closure of an intrinsically normal ductus arteriosus; in these cases the empiric risk for first degree relatives is approximately 3.4% (Nora et al, 1970), which is compatible with multifactorial inheritance. Autosomal dominant inheritance in some families is likely (McKusick, 1978; #16910). PDA is one of the most common cardiac defects due to congenital rubella (Dudgeon, 1967). Other intrauterine environmental factors that can result in PDA include maternal phenylketonuria (Fisch, 1969) and systemic lupus erythematosus (Chameides et al, 1977), and possibly prenatal exposure to oral contraceptive agents (Heinonen, 1977).

Hypoplastic left ventricle

The incidence of hypoplastic left ventricle is 36.5 per 100 000 births, and approximately 70% of cases include aortic and/or mitral valve atresia (Brownell & Shokier, 1976). Multiple affected sibs and parental consanguinity have been reported in some families raising the possibility of autosomal recessive inheritance in these cases (McKusick, 1978; #24155). However, the empiric recurrence risk for first degree relatives is 2 % (Brownell & Shokier, 1976), which is compatible with multifactorial inheritance in the majority of cases. Mothers with

phenylketonuria have had offspring with hypoplastic left ventricle and other cardiac malformations (Fisch et al, 1969; Huntley & Stevenson, 1969).

Valvular dysplasias

Aortic stenosis (AS) can be subvalvular, valvular or supravalvular. Subvalvular stenosis may be due to a thin membranous diaphragm or a thick fibromuscular obstruction. The aortic valve may be secondarily thickened due to abnormal haemodynamics caused by the obstruction. In other cases, aortic subvalvular obstruction may be a secondary consequence of an abnormally placed papillary muscle and mitral valve. Subaortic stenosis may also be due to diffuse hypertrophy of the left ventricle (hypertrophic subaortic stenosis). This latter condition, as an isolated defect, is ordinarily considered to be due to an autosomal dominant mutation and may be associated with ventricular arrhythmias (McKusick, 1978; #19260). The phenotype is variable and therefore evaluation of at-risk relatives using echocardiography is warranted.

Supravalvular AS is a narrowing that occurs in the aorta just above the coronary arteries; it is infrequent as an isolated lesion and usually occurs as part of the infantile hypercalcaemia syndrome of Williams (Rudolph, 1977). However, supravalvular AS also occurs as an autosomal dominant condition in occasional families (McKusick, 1978; #18550). Valvular AS is usually associated with abnormal development of the valve leaflets. In 85% of cases there is a bicuspid aortic valve, and in 14% there is no apparent separation into leaflets. Only rarely are there three normal leaflets with fusion at the commissures. Severe stenosis can result in secondary effects that include hypoplasia of the ascending aorta, and left ventricular endocardial thickening (Rudolph, 1977). The incidence of AS is 0.21 to 0.26 per 1000 births (Heinonen, 1976) with a recurrence risk of 2 to 4 % in first degree relatives (Nora & Nora, 1978). It has been suggested that isolated AS may occur after intrauterine exposure to oral contraceptive agents (Heinonen, 1977).

It is important to realise that a bicuspid aortic valve without congenital AS is common, occurring in 2 to 3% of the population (Rudolph, 1977). These individuals may be at risk for bacterial endocarditis and/or calcific aortic stenosis later in life. Many patients with valvular or subvalvular AS have some degree of aortic regurgitation. Aortic regurgitation can also exist as a secondary consequence of a subpulmonic VSD in which the muscular support of the normal aortic cusps is defective.

Pulmonic stenosis (PS) can also be valvular, subvalvular, or supravalvular. In valvular stenosis the valve is usually normally formed but the cusps are thickened and fused (Rudolph, 1977). Secondary consequences of PS can include infundibular hypertrophy and hypoplasia of the pulmonary arterial system. Subvalvular PS with a normal valve is rare but may occur because of a discrete subpulmonic fibromuscular ring or aberrant muscular bands that may be associated with a VSD. Supravalvular PS may be caused by discrete diaphragms, diffuse constrictions, or hypoplasia of the major pulmonary arteries. Peripheral branch stenosis is a particularly frequent sequella of congenital rubella. It has also been associated with congenital heart block in offspring of mothers with systemic lupus erythematosus (Chameides et al, 1977). The incidence of PS is 0.66 to 0.71 per 1000 births (Heinonen, 1976) and recurrence risk for first degree relatives is 2 to 3.5 % (Nora & Nora, 1978). Pulmonic atresia accounts for only 1 to 2% CHD in children and the recurrence risk is 1.0 to 1.5 % (Rudolph, 1977). Pulmonic regurgitation due to an absent pulmonic valve is a rare condition; most cases of pulmonic regurgitation are secondary to other cardiovascular lesions.

Mitral stenosis may be associated with abnormal mitral valve cusps or cusps that appear normal but are fused. Obstruction may also result from a parachute mitral valve in which the chordae tendinae are attached to a single papillary muscle. Mitral atresia is usually associated with complex heart defects. Congenital mitral regurgitation is rare, but may occur with abnormal insertion of short chordae tendinae, accessary commissures, or undevelopment of valve leaflets. Cleft of the mitral valve may occur as an isolated lesion but more commonly it is associated with endocardial cushion defect or other lesion. The murmur of congenital mitral regurgitation may appear later in life leading to the erroneous assumption that the lesion is acquired. In the past, rheumatic fever was thought to be the aetiology of many of these congenital lesions. A prolapsing or 'floppy' mitral valve may be the most common human structural cardiac lesion with a frequency of 4% in the the adult population. Although it occurs in childhood, the exact incidence is not known. Autosomal dominant transmission of this condition has been shown (McKusick, 1978; #15770). A family with mitral and aortic regurgitation compatible with X–linked inheritance has been reported, but it is not certain that this represents a single gene defect (McKusick, 1978; #31440).

Isolated tricuspid stenosis is rare and has a 1% recurrence risk in first degree relatives. It is most frequently seen with hypoplastic right ventricle and pulmonic stenosis or atresia. Tricuspid regurgitation may also be associated with hypoplastic right ventricle or with the Ebstein anomaly. In this latter malformation the tricuspid valve is displaced downward and there is anomalous attachment of the posterior and septal leaflets to the right ventricular wall. The recurrence risk for the Ebstein anomaly in first degree relatives is 1.1% (Nora et al, 1970). The increased frequency of this rare anomaly in offspring of mothers taking lithium led to the discovery that lithium is a teratogen with an estimated 10% risk for cardiac anomalies after exposure in the first trimester.

Tricuspid atresia with ASD also has been observed after lithium exposure (Nora & Nora, 1978). The Ebstein anomaly associated with secundum ASD has been observed after intrauterine exposure to contraceptive agents (Heinonen, 1977), although causation is not definitely established. The Ebstein anomaly has also occurred in sibs, which is suggestive of autosomal recessive inheritance in some cases; however these may represent instances of multifactorial inheritance (McKusick, 1978; # 22470).

Conduction defects

Conduction defects may accompany gross cardiac malformations, for example first degree atrioventricular block with endocardial cushion defect. However in many cases there is no underlying gross structural defect. Paroxysmal ventricular fibrillation with a short PR interval has been observed in one family in a pattern suggestive of autosomal dominant inheritance (McKusick, 1978; # 19245). Ventricular fibrillation with prolonged QT interval (Romano-Ward syndrome) is more clearly defined as an autosomal dominant condition which has been reported in several families (McKusick, 1978; #19250). Atrioventricular conduction defect progressing from first to third degree has also been established as an autosomal dominant condition (McKusick, 1978; #14040). Autosomal recessive inheritance of congenital heart block with absent atrioventricular node has been reported (McKusick, 1978; #23470). In other instances of autosomal recessive inheritance of congenital heart block, congenital cardiomyopathy may be the underlying mechanism. The Jervell and Lange-Nielsen syndrome of congenital deafness, prolonged QT interval and sudden death (McKusick, 1978; #22040) warrants special mention since it implies that a congenitally deaf person should have an electrocardiogram as part of his or her evaluation. Audiologic evaluation may be warranted in patients with a prolonged QT interval. The Wolff-Parkinson-White syndrome has been reported more than once in several generations of a family, and the Kent bundles may be present in individuals without electrocardiographic evidence of the syndrome (Gillette et al, 1978).

Conduction defects have been well documented in offspring of mothers with systemic lupus erythematosus (Chameides et al, 1977); complete heart block may be present with or without cardiomyopathy. In at least one case, the block was due to interruption of the conduction system by a thickened annulus fibrosus and absence of a discrete atrioventricular node.

Other congenital heart defects

Many malformed hearts have more than a single anatomic defect, and over 95% of cases in which there is no other organ system involvement are due to multifactorial inheritance. As seen from the examples listed under specific cardiac lesions, it is apparent that single gene defects, teratogens and maternal ill health must be considered as aetiologies.

Endocardial fibroelastosis

Endocardial fibroelastosis (EFE) is a disorder in which the ventricles or atria are lined by a thick membrane resulting from proliferation of collagen and elastic fibres. The condition may be secondary to any CHD, such as AS, that results in severe obstruction. Primary or idiopathic EFE usually occurs in young infants and may be congenital. A viral aetiology has been suggested but not confirmed. Mumps virus was previously considered to be causative but there is no adequate documentation for this (Rudolph, 1977). Autosomal recessive and X–linked recessive inheritance have been well documented in occasional families (McKusick, 1978; #22600; #30530).

Recurrence risks

Recurrence risks for first degree relatives of patients with isolated CHDs having a multifactorial basis are in general 2 to 4%. Some of the rare lesions such as tricuspid atresia, Ebstein anomaly, truncus arteriosus, and pulmonic atresia have a slightly lower risk of approximately 1%. The lesion that occurs in first degree relatives is frequently the same as, or similar to, the lesion occurring in the proband (Nora et al, 1970). For example, a child with tetralogy of Fallot may have a sib with a VSD or PS. Although extensive empiric recurrence risk figures for families with two affected first degree relatives are not available for all cardiac defects, information gathered on other multifactorial defects indicates that the risk approximately doubles when two first-degree relatives are affected. Similarly, the recurrence risk when only a second degree relative is affected is approximately one half that seen for a first degree relative.

CONGENITAL HEART DEFECTS AS PART OF ASSOCIATIONS, COMPLEXES AND SYNDROMES

Aetiology

When all cases of CHDs are considered, approximately 90% are estimated to be due to multifactorial inheritance, and the majority are isolated defects (Nora & Nora, 1978). Multifactorial inheritance often can be excluded if additional major defects are found, although a second defect on a coincidental basis may be impossible to exclude in an individual patient. Since 14% of newborn babies may have a spurious minor anomaly (Smith, 1976, p 434), it would not be uncommon coincidentally to find one minor anomaly among patients with 'isolated' CHDs. Likewise, anomalies representing secondary con-

sequences or field defects would not rule out a multifactorial aetiology.

Approximately 5% of all CHDs are due to a chromosome abnormality, 3% to a single gene defect, and 2% to a recognized environmental factor, most commonly rubella (Nora & Nora, 1976). There is also a significant number of CHDs of unknown aetiology which are not included in these figures. Most defects due to defined aetiologies are associated with defects in other organ systems. Discussion of every chromosome abnormality, single gene defect, or syndrome of unknown aetiology that has a CHD as a component is beyond the scope of this chapter, though the reader can be referred elsewhere for this purpose (Smith, 1976; Nora & Nora, 1978; Yunis, 1977; McKusick, 1978).

Chromosomal disorders

Most of the common, well defined chromosomal aneuploidy syndromes have CHDs as a component in a significant number of cases. Forty per cent of individuals with trisomy 21 have CHDs with the most common being atrioventricular canal, PDA and ASD, in decreasing order of frequency. CHDs found in 50% or more of patients with trisomy 18 include VSD, ASD or PDA. Between 10 and 50% of these patients have bicuspid aortic or pulmonic valves, nodularity of valve leaflets, PS, or coarctation of the aorta, while less than 10% have anomalous coronary arteries, transposition of the great vessels, tetralogy of Fallot, coarctation of the aorta or dextrocardia (Smith, 1976, p 10–11). Trisomy 13 is characterized by CHDs in 80% of patients, with the most frequent lesions being VSD, PDA, ASD, or dextrocardia. Less than 50% of these patients have anomalous venous return, overriding aorta, PS, hypoplastic aorta, mitral or aortic atresia, or bicuspid aortic valve (Smith, 1976, p 14). It is evident from the multitude of heart defects listed for each chromosomal syndrome that a particular heart lesion is not specific for a given chromosome abnormality. However, some chromosomal syndromes, for example monosomy-X, are characterized by a relatively specific heart lesion; 20% of patients with the Turner syndrome have cardiac involvement, and of these patients, 70% have coarctation of the aorta. Not all aneuploidy syndromes are characterized by cardiac defects; XXY Klinefelter syndrome and mosaic trisomy 8 (Warkany syndrome) serve as examples.

Structural chromosome abnormalities such as del(5p) (cri-du-chat syndrome) may also result in CHDs. In these patients approximately 30% have a cardiac defect which is variable in type (Smith, 1976, p 24).

It is not understood why a given chromosome abnormality can result in cardiac defects in some individuals and not in others, or why the heart defect is variable in type. Therefore every individual patient with a chromosome abnormality must have careful evaluation to determine whether or not a CHD is present, and if present to determine the exact type of lesion. Conversely, the presence of a CHD should lead the examiner to look for other anomalies that might lead one to suspect a chromosome abnormality as the aetiology. It is also reasonable to obtain blood for chromosome analysis from all patients with a CHD who have unexplained mental retardation. Moribund neonates with a CHD also warrant karyotype analysis, even if no other anomalies are readily apparent. This approach will ensure that a chromosome abnormality is not missed in an infant who has unsuspected internal malformations, and will facilitate genetic counselling for the family.

Autosomal dominant disorders

A single autosomal dominant gene can have a pleiotropic effect that results in a structural CHD as well as other malformations. The prototype for this type of inherited disease is the Holt-Oram syndrome. ASD is the most common cardiac lesion, and hypoplasia and proximal placement of the thumb is the most frequent skeletal defect. However, other cardiac defects including VSD, and other abnormalities of the upper extremity have been observed even within the same family. Because expression can be highly variable, careful examination of other family members should be performed to detect previously unsuspected cases. Variable expression should also be taken into account when genetic counselling is given since future family members may be more or less severely affected. Other examples of autosomal dominant conditions that include a CHD as a consistent or occasional feature are the Leopard syndrome (PS), Apert syndrome (PS, overriding aorta, VSD), Treacher Collins syndrome (VSD or ASD, PDA), and Waardenberg syndrome (VSD). The 'Noonan syndrome' is a frequently applied eponym that is used to refer to an aetiologically heterogeneous group of patients with similar phenotypes. Although most cases are sporadic, an autosomal dominant form does exist. Pulmonic stenosis, septal defects and hypertrophic subaortic stenosis are the most commonly seen lesions. CHDs have been reported as rare components of some relatively common autosomal dominant disorders; for example, PS in a patient with neurofibromatosis (Neiman et al, 1974). It should not necessarily be assumed that the heart defect is due to the neurofibromatosis gene since the association may be coincidental. There are many other autosomal dominant diseases, such as Ehlers-Danlos syndrome, that have cardiac involvement but that are not associated with developmental structural cardiac defects.

Autosomal recessive disorders

Autosomal recessive genes can also be responsible for CHDs as part of multisystem disorders. The Ellis-van Creveld syndrome is a well known example in which approximately 50% of patients have a cardiac defect, most commonly ostium primum ASD. Some other autosomal recessive disorders that may be associated with CHDs include the Carpenter syndrome (PDA, VSD, PS, TGA), Kartagener syndrome (dextrocardia with ASD or VSD), Fanconi pancytopenia syndrome (ASD, PDA), Meckel-Gruber syndrome (PDA, septal defects, coarctation of aorta, PS), Smith-Lemli-Optiz syndrome, Thrombocytopenia-Absent Radius syndrome, Zellweger syndrome, and some cases of the Ivemark syndrome (McKusick, 1978; #20853). Several lysosomal storage diseases such as Pompe disease and Hunter mucopolysaccharidosis involve the heart as part of a generalized disease process, but are not associated with primary developmental aberrations.

X-linked disorders

X-linked recessive disorders that include cardiac and other anatomic defects are not very common. The Aase syndrome with VSD may be an example. X-linked dominant disorders that are sometimes associated with CHDs are incontinentia pigmenti and focal dermal hypoplasia.

Teratogens

Infectious teratogens

Infectious teratogens have already been discussed as a cause of isolated CHDs. The only well-documented infectious teratogen is the rubella virus, which can result in many different cardiac defects including PDA, PBS, VSD, ASD, and tetralogy of Fallot. Most affected infants have additional non-cardiac abnormalities. Rubella should not be accepted as the aetiology for a CHD without adequate documentation in the form of serum viral antibody titres, or preferably positive viral cultures. When this is not possible, other signs such as deafness, cataract, chorioretinitis or haematologic findings may lead to a presumptive diagnosis.

Pharmacologic teratogens

Thalidomide is notorious for its induction of limb defects in exposed fetuses. Five to ten% of exposed patients also had CHDs, especially tetralogy of Fallot, VSD, ASD, and truncus arteriosus. The failure of this agent to induce birth defects in many animals serves as a constant reminder that no drug should be considered totally safe in pregnancy on the basis of negative animal data, and that therefore no drug should be given to a pregnant woman unless absolutely necessary for her own health or the health of the fetus. This mandate also applies to drugs that have been used in humans for many years without documented teratogenic effects. Variable susceptibility to a given agent is well documented among inbred strains of laboratory animals and similar variation in susceptibility may also exist in humans. In some cases the overall incidence of induced defects may be so low that teratogenicity would be difficult to document. In addition, combinations of drugs could have a teratogenic effect that may not be present when either drug is tested alone.

On the other hand, some therapeutic agents cannot be withdrawn safely during pregnancy in spite of suspected or known teratogenicity. The anticonvulsants hydantoin and trimethadione are two such agents. Trimethadione results in cardiac defects (TGA, tetralogy of Fallot, hypoplastic left heart) along with other characteristic features in 15 to 30% of exposed fetuses (Nora & Nora, 1978). This agent can often be replaced by a safer anticonvulsant, and ideally this should be done in post-pubertal females prior to childbearing. This approach can prevent exposure of the fetus in an unplanned or unsuspected pregnancy. Hydantoins pose a two to threefold increased risk of CHD over the general population (Committee on Drugs: American Academy of Pediatrics, 1978), although other features of the fetal hydantoin syndrome may be present in 10% or more of exposed infants. Frequently this drug is essential for seizure control, and it is generally accepted that the ill effects of seizures on mother and fetus are probably greater than the teratogenic risks of the drug. Women of childbearing age who are taking hydantoin should be counselled about its possible teratogenic effects before a pregnancy is undertaken.

Coumarin derivatives result in abnormal liveborn infants in approximately 17% of pregnancies; PDA and PBS have been observed in affected infants. It should be noted in this regard that a CHD in the mother may be an indication for anticoagulant therapy, and the fetus is therefore not only at risk for CHD on a teratogenic basis but also on a multifactorial basis (Hall et al, 1980).

Alcohol may be the non-therapeutic drug most frequently taken by pregnant women. Alcohol appears to induce CHDs in some exposed fetuses; ASD is most commonly seen but VSD, tetralogy of Fallot, and other defects can also occur. The overall incidence of the fetal alcohol syndrome may be 0.2 to 0.4% (Smith, 1979), with CHD present in 30 to 50% of affected infants (Loser & Majewski, 1977). Heavy drinkers, defined as women consuming a daily average equivalent of 45 ml or more absolute alcohol, had offspring with a 17% incidence of major anomalies compared to a 2 to 3% incidence in more moderate drinkers (Ouellette et al, 1977). A 'safe' level of alcohol intake during pregnancy has not been established.

Other pharmacologic agents that have been suggested to induce CHDs in humans include phenobarbital, amphetamines, meprobamate (Milkovich & van den Berg, 1974), cyclophosphamide (Toledo et al, 1971) and oral contraceptive agents when taken during pregnancy;

however none of these agents has conclusively been shown to cause birth defects. In some cases, such as for example meprobamate (Hartz et al, 1975) and amphetamines (Milkovich & van den Berg, 1977), recent large studies have refuted the original reports of teratogenicity.

Other teratogens

Non-pharmacologic chemical teratogens may exist in the environment, although none has been specifically linked with CHD to date. Prenatal exposure to methylmercury appears to cause microcephaly and cerebral palsy (Amin-Zoki et al, 1979). It is not inconceivable that chemical pollutants or chemical exposure in the workplace may some day be shown to be teratogenic.

Maternal disease states such as phenylketonuria, systemic lupus erythematosus, and diabetes mellitus may adversely influence the developing heart. It has been suggested that optimal control of the diabetic state may minimize these adverse effects, but controlled studies have not yet been performed. Similarly, institution of a low phenylalanine diet prior to conception may reduce the risk for offspring of mothers with phenylketonuria (Lenke & Levy, 1980).

Unknown aetiology

There are many infants with cardiac defects as part of multiple malformation disorders of unknown aetiology. Some patterns of malformations are recognized as particular syndromes, for example the Cornelia de Lange syndrome, or are seen more commonly than expected by chance alone, as in the VATER or VACTERL association. Other malformation complexes may not fall into currently recognized patterns of malformations which allow for accurate prediction of recurrence risks. The aetiology of the multiple malformations in many of these infants is unknown, and when no specific chromosome abnormality, teratogen or single gene defect is identified, most occur on a sporadic basis with a recurrence risk of 1% or less in sibs.

PRENATAL DIAGNOSIS

The most recent advance in the management of CHDs that has great potential from the vantage point of genetic counselling is in the area of prenatal diagnosis. At the time of writing, M-mode and real-time two-dimensional echocardiographic studies have been applied to fetuses ranging from 18 to 41 weeks gestation (Kleinman et al, 1980). Studies are geared mainly to gathering information on the fetus that will be helpful for obstetric and postnatal paediatric care. However, refinement of technique and equipment may allow earlier, definitive diagnosis of CHD that would give parents the option of terminating affected fetuses. Fetoscopy and/or ultrasound have been used to diagnose affected fetuses with syndromes, such as Ellis-van Creveld dwarfism (Makoney & Hobbins, 1977) which is commonly associated with CHD; however skeletal abnormalities served as the basis for the diagnoses in these cases.

SUMMARY

In the evaluation of a patient with a CHD, it is important to establish whether the heart defect is the only abnormality present, or if other major and/or minor anomalies exist. The majority of isolated CHDs are due to multifactorial inheritance, while less than 5% are due to a single gene defect or an identifiable teratogen. When CHDs coexist with other anomalies the aetiology is more likely to be chromosomal, Mendelian, teratogenic or unknown.

The recurrence risk for first degree relatives of patients with CHD having a multifactorial basis is generally 2 to 4% and this risk figure approximately doubles when two first degree relatives are affected. Recurrence risks in single gene disorders are in accordance with the rules of Mendelian inheritance, allowing for new mutations, incomplete penetrance and variable expression.

In many instances the cause of a CHD in association with other anomalies is unknown, but chromosome abnormalities, teratogens, poor maternal health, and rare single gene syndromes must always be considered. When no such cause is identifiable, counselling on the basis of a sporadic event with a recurrence risk of 1% or less for sibs may be given. It is important for the family to understand the basis for this counselling, since rarely the birth of a second affected infant will occur and may suggest a new autosomal recessive syndrome with 25% recurrence risk.

The potential for early prenatal diagnosis of CHDs is increasing rapidly, both in terms of detection of associated anomalies and/or the cardiac defect itself.

ACKNOWLEDGEMENT

Thanks to Ms Catherine Umeh for devoted assistance in manuscript preparation.

REFERENCES

Amin-Zaki L, Majeed M A, Elhassani S B, Clarkson T W, Greenwood M R, Doherty R A 1979 Prenatal methylmercury poisoning. American Journal of Diseases in Childhood 133: 172–177

Anderson R C 1977 Congenital heart malformations in North American Indian children. Pediatrics 59: 121–123

Bergsma D (ed) 1979 Birth defects compendium, 2nd edn. Alan R Liss, Inc., N.Y. p 768–69

Boon A R, Farmer M B, Roberts D F 1972 A family study of Fallot's tetralogy. Journal of Medical Genetics 9: 179–192

Brownell L G, Shokier M H K 1976 Inheritance of hypoplastic left heart syndrome (HLHS): further observations. Clinical Genetics 9: 245–49

Cascos A L 1972 Genetics of atrial septal defect. Archives of Diseases in Childhood 47: 581–87

Chameides L, Truex R C, Vetter V, Rashkind W J, Galioto F M, Noonan J A 1977 Association of maternal systemic lupus erythematosus with congenital complete heart block. New England Journal of Medicine 297: 1204–1207

Committee on Drugs: American Academy of Pediatrics 1978. Anticonvulsants and pregnancy. Pediatrics 63: 331–33

Dudgeon J A 1967 Maternal rubella and its effect on the fetus. Archives of Diseases in Childhood 42: 110–125

Fisch R O, Doeden D, Lansky L L, Anderson J A 1969 Maternal phenylketonuria: detrimental effects on embryogenesis and fetal development. American Journal of Diseases in Childhood 118: 847– 858

Gillette P C, Freed D, McNamara D G 1978. A proposed autosomal dominant method of inheritance of the Wolff-ParkinsonWhite syndrome and supraventricular tachycardia. Journal of Pediatrics 93: 257–58

Greenwood R D, Rosenthal A, Parisi L, Fyler D C, Nadas A S 1975 Extracardiac abnormalities in infants with congenital heart disease. Pediatrics 55: 485–92

Greenwood R D, Rosenthal A 1976 Cardiovascular malformations associated with tracheoesophageal fistula and esophageal atresia. Pediatrics 57: 87–91

Hall J G, Pauli R M, Wilson K M 1980 Maternal and fetal sequelae of anticoagulation during pregnancy. American Journal of Medicine 68: 122–140

Hartz S C, Heinonen O P, Shapiro S, Siskind S, Slone D 1975 Antenatal exposure to mebromabate and chlordiazepoxide in relation to malformations, mental development, and childhood mortality. New England Journal of Medicine 292: 726–728

Heinonen O P 1976 Risk factors for congenital heart disease: a prospective study. In: Kelly S, Hood E B, Janerich D T, Porter I H (eds) Birth defects: risks and consequences, Academic Press, Incorporated, New York, p 221–264

Heinonen O P, Slone D, Monson R R, Hook E B, Shapiro S 1977 Cardiovascular birth defects and antenatal exposure to female sex hormones. New England Journal of Medicine 296: 67–70

Huntley C C, Stevenson R E 1969 Maternal phenylketonuria: course of two pregnancies. Obstetrics and Gynecology 34: 694–700

Jackson B T 1968 The pathogenesis of congenital cardiovascular anomalies. New England Journal of Medicine 279: 80–89

Kahler R L, Baunwald E, Plauth W H, Morrow A G 1966 Familial congenital heart disease. American Journal of Medicine 40: 384–99

Kleinman C S, Hobbins, J C, Jaffe C C, Lynch D C, Tainer N S 1980 Echocardiographic studies of the human fetus: prenatal diagnosis of congenital heart disease and cardiac dysrhythmias. Pediatrics 65: 1056–1067

Lenke R R, Levy H L 1980 Maternal phenylketonuria and hyperphenylalaninemia: an international survey of the outcome of untreated and treated pregnancies. New England Journal of Medicine 303: 1202–1208

Loser H, Majewski F 1977 Type and frequency of cardiac defects in embryofetal alcohol syndrome; report of 16 cases. British Heart Journal 39: 1374–79

Mahoney M J, Hobbins J C 1977 Prenatal diagnosis of chondroectodermal dysplasia (Ellis–van Creveld syndrome) with fetoscopy and ultrasound. New England Journal of Medicine 297: 258–60

McKusick V A (ed)1978 Mendelian inheritance in man, 5th edn. The Johns Hopkins University Press, Baltimore, p 38–806

Milkovich L, van den Berg B J 1974 Effects of prenatal mebromate and chlordia-zepoxide hydrochloride on human embryonic and fetal development. New England of Medicine 291: 1268–1270

Milkovich L, van den Berg B J 1977 Effects of antenatal exposure to anorectic drugs. Obstetrics 129: 637–42

Miller M E, Smith D W 1979 Conotruncal malformation complex: examples of possible monogenic inheritance. Pediatrics 63: 890–892

Miller R W 1971 Studies in childhood cancer as a guide for monitoring congenital malformations. In: Hook E B, Janervich D T, Porter I H (eds) Monitoring, birth defects and environment: the problem of surveillance. Academic Press, New York. p 97–117

Mitchell S C, Korones S B, Berendes H W 1971 Congenital heart disease in 56, 109 births; incidence and natural history. Circulation 43: 323–332

Neiman H L, Mens E, Holt J F, Stern P B L 1974 Neurofibromatosis and congenital heart disease. American Journal of Roentgenology 122: 146–149

Nora J J, Meyer T C 1966 Familial nature of congenital heart diseases. Pediatrics 37: 329–334

Nora J J, McNamara D G, Fraser F C 1967 Hereditary factors in atrial septal defect. Circulation 35: 448–456

Nora J J, Sommerville R J, Fraser F C 1968 Homologies for congenital heart diseases: murine models influenced by dextroamphetamine. Teratology 4: 413–416

Nora J J, McGill C W, McNamara D G 1970 Empiric recurrence risks in common and uncommon congenital heart lesions. Teratology 3: 325–330

Nora J J, Nora A H, Toews W H 1974 Lithium, Ebstein's anomaly and other congenital heart defects. Lancet 2: 594–97

Nora J J, Nora A H 1978 The evolution of specific genetic and environmental counselling in congenital heart diseases. Circulation 57: 205–213

Ouellette E M, Rosett H L, Rosman N P, Weiner L 1977 Adverse effects on offspring of maternal alcohol abuse during pregnancy. New England Journal of Medicine 297: 528–30

Patterson D F, Pyle R L, Van Mierop L, Melbin J, Olson M 1974 Hereditary defects of the conotruncal septum in Keeshond dogs: pathologic and genetic studies. Pediatric Cardiology 34: 187–205

Pitt D B 1962 A family study of Fallot's tetrad. Austrian Annals of Medicine 11: 179–183

Hoffman J I E 1977 Circulatory system. In: Rudolph A M (ed) Pediatrics, 16th edn. Appleton-Century-Crofts, New York, ch 27, p 1404–1469

Smith D W (ed) 1976 Recognizable patterns of human malformation; genetic, embryologic, and clinical aspects. 2nd edn. W B Saunders Co, Philadelphia. p 3–434

Smith D W 1979 The fetal alcohol syndrome. Hospital Practice 11 121–128

Toledo T M, Harper R C, Moser R H 1971 Fetal effects during cyclophosphamide and irradiation therapy. Annals of Internal Medicine 74: 87–91

Van Mierop L H S, Patterson D F, Schnarr W R 1977 Hereditary conotruncal septal defects in Keeshond dogs: embryologic studies. Pediatric Cardiology 40: p 936–950

Warkany J (ed) 1971 Congenital malformations, Year Book Medical Publishers, Incorporated, Chicago, ch 8 p 64, 459–484

Yao J, Thompton M W, Trusler G A, Trimble A S 1968 Familial atrial septal defect of the primum type: a report of four cases in one sibship. Canadian Medical Association Journal 98: 218–219

Yunis J J (ed) 1977 New chromosomal syndromes. Academic Press, New York

69

Coronary heart disease

G. Utermann

CLINICAL DESCRIPTION – COMPLICATIONS – NATURAL HISTORY – PATHOGENESIS

Cardiovascular diseases have attained the first position in the statistics of morbidity and mortality in all highly industrialised countries. Roughly half of all cardiovascular deaths are due to coronary heart disease. Coronary heart disease results from atherosclerosis of the coronary arteries and accounts for 40% of the total mortality in men aged from 45–75 years in the USA and for 30% in western Europe.

Among the clinical expressions of coronary heart disease are congestive heart failure, conduction defect, arrhythmia, angina pectoris and myocardial infarction. Most cases of sudden unexpected death also result from coronary heart disease. Before clinical symptoms have evolved the diagnosis of coronary heart disease is difficult because coronary sclerosis may be masked by the coronary reserve. It is important to realise that coronary insufficiency signifies the result of a disequilibrium between demand and supply of blood and oxygen.

Coronary heart disease is a consequence of atherosclerosis of coronary arteries. Therefore understanding the contribution of genetic factors on the development of coronary heart disease means understanding the role of genetic factors in the atherosclerotic process. According to a WHO definition atherosclerosis is:

a variable combination of changes in the arterial wall consisting of the focal accumulation of lipids, complex carbohydrates, blood and blood products, fibrous tissue and calcium deposits associated with changes in the media (Classification of Atherosclerosis lesions, Report of Study Group on Definition of Terms, 1958).

The fundamental element of atherosclerosis is the atherosclerotic plaque. Three classic types of lesion are recognised: the fatty streak, the fibrous plaque, and the so-called 'complicated lesion' (McGill et al, 1963; Wissler, 1974). The relation between the fatty streak and the fibrous plaque is still a matter of controversy. It has been suggested that fatty streaks are precursors of fibrous plaques. However, this view is not any longer generally accepted (Ross & Glomset, 1976). Probably there exist different types of fatty streaks, only some of which are associated with atherosclerosis (Smith, 1975). The yellow colour of these lesions is due to the presence of lipid deposits found primarily within smooth muscle cells and macrophages. (Smith & Smith, 1976)

The lesions of atherosclerosis are characterised by intimal proliferation of smooth muscle cells, accumulation of large amounts of connective tissue matrix including collagen, elastic fibres, and proteoglycans, and deposition of intra- and extra-cellular lipid. Many factors are involved in this process and different hypotheses have been advanced to explain how an atherosclerotic plaque starts. One of these, the response-to-injury hypothesis, dates back to the pioneering work of Virchow (1856). This hypothesis still is in the conceptual framework for most recent hypotheses on atherogenesis and has been modified and extended by many investigators (Duguid, 1949; Mustard & Packham, 1975; Ross & Glomset, 1973; 1976). According to the injury hypothesis, the primary event in the pathogenesis of atherosclerosis is endothelial damage as a result of mechanical, chemical, immunologic or toxic sources of injury. Factors such as hyperlipidemia, the increased shear stress in hypertension or toxic agents contained in cigarette smoke may injure the endothelium and alter the nature of the endothelial barrier to the passage of blood constituents into the arterial wall (Getz et al 1969, Glagov 1972, Smith and Slater 1972). The fundamental response following some form of injury to the endothelium is intimal smooth muscle cell proliferation. Ross and Glomset (1976) have postulated that this process is platelet – mediated. According to these authors endothelial damage is a prerequisite for smooth muscle cell proliferation and anything which increases platelet agglutination and platelet sticking on the arterial intima can open up the endothelium and accelerate the entry and accumulation of low density lipoproteins or fibrinogen deep into the arterial wall. The arterial smooth muscle cell is the predominant cell type involved in lipid uptake, proliferation and necrosis. The lipid material which accumulates in the intima has the physicochemical and immunochemical properties of lipoproteins. There are rather remarkable quantities of intact low-density lipoproteins (LDL) in the diseased artery wall (Kao & Wissler 1965; Scott & Hurley 1970; Smith, 1975; Walton & Williamson, 1968). This may reflect the importance of chronic hyperlipidemia, especially elevated LDL in the process of atherosclerosis (Smith & Slater, 1972).

The effect of LDL may be twofold. First, it has been suggested that chronic hypercholesterolaemia injuries the endothelium and leads to focal desquamation. The interruption of the intact endothelial barrier is followed by a platelet response and also by cellular responses involving smooth muscle cells and endothelial cells (Ross & Glomset, 1976). Second, it results in lipid accumulation in preexisting atheromatous lesions (Ross & Harker, 1976). Once the endothelial barrier is broken, the lipoproteins can either be taken up by smooth muscle cells by receptor-mediated endocytosis (Bierman & Albers, 1975) or may be trapped in the intracellular matrix by glycosaminoglycans produced by the smooth muscle cells. LDL and also VLDL have been shown to bind to specific connective tissue elements of the arterial intima, such as glycosaminoglycans and elastic fibres, and moreover LDL provides the excessive amounts of cholesterylester which accumulate in the lesion.

There may be an element of cell transformation in the neoplastic sense, at the beginning of plaque formation. Benditt and Benditt (1973) have provided evidence that smooth muscle cells in one plaque are monoclonal. Moreover they have some of the characteristics of transformed cells. It is however not known what it is that makes these cells mutate and become nodules of monoclonal proliferating cells. Even though a uniform hypothesis to explain the cause and pathogenesis of atherosclerosis does not exist, some actors in the complex interplay have been identified. One of these is plasma cholesterol, or more precisely plasma lipoproteins. The reason for this is that a number of mutations involving the lipoproteins of blood plasma are known in man and some of these have a remarkably high frequency in the population (Goldstein et al, 1973). These mutations include some unique monogenic dominant disorders of lipoprotein metabolism that are all associated with a considerably increased risk for premature coronary heart disease. Moreover a single polymorphic gene locus has recently been identified that participates in the control of plasma lipid levels in man (Utermann et al, 1977b; 1979a). For this reason this chapter will mainly be concerned with the genetic control of plasma lipids and its disturbances – the genetic hyperlipidaemias.

RISK FACTOR CONCEPT

A series of large epidemiological studies throughout the world have established what is called the risk factor concept (Albrink et al, 1961; Cassel, 1971; Chapmen et al, 1964; Dawber et al, 1971; Doyle, 1963; Epstein et al, 1965; Kannel et al, 1964; 1966; Keys et al, 1971; Paul et al, 1963; Stamler, 1967). According to this concept, hypercholesterolemia, high consumption of cigarettes and hypertension are first-order independent risk factors for coronary heart disease. They are attributed with a causal relation to atherosclerosis. For some time each of these risk factors was looked at seperately. However it soon became evident that these factors are not simply additive. Multivariate analysis therefore has proved extremely useful in the prediction of relative risk for coronary heart disease (Keys, 1972 a and b; Keys et al, 1972). A second, less significant risk factor category, includes diabetes mellitus, gout, adiposity, lack of exercise and stress. Epidemiologic studies by themselves can not establish causal relationships, but the role of risk factors in atherosclerosis has been validated from the combined approaches of epidemiology, experimental pathology and clinical investigation. The study of mutations in humans involving the plasma lipoproteins have shed light on the role of lipoproteins in atherosclerosis. While there is general agreement on the positive correlation between cholesterol levels and the incidence of coronary heart disease, the role of triglycerides is still a matter of controversy. Cholesterol is present in different kinds of lipoprotein particles in plasma (see lipoproteins) and these are not equivalent with respect to coronary risk. Whereas, cholesterol in LDL is positively correlated with premature coronary heart disease, a negative correlation of cholesterol in HDL with coronary atherosclerosis has been established in epidemiological studies (Castelli et al, 1975; Gofman et al, 1966; Gordon et al, 1977; Medalie et al, 1973; Rhoads et al, 1976), and a protective effect against coronary heart disease has been attributed to HDL (Miller & Miller, 1975). Conventionally plasma lipids and lipoproteins are analysed in the fasting state; but humans are not fasting for most of their lives. Zilversmit (1979) has postulated that degradation products of triglyceride-rich lipoproteins (remnants) present in postprandial plasma may have a pronounced atherogenic effect. Indeed, one human disorder of lipoprotein metabolism (type III hyperlipoproteinaemia) where remnant like lipoproteins accumulate even in the fasting state, is associated with premature atherosclerosis.

GENETICS OF CORONARY HEART DISEASE — GENERAL ASPECTS

As early as 1897, Osler realized the familial aggregation of heart attacks. Present days knowledge suggests that this aggregation is largely due to clustering of genetically determined risk factors in certain families. The contribution of genetic factors to the development of coronary heart disease has been documented by several studies during the last decades (Gertler & White, 1954; Robertson & Cumming, 1979; Slack, 1969; Slack & Evans, 1966; Thomas & Cohen, 1955). These studies suggested that coronary heart disease is a heterogeneous group of disorders. Different environmental and genetic factors interact in a highly complex and poorly understood fashion in the pathogenesis of coronary atherosclerosis. Moreover the interaction-patterns are different in different individuals. Whereas heavy smoking may be the major precipitating agent in one individual, genetically determined hypercholesterolaemia is the major cause for premature coronary heart disease in others. Nora et al, (1980) have calculated that the heritability of ischaemic heart disease that produces myocardial infarction before 55 years of age, is 0.63. In their series of patients, the risk ratio was greater for a family history of ischaemic heart disease then for the highest quintile of cholesterol levels. 15% of patients in their study had a monogenic hyperlipidemia. However even when families with monogenic lipid disorders were eliminated heritability was still 0.56, indicating that genetic control of other factors that do not operate through lipoprotein pathways are also important.

Genetic factors affecting the susceptibility to coronary heart disease operate though such risk factors as blood lipid concentrations and blood pressure. The results of search for genetic factors in hypertension are still limited. It has been demonstrated by family and twin studies that hereditary factors are involved in hypertension (Miall & Oldham, 1958; Pickering, 1959; Platt, 1959; 1963; Thomas & Cohen, 1955). Although most data favour the assumption of multifactorial inheritance of blood pressure, single gene diseases have recently been implicated. Genetic disorders of plasma lipid metabolism have been delineated (Table 69.1).

PLASMA LIPOPROTEINS

Only a brief general description of the major human lipoproteins and of the metabolism of lipoproteins can be given here. Several recent reviews covering the topic are available for more detailed information (Eisenberg & Levy, 1976; Fredrickson et al, 1978; Havel, 1975; Schaefer et al, 1978; Smith et al, 1978).

Three major lipoprotein classes, different in particle size, chemical composition and physicochemical properties, are present in the plasma of healthy fasting sub-

Table 69.1 Genetic dyslipoproteinaemias

	Primary defects
I Autosomal recessive forms	
(a) Lecithin-cholesterol-acyltransferase deficiency	enzyme deficiency
(b) Familial Hyperchylomicronaemia	
1. Lipoprotein Lipase Deficiency	enzyme deficiency
2. Apolipoprotein C-II Deficiency	cofactor deficiency
(c) Tangier Disease	unknown
(d) Abetalipoproteinaemia	unknown
(e) Fish-eye-disease	unknown
(f) Primary Dysbetalipoproteinaemia	apoprotein E-structure
II Autosomal dominant forms	
(a) Fam. Hypercholesterolaemia	1. LDL-Receptor deficiency
	2. LDL-Receptor defect
	3. Internalisation defect
(b) Fam. Hypertriglyceridaemia	unknown
(c) Fam. Combined Hyperlipidaemia	unknown
(d) Fam. Hypobetalipoproteinaemia	unknown
(e) Hypoalphalipoproteinaemia Type Milano	Apo A-I-Structure
Homozygous for autosomal dominant forms	
(a) Homozygous fam. Hypercholesterolaemia	
(b) Homozygous Hypobetalipoproteinaemia	
III Polygenic forms	
(a) Polygenic Hypercholesterolaemia	multiple, unknown
(b) Broad-Beta-Disease	apo E-structure plus
(Hyperlipoproteinaemia Type III)	independent factor(s)
(c) Fam. Hyperalphalipoproteinaemia	unknown, one major gene?

For reference see Fredrickson et al (1978), Gjone et al (1978), Herbert et al (1978), Carlson and Philippson (1980), Utermann et al (1977b), Franceschini et al (1980), Siervogel et al (1980), Breckenridge et al (1979)

jects and can be separated by ultracentrifugation. These are the very-low-density lipoproteins (VLDL, d<1.006 g/ml), the low-density lipoproteins (LDL, d=1.019–1.063 g/ml) and the high-density lipoproteins (HDL, d=1.063–1.21 g/ml). These fractions, in general, correspond to pre-beta lipoproteins (VLDL), beta lipoproteins (LDL) and alpha-1 lipoproteins (HDL), as separated by electrophoretic methods. In certain forms of dys- or hyperlipoproteinaemia other lipoproteins may occur in fasting plasma, including chylomicrons and intermediate density lipoproteins (IDL d = 1.006–1.019 g/ml). The electrophoretic system has been used for the classification of hyperlipidaemias into phenotypes I (hyperchylomicronaemia), IIa (hyperbetalipoporteinaemia), IIb (hyperbeta-plus hyperprebetalipoproteinaemia), III (dysbetalipoproteinaemia), IV (hyperprebetalipoproteinaemia) and V (hyperprebeta-plus hyperchylomicronaemia), each characterized by elevation of one or more distinct lipoprotein fractions (Beaumont et al, 1970; Fredrickson et al, 1968; 1967).

The major constituents of lipoproteins are cholesterol (free and esterified), triglyceride, phospholipid and protein. All lipoproteins contain the major lipid classes, but in different concentrations. The various protein moieties, or apolipoproteins, are preferentially present in certain lipoproteins. Several apolipoproteins have been described and characterised in recent years and will be designated here according to the ABC nomenclature proposed by Alaupovic (1971). HDL contains Apo A-I and apo A-II as major protein constituents. Minor proteins in HDL are apo C-I, apo C-II, apo C-III, apo D and apo E. Apo A-I, the most abundant apoprotein in HDL, acts as a cofactor for the plasma enzyme lecithin-cholesterol acyltransferase (LCAT). LDL contains almost exclusively apo B. Apo B is also a major protein constituent of VLDL, together with apo C-I, C-II, C-III and apo E. Plasma chylomicrons have a protein composition similar to VLDL, but lymph chylomicrons have a remarkably different composition containing apo B, apo A-I and apo A-IV as major apoproteins (Green et al, 1979; Utermann & Beisiegel, 1979). Apo E and apo B are both recognized by a specific high affinity cell surface receptor and are involved in the catabolism of lipoproteins by cells (Goldstein & Brown, 1974; Mahley, 1978; Mahley et al, 1977; Sherrill et al, 1980).

The plasma lipoproteins represent a highly dynamic system in which the different lipoprotein particles are metabolically interrelated. Lipoproteins are secreted as precursor molecules of circulating plasma lipoproteins, primarily by the liver (VLDL and apo E-rich nascent HDL, Felkner et al, 1977; Hamilton, 1978) and by the intestine (chylomicrons and nascent apo A-I rich HDL, Green et al, 1978). In plasma, precursor lipoproteins are rapidly converted to mature lipoproteins by the combined action of enzymes (lipases, LCAT), by exchange

of apolipoproteins and lipids and by interaction with cells. One of the most important metabolic pathways is the conversion of endogenous VLDL to LDL (α_2- pathway, Eisenberg et al, 1978; 1973). Upon entry into the plasma compartment, VLDL accepts apo C's from HDL. One of the C apoproteins (apo C-II) is an activator of lipoprotein lipase (LPL). In the first step of the α_2-pathway, the core triglycerides of VLDL are hydrolysed at the capillary endothelium by the action of apo C-II activated lipoprotein lipase and apo C's are transferred back to HDL. The triglyceride and apo C poor particles generated have the density of IDL and are called remnants. In a second step, that possibly involves interaction with a specific hepatic receptor for apo E, remnants are further degraded to LDL. Most or all LDL in normal human plasma represents a catabolic product of VLDL. A similar pathway exists for the chylomicrons that are the transport vehicles for exogenous fat and are assembled in the intestine and released into the lymph. Upon entry into the plasma compartment, lymph chylomicrons lose apo A-I and apo A-IV. Apo A-I is transferred to HDL (Schaefer et al, 1978) and apo A-IV in humans occurs as 'free apoprotein' in the fraction d >1.21 g/ml (Beisiegel & Utermann, 1979). In exchange, chylomicrons acquire apo C from HDL and apo E. These plasma chylomicrons then are attacked by lipoprotein lipase and degraded to remnants. Finally, chylomicron remnants are taken up and degraded by liver cells through an apo E receptor mediated mechanism (Sherrill et al, 1980). Thus both VLDL and chylomicrons have to pass through the same degradation pathway. The degradation of triglyceride-rich lipoproteins is tightly bound to the metabolism of HDL. There is not only the described transfer of surface components (apoproteins, phospholipids) to HDL during lipolysis and upon entry of chylomicrons into the plasma, but there is also a bi-directional exchange of cholesteryl-ester between HDL and LDL. Most of this core lipid is present in LDL in human plasma, but it is formed by the LCAT mediated esterification of HDL-cholesterol (Glomset and Norum 1973). The metabolic interrelationships between the different classes of lipoproteins explain the multiple lipoprotein abnormalities that may emerge as a consequence of a single gene mutation in several lipoprotein disorders (Gjone et al, 1978; Herbert et al, 1978).

GENETIC CONTROL OF PLASMA CHOLESTEROL

Elevated plasma cholesterol concentration, particularly an elevation of cholesterol in the low-density-lipoproteins, is a major independent risk factor for coronary heart disease. There is considerable variance of cholesterol concentrations within and in between populations.

The Dutch physician De Lange (1933) was one of the first to note this and correlate it with the incidence of coronary heart disease. Differences between ethnic groups seem to be largely due to different environmental factors, e.g. nutrition, rather than to genetic differences (Keys, 1975). A significant genetic influence on serum lipid and lipoprotein levels, including cholesterol, triglycerides, phospholipids, and the major lipoprotein classes (VLDL, LDL, HDL) has been observed in twin studies (Adlersberg et al, 1957; Blomstrand & Lundman, 1966; Christian et al, 1976; Gedda and Poggi, 1960; Heiberg, 1974; Jensen et al, 1965; Kang et al, 1971; McDonough et al, 1962; Meyer, 1962; Osborne et al, 1959; Pikkarainen et al, 1966). The genetic effect is particularly pronounced for cholesterol. Moreover significant correlations of cholesterol levels were found in several family studies (Johnson et al, 1965; Martin et al, 1973; Mayo et al, 1969; Robertson et al, 1980; Schaeffer et al, 1958; Sing et al, 1975; Weinberg et al, 1976). Familial factors influencing lipid levels have a fairly high degree of specificity for cholesterol and triglycerides. Familial correlations tend to be stronger for blood relatives than for unrelated members of the same household and stronger for cholesterol than for triglycerides (Hewitt et al, 1979). Sing and Orr (1978) have estimated that only approximately 20% of the observed correlation between sibs living in the same household is attributable to shared environments. This argues for a high quantitative contribution of genetic factors. However, quantitative data on the contribution of genetic factors to plasma cholesterol or lipoprotein levels should be considered with great reservation. Several workers have tried to identify 'major genes' acting on either cholesterol to triglyceride by statistical methods (Ott, 1979). The inherent difficulties of such an approach have been discussed by Hewitt et al (1979).

GENES AFFECTING THE NORMAL VARIANCE OF PLASMA LIPOPROTEIN LEVELS: POLYMORPHISM OF APOLIPOPROTEIN E AND LP(a)-VARIATION

Any genetic factor affecting the concentration or possibly even the relative distribution of plasma lipids and lipoproteins could contribute to the susceptibility or resistence to coronary heart disease. The dependence of coronary heart disease risk on lipid level may be approximately linear (Carlson & Böttiger, 1972; Kannel et al, 1964). Under these circumstances the contribution made by a genetic factor to population variance of lipid level would be a reasonable index of it's importance from a public health standpoint. One such genetic system has recently been discovered, namely the polymorphism of apolipoprotein E. This protein is a major constituent of VLDL and of a subfraction of HDL. Apo E is involved in the receptor mediated catabolism of lipoproteins. The protein exhibits genetic polymorphism that may be demonstrated by isoelectric focusing or two-dimensional electrophoresis (Fig. 69.1). The polymorphism originally was believed to be under the control of two independent but closely linked gene loci (haplotypes), where two alleles $apo\ E^n$ and $apo\ E^d$ at the apo E-N/D locus, specify for the isoproteins E-2 and E-3 and a separate gene locus specifies for isoprotein E-4 (Utermann et al, 1980a). There is now good evidence that the gene specifying isoprotein E 4 (apo E^4) is allelic to the $apo\ E^n$ and $apo\ E^d$ genes (Utermann et al, 1982; Zannis et al, 1981). Hence the polymorphism is under the control of three alleles at one gene locus. These alleles determine the six phenotypes apo E-4/4, apo E-N/N, apo E-D/D, apo E-N/4, apo E-N/D and apo E-D/4 (Table 69.2, Fig. 69.1). The interest in this polymorphism was stimulated by the observation that the homozygous apo E−D/D phenotype, that has a frequency of 1% in the German population, is associated with a specific form of dyslipoproteinemia. This form has been termed primary dysbetalipoproteinemia and is characterised by elevation of cholesterol-rich VLDL, presence of a so-called beta-VLDL fraction and low concentration of LDL. Primary dysbetalipoproteinemia is the most frequent monogenic dyslipoproteinemia known in man and is transmitted as an autosomal recessive trait (Utermann et al, 1977). Due to the high frequency of the $apo\ E^d$ allele, vertical transmission of the dyslipoproteinemia is observed in many kindreds (Utermann et al, 1977b; 1979b). With few exceptions (see type III hyperlipoproteinaemia), homozygous apo E-D/D subjects have sub-normal total cholesterol concentrations (mean $\pm$ SD 161 $\pm$ 51 mg/dl) when compared with individuals that do not have the $apo\ E^d$ allele (mean $\pm$ SD 204 $\pm$ 41 mg/dl). Heterozygous carriers of the $apo\ E^d$ allele exhibit plasma cholesterol levels intermediate between the homozygotes for the apo E^d gene and those that do not have the $apo\ E^d$ allele (mean $\pm$ SD 186 $\pm$ 32 mg/dl). Hence the gene $apo\ E^d$ has a hypocholesterolemic effect even in single dose and the alleles at the $apo\ E^d$ gene locus determine three overlapping cholesterol distributions in the population (Fig. 69.2). In contrast plasma triglyceride, VLDL-triglyceride and VLDL-cholesterol concentrations are highest in homozygotes for the $apo\ E^d$ allele, intermediate in heterozygotes with one copy of the $apo\ E^d$ gene and lowest in individuals that lack the $apo\ E^d$ allele, (Utermann et al, 1979a). The significant effect of the $apo\ E^d$ alleles on plasma lipids implies a major role of the $apo\ E^d$ gene locus on the development of human arteriosclerosis and coronary heart disease. The typical lipoprotein distribution seen in apo E−D/D subjects corresponds to the lipoprotein pattern seen in subjects with hyperlipoproteinemia type III. In fact, all patients with the clas-

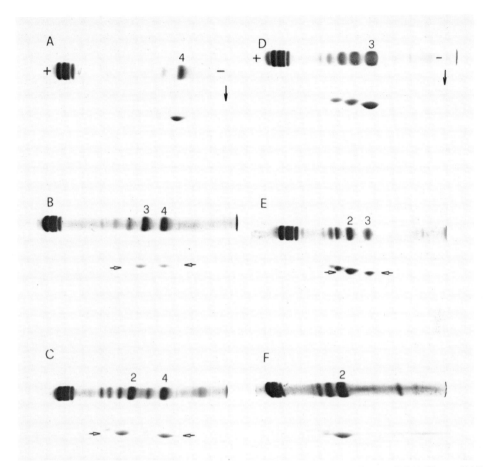

Fig. 69.1 Demonstration of the six common apo E phenotypes: apo E 4/4 (A), apo E-N/4 (B), apo E-D/4 (C), apo E-N/N (D), apo E-N/D (E) and apo E-D/D (F) by one-dimeonal isoelectric focusing and two-dimensional gel electrophoresis. One-dimensional gels are positioned horizontally to allow comparison with two – dimensional gels and major apo E bands in the focusing gels are labelled 2–4 from acidic to basic (Utermann et al, 1977b). Open arrows indicate the two major isoforms in the heterozygous phenotypes and solid arrows the direction of the second dimension electrophoresis.

sical type III disorder reported to date are of phenotype apo E−D/D (Utermann et al, 1975; 1977a; 1979b; Pagnan et al, 1977; Warnick et al, 1979; Weidman et al, 1979; Zannis & Breslow, 1980). This intriguing observation has raised the question as to what factors determine whether a homozygous apo E−D/D individual will be hypocholesterolemic or develop type III hyperlipo-

Table 69.2 Apo E-phenotypes and gene frequencies in 489 blood donors

Phenotype	Observed (%)	Expected	Gene frequency
Apo E-N/N	289 (59,1)	287	$E^n = 0.7658$
Apo E-N/4	107 (21,9)	110	
Apo E-4/4	14 (2,9)	11	$E^4 = 0.1480$
Apo E-N/D	64 (13,1)	64	$E^d = 0.0858$
Apo E-D/4	10 (2,0)	13	
Apo E-D/D	5 (1,0)	4	

Data reevaluated from Utermann et al, 1977b, 1980

proteinaemia. This question will be discussed later (see hyperlipoproteinaemia type III).

A further genetic system that possibly has implications for human atherosclerosis is the Lp(a)− system. The Lp (a)− antigen was first described by Berg (1963) as part of the LDL fraction and was found in about 35% of persons in north-west Europe. The original population and family studies suggested that the polymorphism is under the control of a single autosomal gene locus with one dominant allele Lp^a and a silent allele L_p. More recent data suggest that Lp(a) is a quantitative trait and is under polygenic control, but with a major gene effect (Albers et al, 1974; Sing et al, 1974). The Lp(a) lipoprotein that has been designated pre-beta-1-lipoprotein or sinking-prebeta-lipoprotein has a density of 1.05–1.08 g/ml and is rich in carbohydrate (Ehnholm et al, 1972; Simons et al 1970). An increased frequency of Lp(a)-positive individuals in patients with myocardial infarction was observed as early as 1965 by Renninger et al. There

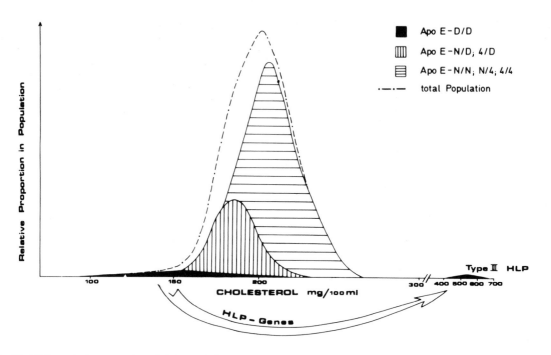

Fig. 69.2 Schematic demonstration of cholesterol distributions in apo E phenotypes (Modified from Utermann et al, 1979a).

is growing evidence that the Lp(a)-lipoprotein is associated with coronary heart disease (Berg et al, 1974; Dahlen et al, 1976; Rhoads et al, 1978), and that metabolic differences exist between individuals with high and low levels of Lp(a)-lipoprotein (Dahlen & Berg, 1976a; b). Presence of the Lp(a)-antigen within arteriosclerotic plaques has been demonstrated by Walton et al, (1974).

GENETIC HYPERLIPIDEMIAS

Autosomal recessive forms

There are several autosomal recessive inborn errors of plasma lipoprotein metabolism known to occur in humans (Table 69.1). Most of these are rare and only some have been reported to be associated with premature atherosclerosis. Among those believed to be associated with premature atherosclerosis are Tangier disease (hereditary deficiency of HDL) (Fredrickson 1964) and familial lecithin-cholesterol acyltransferase deficiency (Gjone et al, 1978). The major clinical findings and lipoprotein abnormalities in these disorders are summarized in Table 69.3.

The Tangier disorder is of particular interest in view of the postulated protective effect of HDL against coronary atherosclerosis. The primary biochemical defect in Tangier disease is unknown but probably relates to the structure or metabolism of apolipoprotein A-I. The disorder is characterized by a deficiency of HDL. There are virtually no normal HDL particles in the plasma of affected individuals. Total plasma cholesterol levels usually are below 120 mg/100 ml, whereas triglycerides tend to be elevated. The chemical composition and physicochemical properties of d < 1.006 g/ml lipoproteins and of LDL are abnormal. The d < 1.006 g/ml fraction contains lipoproteins that are considered abnormal chylomicron remnants.

LDL are triglyceride-rich and have an enhanced electrophoretic mobility in gel electrophoresis. The concentration of apo A-I, the major apoprotein of normal HDL, usually is less than 2% of controls and most of the residual apo A-I is not associated with lipoproteins but sediments at density 1.21 g/ml (Herbert et al, 1978). Patients with Tangier disease have deposits of cholesteryl-esters in tonsils, bone marrow, liver, spleen, peripheral nerves and arterial wall (Ferrans & Fredrickson, 1975).

Due to the complete absence of HDL from the plasma, a high incidence of coronary heart disease should be expected. However only a small number of adult patients have been studied and it is not possible to conclude whether or not there is an increased risk for premature atherosclerosis in Tangier disease. Heterozygous carriers of the Tangier gene that have roughly half normal HDL levels do not develop premature atherosclerosis (Assmann et al, 1978).

Table 69.3 Major clinical and laboratory findings in the autosomal recessive dyslipoproteinemias

Form	Lipid- and lipoprotein abnormalities	Characteristic clinical and laboratory findings	Premature coronary heart disease
Lecithin-cholesterol acyltransferase deficiency	Deficiency of cholesteryl-esters in plasma; abnormal chemical and physicochemical properties of all major lipoproteins. HDL contains discoidal particles	Corneal opacities, anemia, proteinuria, late nephropathy. Sea blue histiocytes in spleen and bone marrow.	present in many patients
Familial hyperchylomicronaemia	Triglycerides grossly elevated; low total plasma cholesterol; severe hyperchylomicronemia; low LDL- and HDL-levels	Eruptive xanthomas, pancreatitis	none
Tangier disease	Low plasma total cholesterol; deficiency of HDL, apo A-I and apo A-II. Abnormal LDL; abnormal chylomicron remnants	Hypoplastic orange tonsils, splenomegalie, storage of cholesterylester in RES; relapsing neuropathy; corneal opacities	unclear
Abetalipoproteinaemia and homozygous hypobetalipoproteinaemia	Extremely low plasma total cholesterol and triglyceride; chylomicrons, VLDL and LDL absent from plasma; deficiency of apo B	Fat malabsorption, retinitis pigmentosa acanthocytosis, ataxic neuropathy	none
Fish eye disease	Reduced levels of HDL	corneal opacities	late atherosclerosis
Primary dysbetalipoproteinaemia	Low or normal plasma total cholesterol; mild hypertriglyceridemia; cholesterol-rich VLDL; presence of beta-VLDL; low LDL	none	none

For references see Gjone et al (1978), Fredrickson et al (1978), Herbert et al (1978), Carlson and Philippson (1980), Utermann et al (1977b)

A second autosomal recessive disorder that has had a considerable impact on the understanding of the role of HDL in the atherosclerotic process is familial LCAT-deficiency.

Lecithin-cholesterol-acyltransferase is an enzyme present in human plasma that catalyses the preferential transfer of a fatty acid residue from the β-position of phosphatidylcholine to the hydroxyl group of cholesterol (Glomset, 1968). Patients with a familial deficiency of the enzyme exhibit multiple lipoprotein abnormalities (Gjone et al, 1978). HDL, which is the main site of acyltransferase catalysed cholesteryl-ester formation in human plasma is anomalously heterogeneous and contain a population of cholesteryl-ester-poor disc-shaped particles. These are considered precursors of the spherical HDL in normal plasma (Hamilton et al, 1976; Utermann et al, 1980b).

The lipoprotein abnormalities in familial LCAT-deficiency result in storage of cholesterol in several tissues. This may be the result of impaired removal of cholesterol from cells due to the disturbed HDL metabolism. Clinically, the disorder is characterised by anaemia, corneal opacity and proteinuria with late renal insufficiency. Many of the hitherto described patients had atherosclerosis (Gjone et al, 1978).

Autosomal dominant forms

The dominant forms of familial hyperlipidaemia are among the most common genetic disorders in man and they are associated with the occurance of premature coronary heart disease. The present genetic classification of dominant familial hyperlipidemia is based primarily on the pioneering work of Goldstein and coworkers (1973). Several studies in different countries have confirmed their findings (Fredrickson et al, 1978; Glueck et al, 1973a; b; Nikkilä & Aro, 1973; Rose et al, 1973). Three frequent monogenic familial disorders of lipoprotein metabolism were delineated by family studies in survivors of myocardial infarction; 20% of survivors under age 60 years had one of these disorders. These are familial hypercholesteroleamia, familial hypertriglyceridaemia and familial combined hyperlipidaemia. Ascertainment of affected kindreds in the work of Goldstein et al has been criticised repeatedly (Hewitt et al, 1979; Ott, 1979), since the selection and classification procedure used would tend to produce results suggestive of major gene effects even when no such genes operate. The appearance of monogenic segregation of cholesterol (LDL-cholesterol) with or without associated xanthomatosis however is undisputed and the discovery of the primary genetic defect in familial hypercholesterolaemia has provided unequivocal evidence for the monogenic causation of this disease (Brown & Goldstein, 1974a; Goldstein & Brown, 1974; Goldstein et al, 1975). The data providing evidence for a monogenic mechanism in familial combined hyperlipidaemia and familial hypertriglyceridaemia are less convincing, especially since there is lack of any specific biochemical marker for these disorders. However, the grouping the disorders as proposed by Goldstein et al (1973) seems the most satisfactory solution at present and provides a conceptual framework for further studies.

Familial hypertriglyceridaemia

Familial hypertriglyceridaemia is a disorder of the adult. Only 10–20% of individuals that carry the gene for familial hypertriglyceridaemia develop hypertriglyceridaemia before the age of 20 years and expression of the disorder in children is extremely rare. A moderate elevation of triglycerides in VLDL is characteristic of the disorder (Goldstein et al, 1973).

Hyperchylomicronaemia is rare. Lipoprotein electrophoresis exhibits a type IV or rarely a type V pattern (Hazzard et al, 1973). Xanthomas usually do not develop. Familial hypertriglyceridaemia is associated with diabetes mellitus and obesity. Family studies on probands with familial hypertriglyceridaemia and diabetes mellitus have provided evidence that the hyperlipidaemia is transmitted independently from diabetes mellitus. However patients that have both familial hyperlipidaemia and diabetes mellitus are more severely affected. A similar relationship may exist between hypertriglyceridaemia and pancreatitis (Brunzell et al, 1973). Besides untreated diabetes, several other factors including alcohol abuses and estrogen therapy, may lead to gross elevation of triglycerides, hyperchylomicronaemia and pancreatitis in patients with familial hypertriglyceridaemia (Fredrickson et al, 1978). Acquired severe hypertriglyceridaemia sometimes represents an exercerbation of a mild preexisting familial hypertriglyceridaemia. However in most individual cases it is impossible to differentiate, since there is no specific biochemical marker for familial hypertriglyceridaemia. The most severe clinical consequence of the familial hyperlipidaemia is atherosclerosis, leading to cerebral vascular disease and coronary heart disease. The role of triglyceride as an independent risk factor for atherosclerosis is still disputed. However, the fact that 5% of unselected survivors of myocardial infarction under age 60 years have familial hypertriglyceridaemia demonstrates that this form of hypertriglyceridaemia is associated with a high risk for premature coronary artery disease (Brunzell et al, 1976).

Family data on the inheritance of familial hypertriglyceridaemia are compartible with an autosomal dominant mode of transmission (Glueck et al, 1973; Goldstein et al, 1973). About 40% of first degree and 25% of second degree adult blood relatives of probands also have hypertriglyceridaemia. The frequency of the disorder has been estimated to be in the order of 2–3/1000 (Goldstein et al, 1973). Another study claims that this figure underestimates the frequency of familial hypertriglyceridaemia (Motulsky & Bowman, 1975; Motulsky 1976). On the basis of this high frequency, homozygotes for familial hypertriglyceridaemia should be expected. However such homozygotes have not yet been identified. One reason for this may be biochemical heterogeneity. The primary biochemical defect in familial hypertriglyceridaemia is unknown. Overproduction of endogenous triglycerides as well as delayed catabolism of VLDL both have been observed in patients with familial hypertriglyceridaemia. Mean LPL levels are lower than in controls but there is no deficiency of LPL (Krauss et al, 1974). Familial hypertriglyceridaemia probably represents a heterogenous group of biochemically distinct disorders that have an elevation of VLDL in common. The recent discovery of genetic variant of apo A-I that is associated with hypertriglyceridaemia and low HDL-cholesterol concentration (Franceschini et al, 1980) may represent an example of such a specific biochemical entity in the heterogenous group collectively designated as familial hypertriglyceridaemia.

Since most patients with familial hypertriglyceridaemia are obese, initial therapy should be dietary, which may result in a fall in triglyceride levels. Simple carbohydrates should be restricted and ethanol intake avoided. Failure of dietary intervention to lower plasma triglycerides is an indicator for drug therapy.

Clofibrate, clofibrate derivatives and nicotinic acid are most effective in the management of hypertriglyceridaemia (Carlson & Olsson, 1979). In patients with a type V pattern, where chylomicrons are also elevated, fat restriction is the most important therapeutic intervention. Norethindrone acetate and nicotinic acid both have been reported to be effective in otherwise untreated patients with type V.

Isolated hypertriglyceridaemia is also seen in $\frac{1}{3}$ of patients with monogenic familial combined hyperlipidaemia (Goldstein et al, 1973). Moreover 'sporadic hypertriglyceridaemia' has been differentiated from the familial disorder by family studies. This latter group is poorly defined and may include non-genetic, polygenic and recessive forms, or isolated cases of familial hypertriglyceridaemia or familial combined hyperlipidaemia. No specific criteria exist to diagnose familial hypertriglyceridaemia in a single patient. Hence differentiation of the familial hypertriglyceridaemia from other genetic or non-genetic forms of hypertriglyceridaemia is not possible except by family studies. If a patient presents with a combination of hypertriglyceridaemia and premature vascular disease a family study is indicated to possibly identify family members at risk.

Familial hypercholesterolaemia

Familial hypercholesterolaemia is the best example of a monogenic disorder in which the mutant gene produces both hypercholesterolaemia and atherosclerosis. The disease exists in two forms, the heterozygous form that has a frequency of about 1/500 in the population and the rare homozygous form that is present in about 1/1 000 000 newborn children.

Heterozygous familial hypercholesterolaemia

The triad of hypercholesterolaemia, xanthomatosis and angina pectoris has been recognized as a dominant inherited syndrome since the work of Müller (1939).

Familial hypercholesterolaemia is characterised chemically by a 2 fold elevation of cholesterol in LDL. Mean plasma cholesterol concentrations are about 350 mg/100 ml, but range from 270 to 550 mg/100 ml. VLDL cholesterol and triglyceride occasionally may also be elevated but this seems to be unrelated to the gene defect. Electrophoresis of plasma followed by staining for lipids results in a type IIa or less frequently IIb phenotype. The elevation of LDL-cholesterol is seen in childhood and is the earliest detectable manifestation of the gene, usually being present at birth (Kwiterovich et al, 1973, 1974).

Clinical symptoms of the disorder are tendonous xanthomas, preferentially of the achilles tendon, xanthelasma, arcus lipoides corneae and coronary atherosclerosis. These symptoms usually develop in second, third and fourth decades of life. By the third decade, arcus corcea and tendon xanthomas are present in about half of heterozygotes. Tuberous xanthomas may be present, but are rare. However none of these symptoms is obligatory, even though as many as 80 per cent of affected subjects ultimately develop xanthomas. In contrast to the other forms of familial hyperlipidaemia, patients with familial hypercholesterolaemia are not obese and do not have glucose intolerance or hyperuricaemia. The fatal complications of the progressive atherosclerosis are myocardial and cerebral infarction. Large family studies have shown that coronary heart disease does occur at an earlier mean age and is much more frequent in affected than in unaffected family members. The largest of this kind by Stone et al (1974) investigated over 1000 subjects from 116 kindreds. In their study, the cumulative probability of coronary heart disease by age 60 years was 52% in affected males and 33% in affected females; the risk for coronary heart disease was about 3–4 times higher in affected subjects compared to intrafamilial controls. The mean age of onset of symptomatic coronary heart disease is about 45 years in affected males and 53 years in females (Harlan et al, 1966). The high risk for premature atherosclerosis for carriers of the gene for familial hypercholesterolaemia is also evident from studies in survivors of myocardial infarction. Independent studies in Finland, Great Britain and the USA have

shown that in unselected survivors the frequency of familial hypercholesterolemia is 3–6%, compared to 0.1–0.2% in the general population (Goldstein et al, 1973; Nikkilä & Aro, 1973, Patterson & Slack, 1972).

The primary biochemical defect in familial hypercholesterolaemia has been elucidated by cell culture studies, using fibroblasts from homozygotes for the disease and from normal controls. In normal humans, LDL is degraded by different mechanisms, one of which involves a high affinity cell surface receptor present on several extrahepatic tissues. This receptor is deficient or functionally abnormal in homozygotes for familial hypercholesterolaemia (Brown & Goldstein 1974a; 1976a; Goldstein & Brown, 1974; Goldstein et al, 1975). The accumulation of LDL in plasma of homozygotes is caused by the absence of functionally normal receptors for LDL on their cell membranes. Heterozygotes for familial hypercholesterolaemia have one normal allele specifying for functionally normal receptors and one abnormal allele at the LDL receptor gene locus. Presence of only half the number of functionally normal receptors results in impaired degradation of LDL and accumulation of LDL in the plasma compartment (Bilheimer et al, 1978, 1979, Brown and Goldstein 1974b). Kinetic studies have demonstrated a delay in catabolism, as well as enhanced synthesis, of apo B in patients with familial hypercholesterolaemia, where the latter represents a secondary response to the primary catabolic lesion (Bilheimer et al, 1979; Langer et al, 1972).

Familial hypercholesterolaemia is transmitted as an autosomal dominant trait (Harlan, 1966; Heiberg, 1976; Heiberg & Berg, 1976; Khatchadurian, 1964; Müller, 1939; Schrott et al, 1972). The dominant gene is highly penetrant at all ages (from 90–100%) when either total cholesterol or LDL-cholesterol is used as a genetic marker for the disease. In affected families a bimodal distribution of cholesterol and LDL-cholesterol is observed. There is, however, some overlap between normal and affected family members. Measurement of LDL-receptor activity on fibroblasts or lymphocytes also shows a bimodal distribution and may be used as an additional criterion to establish the diagnosis (Bilheimer et al, 1978; Fredrickson et al, 1978).

The gene locus for familial hypercholesterolaemia is closely linked to the gene locus for the third complement component (Berg & Heiberg, 1979; Elston et al, 1976; Ott et al, 1974).

Treatment of familial hypercholesterolaemia should begin with a fat-modified diet (Levy et al, 1971). A diet low in cholesterol and with a ratio of polyunsaturated to saturated fatty acids close to 2 is recommended. However, such a diet alone usually is not sufficient for effectively lowering LDL-cholesterol levels and therefore drugs are commonly added to the dietary regime. Clofibrate, nicotinic acid and D-thyroxin have been used either alone or in different combination (Levy et al, 1972). The most effective drugs, however, for lowering plasma cholesterol levels in familial hypercholesterolemia are the bile acid sequestring agents: cholestyramine and cholestipol, that may reduce plasma cholesterol by 30% or more (Fallon & Woods, 1968; Farah et al, 1977; Howard et al, 1966; Lees & Lees, 1976; Levy et al, 1973). When the disease process is severe, patients can still be treated by surgical approaches using Dacron protheses, coronary bypass or endarterectomy.

In the differential diagnosis of the disorder other forms of hypercholesterolaemia have to be considered. These are secondary hypercholesterolaemia, polygenic hypercholesterolaemia and the hypercholesterolaemia seen in $\frac{1}{3}$ of patients with familial combined hyperlipidaemia. Patients with these disorders rarely develop xanthomas, in particular no xanthomas of the achilles tendon. Even in the absence of visible or palpable xanthomas, thickening of the achilles tendon has turned out as a valuable clinical criterion for the differential diagnosis of familial hypercholesterolaemia (Blankenhorn & Mayers, 1969; Mabuchi et al, 1977). Tendon xanthomas that are clinically indistinguishable from those in familial hypercholesterolaemia may develop in patients with autosomal recessive cerebrotendinous xanthomatosis. However, these individuals have normal LDL-cholesterol and may be distinguished by other clinical features, such as cataracts and mental deterioration. Similarly xanthelasma and arcus corneae can also be observed in patients with normal cholesterol levels and may occur as a familial trait.

As a consequence of the autosomal dominant mode of transmission, every first degree relative of a propositus with familial hypercholesterolaemia has a risk of 50% to have inherited the mutant gene and be at risk for premature atherosclerosis and coronary heart disease. Therefore, once the diagnosis of familial hypercholesterolaemia has been established in a patient, a family study is indicated to identify affected relatives before they manifest clinical complications. The potential of such an approach has been demonstrated by a large Norwegian population genetic study on xanthomatosis and hypercholesterolaemia. In this study 30% of patients ascertained by a propositus with xanthomatosis came from only 7 large kindreds, each showing classical dominant inheritance of the trait (Heiberg, 1976).

Homozygous familial hypercholesterolaemia

Rarely, two heterozygotes for familial hypercholesterolaemia marry and produce a homozygous child (Fig. 69.3). This condition is much more devastating than the heterozygous form of the disease. Plasma LDL levels are elevated roughly 6 fold in these children as compared to controls. Total plasma cholesterol levels range from 600–1200 mg/100ml. There is massive deposition of cho-

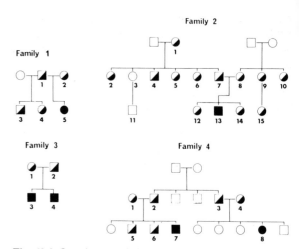

Fig. 69.3 Genetic transmission of familial hypercholesterolaemia. Black filled symbols denote homozygotes and half filled symbols heterozygotes for the disease (From Mabuchi et al, 1978; with permission of the publishers).

lesterol in tissues and myocardial infections generally occur in the first two decades of life (Fredrickson et al, 1978; Khatchadurian & Uthman, 1973; Mabuchi et al, 1978). Gross hypercholesterolaemia is present at birth and persists throughout life. Cutaneous xanthomas, which have a unique yellow-orange colour may be present at birth and have been found by age 4 in virtually every patient. Tendon xanthomas and arcus corneae develop in childhood. A typical form of the xanthomatous infiltration of the aortic valve may result in aortic valvular stenosis. Occasionally, mitral regurgitation and mitral stenosis have been observed due to xanthomatous plaquing and thickening of the endocardial surfaces of the mitral valve. Further clinical and laboratory findings are painfull and inflamed joints, cardiac murmurs and persistently elevated sedimentation rate. Generalised atherosclerosis results in death from myocardial infarction before 30 years of age. However in a large series of patients from Japan six exceeded the third decade (Mabuchi et al, 1978). The cholesterol in the xanthoma is present within histiocytic foam cells mostly in the form of cytoplasmic droplets that are not bound to membranes. Upon autopsy, typical atherosclerotic plaques are found in the arteries; in addition there are intimal infiltrations of xanthomatous foam cells similar in histologic appearance to those in the tuberous xanthomas. Severe atherosclerosis occurs not only in the coronary arteries but in the thoracic and abdominal aorta and in the major pulmonary arteries as well.

The homozygotes held the key to solving the primary biochemical defect in familial hypercholesterolaemia and thus the biochemical mechanism underlying a dominantly inherited disorder (heterozygous familial hypercholesterolaemia, Brown & Goldstein 1974b). By studying fibroblasts from homozygous children Goldstein and Brown (1974) were able to demonstrate a genetic defect in the LDL-receptor in familial hypercholesterolaemia. This defect leads to deficient binding, uptake and degradation of LDL by body cells and this results in accumulation of LDL in massive levels in plasma with the ultimate development of xanthomas and atherosclerosis. Elucidation of this defect has led to the detection of an important biochemical pathway. The LDL-pathway and its relation to human atherosclerosis has been described in several recent reviews (Brown & Goldstein, 1976b; c; d; Goldstein & Brown 1977b, Goldstein et al, 1979). The sequential steps in this LDL-pathway are shown in Figure 69.4

In the course of their studies, Goldstein and Brown identified three different mutant alleles at the LDL-receptor locus (Anderson et al, 1977; Goldstein et al, 1975; Goldstein & Brown, 1977a). The one allele most frequently observed in their material specifies a receptor that is not able to bind LDL and has been termed R^{b^o}. A second allele is termed R^{b^-}. This allele specifies a receptor that still is able to bind LDL, but the amounts of LDL bound are only 1–10% of normal controls. A very rare third allele was detected in only one patient who turned out to be a compound. He had one R^{b^o} allele and one allele designated R^{b^+,i^o}. This allele specifies a receptor that is able to bind LDL normally, but is not able to internalize the LDL. This mutant receptor has lost the

ability to become localized to coated pits. From 43 patients studied by Brown and Goldstein, 24 were homozygous for the R^{bo} allele. 18 patients were either homozygous R^{b-}/R^{b-} or $R^{b^{\prime\prime}}/R^{b-}$ compounds. These two types can not be differentiated by the present biochemical assays. One patient was the above mentioned $R^{b^o}/R^{b,i^o}$ compound. The parents of homozygous propositi are obligate heterozygotes and have the dominant form of familial hypercholesterolaemia. The frequency of parental consanguinity was at least 33% in a study from Japan (Mabuchi et al, 1978).

A form of severe hypercholesterolaemia associated with xanthomatosis and premature atherosclerosis has been described in some children, where both parents had normal plasma lipid and lipoprotein levels. This form has been designated 'pseudo-homozygous hypercholesterolaemia' (Mishkel, 1976; Morganroth et al, 1974). The primary defect, aetiology and genetics of this disorder are unknown. It can be differentiated from homozygous familial hypercholesterolaemia by demonstration of uneffected parents and more specifically by the LDL-receptor assay.

Therapy for homozygous familial hypercholesterolaemia is still far from being optimal. Drugs like cholestyramin may reduce plasma cholesterol levels by 20–30% However this reduction is not sufficient to prevent myocardial infarction and many of the children do not tolerate the drug regime. In this situation portocaval shunt and plasma exchange therapy have been used

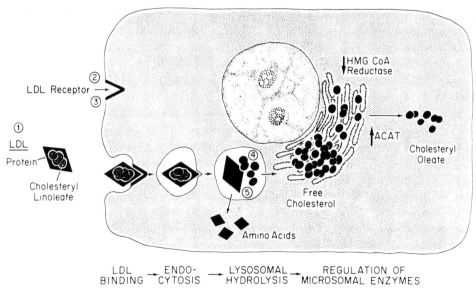

LDL → ENDO- → LYSOSOMAL → REGULATION OF
BINDING   CYTOSIS   HYDROLYSIS   MICROSOMAL ENZYMES

Fig. 69.4 LDL-pathway in human cultured fibroblasts. The sequential steps in the pathway are binding of LDL to the receptor, uptake of LDL, lysosomal hydrolysis of protein and cholesteryl esters and regulation of cellular cholesterol synthesis and cholesteryl ester formation. The numbers indicate the sites in the pathway at which mutations have been identified: (1) abetalipoproteinaemia; (2) familial hypercholesterolaemia, receptor-binding negative and receptor-binding defective types; (3) familial hypercholesterolaemia internalisation defect; (4) Wolman disease; (5) cholesteryl ester storage disease (Adopted from Brown and Goldstein 1974b, with the permission of the publishers).

either alone, or in combination, as the most effective therapeutic intervention in homozygous familial hypercholesterolaemia (Bilheimer et al, 1975; King et al, 1980; Starzel et al, 1973; 1974; Thompson et al, 1975; 1977). Ileal bypass has also been recommended, seems to meet with little success (Burchwald et al, 1975; Thomson & Gotto, 1973). The LDL-receptor is expressed on amniotic cells in early pregnancy (Goldstein et al, 1974; Wienker et al, 1976). This has made possible the successful prenatal diagnosis of homozygous familial hypercholesterolaemia in one case at risk (Brown et al, 1978).

Familial combined hyperlipidemia
Familial combined hyperlipidaemia (multipe type hyperlipidaemia) is the most frequent monogenic familial hyperlipidaemia occurring, in 3–15/1000 subjects in the population, but had not been recognized as a distinct genetic entity until 1973 (Glueck et al, 1973; Goldstein et al, 1973; Nikkilä & Aro, 1973; Rose et al, 1973). The disorder is inherited as an autosomal dominant trait. A characteristic features of familial combined hyperlipidaemia is its pleomorphic manifestation, even among relatives in the same family. Roughly, 1 in 3 of affected individuals have hypercholesterolaemia (evelated LDL), 1 in 3 have hypertriglyceridaemia (evelated VLDL) and 1 in 3 have both hypercholesterolaemia and hypertriglyceridaemia (evelated LDL and VLDL). Accordingly patients may present with a type IIa, IIb, IV or rarely a type V phenotype (Hazzard et al, 1973). In a given individual, the type of hyperlipoproteinaemia may change spontaneously. Mean plasma lipid levels are significantly increased, but tend to show a lesser degree of elevation than either in familial hypercholesterolaemia or familial hypertriglyceridaemia. However, lipid levels may be in the normal range at one time and abnormal at another time. Elevation of plasma lipids is not seen in children of adults affected with familial combined hyperlipidemia. Rarely is the lipid abnormality expressed before the age of 25 years.

The disorder is associated with obesity, hyperinsulinaemia and glucose intolerance. Xanthomas do not occur. Patients with excessive hypertriglyceridaemia may develop pancreatitis. The most severe complication of combined hyperlipidaemia is coronary atherosclerosis. In independent studies from Finland and the USA, 11–20% of survivors of myocardial infarction under age 60 years had this disorder (Goldstein et al, 1973; Nikkilä & Aro, 1973). There are, at present, no good incidence figures available on patients randomly selected from the population. The occurance of phenotypically different lipoprotein patterns in familial combined hyperlipidaemia is believed to be the expression of one single dominant gene. In a study of 47 families with combined hyperlipidaemia, identified among survivors of myocardial infarction, 50% of first degree relatives above age 25

years had hyperlipidaemia, consistent with a dominant mechanism. It has been concluded from the analysis of lipid distribution in those families that the gene primarily affects triglyceride metabolism, but has secondary effects on cholesterol metabolism. The primary biochemical lesion underlying the disorder is unknown and its pathophysiology is unclear. Subjects with hypercholesterolaemia from kindreds with combined hyperlipidaemia have a functionally normal LDL-receptor. To data no specific biochemical test exists for the diagnosis of familial combined hyperlipidaemia. Due to this lack of a specific marker for the disorder, the diagnosis is not possible in an individual patient. The only method available to make the diagnosis and to differentiate combined hyperlipidaemia from the other forms of primary hyperlipidaemia is by family studies. This approach for identification had also been used in the original delineation of the disorder and this has necessarily biased the subsequent genetic analysis. Hence the single-gene inheritance of familial combined hyperlipidaemia cannot be considered proven. However, four large pedigrees each showing vertical transmission over three generations and the expected 1:1 segregation ratio have been reported in the literature. The data from these kindreds are most easily explained by single-gene inheritance. In any event, suspicion of familial combined hyperlipidaemia in a given patient should lead to determinations of plasma lipids in all first degree adult relatives since the risk for first degree relatives of a proband with familial combined hyperlipidaemia to also have the disorder is 50%.

Treatment of combined hyperlipidaemia depends on the phenotypic expression of the disease. For individuals with pure hypercholesterolaemia (Type IIa) or pure hypertriglyceridaemia (type IV) the same rules as described for familial hypercholesterolaemia or familial hypertriglyceridaemia, respectively, may be used as a guide. In obese probands with the IIb phenotype, treatment begins with the prudent diet, emphasizing weight reduction as well as fat modification. With the exception of bile-sequestring agents, the same drugs mentioned for the therapy of familial hypercholesterolaemia (clofibrate, D-thyroxin, nicotinic acid) are appropriate for treatment. Sometimes a combination of resin and clofibrate may be required to correct both the hypercholesterolaemia and the hypertriglyceridaemia (Fredrickson, 1972; Havel, 1972; Levy et al, 1972).

Polygenic hyperlipidemia

Familial type III hyperlipoproteinaemia
Familial type III hyperlipoproteinaemia (broad-beta-disease) is a disorder of lipoprotein metabolism associated with grossly elevated plasma concentrations of both cholesterol and triglycerides. Lipid levels are extremely sensitive to caloric intake and consequently there is

considerable variability of cholesterol and triglyceride levels in a given patient. Usually however cholesterol concentrations are over 300 mg/100 ml and triglyceride levels tend to exceed those of cholesterol. Chylomicrons that are rich in cholesterol may be present in fasting plasma. The characteristic lipoprotein abnormality of the type III disorder is the accumulation in plasma of lipoprotein particles that are intermediate in density, size, chemical composition and electrophoretic mobility between VLDL and LDL (Fredrickson et al, 1968; 1978; Hazzard et al, 1972; Mishkel et al, 1975; Morganroth et al, 1975; Patsch et al, 1975). Electrophoresis of type III plasma followed by staining for lipids frequently reveals a broad unresolved band extending between beta- and prebeta lipoproteins. Analytical ultracentrifugation of type III lipoproteins results in a pattern characterised by an elevated concentration of S_f 12–100 lipoproteins (VLDL and IDL) and a decrease in S_f 0–12 lipoproteins (LDL) (Fredrickson et al, 1968). Upon preparative ultracentrifugation the abnormal lipoproteins in part float with VLDL and are demonstrated by electrophoresis as a beta migrating subfraction. The abnormal lipoprotein therefore is called 'floating-beta lipoprotein' or beta-VLDL. It differs from normal VLDL in a higher proportion of cholesterol relative to triglyceride and in apoprotein composition. Beta-VLDL is absolutely or relatively enriched in apo E and depleted of apo C (Havel & Kane 1973). Apo E exhibits a structural abnormality designated as the apo E-D/D phenotype (Utermann et al, 1975; 1977a; 1979b).

Hyperlipoproteinaemia type III is a disorder of the adult and is rarely seen before the age of 20 years. There are only few documented cases where type III hyperlipoproteinaemia existed in childhood. Clinically, the disorder is associated with xanthomatosis, coronary heart disease and peripheral vascular disease (Borrie, 1969; Mishkel et al, 1975; Morganroth et al, 1975; Moser et al, 1974). The most typical clinical feature seen in about 60% of patients are planar yellowish lipid deposits in the creases of the palm (xanthoma striata palmaris). Tuberous xanthomas are present in about 70% of type III subjects and tendon xanthomas in 25%. Eruptive xanthomas, xanthelasma and arcus corneae may occur but are comparatively rare. 33% of patients have coronary heart disease and 27% exhibit peripheral vascular disease. About 50% of patients have glucose intolerance. These data, however, are biased by the selection of patients exclusively from clinical material. Thus 100% of patients acertained by a dermatologist will present with xanthomas (Borrie, 1969). There exist no data on patients randomly selected from the population. The increased risk for premature coronary heart disease is evident from the frequency of type III hyperlipoproteinaemia among survivors of myocardial infarction. In this group, the frequency is about 1 per 100 (Utermann 1980)

compared to $\sim$ 1 per 5000 in the general population (Fredrickson et al, 1978). Men tend to present with clinical symptoms earlier than women. In a large series of patients from the NIH, ischaemic vascular disease was diagnosed at a mean age of 39 years in men, but 10 years later in women. The familial occurance of type III disorder has been known since the early pioneering work of Fredrickson and coworkers (1967), but for many years there were conflicting results on its genetic mode of transmission (Fredrickson et al, 1978; Hazzard et al, 1975; Morganroth et al, 1975; Moser et al, 1974). The key to the clarification of the complicated genetics of type III hyperlipidaemia came from the recent discovery of a polymorphism of apolipoprotein E, which is determined by three autosomal alleles apo E^n, apo E^4 and apo E^d (see polymorphism of apo E). Virtually every patient with classical type III studied to date was homozygous for the gene apo E^d (phenotype apo E−D/D), suggesting an autosomal recessive mode of inheritance. However 1% of unselected German blood donors are homozygous apo E-D/D whereas the frequency of classic type III is only about 1 in 5000. Moreover, most individuals of phenotype apo E-D/D present with hypo- rather than hypercholesterolaemia; but all have in common the same type of dyslipoproteinaemia characterised by the presence of beta-VLDA and designated primary dysbetalipoproteinaemia (Utermann et al, 1977b). No more than 2% of apo E-D/D individuals ever develop clinical signs of the type III disorder and an additional mechanism resulting in the hyperlipidaemia in type III patients had to be anticipated. Therefore it was proposed that type III hyperlipoproteinaemia is caused by the simultaneous but independent inheritance of the apo E^d genes and of other defects that produce hyperlipidaemia. Comparative studies of 19 kindreds ascertained through a proband of phenotype apo E-D/D gave direct support for this two−factor-hypothesis. Probands with type III hyperlipoproteinaemia came from families where various phenotypic forms of hyperlipidaemia were present in about 50% of all adult first degree relatives of propositi (Utermann et al, 1979a and Fig. 69.5). Hyperlipidaemia and apo E-phenotypes segregated independently in the families and some kindreds showed evidence for coexistence of monogenic combined hyperlipidaemia. On the contrary, hyperlipidaemia was not observed in kindreds where the probands were normocholesterolaemic. From these observations it has been concluded that type III hyperlipoproteinaemia is caused by at least two non allelic genes. Depending on the form of the coinherited hyperlipidaemia the disorder will be dimeric in some and polygenic in other patients. Vertical transmission of the dyslipoproteinaemia has been observed in many kindreds and previously had been taken as evidence for a monogenic dominant mechanism (Hazzard et al, 1975). However, this phenomenon represents pseudodominance that

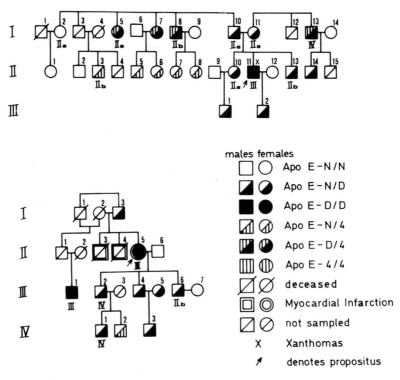

Fig. 69.5 Inheritance of apo E phenotypes and hyperlipoproteinaemia type III in two families. Roman numerals under the symbols denote the lipoprotein phenotypes of hyperlipidaemic subjects (From Utermann et al, 1979b, modified)

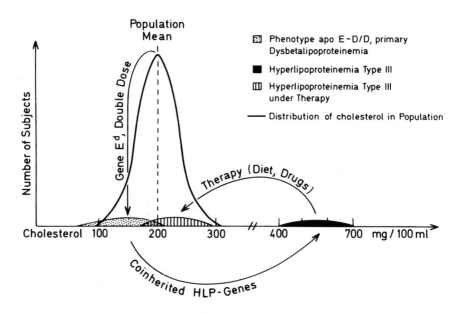

Fig. 69.6 Hyperlipidaemia type III as a multifactorial disorder: Schematic representation of the genetic two-factor hypothesis (Utermann et al, 1979b) and of the interaction of genetic and environmental factors in producing differences in the phenotypic expression of the hyperlipidaemia. HLP genes denotes hyperlipidaemic genes e.g. any single gene or polygenes that result in hyperlipidaemia.

is due to the high frequency of the *apo E*^{d} allele (~ 0.09) in the population (Utermann et al, 1977b).

As mentioned earlier, lipid levels in type III patients are very sensitive to caloric intake. Most patients respond well to dietary or drug therapy. On a strict regime, cholesterol concentration may be lowered to a normal level and xanthomas may disappear. Moreover, hormonal factors such as hyperthyroidism, and oestrogen treatment can completely eliminate the hyperlipidaemia, whereas hypothyroidism markedly exaggerates the lipoprotein abnormalities (Falko et al, 1979; Hazzard & Bierman, 1972; Kushwaha et al, 1977). Hypothyroidism as well as severe nephropathy possibly are among the exogenous factors that may precipitate type III hyperlipoproteinemia in a subject of *apo E*^{d}/*E*^{d} genotype, a phenomenon previously described as secondary type III hyperlipoproteinaemia. Since the degree of hyperlipidaemia and clinical symptoms are under the control of different genes interacting with endogenous and environmental factors, type III hyperlipoproteinaemia ultimately has to be defined as a multifactorial disorder (Fig. 69.6). The genetic two factor concept of type III hyperlipoproteinaemia predicts that more than one defect operates in subjects with classical type III disorder. One of these is shared by all type III subjects and also operates in subjects with simple uncomplicated dysbetalipoproteinaemia. This defect relates to the structural abnormality of apo E.

The abnormal beta-VLDL and the cholesterol-rich chylomicrons present in type III plasma are considered degradation products (remnants) of triglyceride-rich lipoproteins that accumulate due to a defect in the catabolism of remnants (Chait et al, 1977; 1978; Hazzard & Bierman, 1971; 1976). Apo E normally plays a key role in the degradation of remnants. There is evidence that apo E is recognized by a hepatic remnant receptor and by the LDL (B/E)-receptor (Sherill et al, 1980). These receptors are probably required for the removal of remnants by the liver. The accumulation of remnant lipoproteins in familial dysbetalipoproteinaemia and in type III hyperlipoproteinaemia may be caused by lack of functionally normal apo E. The apo E-D form of the protein from some patients with type III hyperlipoproteinaemia indeed represents a non-functional mutant that is not recognized by the LDL (B/E)-receptor, thus explaining the accumulation of remnants and the reduced concentration of LDL (Schneider et al, 1981). Moreover this mechanism could also explain the mild dyslipoproteinaemia seen in subjects heterozygous for the *apo E*^{d} allele. (Havel et al, 1980.) The metabolic block at the remnant removal step, however, usually does not result in hyperlipoproteinaemia type III, but a second independent defect is required for the development of hyperlipidaemia. Kinetic studies performed on patients with classical type III disorder have shown that

in addition to a delay in the catabolism of remnants there exists an enhanced synthesis of VLDL. Hence the development of gross hyperlipidaemia seems to result from an overload of the defective alpha$_2$-path by overproduction of VLDL. In addition to overproduction of VLDL, a direct secretion of beta-VLDL by the liver and conversion of these particles to LDL has been postulated to occur in subjects with type III hyperlipidaemia (Berman et al. 1978). However, this alternative pathway (β-path) bypassing the normal alpha$_2$-path in type III subjects is difficult to understand on the basis of the present concept of the functional abnormality of apo E in type III subjects. Whereas apo E from some type III subjects is not recognized by the LDL (B/E)-receptor, leading to the accumulation of beta-VLDL it has been demonstrated that a specific receptor for beta-VLDL, exists on macrophages (Mahley et al, 1980). These cells may bind and internalise the beta-VLDL and become overloaded with cholesteryl-ester in type III hyperlipoproteinaemia and develop into foam cells. Foam cells that probably are derived from macrophages form the basis of xanthomas and have been found on autopsy in coronary vessels, on the endocardial surface, the spleen and the bone marrow of patients with type III disorder. It may be that the abnormal beta-VLDL leads to an unusual response of the vascular wall with formation of foam cells that may greatly accelerate the development of atherosclerosis.

Demonstration by electrophoresis of beta-VLDL was the original diagnostic test for the type III disorder. However this lipoprotein abnormality is not pathognomonic for hyperlipoproteinaemia type III and alternative clinical-chemical tests have been proposed that are based on the abnormal lipid-chemical composition of VLDL in the type III disorder (Fredrickson et al, 1975; 1978; Havel, 1977; Hazzard et al, 1972; Mishkel et al, 1975). In all of these tests arbitrary cut points were used to define the abnormal composition and none was specific. The observation of the structural apo E abnormality in type III hyperlipoproteinaemia provides the basis for the specific diagnosis of the disorder by electrofocusing of apo-VLDL. Demonstration of the apo E-D/D phenotype in a hyperlipidaemic individual unequivocally proves the diagnosis of the type III disorder (Pagnan et al, 1977; Utermann et al, 1975; 1977a; Warnick et al, 1979; Weidman et al, 1979, Zannis & Breslow, 1980).

An excellent response to therapy is the rule in most patients with type III hyperlipoproteinaemia. Upon weight reduction there is frequently a dramatic decrease in plasma lipid levels. A diet high in poly-unsaturated fat and low in cholesterol is recommended but it should contain 50% of the calories as fats. In cases where plasma lipid levels remain elevated, even after ideal weight is achieved, clofibrate is the drug of choice to reduce them to normal. Regression of xanthomata and of peripheral vascular disease has been reported as a consequence of hypolipidemic therapy (Zelis et al, 1970).

Genetic counselling in hyperlipoproteinaemia type III can help to recognize family members at risk. The risk for relatives of propositi is twofold. Given that the coexisting hyperlipidaemia is one of the monogenic dominant forms, the risk for a first degree relative to also have inherited the 'hyperlipidaemic gene' is 1 in 2. The risk for the development of the type III disorder is different for sibs and for children of a proband. In the most frequent situation both parents of a proband will be heterozygous carriers of the *apo E^d* allele and the risk for any of their children to be homozygous *apo E^d/E^d* will be 1 in 4. The combined risk to coinherit both *apo E^d* alleles and the hyperlipidemic gene then will be $\frac{1}{4} \times \frac{1}{2} = \frac{1}{8}$. The risk for children of a proband can be calculated from the known frequency of the *apo E^d* allele in the population. A proband with type III disorder has a chance of about 16% to have a spouse heterozygous for the apo E^d allele and any child from this mating has a risk of 1 in 2 to be homozygous *apoE^d/E^d*, and, independently, 1 in 2 to inherit the 'hyperlipidaemic gene'. Hence the risk for children of a proband to develop hyperlipoproteinaemia type III in later life is about 4%. Actually the risk is even higher, since there is a 1% chance of the spouse being homozygous *apo E^d/E^d*, and, furthermore, the spouse may also contribute 'hyperlipidaemic genes' due to the high frequency of these genes in the population. Therefore apo E-phenotyping is recommended in families of type III probands. This permits the early detection of apo E-D/D relatives that are at risk to develop type III hyperlipoproteinaemia in later life. A follow up of the at risk individuals then permits early therapeutic intervention in those that start to develop the disorder.

Polygenic hypercholesterolaemia
Plasma cholesterol levels are under the control of many different genes and environmental factors that together result in a nearly gaussian distribution of cholesterol levels in the population. Clustering of several genes in one individual that all tend to moderately elevate plasma cholesterol levels theoretically should result in polygenic hypercholesterolaemia. Indeed, Goldstein and coworkers (1973), in a study of survivors of myocardial infarction, were able to identify a group of patients with elevated plasma cholesterol levels, but with no evidence for bimodality of plasma cholesterol concentrations in the families of affected probands. Instead, the distribution of cholesterol in these families is unimodal but shifted towards a higher mean level. This form was defined as polygenic hypercholesterolaemia and by definition is caused by several independent genes clustering in one individual. Several other studies have provided evidence for the occurrance of polygenic hypercholesterolaemia (Carter et al, 1971; Robertson et al, 1979; Slack, 1975).

The disorder can be delineated only by family studies. The classic clinical features of familial hypercholesterolaemia such as xanthomas and corneal arcus do not occur in polygenic hypercholesterolaemia, but the disorder is likely to be associated with premature atherosclerosis. There are, however, no studies on the prevalence of clinical symptoms in this groups of patients. The frequency of polygenic hypercholesterolaemia can not be given since it depends on the arbitrary definition of upper limits for normal cholesterol levels.

Familial hyperalphalipoproteinemia
The familial aggregation of hyperalphalipoproteinemia was first observed by Glueck et al (1975). These authors arbitrarily defined a concentration of cholesterol in HDL exceeding 70 mg/100 ml as hyperalphalipoproteinaemia and noticed that among blood relatives of probands, about 50% had elevated HDL-cholesterol levels. Familial hyperalphalipoproteinaemia is not a disorder, but rather the opposite. In families affected with hyperalphalipoproteinaemia, Glueck and colleagues observed a significantly lower degree of coronary atherosclerosis; the mean age at death of individuals with the trait was higher than the population mean. From these data it was concluded that hyperalphalipoproteinaemia is a longevity syndrome (Glueck et al, 1976). This interpretation is consistent with and complementary to the present hypothesis that HDL has a protective effect against coronary atherosclerosis. No other lipoprotein, laboratory or clinical abnormalities were observed in patients with familial hyperalphalipoproteinaemia. The mechanism resulting in the elevated HDL-cholesterol in familial hyperalphalipoproteinaemia is completely unclear. From the segregation of the trait in families, an autosomal dominant mode of inheritance could be anticipated. However this assumption is not consistent with the correlation of HDL-cholesterol levels between family members (Glueck et al, 1976). At present the genetics of familial hyperalphalipoproteinaemia are unclear but most probably the trait is under polygenic control. Moreover, there seem to exist different forms of hyperalphalipoproteinaemia in Caucasians and Blacks. Whereas hyperalphalipoproteinaemia occurred as a familial trait with evidence for a major gene effect in Caucasians, most cases among American Blacks were sporadic (Siervogel et al, 1980).

REFERENCES

Adlersberg D, Schaeffer L E, Steinberg A G 1957 Studies on genetic and environmental control of serum cholesterol level (Abst.). Circulation 16: 487–488

Alaupovic P 1971 Conceptual development of the classification systems of plasma lipoproteins, In: Peeters H (ed) Protides of the biological fluids. Pergamon, Oxford. p. 9

Albers J J, Wahl P, Hazzard W R 1974 Quantitative genetic studies of the human plasma Lp(a) lipoprotein Biochemical Genetics 11: 475–486

Albrink M J, Mergs J W, Man E B 1961 Serum lipids, hypertension and coronary artery disease. American Journal of Medicine 31: 4–23

Anderson R G W, Goldstein J L, Brown M S 1977 A mutation that impairs the ability of lipoprotein receptors to localize in coated pits on the cell surface of human fibroblasts. Nature 270: 695–699

Assmann G, Simantke O, Schaefer H E, Smootz E 1977 Characterization of high density lipoproteins in patients heterozygous for Tangier disease. Journal of Clinical Investigation 60: 1025–1035

Beaumont J L, Carlson L A, Cooper G R, Fejfar Z, Fredrickson D S, Strasser T 1970 Classification of hyperlipidemias and hyperlipoproteinemias. Bulletin of the World Health Organisation 43: 891–908

Beisiegel U, Utermann G 1979 An Apolipoprotein Homolog of Rat Apolipoprotein A-IV in Human Plasma. Isolation and Partial Characterisation. European Journal of Biochemistry 93: 601–608

Benditt D P, Benditt J M 1973 Evidence for a monoclonal origin of human atherosclerotic plaques. Proceedings of the National Academy of Sciences USA 70: 1753–1756

Berg K 1963 A new serum type system in man: The Lp system. Acta Pathologica and Microbiologica Scandinavica 59: 369–382

Berg K, Dahlean G, Frick M H 1974 Lp(a) lipoprotein and pre-β-1-lipoprotein in patients with coronary heart disease. Clinical Genetics 6: 230–235

Berg K, Heiberg A 1979 Confirmation of linkage between familial hypercholesterolemia with xanthomatosis and the C 3 polymorphism. In: Winnipeg Conference (1977): Fourth International Workshop on Human Gene Mapping. Birth Defects: Original Article Series. The National Foundation, New York

Berman M, Eisenberg S, Hall M H, Levy R J, Bilheimer D W, Phair R D, Goebel R H 1978 Metabolism of apo B and apo C lipoproteins in man: Kinetic studies in normals and hyperlipoproteinemics. Journal of Lipid Research 19: 38–56

Bierman E L, Albers J J 1975 Lipoprotein uptake by cultured human arterial smooth muscle cells. Biochimica Biophysica Acta 388: 198–202

Bilheimer D W, Goldstein J L, Grundy S M, Brown M S 1975 Reduction in cholesterol and low density lipoprotein synthesis after portocaval shunt surgery in a patient with homozygous familial hypercholesterolemia. Journal of Clinical Investigation 56: 1420–1430

Bilheimer D W, Ho Y K, Brown M S, Anderson R G W, Golstein J L 1978 Genetics of the low density lipoprotein receptor. Journal of Clinical Investigation 61: 678–696

Bilheimer D W, Stone N J, Grundy S M 1979 Metabolic Studies in familial hypercholesterolemia. Evidence for a gene-dosage effect in vivo. Journal of Clinical Investigation 64: 524–533

Blankenhorn D H, Mayers H J 1969 Radiographic determination of Achilles tendon xanthoma size. Metabolism 18: 882–886

Blomstrand R, Lundman T 1966 Serum lipid, smokind and heredity. Acta medica scandinavica supplement 455, 180: 51–60

Borrie P 1969 Type III hyperlipoproteinemia. British Medical Journal 2: 665–667

Breckenridge W C, Little J A, Steiner G, Chow A, Poapst M 1978 Hypertriglyceridemia associated with deficiency of apolipoprotein C-II. New England Journal of Medicine 298: 1265–1273

Brown M S, Goldstein J L 1974a Familial hypercholesterolemia: Defective binding of lipoproteins to cultured fibroblasts associated with impaired regulation of 3-hydroxy-3-methyl-glutaryl coenzyme A reductase activity. Proceedings of the National Academy of Sciences of the USA 71: 788–792

Brown M S, Goldstein J L 1974b Expression of the familial hypercholesterolemia gene in heterozygotes: mechanism for a dominant disorder in man. Science 185: 61–63

Brown M S, Goldstein J L 1976a Analysis of a mutant strain of human fibroblasts with a defect in the internalisation of receptor-bound low density lipoprotein. Cell 9: 663–674

Brown M S, Goldstein J L 1976b Familial hypercholesterolemia: A genetic defect in the low-density lipoprotein receptor. New England Journal of Medicine 294: 1386–1390

Brown M S, Goldstein J L 1976c Receptor-mediated control of cholesterol metabolism. Science 191: 150–154

Brown M S, Goldstein J L 1976d Receptor-mediated control of cholesterol metabolism: study of human mutants has disclosed how cells regulate a substance that is both vital and lethal. Science 191: 150–154

Brown M S, Goldstein J L, Vandenberghe K, Fryns J P, Kovanen P T, Eckels R E, van den Berghe H, Cassiman J J 1978 Prenatal diagnosis of homozygous familial hypercholesterolemia: Expression of a genetic receptor disease in utero. Lancet I, 526–529

Brunzell J D, Schott H G 1973 The interaction of familial and secondary causes of hypertriglyceridemia: Role in pancreatitis. Transactions of the Association of American Physicians 86: 245–253

Brunzell J D, Schott H G, Motulsky A G, Bierman E L 1976 Myocardial infarction in the familial forms of hypertriglyceridemia. Metabolism 25: 313–320

Buchwald H, Moore R B, Varco R L 1975 The partial ideal bypass operation in treatment of the hyperlipidemias. In: Lipids, Lipoproteins and Drugs (Proceedings of the 5th International Symposium on drugs affecting lipid metabolism, Milan), Plenum Press New York, pp 221–239

Carlson L A, Böttiger L E 1972 Ischaemic heart – disease in relation to fasting values of plasma triglycerides and cholesterol. Stockholm prospective study. Lancet I: 865–868

Carlson L A, Olsson A G 1979 Effect of hypolipidemic drugs on serum lipoproteins. In: Eisenberg S (ed) Progress in Biochemical Pharmacology Vol. 15, Lipoprotein Metabolism, Karger S AG, Basel, 238–257

Carlson L A, Philipson B 1979 Fish-eye disease: a new familial condition with massive corneal opacities and dyslipoproteinemia. Lancet: 921–924

Carter C O, Slack J, Myant N M 1971 Genetics of hyperlipoproteinaemias. Lancet I: 400–401

Cassel J C 1971 Summary of major findings of the Evans County cardiovascular studies. Archives of Internal Medicine 128: 887–889

Castelli W P, Doyle J T, Gordon T, Hames C, Hulley S B, Kagan A, McGee D, Vicic W J, Zukel W J 1975 HDL cholesterol levels (HDL-C) in coronary heart disease. A cooperative lipoprotein phenotyping study. Circulation 52: Suppl. II–97

Chait A, Albers J J, Brunzell J P, Hazzard W R 1977 Type III hyperlipoproteinemia ('remnant removal disease'). Insight into the pathogenic mechanism. Lancet I: 1176–1178

Chait A, Hazzard W R, Albers J J, Kushwaha R P, Brunzell J D 1978 Impaired very low density lipoprotein and triglyceride removal in Broad Beta Disease: Comparison with endogenous hypertriglyceridemia. Metabolism 27: 1055–1066

Chapman J M, Massey F J 1964 The interrelationship of serum cholesterol, hypertension, body weight and risk of coronary heart disease – Results of the first ten years 'follow-up' in the Los Angeles Heart Study. Journal of Chronic Disease 17: 933–949

Christian J C, Cheung S W, Kang K, Harmath F P, Huntzinger D J, Powell R C 1976 Variance of plasma free and esterified cholesterol in adult twins. American Journal of Human Genetics 28: 174–000

Dahlen G, Berg K 1976a Pre-beta-1-lipoprotein and Lp(a) antigen in relation to triglyceride levels and insulin release following on oral glucose load in middle-age males. Acta Medica Scandinavica 199: 413–419

Dahlen G, Berg K 1976b Further evidence for the existance of genetically determined metabolic differences between Lp(a+) and Lp(a–) individuals. Clinical Genetics 9: 357–364

Dahlen G, Berg K, Frick M H 1976 Lp(a) lipoprotein/pre-beta-1-lipoprotein, serum lipids and atherosclerotic disease. Clinical Genetics 9: 558–566

Dawber T R, Kannel W B, McNamara P M 1971 The prediction of coronary heart disease. Transactions of the Association of Life Insurance Medical Directors of America 47: 70–104

De Lange C D 1933 Significance of geographic pathology in race problems in medicine. Geneeskundig tijdschrift voor Nederlandsch-Indie 73: 1026

Doyle J T 1963 Risk factors in coronary heart disease. New York Journal of Medicine 1317–1320

Duguid J B 1949 Pathogenesis of arteriosclerosis. Lancet II: 925–927

Ehnholm C, Garoff H, Renkonen O, Simons K 1971 Proteins and carbohydrates composition of Lp(a) lipoprotein from human plasma. Biochemestry 11: 3229–3232

Eisenberg S, Levy R J 1976 Lipoprotein metabolism. Advances in Lipid Research 13: 1–89

Eisenberg S, Bilheimer D N, Levy R J, Lindgren F T 1973 On the metabolic conversion of human plasma very low density lipoprotein to low density lipoprotein. Biochimica Biophysica Acta 326: 361–000

Eisenberg S, Chajek T, Deckelbaum R 1978 Molecular aspects of lipoproteins interconversion. Pharmacological Research Communications 10: 729–738

Elston R C, Namboodiri K K, Go R C P, Siervogel R M, Glueck C P 1976 Possible linkage between essential familial hypercholesterolemia and third complement component (C3). In: Baltimore Conference (1975): Third International Workshop on Human Gene Mapping. Birth defects: Original article series XII: 7. The National Foundation, New York

Epstein F H, Ostrander jr. L D, Johnson B C, Payne M W, Hayner N S, Keller J B, Francis jr T 1965 Epidemiological studies of cardiovascular disease in a total community –
Tecumseh, Michigan Annals of Internal Medicine 62: 1170–1187

Falko J M, Schonfeld G, Witzum J L, Kolar J, Weidman S W 1979 Effects of estrogen therapy on apolipoprotein E in type III hyperlipoproteinemia. Metabolism 28: 1171–1177

Fallon H J, Woods J W 1968 Responses of hyperlipoproteinemia to Cholestyramine renin. Journal of the American Medical Association 204: 1161–

Farah J R, Kwiterowich P O Jr, Neill C A 1977 Dose-effect relation of cholestyramine in children and young adults with familial hypercholesterolemia. Lancet I: 59–63

Felkner T E, Fainaru M, Hamilton R L, Havel R J 1977 Secretion of the arginine-rich and A-I apolipoproteins by the isolated perfused rat liver. Journal of Lipid Research 18: 465–00

Ferrans V J, Fredrickson D S 1975 The pathology of Tangier disease. A light and election microscopic study. American Journal of Pathology 78: 101–158

Franceschini G, Sirtori C R, Capurso A, Weisgraber K H, Mahley R W 1980 A-I Milano Apoprotein. Journal of Clinical Investigation 66: 892–900

Fredrickson D S 1972 A physician's guide to hyperlipidemia. Modern Concepts in Cardiovascular Disease 41: 31–36

Fredrickson D S 1964 Inheritance of high density lipoprotein deficiency (Tangier Disease). Journal of Clinical Investigation 43: 228–236

Fredrickson D S, Goldstein J L, Brown M S 1978 The familial hyperlipoproteinemias. In: Stanbury J B, Wyngaarden J B, Fredrickson D S (eds) Metabolic Basis of Inherited Disease 4th edn. McGraw Hill, New York pp 604–605

Fredrickson D S, Levy R J, Lees R S 1967 Fat transport in lipoproteins: an integrated approach to mechanisms and disorders. New England Journal of Medicine 276: 34–44, 94–103, 148–156, 215–225, 273–281

Fredrickson D S, Levy R J, Lees R S 1968 A comparison of heritable abnormal lipoprotein patterns as defined by two different techniques. Journal of Clinical Investigation 47: 2446–2457

Fredrickson D S, Morganroth J, Levy R J 1975 Type III hyperlipoproteinemia: an analysis of two contemporary definitions. Annals of Internal Medicine 82: 1501–57

Gedda L, Poggi D 1960 Sulla regolazione genetica del colesterolo ematico. Acta Geneticae Medicae et Gemellologiae 9: 135–153

Gertler M M, White P D 1954 Coronary heart disease in young adults: A multidiciplinary study. Cambridge, Massachussets, Harvard University Press

Getz G S, Vesselinovitch D, Wissler R W 1969 A dynamic pathology of atherosclerosis. American Journal of Medicine 46: 657–673

Gjone E, Norum K R, Glomset J A 1978 Familial lecithin-cholesterol acyltransferase deficiency. In: Stanbury J B, Wyngaarden J B, Fredrickson D S, (eds) The metabolic basis of inherited disease 4th edition. McGraw-Hill, New York: pp 589–603

Glagov S 1972 Hemodynamic risk factors: mechanical stress, mural architecture, medial nutrition and the vulnerability of arteries to atherosclerosis. In: Wissler R W, Geer J C, (eds) The pathogenesis of atherosclerosis. Williams and Wilkins Baltimore p 164

Glomset J A 1968 The plasma lecithin-cholesterol acyltransferase reaction. Journal of Lipid Research 9: 155–167

Glomset J A, Norum K R 1973 The metabolic role of lecithin– cholesterol acyltransferase: Perspectives from pathology, Advances in Lipid Research 11: 1–

Glueck C J, Fallat R, Buncher C R, Tsang R, Steiner P 1973 Familial combined hyperlipoproteinemia. – Studies in 91 adults and 95 children from 33 kindreds. Metabolism 22: 1403–1428

Glueck C J, Fallat R W, Millet F, Gartside P, Elston R C, Go R C P 1975 Familial hyperalphalipoproteinemia: Studies in eighteen kindreds. Metabolism 52: 1544–1568

Glueck C J, Gartside P, Fallat R W, Sielski J, Steiner P M 1976 Longevity syndromes: familial hypobeta and familial hyperalphalipoproteinemia. Journal of laboratory and clinical Medicine 88: 941–957

Glueck C J, Tsang R, Fallat R W 1973b Familial hypertriglyceridemia: Studies in 130 children and 45 siblings of 36 index cases. Metabolism 22: 1287–1309

Gofman J W, Young W, Tandy R 1966 Ischemic heart disease, atherosclerosis and longevity. Circulation 34: 679–000

Goldstein J L, Anderson R G W, Brown M S 1979 Coated pits, coated vericles, and receptor – mediated endocytosis. Nature 279: 679–685

Goldstein J L, Brown M S 1974 Binding and degradation of low density lipoproteins by cultured human fibroblasts. Journal of Biological Chemistry 249: 5153–5162

Goldstein J L, Brown M S 1977a Genetics of the LDL receptor: Evidence that the mutations affecting binding and internalisation are allelic. Cell 12: 629–641

Goldstein J L, Brown M S 1977b The low-density lipoprotein pathway and its relation to atherosclerosis. Annual Review in Biochemistry 46: 897–930

Goldstein J L, Dana S E, Brunschede G Y, Brown M S 1975 Genetic heterogeneity in familial hypercholesterolemia: Evidence for two different mutations affecting functions of low–density lipoprotein receptor. Proceedings of the National Academy of Sciences USA 72: 1092–1096

Goldstein J L, Harrod M J E, Brown M S 1974 Homozygous familial hypercholesterolemia: Specificity of the biochemical defect in cultured cells and feasibility of prenatal detection. American Journal of Human Genetics 26: 199–206

Goldstein J L, Schrott H G, Hazzard W R, Bierman E L, Motulsky A G 1973 Hyperlipidemia in coronary heart disease. I. Genetic analysis of lipid levels in 176 families and delineation of a new inherited disorder, combined hyperlipidemia. Journal of Clinical Investigation 52: 1544–1568

Gordon T, Castelli W P, Hjortland M C, Kannel W B, Dawber T R 1977 High density lipoproteins as a protective factor against coronary heart disease. American Journal of Medicine 62: 707–714

Green P H, Glickman R M, Saudek C D, Blum C B, Tall A R 1979 Human intestinal lipoproteins – studies in chyluric subjects. Journal of Clinical Investigation 64: 233–

Green P H R, Tall A R, Glickman R M 1978 Rat intestine secretes discoid high density lipoprotein. Journal of Clinical Investigation 61: 528–534

Hamilton R L 1978 Hepatic secretion and metabolism of high density lipoproteins In: Dietschy J M, Gotto, A M, Ontko J A (eds) Disturbances in lipid and lipoprotein metabolism. American Physiological Society, Bethesda, Maryland pp 155

Hamilton R L, Williams M C, Fielding C J, Havel R J 1976 Discoidal bilayer structure of nascent high density lipoproteins from perfused rat liver. Journal of Clinical Investigation 58: 667–680

Harlan W R, Graham J B, Estes H 1966 Familial hypercholesterolemia: a genetic and metabolic study. Medicine 45: 77–110

Havel R J 1972 Hyperlipidemias: The significance and management. Modern Medicine and Biology 63: 37–59

Havel R J 1975 Lipoproteins and lipid transport. In Lipids, Lipoproteins, and Drugs, Advances in Experimental Medicine and Biology 63: 37–59

Havel R J 1977 Classification of the hyperlipidemias. Annual Reviews in Medicine 28: 195–209

Havel R J, Chao Y S, Windler E E, Kotite L, Guo L S S 1980 Isoprotein specificity in the hepatic uptake of apolipoprotein E and the pathogenesis of familial dysbetalipoproteinemia. Proceedings of the National Academy of Sciences USA 77: 4349–4353

Havel R J, Kane J P 1973 Primary Dysbetalipoproteinemia: predominance of a specific apoprotein species in triglyceride–rich lipoproteins. Proceedings of the National Academy of Sciences USA 70: 2015–2019

Hazzard W R, Bierman E L 1971 Impaired removal of very low density lipoprotein (VLDL) 'remnants' in the pathogenesis of broad–beta disease (hyperlipoproteinemia type III). Clinical Research 19: 476–

Hazzard W R, Bierman E L 1972 Aggravation of broad–β disease (type III hyperlipoproteinemia) by hypothyroidism. Archives of Internal Medicine 130: 822–828

Hazzard W R, Bierman E L 1976 Delayed clearance of chylomicron remnants following Vitamin A containing oral fat loads in Broad–β–disease (Type III hyperlipoproteinemia). Metabolism 25: 777–801

Hazzard W R, Goldstein J L, Schrott H G, Motulsky A G, Bierman E L 1973 Hyperlipidemia in coronary heart disease. III. Evaluation of lipoprotein phenotypes of 156 genetically defined survivors of myocardial infarction. Journal of Clinical Investigation 52: 1569–1577

Hazzard W R, O'Donell T F, Lee Y L 1975 Broad-beta-disease (type III hyperlipoproteinemia) in a large kindred. Evidence for a monogenic mechanism. Annals of Internal Medicine 82: 141–149

Hazzard W R, Prote D J, Bierman E L 1972 Abnormal lipid composition of very low density lipoproteins in diagnosis of broad–beta disease (type III hyperlipoproteinemia). Metabolism 21: 1009–1019

Heiberg A 1974 The heritability of serum lipoprotein and lipid concentrations. A twin study. Clinical Genetics 6: 307–316

Heiberg A 1976 Inheritance of xanthomatosis and hyper-β-lipoproteinemia: A study of 7 large kindreds. Clinical Genetics 9: 92–111

Heiberg A, Berg K 1976 The inheritance of hyperlipoproteinemia with xanthomatosis: A study of 132 kindreds. Clinical Genetics 9: 203–233

Herbert P N, Gotto A M, Fredrickson D S 1978 Familial lipoprotein deficiency. In: Stanbury J B, Wyngaarden J B, Fredrickson D S (eds) The metabolic basis of inherited disease. 4th edition. McGraw-Hill New York pp 544–588

Hewitt D, Jones G J L, Godin G J, Wraight D, Breckenridge W C, Little J A, Steiner G, Mishkel M A 1979 Nature of the familial influence on plasma lipid levels. Atherosclerosis 32: 381–396

Howard R P, Brusco O J, Furman R H 1966 Effect of cholestyramine administration on serum lipids and on nitrogen balance in familial hypercholesterolemia. Journal of Laboratory and Clinical Medicine 68: 12

Jensen J, Blankenhorn D H, Chin H P, Stugeon P, Ware A G 1965 Serum lipids and serum uric acid in human twins. Journal of Lipid Research 6: 193–205

Johnson B C, Epstein F H, Kjelsberg M O 1965 Distribution and familial studies of blood pressure and serum cholesterol levels in a total community, Tecumseh, Michigan. Journal of Chronic Diseases 18: 147

Kang K W, Taylor G E, Greves J H, Staley H L, Christian J C 1971 Genetic variability of human plasma and erythrocyte lipids. Lipids 6: 595–600

Kannel W B, Castelli W P Gordon T 1966 Serum cholesterol, lipoproteins and risk of coronary heart disease The Framingham study. Annals of Internal Medicine 24: 1

Kannel W B, Dawber T G, Friedman G D, Glennon W C, Mc Namara P M 1964 Risk factors in coronary heart disease. Annals of Internal Medicine 61: 888

Kao V, Wissler R W 1965 A study of the immunohistochemical localization of serum lipoproteins and other plasma proteins in human atherosclerotic lesions. Experimental and Molecular Pathology 4: 465

Keys A 1972a Predicting the risk of coronary disease. Proceedings American Life Convention, Medical Section, May 29–31: 15–43

Keys A, Aravanis C, Blackburn H, van Buchem F S P, Buzina R, Djordjevic B S et al. 1972 The probability of middle-aged men developing coronary heart disease in five years. Circulation 45: 815–828

Keys A 1972 b Predicting coronary heart disease In: G Tibblin, A Keys, L Werkö (eds) Preventive Cardiology. Halsted Press, New York pp 21–32

Keys A 1975 Coronary heart disease – The global picture. Atherosclerosis 22: 149–192

Keys A, Taylor H L, Blackburn H, Brozek J, Anderson J T 1971 Mortality and coronary heart disease among men studied for twenty-three years. Archives of Internal Medicine 128: 201–214

Khachadurian A K 1964 The inheritance of essential familial hypercholesterolemia. American Journal of Medicine 37: 402–407

Khachadurian A K, Uthman S M 1973 Experiences with the homozygous cases of familial hypercholesterolemia. Nutrition and Metabolism 15: 132

King M E E, Breslow J L, Lees R S 1980 Plasma – exchange therapy of homozygous familial hypercholesterolemia. New England Journal of Medicine 302: 1457–1459

Krauss R M, Levy R I, Fredrickson D S 1974 Selective measurement of two lipase activities in post-heparin plasma from normal subjects and patients with hyperlipoproteinemia. Journal of Clinical Investigation 54: 1107–1124

Kushwaha R S, Hazzard W R, Gagne C, Chait A, Albers J J 1977 Type III hyperlipoproteinemia/Paradoxical hyperlipidemic response to estrogen. Annals of Internal Medicine 87: 517–525

Kwitorovich P O, Fredrickson D S, Levy R J 1974 Familial hypercholesterolemia (one form of familial type III hyperlipoproteinemia). A study of its biochemical, genetic and clinical presentation in childhood. Journal of Clinical Investigation 53: 1237–1249

Kwitorovich P O, Levy R J, Fredrickson D S 1973 Neonatal diagnosis of familial type-II hyperlipoproteinemia. Lancet 1: 118–121

Langer T, Strober W, Levy R J 1972 The metabolism of low density lipoprotein in familial type II hyperlipoproteinemia. Journal of Clinical Investigation 51: 1528–1536

Lees R S, Lees A M 1976 Therapy of the hyperlipidemias. Postgraduate Medicine 60: 99–107

Levy R I, Bonnell M, Ernst N D 1971 Dietary Management of hyperlipoproteinemia. Journal of the American Diet Association 58: 406–???

Levy R I, Fredrickson D S, Shulman R, Bilheimer D W, Breslow J L, Stone N J, Lux S E, Sloan H R, Krauss R M, Herbert P N 1972 Dietary and drug treatment of primary hyperlipoproteinemia. Annals of Internal Medicine 77: 267

Levy R I, Fredrickson D S, Stone N J, Gotto A M, Herbert P M, Kwiterovich P O, Langer T, La Rosa J, Lux S E, Rider A K, Schulman R S, Sloan H R 1973 Cholestyramine in type II hyperlipoproteinemia. A double-blind trial of cholestyramine in type II hyperlipoproteinemia. Annals of Internal Medicine 79: 51

Mabuchi H, Ito S, Haba T, Ueda K, Ueda R, Tatami R, Kametani T, Koizumi I, Ohta M, Miyamoto S, Takeda R, Takegoshi T 1977 Discrimination of familial hypercholesterolemia and secundary hypercholesterolemia by Achille's tendon thickness. Atherosclerosis 28: 61–68

Mabuchi H, Tatami R, Haba T, Ueda K, Ueda R, Kametani T, Itoh S, Koizumi I, Oota M, Miyamoto S, Takeda R, Takeshita H 1978 Homozygous familial hypercholesterolemia in Japan. American Journal of Medicine 65: 290–297

Mahley R W 1978 Alterations in plasma lipoproteins induced by cholesterol feeding in animals including man. In: Dietschy J M, Gotto A M, Ontko J A (eds) Disturbances in lipid and Lipoprotein Metabolism American Physiological Society, Bethesda MD, 181–197

Mahley R W, Innerarity T L, Browns M S, Ho Y K, Goldstein J L 1980 Cholesteryl ester synthesis in macrophages: Stimulation by β–very low density lipoproteins from cholestrol-fed animals of several species. Journal of lipid Research 21: 970–980

Mahley R W, Innerarity T L, Pitas R E, Weisgraber K H, Brown J H, Gross E 1977 Inhibition of lipoprotein binding to cell surface receptors of fibroblasts following selective modification of arginyl residues in arginine-rich and B apoproteins. Journal of Biological Chemistry 252, 7279–7287

Martin A O, Kurczynski T W, Steinberg A G 1973 Familial studies of medical and anthropometric variables in a human isolate. American Journal of Human Genetics 25: 581–593

Mayo O, Frazer G R, Stamatoyannopoulos G 1969 Genetic influence in serum cholesterol in two Greek villages. Human Heredity 19: 86–99

Mc Donough J R, Hames C G, Greenberg B G, Griffin L H, Edwards jr A J 1962 Observations on serum cholesterol levels in the twin population of Evans County, Georgia. Circulation 25: 962–969

Mc Gill H G jr, Geer J C, Strong J P 1963 The natural history of human atherosclerosis. In: Sandler M Bourne G H (eds) Atherosclerosis and its origin, Academic Press, New York, Chapt. 2

Medalie J H, Kahn H A, Wenfield H N 1973 Five-year myocardial infarction incidence. I. Association of variables to age and birth place. Journal of Chronic Diseases 26: 329–349

Meyer K 1962 Serum cholesterol and heredity. A twin study. Acta medica Scandinavia 172: 401–404

Miall W E, Oldham P D 1958 Factors influencing arterial blood pressure in the general population. Clinical Sciences 17: 409–444

Miller G J, Miller N E 1975 Plasma-high-density lipoproteine concentration and development of ischemic heart disease. Lancet 1: 16–19

Mishkel M A 1976 Pseudohomozygous and pseudoheterohygous type II hyperlipoproteinemia. American Journal of Disease of Children 130: 991–993

Mishkel M A, Nazir D I, Crowther S 1975 A longitudinal assessment of lipid ratios in the diagnosis of type III hyperlipoproteinemia. Clinica Chimica Acta 53: 121–136

Morganroth J, Levy R I, McMahon A E 1974 Pseudohomozygous type II hyperlipoproteinemia. Journal of Pediatry 85: 639–643

Morganroth J R, Levy R I, Fredrickson D S 1975 The biochemical, clinical and genetic features of type III hyperlipoproteinemia. Annals of Internal Medicine 82: 158–174

Moser H, Slack J, Borrie P 1974 Type III hyperlipoproteinemia: A genetic study with an account of the risk of coronary death in first degree relatives. In: Schettler G, Weizel A (eds), Atherosclerosis III. Springer Berlin, p 854

Motulsky A G 1976 The genetic hyperlipidemias. New England Journal of Medicine 294: 823–827

Motulsky A P, Boman H 1975 Screening for the hyperlipidemias. In: Milunsky A (ed) The prevention of genetic disease and mental retardation. Saunders Philadelphia, pp 303–316

Müller C 1939 Angina pectoris in hereditary xanthomatosis. Archives of internal Medicine 69: 675–700

Mustard J F, Packham M A 1975 The role of blood and platelets in atherosclerosis and the complication of atherosclerosis. Thromb Diath Haemorrh 33: 444–456

Nikkilä E A, Aro A 1973 Family study of serum lipids and lipoproteins in coronary heart disease. Lancet 1: 954–959

Nora J J, Lortscher R H, Spangler R D, Nora A H, Kimberling W J 1980 Genetic – Epidemiologic study of early – onset ischemic heart disease. Circulation 61: 503–508

Osborne R H, Adlersberg D, De George F W, Wang C 1959 Serum lipids, hereditary and environment. A study of adult twins. American Journal of Medicine 26: 54–59

Osler W 1897 Lectures on Angina pectoris and allied states. New York, Appleton-Century Crofts

Ott J 1979 Detection of rare major genes in lipid levels. Human Genetics 51: 79–91

Ott J, Schrott H G, Goldstein J L, Hazzard W R, Allen F H jr., Falk C T, Motulsky A G 1974 Linkage studies in a large kindred with familial hypercholesterolemia. American Journal of Human Genetics 26: 598–603

Pagnan A, Havel R J, Kane P, Kotite L 1977 Characterisation of human very low density lipoproteins containing two electrophoretic populations: double pre-beta lipoproteinemia and primary dysbetalipoproteinemia. Journal of Lipid Research 18: 613–622

Patsch J R, Sailer S, Braunsteiner H 1975 Lipoprotein of density 1.006–1.020 in the plasma of patients with type III hyperlipoproteinemia in the postabsorptive state. European Journal of Clinical Investigation 5: 45–55

Patterson D, Slack J 1972 Lipid abnormalities in male and female survivors of myocardial infarction. Lancet 1: 393

Paul O, Lepper M H, Pehlan W H, Dupertuis G W, MacMillan A, Mc Kean H, Park H 1963 A longitudinal study of coronary heart disease. Circulation 28: 20–31

Pickering G W 1959 The nature of essential hypertension. Lance II: 1027–1028

Pikkarainen J, Takkunen J, Kulonen E 1966 Serum cholesterol in Finnish twins. American Journal of Human Genetics 18: 115–126

Platt R 1959 The nature of essential hypertension Lancet I: 55–57

Platt R 1963 Heredity in hypertension. Lancet I: 899–904

Renninger W, Wendt G G, Nawrocki P, Weigand H 1965 Beitrag zur Problematik des Lp-Systems. Humangenetik 1: 658–667

Rhoads G G, Gulbrandsen C L, Kagan A 1976 Serum lipoproteins and coronary heart disease in a population study of Hawaii Japanese men. New England Journal of Medicine 294: 293–298

Rhoads G R, Morton N E Gulbrandsen C L, Kagan A 1978 Sinking pre-beta lipoprotein and coronary heart disease in Japanese – American men in Hawaii. American Journal of Epidemiology 108: 355–356

Robertson F W, Cumming A M 1979 Genetic and environmental variation in serum lipoproteins in relation to coronary heart disease. Journal of Medical Genetics 16: 85–100

Rose H G, Krantz P, Weinstock M, Juliano J, Haft J I 1973 Inheritance of combined hyperlipoproteinemia: Evidence for a new lipoprotein phenotype. American Journal of Medicine 54: 148–

Ross R, Glomset J A 1973 Atherosclerosis and the arterial smooth muscle cell. Science 180: 1332–1339

Ross R, Glomset J A 1976 The pathogenesis of atherosclerosis. New England Journal of Medicine 295: 369–375, 420–426

Ross R, Harker L 1976 Hyperlipidemia and atherosclerosis. Science 193: 1094–1100

Schaefer E J, Eisenberg S, Levy R I 1978 Lipoprotein apoprotein metabolism. Journal of Lipid Research 19: 667–000

Schaeffer L E, Adlersberg C, Steinberg A G 1958 Heredity, environment and serum cholesterol. A study of 201 healthy families. Circulation 17: 537–542

Schneider W J, Kovanen P T, Brown M S et al 1981 Familial dysbetalipoproteinemia: Abnormal binding of mutant apoprotein E to LDL receptors of human fibroblasts and membranes from liver and adrenal of rats, rabbits, and cows. Journal of Clinical Investigation 68: 1075–1085

Schrott H G, Goldstein J L, Hazzard W R, McGoodwin M M, Motulski A G 1972 Familial hypercholesterolemia in a large kindred. Evidence for a monogenic mechanism. Annals of Internal Medicine 76: 711–720

Scott P J, Hurley P J 1970 The distribution of radioiodinated serum albumin and low-density lipoprotein in tissues and the arterial wall. Atherosclerosis 11: 77–103

Sherrill B C, Innerarity T L, Mahley R W 1980 Rapid hepatic clearance of the canine lipoproteins containing only the E apoprotein by a high affinity receptor. Identity with the chylomicron remnant transport process. Journal of Biological Chemistry 255: 804

Siervogel R M, Morrison J A, Kelly K, Mellies M, Gartside P, Glueck C J 1980 Familial hyper-alpha-lipoproteinemia in 26 kindreds. Clinical Genetics 17: 13–25

Simons K, Ehnholm C, Renkonen O, Bloth B 1970 Characterisation of the Lp(a) lipoprotein in human plasma. Acta Pathologica and Microbiologica Scandinavica 78: 459–466

Sing C F, Chamberlain M A, Block W D, Feiler S 1975 Analysis of genetic and environmental sources of variation in serum cholesterol in Tecumseh, Michigan, Part 1 (Analsis of the frequency distribution for evidence of a genetic polymorphism). American Journal of Human Genetics 27: 333

Sing C F, Orr J D 1978 Analysis of genetic and environmental sources of variation in serum cholesterol in Tecumseh, Michigan. IV. Separation of polygene from common environment effects. American Journal of Human Genetics 30: 491–504

Sing C F, Schultz J S, Shreffler D C 1974 The genetics of the Lp antigen. II. A family study and proposed models of genetic control. Annals of Human Genetics 38: 47–56

Slack J 1969 Risks of ischaemic heart disease in familial hyperlipoproteinaemic states. Lancet II: 1380–1383

Slack J 1975 The genetic contribution to coronary heart disease through lipoprotein concentrations. Postgraduate Medical Journal 51(8): 27–32

Slack J, Evans K A 1966 The increased risk of death from ischaemic heart disease in first degree relatives of 121 men and 96 woman with ischaemic heart disease. Journal of Medical Genetics 3: 239

Smith E 1975 Development of the atheromatous lesion. In: Wolf S, Wethessen N T (eds) The smooth muscle of the artery, Advances in Experimental Biology and Medicine 57. Plenum Press, New York pp 254

Smith E B, Slater R S 1972 Relationship between bw-density lipoprotein in aortic intima and serum lipid levels. Lancet 1: 463–469

Smith E B, Smith R H 1976 Early changes in aortic intima. In: Paoletti R, Gotto A M jr (eds) Atherosclerosis Reviews, Vol. 1 Raven Press, New York pp 119–136

Smith L C, Pownall H J, Gotto A M 1978 The plasma lipoproteins: structure and metabolism. Annual Reviews of Biochemistry 47: 751

Starzl T E, Chase H P, Putman C W, Porter K A 1973 Portocaval shunt in hyperlipoproteinemia. Lancet 2: 940–944

Starzl T E, Chase H P, Putnam C W, Nora J J, Fennel R H Jr., Porter K A 1974 Portocaval shunt in hyperlipidemia. Lancet 2: 1263

Stone N J, Levy R I, Fredrickson D S, Verter J 1974 Coronary artery disease in 116 kindred with familial type II hyperlipoproteinemia. Circulation 49: 476–488

Thomas C B, Cohen B H 1955 The familial occurance of hypertension and coronary heart disease, with observations concerning obesity and diabetes. Annals of Internal Medicine 42: 90–127

Thompson G R, Gotto A M 1973 Ileal bypass in the treatment of hyperlipoproteinemia. Lancet 2: 35–36

Thompson G R, Lowenthal R, Myant N B 1975 Plasma exchange in the management of homozygous familial hypercholesterolemia. Lancet I: 1208–1211

Thompson G R, Spinks T, Ranicar A, Myant N B 1977 Non-steady-state studies of low-density-lipoprotein turnover in familial hypercholesterolemia. Clinical Science and Molecular Medicine 52: 361–369

Utermann G 1980 Polymorphism of apolipoprotein E In: Gotto A M, Smith L C, Allen B (eds), Atherosclerosis V, Springer New York, pp 689–694

Utermann G, Beisiegel U 1979 Apolipoprotein A-IV: A protein occuring in human mesenteric lymph chylomicrons and free in plasma. European Journal of Biochemistry 99: 333–343

Utermann G, Canzler H, Hees M, Jaeschke M, Mühlfellner G, Schoenborn W, Vogelberg K H 1977a Studies on the metabolic defect in broad-β-disease (hyperlipoproteinemia type III). Clinical Genetics 12: 139–154

Utermann G, Hees M, Steinmetz A 1977b Polymorphism of apolipoprotein E and occurance of dysbetalipoproteinemia in man. Nature 269: 604–607

Utermann G, Jaeschke M, Menzel J 1975 Familial hyperlipoproteinemia type III: Deficiency of a specific apolipoprotein (Apo E-III) in the very low density lipoproteins. Federation of the European Biochemical Societies Letters 56: 352–355

Utermann G, Langenbeck U, Beisiegel U, Weber W 1980a Genetics of the apolipoprotein E system in man. American Journal of Human Genetics 32: 339–347

Utermann G, Menzel H J, Adler G, Dieker P, Weber W, 1980b Substitution in vitro of lecithin-cholesterol-acyltransferase. Analysis of changes in plasma lipoproteins. European Journal of Biochemistry 107: 225–241

Utermann G, Pruin N, Steinmetz A 1979a Polymorphism of apolipoprotein E. III. Effect of a single polymorphic gene locus on plasma lipid levels in man. Clinical Genetics 15: 63–72

Utermann G, Steinmetz A, Weber W 1982 Genetic control of human apolipoprotein E polymorphism: Comparison of one- and two-dimensional techniques of isoprotein analysis. Human Genetics in press

Utermann G, Vogelberg K H, Steinmetz A, Schoenborn W, Pruin N, Jaeschke M, Hees M, Canzler H 1979b Polymorphism of apolipoprotein E. II. Genetics of hyperlipoproteinemia type III. Clinical Genetics 15: 37–62

Virchow R 1856 Phlogose und Thrombose im Gefa-β-system, Gesammelte Abhandlungen zur wissenchaftlichen Medizin. Frankfurt am Main, Meidinger Sohn p 458

Walton K W, Hitchens J, Magnani H N, Khan M 1974 A study of methods of identification and estimation of Lp(a) lipoprotein and of its significance in health, hyperlipidaemia and atherosclerosis. Atherosclerosis 20: 323–346

Walton K W, Williamson N 1968 Histological and immunofluorescent studies in the evaluation of the atheromatous plaque. Journal of Atherosclerosis Research 8: 599–

Warnick G R, Mayfield C, Alber J J, Hazzard W R 1979 Gel isoelectric focusing method for specific diagnosis of familial hyperlipoproteinemia type III. Clinical Chemistry 25: 279–284

Weidman W S, Suarez B, Falko J M, Witzum J L, Kolar J, Raben M, Schonfeld G 1979 Type III hyperlipoproteinemia: Development of a VLDL apo E gel isoelectric focusing technique and application in family studies. Journal of Laboratory and Clinical Medicine 13: 549–569

Weinberg R, Avet L M, Gardner M J 1976 Estimates of the heritability of serum lipoprotein and lipid concentrations. Clinical Genetics 9: 588–592

Wienker T F, Utermann G, Ropers H H 1976 Prenatal diagnosis of homozygous familial hypercholesterolemia: Investigation of a case at risk. Clinical Genetics 9: 545–552

Wissler R W 1974 Development of the atherosclerotic plaque. In: Braunwald E (ed) The Myocardium: Failure and Infarction ed. HP Publ. Co New York, pp 155–166

Zannis V I, Breslow J L 1980 Characterization of a unique human apolipoprotein E variant associated with type III hyperlipoproteinemia. Journal of Biological Chemistry 255: 1759–1762

Zannis V I, Just P W, Breslow J L 1981 Human Apolipoprotein E Isoprotein Subclasses are genetically determined. American Journal of Human Genetics 33: 11–24

Zelis R, Mason D R, Braunwald E, Levy R I 1970 Effects of hyperlipoproteinemias and their treatment on the peripheral circulation. Journal of Clinical Investigation 49: 1007

Zilversmit D B 1979 Atherogenesis: A postprandial phenomenon. Circulation 60: 473–485

70

The cardiomyopathies

R. Emanuel and R. Withers

INTRODUCTION

The genetically determined condition now generally known as hypertrophic cardiomyopathy first made its appearance on the clinical scene in 1947 when described by William Evans as Familial Cardiomegaly (Evans, 1949). Little was then heard of this entity until Teare's description in 1958 of Asymmetrical Hypertrophy of the Heart in Young Adults (Teare, 1958). Recognition did not become widespread until the early 1960s, a time when the study of haemodynamics was a primary interest in cardiology; hence the abnormal ventricular function and the mechanism of left ventricular outflow obstruction seen in a percentage of cases became a matter of controversy and received more attention than the fundamental problems of inheritance and pathogenesis (Criley et al, 1965; Ross et al, 1966; White et al, 1967).

An early difficulty encountered with the cardiomyopathies was one of classification which, if based on aetiology as all sound classifications must be, became impossibly cumbersome and of little value (Hudson, 1970; Emanuel, 1970) for the vast majority of cases had to be labelled 'idiopathic'.

Goodwin and his coworkers were much aware of this problem and evolved both a definition and classification which is in use today. A cardiomyopathy is now defined as 'heart muscle disease of unknown cause or association' (Goodwin & Oakley, 1972). Thus, by definition, such conditions as acromegalic heart disease, thyrotoxic heart disease and the end stages of coronary artery disease associated with considerable cardiomegaly and failure are excluded. Goodwin divided the cardiomyopathies into two main types dependent on the pathophysiology of the left ventricle. In the first type, hypertrophic cardiomyopathy (with or without obstruction to left ventricular outflow), the main features were massive hypertrophy of the left ventricle, particularly the interventricular septum, associated with a small left ventricular cavity. The primary haemodynamic fault was in ventricular filling due to decreased compliance of the thickened, abnormal ventricular muscle. In the second type, congestive cardiomyopathy, there was a degree of left ventricular hypertrophy although the salient features were gross dilatation of the left ventricular cavity and normal coronary arteries. In this group the main haemodynamic fault was 'pump failure' with reduction in the ejection fraction. Goodwin's classification recognized two other subgroups, both rare, and designated them 'constrictive' and 'restrictive' (Goodwin, 1970).

By definition, the aetiology of the cardiomyopathies is unknown, but in hypertrophic cardiomyopathy genetic factors are recognised to be important. Familial cases are common (Braunwald et al, 1964; Cohen et al, 1964; Emanuel et al, 1971) and autosomal dominant inheritance has been reported by many authors (Brigden, 1957; Hollman et al, 1960; Walther et al, 1960; Paré et al, 1961; Treger & Blount, 1965; Emanuel, 1971; Emanuel et al, 1971). In the remaining three groups – the congestive, constrictive and restrictive – there is little evidence of a familial tendency. As this chapter is concerned with genetically determined diseases, further comments on the cardiomyopathies will be confined to hypertrophic cardiomyopathy which may occur with or without obstruction to left ventricular outflow.

CLINICAL FEATURES

Clinically, the disease is often asymptomatic and diagnosed at routine examination, which may have been prompted because some other member of the family had been found to be affected, or died suddenly. When symptoms are present they include angina and dyspnoea from left ventricular dysfunction, and arrhythmias, the frequency of which has only been appreciated recently with the advent of ambulatory monitoring (Savage et al, 1979; McKenna et al, 1980). In addition, syncope and sudden death are not uncommon, and evidence is accumulating that these events are generally due to a ventricular tachyarrhythmia, frequently ventricular fibrillation (Goodwin & Krikler, 1976). One of the most difficult tasks which confront the physician in this disease is to identify those cases with an increased risk of unexpected death. There is no sure way of doing this, but sinister features include a short history of paroxysmal arrhythmias and an elevated end diastolic pressure in the left ventricle. It also appears that males with a positive family history are at increased risk. The presence of a gradient across the left ventricular outflow does not increase the hazard of sudden demise; in fact, there is some evidence suggesting that cases without obstruction have a worse prognosis (Frank & Braunwald, 1968; Goodwin, 1970; Maron et al, 1978c; Maron et al, 1978a).

The clinical features of the disease include normal development in infancy and childhood and varying degrees of left ventricular hypertrophy, particularly of the interventricular septum. When there is obstruction to left ventricular outflow, there is an ejection murmur simulating that heard in aortic valve stenosis. The hypertrophic process also involves the papillary muscles to a greater or lesser degree, and mitral valve function may be abnormal, giving rise to mitral valve prolapse and regurgitation. Thus, late systolic or pansystolic murmurs at the apex are not uncommon. In some cases, mitral regurgitation is the dominant feature and may be misdiagnosed, particularly in children, as rheumatic mitral regurgitation. Similarly, if obstruction to left ventricular outflow dominates the clinical picture, the diagnosis of aortic valve disease may be entertained. The quality of the arterial pulse, however, is usually sufficient to lead to the correct diagnosis. In hypertrophic cardiomyopathy, obstruction to left ventricular outflow does not occur until mid or late systole, hence the upstroke of the arterial pulse is normal or sharp, whereas in fixed aortic valve stenosis, obstruction to left ventricular outflow is present throughout systole producing the classical slow rising or plateau pulse (Hardarson et al, 1973; Goodwin, 1974).

Electrocardiography

The electrocardiogram can also be misleading for, in addition to some degree of left ventricular hypertrophy and, not infrequently, left atrial hypertrophy, there may be Q waves with ST and T wave changes in both the anterior and anteroseptal leads, or left bundle branch block (Savage et al, 1978). If, therefore, the patient is a middle-aged male with angina and only slight left ventricular enlargement, it is all too easy to make the erroneous diagnosis of coronary artery disease, missing the underlying hypertrophic cardiomyopathy. Extensive investigations are usually unnecessary to establish the correct diagnosis. Where required, echocardiography and left heart catheterization are the most helpful (Hardarson et al, 1973; Goodwin, 1974).

Pathophysiology

There has been much controversy about the mechanism of the obstruction to left ventricular outflow seen in some cases of hypertrophic cardiomyopathy. The degree of obstruction may vary from beat to beat and can often be provoked by inotropic agents in cases where there is little or no obstruction in the resting state. It is now generally agreed that a number of factors, which include abnormal ventricular contraction, the distorted ventricular cavity with abnormal alignment and contraction of the papillary muscles, systolic anterior movement of the mitral valve and the hypertrophied interventricular septum, all play a part depending on the degree to which each abnormality is present in any particular case (Falicov & Resnekov, 1977). The most important determinant may yet prove to be the amount and distribution of the abnormal myocardial fibres within the heart (Maron et al, 1974; Henry et al, 1974).

Myocardial histology

Histological examination of the myocardium shows complete loss of the normal orderly pattern. In hypertrophic cardiomyopathy the muscle bundles are arranged in a totally disordered fashion and are interspersed with tracts of connective tissue. The myocardial fibres themselves are short in length and run in all directions, often forming small whorls. The fibres are considerably larger in diameter than normal often measuring around 90–100 μm (normal 5–12 μm). An additional histological feature consists of large, bizarre-shaped nuclei, each surrounded by a clear zone, the so-called 'perinuclear halo', which is rich in glycogen. The adjacent myocardial fibrils often have a motheaten appearance (Fig. 70.1). Although the main concentration of abnormal fibres is usually found in the interventricular septum, they are scattered throughout the myocardium involving the walls of all four cardiac chambers to a greater or lesser degree (Van Noorden et al, 1971; Olsen, 1973).

Course & prognosis

Complications which may occur during the course of the disease include arrhythmias, which may be associated with emboli. These can arise from either the left or right side of the heart and therefore present as systemic or pulmonary emboli. Infective endocarditis has been documented in a number of cases, but is rare (Vecht & Oakley, 1968). An increased frequency of mitral ring calcification has been reported (Kronzon & Glassman, 1978) but this observation has not been confirmed by others (Kessler & Rahim, 1979). Hypertrophic cardiomyopathy may be associated with congenital heart disease, particularly bicuspid aortic valve and secundum atrial septal defects (Honey & Gold, 1971; Shem-tov et al, 1971; Block et al, 1973; Somerville & Beçu, 1977; Feizi et al, 1978). There also appears to be an association, which is unexplained, between hypertrophic cardiomyopathy and the systemic myopathies (Meerschwam & Hootsmans, 1971), Friedreich disease (Gach, 1971; Van der Hauwaert & Dumoulin, 1976), Turner syndrome (Nghiem et al, 1972), Noonan syndrome

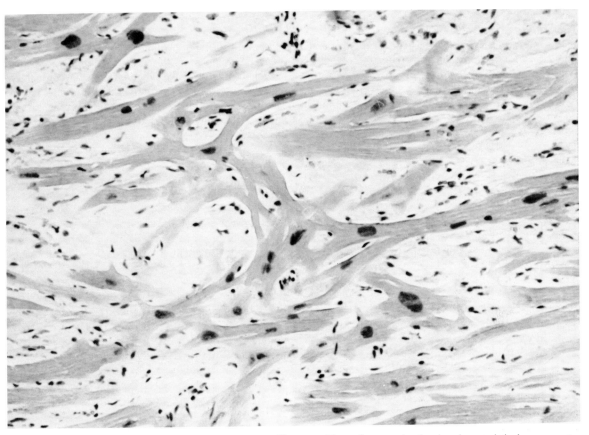

Fig. 70.1 Photomicrograph of the myocardium from a case of hypertrophic cardiomyopathy showing characteristic derangement of normal architecture with marked hypertrophy and branching of myocardial fibres. Many of the nuclei are large and bizarrely shaped. There is also considerable interstitial fibrosis. Haematoxylin and eosin × 124

(Phornphutkul et al, 1973; Hirsch et al, 1975; Jackson et al, 1979) and lentiginosis (Polani & Moynahan, 1972; Somerville & Bonham-Carter, 1972).

The natural history of the disease is extremely variable and the prognosis in any one case difficult to determine. Many affected individuals die unexpectedly in childhood, adolescence or middle life, and a few develop cardiac failure, while others remain asymptomatic for decades. Now that the disease is well recognized and the appropriate investigations more readily undertaken, it is not uncommon to find patients with hypertrophic cardiomyopathy surviving into their 60s and 70s, many such cases having been previously considered to have coronary artery disease or rheumatic heart disease (Hardarson et al, 1973; Goodwin, 1974).

Therapy

Therapy for this disorder is unsatisfactory. Angina and even syncope may be relieved by one of the adrenergic beta blocking drugs but, to date, there is no good evidence that this group of drugs protects against sudden death (Goodwin, 1974; Goodwin, 1979). However, it is possible that until recently, particularly in the case of propranolol, doses used have been sub-optimal (Gilbert et al, 1980). As there is a risk of infective endocarditis, antibiotic cover should be used prior to dentistry or on any other occasion when the patient is exposed to a septic hazard. The maintenance of sinus rhythm is all important, particularly in the elderly, for the loss of atrial transport dramatically reduces the ejection fraction of the myopathic ventricle. In many patients, cardiac failure develops rapidly after the onset of atrial fibrillation. This, therefore, is one of the rare diseases in which repeated cardioversion may be required. In view of the embolic risk, prophylactic anticoagulants should be used prior to restoring sinus rhythm and, if the patient is having frequent paroxysmal arrhythmias, anticoagulants should form a permanent part of treatment.

The question of surgical treatment arises in cases of hypertrophic cardiomyopathy with obstruction to left ventricular outflow, particularly in those patients who suffer from angina or syncope in spite of medical treatment. Morrow et al (1975) considered that 10–15 per cent of all patients with hypertrophic cardiomyopathy required surgical treatment, his study being based on 83 cases treated with left ventriculomyotomy and myectomy. Maron et al (1978b) have reviewed the long term results in 124 patients operated on between 1960 and 1975, and Reis et al (1977) reported excellent results in 30 cases similarly treated. Cooley et al (1973), on the other hand, considered the surgical treatment of choice to be mitral valve replacement. The pros and cons of these different surgical approaches have been discussed by Epstein et al (1973).

GENETICS

As stated above, early studies (Davies, 1952; Campbell & Turner-Warwick, 1956; Brigden, 1957; Bercu et al, 1958; Teare, 1958; Garrett et al, 1959; Hollman et al, 1960; Walther et al, 1960; Brent et al, 1960; Paré et al, 1961; Schrader et al, 1961; Stampbach et al, 1961; Braunwald et al, 1964; Bishop et al, 1962; Wigle et al, 1962; Wood et al, 1964; Estes et al, 1963; Björk & Orinius, 1964; Cohen et al, 1964; Treger & Blount, 1965; Maurice et al, 1966; Horlick et al, 1966; Weber et al, 1966; Meerschwam, 1969) indicated that a familial tendency existed in hypertrophic cardiomyopathy. Many of the studies reported pedigrees in which the disease appeared to be transmitted as an autosomal dominant trait, for example that of Brigden (1957). In some families, however, dominant inheritance could only be entertained if variable expressivity and incomplete penetrance were also assumed. On the other hand, there were many instances where the condition appeared to be sporadic. A glance at the nomenclature used in these early studies reveals a plethora of synonyms due to variable expression of the disorder, many of which are still in current use (Maron & Epstein, 1979b).

Recent family studies

In 1971, we attempted a genetic study (Emanuel et al, 1971), based on clinical findings, of 671 first degree relatives of 97 index patients. Five hundred and fifty-eight of the relatives were clinically examined. Looking at the types of mating which produced the probands, we identified 76 families in which neither parent was affected, 12 families in which one parent was affected, and one family in which both parents were affected. The remaining 8 families were excluded because of doubtful diagnosis in the parents. Analysis of the 12 families with one affected parent was consistent with dominant inheritance. For some of the 67 families in which neither parent was affected the proband could be considered to have received a new mutation, although for other families there was evidence of affected relatives. On the other hand, in those families with only one affected member,

or with affected sibs, recessive inheritance might have been responsible for the condition. Our data seemed to confirm this latter possibility because the number of affected individuals did not differ significantly from that expected on the recessive hypothesis. It is interesting that Yamaguchi et al (1977) studied 67 probands and their families, and found one group of families having 64 per cent consanguinity and giving a segregation ratio of 0.196 which they suggested involved a recessive gene. However, congestive rather than hypertrophic cardiomyopathy seemed to be characteristic of this group.

The advent of echocardiography (which was not available for our study in 1971) led to an attempt to improve the diagnosis of the condition by Henry et al (1973). They showed that asymmetric septal hypertrophy (ASH) was present in every patient falling into the idiopathic hypertrophic subaortic stenosis (IHSS) 'disease spectrum', regardless of the presence or absence of obstruction. (The diagnosis of ASH was used when the ratio between the interventricular septal thickness and the thickness of the posterior free ventricular wall was 1.3 or more). Clark et al (1973) selected patients with IHSS, found that 27/30 had ASH, and examined the incidence of ASH in the relatives. Forty-eight per cent of the parents, 55% of the sibs and 30% of the children showed ASH on echocardiography. However, only 16% of the relatives had classical clinical hypertrophic cardiomyopathy. The sole abnormality in 12% was ASH. On this basis they suggested that the condition was inherited as an autosomal dominant trait with high penetrance. However, it is important to appreciate that their probands were 26 consecutive patients with either ASH or clinical hypertrophic cardiomyopathy admitted for cardiological investigation, to which were added 4 patients from a cardiological out-patient clinic. Thus, some cardiological disorder was suspected, and either cardiac catheterization or echocardiography was used to determine the condition.

Their paper is important, firstly because some subsequent contributions to the genetics of hypertrophic cardiomyopathy (Bingle et al, 1975; Maron et al, 1979a; ten Cate et al, 1979; van Dorp et al, 1976) have assumed that it gives a clear picture of the genetics of either hypertrophic cardiomyopathy or asymmetric septal hypertrophy. Secondly, it has led McKusick (1978) to catalogue two dominant genes: one for Familial Idiopathic Cardiomyopathy (No. 11520), the other for Ventricular Hypertrophy (No. 19260). Moreover, the references he quotes for each are muddled.

However, ASH occurs in some normal adults (Bulkley et al, 1977; Maron et al, 1978d), it is present in congenital heart disease, especially in those cases where the right ventricle is involved (Maron et al, 1975; Larter et al, 1976; Maron et al, 1979a), and is not uncommon in fixed aortic valve stenosis (Maron et al, 1979c).

We have attempted to investigate the association between ASH and hypertrophic cardiomyopathy in two studies. In the first study we examined two types of family (Emanuel et al, unpublished), in both of which the probands had confirmed hypertrophic cardiomyopathy. There were 17 families of the first type in which one of the parents showed clinical signs of the disease. In the second type of family, of which there were 7, both parents of each proband were clinically normal, but one had echocardiographic evidence of ASH. One hundred and forty-eight out of the 150 first degree relatives were examined or, if dead prior to the study, were investigated through necropsy or operation reports to establish the presence or absence of heart disease. In the first type of family, where both the proband and one parent had hypertrophic cardiomyopathy, the matings produced 53 offspring, 30 of whom had hypertrophic cardiomyopathy with ASH and 3 of whom had ASH as the only anomaly. We have called this latter condition isolated asymmetric septal hypertrophy (IASH). In the second type of family, where one of the parents had IASH, 13 out of 24 offspring had hypertrophic cardiomyopathy, and 1 in 24 had IASH. In both types, the numbers of affected offspring do not differ significantly from those expected in dominant inheritance. We concluded that IASH and hypertrophic cardiomyopathy, when they occur in the same family, are different manifestations of the same condition transmitted as an autosomal dominant trait.

In the second study (Marcomichelakis et al, unpublished) we looked at the incidence of ASH in a normal male population. We found that the ratio between the thickness of the interventricular septum and the posterior left ventricular wall increased with age to a level in the region of 1.3, the critical value used to classify ASH. In fact, in this normal group of 100 males there were 5 whose ratio was greater than 1.3. Three of these were probably normal when allowance was made for age, but the remaining 2 had ratios which were clearly unusual for their age. All available first degree relatives of these latter 2 subjects and one of the others with a ratio in excess of 1.3 were examined clinically and echocardiographically. Thirteen out of the 14 living relatives were examined and all were normal. This suggests that a distinction must be made between IASH associated with hypertrophic cardiomyopathy within families, where inheritance is an an autosomal dominant trait, and IASH not associated with hypertrophic cardiomyopathy, where IASH may not be inherited. A larger study of the inheritance of IASH is required to confirm these findings.

HLA studies

The distinction between cardiomyopathic associated ASH and IASH has to be remembered in considering the study carried out by Darsee* et al (1979a, 1979b) on the association between HLA types and the disease. Their patients were symptomatic and had ASH. They compared HLA types in their 70 patients with those in 70 controls and showed an association of B12 in Caucasoids and B5 in Negroids with non-hypertensive hypertrophic cardiomyopathy. Data from 6 families were consistent with close linkage between the presumed non-hypertensive hypertrophic cardiomyopathy locus and the HLA complex on chromosome 6. These results have been discussed by Motulsky (1979) and Hodge et al (1979). Motulsky drew attention to possible alternative explanations for these associations in the two racial groups. The different associations could either reflect a difference of ancestry between the groups, or imply a selective advantage of combinations of particular HLA types with the cardiomyopathy allele, perhaps mediated through a common effect on cardiac development.

Another study of HLA and cardiomyopathy has been reported by Matsumori et al (1979). Twenty-two of their 26 patients were diagnosed following cardiac catheterization, but in the remaining 4 no haemodynamic studies were carried out, the diagnosis of ASH being made following echocardiography. Although Matsumori found no association over his whole group, there was an association between the disease and HLA-B7 within families. Moreover, as MacArthur and McKenna (1980) point out, Matsumori's data indicate a lower incidence of B12 and B5 in the Japanese population as compared with Darsee's findings. Both studies are therefore consistent with linkage between a hypertrophic cardiomyopathy locus and the HLA complex, the different associations simply reflecting differences in ethnic origin.

Biochemical studies

What is lacking at the moment in hypertrophic cardiomyopathy is any knowledge of a fundamental biochemical abnormality associated with the mutant gene. A start on such an investigation has been made by Liew et al (1980). They examined myocardial tissue from the left ventricular septum of patients with hypertrophic cardiomyopathy who were undergoing ventriculomyotomy-myectomy. Six out of 9 patients had a positive family history for hypertrophic cardiomyopathy with a dominant mode of inheritance. They compared the electrophoretic patterns of the histones in these patients with those from patients with normal hearts and from patients with acquired infundibular hypertrophy. The nuclear histones in the three groups were identical but the nuclear non-histone proteins showed distinct differences between the hypertrophic cardiomyopathic group and the other two groups. The altered non-histone proteins did not exhibit the patterns of the major contractile proteins. Furthermore, these nuclear proteins most probably did not come from non-muscle cells, i.e. connective tissue nuclei.

* But see 'Data falsification'. Nature, 1981, 294: 684

The function of these non-histone proteins is not known. One protein (pH 5.1, M_r 54,000) was markedly increased and another (pH 4.9 M_r 58,000) was greatly reduced in the hypertrophic cardiomyopathic hearts. Several other protein fractions were also decreased. These latter fractions were also reduced in the cardiomyopathy of Syrian hamsters. The authors concluded that the electrophoretic patterns in hypertrophic cardiomyopathy and the very early stage of hamster cardiomyopathy are strikingly similar. The fact that several proteins were affected suggests that they are regulated simultaneously, and thus the primary defect may be one of gene regulation. This may account for the variability in expression of the phenotype and the difficulties found in establishing any really clear diagnostic criteria for hypertrophic cardiomyopathy.

ADDENDUM

Since preparing this chapter there has been a report of the World Health Organization and International Society and Federation of Cardiology Task Force on the definition and classification of the Cardiomyopathies (British Heart Journal Vol. 44, Page 672, 1980). The definition now suggested is "Cardiomyopathies are heart muscle diseases of unknown cause". This is slightly different from the one we have used. In addition, the Task Force has suggested that the term 'congestive cardiomyopathy' should be replaced by 'dilated cardiomyopathy'.

REFERENCES

Bercu B A, Diettert G A, Danforth W H, Pund E E, Ahlvin R C, Belliveau R R 1958 Pseudoaortic stenosis produced by ventricular hypertrophy. American Journal of Medicine 25: 814–18

Bingle G J, Dillon J, Hurwitz R 1975 Asymmetric septal hypertrophy in a large Amish kindred. Clinical Genetics 7: 225–61

Bishop J M, Campbell M, Wyn Jones E 1962 Cardiomyopathy in four members of a family. British Heart Journal 24: 715–25

Björk G, Orinius E 1964 Familial cardiomyopathies. Acta Medica Scandinavica 176: 407–24

Block P C, Powell W J, Dinsmore R E, Goldblatt A 1973 Coexistent fixed congenital and idiopathic hypertrophic subaortic stenosis. American Journal of Cardiology 31: 523–6

Braunwald E, Lambrew C T, Rockoff S D, Ross J, Morrow A G 1964 Idiopathic hypertrophic subaortic stenosis. I.A description of the disease based upon an analysis of 64 patients. Circulation 30: Supplement IV: 3–119

Brent L B, Aburano A, Fisher D L, Moran Th L, Myers J D, Taylor J W 1960 Familial muscular subaortic stenosis. Circulation 21: 267–80

Brigden W 1957 Uncommon myocardial diseases: the non-coronary cardiomyopathies. Lancet 2: 1179–84

Bulkley B H, Weisfeldt M L, Hutchins G M 1977 Asymmetric septal hypertrophy and myocardial fiber disarray: features of normal developing and malformed hearts. Circulation 56: 292–8

Campbell M, Turner-Warwick M 1956 Two more families with cardiomyopathy. British Heart Journal 18: 393–402

Clark C E, Henry W L, Epstein S E 1973 Familial prevalence and genetic transmission of idiopathic hypertrophic subaortic stenosis. New England Journal of Medicine 289: 709–14

Cohen J, Effat H, Goodwin J F, Oakley C M, Steiner R E 1964 Hypertrophic obstructive cardiomyopathy. British Heart Journal 26: 16–32

Cooley D A, Leachman R D, Wukasch D C 1973 Diffuse muscular subaortic stenosis: surgical treatment. American Journal of Cardiology 31: 1–6

Criley J M, Lewis K B, White J I Jr, Ross R S 1965 Pressure gradients without obstruction. A new concept of hypertrophic subaortic stenosis. Circulation 32: 881–7

Darsee J R, Nutter D O, Heymsfield S B 1979b Hypertrophic cardiomyopathy and human leucocyte antigen linkage. New England Journal of Medicine 300: 877–82

Darsee J R, Nutter D O, Heymsfield S B 1979b Hypertrophic cardiomyopathy (letter). New England Journal of Medicine 301: 443

Davies L G 1952 A familial heart disease. British Heart Journal 14: 206–12

Emanuel R 1970 A classification for the cardiomyopathies. American Journal of Cardiology 26: 438–9

Emanuel R 1971 Hypertrophic obstructive cardiomyopathy. In: CIBA Study Group No.37, J & A Churchill, London, p 54

Emanuel R, Withers R F J, O'Brien K 1971 Dominant and recessive modes of inheritance in idiopathic cardiomyopathy. Lancet ii: 1065–7

Emanuel R, Marcomichelakis J, Withers R F J, O'Brien K (unpublished) The inheritance of asymmetric septal hypertrophy.

Epstein S E, Morrow A G, Henry W L, Clark C E 1973 The role of operative treatment in patients with idiopathic hypertrophic subaortic stenosis. Circulation 48: 677–80

Estes H, Whalen R E, Roberts S R, McIntosh D D 1963 The electrocardiographic and vectorcardiographic findings in idiopathic hypertrophic subaortic stenosis. American Heart Journal 65: 155–61

Evans W 1949 Familial cardiomegaly. British Heart Journal 11: 68–82

Falicov R E, Resnekov L 1977 Mid ventricular obstruction in hypertrophic obstructive cardiomyopathy. New diagnostic and therapeutic challenge. British Heart Journal 39: 701–5

Feizi O, Farrer-Brown G, Emanuel R 1978 Familial study of hypertrophic cardiomyopathy and congenital aortic valve disease. American Journal of Cardiology 41: 956–64

Frank S, Braunwald E 1968 Idiopathic hypertrophic subaortic stenosis. Clinical analysis of 126 patients with emphasis on the natural history. Circulation 37: 759–88

Gach J V 1971 Hypertrophic obstructive cardiomyopathy and Friedreich's ataxia. British Heart Journal 38: 1291–8

Garrett G, Hay W J, Richards A G 1959 Familial cardiomegaly. Journal of Clinical Pathology 12: 355–61

Gilbert B W, Pollick C, Adelman A G, Wigle E D 1980 Hypertrophic cardiomyopathy: subclassification by M mode echocardiography. American Journal of Cardiology 45: 861–72

Goodwin J F 1970 Congestive and hypertrophic cardiomyopathies. A decade of study. Lancet i: 731–9

Goodwin J F, Oakley C M 1972 The cardiomyopathies. British Heart Journal 34: 545–52

Goodwin J F 1974 Prospects and predictions for the cardiomyopathies. Circulation 50: 210–19

Goodwin J F, Krikler D M 1976 Arrhythmia as a cause of sudden death in hypertrophic cardiomyopathy. Lancet ii: 937–40

Goodwin J F 1979 (unpublished.) 7th Asian Pacific Conference of Cardiology, Bangkok

Hardarson T, De la Calzada C S, Curiel R, Goodwin J F 1973 Prognosis and mortality of hypertrophic obstructive cardiomyopathy. Lancet ii: 1462–7

Henry W L, Clark C E, Epstein S E 1973 Asymmetric septal hypertrophy: echocardiographic identification of the pathognomic anatomic abnormality of IHSS. Circulation 47: 225–33

Henry W L, Clark C E, Roberts W C, Morrow A G, Epstein S E 1974 Differences in distribution of myocardial abnormalities in patients with obstructive and non-obstructive asymmetric septal hypertrophy (ASH): Echocardiographic and gross anatomy findings. Circulation 50: 447–55

Hirsch H D, Gelband H, Garcia O, Gottlieb S, Tamer D M 1975 Rapidly progressive obstructive cardiomyopathy in infants with Noonan's syndrome. Report of two cases. Circulation 52: 1161–5

Hodge S E, Spence M A, Cederbaum S D 1979 Hypertrophic cardiomyopathy (letter). New England Journal of Medicine 301: 442–3

Hollman A, Goodwin J F, Teare D, Renwick J W 1960 A family with obstructive cardiomyopathy (asymmetrical hypertrophy). British Heart Journal 22: 449–56

Honey M, Gold R G 1971 Congenital physiologically corrected transposition with hypertrophic cardiomyopathy. British Heart Journal 33: 214–19

Horlick L, Petkovich N J, Bolton C F 1966 Idiopathic hypertrophic subvalvular stenosis. American Journal of Cardiology 17: 419–25

Hudson R E B 1970 The cardiomyopathies: order from chaos. American Journal of Cardiology 25: 70–7

Jackson G, Anand I S, Oram S 1979 Asymmetric septal hypertrophy and propranolol treatment in a case of Ullrich-Noonan syndrome. British Heart Journal 42: 611–4

Kessler K M, Rahim A 1979 Mitral anular calcification and idiopathic hypertrophic subaortic stenosis (letter). American Journal of Cardiology 44: 579

Kronzon I, Glassman E 1978 Mitral ring calcification in idiopathic hypertrophic subaortic stenosis. American Journal of Cardiology 42: 60–6

Larter W E, Allen H D, Sahn D J, Goldberg S J 1976 The asymmetrically hypertrophied septum: further differentiation of its causes. Circulation 53: 19–27

Liew C C, Sole M J, Silver M D, Wigle E D 1980 Electrophoretic profiles of nonhistone nuclear proteins of human hearts with muscular subaortic stenosis. Circulation Research 46: 513–19

MacArthur C, McKenna W 1980 HL-A and hypertrophic cardiomyopathy (letter). American Heart Journal 99: 542–3

Marcomichelakis J, O'Brien K, Emanuel R, Withers R (unpublished) Echocardiographic changes in the thickness of the interventricular septum and posterior left ventricular wall occurring with age in a normal male population

Maron B J, Ferrans V J, Henry W L, Clark C E, Redwood D R, Roberts W C, Morrow A C, Epstein S E 1974 Differences in distribution of myocardial abnormalities in patients with obstructive and nonobstructive asymmetric septal hypertrophy (ASH): light and electron microscopic findings. Circulation, 50: 436–46

Maron B J, Edwards J E, Ferrans V J, Clark C E, Lebowitz E A, Henry W L, Epstein S E 1975 Congenital heart malformations associated with disproportionate ventricular septal thickening. Circulation 52: 926–32

Maron B J, Lipson L C, Roberts W C, Savage D D, Epstein S E 1978a "Malignant" hypertrophic cardiomyopathy: identification of a subgroup of families with unusually frequent premature death. American Journal of Cardiology 41: 1133–40

Maron B J, Merrill W H, Freier P A, Kent K M, Epstein S E, Morrow A G 1978b Long-term clinical course and symptomatic status of patients after operation for hypertrophic subaortic stenosis. Circulation 57: 1205–13

Maron B J, Roberts W C, Edwards J E, McAllister H A Jr, Foley D D, Epstein S E 1978c Sudden death in patients with hypertrophic cardiomyopathy: characterization of 26 patients without functional limitation. American Journal of Cardiology 41: 803–10

Maron B J, Verter J, Kapur S 1978d Disproportionate ventricular septal thickening in the developing normal human heart. Circulation 57: 520–26

Maron B J, Edwards J E, Moller J H, Epstein S E 1979a Prevalence and characteristics of disproportionate ventricular septal thickening in infants with congenital heart disease. Circulation 59: 126–33

Maron B J, Epstein S E 1979b Hypertrophic cardiomyopathy. A discussion of nomenclature. American Journal of Cardiology 43: 1242–4

Maron B J, Gottdiener J A, Roberts W C, Hammer W J, Epstein S E 1979c Nongenetically transmitted disproportionate ventricular septal thickening associated with left ventricular outflow obstruction. British Heart Journal 41: 345–9

Maurice P, Ben-Ismail M, Penther Ph, Ferrane J, Lenègre J 1966 Les myocardiopathies obstructives. I. Etude clinique et radiologique. Archives des Maladies du Coeur et des Vaisseaux 59: 375–90

Matsumori A, Hirose K, Wakabayashi A, Kawai C, Nabeya N, Sakurami T, Tsuji K 1979 HL-A and hypertrophic cardiomyopathy. American Heart Journal 97: 428–31

McKenna W J, Chetty S, Oakley C M, Goodwin J F 1980 Arrhythmia in hypertrophic cardiomyopathy. Exercise and 48 hour ambulatory electrocardiographic assessment with and without beta-adrenergic blocking therapy. American Journal of Cardiology 45: 1–5

McKusick V A 1978 Mendelian inheritance in man, 5th edn. Baltimore, Johns Hopkins

Meerschwam I S 1969 Hypertrophic obstructive cardiomyopathy. Excerpta Medica (Amsterdam) p 20

Meerschwam I S, Hootsmans W J M 1971 An electromyographic study in hypertrophic obstructive cardiomyopathy. In: Wolstenholme F E W, O'Connor M (eds) Hypertrophic obstructive cardiomyopathy, CIBA Foundation study group No.37, J & A Churchill, London. p 55

Morrow A G, Reitz B A, Epstein S E, Henry W L, Conkle D M, Itscoitz S B, Redwood D R 1975 Operative treatment in hypertrophic subaortic stenosis. Techniques, and the results of pre and postoperative assessments in 83 patients. Circulation 52: 88–102

Motulsky A G 1979 The HLA complex and disease: some interpretations and new data in cardiomyopathy (editorial). New England Journal of Medicine 300: 918–9

Nghiem Q X, Toledo J R, Schreiber M H, Harris L C, Lockhart L L, Tyson K R T 1972 Congenital idiopathic hypertrophic subaortic stenosis associated with a phenotypic Turner's syndrome. American Journal of Cardiology 30: 683–9

Olsen E G J 1973 The pathology of the heart. Intercontinental Medical Book Corporation, New York. p 171–87

Paré J A P, Fraser R G, Pirozynski W J, Shanks J A, Stubington D 1961 Hereditary cardiovascular dysplasia. A form of familial cardiomyopathy. American Journal of Medicine 31: 37–62

Phornphutkul C, Rosenthal A, Nadas A S 1973 Cardiomyopathy in Noonan's syndrome: report of 3 cases. British Heart Journal 35: 99–102

Polani P E, Moynahan E J 1972 Progressive cardiomyopathic lentiginosis. Quarterly Journal of Medicine 41: 205–25

Reis R L, Hannah H, Carley J E, Pugh D M 1977 Surgical treatment of idiopathic hypertrophic subaortic stenosis (IHSS). Postoperative results in 30 patients following ventricular septal myotomy and myectomy (Morrow procedure). Circulation 56: suppl II: II128–II132

Roberts W C 1973 Operative treatment of hypertrophic obstructive cardiomyopathy. The case against mitral valve replacement. American Journal of Cardiology 32: 377–81

Ross J Jr, Braunwald E, Gault J H, Mason D T, Morrow A G 1966 The mechanism of the intraventricular pressure gradient in idiopathic hypertrophic stenosis. Circulation 34: 558–78

Savage D D, Seides S F, Clark C E, Henry W L, Maron B J, Robinson F C, Epstein S E 1978 Electrocardiographic findings in patients with obstructive and nonobstructive hypertrophic cardiomyopathy. Circulation 58: 402–8

Savage D D, Seides S F, Maron B J, Myers D J, Epstein S E 1979 Prevalence of arrhythmias during 24-hour electrocardiographic monitoring and exercise testing in patients with obstructive and nonobstructive hypertrophic cardiomyopathy. Circulation 59: 866–75

Shem-tov A, Deutsch V, Hahini J H, Neufeld H N 1971 Cardiomyopathy associated with congenital heart disease. British Heart Journal 33: 782–93

Schrader W H, Pankey G A, Davis R B, Theologides A 1961 Familial idiopathic cardiomegaly. Circulation 24: 599–606

Somerville J, Beçu L 1977 Congenital heart disease associated with hypertrophic cardiomyopathy. Johns Hopkins Medical Journal 140: 151–62

Somerville J, Bonham-Carter R E 1972 The heart in lentiginosis. British Heart Journal 34: 58–66

Stempbach O, Wyler F, Rentsch M, Schüpbach P 1961 Diagnostische und hämodynamische Probleme bei der Aortenstenose. Cardiologia (Basel) 38: 112–41

Teare R D 1958 Asymmetrical hypertrophy of the heart in young adults. British Heart Journal 20: 1–8

ten Cate F J, Hugenholtz P G, van Dorp W G, Roelandt J 1979 Prevalence of diagnostic abnormalities in patients with genetically transmitted asymmetric septal hypertrophy. American Journal of Cardiology 43: 731–7

Treger A, Blount S G 1965 Familial cardiomyopathy. American Heart Journal 70: 40–53

Van der Hauwaert L G, Dumoulin M 1976 Hypertrophic cardiomyopathy in Friedreich's ataxia. British Heart Journal 38: 1291–8

van Dorp W G, ten Cate F J, Vletter W B, Dohmen H, Roelandt J 1976 Familial prevalence of asymmetric septal hypertrophy. European Journal of Cardiology 4: 349–57

Van Noorden S, Olsen E G J, Pearse A G E 1971 Hypertrophic obstructive cardiomyopathy. A histological, histochemical and ultrastructural study of biopsy material. Cardiovascular Research 5: 118–31

Vecht R J, Oakley C M 1968 Infective endocarditis in three patients with hypertrophic obstructive cardiomyopathy. British Medical Journal ii: 455–9

Walther R J, Madoff I M, Zinner K 1960 Cardiomegaly of unknown cause occurring in a family. New England Journal of Medicine 263: 1104–10

Weber D J, Gould L, Schaffer A I 1966 A family with idiopathic myocardial hypertrophy. American Journal of Cardiology 17: 419–25

White R I, Criley J M, Lewis K B, Ross R S 1967 Experimental production of intracavity pressure differences. Possible significance in the interpretation of human hemodynamic studies. American Journal of Cardiology 19: 806–17

Wigle E D, Heimbecker R O, Gunton R W 1962 Idiopathic ventricular septal hypertrophy causing muscular subaortic stenosis. Circulation 26: 325–40

Wood R S, Taylor W J, Wheat M W, Schiebler G L 1962 Muscular subaortic stenosis in childhood. Pediatrics 30: 749–58

Yamaguchi M, Toshima H, Yamase T, Ikeda Y, Koga Y, Yoshioka H, Ito M, Fujino T, Yasuda H 1977 A family study of idiopathic cardiomyopathy. Proceedings of the Japan Academy 53: Series B 209–14

Congenital and hereditary urinary tract disorders

J. Zonana and J. H. DiLiberti

Congenital and hereditary urinary tract disorders cover a wide spectrum, ranging from gross abnormalities of morphogenesis to more subtle derangements of renal function. The discussion of these disorders is organised as outlined in Table 71.1. Hereditary and congenital urinary tract disorders frequently present during infancy and childhood but some are discovered during adult life and occasionally an affected individual remains asymptomatic for an entire lifetime. The latter situation creates considerable difficulty for genetic analysis. Many renal disorders are clearly hereditary, following well-recognized Mendelian patterns of inheritance. Others, especially those with abnormal structural differentiation, have only recently been shown to have a genetic component. Heterogeneity has been recognized with increasing frequency in most of these disorders.

Table 71.1 Congenital and hereditary urinary tract disorders

I. Structural abnormalities of the urinary tract
   A. Renal
      1. Agenesis
      2. Dysplasia
      3. Cystic (Ch. 72)
   B. Collecting System
   C. Malformation syndromes and associated urinary tract
      anomalies

II. Neoplasia
III. Functional abnormalities of the nephron
   A. Glomerular
      1. Nephrotic syndrome (Ch. 73)
      2. Nephritis
   B. Tubular (Ch. 73)

STRUCTURAL ABNORMALITES OF THE URINARY TRACT

Renal agenesis

Bilateral and unilateral renal agenesis are discussed together, since it now appears that they may have common aetiologies. Bilateral renal agenesis has a reported (Potter, 1965; Ratten et al, 1973; Carter et al, 1979)

incidence of 0.12 to 0.3 per 1000 total births with a male to female ratio of approximately 2.7. Estimates of the incidence of unilateral agenesis range from 1:52 to 1:1286 (Museles et al, 1971; Bernstein, 1975). Bilateral renal agenesis frequently results in stillbirth, with a reported (Potter, 1965) 38% prenatal loss in one series. Severe oligohydramnios is present, with rare exceptions. Liveborn infants are frequently both premature and small for gestational age and most die within hours of birth as the result of respiratory insufficiency.

The central pathological finding is bilateral absence of the kidney, ureters, and renal arteries, with a hypoplastic bladder lacking ureteral orifices (Potter, 1965). Occasionally ureteric remnants may be present but these cases are still classified as bilateral renal agenesis (Carter et al, 1979). Females have associated uterine and proximal vaginal agenesis with normal gonads, while in males the vas deferens and seminal vesicles are absent.

The frequent additional malformations, believed to be secondary to severe oligohydramnios, have been termed (Potter, 1974; Thomas & Smith, 1974) the 'oligohydramnios tetrad'. They are also found in association with severe oligohydramnios of non-renal origin and are absent in rare cases of bilateral renal agenesis without oligohydramnios (Bain & Scott, 1960; Mauer et al, 1974; Hjalmarson & Sabel, 1978). Pulmonary hypoplasia, with arrest of alveolar development at the 12–16 week developmental level, is directly related to the presence of oligohydramnios (Hislop et al, 1979). The characteristic facial appearance of premature senility, broad epicanthal folds, blunt nose, micrognathia, and low set posteriorly rotated ears, as well as the clubfeet and bowed legs are all believed to be deformations secondary to oligohydramnios and uterine constraint.

The majority of cases of bilateral renal agenesis involve only the primary renal and internal genital malformations, with secondary malformations due to oligohydramnios. Some infants, however, display a broader range of malformations with involvement of the anus, external genitalia, or even sirenomelia. These defects are not secondary to the renal agenesis but are considered (Buchta et al, 1973; Cater et al, 1979) an extension of an abnormal 'single developmental' field complex. Another small group of infants have multiple congenital anomalies of distant organ systems, including malformations of the heart or spine. The heterogeneity of associated malformations may help to distinguish distinct aetiologies.

Unilateral renal agenesis involves absence of a single kidney and the ipsilateral ureter and artery. The bladder has no ureteral orifice on the involved side, while the contralateral kidney may be completely normal, but is frequently ectopic (Bernstein, 1975). Abnormalities of hydronephrosis, dysplasia or pyelonephritis have been reported in contralateral kidneys (Holmes, 1972; Carter et al, 1979), however, these series are biased by the inclusion of predominantly hospitalized patients. Many people with unilateral renal agenesis are totally asymptomatic and are only discovered accidentally or by family studies.

A high rate of complete or partial uterine duplication, up to 35 % is associated with unilateral agenesis. Approximately 43% of women with abnormalities of uterine duplication have unilateral renal agenesis (Semmens, 1962; Fried et al, 1978; Magee et al, 1979). Absence of the vas deferens, seminal vesicle cysts or cryptorchidism may be found in males (Knudsen et al 1979; Ogried & Hatteland, 1979). Therefore, absence of the vas deferens in males or a duplicated uterus in females are indications for a renal ultrasound examination. Similarly, discovery of unilateral renal agenesis in a female should prompt the appropriate uterine examinations. Occasional patients with additional non-renal malformations, including imperforate anus, vertebral and sacral defects, demonstrate heterogeneity and may represent distinct disorders (Holmes, 1972; Emanuel et al, 1974).

Discussion of the possible pathogenesis of renal agenesis centers on several key morphogenetic events. The kidney develops from two sources, the mesonephric duct, which gives rise to the ureteric bud, and the metanephric blastema (Potter, 1972). The ureteral bud undergoes multiple divisions and forms the ureter, pelvis, calyces and collecting tubules. It also induces the metanephric blastema to proliferate and develop into nephrogenic cells and stroma. Severe disturbances in development or complete agenesis of the mesonephric duct, or of the subsequent ureteric bud, will result in renal agenesis. This theory has support from both clinical correlations and animal models. Embryologic studies (Cramer & Gill, 1975; Marshall et al, 1978) of the ACI rat, which has a high frequency of spontaneous renal agenesis, and of arsenate-induced renal agenesis (Burk & Beaudoin, 1977) in other rat strains, confirm the postulated pathogenic mechanisms. Abnormalities of the vas deferens and seminal vesicle occur as a consequence of their derivation from the mesonephric duct. Since paramesonephric duct (mullerian duct) formation is also dependent upon normal mesonephric duct development,

associated uterine and vaginal abnormailties can similarly be explained (Marshall & Beisel, 1978).

Renal agenesis has multiple aetiologies (Fitch, 1977). Until recent observations, both bilateral and unilateral renal agenesis were thought to be etiologically unrelated, sporadic, and nongenetic disorders. A number of families with multiple affected members have been reported (Madisson, 1934; Schmidt et al, 1952; Baron, 1954; Arends, 1957; Rosenfeld, 1959; Gorvey et al, 1962; Rizza & Downing, 1971; Buchta et al, 1973; Whitehouse & Mountrose, 1973; Hack et al, 1974). Individuals within the same family have had unilateral or bilateral renal agenesis or dysplasia (Hilson, 1957; Kohn & Borns, 1973; Buchta et al, 1973; Cain et al, 1974; Zonana et al, 1976; Carter et al, 1979). Monozygotic twins have been described, one with unilateral involvement and the other bilateral (Mauer et al, 1974; Carter et al, 1979). Individuals with unilateral agenesis have had dysplasia, duplication or hydronephrosis of the contralateral kidney (Buchta et al, 1973; Zonana et al, 1976; Carter et al, 1979). Renal agenesis, both bilateral and unilateral, can be pathogenetically related, and are at the extreme end of a spectrum of ureteric bud malformations. In the familial cases, many of the pedigrees appear consistent with an autosomal dominant pattern of inheritance, with variable expression.

Family studies have only recently been undertaken utilizing ultrasound examination or IVP to detect subclinical renal anomalies. Close relatices of most previously described 'sporadic' cases have not received adequate renal evaluation. In families purported (Buchta et al, 1973; Bois et al, 1975; Schinzel et al, 1978) to display autosomal recessive or multifactorial inheritance, clinically normal parents have frequently not been adequately examined. A possible sex linked recessive form of bilateral renal agenesis has been postulated (Pashayan et al, 1977) on the basis of one family study. A recent extensive population survey (Carter et al, 1979), not utilizing radiologic methods, found an empiric recurrence risk of 3.5% for bilateral renal agenesis. This rate was considered too high for multifactorial inheritance based on the reported incidence in the general population. This study did confirm the etiologic relationship of agenesis and dysplasia, both unilateral and bilateral. A large number of family studies, utilizing renal ultrasound or pyelography, will be necessary to delineate the complete genetic and non-genetic heterogeneity of renal agenesis.

Most familial cases of bilateral and unilateral renal agenesis have malformations limited to the urinary tract, internal genitalia and those secondary to oligohydramnios. Cases with multiple malformations should be examined for specific syndromes. Although chromosome defects are occasionally observed in patients with renal agenesis and multiple anomalies (Egli & Stadler, 1973) (see Table 71.2) chromosome studies in the majority of

Table 71.2 Urinary tract abnormalities associated with chromosomal disorders. (Warkany, et al, 1966; Egli & Stadler, 1973; Smith, 1976; Bergsma, 1979)

Chromosome abnormality	Renal abnormality	Estimated frequency of urinary tract malformation (Reported renal abnormalities may be coincidental)*
4 p-	Agenesis, hypoplasia	33%
5 p-	Horseshoe kidney, agenesis	Occasional*
8 trisomy	Hydronephrosis	
13 q-	Hydronephrosis, vesicoureteral junction obstruction	Uncommon*
13 trisomy	Cysts, hydronephrosis, horseshoe kidney, ureteral duplication	60–80%
18 q-	Horseshoe kidney, unilateral agenesis, hydronephrosis	40%
18 trisomy	Horseshoe kidney, ectopia, ureteral duplication, cortical cysts	70%
18 ring	Hydronephrosis, tubular dilatation	20%
21 q-	Unilateral agenesis	Uncertain*
21 trisomy	Agenesis, hypoplasia, horseshoe kidney	3–7%
Extra acrocentric chromosome (Iris coloboma, anal atresia)	Agenesis, horseshoe kidney	Common
XO (plus other Turner karyotype abnormalities)	Horseshoe kidney, duplication of collecting system, abnormal rotation	60–80%
XXXXY	Hydronephrosis	10%*
XXXXX	Hypoplasia, dysplasia	Uncertain*
Triploidy	Hydronephrosis	Uncertain*

cases are normal. Several single gene disorders are associated with renal agenesis (see Table 71.3). One example, the branchio-oto-renal dysplasia syndrome, is an autosomal dominant disorder which may have either unilateral or bilateral renal agenesis or dysplasia (Fitch & Srolovitz, 1976; Melnick et al, 1976; Melnick et al, 1978). Associated anomalies include preauricular pits, branchial cleft fistulas and hearing loss. A proband with renal agenesis, along with immediate family members, should be examined for these abnormalities. This syndrome may be responsible for many of the early observations (Hilson, 1957) of associated ear and renal malformations.

Renal agenesis is also associated with multiple malformation syndromes of unknown aetiology. These are outlined in a subsequent section (see Table 71.3). The VATER association of vertebral anomalies, anal atresia, tracheo-esophageal fistula and renal abnormalities is one of the more common of these disorders (Quan & Smith, 1973). It usually occurs sporadically, however, some pedigrees appear to be consistent with an autosomal dominant pattern of inheritance (Kurnit et al, 1978). Patients with renal agenesis and their families, should be examined for possible associated defects.

At the present time it would be reasonable to recommend renal ultrasound or pyelographic examination of all first degree relatives of probands with renal agenesis. The only exception would be cases of known aetiology

with a small risk of recurrence, such as those of chromosomal aetiology. If additional affected members are discovered, the pedigree should be analysed for a distinct pattern of inheritance and additional family members studied as necessary. Bilateral renal agenesis has a significant empiric recurrence risk and prenatal diagnosis should be considered. The risk of bilateral renal agenesis in the offspring of an individual with unilateral renal agenesis is unknown. The counseling is further complicated when there are no other affected family members.

Prenatal diagnosis

The need for a reliable method of prenatal diagnosis for congenital renal abnormalities is apparent. Ultrasound examination has been the major diagnostic approach to date (Kaffe et al, 1977b; Grannum et al, 1980). Using this method, severe oligohydramnios can be identified as early as 16 weeks gestation. Failure to visualize the fetal bladder over a defined period of time may indicate inadequate urine formation. Conversely, detection of a large distended bladder may indicate distal urethral obstruction. Actual identification of the kidneys and abnormal renal structures, such as renal cysts, may also be accomplished (Bartley et al, 1977; Balfour & Lawrence, 1980; Grannum et al, 1980). The kidneys can be visualized as early as 18–20 weeks gestation and at least two cases of bilateral renal agenesis have been diagnosed prior to 20 weeks gestation (Kaffe et al, 1977a; Miskin, 1979). Son-

Table 71.3 Non-chromosomal syndromes and associated urinary tract malformations.

Disorder	Urinary tract abnormality	Inheritance
Acral-renal association (Dieker & Opitz, 1969)	Agenesis, duplication	
Apert syndrome (Smith, 1976)	Hydronephrosis, polycystic kidney	AD
Cerebrohepatorenal (Zellweger) (Danks, 1975)	Cortical cysts, dysplasia	AR
Chondroectodermal dysplasia (Blackburn & Belliveau, 1971)	Renal tubular dilatation	AR
Congenital rubella syndrome (Menser, et al 1967)	Polycystic, duplication, unilateral agenesis	
Cryptophthalmos (Varnek, 1978)	Aplasia	
de Lange syndrome (France, et al 1969)	Hypoplasia, dysplasia, cystic	
Ectrodactyly (EEC syndrome) (Gorlin, et al, 1976)	Aplasia, hydronephrosis	AD
Ectromelia-ichthyosis (Cullen, et al, 1969)	Polycystic kidney, hydronephrosis	AR
Ehlers-Danlos (McKusick, 1972)	Haematuria, hypoplasia, cortical cysts, uretero-pelvic obstruction	AD
Fanconi pancytopenia (McDonald & Goldschmidt, 1959)	Hypoplasia, agenesis, ectopia, horseshoe kidney	AR
Fetal alcohol syndrome (Qazi et al, 1979)	Horseshoe kidney, duplication, hypoplasia	
Fetal trimethadione syndrome (Zackai et al 1975)	Unilateral agenesis	
Hemihypertrophy (Gorlin et al, 1976)	Ipsilateral renal enlargement, cysts, hydronephrosis, Wilms' tumour	
Ivemark (Ivemark et al, 1959)	Dysplasia	AR
Johanson-Blizzard (Johanson & Blizzard, 1971)	Hydronephrosis	
Klippel-Feil (Duncan 1977)	Agenesis, ectopia	
Laurence-Moon-Biedl (Nadjini et al, 1969)	Hydronephrosis, hypoplasia	AR
Lenz microphthalmia (Gorlin et al, 1976)	Uni- and bilateral agenesis, dysplasia, hydroureter	X-L R
Lipodystrophy, generalized congenital (Reed et al, 1965)	Hydronephrosis, hydroureter, enlarged kidney	AR
Lissencephaly (Miller, 1963)	Agenesis	AR
Marfan syndrome (Loughridge, 1959)	Duplication, ectopia	AD
Meckel syndrome (Fried et al, 1971)	Polycystic dysplastic kidney	AR
Multiple lentigenes syndrome (Swanson et al, 1971)	Unilateral agenesis, hydronephrosis	AD
M.U.R.C.S. Association (Duncan et al, 1979)	Agenesis, ectopia	
Myelomeningocele (Cameron; 1956)	Horseshoe kidney, cysts, hydronephrosis	
Neurofibromatosis (Feinman & Yakovac, 1970)	Renal artery stenosis	AD
Oculoauriculovertebral dysplasia (Goldenhar) (Sugiura, 1971)	Aplasia, duplication, ectopia	
Oculorenal associations (several types) (Senior et al 1961; Loken et al, 1961; Fairley et al, 1963)	Dysplasia, cysts, nephronophthisis	AR
Oral-facial-digital (type I) (Doege et al, 1964)	Cortical cysts	X-L R
Oro-cranial-digital (Juberg & Hayward, 1969)	Horseshoe kidney	AR

Table 71.3 (cont'd)

Disorder	Urinary tract abnormality	Inheritance
Osteo-onycho-dysplasia (Cohen & Berant, 1976)	Duplication	AD
Oto-branchial-renal (Melnick, et al 1978)	Unilateral agenesis	AD
Prune belly (Pagon et al, 1979)	Hydronephrosis, hydroureter, posterior urethral valves	
Roberts (Freeman et al, 1974)	Horseshoe kidney, cysts	AR
Rubinstein-Taybi (Rubinstein, 1979)	Agenesis, ureteral duplication, hydronephrosis	
Russell-Silver (Haslan et al, 1973)	Ureteropelvic-junction obstruction, reflux	
Saethre-Chotzen (Bartsocas et al 1970)	Duplication	AD
Thalidomide embryopathy (Warkany, 1971)	Unilateral agenesis, rotation anomalies, hydronephrosis, duplication, horseshoe kidney	
Thanatophoric dysplasia (Smith, 1976)	Horseshoe kidney, hydronephrosis	AD?
Tuberous sclerosis (Anderson & Tanner, 1969)	Cyst, dysplasia	AD
VATER association (Barry & Auldist, 1974)	Unilateral agenesis, hypoplasia, dysplasia	
Von Hippel-Lindau (Simon & Thompson, 1955)	Cyst	AD
Wiedemann-Beckwith (Beckwith, 1969)	Hyperplasia, medullary dysplasia	AR
Williams (Chantler, et al, 1966)	Renal artery stenosis	

ographic measurements of the ratio of kidney to abdominal circumference have recently been published (Grannum et al, 1980). Reports of third trimester diagnosis of renal agenesis, dysplasia or polycystic disease are more numerous (Keirse & Meerman, 1978; Mendoza et al, 1979; Older et al, 1979). Diagnosis late in pregnancy may still aid in obstetrical management and early neonatal care.

Some investigators (Kaffe et al, 1977a; Miskin, 1979) have suggested the use of fetal pyelography to confirm the diagnosis of renal agenesis, however, the rate of successful renal visualization in normal pregnancies is unknown. Maternal serum and amniotic fluid alpha fetoprotein measurements have been examined (Balfour & Laurence, 1980; Seller & Child, 1980) as possible diagnostic aids but the levels may be elevated in the presence of oligohydramnios, whether or not there is a fetal renal abnormality. They have also been elevated in cases of fetal obstructive uropathy (Vinson et al, 1977; Nevin et al, 1978; Dean & Bourdeau, 1980). In contrast, the serum alpha fetoprotein level measured at birth in infants with bilateral renal agenesis were normal (Ainbender & Brown, 1976). Further data about alpha fetoprotein levels and renal agenesis are necessary before the usefulness of this assay is known.

The wide variability of expression of ureteral bud abnormalities in some families must be emphasised when prenatal diagnosis is considered. Less severe forms of renal dysplasia, not detected by present prenatal diagnostic methods, may still present significant renal functional problems to the infant. Prenatal diagnosis of these disorders must be approached cautiously, since diagnostic methods are still being explored.

Renal dysplasia

Renal dysplasia results from abnormal metanephric development, with altered structural organization and ductal differentiation (Bernstein, 1978). Dysplasia is essentially a histologic diagnosis with distinct diagnostic criteria including abnormal ductal and mesenchymal elements, such as cartilaginous metaplasia, primitive glomeruli and ducts which may undergo cystic dilatation (Bernstein, 1971; Risdon et al, 1975; Pardo-Mindan et al, 1978). The histology of dysplasia is thought to be distinct from that found in the polycystic disorders. In the past, there has been a good deal of confusion about the terminology and description of these two groups of disorders. Renal dysplasia is heterogeneous, both in functional and structural involvement. The affected kidney may be cystic or solid; hypoplastic or enlarged.

Associated malformations of the ureters, bladder, or urethra are found in ninety per cent of cases (Bernstein, 1978).

Dysplasia is frequently accompanied by renal hypoplasia, but two forms of hypoplasia not associated with dysplasia occur (Bernstein, 1968). The Ask-Upmark kidneys, with segmental hypoplasia, is congenital but no familial cases have been reported (Arant et al, 1979). The other disorder, oligomeganephronie characterised by extreme glomerular hypertrophy and severe hypoplasia, also does not appear to be inherited.

Renal dysplasia has been separated into three clinical types (Bernstein, 1978). The first type, obstructive renal dysplasia, is frequently bilateral and most commonly associated with posterior urethral valves. Prune belly syndrome, or an ectopic ureterocele can also be associated malformations (Gribetz & Leiter, 1978). The dysplasia is postulated to be secondary to obstruction with increased hydrostatic pressure interfering with normal metanephric differentiation. This type of dysplasia is usually sporadic.

The second category of dysplasia includes the multicystic and aplastic kidney. The multicystic kidney is enlarged and distorted with numerous cysts, while the aplastic kidney is small and solid (Pathak & Williams, 1964; Newman et al, 1972). Either may be unilateral or bilateral, with the contralateral kidney, in unilateral cases, having a high incidence of renal and ureteral ectopia. The multicystic kidney usually lacks renal function, with total ureteropelvic obstruction. Many small aplastic kidneys have a patent renal pelvis and ureter. Theories of pathogenesis are controversial and obstruction has again been postulated to be the primary defect with secondary renal dysplasia. However, abnormal ureteric bud formation could be responsible for both obstruction and abnormal metanephric induction, resulting in dysplasia. Bilateral involvement, if associated with severe oligohydramnios, results in an infant with a phenotype consistent with the 'oligohydramnios tetrad'. Unilateral involvement usually has a good clinical prognosis.

The final clinical category involves the association of renal dysplasia with distinct syndromes (see Table 71.2) which must be considered when dysplasia is associated with unusual non-renal malformations. The Meckel syndrome, an illustrative example, is an autosomal recessive disorder, with variable features of encephalocele, polydactyly, cleft palate and cystic dysplasia of the kidneys (Fried et al, 1971; Mecke & Passarge, 1971). The kidneys may be enlarged or hypoplastic with cysts and fibrosis present secondary to markedly abnormal metanephric differentiation (Bernstein et al, 1974). Prenatal diagnosis of this disorder has been accomplished (Chemke et al, 1977; Kaffe et al, 1977b; Shapiro et al, 1977, Friedrich et al, 1979; Nevin et al, 1979) using both alpha fetoprotein levels, elevated in the presence of an encephalocele, and sonographic detection of oligohydramnios and cystic kidneys. Both techniques should be utilized because of the variable occurrence of encephalocele and detectable renal involvement.

Although most cases of multicystic and aplastic dysplasia appear to the be sporadic, adequate family studies utilizing sonographic or radiographic techniques have not been performed. Families with affected siblings (Cole et al, 1976; Krous & Wenzl, 1980) and also pedigrees consistent with possible autosomal dominant inheritance with variable expression (Buchta et al, 1973; Zonana et al, 1976) have been reported. The gene expression within a family may range from renal duplication to severe dysplasia. Complete renal agenesis is now recognized as the most extreme expression of this abnormal gene influencing ureteric bud development. These familial cases of dysplasia are clinically and pathologically indistinguishable from the sporadic cases.

Further work will be necessary to define the contribution of genetic factors and their heterogeneity in the different types of dysplasia. In the second category, multicystic and aplastic kidneys, an ultrasound investigation of first degree relatives should be recommended. Exact recurrence risks are presently unavailable. Prenatal diagnosis of severe dysplasia has been accomplished by sonography during the second and third trimester (Bartley et al, 1977; Mendoza et al, 1979; Older et al, 1979; Grannum et al, 1980). The kidney to abdominal circumference ratio may be elevated in cases with multicystic kidneys and reduced in those with aplastic or hypoplastic kidneys. Abnormal renal structures, including cysts, may be detectable during the later part of the second trimester.

Structural abnormalities of the ureter

Less severe ureteral malformations also have a hereditary basis. A duplication anomaly of the urinary tract involves a duplex kidney with separate calyceal systems. The two ureters may join, as a bifid ureter, or open independently into the bladder. The reported (Privett et al, 1976) incidence of duplication anomalies varies from 1:50 to 1:300, with approximately 20% bilateral involvement. The overall clinical prognosis for patients with a duplication anomaly is good. It can be associated with hydronephrosis, ureterocele and pyelonephritis, but the great majority of individuals are asymptomatic. Abnormal division during ureteric bud formation can be postulated as the pathogenetic mechanism. Affected females outnumber males by a two to one ratio and several studies (Girsh & Karpinski, 1956; Whitaker & Danks, 1966; Atwell et al, 1974) report an apparent autosomal dominant pattern of inheritance with variable expression. Duplications are a relatively minor ureteric bud abnormality and may be the result of a single gene abnormality. They can be associated with more severe disturbances of uretetic bud morphogenesis, which may be inherited as an apparent autosomal dominant trait and involve either a different gene locus or be allelic disorders (Perlman et al, 1976).

An abnormal vesicoureteral junction may also result from abnormal ureteric bud morphogenesis and cause vesicoureteral reflux. The clinical significance of ureteral reflux has been widely debated. Many pedigress have been published (Miller & Caspari, 1972; Lewy & Belman, 1975; Sengar et al, 1979) and autosomal dominant inheritance with variable expression has been postulated.

MALFORMATION SYNDROMES AND ASSOCIATED URINARY TRACT ABNORMALITIES

Malformations of the urinary tract are observed in association with, or are an integral part of, a wide variety of syndromes. The available data for many syndromes contain bias of ascertainment, making the validity of some associations uncertain. The high frequency of urinary tract anomalies in the general population confounds this issue further, since the incidence of urinary tract malformations in some syndromes does not appear to be significantly higher (Kissane, 1966; Egli & Stadler 1973, Royer et al, 1974). Among the disorders discussed or tabulated below there may be chance associations which are not truly indicative of increased risk for urinary tract malformations. Well-documented syndromes with associated urinary tract malformations have been divided into chromosomal and non-chromosomal categories.

Urinary tract malformations occur with increased frequency in patients with many of the well-defined chromosomal syndromes (see Table 71.2). As more patients are studied some of the less common syndromes will undoubtedly also be shown to have an increase in associated urinary tract malformations. In the two most common syndromes in Table 71.2, the Turner and Down syndromes, urinary tract anomalies are more numerous in the former, with an overall frequency of about 60% (Reveno & Palubinskas, 1966; Hung & Lopresti, 1968; Persky & Owens, 1971; Egli & Stadler, 1973; Litvak et al, 1978). In contrast, the risk for patients with trisomy 21 is about 3-7%, only a modest increase over general population figures (Kissane, 1966; Egli & Stadler, 1973; Royer et al, 1974).

Urinary tract anomalies commonly observed in the Turner syndrome include horseshoe kidney, duplication of the collecting system, positional and rotational anomalies, multicystic kidney, and agenesis (Reveno & Palubinskas, 1966; Hung & Lopresti, 1968; Persky & Owens, 1971; Egli & Stadler, 1973; Litvak et al, 1978). Horseshoe kidneys and duplication are the most common

lesions and each is present in about 20% of patients. In patients with the Turner syndrome there is no clear correlation between the nature of the X–chromosome abnormality and the type or frequency of urinary tract lesions, except perhaps for a slightly lower reported frequency of malformations associated with mosaic XO karyotypes (Egli & Stadler, 1973).

The natural history of urinary tract anomalies in the Turner Syndrome, as well as in the general population, is uncertain. Most patients appear to remain asymptomatic but there has been little information published about older individuals. The apparent increase in urinary tract infections reported in chromosomally normal patients with similar urinary tract malformations suggests the need for careful long-term follow-up (Kunin, 1970; Smellie et al, 1964). Obstructive lesions of the urinary tract should be corrected promptly. Intravenous pyelography along with serum creatinine determinations should be a part of the initial evaluation of all patients with the Turner syndrome. In prepubertal children an excellent estimate of glomerular filtration rate can be obtained by relating height to plasma creatinine level (Schwartz et al, 1976). This generally avoids the need to do bothersome and frequently inaccurate 24-hour creatinine clearance studies. Periodic screening for asymptomatic urinary tract infections should be considered (Kunin, 1971). Several convenient, inexpensive methods have become available (Margileth & Filipesen, 1974; Randolph & Morris, 1974). Patients with the Turner syndrome and urinary tract abnormalities are at increased risk for hypertension (Haddad & Wilkins, 1959). Periodic blood pressure determinations with careful approach to technique and age-related standards should be obtained.

Urinary tract malformations associated with non-chromosomal syndromes are summarized in Table 71.3. The large number of disorders precludes individual discussion. Many of the urinary tract anomalies are similar to those discussed above and the same general diagnostic approach and follow-up methods are appropriate.

NEOPLASTIC DISORDERS

Renal tumours generally occur sporadically but are found with increased frequency in association with some malformation syndromes and inherited diseases. Familial cases without obvious associated underlying diseases have also been reported (Table 71.4).

The most important neoplastic condition affecting the kidney during childhood is Wilms tumour, a solid retroperitoneal tumour with varying degrees of differentiation which arises from embryonic renal tissue. It is one of the most common of the abdominal masses and neoplastic conditions occuring in infancy and childhood.

Table 71.4 Renal tumors associated with hereditary disorders or malformation syndromes.

Tumour type	Syndrome	Inheritance of primary condition	Risk for developing tumour
Hamartoma	Tuberous sclerosis	AD	50–60%
Hamartoma and nephroblastomatosis	Familial syndrome with fetal gigantism, unusual facies, islet cell hyperplasia (Perlman et al, 1976)	AR	100%
Hypernephroma (renal cell carcinoma)	Von Hippel-Lindau	AD	?
	Familial	AD	?
	Chromosomal translocation	Chromosomal	?
Wilms tumour	Wiedeman-Beckwith	?	?
	Hemihypertrophy	?	?
	Familial Wilms'	AD	?
	Aniridia	See text	See text

The first conditions clearly proven to have an increased risk of Wilms tumour were sporadic aniridia and hemihypertrophy (Miller et al, 1964). Subsequently a similar association has been demonstrated with the Wiedemann-Beckwith syndrome of omphalocele, visceromegaly and macroglossia (Beckwith, 1969). The aniridia-Wilms tumour association is better understood since the discovery that a small deletion in the short arm of chromosome 11 (11p 13–14.1) is present in many if not most cases (Francke et al, 1978; Riccardi et al, 1978; Bader et al, 1979; Yunis & Ramsay, 1980). Additional associated anomalies included ambiguous genitalia in males, external ear malformations, microcephaly, coarse, perhaps characteristic, facies and mental retardation. There is a high risk of Wilms tumour in patients with this deletion, but not all affected individuals develop tumours. The risk for Wilms tumour was in the past assumed to be increased only in patients with sporadic aniridia (Smith, 1976). The 11p deletion with Wilms tumour and aniridia was recently reported in 3 members of one family, however, demonstrating that some individuals with familial aniridia are also at risk (Yunis & Ramsay, 1980). For the majority of patients with autosomal dominant aniridia the risk of developing Wilms tumour is presumably not increased. A karyotype with prometaphase banding should be obtained on all patients with sporadic aniridia as part of their individual evaluation. In familial aniridia at least one family member should have prometaphase chromosome studies. No differences in tumour histology between sporadic cases and syndrome associated cases, including the 11p deletion, have been reported.

Wilms tumour also occurs on a familial basis unassociated with other anomalies (Fitzgerald & Hardin, 1955; Brown et al, 1972; Knudson & Strong, 1972; Cordero et al, 1980). The reported frequency of familial Wilms tumour varies greatly with no obvious explanation for the observed differences (Knudson & Strong, 1972; Cordero et al, 1980). Familial Wilms tumour appear to be bilateral more often than expected (Knudson & Strong, 1972; Bond, 1975).

An interesting hypothesis about the aetiology of familial Wilms tumour had been postulated by Knudson and Strong (1972). This two mutation theory of carcinogenesis requires a first mutation to be present on an hereditary basis in the germ cell line. Subsequently a second somatic mutation can induce tumour formation. The histologic appearance of familial Wilms tumour includes subcapsular dysplasia, an abnormality not observed in sporadic or syndrome associated Wilm tumours (Miller 1980).

Screening for early detection of Wilms tumour seems prudent when a patient at increased risk has been identified. There is, however, no agreement on how screening should be done and whether it is efficacious. Intravenous pyelography at frequent intervals is unsatisfactory from the standpoint of radiation exposure, cost, risk and discomfort to the patient. In addition, a large tumour can be observed within a few months of a normal intravenous pyelogram. Use of abdominal ultrasound examination eliminates or diminishes most of these objections. Coupled with frequent, careful abdominal examinations and evaluation for haematuria, the ultrasound technique should be an acceptable screening approach.

A reasonable protocol consists of initial intravenous pyelography, followed by abdominal examination and urinalysis every one to two months, with ultrasound examinations at two to four month intervals during the period of highest risk, birth to four years of age. Other schedules could certainly be proposed and newer imaging techniques such as computerized tomography may prove useful. Surgery, radiotherapy and chemotherapy have dramatically increased survival with cure rates of

50–90% currently reported depending on the state of the tumour (Jenkin, 1976).

Familial cases of renal cell carcinoma are occasionally reported (Rusche, 1953; Guirguis, 1973). It is uncertain how many of these families also have von-Hippel-Lindau disease, which is known to be associated with this tumour (Kaplan et al, 1961). Braun et al, (1975) have suggested an association between HLA-W17 and familial renal cell carcinoma. Of interest in light of the 11pdeletion Wilms tumour association noted above is a report of renal cell carcinoma in 10 members of a family with an apparently balanced translocation involving chromosomes 3 and 8 (Cohen et al, 1979). This may represent an unbalanced rearrangement undetectable by current cytogenetic techniques. Further studies are needed before a decision to recommend karyotyping and HLA analysis for patients with renal cell carcinoma can be made.

Nephritis

Nephritis can occur as part of a heterogeneous group of disorders. Some involve only the kidney, while others affect multiple organ systems. Most of these disorders result in profound impairment of renal function and not infrequently the need for dialysis and/or transplantation. All are characterized by the presence of glomerular lesions but histologic abnormalities in other parts of the kidney are also usually present. Hereditary disorders associated with documented nephritis are summarized in Table 71.5.

The prototype hereditary nephritis is the Alport syndrome, characterised by recurrent haematuria, progressive renal insufficiency and hearing loss (Alport, 1927). Haematuria is usually the earliest manifestation and often occurs during respiratory infections as early as the first few months of life. Both microscopic and gross haematuria occur and small numbers of red blood cells are often found during the intervals between episodes of gross haematuria. Proteinuria is often present but usually is mild early in the course of the disease. Sensorineural hearing loss is an inconstant finding, present in perhaps 30-40% of affected individuals. Unilateral and bilateral hearing loss occurs with deficits often most pronounced for high frequencies. Ocular abnormalities including cataracts are noted in about 15% of cases (Kaufman et al, 1970).

The natural history of the Alport syndrome is extremely variable. For unknown reasons affected males generally have more severe and more rapidly progressive disease than females. Following the onset of haematuria, proteinuria develops and glomerular filtration decreases. Haematuria is sometimes severe enough to induce renal colic. Development of the nephrotic syndrome is unusual. After several years, or as long as decades, progressive renal failure ensues. If gross haematuria does not occur the earliest indications of severe nephritis in the

Table 71.5 Hereditary syndromes with nephritis

Syndrome	Inheritance
Familial progressive nephritis and deafness (Alport) (McKusick, 1978)	XL? AD
Familial progressive nephritis and thrombocytopathy (Parsa et al, 1976)	AD
Familial progressive nephritis (McKusick, 1978)	AD
Familial recurrent hematuria (McConville et al, 1966)	AD
Osteo-dysplasia-onycho (nail-patella) (Bennett, et al, 1973)	AD
Asphyxiating thoracic dysplasia (Gruskin et al, 1974)	AR
C2 Deficiency (Sobel et al, 1979)	AR
Hereditary immune nephritis (Teisberg, et al, 1973)	AD
Charcot-Marie-Tooth (Lemieux & Neemeh, 1967)	AD
Laurence-Moon-Biedl (Hurley, et al, 1975)	AR
Wiskott-Aldrich (Spitler, et al, 1980)	X-L R
Fabry (Desnick, et al, 1978)	X-L R

child are often decreased appetite and activity, poor growth, and pallor. Occasionally hypertensive encephalopathy and seizures are the first signs of nephritis. Affected males usually have end-stage renal disease by the third or fourth decades and if untreated die of uraemia. Females rarely progress to uraemia, the usual course involving intermittent episodes of haematuria with perhaps mild to moderate decrease in glomerular filtration rate. The course in women can occasionally be as severe as in affected males, emphasizing the need for regular medical follow-up.

The complications observed in the Alport syndrome and other forms of familial nephritis are in essence those seen in other forms of end-stage renal diase. Many can be ameliorated if patients are identified before a severely uraemic state develops. Particular attention must be paid to metabolic derangements and blood pressure determination. The interval between evaluations depends upon the degree of renal impairment but should probably be no more than 6–12 months in asymptomatic individuals.

Unfortunately, no specific therapy for progressive familial nephritis exists. Patients with end stage renal disease currently have two options: dialysis or transplantation. Each has significant associated morbidity but also the potential for adding productive years of life. Recent developments in chronic ambulatory peritoneal dialysis have allowed patients, who for various reasons are not good candidates for haemodialysis or transplantation, the chance to lead reasonably normal lives.

In the absence of a positive family history it can be quite difficult to differentiate familial progressive nephritis from sporadic forms. Numerous causes of recurrent haematuria including infections, calculi, tumours, non-familial benign recurrent haematuria and other types of nephritis must be considered. The urine sediment must be searched carefully for red blood cell casts to prove a glomerular origin of the haematuria. If any abnormalities are found a renal biopsy will generally confirm the diagnosis but the findings may not be pathognomonic. The decision to perform a biopsy depends on the extent of the abnormalities detected and the need to have a definitive diagnosis for counselling. The most characteristic renal biopsy findings in familial progressive nephritis are split, lamellated glomerular basement membranes and interstitial foam cells (Bernstein, 1979). After glomerular disease is established other conditions associated with familial disease must be sought, in particular high frequency hearing loss, ocular abnormalities, and abnormalities of platelet size and function.

Several distinct varieties of progressive nephritis apparently exist. The Alport syndrome includes families with nephritis and hearing loss but individuals may have either or both. Convincing evidence exists supporting a distinct variety of familial progressive nephritis without hearing loss. Descriptions of families with progressive nephritis and hyperprolinaemia appear to represent the chance observation of concordance for two distinct disorders (Kopelman et al, 1964; Efran, 1965). This does not appear to be the case, however, for the association of nephritis with large platelets that are defective in function, and appears to be a distinct syndrome. Deafness is also observed in these patients.

The pathogenesis of the Alport syndrome is unknown. Available data supports the hypothesis of a primary basement membrane defect. No primary immune-mediated abnormalities have been demonstrated, but some glomeruli have secondary deposition of immunoglobulins and complement (Spear et al, 1970). Abnormal disulfide bond cross-linking in basement membrane collagen has been proposed as the initiating event in development of the renal lesions (Spear et al, 1970).

An autosomal dominant mode of inheritance is well established for the majority of cases of familial progressive nephritis (See Table 71.5). Alternative mechanisms have been proposed to explain several statistical anomalies such as the apparently increased transmission rate from heterozygous mothers to daughters and decreased

transmission by affected fathers to sons (Shaw & Glover, 1961). In a syndrome with great variability more than one mode of inheritance may be present but difficult to ascertain. An X–linked variety may in fact exist (McKusick, 1978).

Genetic counselling for progressive nephritis depends greatly upon careful evaluation of other family members. Approximately 1 in 5 of all cases are presumed to result from new mutations. Most affected individuals will therefore have one or more family members with some demonstrable evidence of the Alport syndrome. All individuals at risk should have audiologic and ocular examinations, urinalysis and serum creatinine determinations.

In most families an autosomal dominant pattern will be evident and a recurrence risk of 50% may be given. Variability of expression must be emphasized, particularly the differences between affected males and females. No capability of prenatal diagnosis currently exists but some families might choose to identify fetal sex and carry only female fetuses to term. The small but definite risk of severe nephritis in affected females must be clearly understood in this situation.

In addition to the progressive familial nephritides discussed above several other disorders should be mentioned. Patients with familial benign recurrent haematuria have haematuria and occasionally proteinuria associated with respiratory tract infections but renal failure rarely, if ever, occurs. The biopsy has a small amount of focal sclerosis but ultrastructural changes in the glomerular basement membrane are generally distinguishable from progressive familial nephritis (McConville et al, 1966). Three hereditary disorders with immunologically mediated nephritis have been reported. Hereditary immune nephritis is distinguished from the Alport syndrome by earlier development of proteinuria and sudden onset of oliguric renal failure with evidence of consumption coagulopathy and low levels of the third component of the complement system (Teisberg et al, 1973). Patients with familial deficiency of the second component of complement (C2) develop mild mesangial nephritis without evidence of systemic disease (Sobel et al, 1979).

Progressive glomerulonephritis, leading to uraemia, can occur in association with two familial skeletal disorders, the nail-patella syndrome (osteo-onycho-dysplasia) and asphyxiating thoracic dysplasia. Of particular concern is the extremely rapid progression to end-stage disease seen occasionally in the nail-patella syndrome (Bennett et al, 1973). Transplantation has been successful in patients with each disorder.

REFERENCES

Ainbender E, Brown E 1976 Bilateral renal agenesis and serum α fetoprotein. The Lancet 1 (1 January): 99

Alport A C 1927 Hereditary familial congenital haemorrhagic nephritis. British Medical Journal 1: 504–506

Anderson D, Tanner R L 1969 Tuberous sclerosis and chronic renal failure. American Journal of Medicine 47 (July): 163–168

Arant B S Jr, Sotelo-Avila C, Bernstein J 1979 Segmental 'hypoplasia' of the kidney (Ask-Upmark). The Journal of Pediatrics 95 (6 December): 931–939

Arends N W 1975 Bilateral renal agenesis in siblings, Journal of American Osteropathic Association 56: 681

Atwell J D, Cook P L, Howell C J, Hyde I, Parker B C 1974 Familial incidence of bifid and double ureters. Archives of Disease in Childhood 49: 390–393

Bader J L, Li F P, Gerald P S, Leikin S L, Randolph J G 1979 11p chromosome deletion in four patients with aniridia and Wilm's tumor (Abstract 850) Proceedings of the American Association of Cancer Research 20: 210

Bain A, Scott J 1960 Renal agenesis and severe urinary tract dysplasia, British Medical Journal 1:841

Balfour R P, Laurence K M 1980 Raised serum AFP levels and fetal renal agenesis. The Lancet 1 (1 February): 317

Baron C 1954 Bilateral agenesis of the kidneys in two consecutive infants. American Journal of Obstetrics and Gynecology 67: 667

Barry J E, Auldist A W 1974 The VATER association. American Journal of diseases of Children 128: 769–771

Bartley J A, Golbus M S, Filly R A, Hall B D 1977 Prenatal diagnosis of dysplastic kidney disease. Clinical Genetics 11: 375–378

Bartsocas C S, Weber A L, Crawford J D 1970 Acrocephalosyndactyly type III Chotzen's syndrome. Journal of Pediatrics 77: 267-272

Beckwith J B 1969 Malformation syndromes. Birth Defects: Original Article Series V (2): 188–196

Bennett W M Musgrave J E, Campbell R A et al 1973 The nephropathy of the nail-patella syndrome. American Journal of Medicine 54(3): 304–319

Bergsma D (ed) 1979 Birth defects compendium, 2 edn. Alan R Liss, Inc, New York

Bernstein J 1968 Developmental abnormalities of the renal parenchyma – renal hypoplasia and dysplasia. In Sommers S C (ed) Pathology Annual, Appleton Century-Crofts, New York, ch 3, p 213–247

Bernstein J 1971 The morphogenesis of renal parenchymal maldevelopment (renal dysplasia). Pediatric Clinics of North American 18 (2 May): 395–407

Bernstein J 1978 Renal hypoplasia and dysplasia. In: Edelmann C M Jr (ed) Pediatric Kidney Disease, Little Brown and Company, Boston, Vol II, ch 39, p. 541

Bernstein J 1979 Hereditary renal disease. Monographs of Pathology, ch 13, 295–326

Bernstein J, Brough A J McAdams A J 1974 The renal lesion in syndromes of multiple congenital malformations. Birth Defects: Original Article Series X(4): 35–43

Bernstein J, Fleischmann L E, Risdon R A Crocker J F S, Schimke R N 1975 Structural Maldevelopment of the kidney. In: Rubin M I (ed) Pediatric nephrology. The Williams and Wilkins Company, Baltimore, ch 13, p 337–373; 670; 721–728

Blackburn M G, Belliveau R E 1971 Ellis-van Creveld syndrome. The American Journal of Diseases of Children 122: 267–270

Bois E, Feingold J, Benmaiz H, Briard M L 1975 Congenital urinary tract malformations: epidemiologic and genetic aspects. Clinical Genetics 8: 37–47

Bond J V 1975 Bilateral Wilms's tumour: age at diagnosis, associated congenital anomalies and possible pattern of inheritance. The Lancet 2: 482–484

Braun W E, Strimlan C V, Negron A G et al 1975 The association of W17 with familial renal cell carcinoma. Tissue Antigens 6 (2 Aug): 101–104

Brown W T, Puranik S R, Altman D H et al 1972 Wilms tumor in three successive generations. Surgery 72: 756–761

Buchta R M, Viseskul C, Gilbert E F, Sarto G E, Opitz J M 1973 Familial bilateral renal agenesis and hereditary renal adysplasia. Zeitschrift Kinderheilk 115: 111–129

Burk D, Beaudoin A R 1977 Arsenate-induced renal agenesis in rats Teratology 16: 247–260

Cain et al 1974 Familial renal agenesis and total dysplasia, American Journal of Diseases of Children 128: 377

Cameron A H 1956 The spinal cord lesion in spina bifida cystica. The Lancet 2 (July): 171–174

Carter C O, Evans K, Pescia G 1979 A family study of renal agenesis. Journal of Medical Genetics 16: 176–188

Chantler C, Davies D H, Joseph M C l966 Cardiovascular and other associations of infantile hyperglycemia. Guy's Hospital Reports 115: 221–241

Chemke J, Miskin A, Rav-Acha Z Porath A Sagiv M, Katz Z 1977 Prenatal diagnosis of Meckel syndrome: alpha-feto protein and beta-trace protein in amniotic fluid. Clinical Genetics 11: 285–289

Cohen A J, Li F P, Berg S et al 1979 Hereditary renal cell carcinoma associated with chromosomal translocation. New England Journal of Medicine 301: 592–595

Cohen N, Berant M l976 Duplications of the renal collecting system in the hereditary osteo-onycho-dysplasia syndrome. The Journal of Pediatrics 89 (2 August): 261–263

Cole B R, Kaufman R L, McAlister W H, Kissane J M 1976 Bilateral renal dysplasia in three siblings: report of a survivor. Clinical Nephrology 5(2): 83–87

Cordero J F, Li F P, Holmes L B, Gerald P S 1980 Wilms tumor in five cousins. Pediatrics 66(5): 716–719

Cramer D V, Gill T J l975 Genetics of urogenital abnormalities in ACI inbred rats. Teratology 12: 27–32

Cullen S I, Harris D E, Carter C H, Reed W B 1969 Congenital unilateral ichthyosiform erythroderma. Archives of Dermatology 99 (June): 724–729

Danks D M 1975 Cerebrohepatorenal syndrome of Zellweger. Journal of Pediatrics 86 (3): 382–387

Dean W M, Bourdeau E J 1980 Amniotic fluid ∝fetoprotein in fetal obstructive uropathy. Pediatrics 66 (4 October): 537–539

Desnick R J, Klionsky B, Sweeley C C 1978 Fabry's disease. In:Stanbury J B (ed) The Metabolic Basis of Inherited Disease, McGraw-Hill, New York, P 810–840

Dieker H, Opitz J M 1969 Associated acral and renal malformations. Birth Defects: Original Article Series V (3: 68–77

Doege T C, Thuline H C, Priest J H, Norby D E, Bryant J S l964 Studies of a family with the oral facial digital syndrome. New England Journal of Medicine 271 (November): 1073–1080

Duncan P A 1977 Embryologic pathogenesis of renal agenesis associated with cervical vertebral anomalies (Klippel-Feil phenotype). Birth Defects: Original Article Series XIII (3D): 91–101

Duncan P A Shapiro L R, Stangel J J, Klein R M, Addonizio J C 1979 The MURCS associations: Mullerian duct aplasia, renal aplasia, and cervicothoracic somite dysplasia. The Journal of Pediatrics 95 (3 September): 399–402

Edelmann C M Jr (ed) 1978 Pediatric kidney disease, Vol II, Little Brown and Company, Boston, P 537–586

Efron M L 1965 Familial hyperprolinemia. New England Journal of Medicine 272 (June): 1243–1254

Egli F, Stalder G 1973 Malformations of kidney and urinary tract in common chromosomal aberrations. Humangenetik 18: 1–32

Emanuel B, Nachman R, Aronson N, Weiss H 1974 Congenital solitary kidney. American Journal of Diseases of Children 127 (January):17–19

Fairley K F, Leighton P W, Kincaid-Smith P 1963 Familial visual defects associated with polycystic kidneys and medullary sponge kidney. British Medical Journal 1: 1060–1063

Feinman N L, Yakovac W C 1970 Neurofibromatosis in childhood. Journal of Pediatrics 76 (3): 339–346

Fitch N 1977 Heterogeneity of bilateral renal agenesis. Canadian Medical Association Journal 116 (February): 381–382

Fitch N, Srolovitz H 1976 Severe renal dysgenesis produced by a dominant gene. American Journal of Diseases of Children 130 (December): 1356–1357

Fitzgerald W L, Hardin H C Jr 1955 Bilateral Wilms Tumor in Wilms Tumor family: case report. Journal of Urology 73: 468–474

France N E, Crome L, Abraham J M 1969 Pathological features in the deLange syndrome. Acta Paediatrica Scandinavica 58: 470–480

Francke U, Holmer L B, Atkins L, Riccardi V M 1979 Aniridia-Wilms' tumor association: evidence for specific deletion of 11p13. Cytogenetics Cell Genetics 24: 185–192

Francke U, Riccardi V, Hittner M, Barges W 1978 Interstitial del (11p) as a cause of the aniridia-Wilms tumor association: band localization and a heritable basis. American Journal of Human Genetics 30: 81a

Freeman M V R, Williams D W, Schimke R N et al 1974 The Roberts syndrome. Clinical Genetics 5: 1–16

Fried A M, Oliff M, Wilson E A, Whisnant J 1978 Uterine anomalies associated with renal agenesis: role of gray scale ultrasonography. American Journal of Roentgenology 131 (December): 973–975

Fried K, Liban E, Lurie M, Friedman S, Reisner S H 1971 Polycystic kidneys associated with malformations of the brain, polydactyly and other birth defects in newborn sibs. Journal of Medical Genetics 8 (September): 285–290

Friedrich U, Hansen K B, Hauge M, Hagerstrand I, Kristoffersen K, Ludvigsen E, Merrild U, Norgaard-Pedersen B, Petersen G B, Therkelsen A J 1979 Prenatal diagnosis of polycystic kidneys and encephalocele (Meckel-syndrome). Clinical Genetics 15: 278–286

Girsh L S, Karpinski F E Jr 1956 Urinary tract malformations: their familial occurrence, with special reference to double ureter, double pelvis and double kidney. The New England Journal of Medicine 254 (18 May): 854–855

Gorlin R J, Pinborg J J, Cohen M M 1976 Syndromes of the head and neck, 2nd edn, McGraw-Hill, New York

Gorvoy J D, Smulewiez J et al 1962 Unilateral renal agenesis in two siblings. Pediatrics 29: 270

Grannum P, Bracken M, Silverman R, Hobbins J C 1980 Assessment of fetal kidney size in normal gestation by comparison of ratio of kidney circumference to abdominal circumference. American Journal of Obstetrics and Gynecology 136 (2 January): 249–254

Gribetz M E, Leiter E 1978 Ectopic ureterocele, hydroureter, and renal dysplasia. Urology XI (2 February): 131–133

Gruskin A B, Baluarte H J, Cote M L, Elfenben I B 1974 The renal disease of thoracic asphyxiant dystrophy, Birth Defects: Original Article Series X(4): 44–50

Guirguis A B 1973 Renal cell carcinoma: unusual occurrence in four members of one family. Urology 2: 283–285

Hack M Jaffe J, Blankstein J, Goodman R M, Brish M 1974 Familial aggregation in bilateral renal agenesis. Clinical Genetics 5: 173–177

Haddad H M, Wilkins L 1959 Congenital anomalies associated with gonadal aplasia: review of 55 cases. Pediatrics 23: 885–902

Haslam R H A, Berman W, Heller R M 1973 Renal abnormalities in the Russel-Silver syndrome. Pediatrics 51 (2): 216–222

Hilson D 1957 Malformation of ears as sign of malformation of genito-urinary tract. British Medical Journal 2 (October): 785–789

Hislop A, Hey E, Reid L 1979 The lungs in congenital bilateral renal agenesis and dysplasia. Archives of Disease in Childhood 54: 32–38

Hjalmarson O, Sabel K G 1978 Bilateral renal aplasia without Potter's syndrome. Acta Paediatrica Scandinavica 67: 212–213

Holmes L B 1972 Unilateral renal agenesis: common, serious, hereditary Pediatric Research 6(4): 419

Hung W, Lorpresti J 1968 The high frequency of abnormal excretory urograms in young patients with gonadal dysgenesis. Journal of Urology 98: 697–700

Hurley R M, Dery P, Nogrady M B, Drummond K N 1975 The renal lesion in the Laurence-Moon-Biedl syndrome. Journal of Pediatrics 87: 206–209

Ivemark B I, Oldfelt V, Zetterstrom R 1959 Familial dysplasia of kidneys, liver and pancreas: a probably genetically determined syndrome. Acta Paediatrica Scandinavica 48: 1–11

Jenkin R D T 1976 The treatment of Wilms' tumor. Pediatric Clinics of North America 23: 147–160

Johanson A, Blizzard R 1971 A syndrome of congenital aplasia of the alae nasi, deafness, hypothyroidism, dwarfism, absent permanent teeth and malabsorption. Journal of Pediatrics 79: 982–987

Juberg R C, Hayward J R 1969 A new familial syndrome of oral, cranial and digital anomalies. Journal of Pediatrics 74 (May): 755–762

Kaffe S, Godmilow L, Walker B A, Hirschhorn K 1977a Prenatal diagnosis of bilateral renal agenesis. Obstetrics and Gynecology 49 (4 April): 478–480

Kaffe S, Rose J S, Godmilow L, Walker B A, Kerenyi T, Beratis N, Reyes P, Hirschhorn K 1977b. Prenatal diagnosis of renal anomalies. American Journal of Medical Genetics I: 241

Kaplan C, Sayre G P, Greene L F 1961 Bilateral nephrogenic carcinomas in Lindau-von Hippel disease. Journal of Urology 86: 36–42

Kaufman D B, McIntosh R M, Smith F G Jr, Vernier R L 1970 Diffuse familial nephropathy: a clinicopathologic study. Journal of Pediatrics 77 (1): 37–47

Keirse M J N C, Meerman R H 1978 Antenatal diagnosis of Potter syndrome. Obstetrics and Gynecology 52 (1 July): 64s–67s

Kissane J M 1966 Congenital malformations. In: Heptinstall R H (ed) Pathology of the kidney, Little, Brown and Company, Boston

Knudsen J B, Brun B, Hans C E 1979 Familial renal agenesis and urogenital malformations. Scandanavian Journal of Urology and Nephrology 13: 109–112

Knudson A G Jr, Strong L C 1972 Mutation and cancer: a model for Wilms tumor of the kidney. Journal of the National Cancer Institute 48: 313

Kohn G, Borns P F 1973 The association of bilateral and unilateral renal aplasia in the same family. The Journal of Pediatrics 83 (1 July): 95–97

Kopelman H, Asatoor A W, Milne M D 1964 Hyperprolinemia and hereditary nephritis. Lancet 2 (November): 1075–1079

Krous H F, Wenzl J E 1980 Familial renal cystic dysplasia associated with maternal diabetes mellitus. Southern Medical Journal 73 (1 January): 85–86

Kunin C M 1971 Epidemiology and natural history of urinary tract infection in school age children. Pediatric Clinics of North America 18 (2 May): 509–528

Kunin C, Southall I, Paquin A J 1960 Epidemiology of urinary tract infections. New England Journal of Medicine 263: 817–823

Kurnit D M, Steele M W, Pinsky L, Dibbins A 1978 Autosomal dominant transmission of a syndrome of anal, ear, renal, and radial congenital malformations. The Journal of Pediatrics 93 (2 August) 270–273

Lemieux G, Neemeh J A l967 Charcot-Marie-Tooth disease and nephritis. Canadian Medical Association Journal 96 (November): 1193–1198

Lewy P R, Belman A B 1975 Familial occurrence of nonobstructive, noninfectious vesicoureteral reflux with renal scarring. The Journal of Pediatrics 86 (6 June): 851–856

Litvak A S, Rousseau T G, Wrede L D, Mabry C C, McRoberts J W 1978 The association of significant renal anomalies with Turner's syndrome. The Journal of Urology 120 (December): 671–672

Loken A C, Hansson O, Halvorsen S, Jolstor N J 1961 Hereditary renal dysplasia and blindness. Acta Paediatrica Scandinavica 50 (March): 177–184

Loughridge L W 1959 Renal abnormalities in the Marfan syndrome. Quarterly Journal of Medicine 28: 531–547

Madisson V H 1934 Ueber das fehler beider nieren. Zentralblatt der Allemeinen Pathologie 60: 1

Magee M C, Lucey D T, Fried F A 1979 A new embryologic classification for uro-gynecologic malformations: the syndromes of mesonephric duct induced Mullerian deformities. The Journal of Urology 121 (March): 265–267

Margileth A M, Filipesen N 1974 Initial urinary tract bacterial infection: and overview of clinical features, management and outcome in 64 children. Clinical Proceedings of Children's Hospital National Medical Center 30: 175

Marshall F F, Beisel D S 1978 The association of uterine and renal anomalies. Obstetrics and Gynecology 51 (5 May): 559–562

Marshall F F, Garcia-Bunuel R, Beisel D S 1978 Hydronephrosis, renal agenesis, and associated genitourinary anomalies in ACI rats. Urology XI (1 January): 58–61

Mauer S M, Dobrin R S Vernier R L 1974 Unilateral and bilateral renal agenesis in monoamniotic twins. The Journal of Pediatrics 84 (2 February): 236–238

McConville J M, West C D McAdams A J 1966 Familial and nonfamilial benign hematuria. Journal of Pediatrics 69 (August): 207–214

McDonald R, Goldshmidt B 1959 Pancytopenia with congenital defects (Fanconi's anaemia). Archives of Diseases of Children 34: 367–372

McKusick V A 1972 Heritable disorders of connective tissue, 4th edn. C V Mosby Company, St. Louis

McKusick V A 1978 Mendelian inheritance in man. The Johns Hopkins University Press, Baltimore

Mecke S, Passarge E 1971 Encephalocele, polycystic kidneys, and polydactyly as an autosomal recessive trait simulating certain other disorders: the Meckel syndrome. Annales de Génétique 14 (2): 97–103

Melnick M, Bixler D, Nane W E, Silk K, Yune H 1976 Familial branchio-oto-renal dysplasia: a new addition to the branchial arch syndromes. Clinical Genetics 9: 25–34

Melnick M, Hodes M E, Nance W E, Yune H, Sweeney A 1978 Branchio-oto-renal dysplasia and branchio-oto dysplasia: two distinct autosomal dominant disorders. Clinical Genetics 13: 425–442

Mendoza S A, Griswold W R, Leopold G R, Kaplan G W 1979 Intrauterine diagnosis of renal anomalies by ultrasonography. American Journal of Diseases of Children 133 (October): 1042–1043

Menser M, Robertson S E J, Dorman D C, Gillespie A M, Murphy A M 1967 Renal lesions in congenital rubella. Pediatrics 40 (November): 901–904

Miller H C, Caspari E W 1972 Ureteral reflux as genetic trait. Journal of the American Medical Association 220 (6 May): 842–843

Miller J Q 1963 Lissencephaly in two siblings. Neurology 13 (October): 841–850

Miller R W 1980 Birth defects and cancer due to small chromosomal deletions. Journal of Pediatrics 96: 1031

Miller R W, Franmeni J F Jr, Manning M D 1964 Association of Wilms tumor with aniridia hemihypertrophy and other congenital malformations. New England Journal of Medicine 270: 922–927

Miskin M 1979 Prenatal diagnosis of renal agenesis by ultrasonography and maternal pyelography. American Journal of Roentgenology 132 (June): 1025

Museles M, Gaudry C L Jr, Bason W M 1971 Renal anomalies in the newborn found by deep palpation. Pediatrics 47: 97–100

Nadjini B, Flanagan M J, Christian J R 1969 Laurence-Moon-Biedl syndrome. American Journal of Diseases of Children 117: 352–356

Nevin N C, Ritchie A, McKeown F, Roberts G 1978 Raised alpha-fetoprotein levels in amniotic fluid and maternal serum associated with distension of the fetal bladder caused by absence of the urethra. Journal of Medical Genetics 15: 61–78

Nevin N C, Thompson W, Davison G, Horner W T 1979 Prenatal diagnosis of the Meckel syndrome. Clinical Genetics 15: 1–4

Newman L, Simms K Kissane J, McAlister W H 1972 Unilateral total renal dysplasia in children. American Journal of Roentgenology Radiotherapy and Nuclear Medicine 116 (December): 778–784

Ogreid P, Hatteland K 1979 Cyst of seminal vesicle associated with ipsilateral renal agenesis. Scandanavian Journal of Urology and Nephrology 13: 113–116

Older R A, Hinman C G, Crane L M, Cleeve D M, Morgan C L 1979 In utero diagnosis of multicystic kidney by gray scale ultrasonography. American Journal of Roentgenology 133 (July): 130–131

Pagon R A, Smith D W, Shepard T H 1979 Urethral obstruction malformation complex: a cause of abdominal muscle deficiency and the 'prune belly'. Journal of Pediatrics 94: 900–906

Pardo-Mindan F J, Pablo C L, Vazquez J J 1978 Morphogenesis of glomerular cysts in renal dysplasia. Nephron 21: 155–160

Parsa K P, Lee D N, Zamboni L, Glassock R J 1976 Hereditary nephritis, deafness and abnormal thrombopoiesis: study of a new kindred. American Journal of Medicine 60 (5): 665–672

Pashayan H M, Dowd T, Nigro A V 1977 Bilateral absence of the kidneys and ureters. Journal of Medical Genetics 14: 205–209

Pathak I G, Williams D I 1964 Multicystic and cystic dysplastic kidneys. British Journal of Urology 36: 318–331

Perlman M, Williams J, Ornoy A 1976 Familial ureteric bud anomalies. Journal of Medical Genetics 13: 161–163

Persky L, Owens R 1971 Genitourinary tract abnormalities in Turner's syndrome. Journal of Urology 105: 309–313

Pilepich M V, Berkman E M, Goodchild N T 1978 HLA typing in familial renal carcinoma. Tissue Antigens 11: 487–488

Potter E L 1965 Bilateral absence of ureters and kidneys: a report of 50 cases. Obstetrics and Gynecology 25 (1 January): 3–12

Potter E L 1972 Normal and abnormal development of the kidney. Year Book Medical Publishers, Chicago, 3–24

Potter E L 1974 Oligohydramnios: further comment. The Journal of Pediatrics 84 (6 June): 931–932

Privett J T J, Jeans W D Roylance J 1976 The incidence and importance of renal duplication. Clinical Radiology 27: 521–530

Qazi Q, Masakawa A, Milman D, McGann B, Chua A, Haller J 1979 Renal anomalies in fetal alcohol syndrome. Pediatrics 63 (6 June): 886–889

Quan L, Smith D W 1973 The VATER association. Journal of Pediatrics 82: 104

Randolph M F, Morris K 1974 Instant screening for bacteriuria in children: analysis of dipstick. Journal of Pediatrics 84(2): 246–248

Ratten G J, Beischer N A, Fortune D W 1973 Obstetric complications when the fetus has Potter's syndrome. I. Clinical considerations. American Journal of Obstetrics and Gynecology 115 (7 April): 890–896

Reed W B, Dexter R, Corley C, Fish C 1965 Congenital lipodystrophic diabetes with acanthosis nigricans. Archives of Dermatology 91: 326–334

Reveno J, Palubinskas A J 1966 Congenital renal abnormalities in gonadal dysgenesis. Radiology 86: 49–51

Riccardi V M, Sujansky E, Smith A C, Francke U 1978 Chromosomal imbalance in the aniridia-Wilms' tumor association: 11p interstitial deletion. Pediatrics 61 (4): 604–610

Risdon R A, Young L W, Chrispin A R 1975 Renal hypoplasia and dysplasia: a radiological and pathological correlation. Pediatric Radiology 3: 213–225

Rizza J M, Downing S E 1971 Bilateral renal agenesis in two female siblings. American Journal of Diseases of Children 121: 60

Rosenfeld L 1959 Renal agenesis. Journal of the American Medical Association 170: 1247

Royer P, Habib R, Mathieu H, Broyer M 1974 Pediatric nephrology, W B Saunders Company. Philadelphia

Rubinstein J H 1979 Broad thumb-hallux syndrome. In: Bergsma D (ed), Birth defects Compendium, 2nd edn, Alan R Liss, Inc, New York, P 157

Rusche C 1953 Silent adenocarcinoma of the kidneys with solitary metastases occurring in brothers. Journal of Urology 70 (August): 146–151

Schinzel A, Homberger C, Sigrist T 1978 Bilateral renal agenesis in 2 male sibs born to consanguineous parents. Journal of Medical Genetics 15: 314–316

Schmidt E C, Hartley A A, Bower R 1952 Renal aplasia in sisters. Archives of Pathology 54: 403

Schwartz G J, Haycock G B, Edelman C M Jr, Spitzer A 1976 A simple estimate of glomerular filtration rate in children derived from body length and plasma creatinine. Pediatrics 58 (2): 259–263

Seller M J, Berry A C 1978 Amniotic fluic alpha-fetoprotein and fetal renal agenesis. The Lancet 1 (1 March): 660

Seller M J, Child A H 1980 Raised maternal serum alpha-fetoprotein, oligohydramnios and the fetus. The Lancet 1 (1 February): 317

Semmens J P 1962 Congenital anomalies of the female genital tract: functional classification based on review of 56 personal cases and 500 reported cases. Obstetrics and Gynecology 19: 328

Sengar D P S, Rashid A, Wolfish N M 1979 Familial urinary tract anomalies: association with the major histocompatibility complex in man. The Journal of Urology 121 (February): 194–197

Senior B, Friedman A I, Brando J L 1961 Juvenile familial nephropathy with tapeto retinal degeneration. American Journal of Ophthalmology 52 (November): 625–633

Shapiro L J, Kaback M M, Toomey K E, Sarti D, Luther P, Cousins L 1977 Prenatal diagnosis of the Meckel syndrome. Birth Defects: Original Article Series XIII (3): 267–272

Shaw R F, Glover R A 1961 Abnormal segregation in hereditary renal disease with deafness. American Journal of Human Genetics 13 (March): 89–97

Simon H B, Thompson G J 1955 Congenital renal polycystic disease: clinical and therapeutic study of 366 cases. Journal of the American Medical Association 159 (October): 657–662

Smellie J M, Hodson C J, Edwards D, Normand I C S 1964 Clinical and radiological features of urinary infection in children. British Medical Journal 2: 1222–1226

Smith D W 1976 Recognizable patterns of human malformation: genetic embryologic and clinical aspects, 2nd edn, W B Saunders Company, Philadephia

Sobel A T, Moisy G, Hirbec G et al 1979 Hereditary C2 deficiency associated with non-systemic glomerulonephritis. Clinical Nephrology 12(3): 132–136

Spear G S 1973 Alport's syndrome: a consideration of pathogenesis Clinical Nephrology I (November-December): 336–337

Spear G S, Whiworth J M, Konigsmark B W 1970 Hereditary nephritis with nerve deafness: immunofluorescent studies on the kidney with a consideration of discordant immunoglobulin-complement immunofluorescent reactions. American Journal of Medicine 49 (1) 52–63

Spitler L E, Wray B B, Mogerman S, Miller J J, O'Reilly R J, Lagios M 1980 Nephropathy in the Wiskott-Aldrich syndrome. Pediatrics 66 (3): 391–398

Sugiura 1971 Congenital absence of the radius with hemifacial microsomia, ventricular septal defect and crossed renal ectopia. Birth Defects: Original Article Series VII(7): 109–116

Swanson S L, Santen R J, Smith D W 1971 Multiple lentigenes syndrome: new findings of hypogonadotrophism, hyposomia and unilateral renal agenesis. Journal of Pediatrics 78 (6 June): 1037–1039

Teisberg P, Grottom K A, Myhre E, Flatmark A 1973 In vivo activation of complement in hereditary nephropathy. Lancet 2: 356–358

Thomas I T, Smith D W 1974 Oligohydramnios, cause of the nonrenal features of Potter's syndrome, including pulmonary hypoplasia. The Journal of Pediatrics 84 (6 June: 811–814

Varnek L 1978 Cryptophthalmos, dyscephaly, syndactyly and renal aplasia. Acta Ophthalmologica 56: 302–313

Vinson P C, Goldenberg R L, Davis R O, Finley S C 1977 Fetal bladder neck obstruction and elevated amniotic alpha-fetoprotein. New England Journal of Medicine 297: 1351

Warkany J, Passarge E, Smith L B 1966 Congenital malformations in autosomal trisomy syndromes. American Journal of Diseases of Children 112 (December): 502–517

Warkany J 1971 Congenital malformations. Year Book Medical Publishers, Inc, Chicago, P 92

Whitaker J, Danks D M 1966 A study of the inheritance of duplication of the kidneys and ureters. The Journal of Urology 95 (February): 176–178

Whitehouse W, Mountrose U 1973 Renal agenesis in nontwin siblings. American Journal of Obstetrics and Gynecology 116: 880

Yunis J J, Ramsay N K C 1980 Familial occurrence of the aniridia-Wilms tumor syndrome with deletion 11p13–14.1. Journal of Pediatrics 96 (6): 1027—1030

Zackai E, Mellman W J, Neiderer B, Hanson J 1975 The fetal trimethadione syndrome. Journal of Pediatrics 87: 280–284

Zonana J, Rimoin D, Lachman R, Sarti D, Kaback M 1976 Renal agenesis – a genetic disorder? Pediatric Research 10: 420

72

Cystic diseases of the kidney

J. Friedman

ADULT POLYCYSTIC KIDNEY DISEASE

Adult polycystic kidney disease (APKD) was first described in the 19th century (Lejars, 1888). Infantile polycystic kidney disease and other cystic renal diseases have been frequently confused with APKD in the literature. Much of the confusion results from older literature, including reports which were based solely on autopsy data and retrospective review of cases at a time when these different cystic diseases were pathologically not easily separable (Anonymous, 1979; Bernstein, 1979). More recent pathologic study including the use of microdissection techniques has further delineated pathologically the differences between adult polycystic kidney disease and infantile polycystic kidney disease (Baert, 1978). The heterogeneity of these two major cystic renal diseases each of which can occur in unusual age groups; i.e., APKD presenting in an infant (Shoker, 1978) has also contributed to the problem of improper reporting of case materials especially in the older literature. The most comprehensive review of APKD was done by Dalgaard, covering approximately 300 cases. This initial major study delineated the clinical patterns of this disease.

Clinical description

The mean age of presentation was 40.7 years in Dalgaard's series. Patients presented with many different signs and symptoms. The most frequent presentation at onset was pain, including both flank pain and renal colic (Kissane, 1980; Segal et al, 1977; Dalgaard, 1957). In one recent series, 20% of cases at presentation had calculi, 10% had pelvo-calyceal system obstruction, and 7% had segmental obstruction (Segal et al, 1977). Dalgaard also noted that patients at presentation or during their course frequently had, in addition to pain, the findings of haematuria, hypertension or signs of cardiac failure, uraemia, flank masses, proteinuria, pyuria or bacteruria, and chronic renal failure. Tubular dysfunction characterized by concentrating defects, inability to decrease the urinary pH after acid loading, and impaired ammonia excretion have now been documented in patients with APKD (Preuss et al, 1979). In Dalgaard's series, the mean survival time after diagnosis was approximately 7 years. The causes of death were uraemia in approximately 60% of cases, CNS bleed in 13%, heart failure in 6%, and the remaining deaths were attributed to multiple other causes. Dalgaard's work was prior to the widespread establishment of centers for haemodialysis and renal transplantation, permitting survival after end stage renal disease supervened. Dalgaard also observed that survival in patients who had the onset of disease at greater than 50 years of age was approximately ten years, while those patients diagnosed at an age less than fifty had a mean survival of approximately 2½ years. This observation clearly suggested that disease of early onset had a worse prognosis. Occasional patients do not have documentable disease present until the 8th or 9th decade (Kissane, 1980).

APKD is clearly associated with several other abnormalities. Approximately one-third to one-half of patients have associated cysts in the liver (Dalgaard, 1957; Kissane, 1980; Bernstein 1979). These cysts are usually few in number, spherical and rarely greater than a few centimeters in diameter. Microscopically, hepatic cysts are usually lined by a single layer of columnar epithelial cells (Kissane, 1980). These hepatic cysts are almost always asymptomatic and virtually never associated with hepatic failure, except in some patients on long-term haemodialysis (Chester et al, 1978; DelGuercio et al, 1973). Associated cystic disease of the pancreas, spleen, ovary and seminal vesicles has also been described (Kissane, 1980). The most significant association with APKD is sacular aneurysms of the cerebral arteries (berry aneurysms) (Pontasse et al, 1954). They occur in 10–15% of patients and are a major cause of death (Kissane 1980; Bernstein, 1979). Conversely, approximately 3% of patients who die from ruptured cerebral aneurysms have adult polycystic kidney disease (Kissane, 1980). Several hereditary conditions have been seen in association with APKD. These include myotonic dystrophy (Emery et al, 1967), Peutz-Jeghers syndrome (Kieselstein), oro-facial-digital syndrome (Harrod et al, 1976), lobster claw deformity (Cameron), and spherocytosis (Chanmugam et al, 1968).

Differential diagnosis

Differential diagnoses vary greatly with the initial presentation. Patients presenting with asymptomatic haematuria, or hypertension will generally receive a standard workup for haematuria or hypertension, as had been well described in many texts. The intravenous urogram will demonstrate a normal pelvocalyceal system which is distorted bilaterally by intrarenal cysts making the diagnosis (Bernstein, 1979). Other patients are evaluated when they are asymptomatic because the diagnosis of APKD has been made in a family member. Patients presenting with flank masses always receive radiographic studies, including intravenous pyelography or nephrosonography, and even occasionally angiography, to rule out neoplastic processes. Patients who present with colic frequently receive an evaluation compatible with stone disease or tumour.

The differential diagnosis is usually made somewhat clearer by the presence of bilateral renal enlargement on physical examination, which on sonography or intravenous pyelography is demonstrated to consist of bilateral cysts distorting the pelvocalyceal system. Renal involvement is virtually always bilateral (Hutchins et al, 1972), however, it may be much more marked on one side than the other, leading to renal asymmetry which requires a more vigorous evaluation to eliminate the possibility of renal neoplasma.

Pathogenesis

The pathogenesis of adult-type polycystic kidney disease has remained elusive. Pathologic studies have more recently characterized the entity as multiple cysts of columnar epithelium which appear to arise from all portions of the nephron as demonstrated by microdissection studies (Baert, 1978). Kidneys are very large with numerous cysts but remain reniform in shape (Kissane, 1980). Some authors have favoured the possibility that there is nephron dilatation primarily rather than primary cyst formation. This disorder is a genetically inherited disease with an autosomal dominant inheritance pattern having a penetrance that approaches 100% in patients who reach the 9th or 10th decade of life (Dalgaard, 1957). This increasing penetrance as life progresses has led many authors to speculate that there is an intrinsic defect within the renal tubules which takes a variable period for expression (Anonymous, 1979; Eulderink & Hogewind, 1978). Support for this proposal may be derived from a report documenting small cysts (100 microns) in kidneys from premature abortuses in a family with APKD (Eulderink & Hogewind, 1978). Others have postulated that a metabolic abnormality is present which eventually induces tubular damage and expresses itself as this cystic disease (Anonymous, 1979). Given the current knowledge available, the pathophysiology remains unknown and is a topic in need of much further study.

Therapy

Management of patients with adult type polycystic kidney disease is similar to patients with any other type of renal disease with similar clinical problems. Patients with chronic renal failure are treated in a standard manner. Those patients with APKD who have renal infection or calculi again receive standard therapy for these problems. Hypertension is also treated in a standard manner. Recently, one group has reviewed its experience with dialysis and renal transplantation in patients with cystic kidney disease and observed that these patients do as well as or better than any other group of patients, or the overall group of patients reaching end stage renal disease (ESRD) (Chester et al, 1978). Approximately 5% of all patients who reach ESRD have polycystic kidney disease (Bernstein, 1979).

Genetics

Many pedigrees have now been studied after the initial work by Dalgaard. Studies appear to have now clearly demonstrated that this disease is of autosomal dominant inheritance. In Dalgaard's series, compiled from Scandinavia, where the population is relatively inbred, the incidence of cases with a documented family history was 67%, while one-third of cases appeared to have no documentable family history and were called sporadic. Other series have suggested that there is a much lower incidence of familial cases. The lack of family history has been used in studies to suggest that there is a relatively high rate of spontaneous mutations which has been estimated at between $6.5-12 \times 10^{-5}$ mutations/gene/generation (Dalgaard). There has also been a large discrepancy in the reported incidence of APKD in autopsy series ($1/350-1/500$) and clinical reports ($1/3000$ and $1/3500$). Some of this discrepancy is probably related to the improper diagnosis of APKD rather than a correct diagnosis of other cystic kidney disease or simple cysts of the kidney, as well as non-recognition of the disease in patients prior to presentation with ESRD or death. There have been a few cases of APKD presenting in infants (Kaye & Lewy, 1974). These have been isolated and rare and prenatal diagnosis is not something one is called upon frequently to consider and it consequently has not been reported. Prenatal diagnosis of infantile polycystic kidney disease by ultrasonography has been attempted (Mendosa et al, 1979; Older et al, 1979; Reilly et al, 1979; Thomas et al, 1978) and could be attempted for APKD if an appropriate family history were present for a symptomatic infant. Since this is an autosomal dominant disorder, when a propositus is discovered, screening of first generation family members, including parents, should be rapidly initiated. This should be continued throughout preceding generations if any evidence of polycystic kidney disease is found. The purpose of this screening is to provide genetic counselling information, as well as guidance in managing the unsuspecting patient who may have some degree of impaired renal function or hypertension. Screening should include a physical examination including determination of blood pressure, urinalysis, serum creatinine, and an intravenous pyelogram or nephrosonogram.

INFANTILE POLYCYSTIC KIDNEY DISEASE

Classically, infantile polycystic kidney disease (IPKD) refers to a group of disorders characterised by varying combinations of bilateral cystic renal disease associated with hepatic fibrosis (Lieberman et al, 1971). This entity can present beyond infancy (Piering et al, 1977), resulting in confusion in the older literature.

Clinical description
Blythe and Ockenden (1971) attempted to divide patients into four groups: those presenting in the perinatal period (at birth), as neonates (one day–1 month of age), infants (3–6 mos.), and juveniles (6 mos.–5 yrs.). These authors stressed that the presence of severe renal disease, usually characterised by oliguria and anuria, and massive renal enlargement being present at birth, was associated with early progression to end stage renal disease. Patients who presented at older ages usually had less severe renal disease; however, they had more severe hepatic disease characterised by hepatomegaly and/or splenomegaly, with portal hypertension and its attendant complications, including varices, bleeding, and hematemasis (Blythe & Ockenden, 1971; Lieberman et al, 1971). In pathologic material, these authors observed that patients presenting at an older age had smaller percentages of renal tubules with ductal ectasia, the major pathologic lesion. Clinically, patients with severe early disease are also noted to have pulmonary hypoplasia, a frequent cause of pneumothorax in the newborn (Lieberman, 1971). The newborn patients with oliguria or anuria also usually had Potter facies. Frequently, patients also had a history of prolonged maternal labour, presumably associated with large distended kidneys. Arthrogryposis as well as oligohydramnios were frequent concomitants as well (Bernstein, 1979; 1980; Lieberman et al 1971). Lieberman et al have reported that patients with the neonatal type of disease frequently had hypertension, and signs of chronic renal failure often developed rapidly, while patients with the infantile type of presentation often had a mixed combination of hepatic and renal disease. Those patients falling into the juvenile group usually had predominantly hepatic involvement. Patients with the earlier age presentations usually were noted to have only a minimal amount of hepatic fibrosis at the time of autopsy. The usual cause of death in patients from the juvenile group was complications of portal hypertension (Lieberman et

al, 1971). Clinically, IPKD patients usually had some haematuria or pyuria, but no increased propensity for urinary tract infections. Anaemia and hypertension were fairly common, and in the neonatal and perinatal forms of the disease, liver function tests are usually normal. Vuthibhagdee has observed more recently a longer survival in some patients presenting at early ages, and this report awaits further confirmation.

Differential diagnosis
Infants presenting with bilateral flank masses and also with oliguria or anuria (with or without haematuria, pyuria, or hypertension) the commonest presentation of IPKD, are statistically most likely to have obstructive uropathy, whether bilateral uretero-pelvic junction obstruction, primary megacystis-megaureter syndrome or posterior urethral valves. Patients with flank masses may also have bilateral cystic dysplasia, which, however, rarely has massively bilateral renal enlargement as seen frequently with infantile polycystic kidney disease. Nephrosonography is the initial test of choice in an attempt to make a differential diagnosis of renal masses in infancy (Rabinowitz et al, 1978). Large, dilated hydronephrotic or obstructed kidneys, obstructed ureters, or large bladders can easily be delineated by this technique. The multicystic dysplastic kidney is characterised by bilateral cysts without the presence of ureters and no recognizable pelvocalyceal system. Infantile PKD on sonography may be characterised by many echoegenic areas but one does not find the presence of cysts, as the individual cysts are rarely greater than 1 cm in diameter and most are on the order of 1 mm in size (Lieberman et al, 1971), which is beyond the resolution of sonography. IPKD patients will have normally appearing pelvocalyceal systems by sonography, as contrasted to the other conditions in the differential diagnosis. Intravenous urography is usually of little value in infants with impaired renal function; however, in the older patients, delayed IVP films showing dye in the dilated tubular structures has been seen in infantile PKD and called characteristic (Bernstein, 1980). Renal scans or angiography are also usually of little value in differential diagnosis. History, physical exam, and ultrasonography are almost always sufficient for the experienced physician, frequently the pediatric nephrologist, to make a diagnosis. Meckel syndrome has been associated with IPKD (Fried et al, 1971, Friedrich et al, 1979).

Therapy
The management of end stage renal disease (ESRD) in patients less than 2 years of age has been extremely unsuccessful. Data from the Transplant Registry as well as recent experience at our and other institutions has shown that dialysis and transplant in this age group has limited success. The technical difficulties attendant to

the small size of the patient has lead to a practice where patients with this disease presenting with ESRD before age 2 have been allowed to die. Patients with IPKD who present at older ages do not usually develop ESRD but succumb to the consequences of portal hypertension (Lieberman et al, 1971, Anand et al, 1975). Therapy for portal hypertension resulting from IPKD remains similar to that of patients with hepatic fibrosis for any reason. The long-term survival of patients with hepatic disease as the major presentation also remains very guarded. Patients who develop renal insufficiency beyond age two should be treated as other children with ESRD provided hepatic impairment is not marked, since the prognosis of patients reaching ESRD at young ages without major hepatic disease if supported by dialysis and transplantation remains unknown.

Pathogenesis

IPKD is characterized pathologically by cystic dilatation of the distal collecting ducts usually of approximately 1 mm in size (Bernstein, 1980). Renal pelves and calyces are usually small and compressed but structurally normal (Bernstein, 1980). This has been variously called ductal ectasia and is also present in the medulla, being similar pathologically to medullary sponge kidney (Bernstein, 1980). Hepatic involvement consists of increased portal bile ducts, with increased connective tissue and fibrosis. There has been some recent excitement in this area with the work of Evan and Gardner (1979). These investigators have been working with an animal model, whereby with administration of agents they produce a renal tubular lesion which appears to be cystic in nature. In this model, by the use of micropuncture techniques measuring single nephron glomerular filtration rates and with the use of scanning and transmission electron microscopy they have proposed that the dilatation of renal tubules may result, in part, from intratubular obstruction due to papillary-like structures (Evan et al, 1979). The relationship of this animal model to PKD is not certain; however, this type of approach may yield much understanding of this disease entity, for which at present the pathogenesis is unclear.

Genetics

Infantile PKD appears to have an autosomal recessive inheritance pattern (Lieberman et al, 1971). There usually is little variability within a family, in that if one child in the family has presented with the neonatal type of disease, this type tends to recur in subsequently affected children (Lieberman et al, 1971; Bernstein, 1980). Since the genetics of this disorder are fairly well understood, genetic counselling may be entered into as for any autosomal recessive disorder which will almost certainly be fatal within the first several years of life.

Recently, several groups have attempted to make the

prenatal diagnosis of IPKD. Some groups have been analyzing various enzymes which are present in renal tubular membranes, obtained from amniotic fluid. The studies are currently still in the preliminary stages but may in the future yield an effective prenatal diagnostic test for IPKD. Currently, nephrosonography appears to be the test of choice to diagnose IPKD prenatally (Mendosa et al, 1979; Older et al, 1979; Reilly et al, 1979; Thomas et al, 1978). The problems encountered include that the fetus must develop to sufficient size so that sonography will be reliable. Kidney size may clearly be delineated, however, and during the second trimester size should become adequate for diagnosis, and this technique, if further experience develops, should become reliable.

NEPHRONOPHTHISIS AND MEDULLARY CYSTIC DISEASE

Many names have appeared in the literature describing this spectrum of diseases including: salt-losing nephritis, renal-retinal dysplasia, medullary sponge kidney, cystic disease of the renal medulla, among others (Bernstein & Gardner, 1979). The confusion in nomenclature, in addition to the many incomplete and anecdotal reports in the literature, has generated many of the misconceptions about this disease entity. Gardner and co-workers (Gardner & Evan, 1980, Bernstein & Gardner, 1979) as well as others (von Collenburg et al, 1978) have more recently classified this group of diseases into four types: (a) childhood onset; (b) adult onset; (c) renal-retinal dysplasia type; and (d) sporadic. These workers compiled all reported cases in the literature, and analysed this body of data to determine the characteristics of each variant of this disease.

Clinical description

The most frequently observed variant of the nephron-ophthisis-medullary cystic disease complex (NMCD) is with onset in childhood. This pattern accounts for approximately two thirds of cases. The sporadic forms, as well as the renal-retinal dysplasia variant, also occur predominantly in childhood. The remaining 25% of cases usually present with adult onset.

The onset in all the variants except the adult onset type of disease has been established to be at a mean age of approximately 10 years (Gardner & Evan, 1980). After diagnosis progression to end stage renal disease occurs, on average, over a 3-year period. In the adult onset disease, the average age at presentation in these series was 30 years, with progression to end stage occurring over the next 4 years. Several parameters are remarkable for their usual absence in NMCD.

Hypertension is present in only 1 in 3 patients. UTIs are very infrequent, as is renal lithiasis. One of the most important points in the differential diagnosis is that the urinalysis in almost always without abnormality of the sediment. However, the specific gravity is uniformly low, due to a defect in renal concentrating ability. Salt-wasting, which is frequently present, may be causally related to the low incidence of hypertension, and often is not present as chronic renal failure worsens. Many authors have stressed the fact that the anemia may be significantly out of proportion to the degree of renal failure present. This idea has been recently brought into question (Gardner & Evan, 1980). Table 72.1 gives presenting symptoms and laboratory findings in NMCD.

Table 72.1 Presenting symptoms and laboratory observations in patients with nephronophthisis-medullary cystic disease

Symptoms or finding	Approximate frequency
Polyuria and polydipsia	80%
Azotemia	75%
Anemia	60%
Tiredness	60%
Growth retardation	40%
Hypertension	30%
Retinal abnormalities	15%
Red or blond hair	?

Differential diagnosis

The definitive diagnosis of this disease entity is at times extremely difficult. NMCD, as per its name, is a histologic diagnosis. Patients who present with polyuria, polydipsia, normal urinalyses except for inability to concentrate the urine, and affected family members with renal disease who have histologic specimens are easily diagnosable. However, if histologic specimens are not available, diagnosis then becomes much more difficult (Gardner & Evan, 1980). A family history of renal failure with the absence of hypertension, hematuria, or other associated findings may strongly suggest the diagnosis. One often attempts renal biopsy to make a definitive pathologic diagnosis. There appears to be no significant advantage of open vs. closed renal biopsy for this purpose (Bernstein & Gardner, 1979). However, biopsy provides definitive diagnosis in at most 30% of cases, and should be attempted knowing this limitation, as cysts are located only in the medulla and deeper cortex.

The pathologic findings in medullary cystic disease-nephronophthisis are characterised by a kidney which is grossly uniformly shrunken and finely scarred. A greatly variable number of corticomedullary and medullary cysts, varying in size between less than 1 mm and rarely greater than 1 cm, filled with translucent fluid are found upon sectioning the kidney (Gardner & Evan, 1980). Microdissection studies have demonstrated that cysts arise only from the medullary collecting ducts (Gardner

& Evan, 1980). Light microscopic examination demonstrates predominantly findings of tubulointerstitial nephritis, namely interstitial fibrosis, with infiltration by lymphocytes, macrophages and plasma cells being common. Tubular atrophy in addition to periglomerular fibrosis and varying amounts of glomerular obsolescence or sclerosis are present depending upon the degree of renal functional loss at the time of histologic study.

Without evidence on biopsy of the classical cystic lesions, the diagnosis may be suspected and one may carry a patient with a presumed clinical diagnosis of NMCD; however, one must realize that the diagnosis always remains open to question. Some authors have advocated pretransplant nephrectomies in order to make definitive histologic diagnoses and provide genetic counselling information and information concerning potential sibling or parental donors, especially in the adult onset type of disease (Avasthi et al, 1976). Other laboratory investigations including intravenous pyelography or nephrosonography are usually not of significant value since cyst size is generally much less than 1 cm, beyond their resolution, and patients at the time of presentation usually have a significantly diminished GFR making IVP resolution poor.

In the absence of a family history, or with a biopsy not demonstrating the classical cysts, careful evaluation for other causes of tubulointerstitial nephritis must be made since only by histologic specimens can a definitive diagnosis be made. In the presence of a positive family history biopsy may rule out other entities such as hereditary nephritis (Alport disease) which is associated frequently with abnormalities of the renal basement membrane by histologic evaluation, and deafness, or chronic glomerulonephritis.

NMCD is also associated with several other syndromes. It is the most frequent cause of death in the Laurence-Moon-Biedl (Bardet-Biedl) syndrome (Alton & McDonald, 1973, Hurley et al, 1975). It is seen with skeletal abnormalities (Mainzer et al, 1970), the Alstrom Syndrome (Goldstein et al, 1971), and hyperuricemia (Thompson et al, 1978).

Therapy

Specific therapy for NMCD is lacking. One provides general care as for any patient with chronic renal failure. Generally, the physician should allow for maintenance of normal body electrolytes, CO_2, calcium and phosphorus to avoid metabolic derangements, bone disease (osteodystrophy and growth failure), and manage hypertension if present. At our institution we have seen over 10 children with NMCD progress to end stage. We have successfully performed renal allografts (cadaveric and living related donor grafts) in this group of patients. There is no report of recurrence of this disease in a transplanted kidney. There is, however, one report where a sibling recipient redeveloped end stage renal disease over several years, which was presumptively the natural course of NMCD that would have supervened in the donor due to the presence of this heritable disease (NMCD) that was not diagnosed at the time of the transplant (Avasthi et al, 1976). Patients with NMCD receiving renal transplants have results not different from other patients with end stage renal disease, and are appropriate candidates for dialysis and transplantation.

Pathogenesis

The pathogenesis of this disease entity remains essentially unknown. The lack of recurrence of disease in patients who have received renal allografts does suggest, however, that a circulating factor is not responsible for the cystic disease, and loss of renal function. Microdissection studies, which have demonstrated a specifically localized dilatation in the medullary collecting ducts, have as yet to provide any further clue to the pathogenesis of this disease (Gardner & Evan, 1980). The most promising animal model is currently that of Evan and Gardner (1979) who by administration of chemical substances have produced isolated cystic dilatation of rat nephrons. They have postulated that intralumenal obstruction produces subsequent alterations in renal function. The applicability of this work to pathogenesis of human medullary cystic disease, however, remains unclear.

Genetics

Recent reviews of NMCD appear to have now placed the genetics on a sound basis. Approximately 2/3 of well-studied cases have had an autosomal recessive mode of inheritance (Gardner & Evan, 1980). This group includes both the isolated juvenile or onset in childhood pattern of the disease, as well as those cases associated with retinal lesions. Approximately 1/4 of cases have an autosomal dominant pattern of inheritance (Gardner & Evan, 1980). The incidence of disease in both males and females is approximately equal in all types of NMCD. The remainder of cases, approximately 10%, appear to be sporadic, that is, without a documentable family history. There appear to be at present no studies of the incidence of this disease complex or of the gene frequency in the population as a whole.

There have been preliminary reports that heterozygotes of the autosomal recessive type have had a partial defect in concentrating ability, but these are yet to be confirmed in larger series. There are currently no methods available for diagnosing heterozygotes. Prenatal diagnosis in a family with previously affected children is not possible. One can only follow a child or adult suspected of having medullary cystic disease by measuring renal function, following concentrating ability periodically, and observing for symptoms of polyuria and polydypsia.

MEDULLARY SPONGE KIDNEY

The first description of medullary sponge kidney (MSK) was made about 40 years ago (Lenarduzzi, 1939; Thorne, 1944). MSK is characterised pathologically by dilatation and/or cystic malformations of the medullary collecting ducts within the renal pyramids, especially at the papillary tips. This entity may be unilateral or bilateral and involve all or only some of the renal pyramids. Its incidence is not well-established, as the diagnosis is usually made only by intravenous urography. Consequently, many asymptomatic patients with this disease never have a definitive diagnosis made. The incidence of MSK was approximately 0.5% when estimated by radiographic criteria on a series of 2600 consecutive urograms (Mayall, 1959).

Clinical description

The vast majority of patients present with renal colic, urinary tract infections (UTI), or gross haematuria (Harrison, 1979, Eckstrom et al, 1959). These presenting factors are attributable to either urinary tract infection or calculi. A small number of patients in some series have also presented with painless microscopic haematuria, while asymptomatic patients are often diagnosed when an intravenous urogram is done for other indications. Presenting symptoms usually occur between the third and sixth decades, although MSK has been diagnosed in a child 5 years old. Progressive loss of renal function, hypertension, as well as other significant management problems, were frequently reported in the early series appearing in the literature (Eckstrom). However, more recently, others have reported that patients with MSK have little progressive loss of renal function (Harrison & Rose, 1979). Renal parenchymal stones, of any aetiology, including MSK, predispose to infection. Patients with MSK often remain symptomatic for years with recurrent calculi and UTI in the majority of cases. Approximately one-half of all patients have hypercalciuria, the aetiology of which is presently unknown (Harrison & Rose, 1979).

More common complications include papillary necrosis, pyelonephritis, and hypertension. These usually occur if either renal parenchymal scarring is present at the time of diagnosis, or if urinary tract obstruction secondary to stones has been present (Eckstrom et al, 1959, Harrison & Rose, 1979). Many patients do require surgical procedures, including pyelolithotomies, ureteral lithotomies, and endoscopy with basketing of stones, but rarely partial or total nephrectomy.

Differential diagnosis

Many patients with MSK have been referred to stone clinics with a diagnosis of nephrocalcinosis, but after a careful history and review of radiographic material, are reclassified as MSK. The radiographic findings are pooled contrast material and cysts or dilated tubules in the renal papillae or deep medullary rays (Lalli, 1969). These pools of contrast usually appear early in the urogram and are persistent after parenchymal opacification has cleared (Lalli, 1969). A diagnostic dilemma is often present in the patient who has papillary necrosis, or pyelonephritis with significant damage to the renal papilla, since the resultant radiographic findings may mimic MSK, especially when stones are present in the renal papillary region (MacDougall & Prout, 1968). In patients who already have somewhat compromised renal function, visualisation on intravenous urography is often poor, again obfuscating the diagnosis.

Other entities which must be considered in the differential diagnosis are papillary tuberculosis, now rarely seen; infantile PKD, usually easily distinguishable by the patient's age; calyceal diverticuli or cysts, which are usually solitary; pyelonephritic scars or cavitation and microabscesses, usually accompanied by cortical loss; renal papillary necrosis, often associated with diabetes; and nephrocalcinosis, which usually has renal cortical involvement as well (MacDougall & Prout, 1968). Differentiation of MSK from these other disease entities is usually not difficult except when pyelonephritis is present with scarring and infection.

There appears to be significant variability and heterogeneity within this disorder. On radiographs an initial finding may be a slightly increased amount of contrast remaining in the papillary tips, without cystic dilatation, which has been described in 1% of urograms (Palubinsakis, 1963). As cited above a 0.5% incidence of MSK has been reported. Whether this intermediate pyelographic finding is a form fruste of the disease, or whether it is an early form which will progress to full MSK, is unknown. This radiographic finding may also be a variant of normal. Further research is needed in order to define these points.

Therapy

There is no specific therapy for MSK, other than management of the complications and problems which occur. The management of chronic UTIs with or without renal calculi can be found in many texts or reviews on the subject. Patients who have hypercalciuria can also be evaluated and treated as any other patient.

Pathogenesis

The pathogenesis of this disease remains entirely unclear. However, several theories have emerged. Since the distal collecting ducts arise embryologically from the ureteric bud during its early branching, several investigators have theorized that a hereditary defect exists in these structures, but that only during development of further life do the tubules manifest cystic dilatations and abnormalities. There are no animal models for study and one can truly only speculate presently about its pathogenesis.

Genetics

There have been multiple reports of MSK in the literature and the overwhelming majority of cases appear to be sporadic. There have, however, been several reports of MSK occurring in multiple family members. Copping reported an occurrence in father and daughter. The most convincing report is that from Kuiper (1971), where he documents four cases of MSK in three generations, and has suspected evidence for 3 more cases in another generation. Currently first order relatives of patients with MSK are not routinely investigated. The above cited case reports do suggest, however, that a certain percentage of MSK may have a familial pattern. This entity may be similar to nephronophthisis-medullary cystic disease complex where there are clearly several type of inheritance and it is impossible to classify the sporadic cases. The vast majority of cases of MSK are sporadic, and radiographs of other family members are not routinely justified. However, one should obtain a family history to be aware of any possible familial disease.

RENAL CYSTS ASSOCIATED WITH OTHER SYNDROMES

Many syndromes have been associated with renal cysts. The most frequently found type of cystic disease in small newborn children is cystic dysplasia. This entity is usually unilateral although it may be bilateral, and is not familial. Frequently, syndromes with multiple malformations are also seen with renal cysts, the most well-known being tuberous sclerosis, Von Hippel-Lindau disease, Jeune syndrome, and the trisomies D and E. A more complete list and a fuller description of these entities can be found in the discussion of congenital renal disorders in this text.

REFERENCES

Alton D J, McDonald P 1973 Urographic findings in the Bardet-Biedl syndrome. Radiology 109: 659–663

Anand S K, Chan J C, Lieberman E 1975 Polycystic disease and hepatic fibrosis in children: Renal function studies. American Journal of Diseases of Childhood 129: 810–813

Anonymous 1979 Polycystic disease of the kidneys. British Medical Journal 1: 291–292

Avasthi P S, Erickson D G, Gardner K D 1976 Hereditary renal-retinal dysplasia and the medullary cystic disease-nephronophthisis complex. Annals of Internal Medicine 84: 157–161

Baert L 1978 Hereditary polycystic kidney disease (adult form): A microdissection study of two cases at an early stage of the disease. Kidney International 13: 519–525

Bernstein J 1979 Polycystic disease. In: Edelmann Jr. C M (ed) Pediatric Kidney Disease, vol II. Little Brown and Company, Boston. ch 40, pp 557–570

Bernstein J 1980 Infantile polycystic disease. In: Hamburger J, Crosnier J. Grunfeld J-P (eds) Nephrology, Wiley-Flammarion, New York and Paris, ch 73, pp 1023–1031

Bernstein J, Gardner Jr. KD 1979 Familial Juvenile nephronophthisis – medullary cystic disease. In: Edelmann Jr. C M (ed) Pediatric Kidney Disease, vol II. Little Brown and Company, Boston. ch 42, pp 580–586

Blyth H, Ockenden B G 1971 Polycystic disease of kidneys and liver presenting in childhood. Journal of Medical Genetics 8: 257–284

Boichis H, Passwell J, David R, Miller H 1973 Congenital hepatic fibrosis and nephronophthisis. Quarterly Journal of Medicine, New Series, XLII 165: 221–229

Cameron J R 1961 Bilateral "hereditary" polycystic disease of the kidneys associated with bilateral teratodactyly of the feet. British Journal of Urology 33: 473–477

Chanmugam D, Rasaretnam R, Karunaratne K E de S 1968 Genetic intelligence: hereditary spherocytosis and polycystic disease of the kidneys in four members of a family. American Journal of Human Genetics 23: 66

Chester A C, Argy Jr W P, Rakowski T A, Schreiner G E 1978 Polycystic kidney disease and chronic hemodialysis. Clinical Nephrology 10: 129–133

Collan Y, Sipponen P, Haapanen E, Lindahl J, Jokinen E J, Hjelt L 1977 Hereditary nephronophthisis with a life span of three decades: Light and electron microscopical, immunohistochemical, clinical and family studies. Virchows Archives of Pathology Anatomy and Histology 376: 195–208

Copping G A, 1967 Medullary sponge kidney: Its occurrence in a father and daughter. Canadian Medical Association Journal 96: 608–611

Dalgaard O Z 1957 Polycystic disease of the kidneys: A follow-up study of 284 patients and their families. Acta Medica Scandinavia 158, Sup 328

Del Guercio E, Greco J, Kim K E, Chinitz J, Swartz C 1973 Esophageal varices in adult patients with polycystic kidney and liver disease. New England Journal of Medicine 289: 678–682

Eckstrom T, Engfeldt B, Lagergren C, Lindrall N 1959 medullary sponge kidney. Almqvist and Wiksell, Stockholm

Emery A E H, Oleesky S, Williams R T 1967 Myotonic dystrophy and polycystic disease of the kidneys. Journal of Medical Genetics 4: 26–28

Eulderink F, Hogewind B L 1978 Renal cysts in premature children: Occurrence in a family with polycystic kidney disease. Archives of Pathology and Laboratory Medicine 102: 592–595

Evan A P, Gardner K D, Bernstein J 1979 Polypoid and papillary epithelial hyperplasia: A potential cause of ductal obstruction in adult polycystic disease. Kidney International 16: 743–750

Fried K, Liban E, Lurie M, Friedman S, Reisner S H 1971 Polycystic kidneys associated with malformations of the brain, polydactyly, and other birth defects in newborn sibs. Journal of Medical Genetics 8: 285–290

Friedrich U, et al 1979 Prenatal diagnosis of polycystic kidneys and encephalocele (Meckel syndrome). Clinical Genetics 15: 278–286

Gardner K D, Evan A P 1980 The nephronophthisis-cystic renal medulla complex. In: Hamburger J, Crosnier J, Grunfeld J-P (eds) Nephrology, Wiley-Flammarion New York and Paris, ch 63, pp 893–907

Goldstein J L, Rialkow P J 1973 The alstrom syndrome. Medicine 52: 53–71

Harrison A R, Rose G A 1979 Medullary sponge kidney. Urological Research 7: 197–207

Harrod M J E, Stokes J, Peede L F, Goldstein J L 1976 Polycystic kidney disease in a patient with the oral-facial-digital syndrome – Type 1. Clinical Genetics 9: 183–186

Hayslett J P 1979 Medullary sponge kidney. In: Edelmann Jr C M (ed), Pediatric kidney disease, vol II, Little, Brown and Company, Boston, ch 72, pp 889–893

Heggo O, Natvig J B 1965 Cystic disease of the kidneys. Acta Pathologica et Microbiologica Scandinavia 64: 459–469

Hurley R M, Dery P, Nogrady M B, Drummond K N 1975 The renal lesion of the Laurence-Moon-Biedl syndrome. Journal of Pediatrics 87: 206–209

Hutchins K R, Mulholland S G, Edson M 1972 Case report: Segmental polycystic disease. New York State Journal of Medicine, 72: 1850–1852

Kaye C, Lewy P R 1974 Congenital appearance of adult-type (autosomal dominant) polycystic kidney disease: Report of a case. Journal of Pediatrics 85: 807–808

Kieselstein M, Herman G, Wahrman J, Voss R, Gitelson S, Feuchtwanger M, Kadar S 1969 Mucocutaneous Pigmentation and intestinal polyposis (Peutz-Jeghers syndrome) in a family of Iraqi Jews with polycystic kidney disease. Isreal Journal of Medical Science 5: 81–90

Kissane J M 1980 Adult polycystic disease. In: Hamburger J, Crosnier J, Grunfeld J-P (eds) Nephrology. Wiley-Flammarion, New York and Paris, ch 62, pp 887–892

Kuiper J J 1971 Medullary sponge kidney in three generations. New York State Journal of Medicine, 71: 2665–2669

Lalli A F 1969 Medullary sponge kidney disease. Radiology 92: 92–96

Le Jars F 1888 Du gros rein polykystique de l'adulte. Steinheill, Paris, pp 5, 55

Lenarduzzi G 1939 Reporto pielografico poca commune dialazione della vie urinaire intrarenali. Radiologica Medica 26: 346

Lieberman E, Salinas-Madrigal L, Gwinn J L, Brennan L P, Fine R N, Landing B H 1971 Infantile polycystic disease of the kidneys and liver: Clinical, pathological and radiological correlations and comparison with congenital hepatic fibrosis. Medicine 50: 277–318

Lundin P M, Olow I 1961 Polycystic kidneys in newborns, infants and children: A clinical and pathological study. Acta Paediatrica 50: 185–200

MacDougall J A, Prout W G 1968 Medullary sponge kidney: Clinical appraisal and report of twelve cases. British Journal of Surgery 55: 130–133

Mainzer F, Saldino R M, Ozonoff M B, Minagi H 1970 Familial nephropathy associated with retinitis pigmentosa, cerebellar ataxia and skeletal abnormalities. American Journal of Medicine 49: 556–562

Mayall G F 1959 Roentgenologic diagnosis of medullary sponge kidney. Acta Radiologica 51: 193–199

Mendoza S A, Griswold W R, Leopold G R, Kaplan G W 1979 Intrauterine diagnosis of renal anomalies by ultrasonography. American Journal of Diseases of Childhood 133: 1042–1043

Older R A, Hinman C G, Crane L M, Cleeve D M, Morgan C L 1979 In utero diagnosis of multicystic kidney by gray scale ultrasonography. American Journal of Radiology 133: 130–131

Palubinskas A J 1963 Renal pyramidal structure opacification in excretory urography and its relation to medullary sponge kidney. Radiology 81: 963–970

Piering W F, Hebert L A, Lemann Jr J 1977 Infantile polycystic kidney disease in the adult. Archives of Internal Medicine 137: 1625–1626

Pontasse E F, Gardner W J, McCormack L J 1954 Polycystic kidney disease and intracranial aneurysms. Journal of American Medical Association 159: 741–749

Preuss H, Geoly K, Johnson M, Chester A, Kliger A, Schreiner G 1979 Tubular function in adult polycystic kidney disease. Nephron 24: 198–204

Rabinowitz R, Segal A J, Mohan Rao H K, Pathak A 1978 Computed tomography in diagnosis of infantile polycystic kidney disease. Journal of Urology 120: 616–617

Rayfield E J, McDonald F D 1972 Red and blonde hair in renal medullary cystic disease. Archives of Internal Medicine 130: 72–75

Reilly K B, Rubin S P, Blanke B G, Yeh M-N 1979 Infantile polycystic kidney disease: A difficult antenatal diagnosis. American Journal of Obstetrics and Gynecology 133: 580–582

Schimke R N 1969 Hereditary renal-retinal dysplasia. Annals of Internal Medicine 70: 735–744

Segal A J, Spataro R F, Barbaric 1977 Adult polycystic kidney disease: A review of 100 cases. Journal of Urology 118: 711–713

Senior B 1973 Familial renal-retinal dystrophy. American Journal of Diseases of Childhood 125: 442–447

Shoker M H K 1978 Expression of "adult" polycystic renal disease in the fetus and newborn. Clinical Genetics 14: 61–72

Thomas J L, Sumner T E, Crowe J E 1978 Neonatal detection and evaluation of infantile polycystic disease by gray scale echography. Journal of Clinical Ultrasound 6: 343–344

Thompson G R, Weiss J J, Goldman R T, Rigg G A 1978 Familial occurrence of hyperuricemia, gout, and medullary cystic disease. Archives of Internal Medicine 138: 1614–1617

Thorn G W, Koepf G F, Clinton M 1944 Renal failure simulating adrenocortical insufficiency. New England Journal of Medicine 231: 76–78

van Collenburg J J M, Thompson M W, Huber J 1978 Clinical, pathological and genetic aspects of a form of cystic disease of the renal medulla: familial juvenile nephronophthisis (FJN). Clinical Nephrology 9: 55–62

Vuthibhagdee A, Singleton E B 1973 Infantile polycystic disease of the kidney. American Journal of Diseases of Childhood 125: 167–170

73

The nephrotic syndromes

R. Norio

INTRODUCTION

The nephrotic syndrome (NS) is a *clinical* diagnosis. It is characterised by oedema, proteinuria, hypoalbuminaemia and hyperlipaemia, and sometimes by microscopic haematuria and arterial hypertension. Response to treatment with steroids or cytotoxic drugs and survival time in the nonresponders vary greatly. Several pathogenetic pathways may lead to NS. Their common denominator is the altered permeability of the glomerular filtration barrier; its details are poorly known.

The classification of NS is largely based on renal histology. This has produced a variety of *descriptive* diagnoses. Clinical genetics, however, endeavours to find an *aetiological* diagnosis. This is difficult for renal disease in general and for the nephrotic syndromes in particular. An essential prerequisite is to take all the findings into account, not only one or two details, however important. Also the microscopic picture alone seldom provides a specific aetiological diagnosis. Very few histological renal findings are pathognomonic for a particular disease; they indicate the progression of the disease rather than give an accurate aetiological diagnosis. This is obvious if several specimens can be studied from the same patient at different ages. In fact, naming a renal disease only by aid of the microscope has led to a confusing diversity in the nomenclature, not only in the descriptions of individual patients but also in classifications.

The main interest of this chapter is directed toward the primary nephrotic syndromes, often without known cause. They mostly affect the paediatric age groups. NS may be called secondary if it occurs as a part of a renal or some other disease entity or is caused by a known exogenous factor. Most adult NS patients belong to this group. Thus, NS occurs associated with many systemic diseases such as anaphylactoid purpura, amyloidosis, diabetes, lupus erythematosus, and sickle cell disease. Known or assumed causes for NS are infections such as maternal syphilis (Hill et al, 1972; Kaschula et al, 1974) and toxoplasmosis (Shahin et al, 1974), cytomegalovirus (de Luca et al, 1964) or E. coli (Flatz, 1964). In Africa the epidemiology of NS differs greatly from that in nontropical countries, being apparently caused by malaria and possibly also by other infections (see the Editorial 'Nephrotic syndrome in the tropics', Lancet 1980: 2:461). Cases of NS have been attributed to toxic agents like mercury (Worthen et al, 1959), bee sting, or maternal steroid-chlorpheniramine treatment (Anand et al, 1979). Among the renal diseases reported to be associated with or complicated by NS, several 'nephritic' disorders, at least in their advanced phases, are common, and nephroblastoma (Zunin & Soave, 1964) and nail-patella syndrome (Similä et al, 1970) are rare. Renal vein thrombosis is nowadays regarded not as a cause but a complication of NS (Kaplan et al, 1978). For further details of secondary NS as well as for other specific features of NS, the reader is referred to textbooks of nephrology.

It is difficult to find a practical grouping for primary NS for the purposes of clinical genetics. Only a few aetiological groups are known. Any attempt at too strict and systematic a classification would lead to confusion and unwarranted conclusions. A suitable balance between nosological splitting and lumping (McKusick, 1969) must be found. A few clearly defined aetiological entities can be split off, whereas other nephrotic syndromes might be left lumped together as heterogeneous but clinically useful groups, until such time as additional knowledge allows for further splitting.

In this chapter the following grouping according to age at onset of NS is used:

Congenital nephrotic syndromes (CN)
— congenital nephrotic syndrome of Finnish type (CNF)
— other types (CNO)
Infantile nephrotic syndromes (IN)
— diffuse mesangial sclerosis (DMS)
— other types (INO)
Nephrotic syndromes of later onset (LN)

This grouping, modified from the terms used by White (1973), is a relative one, with compromises and overlapping among the groups. It may, however, be useful as regards treatment, prognosis, genetic counselling and prenatal diagnosis. Before placing a patient in any of the groups, the possibility of a 'secondary' causative factor must be taken into account.

CONGENITAL NEPHROTIC SYNDROMES (CN)

Congenital nephrotic syndromes are apparently present at birth, at least latently, and become manifest by the age of three months. In this group the congenital nephrotic syndrome of Finnish type is the only distinct aetiological entity known.

Congenital nephrotic syndrome of Finnish type (CNF)
Since the 1950s (Hallman et al, 1956) this disease has raised active interest among Finnish paediatricians because it has proved to be exceptionally common in Finland. By 1973, 151 patients were known, and the number now exceeds 200. The incidence in Finland is about 1 in 8000 (Huttunen, 1976). However, CNF has been reported from all over the world (Norio, 1966; Hallman et al, 1970), most cases among the Caucasians, but also among Negroes (Eiben et al, 1954; George et al, 1976), American Indians (George et al, 1976), Japanese (Kobayashi et al, 1961; Yamamoto et al, 1961), Indians (Rajamma et al, 1974) and Maoris (Kendall-Smith et al, 1968). About 150 CNF or CNF-like cases have been published outside Finland. Of the cases of NS manifesting in the first year of life, one half in North America (according to George et al, 1976) and one third in France (judging by the series of Habib & Bois, 1973) may have CNF.

The clinical picture of CNF varies only slightly (Hallman et al, 1970, 1973; Huttunen, 1976; Hallman & Rapola, 1978). As proof of the congenital character of CNF, the placenta is obviously always abnormally large, amounting to more than 25% of the birth weight (Fig. 73.1). The majority of patients are born prematurely – 90% of them before the 39th week of gestation – and are small for dates. Signs of perinatal asphyxia, such as meconium-stained amniotic fluid, low Apgar score and respiratory distress, are common; some patients die perinatally before the diagnosis of CNF has been made. Malformations are not a part of CNF; broad cranial sutures may be a sign of delayed ossification, and flexed ankles may indicate muscular weakness.

Proteinuria probably always exists from birth. Oedema is detectable from birth in one fourth of the cases, during the first week of life in half, and by the age of three months in all cases.

The patients fail to thrive; they never learn to walk or speak. Distension of the abdomen, due to meteorism and ascites, is a very characteristic sign; herniae are common. After the first few months the appearance is dystrophic rather than oedematous (Fig. 73.2).

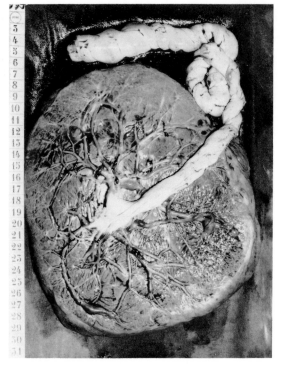

Fig. 73.1 Large placenta of newborn CNF infant; weight 1850 g, measurements 25 × 22 × 6 cm.

High susceptibility to infections and complete resistance to corticosteroids and antimetabolites are a rule. The outcome is always fatal, in half the cases by 6 months, in 75% by 12 months and always by 4 years of age. The cause of death is often infections, never uraemia, but the precise cause of death remains unknown in nearly half of the cases. Thromboembolic complications have been found at autopsy in a fifth of the recent cases. The laboratory findings are similar to those of NS in general. Proteinuria is massive and in most patients selective (Huttunen et al, 1980b). Microscopic haematuria occurs often; leucocytes, amino acids and glucose may also be found in the urine. The values of blood urea nitrogen are in general normal, sometimes slightly raised but never grossly elevated.

The kidneys are large as compared to the weight of the patient. The histological alterations are polymorphic and progressive; no single finding is pathognomonic or necessary for the diagnosis (Hallman et al, 1973; Hallman & Rapola, 1978; Huttunen et al, 1980a). Dilatations of the proximal, but sometimes also distal, tubules are the most characteristic findings. Their amount varies greatly, from an occasional dilatation to a universal dispersion throughout the renal cortex. The tubular epithelium is tall in the beginning, but flat and atrophic in advanced cases. In the glomeruli, proliferation of mesangial cells and increase of PAS- and silver-positive matrix are char-

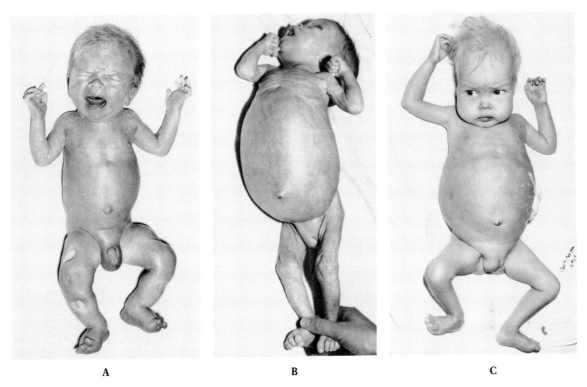

Fig. 73.2 Three infants with CNF.
A. A boy, age 2 weeks, with oedema of the face and particularly of the lower limbs.
B. A severely affected girl, age 7 months, with a typical opisthotonic position, greatly distended abdomen, dystrophic but not oedematous appearance, and right inguinal hernia.
C. A girl, age 2 years 2 months, with milder course and longer survival than average.

acteristic; this mesangial sclerosis does not cause narrowing of the capillaries except in the very advanced cases. In a part of the glomeruli, periglomerular onion-like fibrosis gradually leads to obstruction and total hyalinization. Immature glomeruli with condensed tufts and wide Bowman's space are often seen in young patients, but according to the latest investigation (Huttunen et al, 1980a) they are also seen in normal infants of the same age, even more frequently than in CNF. In the interstitium, round cell infiltration and fibrosis increase with age. For electron microscopic findings see Rapola and Savilahti (1971) and Hallman and Rapola (1978).

Because of the complete resistance to corticosteroids or antimetabolites, treatment is purely symptomatic. Attempts at renal transplantation in nine Finnish patients have failed; in the small and chronically 'undernourished' patients both technical and postoperative difficulties are immense. From other countries there are two reports of successful renal transplantation: for three patients aged 4, $2\frac{1}{2}$ and $2\frac{1}{2}$ years of Hoyer et al (1973) and for one infant aged 2 years and 4 months reported by Floret et al (1976). The patients of Hoyer et al were from Minnesota – a state abundant with Finnish immig-

rants – and one of them had pure Finnish ancestry. In spite of this, none of the case reports gave a completely typical picture of CNF; thus the aetiology remains uncertain.

CNF is an autosomal recessive disease. In a series of 57 Finnish families (Norio, 1966) the sex ratio was 1.07 and the proportion of affected sibs very close to 0.25. 16 parental marriages were shown to be consanguineous, even if remotely in most cases. 43 parents (38%) were related to parents of other CN families.

The ancestry was distributed unevenly in a large area which has been permanently populated for less than 500 years. In fact, CNF was the first of the rare recessive disorders (there are now over 20) discovered to be overrepresented among the Finns. This concentration of recessive disorders is due to the peculiar population structure of Finland (Norio et al, 1973; Norio & Nevanlinna, 1980; Norio, 1981).

Heterozygous manifestations are not known. True, Kniker and Prindiville (1969) and Kniker and Sweeney (1972) reported having found slightly increased amounts of glomerular basement membrane-like material in the urine of relatives of CNF patients but this finding could not be substantiated in Finnish patients (Huttunen et al, 1976).

Although the prognosis of CNF patients is poor, the families can be helped by prenatal diagnosis since alpha-fetoprotein (AFP) concentration is very high in the amniotic fluid and often also in maternal serum (Aula et al, 1978), apparently due to fetal proteinuria even by the second trimester. Up to 1980, 43 pregnancies of families with a previous CN baby have been monitored in Finland without a single false result (P. Aula, personal communication). In the AFP-screening of maternal serum of 10 504 Finnish pregnancies, 4 fetuses with confirmed CNF and 2 suspected cases have been found (Ryynänen et al, 1982). CNF is one possibility to be taken into account in pregnancies with a 'false-positive' AFP-result; this diagnosis can be confirmed from ultrastructural and recently also from light microscopic findings of the fetal kidneys (Rapola, 1981). Whenever CNF is to be expected, the pregnancy should be terminated by hysterotomy, because autolysis greatly hampers the interpretation of renal histology in prostaglandin or saline induced abortions (Aula et al, 1978). Prenatal diagnosis may not be possible in other forms of congenital or infantile nephrosis (Spritz et al, 1978; Rapola & Hallman, 1979).

The pathogenesis of CNF is unknown. The reported immunological abnormalities of earlier studies (Lange et al, 1963; Kouvalainen, 1963) have not been confirmed (Hoyer et al, 1967; Rapola & Savilahti, 1971; Griswold & McIntosh, 1972) and are thus apparently secondary. The increased permeability of the glomerular basement membrane could be due to a genetically determined failure in its synthesis (Norio, 1966), but studies of the basement membrane have not solved the question so far (Mahieu et al, 1976; Tryggvason, 1977). Glomeruli are present in nearly twice the normal number (Tryggvason & Kouvalainen, 1975).

Other kinds of congenital nephrotic syndrome(CNO)
An undisputed diagnosis of CNF brings with it very decisive consequences for the infant and his family: the disease leads to a rapid and certain death, has a recurrence risk of 25% for sibs, and prenatal diagnosis is possible. Therefore, a definite diagnosis of CNF should not be made on uncertain grounds. According to the Finnish experience, the disease is very unlikely to be CNF if the weight of the placenta is normal, if age at onset is more than 3 months, if psychomotor development is within normal limits, if the patient shows overt uraemia or is alive at the age of 4 years or more. A 'congenital' manifestation of NS need not necessarily imply CNF but may also be due to either an exogenous or an unknown 'idiopathic' aetiology. Because of considerable overlap with related disorders they will be discussed together with 'Infantile nephrotic syndromes'.

INFANTILE NEPHROTIC SYNDROMES (IN)

Diffuse mesangial sclerosis (DMS)
In the group of NS manifesting at 3 to 12 months of age, the histopathological diagnosis of diffuse mesangial sclerosis (DMS) probably delineates a clinically and possibly also an aetiologically distinct entity. Habib and Bois (1973) introduced the idea when reporting six patients from France. At least 13 other patients with possible DMS have been described (Rossenbeck et al, Family 1, 1966; Hallman et al, 1973; Kaplan et al, 1974; Richard et al, 1975; Seelig et al, 1975; Gonzales et al, 1977; Rumpelt & Bachmann, 1980).

Nothing exceptional is known about the pregnancy or perinatal features; the placenta, in particular, has not been reported to be abnormally large (a possible exception is patient 1 described by Rossenbeck et al, 1966). Age of manifesting oedema or proteinuria has mostly been 1 to 13 months, though in one case at 2 weeks (Rumpelt & Bachmann, 1980). The patients develop progressive renal insufficiency, which is often also the cause of death. The disease is resistant to steroids or cytotoxic drugs, and the outcome is always fatal, usually by the age of 4 years.

The histological picture is characteristic, perhaps pathognomonic, and differs distinctly from that seen in CNF. All glomeruli are affected. The capillary tufts are small and contracted, and Bowman's space seems correspondingly wide. The number of glomerular cells is not increased. Instead, mesangial PAS- and silver-positive sclerosing fibrils are a constant finding, and the capillaries are severely occluded. Epithelial crescents may be present. Tubular atrophy and dilatations are common, as is interstitial fibrosis. Rumpelt and Bachmann (1980) have described a 'cloudy pattern' alteration of the glomerular basement membrane by electron microscopy.

In two families reported by Habib and Bois and in three other probable DMS families (Rossenbeck, Gonzales) two or three sibs have been affected. This suggests autosomal recessive inheritance. Attempts at prenatal diagnosis have not been reported; it may not be possible.

Other kinds of infantile nephrotic syndrome (INO)
Nephrotic syndrome is a rare disease during the first year of life. At that age also the cause may be exceptional. If an individual patient does not fit into the narrow limits of CNF or DMS or if an undisputed exogenous cause cannot be traced, very little can be said about the clinical course, response to treatment, prognosis, aetiology, and risk of recurrence in subsequent sibs. It seems that INO is often associated with overt histological glomerular changes and poor prognosis, and is often familial. The clinical features may appear in all possible combinations. A congenital manifestation – even with a large placenta

– may, in contrast to CNF, be compatible with normal growth and development, considerably longer survival (Vernier et al, 1957; Gantner, 1965; Habib & Bois, 1973) and even complete recovery (Anand et al, 1979). Moreover, the onset may be 'late' but the course rapidly fatal (Nagi & Nouri, 1974). In familial cases, affected members of a sibship may show wide variation as concerns age at onset, course, prognosis and survival (Mehls & Schärer, 1970). An unanswered question is, whether the CNF gene in a non-Finnish genetic background might, in a proportion of cases, cause a milder disorder with longer survival (and terminal renal failure) (Hoyer et al, 1973; Moncrieff et al, 1973, Family 2) than is the rule in Finland. However, different recessive genes are probably responsible for many cases of INO.

Many attempts at a histological classification may in the clinical sense be confusing rather than helpful. However, the classifications of Habib & Bois (1973) and Kaplan et al (1974) are also useful clinically. Many authors use the word 'microcystic' when speaking of the tubular dilatations typical of CNF. When Oliver (1960) introduced this term, he did not give detailed clinical data on his patients nor did he use it as a synonym for CNF. Unfortunately the term has come to have various meanings. As a histological term, 'microcystic' may lead to confusion with 'true' polycystic diseases of the kidney. Tubular dilatations are not seen in every renal biopsy specimen of CNF patients. Instead, they can be found in many other entities, e.g. DMS. Oliver himself reported patients who died 'in many instances of terminal renal failure'. The term microcystic renal disease should obviously be abandoned as the synonym for CNF (Hallman et al, 1973).

It is reasonable to try conventional treatment of NS in cases of INO, although the results are uncertain. Genetic counselling in families with INO must be done cautiously, bearing in mind the possibility of autosomal recessive transmission.

NEPHROTIC SYNDROMES OF LATER ONSET (LN)

'Idiopathic' nephrotic syndrome usually manifests after the first year of life. The majority, about 80% or more of the cases, belong histologically to the group with 'minimal (glomerular) changes'; of these, over 90% respond to varying degrees to treatment with steroids or cytotoxic agents. The rest show various histological glomerular changes and their prognosis is distinctly poorer.

It is usually assumed that 'idiopathic' nephrotic syndrome, here called nephrotic syndrome of later onset (LN), is a non-familial disease. However, surprisingly many familial cases have been reported. By 1968 I had found 79 familial cases in the literature (Norio, 1969). In the series of their own patients Mehls and Schärer (1970) from Germany described 12 familial cases out of 135 (?) (9%), Bader et al (1974a,b) from Indiana, USA, 14 out of 70 (20%), and Gekle et al (1975) from Germany 4 out of 73 (5%). Moncrieff et al (1973) reported at least 20 familial cases from Great Britain, Gonzales et al (1977) 24 cases from France, and White (1973) 40 cases out of about 1850 (2%) through an inquiry in 24 European paediatric departments. The majority of the familial cases are pairs of sibs, including 13 pairs of twins, all apparently monozygous (those reported by 1968, see Norio, 1969; Roy & Pitcock, 1971; Bader et al, 1974a,b). As yet, no familial LN cases are known in Finland.

The clinical data on familial LN found in the literature are fragmentary, difficult to combine and, in part, even contradictory. Without presenting a detailed analysis of them, some conclusions, even if uncertain, may be justified:

Marked histological glomerular alterations are observed in a far greater proportion of patients (about a half of those reported by White, 1973) than in the non-familial cases; prognosis is worse than average in these cases.

The prognosis for patients with minimal changes is similar to that in non-familial cases.

The histological grouping of an individual patient may change during the course of the disease.

The clinical features (age at onset, histological picture and prognosis) are often similar in affected sibs, but there are numerous exceptions to this rule, even in identical twins (Bader et al, 1974a,b).

A male preponderance is also evident in familial LN.

Aetiologically LN certainly is heterogeneous. As in most common disorders, the exact role of heredity has not been discovered. The familial cases of 'usual' LN have occurred mostly in pairs, i.e. only two affected sibs per family. Monozygous twins, all concordantly affected, have been overrepresented and no dizygous concordant twin pairs with LN have been reported. Some cases of LN in two consecutive generations or in near collateral relatives are also known (Norio, 1969; White, 1973; Gekle et al, 1975). Based on these facts I suggested the possibility of a polygenic basis for at least a proportion of LN cases (Norio, 1969). The analysis of Bader et al (1974 a,b) gives support to this assumption.

Besides the 'usual' familial LN there are several reports of 'unusual' families with juvenile and infantile, or even congenital cases in the same sibship (Moncrieff et al, 1973, Families V & VI). Also the course of the disease may vary greatly between sibs, ranging from symptomless proteinuria to a rapidly fatal outcome, and from minimal glomerular changes to severe histological alterations. In these exceptional cases, sibships with more than two affected sibs have been reported, and sometimes also parental consanguinity (Fanconi & Illig, 1960; Devin, 1960; Fournier et al, 1963). Probably different autosomal recessive genes are responsible in these cases.

The treatment of familial LN patients is similar to that of non-familial cases. Renal biopsy may give valuable clues to the course and prognosis. For genetic counselling, Bader et al (1974a,b) have estimated a surprisingly high recurrence risk of 6% for the sibs of a patient. A convenient figure for general use is perhaps less than 5% though many nephrologists might even be inclined towards a smaller risk figure, say less than 2%. However, overt glomerular alterations in a renal biopsy might indicate a greater risk of recurrence than in cases with minimal changes because patients with overt glomerular changes are particularly frequent among familial cases. Further, in many hereditary disorders the majority of patients are sporadic and only the minority are familial. Hence a proportion of non-familial LN patients with overt glomerular changes may in fact be genetic.

CONCLUSIONS

The nephrotic syndrome is aetiologically heterogeneous.

To achieve an accurate diagnosis the patient should be evaluated on a broad basis rather than concentrating on one or two features only (e.g. renal histology). If a distinct exogenous aetiology is not demonstrable, age at onset may serve as a first criterion for further grouping.

In cases manifesting congenitally (or during the first 3 months of life) the congenital nephrotic syndrome of Finnish type, and in those manifesting during the first year of life diffuse mesangial sclerosis must be taken into consideration. The former diagnosis must be made on strict criteria only, because it means a hopeless prognosis, a recurrence risk of 25% in sibs and the possibility of prenatal diagnosis. In other, rare and poorly understood nephrotic syndromes during the first year of life, course and prognosis may vary greatly, being often severe. Familial occurrence is not unusual and autosomal recessive inheritance is possible, if not probable.

The 'usual' or 'idiopathic' nephrotic syndrome usually manifests after the first year of life. In at least some of these patients heredity may play an important role in aetiology, probably in some polygenic manner. The recurrence risk in sibs is greater than is universally assumed: perhaps less than 5% in general but greater in cases with overt histological glomerular alterations.

REFERENCES

Anand S K, Northway J D, Bernier R L 1979 Congenital nephrotic syndrome: report of a patient with cystic tubular changes who recovered. Journal of Pediatrics 95: 265

Aula P, Rapola J, Karjalainen O, Lindgren J, Hartikainen A L, Seppälä M 1978 Prenatal diagnosis of congenital nephrosis in 23 high-risk families. American Journal of Diseases of Children 132: 984

Bader P I, Grove J, Trygstad C W, Nance W E 1974a Familial nephrotic syndrome. American Journal of Medicine 56: 34

Bader P I, Grove J, Nance W E, Trygstad C W 1974b Inheritance of idiopathic nephrotic syndrome. Birth Defects: Original Article Series, Vol X, No 4: 73

Devin P 1960 Syndromes néphrotiques familiaux et congénitaux. Thèse médicale Nancy No. 27

Eiben R M, Kleinerman J, Cline J C 1954 Nephrotic syndrome in a neonatal premature infant. Journal of Pediatrics 44: 195

Fanconi G, Illig R 1960 Das familiäre Vorkommen der Lipoid-nephrose und der Nephronophthise. Moderne Probleme der Pädiatrie 6: 298

Flatz G 1964 Nephrotisches Syndrom und Pyknocytose bei einem jungen Säugling. Monatsschrift für Kinderheilkunde 112: 102

Floret D et al 1976 Transplantation rénale à l'age de 2 ans 4 mois pour syndrome néphrotique congénital. La Nouvelle Presse Médicale 5: 2701

Fournier A, Paget M, Pauli A, Devin P 1963 Syndromes néphrotiques familiaux. Syndrome néphrotique associé à une cardiopathie congénitale chez quatre soeurs. Pédiatrie 18: 677

Gantner J 1965 Das idiopathische nephrotische Syndrom im Säuglingsalter an Hand von vier eigenen Beobachtungen. Helvetica Paediatrica Acta 20: 374

Gekle D, Buchinger G, Könitzer I 1975 Untersuchungen zur Familiarität des nephrotischen Syndroms. Monatsschrift für Kinderheilkunde 123: 106

George C R P, Hickman R O, Stricker G E 1976 Infantile nephrotic syndrome. Clinical Nephrology 5: 20

Gonzales G, Kleinknecht C, Gubler M C, Lenoir G 1977 Syndromes néphrotiques familiaux. La Revue de Pédiatrie 13: 427

Griswold W, McIntosh R M 1972 Immunological studies in congenital nephrosis. Journal of Medical Genetics 9: 245

Habib R, Bois E 1973 Hétérogénéité des syndromes néphrotiques a debut précoce du nourisson (syndrome néphrotique 'infantile'). Etude anatomoclinique et génétique de 37 observations. Helvetica Paediatrica Acta 28: 91

Hallman N, Hjelt L, Ahvenainen E K 1956 Nephrotic syndrome in newborn and young infants. Annales Paediatriae Fenniae 2: 227

Hallman N, Norio R, Kouvalainen K, Vilska J, Kojo N 1970 Das kongenitale nephrotische Syndrom. Ergebnisse der Inneren Medizin und Kinderheilkunde 30: 3

Hallman N, Norio R, Rapola J 1973 Congenital nephrotic syndrome. Nephron 11: 101

Hallman N, Rapola J 1978 Congenital nephrotic syndrome. In: Edelman C M Jr (ed) Pediatric kidney disease, Little Brown and Company, Boston, Vol. 2, ch 54, 711

Hill L L, Singer D B, Falletta J, Stasney R 1972 The nephrotic syndrome in congenital syphilis. An immunopathy. Pediatrics 49: 260

Hoyer J R, Michael A F Jr, Good R A, Vernier R L 1967 The nephrotic syndrome of infancy: clinical, morphologic, and immunologic studies of four infants. Pediatrics 40: 233

Hoyer J R et al 1973 Successful renal transplantation in 3 children with congenital nephrotic syndrome. Lancet 1: 1410

Huttunen N–P 1976 Congenital nephrotic syndrome of Finnish type: study of 75 patients. Archives of Diseases in Childhood 51: 344

Huttunen N–P, Hallman N, Rapola J 1976 Glomerular basement membrane antigens in congenital and acquired nephrotic syndrome in childhood. Nephron 16: 401

Huttunen N–P, Rapola J, Vilska J, Hallman N 1980a Renal pathology in congenital nephrotic syndrome of Finnish type: a quantitative light microscopic study on 50 patients. International Journal of Pediatric Nephrology 1: 10

Huttunen N–P, Vehaskari M, Viikari M, Laipio M–L 1980b Proteinuria in congenital nephrotic syndrome of the Finnish type. Clinical Nephrology 13: 12

Kaplan B S, Bureau M A, Drummond K N 1974 The nephrotic syndrome in the first year of life: is a pathologic classification possible? Journal of Pediatrics 85: 615

Kaplan B S, Chesney R W, Drummond K N 1978 The nephrotic syndrome and renal vein thrombosis. American Journal of Diseases of Children 132: 367

Kaschula R O C, Uys C J, Kuijten R H, Dale J R P, Wiggelinkhuizen J 1974 Nephrotic syndrome of congenital syphilis. Archives of Pathology 97: 289

Kendall-Smith I M, Pullon D H H, Tomlinson B E 1968 Congenital nephrotic syndrome in Maori siblings. New Zealand Medical Journal 68: 156

Kniker W T, Prindiville T 1969 Increased urinary glomerular basement membrane products: a measure of renal inflammation or altered metabolism. Pediatric Research 3: 513

Kniker W T, Sweeney M J 1972 Increased urinary basement membrane-like products (BMP) in infants with congenital nephrosis (CN) and their healthy relatives. Clinical Research 20: 115

Kobayashi N, Imahori K, Wakao H 1961 The congenital nephrotic syndrome, a case report and a review. Paediatria Universitatis Tokyo 6: 27

Kouvalainen K 1963 Immunological features in the congenital nephrotic syndrome. A clinical and experimental study. Annales Paediatriae Fenniae, Suppl 22

Lancet (editorial) 1980. Nephrotic syndrome in the tropics. Lancet 2: 461

Lange K, Wachstein M, Wasserman E, Alptekin F, Slobody L B 1963 The congenital nephrotic syndrome, an immune reaction? American Journal of Diseases of Children 105: 338

de Luca G, Delendi N, D'Andrea S 1964 Un raro caso di nefrosi congenita e malattia da inclusioni citomegaliche. Nota I. Minerva Pediatrica 16: 1164

Mahieu P, Monnens L, van Haelst U 1976 Chemical properties of glomerular basement membrane in congenital nephrotic syndrome. Clinical Nephrology 5: 134

McKusick V A 1969 On lumpers and splitters, or the nosology of genetic disease. Birth Defects: Original Article Series Vol 5 No 1: 23

Mehls O, Schärer K 1970 Familiäres nephrotisches Syndrom. Monatsschrift für Kinderheilkunde 118: 328

Moncrieff M W, White R H R, Glasgow E F, Winterborn M H, Cameron J S, Ogg C S 1973 The familial nephrotic

syndrome: II. A clinicopathological study. Clinical Nephrology 1: 220

Nagi N A, Nouri L 1974 Infantile nephrotic syndrome. Postgraduate Medical Journal 50: 237

Norio R 1966 Heredity in the congenital nephrotic syndrome. A genetic study of 57 Finnish families with a review of reported cases. Annales Paediatriae Fenniae 12: suppl 27

Norio R 1969 The nephrotic syndrome and heredity. Human Heredity 19: 113

Norio R 1981 Diseases of Finland and Scandinavia. In: Rothschild H (ed) Biocultural aspects of disease. Academic Press, New York, p 359

Norio R, Nevanlinna H R, Perheentupa J 1973 Hereditary diseases in Finland; rare flora in rare soil. Annals of Clinical Research 5: 109

Norio R, Nevalinna H R 1980 Rare hereditary diseases and markers in Finland. In: Eriksson A W, Forsius H R, Nevanlinna H R, Workman P L, Norio R (eds) Population structure and genetic disorders. Academic Press, London, p 567

Oliver J 1960 Microcystic renal disease and its relation to 'infantile nephrosis'. American Journal of Diseases of Children 100: 312

Rajamma K, Balasundaram D, Rao B N 1974 Congenital nephrotic syndrome: a case report. Indian Pediatrics 11: 149

Rapola J 1981 Renal pathology of fetal congenital nephrosis. A light microscopic study of 15 cases. Acta Pathologica et Microbiologica Scandinavica Sectio A 89: 63

Rapola J, Savilahti E 1971 Immunofluorescent and morphological studies in congenital nephrotic syndrome. Acta Paediatrica (Uppsala) 60: 253

Rapola J, Hallman N 1979 AFP and congenital nephrosis Finnish type. Lancet 1: 274

Richard P, Déchelette E, Gilly J, Bouvier R, Larbre F 1975 Syndrome néphrotique infantile. A propos de 14 observations. Pédiatrie 30: 581

Rossenbeck H G, Margraf O, Hofmann D 1966 Über das infantile nephrotische Syndrom bei kongenitaler Glomerulonephritis. Deutsche Medizinische Wochenschrift 91: 348

Roy S III, Pitcock J A 1971 Idiopathic nephrosis in identical twins. American Journal of Diseases in Children 121: 428

Rumpelt H J, Bachmann H J 1980 Infantile nephrotic syndrome with diffuse mesangial sclerosis: a disturbance of glomerular basement membrane development? Clinical Nephrology 13: 146

Ryynäen et al 1982 Antenatal screening of maternal serum alpha-fetoprotein for congenital nephrosis in Finland. British Journal of Obstetrics and Gynaecology, in press

Seelig H P, Seelig R, Schärer K 1975 Immunhistologische Untersuchungen bei der diffusen mesangialen Sklerose mit nephrotischen Syndrom im Säuglingsalter. Zeitschrift für Kinderheilkunde 120: 111

Shahin B, Papadopoulou Z L, Jenis E H 1974 Congenital nephrotic syndrome associated with congenital toxoplasmosis. Journal of Pediatrics 85: 366

Similä S, Vesa L, Wasz-Höckert O 1970 Hereditary onycho-osteodysplasia (the nail-patella syndrome) with nephrosis-like renal disease in a newborn boy. Pediatrics 46: 61

Spritz R A, Soiffer S J, Siegel N J, Mahoneu M J 1978 False-negative AFP screen for congenital nephrosis Finnish type. Lancet 2: 1251

Tryggvason K 1977 Composition of the glomerular basement membrane in the congenital nephrotic syndrome of the

Finnish type. European Journal of Clinical Investigation 7: 177

Tryggvason K, Kouvalainen K 1975 Number of nephrons in normal human kidneys and kidneys of patients with the congenital nephrotic syndrome. A study using a sieving method for counting of glomeruli. Nephron 15: 62

Vernier R L, Brunson J, Good R A 1957 Studies on familial nephrosis. American Journal of Diseases of Children 93: 469

White R H R 1973 The familial nephrotic syndrome: I. A European survey. Clinical Nephrology 1: 216

Worthen H C, Vernier R L, Good R A 1959 Infantile nephrosis. American Journal of Diseases of Children 98: 731

Yamamoto Y, Kuroda T, Kanamura S, Sawada S 1961 A case of 'congenital nephrotic syndrome'. Annales Paediatrica Japonica 7: 391

Zunin C, Soave P 1964 Association of nephrotic syndrome and nephroblastoma in siblings. Annales Paediatriae (Basel) 203: 29

Haemoglobinopathies and thalassaemias

J.A. Phillips and H.H. Kazazian

INTRODUCTION

The biosynthesis of haemoglobin in the erythrocyte is one of the most striking examples of cellular specialization known in nature. Inherited disorders of haemoglobin synthesis, such as the haemoglobinopathies and the thalassaemia syndromes, are common and significant clinical conditions. The purpose of this chapter is to summarize briefly current knowledge of the structure, function, and biosynthesis of normal haemoglobin, then to discuss clinical diseases which result from qualitative (haemoglobinopathies) or quantitative (thalassaemia syndromes) defects in globin synthesis.

NORMAL HUMAN HAEMOGLOBIN

Haemoglobin is a tetramer with a molecular weight of 64 500. It consists of two α and two non-α globin polypeptide chains, each of which has a single covalently bound haem group. Each of the four haem groups is made up of an iron atom bound within a protoporphyrin IX ring.

In man, the six known different globin polypeptide chains are designated α, β, γ, δ, ϵ, and ζ. Each chain consists of a specific sequence of amino acids linked by peptide bonds. The α-chains contain 141 amino acids, while the β, γ, δ, and ϵ-chains have 146 residues. The ϵ, γ, and δ-chains are more similar to β-chains than to α-chains, differing from β at 36, 39, and 10 positions, respectively (Bunn et al, 1977a; Baralle et al, 1980). The two globins, ϵ and ζ, are found in embryonic erythrocytes; and while the ζ sequence is is incompletely known, it appears to be an analogue of the α-chain.

The haemoglobin composition of erythrocyte lysates can be quantified by zone electrophoresis. Different haemoglobin tetramers, their structure, percentage in normal adult lysate, and conditions in which levels are increased, are seen in Table 74.1 (Bunn et al, 1977a). Haemoglobin A ($\alpha_2\beta_2$) is usually 92% of the total haemoglobin in normal adults. Haemoglobin A_2 ($\alpha_2\delta_2$) constitutes about 2.5%, and it is evenly distributed in normal red cells; it may be increased in β-thalassaemias and megaloblastic anaemia and decreased in iron deficiency and sideroblastic anaemias.

Hb A_{1c} differs from Hb A by the post-translational addition of a glucose at the NH_2-terminus of the β chain, hence the tetramer's structure is $\alpha_2(\beta$-N-glucose$)_2$. The percentage of Hb A_{1c} (5% in normals) is related to the intracellular concentration of glucose and the red cell lifespan. In diabetic patients, the concentration of Hb A_{1c} is increased about two-fold because of the ele-

Table 74.1 Human haemoglobins

Hb name	Synonym	Structure	% in adults	Conditions in which increased
A	Adult Hb	$\alpha_2\beta_2$	92	
A_{1c}		$\alpha_2(\beta$-N-glucose$)_2$	5	Diabetes mellitus
A_2		$\alpha_2\delta_2$	2.5	β-thalassemia
F	Fetal Hb	$\alpha_2\gamma_2$	< 1	Newborn, β-thalassemia, and marrow stress
H		β_4	0	Some α-thalassemias
Barts		γ_4	0	Some α-thalassemias
Gower 1	Embryonic Hb	$\zeta_2\epsilon_2$	0	Early embryos (< 8 weeks)
Gower 2	Embryonic Hb	$\alpha_2\epsilon_2$	0	Early embryos (< 8 weeks)
Portland	Embryonic Hb	$\zeta_2\gamma_2$	0	Early embryos (< 8 weeks) and α°-thalassemia (hydrops fetalis)

Data from Bunn HF, et al: Human Hemoglobins. Philadelphia: Saunders, 1977.

vated glucose concentration in their red cells (Bunn et al, 1977a).

While Hb F ($\alpha_2\gamma_2$) comprises the bulk of haemoglobin (50–85%) in human newborns, it declines rapidly after birth, reaching concentrations of 10–15% by four months of age. Subsequently, the decline is slower; and adult levels of <1% are reached by three to four years of age. Fetal haemoglobin may be increased in β- and δβ-thalassaemia, hereditary persistence of fetal haemoglobin, D_1 trisomy, some cases of thyrotoxicosis, megaloblastic and aplastic anaemia, leukaemia and various malignancies involving marrow, sickle cell anaemia, and during pregnanacy (Cooper & Hoagland, 1972). Hb F is measured by resistance to alkali, electrophoresis, or column chromatography.

Hbs Gower I ($\zeta_2\epsilon_2$), Gower II ($\alpha_2\epsilon_2$), and Portland ($\zeta_2\gamma_2$) are embryonic haemoglobins found in fetuses before 7 to 10 weeks of gestation. At 4 to 5 weeks of gestation, a simultaneous decrease in ζ- and ϵ-chain production and an increase in α- and γ-chain production occur (Kazazian, 1974). β-chain synthesis in reticulocytes accounts for 4% of non-α synthesis at 5 weeks of gestation and gradually increases thereafter (Kazazian & Woodhead, 1973). While the time of the decrease in ϵ- and ζ-chains coincides with the switch from yolk sac to hepatic-derived erythrocytes, the restriction of embryonic chain synthesis to yolk sac cells and the converse restriction of γ- and β-chains to hepatic cells have not been proven.

Hbs H and Barts are tetramers of β- and γ-chains, respectively, and both function very poorly in transporting oxygen. These two haemoglobins may be increased in some types of α-thalassaemia.

Primary and secondary structures

The primary structure of each globin chain is its amino acid sequence; 141 amino acids in α-chains and 146 amino acids in β-, γ-, δ-, and ϵ-chains. The primary structure of α- and β-chains is seen in Figure 74.1.

The relationship between adjacent amino acids along the chain enables interactions which can result in one of two basic configurations of secondary structure: the α-helix or β-pleated-sheet. The α-helix, stabilized by hydrogen bonding between carbonyl and amino groups, has 3.6 amino acid residues per turn. About 75% of haemoglobin in its native state is in the α-helix form, as shown in Figure 74.1. The β-pleated-sheet configuration predominates in other molecules, such as immunoglobulins and chymotrypsin.

At specific locations in the haemoglobin subunits, the rodlike α helix is interrupted by nonhelical segment which allow folding. On X–ray crystallography, the confirmations of α and β haemoglobin subunits are seen to be similar. The β-globin chain has eight helical segments, A through H, and the secondary structure of the α-globin

corresponds to that of the β-globin except for the absence of residues forming the D helical region (Fig. 74.1). The histidine residue at position 8 of the F helical segment (F8) is linked covalently to the haem iron molecule. This histidine residue is located at position 87 in the α-chain and 92 in the β-chain, and mutations altering it have important pathological consequences. Amino acids with charged side groups; e.g., lysine, arginine, and glutamic acid, lie on the external surface, while uncharged residues tend to be oriented toward the interior of the molecule (Rieder, 1974).

Tertiary and quaternary structures

Tertiary structure refers to the configuration of a protein subunit in three-dimensional space, while quaternary structure refers to the relationships of the four subunits of haemoglobin to each other. The haaemoglobin tetramer has been shown by X–ray crystallography to be an oblate spheroid with a diameter of 55 Å and a single axis of symmetry. The globin chains are folded so that the four haem groups are in surface clefts equidistant from each other. The four subunits forming the tetramers are labeled α_1, α_2, β_1, and β_2. While there is no contact between the two β-chains, each α-chain touches both β-chains. Bonds across the $\alpha_1\beta_1$ interface are firmer than those at the $\alpha_1\beta_2$ interface and changes from oxy- to deoxyhaemoglobin involve more extensive movement at the $\alpha_1\beta_2$ interface. The quaternary structure changes markedly in going from oxy- to deoxyhaemoglobin, and this accounts for many of the observed changes in physical properties. Haemoglobin mutations resulting in amino acid substitutions at these points can markedly alter specific functional properties (Rieder, 1974).

Functional properties

For haemoglobin to fulfill its physiologic role, it must bind oxygen with a certain affinity. One measure of oxygen affinity is P_{50}, or the partial pressure of oxygen in mm Hg which is required for 50% saturation of haemoglobin: a haemoglobin with increased P_{50} has decreased oxygen affinity (Fig. 74.2). Oxygen affinity is also affected by a number of environmental factors including temperature, pH, organic phosphate concentration, and pCO_2 (see Fig. 74.2) (Bellingham, 1976).

The sigmoid shape of the oxyhaemoglobin dissociation curve reflects haem-haem interaction; i.e., successive oxygenation of each haem group in the tetramer increases the oxygen affinity of the remaining unoxygenated haem groups. The basis of haem-haem interaction is the decrease in the atomic radius of the haem iron that occurs with oxygenation allowing the iron atom to fit into the plane of the porphyrin ring. This alteration is amplified by a series of conformational changes which affect the other haem groups (Bellingham, 1976). The resulting sigmoid oxyhaemoglobin dissociation curve has great

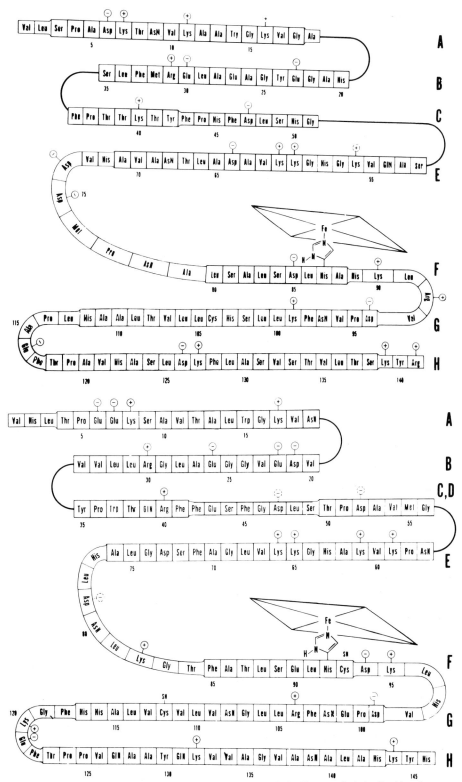

Fig. 74.1 The primary and secondary structures of globin chains. Top: α-chain. Bottom: β-chain. Residues in squares are in α-helix configuration and nonhelical residues are in rectangles. (From Murayama M 1971 In: Nalbandian R M (ed) Molecular aspects of sickle cell hemoglobin. Charles Thomas, Springfield, IL. By permission of Charles C. Thomas, Publisher.)

physiologic importance because it enables large amounts of oxygen to be bound or released with a small increase or decrease in oxygen tension. In contrast to Hb A, Hb H (β_4) and Hb Barts (γ_4) lack subunit interaction and have a hyperbolic rather than sigmoid oxyhaemoglobin dissociation curve which prevents oxygen release at physiologic oxygen tensions.

The Bohr effect is a change in oxygen affinity of haemoglobin with a change in pH. This effect is beneficial at the tissue level where the lower pH decreases the oxygen affinity and promotes oxygen release (Fig. 74.2). Oxygen uptake in the lungs is enhanced by the opposite changes in pH and pCO_2.

Red cells have unusually high concentrations of 2,3-diphosphoglycerate (2,3-DPG). One molecule of 2,3-DPG sits in a pocket in deoxyhaemoglobin bound to specific β-chain residues (1, 2, 82, and 143 of both β-chains). The importance of the binding is that 2,3-DPG stabilizes the deoxy form of haemoglobin in preference to the oxy form, thereby lowering the oxygen affinity of the molecule. The γ chain of Hb F lacks the β^{143} histidine residue, and the resultant decrease in binding of 2,3-DPG to Hb F accounts for the increased oxygen affinity of fetal red cells compared to that of adult red cells (Bellingham, 1976).

HAEMOGLOBIN BIOSYNTHESIS

Genetics

In man there are nine different genetic loci which code for the six globin genes (Bernards et al, 1979; Lawn et al, 1978; Proudfoot & Baralle, 1979; Orkin, 1978; Lauer et al, 1980; Baralle et al, 1980). In addition, there are at least three pseudogenes which have sequences similar to other globin genes but which differ in that they are not expressed into globin proteins (Fritsch et al, 1980; Proudfoot & Maniatis, 1980). Normally, globin tetramers are formed of two α or α-like chains and two non-α-chains; a schematic representation of the interaction of the products of these genes is shown in Figure 74.3. Since humans are diploid; i.e., have a pair of each non-sex chromosome or autosome, they have two genes for each autosomal locus. For example, there are two loci encoding the structure of the α-chain; thus, there are four α-chain genes. In contrast, there is only a single β-globin locus; therefore, two β genes (Fig. 74.3). The relative numbers of α and β loci are important in understanding the different inheritance patterns of α- and β-thalassemias, as well as the different relative amounts of variant hemo-

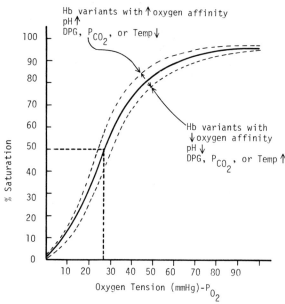

Fig. 74.2 The oxyhaemoglobin dissociation curve and effect of different factors on oxygen affinity.

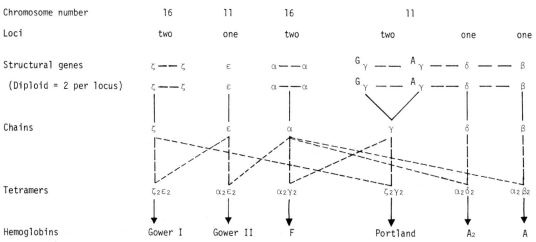

Fig. 74.3 Schematic representation of the various globin genes and their products.

globins in individuals carrying a variant α- or β-globin gene. These quantitative differences correlate directly with the clinical severity of the various disorders.

The region of chromosome 11 (11p 1205-8) (Gusella et al, 1979) containing the β-like genes (ε, ^{G}γ, ^{A}γ, δ, β) has been thoroughly mapped by restriction endonuclease analysis (Fig. 74.4A). In addition, the ε, ^{G}γ, ^{A}γ, δ, and β-globin genes have been sequenced (Baralle et al, 1980; Slighton et al, 1980; Spritz et al, 1980a; Lawn et al, 1980; Efstradiadis et al, 1980). Each of these genes contains two intervening sequences (IVSs) which interrupt the coding sequence at the junctions of the codons for amino acids 30–31 and 104–105. The first IVS is 122–130 base pairs (bp), while the second is 850–904 bp in length. The entire β-gene cluster spans about 50 kilobases (kb) and contains one ε, two γ, one δ, and one β locus, plus two pseudogene loci (Fritsch et al, 1980). These pseudogenes have sequences which are similar to β-gene sequences, but differ in having altered sequences which prevent production of functional globin chains. Pseudogenes comprise a minority of the single gene sequences in both the α- and β-gene regions. Single gene sequences, in turn, comprise only about 7 kb of the 60 kb of DNA in the β-gene region, while the remaining 43 kb are flanking sequences, presumably having some unknown regulatory role. In this regard, nucleotides within the 4 kb 5' to the δ locus have been suggested to be important in γ-gene regulation, since their deletion in some forms of hereditary persistence of fetal haemoglobin is associated with increased γ-gene expression (Fritsch et al, 1979).

The α-gene complex contains two α loci which have 3.6 kb between their centers, two ζ loci, and at least one pseudo-α locus (ψα₁). Figure 74.4B depicts this complex which is on chromosome 16; and it should be noted that in each case about 4 kbs separate the ζ₁, ψα₁, α₂, and α₁ loci, suggesting the existence of discrete duplication units in the DNA (Proudfoot & Maniatis, 1980). α-genes have smaller intervening sequences than are found in the β-like genes; IVS I contains 114 bp, while IVS II contains 132 bp (Liebhaber et al, submitted).

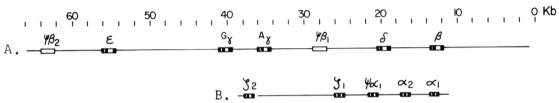

Fig. 74.4 Globin genes complexes. (A) β-gene complex on chromosome 11. (B) α-gene complex on chromosome 16. Distances along the chromosome are measured in kilobases (kb) at top.

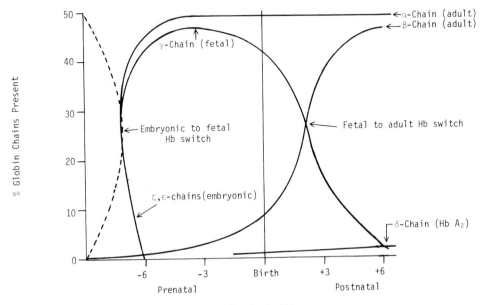

Fig. 74.5 Qualitative and quantitative changes in globin chains during human development. Note that the percentage of β-chains accumulated in early fetal development is much less than the percentage of β-chains synthesized during fetal development. Modified from Bunn H F, Forget B G, Ranney H M 1977 In: Human haemoglobins. Saunders, Philadelphia, ch 1, p 4)

Ontogeny

The globin genes are expressed at different times and in different relative amounts during human development (Fig. 74.5). The sequence of appearance of the various globin chains is helpful in understanding the timing of onset of clinical manifestations of the haemoglobinopathies and thalassaemias. For example, a deficiency of α- or γ-chain synthesis and α- or γ-variants with abnormal functions should be observed at birth, while a deficiency of β chains may not cause symptoms until several months of age. Finally, levels of β-chain variants, such as Hb S, progressively increase over the first months, so that the onset of clinical manifestations may be delayed until the latter half of the first year of life.

Globin biosynthesis

The genetic information for every normal and abnormal globin chain is encoded in the nucleotide sequence of the DNA. These sequences, or genes, are located at specific loci on chromosomes 16 and 11 (Deisseroth et al, 1977; Scott et al, 1979; Gusella et al, 1979; Deisseroth et al, 1978).

As mentioned above, IVSs reside between the portions of the globin genes that are translated into protein. These IVSs are present in the gene and in the RNA transcribed from the gene which is called messenger RNA precursor (pre-mRNA) (Fig. 74.6). Pre-mRNA undergoes excision of the intervening sequences and splicing of the translated portions (Tilghman et al, 1978). Studies of the function of hybrid SV 40-β-globin genes in cultured monkey kidney cells suggest that IVS excision is crucial to mRNA transport from the nucleus to the cystoplasm (Hamer & Leder, 1979).

Further processing occurs at each end of this RNA molecule (Kazazian et al, 1977). At the 5′-end, guanosine is added in a special triphosphate linkage, and this guanosine and the next two nucleotides are then methylated. These 5′-end modifications are called capping and meth-

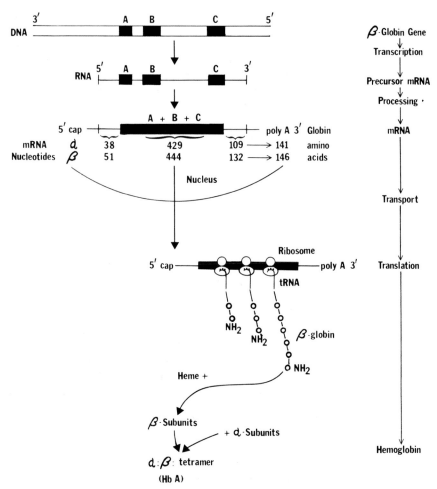

Fig. 74.6 Steps involved in haemoglobin biosynthesis. Understanding of the order and function of various steps is incomplete.

ylation; and while their function is not completely known, they have been shown to be vital for initiation of translation of many mRNAs, including globin mRNAs. The 3'-end modification involves the addition of about 150 adenylic acid nucleotides [poly(A)]. Poly(A) addition may also be important for the transport of mRNA to the cytoplasm and its subsequent stability. With ageing of the mRNA, the poly (A) 'tail' shortens (Merkel et al, 1976).

Once the processed mRNA has been transported to the cytoplasm, it binds to ribosomes. The first step in translation (initiation) requires the binding of mRNA to the two ribosome subunits, amino acyl-tRNA, guanosine triphosphate, and protein initiation factors. Initiation occurs at the 5', or capped, end of mRNA which corresponds to the NH_2-terminal end of the globin chain. Protein synthesis then proceeds toward the COOH-terminal end. Four to six chains of varying length (nascent chains) undergo translation on the same mRNA simultaneously. When these nascent chains have attained full length, a termination codon is reached. Since no tRNA is available for decoding this codon, polypeptide synthesis stops and, with the assistance of protein termination factors, the polypeptide chain is released from the ribosome and its mRNA. About one third of the mature mRNA sequence is not used for translation, but these untranslated nucleotides which are located at both ends of the molecule probably have other regulatory functions (Kazazian et al, 1977).

The protein chain assumes its secondary and tertiary structures due to interactions resulting from its amino acid sequence. Next, haem is bound and, in combination with other polypeptide subunits, the quarternary haemoglobin molecule is formed. These steps are shown in Figure 74.6.

HUMAN HAEMOGLOBIN VARIANTS

Molecular aetiology

Abnormal haemoglobins result from mutations which change the sequence or number of nucleotides within the globin gene involved or from mispairing during meiosis giving fusion of two different genes. Mutation can cause substitution, addition, or deletion of one or more amino acids in the polypeptide sequence of the affected globin (Table 74.2).

Single base changes can result in single amino acid substitutions; e.g., Hb S (β^6 Glu→Val), shortened chains due to premature termination of translation; e.g., Hb McKees Rock [$\beta^{145 \, (Tyr \to Term)}$], or elongated chains. Elongated chains result when the terminator codon undergoes a mutation to a codon for an amino acid such as UAA → CAA in Hb Constant Spring. Two other elongated α chains are Hb Icaria and Hb Koya Dora, both of which also have 31 additional residues and differ from Hb Constant Spring only at residue 142 (Bunn et al, 1977b).

Single base deletions or additions can cause a frame shift in the normal reading process (Seid-Akhavan et al, 1976). For example, in the α^{Wayne} variant a single base deletion (A) causes the following codons to be read out of phase:

Table 74.2 Molecular basis of haemoglobinopathies

Mutation	Example	Clinical manifestation
Nucleotide base substitutions to a codon for		
Another amino acid	Hb S ($\beta^{6Glu \to Val}$)	Sickling
	Hb C_{Harlem} ($\beta^{6Glu \to Val} + \beta^{73 \, Asp \to Asn}$)	Sickling
Termination	Hb McKees Rock ($\beta^{145 \, Tyr \to Termination}$)	Increased oxygen affinity and polycythemia
Amino acid instead of termination	Hb Constant Spring ($\alpha^{Termination \to Gln}$)	Decreased synthesis (thalassemia-like)
Nucleotide base deletions		
Single base deletion → frame shift	Hb Wayne ($\alpha^{139-141 \, [Lys-Tyr-Arg]} \to Asn-Thr-Val...]$)	Normal
Triplet deletion → single amino acid	Hb Leiden ($\beta^{6 \, or \, 7 \, Glu \to O}$)	Unstable
Multiple codon	Hb Gun Hill ($\beta^{91-95 \, [Leu-His-Cys-Asp-Lys]} \to 0$)	Unstable
Crossover	Hb Lepore (δβ-fusion with segments of δ and β lost)	Decreased synthesis (thalassemia-like)
Whole gene	α-Thalassemia$_1$ and α-thalassemia$_2$ combination	Hb H disease
Nucleotide base additions		
Two bases added → frame shift	Hb Cranston ($\beta^{144[Tyr-His]} \to [Ser-Ile-Thr...]$)	Unstable
Multiple codon	Hb Grady (9 bases → 3 additional amino acids)	Normal

Lys   Tyr   Arg   Term
(AAA – UAC – CGU) – UAA

     Asn   Thr   Val
→ (AAU – ACC – GUU) . . .

Deletions of three, or multiples of three, nucleotides in the DNA cause deletions of one or more amino acids. It is interesting that of 13 examples of this type, all are β-chain variants, including Hb Leiden ($\beta^{6 \text{ or } 7 \text{ Glu}\to 0}$) and Hb Gun Hill [$\beta^{91-95 \text{ (Leu-His-Cys-Asp-Lys)}} \to 0$]. Deletions of segments of genes may be due to nonhomologous crossing-over after mispairing in meiosis. This mechanism accounts for the Lepore globins (δβ fusion chains), anti-Lepore globins (βδ fusion chains), and Kenya globin (γβ fusion chain) (Kazazian et al, 1977).

Known variants

The number of known haemoglobin variants resulting from changes in the nucleotide base number or sequence in DNA is now 322 (Table 74.3) (Internat. Hbg. Info. Ctr., 1980). Most of these mutants were detected by zone electrophoresis which separates haemoglobins on the basis of charge differences resulting from the amino acid substitutions. Since many mutations which do not change the protein's charge are not detected by this method, many undetected haemoglobin variants must

still exist in the population. The number of β variants (194) is approximately twice that of α variants (102), even though there are two α loci and a single β locus. Also, the percentage of β-chain variants which have abnormal physical properties (60%) is nearly twice that of the α chain variants (34%). The great majority of these mutants arise from a single base substitution which results in a single amino acid substitution. Many of these substitutions, even some of those which produce abnormal physical properties in the variant haemoglobin, are clinically silent and were detected only by population screening. Other substitutions cause 1) instability of the tetramer; 2) deformity of the 3-dimensional structure; 3) inhibition of ferric iron reduction; 4) alteration of the residues which interact with haem, with 2,3 DPG, or at the α-β subunit contact site; or 5) abnormality of other properties of the molecule resulting in a variety of clinical phenotypes (Table 74.4).

The location of the amino acid changed by the mutation can often be correlated with the resultant phenotype. Unstable haemoglobin variants are caused by several types of changes in the primary sequence which affect the secondary, tertiary, or quaternary structure. These substitutions tend to be at residues in the interior of the molecule, at contact points between chains, at residues which interact with the haem groups (Rieder, 1974), or

Table 74.3 Known haemoglobin variants (1980)*

Globin chain	Total variants	Clinically silent	Unstable	Abnormal properties		Ferric Hb
				Abnormal oxygen affinity		
α	102	67 (66%)	12 (12%)	22 (22%)		2 (2%)
β	194	78 (40%)	59 (30%)	77 (40%)		5 (3%)
γ	16	14 (88%)	2 (13%)	–		–
δ	10	10 (100%)	–	–		–
Totals	322	169 (52%)	73 (23%)	99 (31%)		7 (2%)

*Fusion variants are not included. Compiled from information supplied by the Director of the International Hemoglobin Information Center, Augusta, Georgia.
(Note: The percentages may be greater than 100 because some variants have more than one abnormal property.)

Table 74.4 Clinical manifestations of haemoglobin mutants

Type	Example	Clinical manifestation
Sickling	Hb S	Sickling due to decreased solubility
Unstable	Hb Bristol	Anaemia with Heinz body formation
Abnormal oxygen affinity		
Decreased	Hb Kansas	Mild anaemia possible
Increased	Hb Chesapeake	Polycythaemia due to decreased oxygen transport
M haemoglobin	Hb M$_{Boston}$	Cyanosis due to ferric haemoglobin
Decreased synthesis	Hb Lepore	Thalassaemia

when a proline residue replaces another amino acid within an α helical region (Hb Genova [β^{28}(B10)$^{Leu \to Pro}$], Hb Abraham Lincoln [β^{32}(B14)$^{Leu \to Pro}$]), resulting in disruption of the helix. Hb Philly [β^{35}(C1$^{Tyr \to Phe}$] is also unstable secondary to a missing hydrogen bond normally found between the α_1 and β_1 subunits. Many other unstable haemoglobins are the result of mutations affecting residues which bind haem or are in the hydrophobic haem cleft; e.g., Hb Gun Hill [$\beta^{91-95 \ (Leu-His-Cys-Asp-Lys) \to 0}$] and Hb Hammersmith ($\beta^{42 \ Phe \to Ser}$).

Substitutions on the surface of the molecule usually do not affect tertiary structure or haem-haem interaction, but they may permit molecular interactions which decrease solubility under certain conditions [Hb S (β^6 $^{Glu \to Val}$]. Substitution of tyrosine for either of the histidines which bind the iron molecule (E7 or F8) results in increased stability of the ferric (oxidized) iron state seen in M haemoglobins, M-Boston [α^{58}(E7)$^{His \to Tyr}$] and M-Iwate [β^{87}(F8)$^{His \to Tyr}$]. Substitution at an $\alpha_1\beta_1$ subunit contact point, such as β^{99}, can disturb haem-haem interactions causing increased oxygen affinity and polycythemia, as with Hb Kempsey [β^{99}(G1)$^{Asp \to Asn}$] (Rieder, 1974).

Inheritance of haemoglobinopathies

Variants of α, β, γ, or δ globins result from mutations affecting their respective genes. All of the variants for β chains, for example, are coded by alleles since they result from different genes found at the single β-chromosomal locus. Heterozygotes for a haemoglobin containing an abnormal β globin have an abnormal as well as a normal β gene at that locus, and their status is often described by the term 'trait.' Since most variants are rare, they usually occur in the heterozygous state and, if they cause clinical symptoms, are examples of autosomal dominant conditions. When both alleles code for the same common β variant, the individual is then homozygous and is said to have the 'disease' state. However, the term 'sickle cell disease' is often used to describe a similar phenotype that is seen when any of several genotypes (SS, SC, S/β-thal, SD$_{Punjab}$, or SO$_{Arab}$) are exposed to a certain environment (hypoxia). Furthermore, under conditions of severe hypoxia a person with the AS genotype or 'trait' can also manifest symptoms of the sickle cell 'disease' phenotype. This distinction between the genotype (homozygous and heterozygous) and the phenotype (trait and disease) is an important one. Also, it should be noted that patterns of inheritance of haemoglobin variants are more precisely expressed in terms of genotypes than in terms of phenotypes.

Inheritance risks from matings of individuals who are normal, heterozygous, or homozygous for variant haemoglobins are shown in Table 74.5. Since there are multiple alleles for each locus, a person heterozygous for two alleles at the same locus (usually referred to as a genetic compound) may be seen; e.g., Hb SC individual. A mating between an AA and an SC individual can result in AS or AC, but not AA or SC, offspring. However, a mating of an AS and an AC individual can result in offspring who are AA, AS, AC, or SC. This pattern of Mendelian inheritance is called codominant inheritance.

SICKLE CELL ANAEMIA AND RELATED DISORDERS

Molecular basis

The sickle cell gene results from a point mutation which causes the amino acid substitution $\beta^{6 \ Glu \to Val}$; therefore, Hb S is $\alpha_2^A\beta_2^{6 \ Glu \to Val}$. The frequency of sickle trait (Hb AS) among United States blacks at birth is about 8%, and the incidence of sickle cell anaemia at birth should be around 0.16%, or 1 per 625 births (Motulsky, 1973). This contrasts with the higher carrier frequencies seen in some areas of Africa (up to 30%) which are due to the protective advantage conferred by the carrier state against falciparum malaria. As expected, the prevalence of sickle cell anaemia differs in these two populations. The prevalence of sickle cell anaemia among all blacks in the United States is about 1 per 1875, considerably lower than expected from the incidence at birth. It is still lower in some underdeveloped regions of Africa, despite the higher incidence of the trait, due to higher mortality in infancy (Motulsky, 1973).

Pathophysiology of sickling

Substitution of valine for glutamic acid at the β^6 residue causes a change on the surface of the deoxygenated β^s

Table 74.5 Inheritance risks for a haemoglobin variant

Parents	Homozygous normal (%)	*Offspring* Heterozygous (%)	Homozygous affected (%)
Both normal	100	0	0
Normal/Heterozygous	50	50	0
Normal/Homozygous	0	100	0
Both heterozygous	25	50	25
Heterozygous/Homozygous	0	50	50
Both homozygous	0	0	100

chain which allows it to interact in a special way with other β chains. This interaction results in the formation by $\alpha_2^A\beta_2^S$ tetramers of a 14-stranded helical polymer with a diameter of 150–170 angstroms. The parallel alignment of these rod-like polymers in turn causes the deformation seen in sickled erythrocytes. In sickle cell anaemia, the sickling process may begin when the oxygen saturation of Hb S is decreased to 85%, but it does not occur in heterozygotes (Hb AS) until the oxygen saturation of haemoglobin is decreased to 40% (Nathan & Pearson, 1974). In addition to a decrease in oxygen tension, a reduction in pH or an increase in 2,3-DPG also promotes sickling. These factors probably interact in patients with sickle cell anaemia since their blood normally has an increased 2,3-DPG concentration.

The viscosity of oxygenated sickle cell blood is increased primarily due to irreversibly sickled cells, but also due to increased gamma globulin levels. When the blood becomes deoxygenated, viscosity increases further due to the cellular rigidity which occurs with sickling. This, in turn, increases the exposure time of erythrocytes to a hypoxic environment, and the lower tissue pH decreases the oxygen affinity which further promotes sickling. The end result is occlusion of capillaries and arterioles and infarction of surrounding tissues. Haemolysis probably occurs secondary to increased mechanical fragility of deformed cells and membrane damage.

Clinical aspects of sickle cell disease

As can be seen from Figure 74.5, β-chain production usually does not reach sufficient levels to cause symptoms until the second half of the first year of life. As higher concentrations of Hb S are reached in erythrocytes, the cells become susceptible to haemolysis and a progressive haemolytic anaemia with splenomegaly is seen. The increased rate of erythropoiesis leads to erythroid marrow expansion and increased folic acid requirements. However, the two major problems for young children with SS disease are infections and vaso-occlusive crises.

Children with sickle cell anaemia have increased susceptibility to potentially life-threatening bacterial infections including sepsis and meningitis caused by *Streptococcus pneumoniae* and *Haemophilus influenzae*. The relative risk of sickle cell anaemia patients compared with that of normals for pneumococcal, *H. influenzae*, and all bacterial meningitis is 579:1, 116:1, and 309:1, respectively (Barrett Connor, 1971). These patients are also susceptible to bacterial pneumonia (often pneumococcus), osteomyelitis (*Salmonella* and *Staphylococcus*) (Fig. 74.7), and urinary tract infections (*Escherichia coli* and *Klebsiella*). Increased susceptibility is also seen for *Shigella* and *Mycoplasma pneumoniae*. Several factors that contribute to this susceptibility are functional hyposplenism, impaired antibody response, decreased opsonization, impaired complement activation in the properdin pathway, and abnormal chemotaxis.

Bacterial infection is the most common reason for hospitalisation of paediatric sickle cell anaemia patients and often leads to the diagnosis (Barrett-Connor, 1971). Serious bacterial infections are seen in approximately one-third of children with sickle cell anaemia before four years of age. Infection, and not crisis, is the most com-

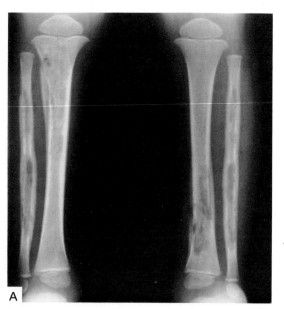
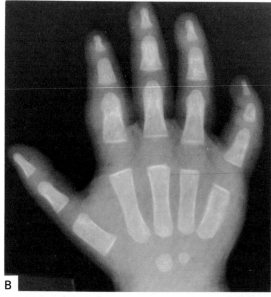

Fig. 74.7 Radiographic changes in sickle cell anemia. (A) Changes in the tibias and fibulas secondary to *Salmonella* osteomyelis. (B) Hand-and-foot syndrome with soft tissue swelling and focal areas of cortical destruction and periosteal new bone formation. (Courtesy of Dr John Dorst)

mon cause of death in these children, although infections often precipitate crises.

Vaso-occlusive crises begin in infancy with dactylitis, or hand-and-foot syndrome (Fig. 74.7). Later crises may involve the periosteum, bones, or joints, resulting in infarction which must be differentiated from osteomyelitis and septic arthritis. Vaso-occlusive crises and sepsis are diffcult to differentiate and often coexist in younger children.

Pulmonary crises with pleural pain and fever may be due to either infection, in situ thrombosis, or embolism. Other clinical manifestations include splenic sequestra-

tion, abdominal and aplastic crises, cholelithiasis, hepatic infarcts, occlusion of cerebral vessels, ocular changes, haematuria, hyposthenuria, hyponatremia, priapism, and skin ulcers (Nathan & Pearson, 1974; Cooper & Hoagland, 1972).

Diagnosis

The peripheral blood smear of sickle cell anaemia patients may have normal, irreversibly sickled, target, and nucleated red cells. Howell-Jolly bodies and red cell fragments are also present, especially after functional asplenia develops (Fig. 74.8A). The clinical history of

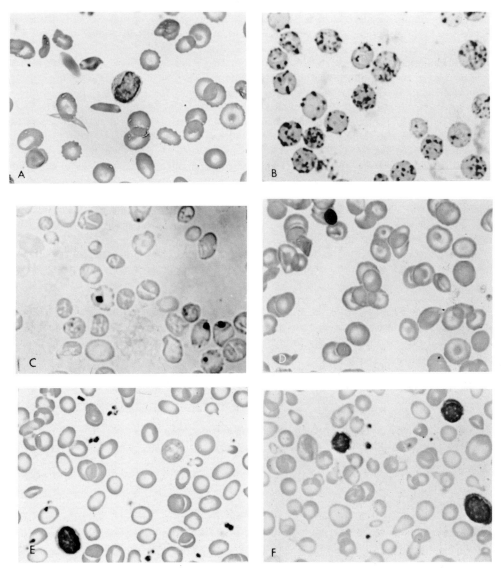

Fig. 74.8 Peripheral blood smears from patients with various disorders of globin synthesis. (A) Homozygous sickle cell anemia. (B) Unstable Hb Zurich with Heinz bodies. (C) Hb H disease. (D) Sickle/β-thhalassaemia.(E) β-thalassaemia trait. F: Homozygous β-thalassaemia. (B) and (C) were prepared as follows: whole blood with EDTA was incubated at 41°C for 3 to 6 hours, than a 1:1 mixture of blood and 0.5% rhodanile blue in 0.9% saline was made and immediately smeared. Haemoglobin precipitates formed secondary to heating are seen. (Courtesy of Dr William Zinkham)

crises or severe infections with anaemia, abnormal red cell morphology on peripheral smear with a normal or elevated mean corpuscular volume, positive sickling test, and Hb S (greater than 80%) and Hb F on haemoglobin electrophoresis, makes the diagnosis of sickle cell anaemia probable. However, family studies indicating that both parents have sickle cell trait are helpful to exclude S/β-thalassaemia and S/hereditary persistence of fetal haemoglobin. In addition, siblings should also be tested to identify and treat previously undiagnosed cases.

Treatment

At present there is no safe drug to ameliorate the condition, but a number of antisickling agents are under trial (Dean & Schechter, 1978). Infections should be treated promptly with antibiotics, and some centers advocate prophylactic antibiotic treatment. A polyvalent pneumococcal polysaccharide has been shown to afford some protection against systemic infections due to *Streptococcus pneumoniae* in sickle cell disease and in splenectomized patients (Ammann et al, 1977); however, multiple clinical failures as well as side effects have been reported (Akhonkhai et al, 1979; Giebiuk et al, 1979).

The associated anaemia is usually tolerated well; but if folate deficiency occurs, the anaemia becomes more severe and is associated with macrocytosis, hypersegmented granulocytes, and a decrease in percentage of reticulocytes. Folate deficiency is prevented easily by daily folic acid supplement. Transfusions are seldom indicated for uncomplicated anaemia, but exchange transfusions can be effective for life-threatening vaso-occlusive crises (cerebral) or in preparation for surgery. Crises should be managed with vigorous hydration because of the patient's inability to concentrate urine and the increased viscosity of his blood. Acidosis and hypoxia should be treated, and analgesics should be given for the accompanying severe pain.

Prevention

During genetic counselling, $AS \times AS$ couples are advised of their 25% risk for having children with sickle cell disease; certain couples may request prenatal diagnosis. In the past two years, methods for the prenatal detection of sickle cell anaemia have been improved to the point that they are now applicable to nearly all couples at risk.

Between 1975 and 1979, about 50 couples at risk for sickle cell anaemia had prenatal diagnosis using fetal blood obtained by techniques of fetoscopy or placental aspiration (Hobbins & Mahoney, 1974; Alter et al, 1976). Synthetic studies were used to detect the types of β-chains produced in fetal red cells. The significant risk of fetoscopy (6% fetal mortality), its limited availability, and the variable clinical course of the disease have com-

bined to limit widespread use of these methods (Alter, 1979).

In 1978, Kan discovered that restriction endonuclease studies of DNA from fetal amniocytes could also enable prenatal diagnosis of sickle cell anaemia in a substantial proportion of cases (Kan & Dozy, 1978). The applicability of this test has been expanded (Phillips et al, 1980a) through the use of other polymorphic restriction endonuclease sites near the β locus. When family studies can be carried out to assign DNA 'markers' to the respective β^A- and β^S-bearing chromosomes of both parents, prenatal diagnosis can now be accomplished in 90% of pregnancies by amniocentesis alone (Phillips et al, 1980a). The remaining 10% of pregnancies in which the disease cannot be excluded still require fetoscopy after amniocentesis.

Interactions with sickle haemoglobin

Heterozygotes for Hb S (AS) generally are asymptomatic; however, severe hypoxia (oxygen saturation less than 40%) can induce sickling. The loop of Henle provides an environment in which both the pH and oxygen tension are decreased sufficiently to cause sickling resulting in microinfarctions, haematuria, and hyposthenuria. Exposure to hypoxia can also cause splenic and other organ infarcts in sickle trait individuals.

Hb C trait is found in about 3% of American blacks at birth, Hb SC disease in 1 per 833, and Hb C disease in about 1 per 1250 (Motulsky, 1973). Patients with SC disease tend to have a variable course with most of the complications occurring less frequently than in SS disease. Other haemoglobin variants which interact with S are D_{Punjab}, O_{Arab}, C_{Harlem} and β-thalassaemia. Clinical manifestations tend to be severe in patients with Hb SS, Hb SD$_{Punjab}$, and Hb SO$_{Arab}$; moderate in those with Hb SC, Hb S/β-thal, and Hb CC; and mild or absent in individuals with Hb AS and Hb AC trait.

UNSTABLE HAEMOGLOBIN VARIANTS

Molecular basis

At least 73 unstable haemoglobin variants are known (Table 74.3). Among these, β-variants are five times more frequent than α-variants (59:12), a discrepancy which may be due to the smaller percentage of unstable haemoglobin and hence milder clinical symptoms associated with the α-chain variants. An individual with a single variant α gene has three normal α genes, so that the percentage of unstable haemoglobin in his red cells is very small (5 to 20%). In contrast, an individual with a variant β gene has only a single normal β gene; so the unstable haemoglobin containing the variant β chain makes up a greater proportion of the total cellular haemoglobin synthesized (20 to 40%) (Bunn et al, 1977c). Because the gene frequencies for these variants are extremely low, almost all affected individuals seen are heterozygotes.

The increased propensity of unstable haemoglobins to denature can result from several types of mutations. As mentioned previously, the α-helix of α- or β-globin can be disrupted by proline replacing another amino acid within the helix. There are at least ten examples of this type of disruption of primary and secondary structure, including Hb Bibba ($\alpha^{136\ \text{Leu}\to\text{Pro}}$) and Hb Genova ($\beta^{28\ \text{Leu}\to\text{Pro}}$) (Rieder, 1974). Deletions of amino acid residues alter primary and secondary structures as well as conformation of the haemoglobin molecules, and eight of the ten variants of this type are unstable; for example, Hb Leiden ($\beta^{6\ \text{or}\ 7\ \text{Glu}\to 0}$) and Hb Gun Hill [$\beta^{91-95\ (\text{Leu-His-Cys-Asp-Lys})\to 0}$] (Bunn et al, 1977c). Interference with interchain contacts permits the αβ dimers to dissociate into monomers; for example, Hb Philly ($\beta^{35\ \text{Tyr}\to\text{Phe}}$) and Hb Tacoma ($\beta^{30\ \text{Arg}\to\text{Ser}}$) lack hydrogen bonds normally linking the α and β subunits. Substitutions which affect haem binding or disturb the hydrophobic haem pocket (certain non-polar residues in the CD, E, F, and FG regions) decrease the molecule's stability (Fig. 74.1). There are over 30 such mutations, and most result in unstable haemoglobins, such as Hb Bristol ($\beta^{67\ \text{Val}\to\text{Asp}}$) and Hb Köln ($\beta^{98\ \text{Val}\to\text{Met}}$) (Rieder, 1974). Finally, globin chain elongation can result in instability due to hydrophobic properties of the extended chain; e.g., Hb Cranston ($\beta^{144-157}$) (Bunn et al, 1977c).

These variant haemoglobins tend to denature spontaneously; and the globin subunits precipitate in the red cell, forming aggregates or Heinz bodies. The Heinz bodies adhere to the red cell membrane and result in decreased pliability of the cell. Inflexible erythrocytes are then selectively trapped by the reticuloendothelial system.

Clinical aspects of unstable haemoglobins

Patients often present in infancy or early childhood with a haemolytic anaemia, jaundice, and splenomegaly, or later with cholelithiasis. Some variants also cause cyanosis due to their abnormal properties; i.e., propensity to form methaemoglobin or decreased oxygen affinity. Clinical severity varies with different unstable variants; for β-variants, symptoms appear after the γ to β transition in haemoglobin synthesis (Fig. 74.5).

Diagnosis

The peripheral smear may be normal or hypochromic. Staining with a supravital stain, such as 1% methyl violet, demonstrates preformed Heinz bodies (Fig. 74.8B). Heat instability of the variant haemoglobin is demonstrated by the formation of a haemoglobin precipitate when a haemolysate is incubated at 50°C or higher, or

at 37°C in 17% isopropanol. Haemoglobin electrophoresis by usual methods may detect only about one half of unstable variants since the charge of these variants is often unaltered by the substitutions. Oxygen saturation curves of whole blood may indicate normal (20% of the unstable variants), decreased (30%), or increased (50%) oxygen affinity (Bunn et al, 1977c).

Treatment

Treatment is generally supportive. If haemolysis is severe, prophylactic folate may be indicated. Oxidant drugs, such as sulfonamides, increase haemolysis in some patients and should be avoided. Transfusions are indicated only in the treatment of aplastic crises. While splenectomy may result in improvement of the anaemia, it also increases the risk of septicaemia, especially in young patients. Because of the mortality associated with septicaemia in splenectomized patients, the physician should reserve splenectomy for selected patients. Splenectomy should be postponed until the patient is at least six years of age, and the administration of pneumococcal vaccine and prophylactic antibiotics should be considered (Bunn et al, 1977c).

HAEMOGLOBIN VARIANTS WITH ALTERED OXYGEN AFFINITY

Molecular basis

The oxygen dissociation curve shown in Figure 74.2 is sigmoid shaped due to haem-haem interactions. Mutations whhich affect haem-haem interaction, the Bohr effect, or deoxyhaemoglobin-2,3-DPG interaction can change the shape or position of the oxygen dissociation curve. Mutations affecting the $\alpha_1\beta_2$ subunit contact point can alter haem-haem interaction by causing the deoxyhaemoglobin conformation to be less stable. These mutations result in increased stability of the oxyhaemoglobin conformation and increased oxygen affinity [Hb Kempsey ($\beta^{99\text{Asp}\to\text{Asn}}$)]. Alternatively, the oxyhaemoglobin conformation can be destabilized by mutations affecting the $\alpha^{94}\beta^{102}$-contact point resulting in decreased oxygen affinity [Hb Kansas ($\beta^{102\ \text{Asn}\to\text{Thr}}$)]. Substitutions at the COOH-terminal ends of globin chains can lead to instability of the deoxyhaemoglobin conformations and increased oxygen affinity [Hb Bethesda ($\beta^{145\ \text{Tyr}\to\text{His}}$)] as well as a reduction in the Bohr effect. 2,3-DPG binds to residues $\beta^{1,\ 2,\ 82,\ \text{and}\ 143}$ in the deoxygenated form. Substitutions altering these residues tend to have increased oxygen affinity [Hb F (γ globin has a serine for histidine substitution at position 143)] (Bellingham, 1976).

The variants with increased oxygen affinity cause a shift to the left of the oxygen dissociation curve

(Fig. 74.2), resulting in less oxygen delivery per gram of haemoglobin. To compensate, haemoglobin concentration and/or blood flow increases in order to partially restore oxygen delivery to the tissues (Bellingham, 1976). Some variants with increased oxygen affinity do not cause polycythaemia due to the small fraction of the total haemoglobin they comprise or to compensatory changes in the shape of the oxygen dissociation curve. Variants with decreased oxygen affinity have a shift to the right and increased oxygen delivery per gram of haemoglobin. As a result, the haemoglobin concentration is normal or decreased [Hb Beth Israel ($\beta^{102 \ Asn \rightarrow Ser}$)] (Nagel et al, 1976).

Clinical aspects and diagnosis

Because the gene frequencies for nearly all variant haemoglobins are very low, patients are nearly always heterozygotes. β-chain variants outnumber α-chain variants by 2:1 (Table 74.3). The great majority of patients are asymptomatic; and when oxygen affinity is increased the major finding is polycythaemia with erythrocytosis, normal white blood cell and platelet counts, and absence of splenomegaly. Since about one half of these variants cannot be detected on routine electrophoresis, whole blood oxygen affinity studies are required for diagnosis. Some concern has been raised regarding the risk to fetuses of mothers who have variants with increased oxygen affinity. The little data available regarding the outcome of such pregnancies in general does not seem to indicate increased fetal mortality (Bellingham, 1976).

Treatment

The condition is generally considered benign. It is important to avoid chemical treatment of the compensatory polycythaemia unless haematocrit levels are high enough to cause increased viscosity.

M HAEMOGLOBIN VARIANTS

Molecular basis

There are five known variants of M haemoglobin, four of which result from substitution of tyrosine for histidine at positions α^{58}, α^{87}, β^{63}, and β^{92} [M-Boston ($\alpha^{58 \ His \rightarrow Tyr}$), M-Iwate ($\alpha^{87 \ His \rightarrow Tyr}$), M-Saskatoon ($\beta^{63 \ His \rightarrow Tyr}$) and M-Hyde Park ($\beta^{92 \ His \rightarrow Tyr}$)]. The substituted tyrosine may form a stable bond with the ferric form of the haem iron. This bond prevents interaction of the ferric iron of the affected α or β with oxygen, but it does not render the globin-haem unit unstable. Both α-variants (M-Boston and M-Iwate) have decreased oxygen affinity, two of the β-variants (M-Hyde Park and M-Saskatoon) have normal affinity, and the final β-variant (M-Milwaukee-I) has decreased oxygen affinity (Bellingham, 1976; Bunn, 1974).

Clinical aspects

M haemoglobin variants, like other rare haemoglobin disorders, are inherited in an autosomal dominant pattern. The age of onset of cyanosis differs depending on whether the α- or β-chain is affected. With α-chain variants, cyanosis is seen at birth; while β-globin variants develop cyanosis when γ to β switching is nearly complete, at about six months of age (Fig. 74.5).

Diagnosis

The blood is chocolate brown and does not change colour on exposure to oxygen. Usually there is no anaemia, and routine electrophoresis may be normal. Spectral analysis allows differentiation of M haemoglobins from methaemoglobin secondary to diaphorase I deficiency. The latter is a red cell enzyme deficiency which is inherited as an autosomal recessive (Bunn, 1974). Because the modes of inheritance for M haemoglobins and diaphorase deficiency differ, usually one parent of a patient with the former is affected, while both parents of a patient with the latter disorder are unaffected.

Treatment

No treatment is indicated; however, the diagnosis should be made so that extensive cardiac and pulmonary evaluations can be avoided.

THALASSAEMIAS: QUANTITATIVE DISORDERS OF GLOBIN SYNTHESIS

The thalassaemia syndromes are genetic disorders characterised by absent or deficient synthesis of one or more of the normal globin chains. Absent globin synthesis is designated with an 'o' superscript; e.g., β^0-thalassemia, while the presence of some (but not enough) of the gene product is noted by a '+' superscript; e.g., β^+-thalassaemia. When there is partial synthesis of the affected globin chain, it is usually structurally normal; therefore, the defect is a quantitative one secondary to unbalanced globin synthesis. This contrasts with the haemoglobinopathies in which the variant haemoglobins are qualitatively or structurally abnormal. Thalassaemia is distributed primarily among people of Mediterranean, African, and Asian descent, but sporadic cases have been reported in many ethnic groups (Kazazian et al, 1977; Orkin & Nathan, 1976).

Molecular basis

As discussed previously and shown in Figure 74.6, globin biosynthesis has many steps, each of which has the potential for regulating the amount of globin chains produced. The thalassaemia syndromes provide examples of defects at several different steps. First, deletion of the DNA sequences coding for the structural gene occurs in

Table 74.6 Characteristics of certain thalassaemia states

Condition	Parents	Inheritance risk (%)	Haemoglobin electrophoresis	DNA Sequences	mRNA
Heterozygotes					
Silent carrier (α-thalassaemia$_2$)	α-thal$_2$, normal	50	1–2% γ$_4$ (birth)	3α	Slight ↓ α
α-Thal trait (α-thalassaemia$_1$)	Both α-thal$_2$ or α-thal$_1$, normal	25 50	5% γ$_4$ (birth)	2α	↓ ↓ α
Hb H	α-thal$_1$, α-thal$_2$	25	4–30% β$_4$ (adults) 20–40% γ$_4$ (birth)	1α	↓ ↓ ↓ α
β$^+$-Thalassaemia	β$^+$/β, normal	50	Hb A$_2$ ↑, slight ↑ F, or 5–12% F	2β	↓ β
β°-Thalassaemia	β°/β, normal	50	Hb A$_2$ ↑, slight ↑ F	2β	0 or ↓ β
δβ°-Thalassaemia	δβ°/δβ, normal	50	5–20% Hb F	1β and 1δ	↓ δ and β
δβ-Lepore	Lepore/β, normal	50	Slight ↑ Hb F, normal or ↓ A$_2$, and 5–15% Lepore	1δ, 1β, and 1δβ-Lepore	↓ δβ-Lepore
Hb Constant Spring (CS)	Hb CS heterozygote, normal	50	1–2% γ$_4$ (birth), 0.5–1% Hb CS	3α α^{cs}	↓ CS
Homozygotes					
Hydrops fetalis (α°-thalassaemia$_1$)	Both α-thal$_1$	25	80% γ$_4$ (birth) 10% δ$_2$γ$_2$, 10% β$_4$	0α	0α
β°-Thalassaemia	Both β°/β	25	↑ Hb F + A$_2$, OA	2β	0 or ↓ β
β$^+$-Thalassaemia	Both β$^+$/β	25	↑ Hb F + A$_2$, ↓ A	2β	↓ β
δβ°-Thalassaemia	Both δβ°/δβ	25	100% Hb F, OA, and OA$_2$	0 β, 0 δ	O δ and O β
δβ-Lepore	Both Lepore/β	25	75% Hb F, 25% Lepore	2δβ-Lepore	↓ δβ-Lepore
Hb Constant Spring (CS)	Both Hb CS heterozygotes	25	5–6% Hb CS	2α 2α^{cs}	↓ CS

Data from Orkin SH, Nathan DG: Current topics in genetics: The thalassaemias. N Engl J Med 295:710, 1976 and Weatherall DJ: The molecular basis of thalassaemia. John Hopkins Medical Journal 139:205, 1976.

most α-thalassaemias and in certain rare types of β-thalassaemia (Table 74.6) (Orkin & Nathan, 1976). Evidence has accumulated that the chromosome in most blacks, Filipinos, and some Chinese which has one of the two α genes deleted arose by a mispairing of the 5' α gene of one chromosome 16 with the 3' α gene of its homologue and subsequent unequal crossing-over (Fig. 74.9) (Orkin et al, 1979; Phillips et al, 1980b). The reciprocal chromosome, one containing three α genes, has been observed in Mediterraneans and blacks (Goossens et al, 1980). In Chinese, about one third of chromosome 16s containing a single functional α-globin gene originated from a simple deletion of the 5' α gene, while another third have a nondeletion defect (Embury et al, 1980). Chromosomes lacking both α genes have been studied in Asian subjects, and they have large deletions which remove ζ$_1$,ψα, and both α genes while leaving the ζ$_2$ gene intact (Pressley et al, 1980).

In most β°-thalassaemias, the β DNA sequence or gene is present, but no β mRNA is detectable, suggesting that the mutation may prevent transcription. Certain patients with β-thalassaemias have a chain terminator mutation in the coding region of the β gene which leads to a β

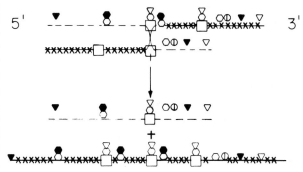

Fig. 74.9 Diagrammatic representation of an unequal crossing-over event. The probable origin of chromosomes with single and triple α-globin genes. Homologous normal chromosome 16s are shown mispairing above, and the resulting chromosomes with a single or triple α-globin genes are shown below. The 5' to 3' orientation is shown from left to right, and the α-globin genes are diagrammatically represented by rectangles or arbitrary size. Small symbols represent the normal locations of restriction endonuclease sites: ▼ = Bam HI, Φ = Eco RI, ○ = Hind II, ▽ = Hind III, and ● = Hpa I.

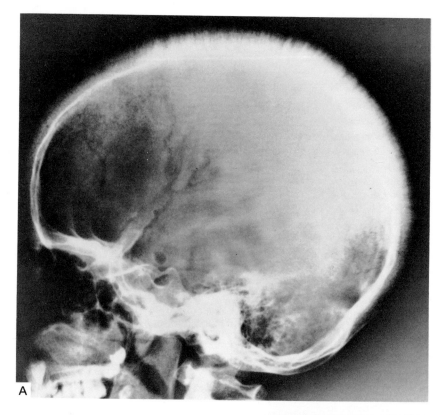

Fig. 74.10 Radiographic changes in homozygous β-thalassaemia (A) Thickened parietal calvaria with outer table destruction and 'hair-on-end' appearance. Note absent pneumatization of maxillary sinuses and coincidental epidermoidoma. (B) Widened medullary cavities, cortical thinning, and coarse trabeculation secondary to intra-medullary hyperplasia. (Courtesy of Dr John Dorst)

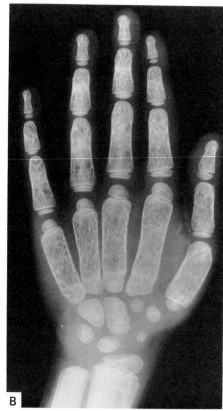

mRNA that cannot be decoded into complete β chains. An example is $\beta^{17\ lys \to term}$ which contains the nucleotide substitution AGG → UAG at the codon for amino acid 17 (Chang & Kan, 1979). Most β⁺-thalassaemia genes lead to decreased β mRNA and commensurate β-globin chain production. Recently it has been shown that some β⁺-thalassaemia patients have defective excision of IVSs from precursor β mRNA (Kantor et al, 1980). One β⁺-thalassaemia gene has been sequenced, and it contains a single nucleotide change from that of the reported sequence of a βᴬ gene. This single substitution near the 3′ end of IVS I may lead to defective splicing of the precursor β mRNA and be responsible for the disorder (Spritz et al, 1980b). Thus, it appears that while deletions account for most α-thalassaemias, the bulk of β-thalassaemia genes have point mutations producing defects in transcription and/or mRNA processing. The heterogeneity seen in the clinical and biochemical manifestations of β-thalassaemias is probably due to different combinations of various β-thalassaemia alleles.

Pathophysiology

In the thalassaemia syndromes there is reduced or absent synthesis of the affected globin chain; the unaffected chain continues to be synthesized at relatively normal levels. The result is an imbalance which causes aggregation and precipitation of excess unpaired chains. In β-thalassaemia, free α-chains aggregate; the aggregates are highly insoluble and form inclusions in nucleated erythroid precursors in the bone marrow. These inclusion bodies cause intramedullary haemolysis (ineffective erythropoiesis). In contrast, in α-thalassaemia the γ_4 (Hb Barts) and β_4 (Hb H) tetramers that form are more soluble. Thus, in severe α-thalassaemias, inclusions are seen in mature erythrocytes and the ineffective erythropoiesis of β-thalassaemia is absent. In any severe thalassaemia, removal of these inclusions from erythrocytes by the reticuloendothelial system damages the cells and produces 'teardrop' forms. Splenomegaly can be secondary to splenic congestion or hypersplenism. After the spleen is removed, cell destruction continues at a decreased rate in the liver, and the number of red cell inclusions may increase greatly. The large number of erythroid precursors expands the marrow cavities, and bone deformities, thinning, and occasional pathologic fractures result (Fig. 74.10) (Nathan, 1972).

Iron accumulation results from increased gastrointestinal absorption stimulated by the anaemia, blood transfusions, and decreased utilization for haemoglobin synthesis. The deposition of excess iron causes damage to the heart, pancreas, and other tissues.

Folic acid requirements are increased in thalassaemia. If deficiencies develop, they may worsen the anaemia.

Clinical features

α-thalassaemia

Patients are often of Mediterranean or oriental descent, but the frequency of mild α-thalassaemia is also high in blacks. When the mutation affects both α loci on the same chromosome 16, the genotype is called α-thal$_1$ (--). When a single locus on only one of the number 16 chromosomes is affected, the genotype is α-thal$_2$ (α-).

Four clinical types are seen depending upon the number of α genes affected. The most severe form is α^0-thal (α-thal$_1$ homozygote) (--/--), or hydrops fetalis with Hb Barts. This condition is found usually in oriental infants who are spontaneously aborted or die of severe hydrops shortly after birth. In the usual case, over 80% of the haemoglobin is Hb Barts (γ_4), which has a very high oxygen affinity causing severe tissue hypoxia; the remainder is Hb Portland ($\zeta_2\gamma_2$) and Hb H (β_4). Both parents carry the α-thal$_1$ trait (Forget & Kan, 1974).

The frequency of HB H disease (--/α-) is high in Southeast Asians, Greeks, and Italians. The anaemia varies with an average range of 8 to 10 gm of haemoglobin per 100 ml of blood, and reticulocytes make up 5 to 10% of red cells. Splenomegaly and, occasionally, hepatomegaly are found. The red cells are microcytic [decreased mean corpuscular volume (MCV)] and their haemoglobin content is decreased [decreased mean corpuscular haemoglobin (MCH)], but the concentration of haemoglobin per cell is normal [normal mean corpuscular haemoglobin concentration (MCHC)]. On the peripheral smear, poikilocytosis, polychromasia, and target cells are seen. The β_4 tetramer (Hb H) inclusions are seen easily following incubation with 1% brilliant cresyl blue, or after splenectomy they can be seen occasionally with methylene blue reticulocyte stain or Wright's stain (Fig. 74.8C) (Forget & Kan, 1974). Studies of globin chain synthesis suggest an α/β ratio of 0.3 to 0.4, rather than 1, and most individuals have a genotype comprised of α-thal$_1$ and α-thal$_2$ (--/α-) (Fig. 74.11). This imbalance causes 20% or higher levels of Hb Barts at birth and Hb H levels of 4 to 30% after the switch from γ- to β-chain synthesis is complete. Both tetramers precipitate causing an inclusion body haemolytic anaemia. Deficient α-chain synthesis causes a drop in Hb A$_2$ ($\alpha_2\delta_2$) levels to 1 to 1.5%. Deficient α-chain synthesis is secondary to a deficiency of α-globin mRNA caused by deletion of three of the four α genes. Usually, one of the parents of such a patient has α-thal$_1$ (--) and the other has α-thal$_2$ (α-). The inheritance risk for Hb H disease in offspring from such matings is 25% with each pregnancy (Table 74.6) (Wasi et al, 1974).

Heterozygous α-thal$_1$ individuals (Fig. 74.11) usually are of oriental or Mediterranean descent. They are relatively asymptomatic, but have a mild microcytic anaemia (10 to 12 gm of haemoglobin per 100 ml of blood) and mild poikilocytosis and anisocytosis. The diagnosis of α-thal trait should be considered seriously when the MCV and MCH are low, the MCHC is relatively normal and the patient is not iron deficient, and the haemoglobin electrophoresis is normal. At birth, Hb Barts may reach 5% in cord blood. The α/β synthesis ratio is 0.6 to 0.75, and the genotype in orientals is usually a single mutation which deletes both α genes on the same chromosome (Fig. 74.11). A second type of α-thal gene which is dysfunctional but not deleted has been found in Chinese and Cypriots (Kan et al, 1977; Orkin et al, 1979). Blacks have mild elevation of Hb Barts (>2%) in 2 to 5% of newborns (Wasi et al, 1974), and such individuals have been shown to have an α-thal trait phenotype. Recent restriction endonuclease studies have shown that the α-thal trait phenotype in blacks is usually due to deletion of a single α gene on both chromosome 16s (trans) (α-thal$_2$ homozygote) (α-/α-), in contrast to the usual oriental genotype [deletion of both α genes on one chromosome 16 (cis, or α-thal$_1$ heterozygote) (αα/--)] (Dozy et al, 1979b).

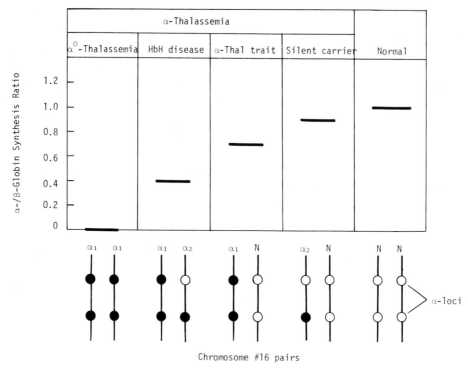

Fig. 74.11 Chain synthesis ratios and proposed genotypes in the different α-thalassemia states. Genotypes: o = normal, N = normal, ● = abnormal, α_1 = α-thal$_1$, α_2 = α-thal$_2$, α_1N could also be $\alpha_2\alpha$s22. (Modified from Nathan DG 1972 Thalassaemia. N Engl J Med 286: 586)

Silent carriers have *α-thal$_2$* genotypes with the deletion of a single α gene ($\alpha\alpha/\alpha$-) in affected orientals, and in 28% of blacks. (Dozy et al, 1979b). The haematologic findings are normal because the reduction of α mRNA is insufficient to produce significant globin chain imbalance ($\alpha/\beta = 0.8$ to 0.9) (Fig. 74.11). Among Southeast Asians there is also a second relatively common α-thal$_2$ allele, the $\alpha^{\text{Constant Spring}}$ gene. This gene encodes an abnormal α chain which has 31 additional amino acids at the COOH-terminal end and which is synthesized at about 3% of the rate of normal α-chains (Bunn et al, 1977b).

β-thalassaemia

In contrast to the α-thalassaemia states in which there are four levels of severity, the β-thalassaemias can be considered as having two degrees of severity: β-thalassaemia major (Cooley's anaemia) results from two β-thalassaemia genes at the β-globin locus; β-thal trait results from a single β-thal gene.

β-thalassaemia major is a severe disease. At birth, affected infants are relatively normal because the change from γ-chain synthesis to β-chain synthesis has not occurred (Fig. 74.5). However, by six months of age the infant develops a severely microcytic hemolytic anemia with aniso- and poikilocytosis, polychromasia, and tear-drop red cells (Fig. 74.8F) (Forget & Kan, 1974). The

failure in β-globin production due to absent or greatly decreased β mRNA leads to imbalance in α- and β-globin synthesis. Subsequent precipitation of free α-chains results in inclusion bodies which damage the erythrocyte membrane and lead to destruction of nucleated red cells in the marrow. The reticulocyte count is usually no greater than 5 to 10% because of massive destruction of erythroid precursors in the marrow. To maintain an adequate haemoglobin level, transfusions are usually required every four to eight weeks. Affected children develop hepatosplenomegaly secondary to extramedullary haematopoiesis and a characteristic oriental facial appearance due to excessive intramedullary haematopoiesis. The bones have expanded marrow cavities resulting in pathologic fractures and a 'hair-on-end' appearance on skull films (Fig. 74.10). Other complications include cholelithiasis, susceptibility to infections, secondary hypersplenism, and delayed growth and maturation (Nathan, 1972; Forget & Kan, 1974).

The major causes of mortality are haemochromatosis and overwhelming infections following splenectomy; the former due to excessive iron deposition as a result of blood transfusions and increased gastrointestinal absorption (Bannerman et al, 1964). Excess iron deposited in the heart, pancreas, liver, and other organs damages tissue and leads to cardiac failure, arrhythmias, diabetes mellitus, and liver failure. Given antibiotic and transfusion therapy, many patients survive until their twenties (Forget & Kan, 1974). Greek and Italian homozygotes generally follow this course.

Affected blacks often have a milder disease (β-thalassaemia intermedia). Transfusions usually are not required in these patients even though α/β synthesis ratios are similar to those observed in Mediterranean homozygotes (Weatherall, 1976).

Individuals with β-thal trait (heterozygous β-thalassaemia) are usually asymptomatic. They have a mild anaemia (10 to 11 gm of haemoglobin per 100 ml of blood) with decreased MCV (55 to 70 μ^3) and MCH (16 to 22 pg). Microcytosis, anisocytosis, poikilocytosis, and targeting and stippling of the red cells can be seen on the blood smear (Fig. 74.8E) (Forget & Kan, 1974). On physical examination there is mild to moderate splenomegaly in about one half of the cases.

Differential diagnosis

In the general practice of medicine, many patients present with a mild microcytic anaemia. Nearly all of them have iron deficiency anaemia or a thalassaemia trait. In heterozygous thalassaemia, the peripheral smear may be more abnormal than that of iron deficiency; and the MCV and MCH are decreased, but the MCHC is normal in contrast to the decreased MCHC seen in advanced iron deficiency anaemia. Also, the MCV in thalassaemia traits tends to be lower in relation to the red cell count than the MCV in iron deficiency. This difference is the basis of the Mentzer index [MCV/red cell count (RBC)]. MCV/RBC values of less than 11.5 suggest thalassaemia trait, while values greater than 13.5 suggest iron deficiency anaemia (Mentzer, 1973). A much more definitive approach is to measure Hb A_2 in patients with microcytosis (Fig. 74.12). Patients with microcytosis and normal Hb A_2 should have serum iron or ferritin determinations; a low value suggests iron deficiency anaemia, while a normal iron or ferritin value suggests α-thal trait (diagnosis is confirmed when documentation is obtained in first-degree relatives). When microcytosis and an increased Hb A_2 are found, β-thal trait is the tentative diagnosis (Pearson et al, 1973). Confirmation of the diagnosis is obtained by family studies and chain synthesis ratios. A possible simple alternative for differentiating iron deficiency from thalassaemia trait in patients with low MCVs is to measure the degree of anisocytosis with an electronic red cell counter. Anisocytosis is significantly greater in patients with iron deficiency than those with thalassaemia trait (Bessman & Feinstein, 1979).

As seen in Table 74.6, β-thal heterozygotes can have

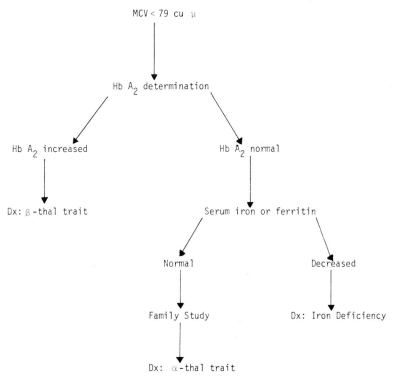

Fig. 74.12 Approach to screening for thalassaemia trait. Note that since this approach was designed as a guide for screening of adults, other causes of microcytosis, such as lead poisoning in children, are not considered. (Modified from Pearson H A, O'Brien R T, McIntosh S 1973 Screening for thalassaemia trait by electronic measurement of MCV. N Engl J Med 288: 351)

different haemoglobin patterns. The most common is that of β^0-thal or β^+-thal with an increased Hb A$_2$ (usually 4 to 6%) and a normal or slightly increased Hb F (2 to 5%). In the rare $\delta\beta$-thal trait, the Hb A$_2$ is normal, but Hb F is usually increased. Finally, Hb Lepore trait has 5 to 15% Hb Lepore, which contains a $\delta\beta$ fusion chain, and a slight elevation of Hb F (Orkin & Nathan, 1976; Forget & Kan, 1974). Chain synthesis studies in most β-thal heterozygotes yield α/β ratios of 1.5 to 2.5.

The term β-thalassaemia intermedia is sometimes used to describe individuals who are either severe β-thal heterozygotes or mild homozygotes; black β^+-thal homozygotes with a mild clinical course are an example. Family studies in some have confirmed that the presumed β^+-thal homozygotes in fact had inherited two different β-thal alleles and thus were actually genetic compounds (Kreimer-Birnbaum et al, 1975). Homozygous $\delta\beta$-thalassaemia also tends to be clinically mild because for unknown reasons Hb F production is higher in this condition than in other β-thal states and compensates for the absent Hb A and Hb A$_2$. One can also find the combination of α-thal and β-thal traits in the same individual. This condition is mild because the resulting α/β synthesis ratio is more normal and there are fewer free α-chains to cause haemolysis.

$\delta\beta$-thalassaemia, or F thalassaemia

Homozygous $\delta\beta$-thalassaemia usually occurs in Greeks and, as stated above, tends to be a mild disorder. The term F thalassaemia is used because homozygotes have 100% Hb F and lack Hb A and Hb A$_2$. The mild anaemia and haemolysis are due to increased γ-chain synthesis, which makes the imbalance between synthesis of α-chains and non-α chains less than that seen in other β-thalassaemias. Patients with heterozygous $\delta\beta$-thalassaemias have mild microcystosis and 5 to 20% Hb F on electrophoresis (Table 74.6).

Hb Lepore thalassaemia

As previously mentioned, Hb Lepore is a variant haemoglobin containing a $\delta\beta$-fusion chain. Originally this chain probably resulted from nonhomologous crossing-over between the linked δ- and β-genes during meiosis. Three different Lepore variants are described which differ in the point at which the $\delta\beta$-fusion occurs. Hb Lepore has an electrophoretic mobility similar to that of Hb S, and it forms 5 to 15% of the total haemoglobin of heterozygotes (Table 74.6). Decreased Hb Lepore synthesis may be secondary to instability of the $\delta\beta$-mRNA. Heterozygotes are clinically similar to β^0-thal heterozygotes and Hb Lepore homozygotes, or Lepore/β^0-thal genetic compounds, are similar to β^0-thal homozygotes (Forget & Kan, 1974).

$\gamma\beta$-thalassaemia

Two full-term newborns with haemolytic, hypochromic anaemia and microcytosis have been described. Hb H and Hb Barts were absent, and globin synthesis studies revealed a deficiency of γ- and β-synthesis in relation to α-synthesis. With time, the peripheral smears and morphology improved and resembled those of the fathers and other relatives with heterozygous β-thal. These cases are probably examples of heterozygous $\gamma\beta$-thalassaemia (Kan et al, 1972; Van der Ploeg et al, 1980). Restriction endonuclease mapping of DNA of one child has shown a large deletion which removes all of the ϵ, $^G\gamma$, $^A\gamma$, and δ genes from one chromosome 11. Interestingly, the deletion ends 2 kb 5' to the β gene, yet that β gene, while present, is not expressed (Van der Ploeg et al, 1980).

δ^0-thalassaemia

Heterozygous and homozygous δ^0-thalassaemia have decreased and absent Hb A$_2$, respectively. However, anaemia and changes in peripheral smears are not seen due to the normal low level of δ-chain production (Fig. 74.5).

Hereditary persistence of fetal haemoglobin

Hereditary persistence of fetal haemoglobin (HPFH) can occur in many different forms due to different mutations. HPFH heterozygotes differ from thalassaemia heterozygotes in that they have no imbalance between the synthesis of α and non-α chains (i.e., γ- and β-chains). The HPFH syndromes are characterised by an asymptomatic heterozygous state without microcytosis. The elevated Hb F ranges from 10 to 15% in the Greek type to 3 to 30% in certain types in blacks. The proportion of γ-chain type ($^G\gamma$ versus $^A\gamma$) varies among patients with different HPFHs and usually, but not always, the Hb F is homogeneously distributed within red cells, in contrast to $\delta\beta$- and other thalassaemias (Kazazian, 1974). In a few cases, HPFH heterozygotes have two populations of cells: one contains Hb F; the other lacks Hb F. These patients are said to have heterocellular HPFH, as opposed to the bulk of patients who have pancellular HPFH (Boyer et al, 1977).

The β and δ genes adjacent to the HPFH gene are often inactive and, in fact, may be deleted in blacks with one HPFH type, but both are present and active in other HPFH cases involving blacks. The differences between HPFH and $\delta\beta$-thallassaemia are subtle, but in $\delta\beta$-thal the clinical picture and blood smears are somewhat more abnormal and the Hb F has a more heterogeneous cellular distribution. HPFH homozygotes have mild hypochromia, microcytosis, and morphologic changes in the red cells; 100% of the haemoglobin is F, and there is no anaemia. In some of these cases, α/γ chain synthesis ratios of 1.5 occur, similar to the α/β ratios seen in milder β-thal trait. It has been hypothesised that a suppression region for γ-chain synthesis is located between the ^{A}γ- and δ-loci and that HPFH, but not δβ-thalassemia mutations, inhibit its function (Kazazian, 1976). In agreement with this concept, the deletions causing HPFH are generally larger than deletions in δβ-thalassaemia (Fritsch et al, 1979).

Interaction of thalassaemia with haemoglobin variants

Thalassaemia and structural variant haemoglobin genes may or may not interact. An interacting thalassaemia gene is one which causes an increased level of the variant haemoglobin chain in the individual heterozygous for the variant gene and a thalassaemia gene at the same locus. When the presence of both the thalassaemia and variant genes does not increase the level of the haemoglobin variant, then the thalassaemia is noninteracting.

α-thalassaemia and α variants

α-thalassaemia$_1$ – Hb Q ($α^{47 \text{ Asp} \rightarrow \text{His}}$). The genetic compound of α-thal$_1$ (--) and Hb Q is found mainly in Thailand. The clinical picture is similar to that of Hb H disease, but there is an absence of Hb A synthesis which is explained by the fact that the $α^Q$ allele occurs on a chromosome from which the second α gene is deleted ($α^{Q}$-) (Lie-Injo et al, 1979).

α-thalassaemia – Hb G-Philadelphia ($p^{68 \text{Asn} \rightarrow \text{Lys}}$). Heterozygotes for Hb G-Philadelphia, the most common α-variant in blacks, have been studied, and the amount of the variant seems to be trimodal (22%, 30%, and 41% of the total haemoglobin) (Baine et al, 1976). Individuals with 30% Hb G have been shown to have chromosomal homologues containing (1) a single $α^G$ gene and (2) two normal $α^A$ genes ($αα/α^G$-); and those with 41% Hb G have one chromosome containing a single $α^G$ gene and another with a single $α^A$ gene ($α$-/$α^G$-) (Sancar et al, 1980). Individuals with 22% Hb G have not yet been studied, but conceivably could have three normal $α^A$ genes in addition to an $α^G$ gene ($αα/α^G α$).

β-thalassaemia and β-variants

In S/β-thalassaemia, the β-thal gene interacts with the $β^S$ gene in the heterozygote to increase the level of Hb S near homozygous SS levels. The S/β-thal heterozygote has a milder clinical course than the SS homozygote, and splenomegaly is a common physical finding. Anaemia is present in S/β-thal and is characterised by microcytic red and target cells with occasional sickled forms (Fig. 74.8). Haemoglobin electrophoresis reveals 60 to 90% Hb S, 0 to 30% Hb A, 1 to 20% Hb F, and increased Hb A$_2$ (Forget & Kan, 1974). The percentages of Hb S and Hb A vary depending on whether the β-thal gene is $β^+$ or $β^0$.

β-*thalassaemia – Hb C* is seen among blacks. Splenomegaly and an increased Hb C level differentiate this genetic compound from that of Hb C heterozygote.

β-*thalassaemia – Hb E* is a common disease in Thailand. It results in a clinical picutre similar to that of homozygous β-thalassaemia.

Management of thalassaemia
Prevention

Matings which can give rise to various types of α- and β-thalassaemias are outline in Table 74.6. The parents of homozygous α- or β-thalassaemia offspring are themselves heterozygotes. As such, with each pregnancy there is a 25% risk of producing another homozygous offspring.

For maximum benefit of genetic counselling, heterozygotes should be identified before they bear affected children. Thalassaemia heterozygotes can be diagnosed tentatively by appropriate studies (MCV, haemoglobin electrophoresis, serum iron) (Fig. 74.12). Once the condition is diagnosed, the heterozygote should be informed of its presence, its inheritance, and the potential for affected children from certain matings so that he or she has an accurate grasp of the risk. In some cases this would result in testing of mates who would be identified as noncarriers, and hence these couples would be at no risk for homozygous offspring. The risk of having a homozygous offspring when both parents are heterozygotes is shown in Table 74.6; other parents might be at risk for genetic compounds in their offspring.

Prenatal diagnosis may be desired by certain heterozygous couples at risk. The procedure is becoming more widely used, but it remains investigative. Also, while the procedure leads to in utero diagnosis, it is not a treatment, but merely a preventive measure. Until recently, prenatal diagnosis of various thalassaemias was done exclusively by analysis of fetal blood. The feasibility of this procedure is based on a number of factors. First, β-chains are synthesized by erythroid precursors as early as five weeks of fetal age (Fig. 74.5). Second, normal standards of β-chain synthesis at 18 to 20 weeks gestation are known. Third, fetal cells can be obtained (with a 6% risk of fetal death at present) by either transabdominal placental puncture under ultrasonography or from fetal vessels visualized by fetoscopy (Alter, 1979). Fourth, small numbers of fetal reticulocytes can be separated from maternal red cells by differential agglutination or by preferential lysis of maternal cells. The fetal blood sample can be incubated with radioactive leucine, and the relative synthesis of α, β (or variant β-chains), and γ-chains can be determined using chromatographic separation (Alter, 1979). Thus, hemoglobinopathies such as sickle cell anaemia can also be diagnosed prenatally. By 1980, about 1000 pregnancies had been tested for β-thalassaemia in this way (Alter, 1979). The procedure has usually resulted in adequate fetal blood samples (>90%) with few technical errors.

Recently, analysis of globin genes by restriction endonuclease mapping of DNA has also been used for prenatal diagnosis of thalassaemias. Fetal amniocytes are obtained for study by amniocentesis, which carries a very low risk of fetal mortality (<0.5%). DNA analysis was first carried out on fetuses at risk for α-thalassaemia and δβ-thalassaemia in whom deletions could be detected (Orkin et al, 1978; Dozy et al, 1979a). Recently, polymorphic restriction endonuclease sites in the β-globin gene complex have been used for prenatal detection of various β-thalassaemias not due to deletions. Kan et al (1980) first showed that a Bam HI site 3' to the β gene was useful for prenatal diagnosis of a certain β⁰-thalassaemia allele in Sardinian couples at risk. Later, Little et al (1980) demonstrated that other polymorphic sites in the γ genes could be valuable in this undertaking in non-Sardinian couples. Using a combination of known DNA polymorphisms and linkage analysis, it has become possible to carry out prenatal diagnosis for various β-thalassaemia states by amniocentesis alone in 75% of pregnancies at risk in which the couple has a previous child (Kazazian et al, 1980). Thus, couples of Greek, Italian, or Indian origin at risk for any of the β-thalassaemias, whether β⁺ or β⁰, have a good chance of avoiding fetoscopy if the coupling phases of their DNA 'markers' can be assigned. To establish the coupling phases, DNA analysis of a previous normal or affected child or of parents of the couple is necessary. Fetoscopy can then be reserved for the 25% of cases in which the disease cannot be excluded by amniocentesis. At present, families in which the coupling phase cannot be established also need fetoscopy.

Therapy

Anaemia. Treatment for severe β-thalassaemia is primarily symptomatic. If anaemia is severe enough, transfusions are required to maintain adequate levels of haemoglobin. There are two approaches. First, transfusion may be given when the patient's haemoglobin drops below 8 gm per 100 ml to avoid symptoms secondary to the anaemia. Second, hypertransfusion, or repeated transfusions, may be given as frequently as needed to maintain the haemoglobin at a minimum of 10 gm per 100 ml. The latter approach may require two to three units every two to four weeks in adults (Forget & Kan, 1974). Some evidence suggests that children maintained on hypertransfusion (haemoglobin greater than 9.5 to 10 gm per 100 ml) are more active, have fewer infections, and have less frequent complications of cardiac dysfunction, hypersplenism, and bone and dental changes. However, evidence is conflicting as to whether this therapy can aid the child to attain normal growth (Forget & Kan, 1974; Weiner et al, 1978).

Iron accumulation. Both methods of transfusion increase the iron overload. Iron chelation therapy with deferoxamine has been used to attempt to prevent this side effect of chronic transfusion. The route of administration is important since 750 mg of deferoxamine IM (with oral ascorbic acid in patients over five years old) resulted in urinary clearance of iron ranging from 2.2 to 44.8 mg per 24 hours (prior to treatment, excretion was 0.1 to 2.5 mg per 24 hours). Subcutaneous infusions of 1.5 gm deferoxamine over 18 hours further increased iron excretion 2.4-fold, and large doses given intravenously increased clearance over that obtained by subcutaneous infusion (Cohen & Schwartz, 1978; Propper et al, 1977). The iron excretion attained following intravenous or slow subcutaneous infusion of deferoxamine is far better than excretion when deferoxamine is injected intramuscularly. Other data suggest that in children, while 20 mg of deferoxamine B per kg of body weight given daily by IM injection might reduce the daily iron accumulation somewhat, if the deferoxamine is given by overnight infusion, it may allow iron balance to be reached even when the child has large transfusion requirements (Weiner et al, 1978). The relative effectiveness of different doses in thalassaemia patients of different ages has been reported (Graziano et al, 1978). These experimental data all suggest that chelation therapy may soon be applicable to clinical practice.

Other side effects of transfusions include hepatitis and cytomegalovirus infections. Also, isoimmunization to minor blood groups may occur, but careful selection of donors may decrease this risk. Sensitization to white cell or plasma antigens may be decreased by using blood with the white cells removed. Urticaria may be treated with antihistamines as well as epinephrine prior to and during transfusion. Febrile reactions may require antipyretics and occasionally, if severe, steroids (Nathan, 1972).

Finally, the increased rate of erythropoiesis can lead to increased folic acid requirements. If a folate deficiency occurs, it may cause increased anaemia; however, a deficiency is easily avoided by daily oral administration of folic acid.

Infection. Splenectomy may be avoided by hypertransfusion therapy; however, splenectomy may be necessary to alleviate hypersplenism with worsening of the anaemia or pain due to progressive splenomegaly or infarction of the spleen. As discussed under sickle cell disease, splenectomized children, especially those under six years of age, are at risk for life-threatening infections. Pneumococcal vaccine, as well as prophylactic penicillin, should be used in such children, and suspected infections should be treated aggressively (Ammann et al, 1977; Forget & Kan, 1974).

Future treatment

While bone marrow transplantation has been used successfully in aplastic anaemia and leukaemia, it has not been used for thalassaemia because of the high risk of rejection, morbidity, and death associated with this procedure.

Theoretical approaches to thalassaemia treatment which may become possible include induction of expression of the deficient globin chain, stabilization of the appropriate mRNA, or activation of non-expressed γ genes to reduce the globin chain imbalance. Methods for insertion of DNA into eukaryotic cells are being developed, but technical as well as ethical problems remain. The chances of applying such techniques to the treatment of thalassaemia syndromes or the haemoglobinopathies seem remote at this time.

REFERENCES

Alter B P 1979 Prenatal diagnosis of hemoglobinopathies and other hematologic disorders. Journal of Pediatrics 95: 501

Alter B P, Modell C B, Fairweather D, Hobbins J C, Mahoney M J, Frigoletto F D, Sherman A S, Nathan D G 1976 Prenatal diagnosis of hemoglobinopathies. New England Journal of Medicine 295: 1437

Akhonkhai V I, Landesman S H, Fikrig S M, Schmalzer E A, Brown A K, Cherubin C E, Schiffman G 1979 Failure of pneumococcal vaccine in children with sickle cell disease. New England Journal of Medicine 301: 26

Ammann A J, Addiego J, Wara D W, Lubin B, Smith W B, Mentzer W C 1977 Polyvalent pneumococcal-polysaccharide immunization of patients with sickle-cell anemia and patients with splenectomy. New England Journal of Medicine 297: 897

Baine R M, Rucknagel D L, Dublin P A Jr, Adams J G III 1976 Trimodality in the proportion of hemoglobin G Philadelphia in heterozygotes. Evidence for heterogeneity in the number of human alpha chain loci. Proceedings of the National Academy of Sciences USA 73: 3636

Bannerman R M, Callender S T, Hardisty R M, Smith R S 1964 Iron absorption in thalassaemia. British Journal of Haematology 10: 490

Baralle E F, Shoulders C C, Proudfoot N J 1980 The primary structure of the human ε-globin gene. Cell 21: 621

Barrett-Connor E 1971 Bacterial infection and sickle cell anemia. Medicine 50: 97

Bellingham A J 1976 Haemoglobins with altered oxygen affinity. British Medical Bulletin 32: 234

Bernards R, Little P F R, Annison G, Williamson R, Flavell R A 1979 Structure of the human $^G\gamma$-$^A\gamma$-δ-β globin gene locus. Proceedings of the National Academy of Sciences USA 76: 4827

Bessman J D, Feinstein D I 1979 Quantitative anisocytosis as a discriminant between iron deficiency and thalassemia minor. Blood 53: 288

Boyer S H, Margolet L, Boyer M L, Huisman T H J, Schroeder W A, Wood W G, Weatherall D J, Clegg J B, Cartner R 1977 Inheritance of F cell frequency in heterocellular hereditary persistence of fetal hemoglobin: An example of allelic exclusion. American Journal of Human Genetics 26: 256

Bunn H F 1974 The structure and function of human hemoglobins. In: Nathan D G, Oski F A (eds) Hematology of infancy and childhood. W B Saunders Co, Philadelphia, ch 13, p 412

Bunn H F, Forget B G, Ranney H M 1977a Hemoglobin structure. In: Human hemoglobins. W B Saunders Co, Philadelphia, ch 1, p 4

Bunn H F, Forget B G, Ranney H M 1977b Human hemoglobin variants. In: Human hemoglobins. W B Saunders Co, Philadelphia, ch 6, p 193

Bunn H F, Forget B G, Ranney H M 1977c Unstable hemoglobin variants-congenital Heinz body hemolytic anemia. In: Human hemoglobins. W B Saunders Co, Philadelphia, ch 8, p 282

Chang J C, Kan Y W 1979 β⁰-thalassemia, a nonsense mutation in man. Proceedings of the National Academy of Sciences USA 76: 2886

Cohen A, Schwartz E 1978 Iron chelation therapy with deferoxamine in Cooley anemia. Journal of Pediatrics 92: 643

Cooper H A, Hoagland H C 1972 Subject review. Fetal hemoglobin. Mayo Clinical Proceedings 47: 402

Dean J, Schechter A N 1978 Sickle cell anemia: Molecular and cellular bases of therapeutic approaches. New England Journal of Medicine 299: 863

Deisseroth A, Nienhuis A, Lawrence J, Giles R, Turner P, Ruddle F H 1978 Chromosomal localization of human β globin gene on human chromosome 11 in somatic cell hybrids. Proceedings of the National Academy of Sciences USA 75: 1456

Deisseroth A, Nienhuis A, Turner P, Velez R, Anderson W F, Ruddle F, Lawrence J, Creagan R, Kucherlapati R 1977 Localization of the human α-globin structural gene to chromosome 16 in somatic cell hybrids by molecular hybridization assay. Cell 12: 205

Dozy A M, Forman E N, Abuelo D N, Barsel-Bowers G, Mahoney M J, Forget B G, Kan Y W 1979a Prenatal diagnosis of homozygous α-thalassemia. Journal of the American Medical Association 241: 1610

Dozy A M, Kan Y W, Embury S H, Mentzer W C, Wang W C, Lubin B, Davis J R Jr, Koenig H M 1979b α-globin gene organisation in blacks precludes the severe form of α-thalassemia. Nature 280: 605

Efstradiadis A, Posakony J W, Maniatis T, Lawn R M, O'Connell C, Spritz R A, DeRiel J K, Forget B G, Weissman S M, Slighton J L, Blechl A E, Smithies O, Baralle F E, Shoulders C C, Proudfoot N J 1980 The structure and evolution of the human β-globin gene family. Cell 21: 653

Embury S H, Miller J A, Dozy A M, Kan Y W, Chan V, Todd D 1980 Two different molecular organizations account for the single α-globin gene of the α-thalassemia-2 genotype. Journal of Clinical Investigations 66: 1319

Forget B F, Kan Y W 1974 Thalassemia and the genetics of hemoglobin. In: Nathan D G, Oski F A (eds) Hematology of infancy and childhood. W B Saunders Co, Philadelphia, ch 7, p 450

Fritsch E F, Lawn R M, Maniatis T 1979 Characterisation of deletions which affect the expression of fetal globin genes in man. Nature 279: 598

Fritsch E F, Lawn R M, Maniatis T 1980 Molecular cloning and characterization of the human β-like globin gene cluster. Cell 19: 959

Giebiuk G S, Schiffman G, Krivit W, Quie P G 1979 Vaccine type pneumococcal pneumonia: occurrence after vaccination in an asplenic patient. Journal of the American Medical Association 241: 2736

Goossens M, Dozy A M, Embury S H, Zachariades Z, Hadjiminas M G, Stamatoyannopoulos G, Kan Y W 1980 Triplicated α-globin loci in man. Proceedings of the National Academy of Sciences USA 77: 518

Graziano J H, Markenson A, Miller D R, Chang H, Bestak M, Meyers P, Pisciotto P, Rifkind A 1978 Chelation therapy in β-thalassemia major. I. Intravenous and subcutaneous deferoxamine. Journal of Pediatrics 92: 648

Gusella J, Varsanyi-Breiner A, Kao F-T, Jones C, Puck T T, Keys C, Orkin S, Housman D 1979 Precise localization of the human β-globin gene complex on chromosome 11. Proceedings of the National Academy of Sciences USA 76: 5239

Hamer D, Leder P 1979 Splicing and the formation of stable RNA. Cell 18: 1299

Hobbins J C, Mahoney M J 1974 In utero diagnosis of hemoglobinopathies. New England Journal of Medicine 290: 1065

International Hemoglobin Information Center 1980 List of Hemoglobin Variants. Augusta, Georgia

Kan Y W, Dozy A M 1978 Antenatal diagnosis of sickle cell anemia by DNA analysis of amniotic fluid cells. Lancet ii: 910

Kan Y W, Lee K Y, Furbetta M, Angius A, Cao A 1980 Polymorphism of DNA sequence in the β-globin gene region. New England Journal of Medicine 302: 185

Kan Y W, Dozy A M, Trecartin R, Todd D 1977 Identification of a non-deletion defect in α thalassemia. New England Journal of Medicine 297: 1081

Kan Y W, Forget B G, Nathan D G 1972 Gamma-beta thalassemia. A cause of hemolytic disease of the newborn. New England Journal of Medicine 286: 129

Kantor J A, Turner P H, Nienhuis A W 1980 Beta-thalassemia: Mutations which affect processing of the β-globin mRNA precursor. Cell 21: 149

Kazazian H H Jr 1974 Regulation of human fetal hemoglobin production. Seminars in Hematology 11: 525

Kazazian H H Jr 1976 The hereditary persistence of fetal hemoglobin syndromes: Variations on the thalassemia theme. Johns Hopkins Medical Journal 139: 215

Kazazian H H Jr, Cho S, Phillips J A III 1977 The mutational basis of the thalassemia syndromes. Progress in Medical Genetics 2: 165

Kazazian H H Jr, Phillips J A III, Boehm C D, Vik T A, Mahoney M J, Ritchey A K 1980 Prenatal diagnosis of β-thalassemia by amniocentesis: Linkage analysis of multiple polymorphic restriction endonuclease sites. Blood 56: 926

Kazazian H H Jr, Woodhead A P 1973 Hemoglobin A synthesis in the developing fetus. New England Journal of Medicine 289: 58

Kreimer-Birnbaum M, Edwards J A, Rusnak P A, Bannerman R M 1975 Mild β-thalassemia in Black subjects. Johns Hopkins Medical Journal 137: 257

Lauer J, Shon C-K J, Maniatis T 1980 The chromosomal arrangement of human α-like globin genes: sequence homology and α-globin gene deletions. Cell 20: 119

Lawn R M, Efstradiadis A, O'Connell C, Maniatis T 1980 The nucleotide sequence of the human β-globin gene. Cell 21: 647

Lawn R M, Fritsch E F, Parker R C, Blake G, Maniatis T 1978 The isolation and characterization of linked δ- and β-globin genes from a cloned library of human DNA. Cell 15: 1157

Leibhaber S, Goossens M, Kan Y W Manuscript submitted

Lie-Injo L E, Dozy A M, Kan Y W, Lopes M, Todd D 1979 The α-globin gene adjacent to the gene for Hb Q-α$^{74\ Asp \to His}$ is deleted, but not that adjacent to the gene for Hb G α^{30} $^{Glu \to Gln}$; Three-fourths of the α-globin genes are deleted in Hb Q-α-thalassemia. Blood 54: 1407

Little P F R, Annison G, Darling S, Williamson R, Camba L, Modell B 1980 Model for antenatal diagnosis of β-thalassemia and other monogenic disorders by molecular analysis of linked DNA polymorphisms. Nature 285: 144

Mentzer W C 1973 Differentiation of iron deficiency from thalassemia trait. Lancet 1: 882

Merkel C G, Wood T G, Lingrel J B 1976 Shortening of the poly(A) region of mouse globin messenger RNA. Journal of Biological Chemistry 251: 5512

Motulsky A G 1973 Frequency of sickling disorders in US Blacks. New England Journal of Medicine 288: 31

Nathan D G 1972 Thalassemia. New England Journal of Medicine 296: 586

Nathan D G, Pearson H A 1974 Sickle cell syndromes and hemoglobin C disease. In: Nathan D G, Oski F A (eds) Hematology of infancy and childhood. W B Saunders Co, Philadelphia, ch 14, p 419

Nagel R L, Lynfield J, Johnson J, Landau L, Bookchin R M, Harris M B 1976 Hemoglobin Beth Israel. A mutant causing clinically apparent cyanosis. New England Journal of Medicine 295: 125

Orkin S H 1978 The duplicated human α globin genes lie close together in cellular DNA. Proceedings of the National Academy of Sciences USA 74: 560

Orkin S H, Alter B P, Altay C, Mahoney M J, Lazarus H, Hobbins J C, Nathan D G 1978 Application of endonuclease mapping to the analysis and prenatal diagnosis of thalassemia caused by globin-gene deletion. New England Journal of Medicine 299: 166

Orkin S H, Nathan D G 1976 Current concepts in genetics. The thalassemias. New England Journal of Medicine 295: 710

Orkin S H, Old J M, Lazarus H, Altay C, Gurgey A, Weatherall D J, Nathan D G 1979 The molecular basis of α-thalassemias: Frequent occurrence of dysfunctional α loci among non-Asians with Hb H disease. Cell 17: 33

Pearson H A, O'Brien R T, McIntosh S 1973 Screening for thalassemia trait by electronic measurement of mean corpuscular volumes. New England Journal of Medicine 288: 351

Phillips J A III, Panny S R, Kazazian H H Jr, Boehm C D, Scott A F, Smith K D 1980a Prenatal diagnosis of sickle cell anemia by restriction endonuclease analysis: Hind III polymorphisms in γ-globin genes extend test applicability. Proceedings of the National Academy of Sciences USA 77: 2856

Phillips J A III, Vik T A, Scott A F, Young K E, Kazazian H H Jr, Smith K D, Fairbanks V F, Koenig H M 1980b Unequal crossing-over: A common basis of single α-globin genes in Asians and American Blacks with Hemoglobin H disease. Blood 55: 1066

Pressley L, Higgs D R, Clegg J B, Weatherall D J 1980 Gene deletions in α-thalassemia prove that the 5′ ζ locus is functional. Proceedings of the National Academy of Sciences USA 77: 3586

Propper R D, Cooper B, Rufo R R, Nienhuis A W, Anderson W F, Bunn H F, Rosenthal A, Nathan D G 1977 Continuous subcutaneous administration of deferoxamine in patients with iron overload. New England Journal of Medicine 297: 418

Proudfoot N J, Baralle F 1979 Molecular cloning of the

human ϵ-globin gene. Proceedings of the National Academy of Sciences USA 76: 5435

Proudfoot N J, Maniatis T 1980 The structure of a human α-globin pseudogene and its relationship to α-globin gene duplication. Cell 21: 537

Rieder R F 1974 Human hemoglobin stability and instability. Molecular mechanisms and some clinical correlations. Seminars in Hematology 11: 423

Sancar G B, Tatsis B, Cedeno M M, Rieder R F 1980 Proportion of hemoglobin G Philadelphia ($\alpha_2^{68\ \text{Asn}\rightarrow\text{Lys}}\beta_2$) in heterozygotes in determined by α-globin gene deletions. Proceedings of the National Academy of Sciences USA 77: 6874

Scoot A F, Phillips J A III, Migeon B R 1979 DNA restriction endonuclease analysis for the localization of the human β and δ globin genes on chromosome 11. Proceedings of the National Academy of Sciences USA 76: 4563

Seid-Akhavan M, Winter W P, Abramson R K, Rucknagel D L 1976 Hemoglobin Wayne: A frameshift mutation detected in human hemoglobin alpha chains. Proceedings of the National Academy of Sciences USA 73: 882

Slighton J L, Blechl A E, Smithies O 1980 Human fetal $^G\gamma$ and $^A\gamma$ globin genes: Complete nucleotide sequences suggest that DNA can be exchanged between these duplicated genes. Cell 21: 627

Spritz R A, DeRiel J K, Forget B G, Weissman S M 1980a Complete nucleotide sequence of the human δ-globin gene. Cell 21: 639

Spritz R A, Jagadeeswaran P, Biro P A, Choudary P V, Elder J T, deReil J K, Manley J, Forget B G, Weissman S M 1980b Cloning, structure, and functional analyses of human β^+-thalassemic globin gene. American Journal of Human Genetics 32: 56A

Tilghman S M, Curtis P J, Tiemeier D C, Leder P, Weissmann C 1978 The intervening sequence of a mouse β-globin gene is transcribed within the 15S β-globin mRNA precursor. Proceedings of the National Academy of Sciences USA 75: 1309

Van der Ploeg L H T, Konings A, Oort M, Roos D, Bernini L, Flavel R A 1980 γ-β-thalassemia studies showing that deletion of the γ and δ genes influences β-globin gene expression in man. Nature 283: 637

Wasi D, Na-Nakorn S, Pootrakul S-N 1974 The α thalassemias. Clinical Hematology 3: 383

Weatherall D J 1976 The molecular basis of thalassemia. Johns Hopkins Medical Journal 139: 205

Weiner M, Karpatkin M, Hart D, Seamans C, Vora S K, Henry W L, Piomelli S 1978 Cooley anemia: High transfusion regimen and chelation-therapy, results, and perspective. Journal of Pediatrics 92: 653

75

Hereditary haemolytic, hypoplastic and megaloblastic anaemias

R. M. Bannerman

INTRODUCTION

This section is an *omnium gatherum* of important hereditary disorders of red cell structure, metabolism or production, many of which produce anaemia. They are grouped arbitrarily, but following tradition, into apparent structural anomalies (in which the biochemical basis is not yet generally worked out); red cell enzyme deficiencies; other disorders of red cell production, including the hereditary dyserythropoietic and hypoplastic anaemias; and megaloblastic anaemias. Although data on the genetics of the rarer of these conditions are quite widely scattered, much important clinical information is available in current haematologic texts, especially those of Wintrobe (1974), Williams and co-editors (1972), and Hardisty and Weatherall (1974). *The Red Cell* by Harris and Kellermeyer (1970) is a valuable background source. Some hereditary anaemias in other species will be mentioned. Although many of these have not yet been matched to human analogues they provide useful models of gene action at the pathophysiological level (Bannerman, Edwards & Pinkerton, 1973; Russell, 1980).

RED CELL SHAPE ANOMALIES

These traits are characterised by shape anomalies readily visible in stained blood films or other preparations. Our understanding of red cell morphology has been enhanced by new techniques such as scanning electron microscopy, especially by Bessis, who has proposed new descriptive terms for various red cell shapes (Bessis, 1976). The biconcave shape (Fig. 75.1) is adapted to achieve the most effective surface-volume relationship for oxygen transport and exchange, but the red cell is not a rigid structure and overall cell elasticity or deformability is essential, since red cells $7\mu m$ in diameter have to squeeze through capillary spaces as narrow as $2–3\mu m$ in diameter. Lack of deformability seems to be a major cause of cell trapping and destruction in the spleen in many hereditary haemolytic anaemias (Mohandas, Phillips, & Bessis, 1979). The normal biconcave 'discocyte' can

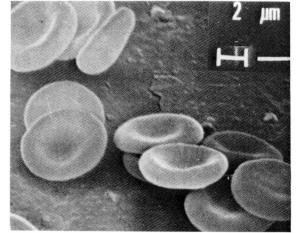

Fig. 75.1 Normal red cells observed by scanning electron microscopy. (By courtesy of H. Kupari-Koby and the Canadian Journal of Medical Technology).

be manipulated to produce spherocytes, as extensively studied by Ponder using hypotonic solutions (Ponder, 1948; Harris & Kellermeyer, 1970). Spherocytes may also appear in small numbers in acquired haemolytic diseases. 'Echinocytes' (i.e. resembling the sea urchin, an echinoderm) can be produced by a variety of means, including prolonged incubation in vitro, and must be distinguished from 'acanthocytes'. 'Stomatocytes' can also be produced in vitro, as well as various other deformations (Weinstein, 1974; Bessis, 1977).

The red cell membrane is a complex and dynamic structure which includes various lipids and a protein framework, especially spectrin which makes up some 20% of membrane protein (Harris & Kellermeyer, 1970; Weinstein, 1974). The membrane's normal integrity has to be maintained by continuous metabolic activity, briefly discussed in the next section of this chapter. Although certain surface active components are concentrated at the membrane (enzymes, antigens), some haemoglobin is also incorporated, and the membrane and the cytoplasm must be regarded as a continuum (Weinstein, 1974).

HEREDITARY SPHEROCYTOSIS

The dominant pattern of inheritance of hereditary spherocytosis (HS) was one of the first described in man, having been reported early in the 20th century. HS has also had many other names, including *microcythémie* from the 1871 report of Vanlair and Masius, Minkowski-Chauffard disease, haemolytic icterus, and later, familial acholuric jaundice (Dacie, 1960, 1980). Early authors observed the small spherocytes (called microcytes) and the characteristic reduced resistance to osmotic lysis in the osmotic fragility test.

The main clinical feature is lifelong chronic haemolysis, often presenting as marked icterus. The degree of anaemia may be slight, and HS is not infrequently an incidental finding in a patient presenting with another disease. Splenomegaly is almost invariably associated. Complications include gallstones and occasionally ankle ulceration (Dacie, 1960).

Blood films show marked variation in morphology with many spherocytes, which appear as smaller, circular and dense erythrocytes (Fig. 75.2 and 75.3). There is usually reticulocytosis and icterus, and urobilinogen and faecal uribilin excretion are increased. Red cell osmotic fragility determination helps to confirm the diagnosis with haemolysis starting at NaCl concentrations of 0.6–0.5 g/dl, and usually becoming complete by 0.5–0.4 g/dl at which level normal red cells are just starting to haemolyse. This important difference can be intensified by incubation of the cells for 24 hours (Harris & Kellermeyer, 1970).

Family study is desirable to support the diagnosis because some spherocytes may be seen in blood films in

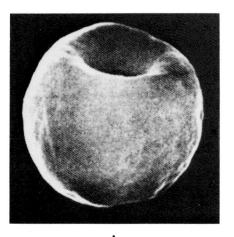

A

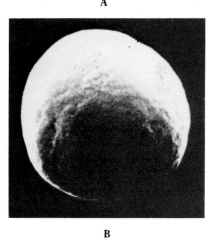

B

Fig. 75.3 Spherocytes observed by scanning electron microscopy, showing (A) a spherocyte II with a remaining central depression; (B) a spherocyte III with negligible remaining depression. (By courtesy of M. Bessis (1977), and Springer International).

other forms of haemolytic disease, including acquired autoimmune haemolytic anaemias. However, some cases of HS may appear to be sporadic (below).

Spherocytosis is clearly associated with reduced red cell deformability and splenic entrapment. This explains the empiric success of splenectomy which was used in this disease as long ago as the last century. Anaemia is usually cured or at least ameliorated by splenectomy. The operation should be considered in any patient with HS with significant haemolysis and is invariably associated with a reduction in the rate of haemolysis. Spherocytes and altered osmotic fragility of the red cells persist after splenectomy, although there are many reports that they may become less marked. However, splenectomy should be delayed in young infants and children until after the age of 5 years, if possible, because of the risk

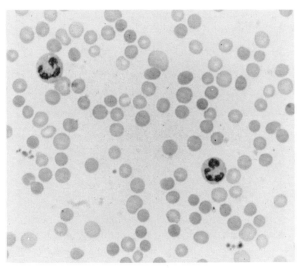

Fig. 75.2 Hereditary spherocytosis. Blood film stained by Wright's stain showing smaller, dense round spherocytes.

of overwhelming septicaemia in asplenic children (Miller et al, 1978).

The red cell and membrane composition in HS have been extensively investigated and various abnormalities discovered, but the primary defect is still not explained (Valentine, 1977; Jandl & Cooper, 1978; Lux, 1979). Thus, HS red cells are unusually permeable to sodium, they are prone to develop surface structural anomalies and to lose fragments of membrane on incubation (Jacob, 1972).

A primary abnormality of structural protein has always been sought, but only recently have there been effective methods to study the proteins of red cell ghosts. Physicochemical abnormalities of microfilamentous protein have been described in HS, but they are heterogeneous. Their possible significance is indicated by the fact that drugs which interfere with microfilament integrity (e.g. vinblastine) also produce spherocytes (Jacob, 1972). However, a specific protein structural abnormality has yet to be defined.

Genetics and heterogeneity

Most families with HS conform to an autosomal dominant pattern of inheritance. However, the condition is probably heterogeneous. Patients with normal blood findings in parents have been reported (e.g. Young, Izzo & Platzer, 1951); these may represent non-penetrance, since considerable variation in severity of red cell changes and haemolysis may exist in affected members of the same family. The possibilities of new dominant mutations or types of HS with recessive inheritance also exist. However, for purposes of genetic counselling, HS should be regarded as an autosomal dominant trait.

The two known animal models are recessively inherited (Pinkerton & Bannerman, 1979). Hereditary spherocytosis in the deermouse, *Peromyscus* (gene symbol *sp*), most closely resembles human HS, with mild anaemia due to chronic haemolysis and decreased red cell osmotic fragility. The spleen is enlarged and haemolysis is alleviated by splenectomy. The tendency to gallstones is also seen in the mouse. HS in *Peromyscus* provides an excellent example of environmental-genotypic interaction. At normal ambient temperature in vivo haemolysis is moderate; if the mouse is maintained at a slightly higher ambient temperature haemolysis is intensified and may then be lethal (Anderson & Motulsky, 1966). Hereditary spherocytosis in the house mouse (gene symbol *sph*) is a very severe condition and homozygotes usually die of anaemia within 24 hours of birth. Studies of membrane proteins in *sp* have shown no specific abnormality. In *sph*, reduction in spectrin and decreased incorporation of phosphate into spectrin have been reported, along with instability of the membrane in red cell ghosts (Greenquist, Shohet & Bernstein, 1978).

HEREDITARY STOMATOCYTOSIS

This condition is characterised by a stomatocyte or 'mouth-like' appearance of the red cells (Lock, Smith & Hardisty, 1961), which are bowl-shaped in three-dimensional view (Fig. 75.4). It is clearly heterogeneous, but in some families is associated with nonspherocytic haemolytic anaemia. There may be increased osmotic fragility, red cell macrocytosis with increased sodium and water content, and reduced potassium, despite greatly

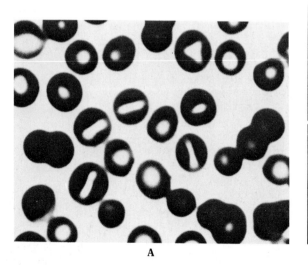 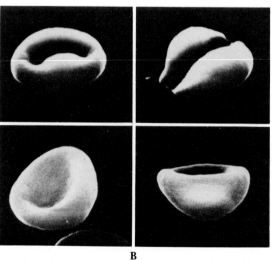

A　**B**

Fig. 75.4 Stomatocytes in man; (A) blood film photographed in the Soret band at 415 nm to demonstrate distribution of haemoglobin; (B) scanning electron microscope appearance showing cup shape. (By courtesy of M. Bessis 1977 and Springer International).

increased activity of the cation pump, suggesting a primary membrane defect (Mentzer et al, 1975). When there is significant haemolysis splenectomy may produce clinical amelioration.

Genetics and heterogeneity

The above mentioned forms are inherited as autosomal dominant traits. However, autosomal recessive inherit-

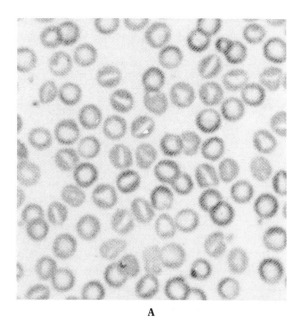

A

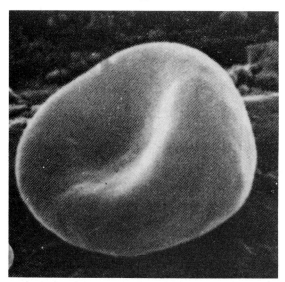

B

Fig. 75.5 Stomatocytes in hereditary stomatocytosis in the Alaskan malamute dog, showing blood film above (A) and scanning electron microscope view below (B). (By courtesy of P. H. Pinkerton et al (1974) and Blood).

ance of rare types of stomatocytosis also exists. One rare but revealing form is that associated with Rh_{null} disease, a recessive trait in which there is mild chronic haemolysis (Sturgeon, 1970). Total lack of Rh antigen activity reflects an underlying membrane defect. Haemolysis and depression of antigenicity, including Rh antigens, are also features of a form of hereditary elliptocytosis (below), but haemolysis does not occur with absence of ABO activity in Bombay blood (Levine et al, 1973).

An animal model, stomatocytosis in the Alaskan malamute dog (Fig. 75.5), is a recessive trait (gene symbol *dan*), associated with mild chronic haemolytic anaemia (Pinkerton et al, 1974). An additional interesting pleiotropic effect is dwarfism due to an abnormality of cartilage growth; no skeletal anomaly has been reported in association with human stomatocytosis.

HEREDITARY ELLIPTOCYTOSIS

This trait has been known for many years, and may be found in about 1 in 3000 individuals of most populations (Bannerman & Renwick, 1962). It is usually a chance finding on examination of a blood film. The elliptocyte (Figs. 75.6 & 75.7) is the most characteristic cell, but a variety of oval forms may also be seen. Sometimes almost all the cells are abnormally shaped, but the proportion varies, though it is often consistent within one family. A minimum of 25–30% of elliptical or oval cells is usually regarded as necessary to make the diagnosis. The hereditary form has to be carefully distinguished from secondary ovalocytosis occurring in anaemias, especially in beta-thalassaemia and in megaloblastic anaemia.

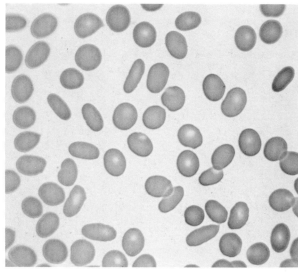

Fig. 75.6 Hereditary elliptocytosis. Blood film stained by Wright's stain showing oval and elliptical forms.

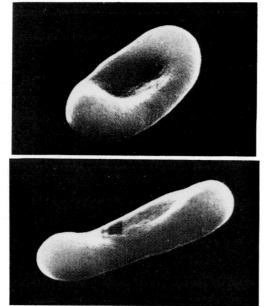

Fig. 75.7 Human elliptocytes observed by scanning electron microscopy. (By courtesy of M. Bessis (1977) and Springer International).

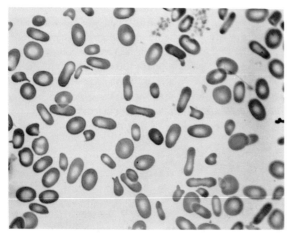

Fig. 75.8 Hereditary elliptocytosis. Blood film from a patient with a haemolytic form showing extreme elliptocytosis and fragmented forms.

In hereditary elliptocytosis, there is usually no haemolysis or other evident pathologic effect associated with the anomaly. However, occasional families show haemolysis which seems to be primarily associated with their elliptocytosis (Cutting et al, 1965). In one example, a mother and several children in a Negro family with elliptocytosis all showed haemolytic anaemia for which no other cause could be found (Bannerman & Renwick, 1962). Their red cells showed extreme morphologic variation (Fig. 75.8), but such an appearance is not necessarily associated with haemolysis in other families, and haemolysis may occur with apparently minor red cell changes. When haemolysis is severe, splenectomy may be effective in reducing it.

The structural or biochemical basis of this anomaly is unknown. The normoblasts are not elliptical, but the elliptical shape of mature red cells is retained by red cell ghosts. Abnormalities of membrane spectrin have been reported but their specificity is uncertain (Lux, 1979).

Genetics and heterogeneity

The usual form of hereditary elliptocytosis in populations of Northern European ancestry is inherited as an autosomal dominant trait with high penetrance. Linkage of hereditary elliptocytosis to Rhesus was one of the earliest autosomal linkages established (Lawler, 1954). The linkage method was then used to demonstrate heterogeneity; one form of hereditary elliptocytosis (El_1) is linked to the *Rh* locus (now known to be an chromosome 1), and the other (El_2) is not (Morton, 1956). The two types are phenotypically indistinguishable; either may apparently be associated with haemolysis. Recent analysis suggests that El_2 may also be on chromosome 1, tentatively linked to the Duffy blood group locus (Keats, 1979). Heterogeneity is further extended by recent observations in Southeast Asia where high frequency of a form of elliptocytosis has been reported. The type seen in coastal Aborigines in Papua is inherited as an autosomal recessive trait, but without anaemia or evidence of significant haemolysis in homozygotes. However, it is consistently associated with impaired antigenic reactivity for many but not all blood group antigens, suggesting an underlying membrane defect (Booth et al, 1977).

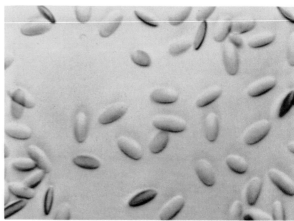

Fig. 75.9 Red blood cells in the llama; unstained wet preparation showing relative symmetry of these physiologically oval cells.

Elliptocytosis is a normal finding in camels and llamas which have small red cells of a very regular oval shape (Fig. 75.9).

HEREDITARY ACANTHOCYTOSIS

This remarkable morphologic anomaly of red cells is included at this point for convenience, since it is not a primary disorder of the red cell itself but results from total or partial failure of betalipoprotein synthesis. There are serious disturbances of function of the central nerv-

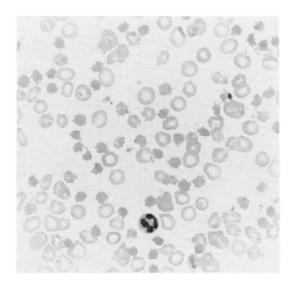

Fig. 75.10 Acanthocytosis in blood film, Wright's stain. (Photographed from blood film of the patient described by Singer, Fisher and Perlstein (1952) by courtesy of Dr. Ben Fisher).

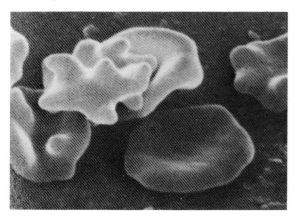

Fig. 75.11 Acanthocytes seen by scanning electron microscopy. (By courtesy of H. Kupari-Koby and the Canadian Journal of Medical Technology).

ous system, and of the bowel, with malabsorption (Herbert, Gotto & Fredrickson, 1978), but the red cell changes are useful in suggesting the diagnosis.

Abetalipoproteinaemia

At least 50% of the red cells of homozygous affected patients show the remarkable spiny appearance illustrated in Figures 75.10, 75.11 (Bassen & Kornzweig, 1950; Singer, Fisher & Perlstein, 1952). Marked autohaemolysis of the red cells on incubation can be corrected by the addition of normal serum, confirming that the primary disorder is not inherent in the red cell itself. However, the membrane lipid content is abnormal, and there are some complex interactions of membrane and serum lipids which are not fully elucidated and in which vitamin E may play a role. Red cell survival in vivo is impaired, with evidence of chronic haemolysis such as reticulocytosis, hyperbilirubinaemia and lowered serum haptoglobin level. The haemolysis is usually compensated in adults so that there is no anaemia. Affected children may be severely anaemic, but the anaemia is partly related to multiple deficiencies caused by intestinal malabsorption.

Abetalipoproteinemia is an autosomal recessive trait. Consanguinity has been present in many of the families, emphasizing the rarity of the trait. While it is reported in different ethnic groups, one quarter of all cases have been Ashkenazi Jews. Heterozygotes cannot readily be detected though some obligate heterozygotes may show minor lipid abnormalities. Their red cells are normal.

Familial hypobetalipoproteinaemia

This milder condition, somewhat paradoxically, is expressed in single gene dose and so is classified as an autosomal dominant trait. Heterozygotes have mild to moderate hypolipidaemia but are usually asymptomatic. They have no serious problems of intestinal absorption or neurological manifestations, and acanthocytes do not occur spontaneously.

A few homozygous affected individuals have been reported to show abetalipoproteinaemia and acanthocytosis. They may have moderate neuromuscular involvement and impaired fat absorption (Herbert, Gotto & Fredrickson, 1978).

HAEMOLYTIC DISORDERS DUE TO RED CELL ENZYME DEFICIENCIES

Background

Although the red cell has been described as 'simple', because of the lack of many of the organelles present in nucleated cells, its metabolic pathways are by no means uncomplicated and have been intensively investigated

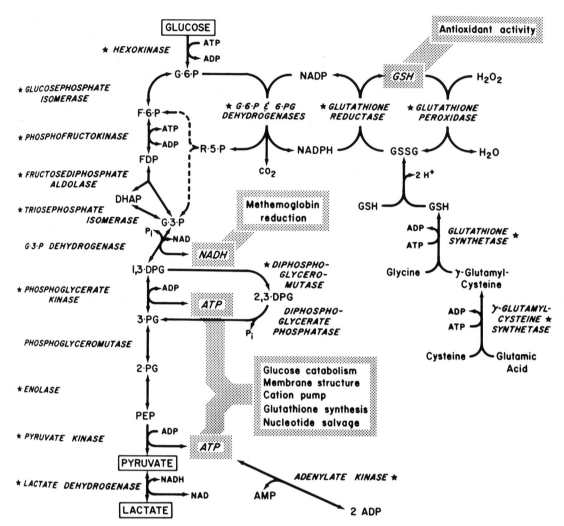

Fig. 75.12 Pathways of glycolysis and glutathione metabolism in the mature erythrocyte. Abbreviations: ATP, adenosine triphosphate; ADP, adenosine diphosphate; G-6-P, glucose 6-phosphate; F-6-P, fructose 6-phosphate; FDP, fructose 1,6-diphosphate; DHAP, dihydroxyacetone phosphate; G-3-P, glyceraldehyde 3-phosphate; NAD, oxidized nicotinamide adenine dinucleotide; NADH, reduced NAD; P_i, inorganic phosphate; 1,3-DPG, 1,3-diphosphoglycerate; 3-PG, 3-phosphoglycerate; 2,3-DPG, 2,3-diphosphoglycerate; 2-PG, 2-phosphoglycerate; PEP, phosphoenolpyruvate; NADP, oxidized nicotinamide adenine dinucleotide phosphate; NADPH, reduced NADP; 6-PG, 6-phosphogluconate; R-5-P, ribose 5-phosphate; GSH, reduced glutathionine; GSSG, oxidized glutathione; AMP, adenosine monophosphate. (From Paglia D E, in Best and Taylor's Physiologic Basis of Medical Practice, 10th ed., Williams and Wilkins, Baltimore, 1979; by permission of the author and publishers.)

(Harris & Kellermeyer 1970). The presence of over one hundred enzymes has been recorded (Surgenor, 1974) and their genetic variation is a major source of our knowledge of human protein polymorphism (Harris, Hopkins & Robson, 1974). Many enzymes are concerned with energy production. The red cell needs energy for several purposes including the sodium pump and other membrane related functions, keeping haemoglobin in reduced form, and maintaining the reduced glutathione

content of the cell. The main source of energy is the breakdown of glucose to lactic acid, with the generation of adenosine triphosphate (ATP), via the Embden-Meyerhof pathway of anaerobic glycolysis (Fig. 75.12).

When investigating patients with red cell enzyme deficiencies it is important to note that during or after a period of active haemolysis immature red cells, sometimes in very high proportions, will be present in the peripheral blood and may have higher relative levels of the enzymes under study, possibly complicating the interpretation of results.

Deficiencies have been described for many of the enzymes known in the red cell, but except for glucose-6-phosphate dehydrogenase (G6PD) deficiency they are rare. Some have so far been reported in only a handful of patients or even single families (Tables 75.1 and 75.2) and only some of the better characterized will be discussed here (Valentine & Tanaka, 1978).

Clinical aspects, natural history and differential diagnosis

The first haemolytic anaemia to be delineated was hereditary spherocytosis, and as others were observed they were distinguished as 'non-spherocytic'. These were further subdivided into types I and II according to whether added glucose did or did not reduce autohaemolysis on incubation (Selwyn & Dacie 1954; Dacie 1960).

Clinically apparent cases of red cell enzyme deficiency usually present as non-spherocytic haemolytic anaemia. Haemolysis is usually chronic, with congenital mild or moderate anaemia and variable evidence of red cell destruction in the form of icterus, reticulocytosis and enlargement of the spleen. Severe forms are usually detected in childhood. Milder examples are sometimes an incidental finding in children or adults who are examined for other reasons. In some cases, especially G6PD deficiency, anaemia may be episodic, resulting from some additional stress.

The exact mechanisms of cell breakdown are not generally worked out. No specific metabolic or drug treatments have been devised for these conditions. Splenectomy is often markedly beneficial in ameliorating anaemia, though it has no effect on the underlying metabolic disorder. The use of splenectomy, blood transfusion or other measures must be decided in each situation. In these, as in other forms of chronic haemolysis with increased erythropoiesis, regular oral folic acid supplementation (1 mg daily) is desirable to prevent the development of relative folate deficiency.

Tissues other than the red cell may express the enzyme deficiency but are usually not otherwise affected, probably because they can utilize other metabolic pathways. Exceptions include certain disorders that affect neurologic and muscle function mentioned below.

The diagnosis must be considered whenever haemolytic disease is found, especially with onset in infancy or childhood. Differential diagnosis includes the haemoglobinopathies, especially unstable haemoglobin syndromes. In adults, acquired forms of haemolytic disease, which are very much more common, have to be excluded by clinical and immunologic investigation. Therefore the diagnosis is partly one of exclusion and may be very difficult to pin down. Proof requires the demonstration of specific enzyme deficiency by enzyme assay, for which both screening and specific methods are available (Beutler, 1971; Grimes & deGrouchy, 1974).

Heredity

The red cell enzyme deficiencies are autosomal recessive traits, except for G6PD and phosphoglycerate kinase deficiency which are X–linked. Consanguinity has been noted in the parents in a number of the rare deficiencies, helping to confirm recessive inheritance. In many instances, partial enzyme deficiency can be demonstrated in heterozygous carriers. Genetic counselling is as for any rare recessive trait, bearing in mind that successive affected sibs are likely to show similar manifestation but later ones will benefit from earlier diagnosis.

Table 75.1 Human red cell enzymes I. Embden-Meyerhof pathway.

Name, common abbreviation	Deficiency	Effect of deficiency	Autohaemolysis type
Hexokinase, HK	AR	Haemolysis, variable	I
Glucosephosphate isomerase, GPI	AR	Haemolysis, variable	I
Phosphofructokinase, PFK	AR	M type: muscle disease, compensated haemolysis	
		L type: chronic haemolysis	
Aldolase	single kindred	Haemolysis	
Triosephosphate isomerase, TPI	AR	Haemolysis	
		Lethal neurologic & cardiac effects	I
Triosephosphate dehydrogenase	not known	–	
Diphosphoglycerate mutase 2,3-DPGase	?AR	Haemolysis	I
Phosphoglycerate kinase, PGK	XR	Haemolysis, severe neurologic effects variable	II
Phosphoglycerate mutase, PGM	not known	–	
Enolase	not known	–	
Pyruvate kinase, PK	AR	Haemolysis only, sometimes severe	usually II
Lactate dehydrogenase, LDH	uncertain		

DEFICIENCIES OF ENZYMES IN THE EMBDEN-MEYERHOF PATHWAY

General

The enzymes in this pathway are listed in Table 75.1. Genetically determined deficiencies and other genetic variation are known for many of them, and linkage sites have been determined for some (McKusick, 1978). None of the variants occurs with the frequency of true polymorphism in any population studied (Giblett, 1975), in contrast to G6PD. Only pyruvate kinase deficiency is sufficiently common to merit full discussion; others will be dealt with very briefly in the order in which they appear in the pathway. Aldolase and lactate dehydrogenase deficiency have been described only in single kindreds (Valentine and Tanaka, 1978).

Hexokinase (HK) deficiency

This deficiency is particularly rare, but apparent recessive inheritance is well documented (Valentine & Tanaka, 1978). Heterogeneity is probable however, and dominant inheritance of deficiency has also been described (Siimes et al, 1979). Investigation is somewhat complicated by the fact that greatly increased levels of HK occur in young erythrocytes and reticulocytes.

Glucosephosphate isomerase (GPI) deficiency

This deficiency is inherited as an autosomal recessive trait and produces moderately severe haemolytic disease without apparent dysfunction of other tissues (Valentine & Tanaka, 1978). There is great heterogeneity, suggesting multiple mutant alleles at the GPI locus determining deficiency (Kahn et al, 1979). The locus is sited on chromosome number 19 (McKusick, 1978).

Phosphofructokinase (PFK) deficiency

The enzyme is complex and includes two types of subunit; M, or muscle type, and L, or liver type (Kahn et al, 1979). Two major forms of deficiency exist (Valentine & Tanaka, 1978). In the first, red cells show partial deficiency, with about 50% enzyme activity and compensated haemolysis, but there is profound enzyme deficiency in muscle, associated with a myopathic syndrome. In this type, the M or muscle subunits appear to be absent; the L subunits persist in red cells and other tissues (Vora et al, 1980). In the second type, muscle enzyme activity and muscle function are normal but enzyme activity is considerably reduced in the red cells, and there is chronic haemolysis.

Triosephosphate isomerase (TPI) deficiency

Though rare, this condition is of some importance because the enzyme deficiency is generalized, involving skeletal and heart muscle as well as red cells and other tissues. Haemolytic anaemia may be severe, but it is the neurologic or cardiac effects which usually lead to death in childhood (Valentine & Tanaka, 1978). Heterozygous carriers show approximately 50% of normal enzyme activity; their frequency in a German population was found to be 1 in 1000 (Eber et al, 1979).

Phosphoglycerate kinase (PGK) deficiency

PGK is the only X–linked enzyme in this pathway. Deficiency is rare, but is manifested as an X–linked recessive trait with severe haemolytic anaemia and neurological symptoms in affected males (Kahn et al, 1979).

Pyruvate kinase (PK) deficiency

PK deficiency is the most common in this rare group. It was first recognized in 1961 in subjects with non-spherocytic haemolytic anaemia (Valentine et al, 1961) and cases have subsequently been reported from many parts of the world.

The anaemia in deficient homozygotes is variable in severity and not well correlated with the degree of deficiency (Valentine, 1977). The anaemia has no specific features other than those of haemolysis, and the diagnosis should be considered in any unexplained haemolytic disorder with onset in childhood. The autohaemolysis test may show marked lysis usually little corrected by the addition of glucose, i.e. type II. Precise diagnosis depends upon enzyme assay (Beutler, 1971). In addition to enzyme deficiency, abnormal accumulation of glycolytic intermediates may be demonstrated, particularly 2, 3-diphosphoglycerate (2,3-DPG). Increased red cell 2,3-DPG reduces the oxygen affinity of haemoglobin and helps to compensate for the anaemia. There is no specific treatment, and severe anaemia, particularly in infants, may have to be managed by blood transfusion. Splenectomy, while having no effect on the underlying process, has sometimes been found to improve the anaemia.

Symptoms occur only in homozygous deficient subjects who have 5 to 20 per cent of normal enzyme activity; various different alterations of K_m values and pH optima have been reported (Kahn, Kaplan & Dreyfus, 1979). Reduced enzyme activity is found in heterozygous carriers.

An animal analogue has been discovered in Basenji dogs in which PK deficiency is an autosomal recessive trait. The anaemia in dogs is severe, with all the complications of chronic haemolysis. The variant enzyme is unstable, and also has a decreased K_m for phosphoenolpyruvate (Standerfer et al, 1975; Black et al, 1978).

DEFICIENCIES OF ENZYMES IN THE HEXOSE MONOPHOSPHATE SHUNT

The shunt pathway (Fig. 75.12), also called the pentose phosphate shunt, accounts for only a fraction of total

Table 75.2 Human red cell enzymes II. Hexose monophosphate pathway.

Name, common abbreviation	Deficiency	Effect of deficiency	Autohaemolysis type
Glucose-6-phosphate dehydrogenase, G6PD	XR	Haemolysis	normal or I
6-phosphogluconate dehydrogenase, 6PGD	AR	Possible haemolysis	–
Glutathione reductase, GSR	usually acquired	Uncertain	II
Glutathione synthetase, GSH	AR	Haemolysis, mild	–
Glutathione peroxidase, GSH-Px	AR	Uncertain, ? none	–
Gamma-glutamyl-cysteine synthetase, GGCS	AR	Haemolysis, mild	–

glycolysis. However, it is important in protecting hae-moglobin against oxidative denaturation, and in gluta-thione metabolism. The enzymes are listed in Table 75.2. Only G6PD deficiency is common, and this enzyme shows a remarkable degree of genetic variation.

Glucose-6-phosphate dehydrogenase deficiency

Glucose-6-phosphate dehydrogenase (G6PD) deficiency is the most common abnormal genetic trait in man, and affects many millions of individuals throughout the world. It is common in Oriental, African, Middle East-ern and Mediterranean groups. Its world distribution corresponds approximately to that of *Plasmodium falci-parum* malaria in the recent past. High gene frequencies may therefore be the result of a selective advantage con-ferred by resistance to this form of malaria (Motulsky, 1975), and there is evidence that parasite rate is lower in G6PD deficient than in normal erythrocytes (Luzzatto, Usanga & Reddy, 1969). X–linkage of G6PD deficiency was initially suggested because of the almost exclusive occurrence of haemolytic reactions in men, and was sub-sequently demonstrated formally (Childs & Zinkham, 1958). There are now known to be many different mutant alleles at the G6PD locus determining a series of variants which will be briefly discussed below. G6PD deficiency has a very important place in human genetics: as the most important marker on the X–chromosome for linkage studies, in elucidating X–inactivation and in understanding allelic variation. The demonstration that G6PD is also X–linked in many other mammals provides evidence of evolutionary conservatisim of the X-chromosome.

The widespread use of primaquine and related agents as substitutes for quinine in malaria prophylaxis in the second world war led to the observation that they might produce acute haemolytic episodes in some individuals, especially Indians in the British forces and Negroes in the American forces, while the majority suffered no such reaction. Similar observations in the U.S. forces in Korea led to the classic investigations at the University of Chi-cago, carried out on volunteer Negro prisoners at a local penitentiary. Beutler (1980) has given an elegant account of these earlier studies, which served to elucidate this reaction and demonstrated its basis in G6PD deficiency.

Pathophysiology

The haemolytic response in G6PD deficient black sub-jects provides the basic model (Beutler, 1972). Under ordinary conditions, the subject shows no manifestation of the trait in adult life. However, when exposed to a sufficient dose of primaquine or one of the series of other drugs or substances listed in Table 75.3, a haemolytic reaction ensues. Infections and fever may have the same

Table 75.3 Drugs causing haemolysis in G6PD deficient subjects.

Clinically significant haemolysis
Acetanilid
Diaphenylsulphon (Dapsone)
Furazolidone
Furmethonol
Naphthalene
Neoarsphenamine
Pentaquine
Pamaquine
Primaquine
Nitrofurazone (Furacin)
Nitrofurantoin (Furadantin)
Phenylhydrazine
Quinocide
Sulphanilamide
N-Acetylsulphanilamide
Sulphapyridine
Sulphamethoxypyridazine (Kynex)
Salicylazosulphapyridine (Azulfidine)
2-Amino-5-sulphanylthiazole (Thiazolsulfone)

Drugs which may cause haemolysis in special circumstances (e.g. in presence of infection)
Acetophenetidin
Acetylsalicylic acid
Chloramphenicol (Chloromycetin)
Chloroquine
Dimercaprol (BAL)
Sulphisoxazole (Gantrisin)
Sulphoxone
Quinacrine (Atabrine)

Modified from Beutler (1971) in which full references are cited

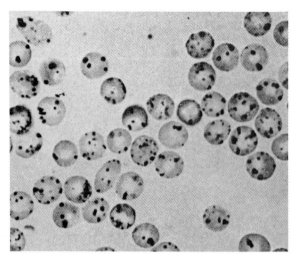

Fig. 75.13 Heinz bodies in a G6PD deficient individual. (From Beutler, Alving and Dern, J. Lab. Clin. Med. 45:40, 1955; by courtesy of Dr. E. Beutler, and the Journal of Laboratory and Clinical Medicine.)

effect. There is a brisk bout of haemolysis of circulating red cells in which the oldest cells are first destroyed. In Negro G6PD deficient subjects the episode is self-limiting even if the offending agent is continued. This occurs because the destroyed older cells are replaced by a wave of new young red cells, which, even in G6PD deficient subjects, have relatively higher levels of the enzyme and are therefore resistant to the action of the agent. Early in the reaction red cells with Heinz bodies can be seen by supravital staining (Fig. 75.13), and the demonstration of Heinz bodies is also the basis of an in vitro test.

Heterogeneity of G6PD deficiency
Heterogeneity was suspected on clinical grounds from the finding of more severe deficiency in affected Mediterranean than Negro subjects and the biochemical basis of this difference was soon made apparent (Boyer, Porter & Weilbacher, 1962). Based on electrophoretic mobility, the normal or 'wild type' form of G6PD was designated type B. Type A is a variant, common in the black population, which migrates slightly more rapidly than type B and may be associated with slight reduction of enzyme activity.

The electrophoretic distinction between these two types provided early direct support for the Lyon hypothesis. It was shown that in heterozygous females carrying one A and one B allele, clones from single skin fibroblasts produced either one or the other type of enzyme (Davidson, Nitowsky & Childs, 1963). The A- variant is the most common deficient type known in Negroes, and over 10% of Negro males have this form of deficiency. The enzyme activity is reduced to 5 to 15% of normal; the residual enzyme is electrophoretically indistinguishable from the normal A variant but is biochemically different.

The most common deficiency in Caucasian populations is due to G6PD Mediterranean and is associated with very low levels of activity, usually less than 1% of normal. When reactions occur in these subjects they tend to be more severe and protracted because even young red cells have very low G6PD activity. Among important precipitating agents in the Mediterranean area is the fava bean. Ingestion of this bean or even, apparently, exposure to its pollen may cause a severe haemolytic reaction, 'favism', with onset 1–2 days after exposure.

The field became extended when it was realized that G6PD deficiency can also be the cause of haemolytic anaemia in the newborn, and of chronic non-spherocytic haemolytic anaemia. Occasional subjects with Mediterranean type deficiency also have chronic haemolysis, and chronic haemolytic anaemia also occurs with rarer variants of G6PD deficiency (Rattazzi et al, 1971). Haemolytic anaemia in the newborn occurs in Mediterranean and Chinese infants with G6PD deficiency, and rarely in A- type enzyme deficiency in Negro infants.

Subsequently, the extent of the heterogeneity has been unfolded. It now appears that there are some 150 variants of G6PD. Most of these have been recognized as causing quantitative or functional deficiency of the enzyme but some are apparently neutral variants with no clinical effect. The active enzyme has a molecular weight of about 100 000 and is composed of four identical subunits, undergoing functional dimer-tetramer association and dissociation. The molecular difference between G6PD B and A is known to be a single amino acid substitution. A brief listing of some important variants is set out in Table 75.4. A complete listing based on that of Yoshida, Beutler and Motulsky (1971) and two subsequent supplements (Beutler & Yoshida, 1973; Yoshida & Beutler, 1978) is given in McKusick (1978). In these tabulations the variants are divided into four classes according to the severity of manifestation:

Class 1 Enzyme deficiency with chronic non-spherocytic haemolytic anaemia

Class 2 Severe red cell enzyme deficiency (less than 10% of normal) but usually not associated with haemolytic anaemia

Class 3 Moderate to mild enzyme deficiency (10–60% of normal)

Class 4 Very mild or no enzyme deficiency (60–100% of normal)

Class 5 Increased enzyme activity (more than twice normal)

A less important subdivision is into four groups of which group I includes all well characterised and distinctive variants, while groups II, III, IV are those for which information is insufficient or which may include variants

Table 75.4 Some important G6PD variants.

Type	G6PD activity %	Class	Population	Complications
G6PD B+	100	4	All	None, normal type
G6PD A+	100	4	African	None, normal type
G6PD A−	10–20	3	African	Haemolysis with drugs, etc. Occasional neonatal haemolysis
G6PD Mediterranean	0–5	2	Greek, Italian, etc.	Haemolysis with drugs, etc. Neonatal haemolysis Favism
G6PD Canton	4–25	2–3	Chinese	Haemolysis with drugs, etc. Neonatal haemolysis Favism
G6PD Albuquerque, Beaujon, Freiburg, New York	0–1	1	very rare	Chronic haemolytic anaemia
G6PD Hektoen	increased	5	very rare	None

duplicating others already listed. Within this classification for example, the Negro deficiency type is in class 3 (moderate to mild deficiency) and is in group I because it has been well characterized.

Deficiencies of other enzymes in the hexose-monophosphate and related pathways

Glutathione reductase (GSR) deficiency is frequently listed as a congenital disorder determining haemolytic and other diseases, but there is now some doubt as to whether such a trait exists. As Beutler (1979) has pointed out, GSR deficiency may result from dietary riboflavin lack, since the enzyme contains flavine-adenine dinucleotide. Furthermore, the role of deficiency of the enzyme in causing red cell haemolysis is in question. 6-phosphogluconate dehydrogenase (6-PGD) deficiency has also been reported in a few families (Valentine & Tanaka, 1978), but is not usually a cause of haemolytic or other disease (Beutler, 1979).

Gamma-glutamyl-cysteine synthetase (GGCS) deficiency may be a very rare cause of mild haemolytic disease. Red cells in the affected individual have about 10% of the normal level of enzyme activity, and very low levels of reduced glutathione (GSH). A defect of GSH levels in sheep, with reduced GGCS activity, has been reported, but its significance as a model is unclear and it is apparently not associated with haemolytic disease (Smith, Lee & Mia, 1973).

Pyrimidine-5′-nucleotidase deficiency

This autosomal recessive trait determines chronic haemolytic anaemia associated with basophilic stippling. Neonatal hyperbilirubinaemia has been reported in this disease; splenomegaly is found but the anaemia is usually mild (Valentine & Tanaka, 1978; Beutler, 1979).

HYPOPLASTIC ANAEMIAS

The following conditions show inadequate production of red blood cells due to a variety of different mechanisms. In Fanconi anaemia, the first one to be well characterized, other cell types are also involved.

FANCONI ANAEMIA (FA)

Fanconi, in 1927, described three brothers of short stature with hyperpigmentation and other physical anomalies associated with pancytopenia (see Fanconi, 1967). Subsequent observations have consolidated the description and confirmed that it is an autosomal recessive trait. In addition to the growth retardation and hyperpigmentation mentioned, various minor malformations, especially of the radius and thumb, and of the kidneys, may also occur (Fanconi, 1967). They may be evident in the newborn, but bone marrow failure usually appears between the ages of 4 and 12, and is progressive. It does not necessarily occur in all the members of a family who show the malformations. Haematologic findings are non-specific, with normocytic or slightly macrocytic anaemia, and moderate leucopenia and thrombocytopenia. Haemoglobin F levels are almost invariably elevated. Bone marrow may appear normal in the early stages but is hypoplastic in the established disease.

Diagnosis is not difficult when more than one case is present in a family, or when characteristic malformations are seen with pancytopenia in a child. However, an isolated case without malformation may present difficulty, and a search for chromosomal aberrations in lymphocytes (below) may be valuable in confirming the diagnosis. The presence of pancytopenia distinguishes this condition from congenital hypoplastic anaemia, and the dyserythropoietic anaemias. The TAR syndrome (thrombocytopenia with absent radii) should be easily distinguishable.

Management is as for other types of bone marrow failure, with minimum use of blood transfusion to avoid or delay the problem of iron overload. Androgen treatment, possibly accompanied by low dose steroids, produces a useful haematologic response in most patients, but the complications of androgen therapy may be troublesome (Beard, 1976). Bone marrow transplantation may become the treatment of choice in the future.

There is an increased risk of malignancy in FA patients, especially acute leukaemia and lymphomas (Swift, 1976; Sandberg, 1980).

Chromosomal aberrations

This was the first disease in which spontaneous chromosomal breaks were observed. Excess breaks and other chromosomal aberrations may be found in 15–74% of lymphocyte metaphases, 10–49% of fibroblasts, and a small proportion of bone marrow cells (Beard, 1976; Sandberg, 1980). They precede the development of pancytopenia suggesting that they represent a secondary component of the primary genetic defect. The chromosomal changes are less marked than in Bloom syndrome, and the increase in sister chromatid exchanges (SCE) found in Bloom syndrome is not present in Fanconi anaemia. However, the cells are more susceptible than normal to many of the chemical and other agents which produce chromosomal aberrations in vitro (Swift, 1976). Fibroblasts from FA patients, and possibly their parents, show increased transformability by SV_{40} virus.

Genetics

Autosomal recessive inheritance is probable, based on the occurrence of multiple affected sibs with normal parents, consanguinity in some families, and usual lack of vertical transmission (Schroeder et al, 1976). As mentioned, heterozygotes may perhaps show minor chromosomal instability. It is suspected that they also have an excess of malignant tumours, including leukaemias (Swift, 1976).

CONGENITAL HYPOPLASTIC ANAEMIA (CHA)

The description of this rare syndrome, or group, characterized by chronically reduced red cell production, has been gradually built up over the last 40 years or more since it was first characterized by Josephs in 1936, and then Diamond and Blackfan (1938). Other names include 'pure red cell aplasia', and the eponymous *Diamond-Blackfan* anaemia; Diamond is co-author of a recent valuable review of some 135 personal and published cases (Diamond, Wang & Alter, 1976).

Most affected children are diagnosed in infancy and show chronic deficiency of red cell production, often with persistent macrocytosis. There are no specific morphologic abnormalities of the red cells, although enzyme levels may be increased, as in a young red cell population. Correspondingly, the fetal 'i' antigen may tend to persist into childhood and even adult life. Persistant mild elevation of Hb F levels may also be found. However, reticulocyte counts are low and there is no evidence of increased red cell destruction. Erythropoietin level is elevated and antibodies to erythropoietin have not been found. Unresponsiveness to erythropoietin, improved by steroid therapy, may be a major part of the underlying pathophysiology (Nathan et al, 1978). White cell and platelet counts are usually normal. Bone marrow examination in untreated patients shows striking deficiency of erythroblasts and normoblasts with otherwise normal bone marrow. In spite of macrocytosis, no megaloblasts are present, serum levels of B_{12} and folate are normal or elevated, and there is no response to treatment with these substances.

Many patients show accompanying anomalies of growth and development. Clinical variability suggests that CHA is also a genetically heterogeneous disorder. Growth failure appears to be more frequent and more severe than can readily be accounted for as a secondary effect of anaemia or of corticosteroid therapy. Associated physical anomalies include triphalangeal thumbs (and other thumb malformations), congenital heart disease and renal malformations. A phenotypic resemblance to the Turner syndrome, with short or webbed neck and broad chest, has been described several times, as in the hitherto unpublished family illustrated in Figure 75.14. Another perhaps nonspecific association is the finding of various chromosome anomalies, especially of chromosome 1. We have found 45,X/46,XX/47,XXX mosaicism in one patient (Fig. 75.14). Abnormalities of tryptophan metabolism described in a few patients have not been confirmed in others and the metabolic basis of CHA is unknown.

Formerly, treatment was by blood transfusion with the many attendant complications, particularly haemosiderosis. Splenectomy is ineffective. More recently, corticosteroid therapy has been found effective in 80% of cases and normal haemoglobin levels can usually be obtained with modest continued doses of prednisone. Many patients show marked dose responsiveness with a prompt fall in haemoglobin level when the dose is reduced. They should be maintained on the lowest possible dose. Refractory cases may be helped by the addition of androgen. Spontaneous remission in adults after years of treatment has been reported. Termination in acute leukaemia has been described once (Wasser et al, 1978), but this appears to be rare, in contrast to Fanconi anaemia. Steroid responsiveness is one of the reasons for suspecting that the primary defect may lie outside the

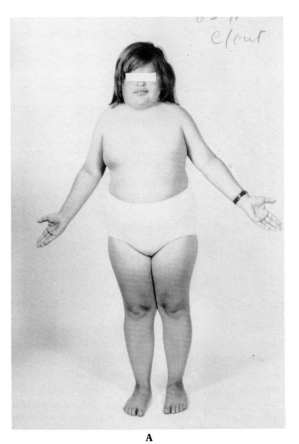

A

red cell precursors themselves, and may be immunologic in nature (Steinberg, Coleman & Pennebaker, 1979).

Genetics and heterogeneity

Sex incidence is 1:1, and this, together with the frequent occurrence of multiple affected sibs of apparently normal parents, strongly suggests autosomal recessive inheritance. However, formal demonstration of this hypothesis is lacking. Several reports describe apparent vertical transmission with an affected parent (usually the mother) and child or children, indicating possible autosomal dominant inheritance.

FAMILIAL DYSERYTHROPOIETIC ANAEMIAS

This group comprises several rare types of hereditary refractory anaemia characterized by marked 'dyserythropoietic' morphologic changes in the red cell series in the bone marrow, including multinuclearity. These changes reflect as yet undetermined metabolic abnormalities of erythropoiesis, such that effective red cell production is impaired and the red cells are abnormal with slightly shortened survival. They have been classified into types I, II and III (Heimpel & Wendth, 1968), of which type II is best characterized. Only I and II will be briefly reviewed here, since III and other possible types are not yet well worked out.

PEDIGREE #1652

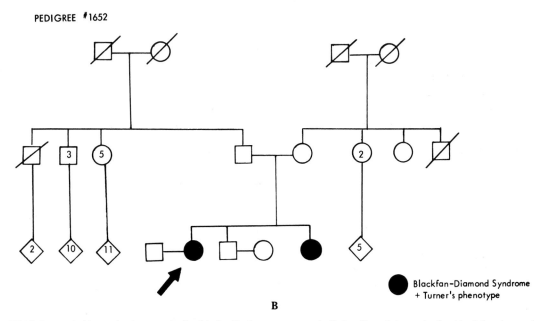

B

Fig. 75.14 Congenital hypoplastic anaemia. In this family there were two similarly affected sisters, both with cleft palate and Turner-like phenotype associated with steroid responsive red cell aplasia. (A) affected 13-year old girl with short neck and broad chest. This patient's karyotype was normal; her identically affected sister showed a 45,X/46,XX/47,XXX karyotype. (B) Pedigree of the family indicating probable autosomal recessive inheritance. Consanguinity not known but the parents' families immigrated to USA from the same area of Poland (Bannerman R M and Marinello M., unpublished, 1980).

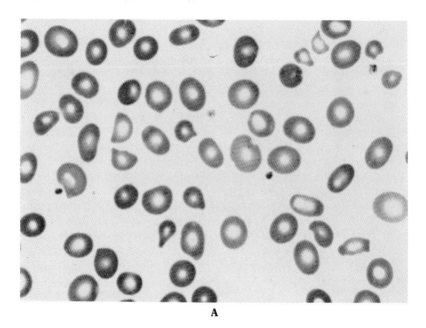

A

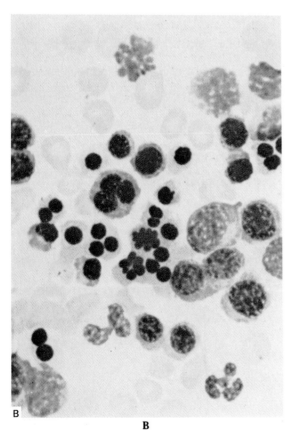

B

Fig. 75.15 Hereditary dyserythropoietic anaemia, type II (HEMPAS), showing (A) blood film with anisocytosis, anisochromasia and poikilocytes; (B) bone marrow with erythroid hyperplasia and binucleated and multinucleated erythroblasts (from Crookston et al (1969), by courtesy of Dr J. H. Crookston and the British Journal of Haematology).

Type I

This very rare condition presents as a mild refractory anaemia with shortened red cell survival and evidence of haemolysis, but without increase in reticulocytes, emphasizing the important element of dyserythropoiesis. Red cells tend to be macrocytic but with no specific changes. Bone marrow shows marked erythroid hyperplasia, megaloblastoid changes, bi- and multinuclear erythroblasts, and other nuclear abnormalities including internuclear chromatin bridges. Haemosiderosis is an important secondary feature even in the absence of blood transfusion (Heimpel & Wendt, 1968).

Type II

Affected patients have usually presented in childhood with anaemia and intermittent jaundice. The red cells show variable aniso- and poikilocytosis (Fig. 75.15A) rather than macrocytosis, but the changes are not diagnostic. However, the red cells show a number of immunologic abnormalities, including sensitivity to anti-I and especially lysis of a significant proportion of the cells in normal acidified serum at 37° C, hence the acronym HEMPAS, for 'Hereditary Erythroid Multinuclearity associated with a Positive Acidified Serum test' (Crookston et al, 1969). The acid serum test is valuable in characterizing this trait. There is some evidence of haemolysis with variable levels of haptoglobin, usually splenomegaly, and variable mild jaundice. However, much of the hyperbilirubinaemia probably results from 'ineffective erythropoiesis' with destruction of haemoglobin in red cell precursors, and red cell survival is only slightly reduced. Splenectomy has been of doubtful benefit. Bone marrow is hyperplastic and over 20% of late erythroblasts show double nuclei or multilobulated or multiple nuclei

(Fig. 75.15B), but megaloblastic changes are not seen. Haemosiderosis is an important secondary feature and removal of iron by chelation or even phlebotomy has been advocated.

Genetics

The two forms which are reasonably well characterized are both autosomal recessive traits. Heterozygotes are symptomless and have no obvious haematologic changes although minor serological abnormalities have been mentioned in some reports. Vertical transmission of a type of dyserythropoietic anaemia (possibly corresponding to type III) has been described in one or two families, including what is perhaps the first description of this type of anaemia (Wolff & Van Hofe, 1951), but there is insufficient evidence to characterize an autosomal dominant form. Presumably this group will be shown to be more heterogeneous and new cases deserve careful family investigation.

REFRACTORY SIDEROBLASTIC ANAEMIAS

The best characterized of these rare forms is an X-linked refractory hypochromic anaemia, described first by Cooley. The family concerned has been followed by other investigators at the University of Michigan (Rundles & Falls, 1946; Rucknagel, 1980) and a few other families have been reported. Affected males show moderate hypochromic anaemia with a markedly pleomorphic

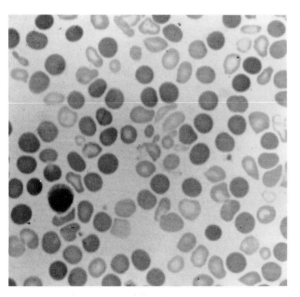

Fig. 75.16 X–linked hereditary hypochromic sideroblastic anaemia. Blood film from a heterozygous female carrier showing marked red cell polymorphism, possibly indicating Lyonization with two red cell populations. (By courtesy of Dr. P. H. Pinkerton, University of Toronto.)

blood picture. The anaemia is not generally severe, although blood transfusion is sometimes needed. Iron overloading is an important feature of the disease even in the absence of transfusion, and sideroblasts are seen in bone marrow.

Carrier females are not anaemic but may show similar red cell changes (Fig. 75.16), suggesting Lyonisation, with two populations of red cells. However, efforts to demonstrate this effect by separating the two cell types have not been entirely successful.

It is possible that a similar, pyridoxine responsive form of anaemia, also occurs as a recessive trait.

The metabolic basis of these disorders is not clear, although inconsistent abnormalities of haem synthesis have been reported. Acquired forms of sideroblastic anaemia are common, resulting from a variety of causes including preleukaemic states, especially in elderly patients (MacGibbon & Mollin, 1964).

ANIMAL MODELS

Several hereditary disorders of stem cell function in the mouse deserve mention here, although none is a precise analogue of a human disease (Pinkerton & Bannerman, 1979). The best known are those associated with mutant alleles at the W locus (Russell, 1980). Some are lethal in the homozygous state, but in others such as the compound heterozygote W/W^v, animals survive with macrocytic, hypoplastic anaemia and pleiotropic effects, including gonadal hypoplasia and deficiency of pigmentation. The bone marrow is hypoplastic and the hypoplasia persists in stem cells transplanted into normal irradiated hosts. In the similar steel (Sl) types of anaemia transplanted stem cells function normally in a normal host, and the defect appears to be in the bone marrow microenvironment. Hertwig anaemia (gene symbol an) is recessively inherited and shows severe hypoplastic anaemia and leucopenia. Transplanted stem cells reproduce the same effects in normal hosts. Another hypoplastic anaemia in the mouse, 'diminutive' (gene symbol dm) is also a recessive trait, and is of particular interest since the anaemia is accompanied by multiple skeletal abnormalities and retarded growth (Russell, 1980).

MEGALOBLASTIC ANAEMIA

Megaloblastic refers to the appearance of bone marrow erythroblasts in which the normal pattern of differentiation is disturbed, so that nuclear activity and cell division lag behind cytoplasmic maturation. It results from impairment of normal DNA synthesis, for which both vitamin B_{12} (cyanocobalamin) and folic acid (pteroylglutamic acid) are essential factors (Beck, 1972a). The megaloblastic appearance in the red cell series is associated with red cell macrocytosis in peripheral blood; there are parallel changes in the granulocyte series, especially giant metamyelocytes in marrow with nuclear hypersegmentation in mature forms. The anaemia is due partly to reduced production of red cells, associated with ineffective erythropoiesis, and partly to shortened red cell survival in peripheral blood, both factors contributing to hyperbilirubinaemia. Anaemia is accompanied by leucopenia, and sometimes thrombocytopenia.

Deficiency of B_{12} or folic acid may arise from multiple causes, including dietary and absorptive defects. Transport and metabolism may also be impaired by genetic and pharmacologic factors. Megaloblastic anaemias which are partly or mainly genetically determined are as follows:

1. Classical (Addisonian) pernicious anaemia (PA)
2. Juvenile PA
3. Congenital PA
4. Disorders of cyanocobalamin and folate transport and metabolism

A brief outline of B_{12} absorption and transport is essential. It is released from complexed forms in food in the stomach and small intestine, and normally binds to a gastric secreted protein, intrinsic factor (IF). The IF-B_{12} complex is absorbed via specific receptors in the distal part of the ileum. B_{12} is then transported by transcobalamins to the liver, via the portal circulation, where it is stored. Transport to tissue sites is also by transcobalamins. The metabolic roles of cyanocobalamin and derivatives, and their interaction with folic acid, are complex and not fully worked out in human tissues. However, at least three systems are impaired in human B_{12} deficiency: (1) methylmalonyl CoA isomerization; (2) deoxyribosyl synthesis and hence DNA synthesis; and (3) methionine methyl synthesis (Beck, 1972b). Methylcobalamin, the derivative directly involved in methionine synthesis, regenerates from methyltetrahydrofolic acid converting it to tetrahydrofolic acid. The latter is required as a cofactor for thymidine synthesis, which may serve partly to explain defective DNA production when either B_{12} or folic acid is seriously deficient.

All forms of B_{12} deficiency require lifelong treatment with intramuscular injections of vitamin B_{12}, usually at least 100 μg monthly, after initial larger loading doses. Much greater doses are needed in some of the rare abnormalities discussed under 'Disorders of cobalamin and folate transport and metabolism' (below).

CLASSICAL PERNICIOUS ANAEMIA (PA)

This most common form of B_{12} deficiency was formerly 'pernicious', leading to death from anaemia and neurological disease, in the period before treatment with liver extracts and subsequently pure vitamin B_{12}. The clinical features are well known (Hardisty & Weatherall, 1974; Williams, 1972; Wintrobe, 1974). Development of manifest disease takes many years of gradual failure of IF production and depletion of B_{12} stores. During this time the patient may be said to have latent or 'pre'-pernicious anaemia, and presumably many potentially affected individuals remain in this state for years and die of other causes without being ascertained as having PA.

The pathophysiology involves: (1) constitutional predisposition to IF production failure, i.e. a genetic factor, discussed further below; (2) progressive gastric atrophy with achlorhydria, to which autoimmune factors contribute; (3) immune factors directly impairing IF function. 90% of PA patients have serum antibodies to the cells which produce IF, the gastric parietal cells (GPC), though these are not entirely specific and occur in other forms of gastritis (Fisher & Taylor, 1971). Blocking and binding antibodies to IF may be found in serum and gastric juice. Thyroid auto-antibodies also occur in the serum of many patients.

Genetic aspects

Earlier descriptions of the disease suggested an ethnic predisposition for Northern Europeans to be affected, and a characteristic habitus. Although there may be a Scandinavian preponderance, the condition occurs worldwide in people of many different ethnic groups. Recent reports document high incidence in relatively young Negro women (e.g. Solanki et al, 1978). There is familial aggregation of PA; about 20% of affected probands also have an affected near relative. There is an association with blood group A, as for carcinoma of stomach, though it has not been found in all studies, and a less marked blood group B association (Mourant, Kopec & Domaniewska-Sobczak, 1978). An apparent association with HLA-B7 has not been sustained by more recent studies (Wright et al, 1977).

Various associations of PA with other diseases, especially carcinoma of stomach and diabetes mellitus, are well documented (Witts, 1963). In addition, patients with PA show an overall increased prevalence of autoimmune phenomena and autoimmune disorders due to them, such as hyperthyroidism and thyroiditis.

Relatives of PA patients tend to have similar disease associations. A proportion of relatives, increasing with advancing age, may have gastritis, the condition of latent PA (Callendar & Denborough, 1957). Relatives also show an increase in prevalence of antibodies to gastric parietal cells, and sometimes IF and thyroid tissue (TeVelde et al, 1964; Doniach, Roitt & Taylor, 1965; Wangel et al, 1968; Whittingham et al, 1969; Varis et al, 1979). Impaired B_{12} absorption, as judged by the Schilling test, may also be found, but it is not always a reliable determination (McIntyre, 1968). Siurala and co-workers found that the most useful single test was low serum pepsinogen (Varis et al, 1979). They and others have been able to discern bimodality in the distribution of results of some of these determinations in relatives, and have been led to propose an autosomal dominant hypothesis. It is suggested that the gene in single dose predisposes to the development of autoimmune reactions, especially against gastric parietal cells, and leads eventually to IF production failure. The hypothetical gene is of low penetrance, and its expression is modified by environmental factors. Pedigree data are limited, but do not provide very clear support for the hypothesis. For instance, in three families with conjugal PA (i.e. both parents of sibships affected) illustrated by Wangel et al (1968) only one out of twelve children had developed PA at the time of observation as adults. A multifactorial explanation appears equally plausible at this time. Although there is no firm basis for genetic counselling, empirically there appears to be a low risk for first degree relatives of patients eventually to develop PA. A larger proportion may have symptomless, progressive atrophic gastritis or latent PA in adult life.

JUVENILE PERNICIOUS ANAEMIA

The juvenile type or childhood PA resembles the adult form in showing autoimmune phenomena and gastric atrophy with IF secretion failure (McIntyre et al, 1965). However, onset is in childhood at around 10 years. Multiple affected sibs suggest the likelihood of autosomal recessive inheritance in some families. Some cases are associated with striking endocrinopathy (Quinto et al, 1964) and some with IgA deficiency (Spector, 1974).

In another type with earlier onset, Immerslund syndrome, gastric function and IF production are normal, but there is a specific defect in B_{12} absorption, often associated with proteinuria (Immerslund & Bjornstad, 1963; Mohamed, McKay & Galloway, 1966). Again, multiple affected sibs with normal parents suggest autosomal recessive inheritance.

CONGENITAL PERNICIOUS ANAEMIA

The onset of this condition is in infancy. There is specific failure of IF production but without other gastric abnormality or the other features of classic PA (Lambert, Prankerd & Smellie, 1961; McIntyre et al 1965; Miller et al, 1966). The occurrence of multiple affected sibs suggests the possibility of autosomal recessive inheritance; no abnormalities have been found in parents or other relatives.

DISORDERS OF COBALAMIN AND FOLATE TRANSPORT AND METABOLISM

Some very rare disorders, usually manifested in infancy, are included under this heading. The metabolic effects may overshadow the anaemia.

Transcobalamin (TC) deficiencies

A severe form associated with absence of TC II, the major transport form, is inherited as an autosomal recessive trait. It is potentially fatal in infancy and best treated with large doses of vitamin B_{12} (Hakami et al, 1971). A partial form of deficiency presenting with persistently low serum B_{12} in adult life has also been reported.

Methylmalonic aciduria

Methylmalonic aciduria is found in all B_{12} deficiencies, and is a useful additional diagnostic test. However, the present heading refers to conditions in which increased excretion of methylmalonic acid is associated with congenital defects in the methylmalonyl CoA mutase system, for which cyanocobalamin is a cofactor. Patients present in infancy with severe acidosis, ketonuria and developmental retardation, but not anaemia (Rosenberg, Lilljequist & Hsia, 1969; Rosenberg, 1978). The condition is heterogeneous. Some cases have been found to respond dramatically to pharmacologic doses of vitamin B_{12}, e.g. 1 mg/day. The genetic basis is uncertain but autosomal recessive inheritance is likely. Prenatal diagnosis can be made by the demonstration of increased amounts of methylmalonic acid in amniotic fluid and in maternal urine, or by enzyme assay of cultured cells (Mahoney, et al, 1975), and prenatal therapy by vitamin B_{12} has been achieved (Ampola et al, 1975).

Disorders of folate metabolism

There are several rare inborn defects which are associated with severe neurologic disorder and megaloblastic anaemia (Rowe, 1978). A specific defect in intestinal folate absorption results in anaemia and neurologic disorder in infancy. Responses to treatment have generally been unsatisfactory; large doses of folic acid given intramuscularly may be required.

The active form of folic acid is tetrahydrofolate, which is maintained by dihydrofolate reductase. Deficiency of this enzyme has been described in a few children, probably as a recessively inherited trait. In a few cases satisfactory treatment has been achieved by intramuscular administration of 5-formyl tetrahydrofolate. Deficiencies of other enzymes involved in the complex metabolism of folic acid include formiminotransferase deficiency associated with severe mental retardation, increased urinary formiminoglutamic acid (FIGLU) excretion, and megaloblastic anaemia in some cases only. The variability suggests that the few cases described are heterogeneous. Tetrahydrofolate methyltransferase deficiency has also been reported, with mild anaemia and severe neurologic disturbance.

Hereditary orotic aciduria

This rare inborn error results from a defect in the normal pathway of uridine synthesis. It produces a syndrome of failure to thrive and mental retardation with megaloblastic anaemia in infancy (Kelley & Smith, 1978). There is no response to vitamin B_{12} or folic acid therapy, but large oral doses of uridine (1500 mg daily) have been successful in managing some cases.

ACKNOWLEDGEMENTS

The writer is grateful to colleagues who have assisted in providing material for this section, and who have criticized the manuscript. Work in his own laboratory has been supported in part by grants from the National Institutes of Health (AM-19424), and the Bureau of Maternal and Child Health Services, Human Genetics Program Project #417.

REFERENCES

Ampola M G, Mahoney M J, Nakamura E, Tonaka K 1975 Prenatal therapy of a patient with vitamin B_{12} responsive methylmalonic acidemia. New England Journal of Medicine 293: 313

Anderson R, Motulsky G 1966 Adverse effect of raised environmental temperature on the expression of hereditary spherocytosis in Deer mice. Blood 28: 365–375

Bannerman R M, Edwards J A, Pinkerton P H 1973 Hereditary disorders of the red cell in animals. In: Brown E (ed) Progress in Hematology. Grune & Stratton, New York. p 131–179

Bannerman R M, Renwick J H 1962 The hereditary elliptocytoses: clinical and linkage data. Annals of Human Genetics London 26: 23

Bassen F A, Kornzweig A L 1950 Malformation of the erythrocytes in a case of atypical retinitis pigmentosa. Blood 5: 381

Beard M E J 1976 Fanconi anaemia. In: Congenital Disorders of Erythropoiesis, Ciba Foundation Symposium 37 new series. p 103–114

Beck W S 1972a General considerations of megaloblastic anemia In: Williams W J, Beutler E, Erslev A J, Rundles R W (eds) Hematology. McGraw-Hill Book Company, New York ch 25, p. 249

Beck W S 1972b Vitamin B_{12} deficiency. In: Williams W J, Beutler E, Erslev A J, Rundles R W (eds) Hematology. McGraw-Hill Book Company, New York ch 26, p 256

Bessis M 1977 Blood Smears Reinterpreted. Brecher G (translated by) Springer International, New York

Beutler E 1971 Abnormalities of the hexose monophosphate shunt. Seminars in Hematology VIII: 311–347

Beutler E 1972 Glucose-6-phosphate dehydrogenase deficiency. In: Williams W J, Beutler E, Erslev A J, Rundles R W (eds) Hematology. McGraw-Hill Book Company, New York. ch 41

Beutler E 1975 Red Cell Metabolism; a Manual of Biochemical Methods. Grune and Stratton, New York

Beutler E 1979 Red cell enzyme defects as nondiseases and as diseases. Blood 54(1): 1–7

Beutler E 1980 The red cell: a tiny dynamo. In: Wintrobe M M (ed) Blood, Pure and Eloquent. McGraw-Hill Book Company, New York. ch 6 p 141

Beutler E, Scott S, Bishop A, Margolis N, Matsumoto F, Kuhl W 1973 Red cell aldolase deficiency and hemolytic anemia: a new syndrome. Transactions of the Association of American Physicians 86: 154

Beutler E, Yoshida A 1973 Human glucose-6-phosphate dehydrogenase variants: a supplementary tabulation. Annals of Human Genetics 37: 151–156

Black J A, Rittenberg M B, Standerfer R J, Peterson J S 1978 Hereditary persistence of fetal erythrocyte pyruvate kinase in Basenji dog. In: Brewer G J (ed) The Red Cells. Alan R Liss, New York. p 275–290

Booth P B, Serjeantson S, Woodfield D G, Amato D 1977 Selective depression of blood group antigens associated with hereditary ovalocytosis among melanesians. Vox Sanguinis 32: 99–100

Boyer S H, Porter J H, Wellbacher R G 1962 Electrophoretic heterogeneity of glucose-6-phosphate dehydrogenase and its relationship to enzyme deficiency in man. Proceedings of the National Academy of Sciences USA 48: 1868

Callender S T, Denborough M A 1957 A family study of pernicious anemia. British Journal of Haematology 3: 88

Childs B, Zinkham W 1958 A genetic study of a defect in glutathione metabolism of the erythrocyte. Johns Hopkins Medical Journal 102: 21–37

Crookston J H, Crookston M C, Burnie K L, Francombe W H 1969 Hereditary erythroblastic multinuclearity associated with a positive acidified serum test: a type of congenital dyserythropoietic anaemia. British Journal of Haematology 17: 11

Cutting H O, McHugh W J, Conrad F G, Marlow A A 1965 Autosomal dominant hemolytic anemia characterized by ovalocytosis. American Journal of Medicine 39: 21

Dacie J V 1960 The Haemolytic Anaemias. Congenital and Acquired. Part I. The Congenital Anaemias. Churchill, London

Davidson R G, Nitowsky H M, Childs B 1963 Demonstration of two populations of cells in the human female heterozygous for glucose-6-phosphate dehydrogenase variants. Proceedings of the National Academy of Sciences 50: 481

Diamond L K, Wang W C, Alter B P 1976 Congenital hypoplastic anemia. Advances in Pediatrics 22: 349–378

Doniach D, Roitt I M, Taylor K B 1965 Autoimmunity in pernicious anemia and thyroiditis: a family study. Annals of the New York Academy of Sciences 124: 605

Eber S W, Dunnwald M, Belohradsky B H, Bidlinsmaier F, Schievelbein, Weinmann H M, Krietsch K G 1979 Hereditary deficiency of triosephosphate isomerase in four unrelated families. European Journal of Clinical Investigation 9(3): 195–202

Fanconi G 1967 Familial constitutional panmyelocytopathy, Fanconi's anaemia (F.A.) I. Clinical aspects. Seminars in Hematology 4: 233–240

Fisher J M, Taylor K B 1971 Annotation: the significance of gastric antibodies. British Journal of Haematology 20: 1

Greenquist A C, Shohet S B, Bernstein S E 1978 Marked reduction of spectrin in hereditary spherocytosis in the common house mouse. Blood 51: 1149–1155

Hardisty R M, Weatherall D J 1974 Blood and Its Disorders. Blackwell Scientific Publications, London

Hakami N, Neiman P E, Canellos G P, Lazerson J 1971 Neonatal megaloblastic deficiency in two siblings. New England Journal of Medicine 285: 1163

Harris H, Hopkinson A, Robson E B 1974 The incidence of rare alleles determining electrophoretic variants: Data on 43 enzyme loci in man. Annals of Human Genetics 37: 237–253

Harris J W, Kellermeyer R W 1970 The Red Cell. Production, Metabolism, Destruction: Normal and Abnormal. Revised edition. Harvard University Press, Cambridge, Mass

Heimpel H, Wendt F 1968 Congenital dyserythropoietic anemia with karyorrhexis and multinuclearity of erythroblasts. Helvetica Medica Acta 34: 103–115

Herbert P N, Gotto A M, Fredrickson D S 1978 Familial lipoprotein deficiency (abetalipoproteinemia, hypobetalipoproteinemia, and Tangier disease) In: Stanbury J B, Wyngaarden J B, Fredrickson D S (eds) The Metabolic Basis of Inherited Disease 4th eds. McGraw-Hill Book Company, New York p 544

Imerslund O, Bjornstad P 1963 Familial vitamin B_{12} malabsorption. Acta Haematologica (Basel) 30: 1

Jacob H S 1972 The abnormal red cell membrane in hereditary spherocytosis: evidence for the causal role of mutant micro-filaments. British Journal of Haematology 23 (suppl): 35–44

Jandl J H, Cooper R A 1978 Hereditary spherocytosis In: Stanbury J B, Wyngaarden J B, Fredrickson D S (eds), The Metabolic Basis of Inherited Diseases. 4th ed. McGraw-Hill Book Company, New York

Kahn A, Kaplan J C, Dreyfus J C 1979 Advances in hereditary red cell enzyme anomalies. Human Genetics 50: 1

Keats B J B 1979 Another elliptocytosis locus on chromosome 1. Human Genetics 50: 227

Kelley W N, Smith L H 1978 Hereditary orotic aciduria In: Stanbury J B, Wyngaarden J B, Fredrickson D S (eds) The Metabolic Basis of Inherited Disease 4th ed. McGraw-Hill Book Company, New York. ch 46 p 1045

Lambert H P, Prankerd T A J, Smellie J M 1961 Pernicious anaemia in childhood: a report of two cases in one family and their relationship to the etiology of pernicious anaemia. Quarterly Journal of Medicine 30: 71

Lawler S D 1954 Family studies showing linkage between elliptocytosis and the Rhesus blood group system. Caryologica 6 (suppl): 26

Levine P, Tripodi D, Struck J Jr, Zmijewski C M, Pollack W 1973 Hemolytic anaemia associated with Rh_{null} but not with Bombay blood. Vox Sanguinis 24: 417–424

Lock S P, Sephton-Smith R, Hardisty R M 1961 Stomatocytosis: a hereditary red cell anomaly associated with haemolytic anaemia. British Journal of Haematology 7: 303–314

Lux S 1979 Spectrin-actin membrane skeleton of normal and abnormal red blood cells. Seminars in Hematology XVI: 21–51

Luzzatto L, Usanga E A, Reddy S 1969 Glucose-6-phosphate dehydrogenase deficient red cells: resistance to infection by malarial parasites. Science 164: 839–842

MacGibbon B H, Mollin D L 1964 Sideroblastic anaemia in man: observations on seventy cases. British Journal of Haematology 11: 59

Mahoney M J, Rosenberg L E, Lindblad B, Waldenstrom J, Zetterstrom R 1975 Prenatal diagnosis of methylmalonic

aciduria. Acta Paediatrica Scandinavica 64: 44

McIntyre P A 1968 Genetic and autoimmune features of pernicious anaemia. I. Unreliability of the Schilling test in detecting genetic predisposition to the disease. Johns Hopkins Medical Journal 122: 181

McIntyre P A, Hahn R, Conley C L, Glass B 1959 Genetic factors in predisposition to pernicious anaemia. Bulletin of the Johns Hopkins Hospital 104: 309

McIntyre O R, Sullivan C W, Jeffries G J, Silver R H 1965 Pernicious anaemia in childhood. New England Journal of Medicine 272: 981

McKusick V A 1978 Mendelian Inheritance in Man. Catalogs of autosomal dominant, autosomal recessive, and X-linked phenotypes. Fifth edition, The Johns Hopkins University Press, Baltimore

Mentzer W C, Smith W B, Goldstone J, Shohet S B 1975 Hereditary stomatocytosis: membrane and metabolism studies. Blood 46: 659–669

Miller D R, Bloom G E, Streiss R R, LoBuglio A F, Diamond L K 1966 Juvenile 'congenital' pernicious anaemia: Clinical and immunologic studies. New England Journal of Medicine 275: 978

Miller D R, Pearson H A, Baehner R L, McMillan C W (eds) 1978 Smith's Blood Diseases of Infancy and Childhood. C V Mosby Company, St. Louis

Mohamed S D, McKay E, Galloway W H 1966 Juvenile familial megaloblastic anaemia due to selective malabsorption of vitamin B_{12}. Quarterly Journal of Medicine 35: 433

Mohandas N, Phillips W M, Bessie M 1979 Red blood cell deformability and hemolytic anemias. Seminars in Hematology XVI: 95–114

Motulsky A G 1975 Glucose-6-phosphate dehydrogenase and abnormal hemoglobin polymorphisms – evidence regarding malarial selection. In: Salzano, F (ed) The Role of Natural Selection in Human Evolution. Amsterdam, North Holland. p 271

Morton N E 1956 The detection and estimation of linkage between the genes for elliptocytosis and the Rh blood type. American Journal of Human Genetics 8: 80

Mourant A E, Kopec A C, Domaniewska-Sobczak K 1978 Blood Groups and Diseases. A study of associations of diseases with blood groups and other polymorphisms. Oxford University Press, New York

Nathan D G, Clarke B J, Hillman D G, Alter B P, Housman D E 1978 Erythroid precursors in congenital hypoplastic (Diamond-Blackfan) anemia. Journal of Clinical Investigation 61: 489–98

Pinkerton P H, Fletch S M, Brueckner P J, Miller D R 1974 Hereditary stomatocytosis with hemolytic anemia in the dog. Blood 44: 557–567

Pinkerton P H, Bannerman R M 1979 Hemolytic disorders of red cell membrane origin. In: Andrews E J, Ward B C, Altman N H (eds) Spontaneous Animal Models of Human Disease, vol 1 American College of Animal Laboratory Medicine, Academic Press, New York. ch 100

Ponder E 1948 Hemolysis and related phenomena. Grune and Stratton, New York. p 29

Quinto M G 1964 Pernicious anemia in a young girl associated with idiopathic hypoparathyroidism. Journal of Pediatrics 64: 241

Rattazzi M C, Corash L M, VanZzanan G E, Jaffe E R, Piomelli S 1971 G-6-PD deficiency and chronic hemolysis: four new mutants – relationships between clinical syndrome and enzyme kinetics. Blood 38: 205–218

Rosenberg L E 1978 Disorders of propionate, methylmalonate, and cobalamin metabolism. In: Stanbury

J B, Wyngaarden J B, Fredrickson D S (eds) The Metabolic Basis of Inherited Disease 4th ed. McGraw-Hill Book Company, New York. ch 21 p 411

Rosenberg L, Lilljequist A C, Hsia Y E 1969 Methylmalonic aciduria: An inborn error leading to metabolic acidosis, long-chain ketonuria and intermittent hyperglycinemia. New England Journal of Medicine 278: 1319

Rowe P B 1978 Inherited disorders of folate metabolism. In: Stanbury J B, Wyngaarden J B, Fredrickson D S (eds) The Metabolic Basis of Inherited Disease 4th ed. McGraw-Hill Book Company, New York. ch 22 p 430

Rucknagel D 1980 Personal communication

Rundles R W, Falls H F 1946 Hereditary (? sex-linked) anemia. American Journal of Medicine and Science 211: 641

Russell E S 1979 Hereditary anemias of the mouse: a review for geneticists. Advances in Genetics 20: 357–459

Sandberg A A 1980 The Chromosomes in Human Cancer and Leukemia. Elsevier, New York

Schroeder T M, Tilgen D, Krüger J, Vogel F 1976. Formal genetics of Fanconi's Anaemia. Human Genetics 32: 257–288

Selwyn J G, Dacie J V 1954 Autohemolysis and other changes resulting from the incubation in vitro of red cells from patients with congenital hemolytic anaemia. Blood 9: 414

Siimes M A, Rahiala E L, Leisti J 1979 Hexokinase deficiency in erythrocytes: a new variant in 5 members of a Finnish family. Scandinavian Journal of Haematology 22(3): 214–8

Singer K, Fisher B, Perlstein M A 1952 Acanthocytosis. A genetic erythrocytic malformation. Blood VII: 577–591

Smith J E, Lee M S, Mia A S 1973 Decreased Y–glutamylcysteine synthetase: The probable cause of glutathione deficiency in sheep erythrocytes. Journal of Laboratory and Clinical Medicine 82: 713–718

Solanki D L, Jacobson R J, McKibbon J, Green R 1978 Racial patterns in pernicious anemia (letter). New England Journal of Medicine 298(24): 1365

Spector J I 1974 Juvenile achlorhydric pernicious anemia with IgA deficiency: A family study. Journal of the American Medical Association 228: 334

Standerfer R J, Rittenberg M B, Chern C J, Templeton J W, Black J A 1975 Canine erythrocyte pyruvate kinase. II. Properties of the abnormal enzyme associated with hemolytic anemia in the Basenji dog. Biochemical Genetics 13: 341–351

Steinbers M H, Coleman M F, Pennebaker J B 1979 Diamond-Blackfan syndrome: evidence for T-cell mediated suppression of erythroid development and a serum blocking factor associated with remission. British Journal of Haematology 41(1): 57–68

Sturgeon P 1970 Hematological observations on the anemia associated with blood type Rh null. Blood 36: 310

Surgenor D MacN 1974 The Red Blood Cell, second ed. vol. 1, Academic Press, Inc, New York

Swift M 1976 Fanconi anaemia: cellular abnormalities and clinical predisposition to malignant disease. In: Congenital Disorders of Erythropoiesis, Ciba Foundation Symposium 37 (new series). p 115–134

TeVelde K, Abels J, Anders G J P A, Arends A, Hoedenaeker P H J, Nieweg H O 1964 A family study of pernicious anemia by an immunologic method. Journal of Laboratory and Clinical Medicine 64: 177

Valentine W 1977 The molecular lesion of hereditary spherocytosis (HS): A continuing enigma. Blood 49: 241–245

Valentine W N, Tanaka K R 1978 Pyruvate kinase and other enzyme deficiency hereditary hemolytic anemias. In: Stanbury J B, Wyngaarden J B, Fredrickson D S (eds) The Metabolic Basis of Inherited Disease 4th ed. McGraw-Hill Book Company, New York. ch 59

Valentine W N, Tanaka K R, Miwa S 1961 A specific erythrocyte glycolytic enzyme defect (pyruvate kinase) in three subjects with congenital non-spherocytic hemolytic anemia. Transactions of the Association of American Physicians 74: 100

Varis K, Ihamaki T, Harkonen M, Samloff I M, Siurala M 1979 Gastric morphology, function, and immunology in first-degree relatives of probands with pernicious anemia and controls. Scandinavian Journal of Gastroenterology 14: 129–39

Vora S, Corash L, Ensel W K, Durham S, Seaman C, Piomelli S 1980 The molecular mechanism of the inherited phosphofructokinase deficiency associated with hemolysis and myopathy. Blood 55: 629–35

Wangel A G, Callender S T, Spray G H, Wright R 1968 A family study of pernicious anaemia. II. Intrinsic factor secretion, vitamin B_{12} absorption and genetic aspects of gastric autoimmunity. British Journal of Haematology 14: 183

Wasser J S, Yolken R, Miller D R, Diamond L 1978 Congenital hypoplastic anemia (Diamond-Blackfan syndrome) terminating in acute myelogenous leukemia. Blood 51(5): 991–5

Weinstein R S 1974 The morphology of adult red cells. In: Surgenor D MacN (ed) The Red Blood Cell ed. second Academic Press, Inc. New York. p 214

Weatherall D J 1975 Fetal haemoglobin synthesis. In: Congenital Disorders of Erythropoiesis, Ciba Foundation Symposium 37 (new series) p 307–328

Whittingham S 1969 The genetic factor in pernicious anaemia. Lancet 1: 951

Williams W J, Beutler E, Erslev A J, Rundles R W 1972 Hematology, McGraw-Hill Book Company, New York

Wintrobe M M 1974 Clinical Hematology, Lea and Febiger, Philadelphia 7th ed.

Witts L J 1963 Pernicious anaemia and endocrine disease. Israel Medical Journal 22: 294

Wolff J A, Van Hofe F M 1951 Familial erythroid multinuclearity. Blood 6: 1274

Wright J P, Callender S T E, Grumet F C, Payne R O, Taylor K B 1977 HLA antigens in Addisonian pernicious anaemia: absence of an HLA and disease association. British Journal of Haematology 36: 15–21

Yoshida A, Beutler E 1978 Human glucose-6-phosphate dehydrogenase variants: a supplementary tabulation. Annals of Human Genetics 41(3): 347–55

Yoshida A, Beutler E, Motulsky A G 1971 Table of human glucose-6-phosphate dehydrogenase variants. Bulletin of the World Health Organization 45: 243–53

Young L E, Izzo M J, Platzer R F 1951 Hereditary spherocytosis I. Clinical, hematologic and genetic features in 28 cases, with particular reference to the osmotic and mechanical fragility of incubated erythrocytes. Blood 6: 1073–1098

76

Defects in coagulation

R. Biggs

During the last century blood coagulation studies have appeared with increasing frequency and as a result a vast and confusing literature exists. From this can be extracted a general appreciation of the very complex reactions which precede the formation of a solid clot in a glass tube. Much of the present insight comes from a comparison of normal blood coagulation with that of patients having disease states. In most instances the defect in clotting is due to the absence or abnormality of a single component of the clotting process. Before describing the disease states and their inheritance it is essential to understand the main outline of the reactions which precede clotting.

When normal blood is collected into a glass tube it is at first liquid but after about 5 minutes is converted quite suddenly into a firm jelly. The jelly is made up of fibrin strands which interlace and adhere to each other, and within this mesh fluid and solid blood constituents are held.

Failure to form fibrin in the normal way is usually associated with haemorrhage after injury and it seems reasonable to suppose that clots play a part in plugging the holes in injured vessels and thus prevent haemorrhage. In reality such a simplistic idea is far too crude. The control of haemorrhage after injury is a complex delicately balanced process in which the contraction of injured vessels, the agglutination of platelets and their adhesion to the vessel wall and blood clotting all play a part. With small injuries such as pinpricks and scratches the contraction of vessels and platelet plugs can control the escape of blood even if blood coagulation is abnormal. When larger injuries occur, normal coagulation is required to control bleeding.

The delay of 5 minutes before blood clots in a glass tube is occupied by a long chain of reactions which may be initiated by contact of the blood with a foreign surface (e.g. glass) or by the presence of damaged tissue. These stimuli lead finally to the liberation from the blood of an enzyme thrombin, which will clot fibrinogen. Thrombin is produced from a precursor, prothrombin. These basic reactions may be expressed:

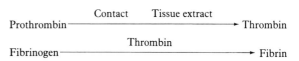

These reactions are certainly complex but accumulated experiments reveal that they are preceded by far more complex reactions to which two partially separate mechanisms contribute. One mechanism involves a long chain of reactions in which a number of coagulation factors all take part. This system is called the 'intrinsic system' since all components are contained within the blood stream. The second mechanism is initiated by tissue extract and is called the 'extrinsic system'. The two mechanisms have a final common pathway. The overall scheme is outlined in Figure 76.1.

It will be seen from Figure 76.1 that the substances which undergo reactions are represented by Roman numerals. This nomenclature was agreed by an International Committee and is now generally accepted. Table 76.1 lists the Roman numerals and the probable incidence of the disease states with which deficiency of these factors may be associated. It will be seen that one factor, factor VI has been deleted, and also that the lack of some factors from the blood does not cause disease states (e.g. factors III, IV and XII). In this chain reaction inactive precursors exist for all of the active intermediate products which are indicated in the scheme by the subscript 'a'. The chain reaction which precedes clotting is immensely powerful. Enough thrombin could be derived from 1 ml of blood to clot all of the fibrinogen in the body. This positive drive to coagulation is normally balanced by the absence of all but traces of active products, by the great instability of intermediate products and by the presence of inhibitors which destroy more stable coagulant products. The most important of these inhibitors is called antithrombin III and it destroys thrombin.

It is not appropriate to discuss the techniques used to study blood coagulation, but since our knowledge of the physiology of normal clotting has evolved through the study of disease states it is found that many laboratory methods may be used to measure degrees of abnormality

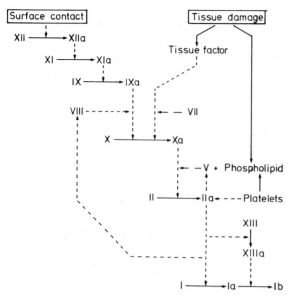

Fig. 76.1 An outline scheme of the complex chain reactions which precede the coagulation of fibrinogen by thrombin in glass tubes. In each component reaction an inactive precursor substance is converted to an active enzyme. The active substances are indicated by the subscript 'a'. It will be seen that coagulation factors VIII (deficiency of which causes haemophilia A) and IX (deficiency of which causes haemophilia B) are closely associated in the chain of reactions. These two diseases of different aetiology have identical clinical features. The diagram is intended as a guide to the discussion of the genetics of the individual factors.

shows no active coagulation factor but that a non-functional protein can be detected using antibodies. Immunological methods have been developed to study many coagulation factors.

Following this introduction it is proposed to deal with the various disease states associated with abnormal coagulation.

FIBRINOGEN (FACTOR I) AND FIBRIN STABILISING FACTOR (FACTOR XIII)

The conversion of fibrinogen to fibrin takes place in at least three stages. First, the thrombin acts on fibrinogen to split off two fibrinopeptides (A and B). Second, the residual fibrin monomer is ready to polymerise to form the characteristic fibrin strands; and third, after polymerisation the strands are crosslinked under the influence of factor XIII:

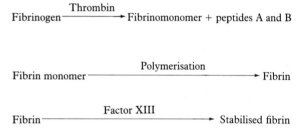

Afibrinogenaemia
A number of patients have been described who have no fibrinogen detectable by clotting or immunological techniques. A comprehensive review of the earlier known cases is given by Kerr (1965) who listed 65 patients. A

in patients who have clotting defects and to prepare concentrates of the various factors from the blood. These separated coagulation factors may be used to make antibodies which in turn may also be used to measure degrees of abnormality. It may happen that the patient's blood

Table 76.1 The nomenclature of blood clotting factors.

Roman numeral	Disease	Inheritance	Incidence per million of the population
I	Afibrinogenaemia	Autosomal	0.1
	Dysfibrinogenaemia	Autosomal	?
II	Prothrombin deficiency	? Autosomal	0.1
III (calcium)	No deficiency		
IV (tissue extract)	No deficiency		
V	Factor V deficiency	Autosomal	0.1
VI (not used)			
VII	Factor VII deficiency	Autosomal	0.1
VIII	Haemophilia A	X–linked recessive	60–70
	Von Willebrand disease	Autosomal dominant	30–50
IX	Haemophilia B	X–linked recessive	7–10
X	Factor X deficiency	Autosomal	0.1
XI	Factor XI deficiency	Autosomal	1.0
XII	Factor XII deficiency	Autosomal	0.1
XIII	Factor XIII deficiency	Autosomal	0.1

more recent study was made by Flute (1977). Many of the patients suffered relatively mild bleeding symptoms which is odd since the total absence of fibrinogen would be expected to produce the most severe abnormality. However some patients must have been severely affected since 14 died from haemorrhage and 16 undiagnosed sibs died in infancy, probably from haemorrhage.

The mode of inheritance of the bleeding condition is autosomal recessive, though from the laboratory point of view asymptomatic carriers may have low levels of fibrinogen. Some earlier reported families seemed to show a preponderance of affected males (Graham, 1957) but the numbers of affected males and females have been about equal in more recent reports. Consanguinity was recorded in 21 of 49 families (Kerr, 1965).

Defective fibrinogen synthesis

In 1958, Imperato and Dettor described a patient who had mild bleeding symptoms and whose blood contained abnormal fibrinogen. Since this time many other patients have been described. In 1973 Ménarché listed 83 cases (37 males and 46 females) in 22 families. In many papers the main interest of those who studied the patients was to discover the biochemical nature of the defective fibrinogen and family studies have been fragmentary. The abnormal fibrinogen was detected by a slow reaction with thrombin (delayed polymerisation) or by delayed or absent release of one or other of the fibrinopeptides. Deviations from normal have also been found by various precipitation methods, by biochemical analysis of the isolated protein and by immunoelectrophoresis. Quantitative estimation of fibrinogen by immunological methods usually gives normal results in these cases.

About 30% of the patients have some slight tendency to bleed more than normal after injury. The majority have no haemostatic defect.

From the information available it seems that the defects (if those which cause no symptoms should be considered as defects) are inherited as autosomal and partially dominant traits. The deviations from normal have been discovered with increasing frequency in recent years and it may be that the structure of fibrinogen is not constant in the normal population and, as there are many different tissue types, so there may be different variants of coagulation proteins which will function adequately in the normal clotting system. The variants are named according to the city in which the patient was studied (e.g. fibrinogen Paris I or Paris II and so on).

Factor XIII

Factor XIII was first reported by Laki and Lorand (1948) as a result of a study of the solubility of fibrin in urea. At the time no natural defects were known. In 1960 Duckert et al described a family in which several members bled abnormally after injury. All of the then available laboratory tests were normal but the patient's fibrin clots dissolved in urea whereas clots from normal plasma were insoluble. They postulated a deficiency of factor XIII as a cause of the abnormality. Since this time a number of other patients have been described. The inheritance seems to be autosomal and partially recessive. Some family members who may be carriers have low factor XIII levels though they have no symptoms of abnormal bleedings.

PROTHROMBIN (FACTOR II)

Prothrombin is the sole precursor of thrombin and as such is essential to normal clotting. Before the true complexity of the clotting system was known, prothrombin was studied using a test called the 'one-stage prothrombin time'. It is now clear that, whereas prothrombin affects the amount of thrombin formed, other factors such as factors V, VII and X affect the speed of thrombin formation. The one-stage prothrombin time is influenced more by the speed of thrombin formation than by the amount of thrombin formed.

The early literature is confused by this technical difficulty and cases of factor V, VII and X deficiency were classed as prothrombin deficiency. It is now clear that true prothrombin deficiency is extremely rare, and to my knowledge no case of complete lack of prothrombin has been described. Both male and female patients are recorded and some families have more than one affected member. It is assumed that the inheritance is autosomal recessive.

FACTOR X DEFICIENCY

Factor X is a central coagulation factor since it is required for prothrombin conversion by both extrinsic and intrinsic clotting systems (see Fig. 76.1). Factor X requires both factor V and a phospholipid to develop its full activity.

There are several methods of measuring factor X clotting activity. When all methods are used on a sample from a patient with factor X deficiency different levels of factor X may be recorded (Denson et al, 1970). Using antibody neutralisation tests it is found that some patients possess a protein resembling factor X whereas in other patients the protein is lacking. These results suggest that there may be a number of molecular defects which interfere with the activity of factor X.

In three families the parents of affected persons were related (Hougie et al, 1957; Graham et al, 1957; Roos et al, 1959; Bachmann, 1959). In the family reported by Graham et al (1957) and Hougie et al (1957) persons who bled excessively had less than 5% of factor X but other family members, who were probably asymptomatic heterozygotes, had levels intermediate between 5 and 100%. It is clear that different molecular variants of factor X cause bleeding and it is probable that the inheritance is autosomal and recessive.

DEFICIENCY OF FACTORS V AND VII

Factors V and VII are both required for the conversion of prothrombin to thrombin by tissue extract. Factor V is also essential for normal prothrombin conversion by the intrinsic clotting system. Both factor V and factor VII deficiencies are rare.

Factor V deficiency may affect males and females. In a family studied by Rush and Ellis (1965) unaffected carriers had low levels of factor V. Three patients are known to have had related parents (Brink & Kingsley, 1952; Kingsley, 1954; Seibert et al, 1958). It seems that the inheritance of factor V deficiency is through an autosomal but incompletely recessive gene.

Factor VII deficiency affects patients of either sex. Hall et al (1964) studied 81 relatives of 3 clinically affected patients. They found reduced factor VII levels in 8 symptomatically normal relatives each of whom had one parent who was a heterozygote. The inheritance seems to be autosomal recessive.

Factor VII deficiency has also been studied using immunological methods by Denson et al (1972). In 9 patients from 6 families they found higher amounts of immunologically detectable protein than of clotting activity. Girolami et al (1979) also found some heterogeneity with respect to clotting activity when different test systems were used. Thus with factor VII it seems likely that different molecular defects are associated with reduced clotting function.

FACTOR VIII DEFICIENCY

There are two distinct diseases associated with deficiency of factor VIII clotting activity (VIII_c). One deficiency causes haemophilia A and the other von Willebrand disease. The two conditions differ from each other in symptomatology, inheritance and the nature of the underlying defect. Whereas haemophilia A patients have deep tissue bleeding and bleeding into joints as the main symptoms, in von Willebrand disease the patients tend to bleed from mucous tissues such as the nose and gastrointestinal tract. The inheritance of haemophilia A is X–linked and recessive whereas that of von Willebrand disease is autosomal and dominant.

The factor VIII molecule can be thought of in two parts, one of which bears the factor VIII clotting activity and the other serving as a carrier protein for this activity. The carrier protein (VIII_{Ag}, factor VIII related antigen) can only be detected immunologically. Haemophilia A patients lack the ability to make VIII_c and von Willebrand disease patients lack VIII_{Ag}. The two components are entirely different in physico-chemical properties. Component VIII_c is heat labile, disappears on storage at room temperature and is used up during clotting. Component VIII_{Ag} on the other hand is relatively stable to heat and storage and is not used up in clotting.

Haemophilia A

Haemophilia A or classical haemophilia has been recognised for many centuries as a familial bleeding disorder affecting males. A full historical review is given by Ingram (1976). Haemophilia is much commoner than the defects so far considered (see Table 76.1).

Inheritance of haemophilia A

Haemophilia A is inherited as an X–linked recessive trait and is thus primarily a disease of males. Female carriers in haemophilic families do sometimes have low enough levels of factor VIII to suffer some bleeding symptoms. Homozygous female bleeders are encountered only in the offspring of a marriage between a female carrier of haemophilia and an affected male. A typical family tree is presented in Fig. 76.2.

The prevalence of haemophilia A

Table 76.2 gives estimates of the prevalence of haemophilia A per 100 000 in various populations. It will be seen that there is a tendency for the prevalence to increase in more recent studies. This increase in the number of known haemophiliacs has considerable social importance and the causes of the increase will be considered.

In the first place, haemophilia A patients now live much longer than in the past. The average age of patients at death used to be 16–20 years (Ramgren, 1962; Andreassen, 1943) whereas it is now nearer to 40 years (Biggs, 1978). Thus the number of patients must increase simply from the accumulation in the population of patients who would previously have died, though the average age of haemophilia A patients recorded in the United Kingdom is still below that of the general population (Biggs, 1974)

In the second place, the recorded number of known haemophilia A patients has increased through better ascertainment. In recent years the treatment of these patients has tended to be concentrated in special centres. In the United Kingdom, for example, 3068 haemophilia A patients were known to attend haemophilia centres in 1975. Detailed enquiries revealed only 108 additional

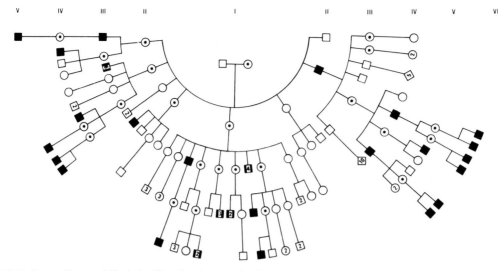

Fig. 76.2 Pedigree of haemophilia A (■ affected male; ⊙ carrier female).

Table 76.2 The prevalence of haemophilia A in various populations.

Author	Country or town	Year	Prevalence per 100 000 of population
Haldane	London	1935	2.0
Andreassen	Denmark	1943	2.2
Sjølin	Denmark	1960	3.6
Ikkala	Finland	1960	3.7
Martin-Villar et al	Spain	1976	3.3
Ramgren	Sweden	1962	3.3
Nilsson	Sweden	1976	6.9
Rosenberg	Brazil	1972	7–10
NHLI	USA	1972	9.0
Biggs	UK	1974	6.0
Mandalaki	Greece	1976	6.2
Mannucci and Ruggeri	Italy	1976	9.8
Brackmann et al	West Germany	1976	9.2
Soulier	France	1976	6.6
Davey	Australia	1976	5.9

haemophilia A patients who were not known at haemophilia centres (Biggs & Spooner, 1978).

In the third place, haemophilia A patients must be added to the population by new mutations. In 1935 and 1947 Haldane pointed out that any gene that caused death before puberty must die out unless it is continually renewed by mutation. The incidence of the disease at birth will represent a balance between loss of genes caused by failure to reproduce and the formation of new genes by mutation. In 1947 Haldane represented this balance:

$$I = \frac{3\mu}{1-f}$$

— Where I is the incidence at birth before selection has occurred by early death. From the fairly complete figures for Denmark (Andreassen, 1943) Haldane took the incidence at birth to be 13.3×10^{-5} live male births.
— Where f is the fitness, which may roughly be considered as the number of children born to affected patients in comparison to those born to normal males at the same era of time. Thus if 1 child is born to a haemophilia A parent where an average of 2 are born to normal males then the fitness is 0.5. From the figures of Andreassen (1943), with the omission of one pedigree which Haldane considered to be 'a truly remarkable dysgenic performance', Haldane calculated the fitness to be 0.286.
— Where μ is the mutation rate per generation, a generation being assumed to be 30 years.

Using these figures in his formula Haldane calculated the mutation rate to be 3.2×10^{-5} males per generation.

This figure for the mutation rate is quite similar to that calculated by other authors: Vogel (1955) 2.7×10^{-5} males per generation; Ikkala (1960) 3.2×10^{-5} males per generation; Ramgren (1962) 2.7×10^{-5} males per generation; Bitter (1964) 4.1×10^{-5} males per generation. Barrai et al (1968) found a much lower figure (1.31×10^{-5} males per generation) but they assumed a very low incidence of haemophilia A which was probably not correct.

Supposing that the mutation rate is as Haldane (1947) suggested then improved fitness of haemophiliacs must lead in the long term to an increased incidence of haemophilia A. Using Haldane's formula, if fitness improved from 0.286 (of Haldane) to 0.5 or 0.8 this could lead to an incidence increase from 13.3×10^{-5} to 19.2 or 48×10^{-5} live male births. Of course much would depend on the average number of children in a family of normal people and on the effectiveness of the whole process of genetic counselling.

The molecular biology of factor VIII
As previously noted the factor VIII molecule consists of 2 components, VIII_c and VIII_{Ag}. When both of these components are measured in normal people there is a fair correlation between the two activities (Fig. 76.3). When a ratio between the two activities is calculated this ratio is on average near 1.0. Thus normal people who have below average VIII_c will tend to have below average VIII_{Ag}. When haemophilia A patients are tested they have low or zero VIII_c but normal or high VIII_{Ag}.

The detection of carriers of haemophilia A
Haemophilia A carriers have on average 50% of the normal VIII_c but they have normal VIII_{Ag}. Some carriers in haemophilia A families (25 to 50%) can be detected from their factor VIII_c levels alone when these are well below normal. However, the VIII_c is very variable in haemophilia A carriers presumably because of random inactivation of the X–chromosome in females (i.e. Lyonisation). In a recent study, Mannucci et al (1978) found that female identical twins who were both carriers of haemophilia A had very different levels of factor VIII_c (4% and 36%). This very large difference must have occurred during development and supports the Lyonisation hypothesis. By measuring both VIII_c and VIII_{Ag} many more carriers can be detected since some carriers with high VIII_c levels have above average VIII_{Ag} and a low ratio of VIII_c to VIII_{Ag}. Using both values 70–94% of carriers in haemophilia A families may be detected (Rizza et al, 1975; Ratnoff & Jones, 1976). The importance of making both measurements is illustrated in Figure 76.3 where it will be seen that there is almost complete separation of normal from carrier values when both VIII_c and VIII_{Ag} are plotted. Had the VIII_c alone been used there would have

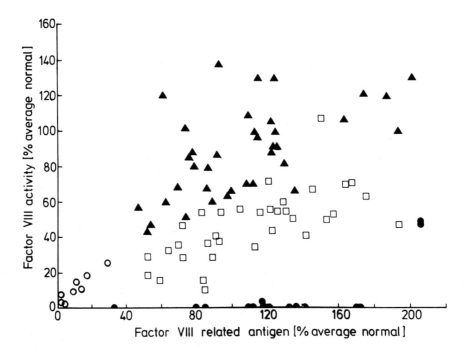

Fig. 76.3 The relationship between factor VIII_c and factor VIII_{Ag} activity.
Normal people ▲   Haemophiliacs ●
Female carriers of Haemophilia □   von Willebrand disease patients ○

been more overlapping values between normals and carriers.

Sporadic cases of haemophilia and the mutation rate in males and females

The improved method for the detection of haemophilia A carriers has been applied to the mothers of sporadic cases of haemophilia A. These families have only one known haemophilia A patient whose condition may be the result of mutation. If some of these sporadic cases represent mutations then a proportion of the mothers of affected sons should be normal women. In fact Biggs and Rizza (1976) found that 39 of 41 mothers of sporadic haemophilia A sons were probably carriers of haemophilia A as judged from laboratory tests. These results suggest that the mutation rate in females may be substantially lower than in males. This suggestion is supported by the findings of Haldane (1947) and Graham (1979) but not by those of Barrai et al (1968) Ratnoff and Jones (1976) and Ananthakrishnan and D'Souza (1979).

Genetic counselling in haemophilia A families

The purpose of genetic counselling must be in the long run to reduce the incidence of haemophilia A by influencing members of haemophilia A familes not to produce affected children. In the first place the person seeking advice must be informed as accurately as possible about the mode of inheritance, about the probability that he or she may produce a haemophilic son and about the steps that may be taken to prevent the birth of an affected male.

From the mode of inheritance certain statements can be made about family members in haemophilia A families. The sons of haemophilia A patients are all normal and cannot transmit haemophilia. The daughters of haemophilia A patients are all certainly carriers. For other female members of haemophilia A families a greater or lesser probability of carrier status exists. The daughters of carriers have a 1 in 2 chance of being carriers, the granddaughters a 1 in 4 chance and so on.

These 'prior' probabilities can be influenced by taking into account the results of laboratory tests (Graham, 1977; 1979). Using statistical analyses (Prentice et al, 1975; Klein et al, 1977) a greater or lesser probability can be deduced from the laboratory results (Bouma et al, 1975; Elston et al, 1976). This probability can be combined with the 'a priori' genetic probability to give an overall probability (Graham 1977; 1979). The importance of the genetic information is obvious. An abnormal laboratory result for a woman randomly selected from the normal population would have less significance than for a female relative of an affected male. In the former, the prior probability that the woman is a haemophilia A carrier is *not* 1 in 4 or 1 in 8 but rather less than 1 in 1000. There are of course some women who are carriers of

haemophilia A unsuspected in the normal population (e.g. Taylor & Biggs, 1957; Graham, 1979). Nevertheless, Graham (1979) calculated that, even with this very low prior probability that a woman without family history is a carrier, the results of laboratory tests could provide acceptable evidence for carrier status.

Experience with haemophilia A families suggests that many interviews may be needed to be certain that the person seeking advice really understands the inheritance of haemophilia and the concept of probability. In fact most women seeking advice simply wish to be told that they are not carriers. Unfortunately this is at present impossible.

Special consideration is needed in counselling potential carriers of haemophilia A who are pregnant. It is now possible to determine the sex of the unborn child and tentatively to determine whether or not a male child has haemophilia A (Mibashan et al, 1979). The selective abortion of affected males would clearly reduce the incidence of haemophilia A in the long and in the short term.

Social implications of haemophilia A

Haemophilia A is socially important out of all proportion to the numbers of patients who exist at any one time. Untreated, each patient would spend much time in hospital and suffer many agonising, life endangering and crippling episodes of haemorrhage. Treatment is now so much improved that it is possible to protect most of the patients by intravenous injections of factor VIII prepared from human blood. For the 3000 to 4000 patients known in the United Kingdom this treatment requires the processing of plasma from the equivalent of about 1 000 000 blood donations annually. This is a high proportion of all blood collected by the United Kingdom Blood Transfusion Service. Such processing would of course produce many other substances of value to patients other than haemophiliacs but the Blood Transfusion Service was not conceived in order to carry out such massive fractionation programmes. Were all of the necessary factor VIII supplied by commercial firms the cost would be likely to exceed £5 000 000 per annum. Nevertheless it can be seen that treated or untreated the patients are a considerable social burden, and therefore the problem of genetic counselling must be pursued with vigour.

Factor VIII deficiency in von Willebrand disease

In this condition both VIII_c and VIII_{Ag} are reduced proportionately (see Fig. 76.3). Von Willebrand disease is inherited as an autosomal dominant trait controlling the production of VIII_{Ag}. The disease was first described by von Willebrand (1926) in a family from an island in the Åland archipelago. It was thought at first to be primarily a disease of the capillary blood vessels but in 1953 Alexander and Goldstein showed that affected patients often had low plasma levels of VIII_c. In 1971 Zimmerman et al showed that patients lacked an antigenically demonstrable component of factor VIII (VIII_{Ag}). This antigenic component can be measured reliably by the Laurel (1972) electroimmunoassay.

Von Willebrand disease varies a good deal in the severity of the bleeding symptoms. In general, patients who have the lowest levels of VIII_c are most severely affected.

The properties of the protein VIII_{Ag} have been studied (Nilsson & Holmberg, 1979). Patients who lack VIII_{Ag} often also lack the ability to agglutinate platelets in the presence of the antibiotic ristocetin. This activity is sometimes called VIIIR:RCF. Also the platelets of von Willebrand disease do not adhere normally to glass. The infusion to patients of VIII_c and VIII_{Ag} in concentrates containing these factors restores all of these test results to normal. Some patients do appear to have normal amounts of VIII_{Ag} by the Laurel technique, but crossed immunoelectrophoresis reveals that the protein is qualitatively different from normal (Holmberg & Nilsson, 1972; Rizza, 1975).

Some of the variable expressions of von Willebrand disease may be associated with homozygosity or heterozygosity for the gene for factor VIII_{Ag} (Nilsson & Holmberg, 1979). At present it must be admitted that there is a good deal of confusion in the genetic interpretation of symptoms and laboratory results in this disease.

FACTOR IX DEFICIENCY HAEMOPHILIA B

Haemophilia B has exactly the same symptomatology and inheritance as haemophilia A. Thus all the literature prior to 1952 (when haemophilia B was described) includes both conditions under the general category haemophilia. Haemophilia B is much less common than haemophilia A. There are probably 5–10 affected males per 1 000 000 of the general population. The lower incidence of haemophilia B is probably due to a lower mutation rate which may be 0.2 to 0.3×10^{-5}, about 10 times less than that for haemophilia A.

Haemophilia B patients have been studied in much the same way as haemophilia A. Immunological tests have been used to detect protein similar to factor IX but lacking in clotting activity. Such a protein has been found in the blood of some patients who are said to be CRM+, positive for cross reacting material (Denson et al, 1968). Some of those who are CRM+ also show an abnormally long clotting time when ox-brain is used in the one-stage prothrombin time (Kidd et al, 1963; Hougie & Twomey, 1967). A multicentre study of 98 kindreds of haemophilia B patients was made by Parekh et al (1978).They found that the patients were CRM− in 52 kindreds. In 16 kindreds the affected males were CRM+ and of these 5 had long clotting times with ox-brain. Other patients had reduced but not absent IX_{Ag}. Kasper et al (1977) made a similar study and divided the 71 kindreds observed by them into 6 subgroups based on the results of laboratory tests. Similar results were obtained by Bertina and Veltkamp (1978).

The carriers of haemophilia B often have low plasma levels of factor IX (Simpson & Biggs, 1962). These authors found that of 53 proven heterozygotes 25 had factor IX levels below 50% of normal whereas of 49 normal females only 2 had levels below 50% of normal. When affected members are CRM+ then the carriers may be found to have less factor IX activity than antigenic protein and this fact may help in genotype assignment (Kaspar et al, 1977; Parekh et al, 1978). On the other hand, in those families whose affected members are CRM− the levels of factor IX antigen correspond with those for the clotting activity.

FACTOR XI DEFICIENCY

Factor XI deficiency was first described by Rosenthal et al (1953). The condition is inherited as an autosomal trait and is probably dominant. Nearly all cases are of Jewish origin and Seligsohn (1978) has found that of 34 kindreds in Israel 33 were of Ashkenazi Jewish origin. There is some difficulty about any discussion of this condition since the haemorrhagic tendency does not seem to be closely related to laboratory results. Patients with very little detectable factor XI may be symptom free and some patients with 20–40% of normal factor XI bleed excessively (Leiba et al, 1965). Seligsohn (1978) using laboratory tests studied 428 healthy Ashkehazi Jewish subjects (372 males and 56 females) of whom 35 had low levels of factor XI (15–49% of normal) and one only 2% of normal factor XI activity. From this study he calculated that the mutant gene frequency among Ashkenazi Jews was from 0.030 to 0.057. The approximate frequency of homozygotes in the population would be 0.1 to 0.3%, and of heterozygotes 5.5 to 11%. The philosophical problem is that these people were normal from the clinical point of view though they had a laboratory deficiency of factor XI.

FACTOR XII (HAGEMAN FACTOR) DEFICIENCY

Factor XII deficiency was first described by Ratnoff and Colopy (1955). The condition is a coagulation paradox. In the laboratory the blood of these patients has a very long clotting time in glass tubes but the patients have no abnormal bleeding even after major surgery. Inheritance is autosomal, and heterozygotes may have a low level of factor XII (Lucia et al, 1979). Saito et al (1979) found that in 47 of 49 affected persons from 42 unrelated families no factor XII like antigen could be detected immunologically. In 2 affected families an antigenic protein related to factor XII was found. The condition thus has at least 2 variants, CRM+ and CRM−.

FLETCHER FACTOR (Hathaway & Alserver, 1970) AND FITZGERALD FACTOR (Waldmann et al, 1975) DEFICIENCIES

Two other inherited asymptomatic plasma factor deficiencies have been described in which the early stages of clotting in glass tubes seems to be defective.

Study of the contact phase in blood coagulation has proved of considerable scientific interest and much of the work is reviewed by Nossel (1972).

COMBINED DEFECTS

A few patients develop defects associated with deficiency or abnormality of more than one coagulation factor. All of these are very rarely encountered but the commonest is probably a combined deficiency of factors V and VIII (Seibert et al, 1958; Jones et al, 1962). The synthesis of factors II, VII, X and IX is influenced by vitamin K, and very rarely patients may have some block in the vitamin K mechanism which leads to combined deficiency of all 4 factors.

ANTITHROMBIN III DEFICIENCY

A number of cases of antithrombin III deficiency have been described (Egeberg, 1965; van de Meer et al, 1973; Marciniak et al, 1974; Sas et al, 1974). In all families the inheritance was autosomal and dominant. The patients all suffered from a tendency for blood to clot in the blood vessels.

CONCLUSION

A general review of the genetics of blood coagulation disorders reveals a number of interesting features. In the early days a coagulation disorder was a clinical condition which might be expressed in severe or mild form. If the carriers of the disease were symptom free then the condition was said to be recessive. With improved laboratory tests it is often found that the average level of the clotting factor in the carriers is about half normal. Thus the gene seems to have a quantitative effect. This is particularly well established for factors VIII and IX in haemophilia A and B.

The improved laboratory tests have also led to the collection of abnormal laboratory results in persons who do not have any notable bleeding tendency. These studies improve our knowledge of biology and protein chemistry but it is difficult to know how much they contribute to our understanding of disease. A laboratory test whose results are not closely related to the clinical manifestations of a disease state cannot be used to control patient treatment, nor can such a test be used to establish the degree of severity of the disease.

In most of the conditions studied it has been found that the disease is not caused by a simple absence of an essential protein but that a number of defects may lead to malfunction of that protein. For example, we cannot know how many different sorts of haemophilia A exist since the chemical structure of factor VIII is still unknown. Where the chemical structure of a protein is better understood (as in fibrinogen) then numerous aberrant forms are known. It seems likely that, like other proteins, the coagulation factors are heterogenous and may be divided roughly into two groups, in one of which the function is within normal limits, and in the other the function falling below normal and the patient manifesting the disease.

In the case of the factor VIII molecule, it seems that complete coagulation activity is assembled by combination in some way of the products of at least 2 genes (VIII_c and VIII_{Ag}). This phenomenon is recognised to occur for other complex substances, such as blood group proteins. The complexity of the factor VIII molecule has a rather strange consequence in that it may be very difficult to determine the mode of inheritance of factor VIII in normal people.

REFERENCES

Alexander B, Goldstein R 1953 Dual hemostatic defect in pseudohemophilia. Journal of Clinical Investigation 32: 551

Ananthakrishnan R, D'Souza S 1979 Some aspects of the occurrence of new mutations in haemophilia. Human Heredity 29: 90

Andreassen M 1943 Haemofili i Danmark opera ex domo biologiae hereditairiae humanae. Universitatis Hafniensis 6 Copenhagen

Bachmann F 1958 Familien Untersuchungen beim kongenitahen Stuart-Prower-Factor-Mangel. Archiv Klaustift Vereb Forsch 33: 27

Barrai I, Cann H M, Cavalli-Sforza L L, de Nicola P 1968

The effect of parental age on rates of mutation for haemophilia and evidence for differing mutation rates for haemophilia A and B. American Journal of Human Genetics 20: 175

Bertina R M, Veltkamp J J 1978 The abnormal factor IX of hemophilia B+ variants. Thombosis and Haemostatis 40: 335

Biggs R 1974 Jaundice and antibodies directed against factors VIII and IX in patients treated for haemophilia and Christmas disease in the United Kingdom. British Journal of Haematology 26: 313

Biggs R 1978 Treatment of haemophilia A and B and von Willebrand's disease. Blackwell Scientific Publications, Oxford. p 92

Biggs R, Rizza C R 1976 The sporadic case of haemophilia A. Lancet 2: 431

Biggs R, Spooner R 1978 National survey of haemophilia and Christmas disease patients in the United Kingdom. Lancet 1: 1143

Bitter K 1964 Erhebungen zur Bestimmungen der Mutationesrate für Hämophilie A and B in Hamburg. Zeitschrift für Menschliche. Vererbungd Konstitutionlehre 37: 251

Bouma B N, van der Klaauw M M, Veltkamp J J, Starkenburg A E, van Tilburg N H, Hermans J 1975 Evaluation of the detection rate of hemophilia carriers. Thrombosis Research 7: 339

Brackmann H-H, Hofman P, Etzel F, Egli H 1976 Home care of haemophilia in West Germany. Thrombosis and Haemostasis 35: 544

Brink A J, Kingsley C S 1952 A familial disorder of blood coagulation due to deficiency of the labile factor. Quarterly Journal of Medicine 21: 19

Denson K W E, Biggs R, Mannucci P M 1968 An investigation of 3 patients with Christmas disease due to an abnormal type of factor IX. Journal of Clinical Pathology 21: 160

Denson K W, Conrad J, Samama M 1972 Genetic variants of factor VII. Lancet 1: 1234

Denson K W E, Lurie A, de Cataldo F, Mannucci P M 1970 The factor X defect: the recognition of abnormal forms of factor X. British Journal of Haematology 18: 309

Duckert F, Jung E, Schmerling D H 1960 A hitherto undescribed congenital haemorrhagic diathesis probably due to fibrin stabilizing factor deficiency. Thrombosis et Diathesis Haemorrhagica 5: 179

Egeberg O 1965 Inherited antithrombin deficiency causing thrombophilia. Thrombosis et Diathesis Haemorrhagica 13: 516

Elston R C, Graham J B, Miller C H, Reisner H M, Brauma B N 1976 Probabilistic classification of hemophilia A carriers by discriminant analysis. Thrombosis Research 8: 683

Flute P F 1977 Disorders of plasma fibrinogen synthesis. British Medical Bulletin 33: 253

Girolami A, Cattarozzi R, Dal Bo Zanon R, Cella G, Toffanin F 1979 Factor VII Padua another factor VII abnormality with defective ox brain thromboplastin activation and a complex hereditary pattern. Blood 54: 46

Graham J B 1977 Genetic counseling in classic hemophilia A. New England Journal of Medicine 296: 996

Graham J B 1979 Genotype assignment (carrier detection) in the haemophilias. Clinics in Haematology 8: 115

Graham J B, Barrow E M, Hougie C 1957 Stuart clotting defect II. Genetic aspects of a 'new' hemorrhagic state. Journal of Clinical Investigation 36: 497

Haldane J B S 1935 The rate of spontaneous mutation of a human gene. Journal of Genetics 31: 317

Haldane J B S 1947 The mutation rate of the gene for haemophilia and its segregation ratio in males and females. Annals of Eugenics 13: 262

Hall C A, Rapaport S J, Arres S B, de Groot J A 1964 A clinical and family study of hereditary proconvertin (Factor VII) deficiency. American Journal of Medicine 37: 172

Hathaway W E, Alsever J 1970 The relation of Fletcher factor to factors XI and XII. British Journal of Haematology 18: 161

Holmberg L, Nilsson I M 1972 Genetic variants of von Willebrand's disease. British Medical Journal 2: 317

Hougie C, Barrow E M, Graham J B 1957 Stuart clotting defect I segregation of an hereditary hemorrhagic state from the heterogenous group heretofore called stable factor (SPCA proconvertin, factor VII) deficiency. Journal of Clinical Investigation 36: 485

Hougie C, Twomey J J 1967 Haemophilia B$_M$ new type of factor IX deficiency. Lancet 1: 698

Ikkala E 1960 Haemophilia a study of its laboratory clinical and social aspects based on known haemophiliacs in Finland. Scandinavian Journal of Clinical and Laboratory Medicine 12: suppl 46

Imperato D C, Dettori A G 1958 Ipofibrinogenemia congenita con fibroastenia. Helvetia Paediatrica Acta 13: 380

Ingram G I C 1976 The history of haemophilia. Journal of Clinical Pathology 29: 469

Jones J H, Rizza C R, Hardisty R M, Dormandy K M, MacPherson J C 1962 Combined deficiency of factor V and factor VIII (antihaemophilic globulin).British Journal of Haematology 8: 120

Kaspar C K, Østarud B, Minami J Y, Shonick W, Rapaport S J 1977 Haemophilia B characterization of genetic variants and detection of carriers. Blood 50: 351

Kerr C B 1965 Genetics of human blood coagulation. Journal of Medical Genetics 2: 221

Kidd B, Denson K W E, Biggs R 1963 The thrombotest reagent and Christmas disease. Lancet ii: 522

Kingsley C S 1954 Familial factor V deficiency; the pattern of heredity. Quarterly Journal of Medicine 23: 323

Klein H G, Aledort L M, Bouma B N, Hoyer L M, Zimmerman T S, De Mets D L 1977 A cooperative study of the detection of the carrier of classic hemophilia. New England Journal of Medicine 296: 959

Laki K, Lorand L 1948 On the solubility of fibrin clots. Science 108: 280

Laurell C B 1972 Electroimmunoassay. Scandinavian Journal of Clinical and Laboratory Investigation 29: suppl 124 21

Leiba H, Ramot B, Many A 1965 Heredity and coagulation studies in the families with factor XI (plasma thromboplastin antecedent) deficiency. British Journal of Haematology 11: 654

Lucia J F, Ercoreca L, Torres M, Giralt M, Rauchis A 1979 Factor XII congenital deficiency. A new family study. Thrombosis and Haemostasis 42: 1009

Mandalaki T 1976 Management of haemophilia in Greece. Thrombosis and Haemostasis 35: 522

Mannucci P M, Coppola R, Lombardi R, Pa M, De Biasi R 1978 Direct proof of extreme Lyonization as a cause of low factor VIII levels in females. Thrombosis and Haemostasis 39: 544

Mannucci P M, Ruggeri Z M 1976 Haemophilia care in Italy. Thrombosis and Haemostasis 35: 531

Marciniak E, Farley C H, de Simone P A 1974 Familial thrombosis due to antithrombin III deficiency. Blood 43: 219

Martin-Villar J, Navarro J L, Ortega F, Yanguas J 1971 The supply and availability of plasma concentrates in the hospital of the Spanish social security. Proceedings of the 1st European meeting of the World Federation of Haemophilia, Milan

Ménaché D 1973 Abnormal fibrinogens. A review. Thrombosis et Diathesis Haemorrhagica 29: 525

Misbashan R S, Thrumpston J K, Singer J D, Rodeck C H, Edwards R J, White J M, Campbell S 1979 Plasma assay of fetal factors VIII$_c$ and IX for prenatal diagnosis of haemophilia. Lancet 1: 1309

National Heart and Lung Institute. Blood Resource Study 1972

Nilsson I M 1976 Management of haemophilia in Sweden. Thrombosis and Haemostasis 35: 510

Nilsson I M, Holmberg L 1979 Von Willebrand's disease today. Clinics in Haematology 8: 147

Nossel H L 1972 The contact system. In: Biggs R (ed) Human Blood Coagulation, Haemostasis and Thrombosis, Blackwell Scientific Publications, Oxford

Parekh V R, Mannucci P M, Ruggeri Z M 1978 Immunological heterogeneity of haemophilia B: a multicentre study of 98 kindreds. British Journal of Haematology 40: 643

Prentice C R M, Forbes C D, Morrice S, McLaren A D 1975 Calculation of predictive odds for possible carriers of haemophilia. Thrombosis and Haemostasis 34: 740

Ramgren O 1962 Haemophilia in Sweden. V. Medical-social aspects. Acta Medica Scandinavica 379: 37

Ratnoff O D, Colopy J E 1955 A familial hemorrhagic trait associated with a deficiency of a clot promoting fraction of plasma. Journal of Clinical Investigation 34: 602

Ratnoff O D, Jones P K 1976 The detection of carriers of classic haemophilia. American Journal of Clinical Pathology 65: 129

Rizza C R 1975 Factor VIII-related antigen and von Willebrand's disease. British Journal of Haematology 31: suppl 231

Rizza C R, Rhymes I L, Austen D E G, Kernoff P B A, Aroni S A 1975 Detection of carriers of haemophilia: a 'blind' study. British Journal of Haematology 30: 447

Roos J, van Arkel C, Verkop M C, Jordan F L J 1959 A new family with Stuart-Prower deficiency. Thrombosis et Diathesis Haemorrhagica 3: 59

Rosenberg I 1972 Hemophilia e estados do Rio Grande do Sul. Frequencia fisiologia et hevanca. Brazilian Journal of Medical and Biological Research 5: 287

Rosenthal R L, Dreskin O H, Rosenthal N 1953 New hemophilia-like disease caused by deficiency of a third plasma thromboplastin factor. Proceedings of the Society for Experimental Biology and Medicine 82: 171

Rush B, Ellis H 1965 Patients with factor V deficiency. Thrombosis et Diathesis Haemorrhagica 14: 14

Saito H, Scott J G, Movat H Z, Scialla S J 1979 Molecular heterogeneity of Hageman trait (factor XII deficiency). Journal of Laboratory and Clinical Medicine 94: 256

Sas G, Blaskó G, Bánhegyi D, Jákó J, Pálos L A 1974 Abnormal antithrombin III (antithrombin III Budapest) as a cause of familial thrombophilia. Thrombosis et Diathesis Haemorrhagica 32: 105.

Seibert R H, Margolius A, Ratnoff O D 1958 Observations on hemophilia, parahemophilia and coexistent hemophilia and parahemophilia. Journal of Laboratory and Clinical Medicine 52: 449

Seligsohn V 1978 High gene frequency of factor XI (PTA) deficiency in Ashkenazi Jews. Blood 51: 1223

Simpson N E, Biggs R 1962 The inheritance of Christmas factor. British Journal of Haematology 8: 191

Sjølin K 1959 Haemophilic Diseases in Denmark. Blackwell Scientific Publications, Oxford

Soulier, J P 1976 Vox Sanguinis International Forum

Taylor K, Biggs R 1957 A mildly affected female haemophiliac. British Medical Journal 1: 1494

van der Meer J, Stoepman-van Dalen E A, Jansen J M S 1973 Antithrombin III deficiency in a Dutch family. Journal of Clinical Pathology 26: 532

Vogel F 1955 Vergleichende Betractungen iiber die Mutationsrate der geschlechts-gebunden-rezessiven Hämophilieformen in der Schweiz und in Dänemark. Blut 1: 91

Vogel F 1977 A probable sex difference in some mutation rates. American Journal of Human Genetics 29: 312

von Willebrand E A 1926 Hereditär pseudohärnofili Finska. Läkasällskapets Handlingar 67: 7

Waldmann R, Araham J P, Rebuck J W, Caldwell J, Saito H, Ratnoff O D 1975 Fitzgerald factor: A hitherto unrecognised coagulation factor. Lancet 1: 949

Zimmerman T S, Ratnoff O D, Powell A E 1971 Immunologic differentiation of classic hemophilia (Factor VIII deficiency) and von Willebrand's disease. Journal of Clinical Investigation 50: 244

77

Leukaemias, lymphomas and related disorders

M. Otter and J.D. Rowley

INTRODUCTION

Chromosome abnormalities were first recognized in cancer cells at the beginning of this century (Boveri, 1914), and their significance has been debated ever since (Mitelman, 1980; Nowell, 1976; Sandberg, 1979). While most researchers have acknowledged that cytogenetic changes of many kinds do occur in malignancies, they usually have preferred to regard them as secondary features of the established tumour itself, having little to do with its origin. In recent years, however, with the advent of technical improvements which allow serial studies of malignant cells (and cell lines) and the identification of individual chromosomes, the field of cancer cytogenetics has progressed substantially. Animal models have demonstrated preferential involvement of specific chromosomes in experimental tumours (Klein, 1979; Levan et al, 1977; Mitelman, 1980), and comparable nonrandom patterns are now being identified in human cancers, most notably in the malignant haematologic diseases (Rowley, 1974, 1980c). This chapter will serve to highlight and summarize the cytogenetic findings currently recognized in human leukaemias, lymphomas, and related disorders. Primary data have been presented in several comprehensive reviews that were recently published on various aspects of cancer cytogenetics (Mitelman & Levan, 1978; Rowley, 1980c, 1980d; Sandberg, 1979).

For chromosomal analysis to be relevant to a malignant disease, karyotypes must be obtained from the tumour cells themselves. Several technical advantages make the study of chromosomal changes somewhat easier in leukaemias than in solid tumours (Meisner, 1975); this may account for the more rapid and extensive progress in cytogenetic investigations of these malignancies.

First, access to the malignant cells is much easier, since obtaining a sample of the leukaemic cell population requires no surgical procedures. A bone marrow aspirate can be processed directly or cultured for a short period of time (Testa & Rowley, 1980a). Also, leukaemic cells can be observed in cultures of peripheral blood under appropriate conditions. If cells are malignant and capable of autonomous growth, they will generally divide in culture without mitogenic stimulation. Therefore, spontaneously dividing cells may be obtained from a 24- or 48-hour culture of peripheral blood from a leukaemic patient whose white count is higher than 15,500 and whose cells consist of at least 10% immature myeloid elements. The karyotypic pattern of these spontaneously dividing cells will resemble that of the bone marrow. Finally, parallel cultures of stimulated and unstimulated blood allow one to compare the patient's constitutional chromosome complement with his leukaemic cell population(s) with relatively little additional laboratory processing. In most cases, the unaffected tissues have normal karyotypes, indicating that the abnormalities of the tumour cells represent somatic mutations in an otherwise normal individual.

Evidence for the presence of an abnormal clone is provided by the observation of at least two 'pseudodiploid' or hyperploid cells or three hypoploid cells, each with the same abnormality identified by banding. When no karyotypic alterations are observed, or when they involve different chromosomes in different cells, the patient is considered to be cytogenetically normal. The isolated changes seen are assumed to be the result of technical artifacts or random mitotic errors; in some lymphoid malignant diseases, they may represent the only dividing malignant cells.

GENETIC AETIOLOGY AND SUSCEPTIBILITY

Our major emphasis in this chapter is on the acquired nonrandom cytogenetic aberrations that characterize human haematologic malignancies and provide compelling evidence for the somatic mutation theory of carcinogenesis. However, the possible role of host genetic factors in the aetiology of human cancer has also long been recognized and has recently been the subject of several comprehensive reviews (Fraumeni, 1975; Knudson et al, 1973; Lynch, 1976; Mulvihill et al, 1977). For leukaemia and lymphoma, these investigations of genetic susceptibility have usually centered on retrospective studies and on studies of twins and pedigrees (Anderson,

1975). Additional evidence for genetic predisposition to leukaemia has been derived from studies of patients with certain syndromes that are associated with constitutional aneuploidy or chromosomal instability and an increased risk of malignancy.

Family and twin studies

Retrospective studies have been used in comparisons of the morbidity and/or mortality rates in first-degree relatives of cancer patients with the rates in control relatives. In one such investigation (Vidabaek, 1947), 17 of 209 patients with leukaemia (8.1%) were found to have at least one leukaemic relative, compared to only one such case among 200 controls (0.5%). Under-reporting of leukaemia in the control group and other methodologic deficiencies make the results of such a study questionable (Gorer & Vidabaek, 1949), and indeed, similar subsequent studies have shown little or only moderately increased familial incidence of leukaemia and lymphoma (Heath, 1976).

Since the earlier studies tended to include all types of leukaemia, a familial clustering of one particular subtype could easily have been missed. In a survey of chronic lymphocytic leukaemia (CLL) in New Zealand, Gunz and Veale (1969) found that 7 of their 54 patients with CLL had sibs with chronic leukaemia (4 CLL, 3 CML), in contrast to an expected family incidence of less than one case, calculated from age-adjusted mortality rates. A case-control study of 459 children with acute leukaemia (Miller, 1963) revealed a significant excess of cases among sibs (six cases observed versus one expected); similar results were obtained in a British study of 1798 paediatric patients with acute leukaemia (Barber & Spiers, 1964). Taken together, these findings may indicate familial susceptibility to certain specific types of leukaemia.

Most instances of familial leukaemia/lymphoma have involved pairs of cases in individual families, although occasional pedigrees with as many as six related cases have been described (Heath, 1976; Zuelzer & Cox, 1969). Concordance, or at least similarity, of cell types tends to prevail within each family, again perhaps suggesting the operation of underlying genetic factors.

Recently, a study in Japan compared the degree of consanguinity among parents of sib leukaemia patients and nonfamilial cases (Kurita et al, 1974). In 20 families with familial leukaemia, 20% of the parents were found to be first cousins, and 10% were first cousins once removed or second cousins. In contrast, only 4.5% of the parents in 200 nonfamilial cases were first cousins.

Twin studies are usually considered to be a powerful means to assess the relative importance of genetic and nongenetic factors in a given disease. Reports that concordance rates among monozygotic (MZ) twins for childhood acute leukaemia far exceed random expectation (MacMahon & Levy, 1964; Miller, 1971) are complicated by the fact that shared placental circulation makes many MZ twins haematopoietic chimeras. As a result, the observed high concordance rates (reported to be 17 to 25%) might simply reflect a single postzygotic prenatal oncogenic event and would not necessarily imply an inherited predisposition to leukaemia (Clarkson & Boyse, 1971). Cytogenetic evidence has, in fact, been presented to support a single intrauterine origin of acute leukaemia in at least one pair of MZ twins (Chaganti et al, 1979).

Constitutional chromosome abnormalities

The increased risk of leukaemia in patients with Down syndrome (47,+21) has been well substantiated in a number of surveys and appears to extend to all age groups (Holland et al, 1962; Jackson et al, 1968; Krivit & Good, 1957; Miller, 1970); these patients do not appear to have an increased risk of solid lymphoreticular tumours (Miller, 1970). Lymphocytic leukaemia has been found to predominate in children with Down syndrome, as in the general pediatric population (Rosner & Lee, 1972), although a recent review of the literature suggested that acute nonlymphocytic leukaemia may predominate (Kaneko et al, 1981). The age peak for leukaemia in Down syndrome occurs somewhat earlier than in childhood leukaemia in general (Miller, 1970), although the greater incidence of transient leukemoid reactions in Down syndrome babies could mimic congenital leukaemia and lead to an exaggerated risk estimate in younger children (Rosner & Lee, 1972).

Leukaemia has also been reported in patients with other constitutional aneuploidies, including several with Klinefelter syndrome (47,XXY and mosaics), Turner syndrome (45,X), trisomy 13 syndrome (47,+13) or other D-group trisomies (Heath, 1976). Most of these associations have been documented as single case reports only, making an accurate risk assessment very difficult. Nevertheless, some evidence supporting a predisposition to leukaemia in nondisjunction conditions can be derived from pedigrees which exhibit both leukaemia/lymphoma and various nondisjunction events in separate family members (Baikie et al, 1961; Conen et al, 1966; Ebbin et al, 1968; Miller et al, 1961; Thompson et al, 1963).

Chromosome instability diseases

Three rare genetic diseases (Bloom syndrome, Fanconi anaemia, ataxia telangiectasia) are characterised by increased rates of chromosome breakage and a predisposition to malignancies of the lymphoreticular system (German, 1972; Hecht and McCaw, 1977). All are inherited as autosomal recessive conditions, and each has a distinctive clinical course and phenotype as well as particular types of chromosome aberrations.

In Bloom syndrome (BS), tthe cytogenetic hallmark is the quadriradial configuration, usually symmetric and involving homologous chromosomes. It is seen in lymphocytes and fibroblasts, along with other types of chromosome breakage and an elevated spontaneous rate of sister chromatid exchange (Brat, 1979; Chaganti et al, 1974). Patients with Fanconi anaemia (FA) show an increased frequency of chromosome breakage and rearrangement in bone marrow and cultured lymphocytes, with no tendency for symmetric quadriradial formation (Schroeder & German, 1974). Cells from patients with ataxia telangiectasia (AT) also show increased levels of chromosome breakage, which may fluctuate over time; pseudodiploid clones containing a marker chromosome No. 14 are another common feature of AT lymphocytes (Cohen et al, 1975; McCaw et al, 1975). In several AT patients who developed leukaemia, this chromosomally abnormal clone has become predominant (McCaw et al, 1975; Saxon et al, 1979).

The autosomal recessive mode of transmission suggests an inherited biochemical (enzymatic) defect, possibly involving DNA metabolism or repair, as in the case of xeroderma pigmentosum, another genetic disorder exhibiting cancer predisposition (basal cell and squamous cell carcinomas, malignant melanomas)and abnormal levels of chromosome damage following exposure to ultraviolet irradiation or alkylating agents (Friedberg et al, 1979). Specific DNA repair defects have, in fact, been demonstrated in AT and FA cells, although there is evidence for genetic heterogeneity within each disease. In any case, these syndromes remain valuable models for examining the interrelationships of genetic background, chromosome abnormalities, and cancer development.

CYTOGENETIC STUDIES IN LEUKAEMIA

Chronic myelogenous leukaemia (CML)

Undoubtedly, the main stimulus for the study of chromosomal changes in human leukaemia came with the report in 1960, by Nowell and Hungerford, of a specific cytogenetic aberration in one type of leukaemia. Named after the city of its discovery, this Philadelphia chromosome (Ph[1]), which appeared to be an unusually small member of the G group, has been found in the bone marrow cells of 85 to 90% of patients with chronic myelogenous leukaemia (First Workshop, 1978a; Sandberg, 1979). Even before being precisely identified, the Ph[1] chromosome served as a useful marker for this disease, and Ph[1]-positive CML has become by far the most extensively studied human malignant disease.

Chronic phase of CML

After the introduction of chromosomal banding techniques, Caspersson et al (1970) and O'Riordan et al (1971) independently identified the Ph[1] chromosome as a 22q-. Its nature was further clarified when Rowley (1973) reported that the abnormality characteristically seen in CML was actually a translocation (usually t(9;22)(q34;q11); Fig. 77.1), with no detectable loss of DNA in the rearrangement (Mayall et al, 1977). Since then, a number of investigators have confirmed this observation, and among 802 Ph[1]-positive CML patients studied with banding techniques, the 9;22 translocation has been observed in 739 cases (93%) (Rowley, 1980a).

Unusual or complex translocations have also been reported, in which the material deleted from the No. 22 is translocated to a single chromosome other than the No. 9, or in which three or more chromosomes (almost always including Nos. 9 and 22) are involved in the Ph[1] rearrangement. Three cases are also known in which no translocation could be detected and a true 22q deletion was apparently present. These exceptions to the 9;22 translocation (summarized in Rowley, 1980a) all indicate that the important change is the partial deletion of the long arm of chromosome No.22. Survival curves for patients with a variant translocation are apparently indistinguishable from those for patients with the usual Ph[1] (Sonta & Sandberg, 1977).

Approximately 10% of patients with Ph[1]-positive CML have additional chromosomal abnormalities in their bone marrow during the chronic phase of their disease (First Workshop, 1978a). The most common changes include an extra No. 8, an isochromosome of the long arm of chromosome No. 17, and second Ph[1], and loss of the Y chromosome. Some evidence indicates that the presence of such changes at the time of diagnosis of the chronic phase confers a worse prognosis than the 46,XX or XY,Ph[1] karyotype (Sakurai et al, 1976).

Acute phase of CML

The terminal acute phase of CML is characterised by additional chromosomal changes (karyotype evolution) in at least 70% of patients (Rowley, 1980a), whereas the others retain the original Ph[1] cell line unchanged. In some instances, the change in the karyotype precedes the clinical signs of blast crisis by two to four months.

Karyotype evolution was observed in 202 of 242 patients (83%) with Ph[1]-positive CML in the acute phase whose chromosomes were analyzed with banding techniques (Rowley, 1980a). The most common changes frequently led to modal chromosome numbers of 47 to 52, with distinctly nonrandom involvement of four particular chromosomes. Among the 202 patients with relatively complete analyses, gain of a No. 8 occurred in 95; gain of a second Ph[1] occurred in 78; an isochromosome 17q occurred in 74; and gain of a No. 19 occurred in 38 patients.

Since nearly all patients studied in the acute phase of CML have been treated, usually with busulfan, it is impossible to determine whether this therapy affects the pattern of abnormalities described earlier. Recent evi-

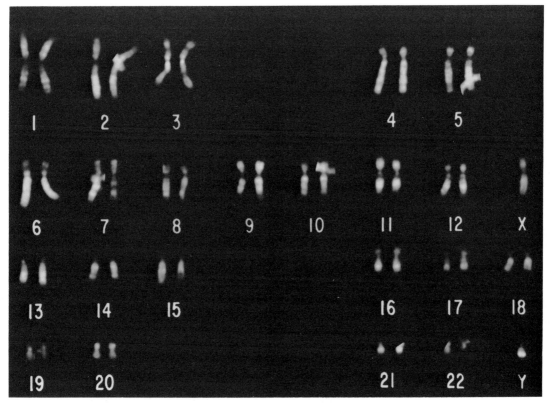

Fig. 77.1 Karyotype of a metaphase cell in a bone marrow aspirate obtained from an untreated male patient with CML. The chromosomes were stained with quinacrine mustard and photographed with ultraviolet fluorescence. In addition to the Ph[1] (22q-) chromosome, the No. 9 on the right (9q+) has an additional pale band that is not present on the normal No. 9.

dence suggests, however, that aggressive chemotherapy in the chronic phase may, in fact, alter the pattern of chromosome abnormalities seen later on (Alimena et al, 1979).

Significance of Ph[1] in diagnosis and prognosis
Even in the pre-banding era, the prognostic significance of the Ph[1] chromosome was recognized (Whang-Peng et al, 1968). A puzzling observation was, and still remains, that patients with Ph[1]-positive CML survived much longer than those with Ph[1]-negative CML (42 versus 15 months, respectively). Furthermore, patients with a Ph[1] chromosome and additional cytogenetic abnormalities during the chronic phase did not have a noticeably poorer prognosis than those with only the Ph[1] chromosome.

Our interpretation of the biologic significance of the Philadelphia chromosome has been modified in recent years, as clinical experience with the marker has increased. Recognition of a Ph[1]-positive acute leukaemia has complicated the classification of patients, and complex interrelationships of the various Ph[1]-positive leukaemias are now becoming apparent (Rowley, 1980a). Clearly, more data are needed; however, in contrast to

the situation in CML, the presence of a Ph[1] in patients with acute leukaemia does not confer a better prognosis (Bloomfield et al, 1977, 1978; Chessells et al, 1979).

Acute nonlymphocytic leukaemia (ANLL)
Included in this classification are cases of acute myelocytic/myeloblastic leukaemia, acute promyelocytic leukaemia, acute myelomonocytic leukaemia, acute monocytic leukaemia, and erythroleukaemia. About 50 per cent of patients with ANLL have clonal karyotypic abnormalities in their bone marrow at the time of diagnosis, most frequently involving chromosomes Nos. 5, 7, 8, and 21 (First Workshop, 1978b; Testa & Rowley, 1980b). In most cases, the material from Nos. 5 and 7 is lost due to partial or complete monosomy, whereas No. 8 is present as extra material and No. 21 may be either lost or gained (Fig. 77.2).

Nonrandom aberrations
The category of ANLL is clinically heterogeneous, and specific cytogenetic abnormalities may be useful for distinction among various subgroups of patients.

An (8;21)(q22;q22) translocation has been reported in

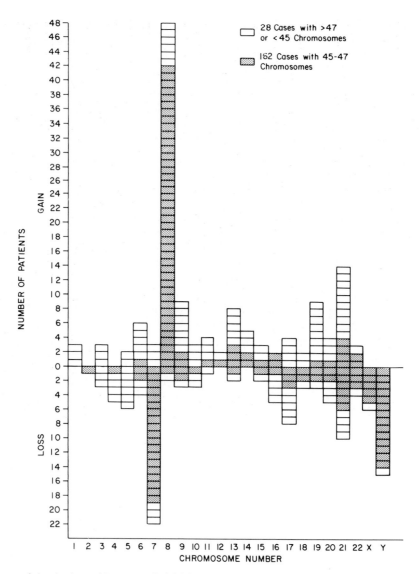

Fig. 77.2 Histogram of clonal gains and losses seen in initial cytogenetic sample from 190 patients with ANLL de novo. The cross-hatched portion indicates the changes observed in the 162 patients who had modal chromosome numbers of 45–47. (Reproduced from Testa and Rowley, 1980b.)

about 8% of all cases of acute myeloblastic leukaemia (AML), and it appears to be restricted to patients with this type (M2 in the French-American-British classification) (Second Workshop, 1980; Fig. 77.3). Kamada et al (1976) reported that all of their patients with this particular translocation showed low levels of leukocyte alkaline phosphatase (LAP), a high percentage (64%) of Auer rods, and a longer median survival (32 weeks) than that of patients with normal or elevated LAP values. Current data on 48 patients with t(8;21) show a median survival of 11.5 months (Second Workshop, 1980). It is also of interest that the 8;21 translocation is frequently

associated with loss of a sex chromosome: 32% of males with t(8;21) are -Y, and 36% of females with t(8;21) are -X (Second Workshop, 1980). Abnormalities of the sex chromosomes are otherwise quite rare in ANLL.

A second highly specific translocation [t(15;17) (q25;q21)] (Fig. 77.4) has been observed in about 40 per cent of patients with acute promyelocytic leukaemia (APL), a unique form of luekaemia characterized by haemorrhagic episodes, disseminated intravascular coagulation, and infiltration of the marrow with 'hypergranular' promyelocytes. Thus far, the 15;17 translocation has not been seen in other types of acute

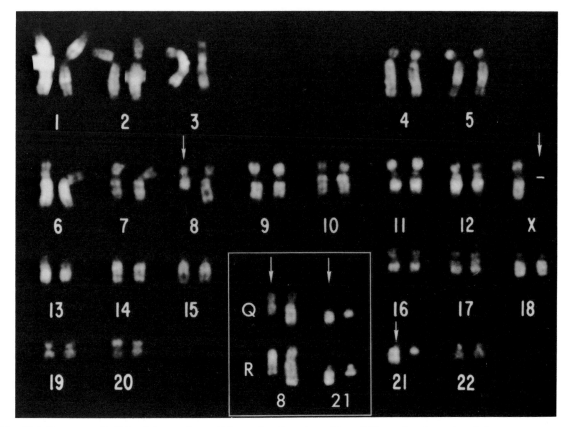

Fig. 77.3 Karyotype of a Q-banded metaphase cell from a female patient with an 8;21 translocation and a missing X–chromosome. The 8q-chromosome (↓) is broken in band q22 and it resembles a No. 16; the 21q+ chromosome (↓) is broken in band q22 and it resembles a No. 14. The inset shows a partial karyotype of pairs No. 8 and No. 21 from another cell that has been sequentially stained for R-banding (bottom) and Q-banding (top).

leukaemia. Since patients with APL should receive heparin along with chemotherapy (Drapkin et al, 1978), detection of the t(15;17) is of great clinical significance, especially in cases of microgranular APL in which the granules may be undetectable at the light-microscope level (Testa et al, 1978).

Karyotype evolution in ANLL
Karyotype evolution occurs in ANLL; approximately 30% of patients develop new aberrations superimposed on the original clone when two or more non-remission samples are studied (Sandberg, 1979; Testa et al, 1979; Testa and Rowley, 1980b). Acquisition of an extra No. 8 is by far the most common additional finding, followed by gain of a No. 18. These changes occur with about equal frequency in patients who were initially cytogenetically normal and those initially abnormal.

Clinical correlations
Sakurai and Sandberg (1976) noted that patients with 100% cytogenetically abnormal cells in their bone mar-

row at the time of diagnosis had a considerably poorer response to therapy than did patients with at least some normal cells. Other studies on large numbers of patients (Nilsson et al, 1977; Golomb et al, 1976, 1978) have confirmed this observation, especially for patients with acute myeloblastic leukaemia. Patients with a normal karyotype have a significantly longer median survival (10 months) than patients with an abnormal karyotype (4 months) (Fig. 77.5). There is one exception to these observations, namely, patients with AML and the t(8;21) have a much better prognosis than patients with other chromosome abnormalities (median survival, 11.5 months).

Secondary ANLL
Acute nonlymphocytic leukaemia as a consequence of therapy for other diseases is currently being diagnosed with increasing frequency. Secondary ANLL has now been observed in patients treated for Hodgkin disease, non-Hodgkin lymphoma, breast and ovarian cancer, as well as nonmalignant diseases. Karyotype analyses of

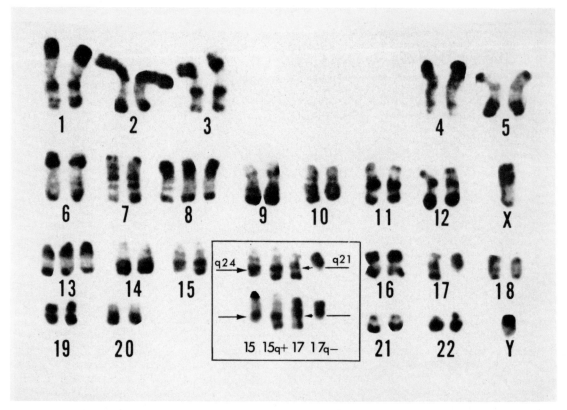

Fig. 77.4 Karyotype of an R-banded metaphase cell obtained from unstimulated PB during relapse. The cell has the t(15;17) and extra chromosomes No. 8 and No. 13 [48,XY,+8,+13,t(15;17)]. The inset shows partial karyotypes of pairs No. 15 and No. 17 from this cell (top row) and another cell. The densely stained band q24 is present both in the normal 15 and in the 15q+, suggesting a translocation breakpoint distal to q24. Two narrow bands in 17q21 are present both in the normal 17 and in the 17q-, suggesting a breakpoint at or near the junction of q21 and q22. Probable breakpoints are identified with arrows, and the number above each arrow identifies the band proximal to the breakpoint [t(15;17) (q25?;q22?)]. (Reproduced from Testa et al, 1978).

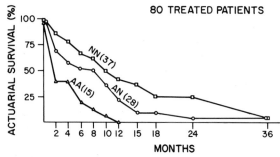

Fig. 77.5 Actuarial survival of all treated patients according to initial chromosome findings. NN denotes normal metaphases only, AN, normal and abnormal metaphases, and AA, abnormal metaphases only. (Reproduced from Golomb et al, 1978).

these patients have revealed a clone of chromosomally abnormal cells in nearly every case, with some highly nonrandom changes now becoming apparent.

Rowley et al (1981) studied the karyotype of 27

patients who developed ANLL either after treatment of a primary malignancy (26 cases) or after a renal transplant (1 case). Fifteen of the patients had previously received both radiotherapy and chemotherapy, eight had had chemotherapy only, and four, radiotherapy only. The median times from diagnosis of the initial disease to the development of ANLL for these treatment groups were 61, 59, and 59 months, respectively. Nineteen of the 27 patients had a clone with a hypodiploid modal number. Twenty-six patients had an abnormal karyotype, with one or both of two consistent chromosomal changes noted in 24 of these patients. Eleven patients had loss of a No. 5; marrow cells from three others were lacking part of the long arm of a No. 5 (5q-); No. 7 was missing from cells of 18 patients; and one patient had a partial deletion of the long arm of a No. 7 (7q-). Although these changes are distinctly different from those seen in lymphomas, they are similar to those seen in about 25 per cent of aneuploid patients with ANLL de novo.

Table 77.1 Frequency of abnormalities of No. 5, No. 7, and No. 8 in patients with acute leukaemia.[a]

| | Number of patients | | | | | |
| | Type of abnormality | | | | | |
Diagnosis	Total[b]	−5	5q−	−7	7q−	+8
ANLL de novo						
Literature review	190	6	9	22	4	48
Childhood[c]	30	0	0	1	5[d]	3
Exposed[e]	19	3	2	3	2	5
Nonexposed[e]	8	0	0	1	0	0
Chicago	44	5	5	8	1	3
ANLL secondary						
Chicago	26	11	3	18	1	5
Literature review	16	3	4	6	3	1

[a] Modified from Rowley (1980c).
[b] Aneuploid patients, all studied with banding.
[c] Data from Benedict et al (1979), Hagemeijer et al (1979) and Morse et al (1979).
[d] Only two patients had the typical del(7)(q22); one other had del(7)(q31).
[e] Data from Mitelman et al (1978).

Thus, the cytogenetic hallmarks of secondary ANLL are an abnormal clone of cells, usually with a hypodiploid modal number, associated with the nonrandom loss of chromosomes 5 and/or 7. The occurrence of these same aberrations in patients with ANLL de novo who may have had occupational exposure to mutagenic agents (Mitelman et al, 1978; 1979b) and the absence of these abnormalities in childhood ANLL (Benedict et al, 1979; Hagemeijer et al, 1979; Morse et al, 1979) provide further support for the proposal that partial or complete loss of Nos. 5 and 7 may identify acute leukaemia associated with exposure to such agents (Rowley, 1980d; Rowley et al, 1981; Table 77.1).

Refractory anaemia and preleukaemia
Some patients with unexplained cytopenias, with or without an increased frequency of blasts in the bone marrow, may develop acute leukaemia. Recent analysis of cytogenetic data on 244 such patients (Second Workshop, 1980) revealed that, as in ANLL, about 50% of such patients had an abnormal karyotype, with the types of chromosomal changes also being very similar to those seen in ANLL. Fifty-two (21%) of these patients had progressed to overt leukaemia at the time of the Workshop. Only 34 of 118 patients (29%) with a normal karyotype had died, roughly half of these having developed ANLL, whereas 66 of 111 patients (60%) with autosomal abnormalities had died, about one half of whom having developed ANLL. None of the seven patients with loss of a sex chromosome developed acute leukaemia. These data indicate that the presence of a chromosome abnormality in patients with cytopenias is a sign of a poor prognosis, since the death rate is higher for such patients than for those with a normal karyotype.

Acute lymphoblastic leukaemia (ALL)
The poor morphology and 'fuzziness' of chromosomes from patients with ALL (Kessous et al, 1975) probably account for the lack of data on their karyotype patterns. At present, reports on only three series of unselected patients studied with banding are available (Cimino et al, 1979; Oshimura et al, 1977; Prigogina et al, 1979).

Nonrandom aberrations
As in ANLL, about 50% of these patients have normal karyotypes; hypodiploidy is quite rare among the abnormal cell lines, hyperdiploidy and pseudodiploidy being much more common and often involving multiple aneuploid clones (Rowley, 1980b; Sandberg, 1979). As shown in Figure 77.6, the chromosome changes in ALL differ from those seen in ANLL. Among 53 chromosomally abnormal patients with ALL, gain of a No. 21 chromosome occurred most frequently, followed by gain of a No. 14 or 13 (Rowley, 1980b). The only chromosome lost with any frequency was one X.

Nonrandom structural rearrangements do occur in ALL, although apparently less often than in ANLL. The most common deletion involves the long arm of No. 6, with breakpoints ranging from 6q11 to 6q25. Recently, a reciprocal translocation [t(4;11)(q21;q23)] has been observed in a number of patients with ALL (Esseltine et al, 1979; Oshimura et al, 1977; Otter, unpublished observations, Prigogina et al, 1979; Van den Berghe et al, 1979a), five of whom had congenital leukaemia. All of these patients responded poorly to therapy and survived at most for six months.

Patients with B-cell ALL constitute a small proportion (about four per cent) of those with ALL; they are identified because their cells express surface immu-

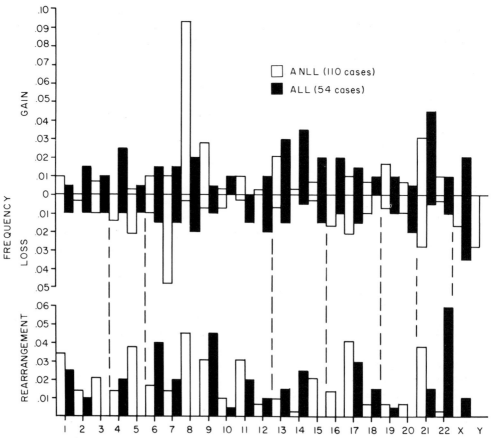

Fig. 77.6 Histogram of chromosome abnormalities (gains, losses, and rearrangements) in 110 cases of ANLL and in 54 cases of ALL, excluding documented cases of secondary karyotypic evolution. The frequency of each abnormality was calculated as a proportion of all abnormalities. (Reproduced from Cimino et al, 1979).
omocytomas being present in any member (key as in Figure 84.6).

noglobulin. With rare exceptions, B-cell ALL is associated with a 14q+ chromosome. The exceptional cases (Berger et al, 1979b; Rowley, unpublished observations) were patients with Burkitt-type ALL whose leukaemic cells had either a t(8;22)(q24;q11) or a t(2;8)(p13;q24), respectively. Both of these translocations have recently been identified as variant translocations in non-endemic Burkitt lymphoma. The donor chromosome involved with No. 14 was identified in 12 of the 17 patients with a 14q+ marker; it was 11q in one case (Roth et al, 1979) and 8q in the remaining cases (Berger et al, 1979a; Mitelman et al, 1979a).

Karyotype evolution
Evolution of the karyotype appears to be a very common phenomenon in ALL, involving a number of different chromosomes (Rowley, 1980b). In one study, addition of a No. 8 was observed in three patients (among eight cases who showed clonal evolution), and an additional No. 3, 6, or 21 was seen, each in two patients (Oshimura et al, 1977). Zuelzer et al (1976), investigating the nature of relapse after prolonged remission, found that, in 80% of the cases, the leukaemic clone seen at relapse was the same as that present at onset of the disease. In many of the remaining cases, the relapse clone was clearly derived from the original one. Marrows obtained in remission on the other hand, were found to be cytogenetically normal, except in five cases where the presence of a few aneuploid cells indicated an impending relapse. Whang-Peng et al (1976) concluded that detection of aneuploid clones at the onset of ALL or later in the disease was not necessarily a bad prognostic sign, but that their persistence and the development of total aneuploidy conferred a poor prognosis. However, recent data obtained with banding have suggested that some types of aneuploidy, particularly hyperdiploidy with more than 50 chromosomes, are not associated with a poor prognosis (Secker Walker et al, 1978). Additional long-term data on patients with ALL are clearly needed before the clinical significance of particular karyotypic patterns can be discerned.

Chronic lymphocytic leukaemia (CLL)

Soon after the discovery of the Philadelphia chromosome, Gunz et al (1962) reported finding a G-group chromosome with deleted short arms in a brother and sister who had CLL, a condition that generally involves neoplastic proliferation of B lymphocytes. Unlike the Ph[1], which is clearly an acquired clonal abnormality, this so-called Christchurch chromosome (Ch[1]) was observed in three unaffected siblings of the original patients. Thus, its presence was interpreted as indicating an increased predisposition to develop CLL (Fitzgerald et al, 1966; Fitzgerald and Gunz, 1964).

Subsequently, however, the aberrant chromosome was found to be a heteromorphic variant of chromosome No. 21, and it has been seen in patients with AML or Down syndrome (Juberg and Jones, 1970) and in normal individuals (Court Brown, 1964), even without banding studies. Today, the Ch[1] is not regarded as a marker for any type of malignancy.

Because CLL patients have a very low mitotic index, contemporary cytogenetic studies on CLL have largely been performed on PHA-stimulated peripheral lymphocytes which probably do not reflect the constitution of the neoplastic cells. Not surprisingly, the vast majority of cases have appeared karyotypically normal (Crossen 1975). More recently, however, a few cases of CLL with chromosome abnormalities have been observed, with chromosomes Nos. 1, 14, and 17 often involved in the rearrangements (Mitelman & Levan, 1978). A preliminary report (Fort et al, 1979) on 10 patients with B-cell CLL indicated that leukocyte cultures stimulated with phytohaemagglutinin had abnormalities which were different from those in cells stimulated with pokeweed mitogen, as might be expected. The former were characterized by gain of chromosomes Nos. 2, 11, or 16 and loss of No. 9, 11, or 7, whereas the latter showed trisomy 4 and monsomy 1, 8, 16, or 20. An extra No. 21 was found in both types of cultures. At least three patients

with CLL have been found to have a 14q+ chromosome (Finan et al, 1978; Gahrton et al, 1979), and an extra No. 12 has been identified in five CLL patients whose cells were stimulated with B-cell mitogens (Autio et al, 1979; Gahrton et al, 1980a).

CYTOGENETIC STUDIES ON OTHER HAEMATOLOGIC MALIGNANCIES

Lymphomas

Chromosomal studies on malignant lymphomas, reviewed recently by Mark (1977), have revealed that the majority of patients have an abnormal karyotype, which is often rather complex with many structural rearrangements (Mark et al, 1979; Rowley & Fukuhara, 1980). Studies completed without banding techniques indicated that the modal chromosome number in the non-Hodgkin lymphomas was usually near-diploid, whereas it was polyploid in more than 50% of the cases of Hodgkin disease. In the lymphomas studied with banding, some recurring types of chromosome changes have been observed, and these will be summarized here.

Burkitt lymphoma

Burkitt lymphoma is a solid tumour affecting immunoglobulin-secreting cells (B lymphocytes). Manolov and Manolova (1972) first reported the presence of an extra band of chromosomal material at the end of the long arm of one chromosome No. 14 (14q+) in fresh tumour samples from five of six patients with African Burkitt lymphoma, and in five of six cell lines established from tumours of other patients. Zech et al (1976) identified the extra material at the end of No. 14 as a translocation from chromosome No.8 [t(8;14)(q24;q32)] in eight of the 10 African Burkitt tumours in which it could be scored. The other two tumours had the 14q+ chromosome, although a translocation from No. 8 could not be established.

Table 77.2 Frequency of 14q+ marker chromosome in lymphoid disorders.[a]

Type of disorder	Number of patients			Donor chromosome						
	Total[b]	Abnormal	With 14q+	1q	8q	11q	14q	18q	Other	Unknown
Burkitt	43	43	35		25					10
Histiocytic	28	28	15	2	2	2	2	0	6	1
Poorly differentiated lymphocytic	28	27	24	0	2	8[c,d]	2	6[c,d]	0	7
T-cell	18	18	9	0	0	1	4	1	3	0

[a] Reproduced from Rowley (1981).
[b] Number of patients on whom a reasonably complete analysis was done.
[c] Identification uncertain in two cases.
[d] One patient had two 14q+ chromosomes.

Since then, the 8;14 translocation has also been consistently reported in cases of American Burkitt lymphoma, both in direct tumour preparations and in cell lines derived from tumour tissue, whether or not the cells were positive for Epstein-Barr virus (Douglass et al, 1980; McCaw et al, 1977; Kakati, 1979; Table 77.2).

Heterogeneity of the translocation in Burkitt lymphoma has also been recognized recently. The cells of several patients with non-African Burkitt lymphoma show a translocation involving the short arm of No. 2 and the long arm of No. 8 [t(2;8)(p12-p13;q24)] (Miyoshi et al, 1979; Van den Berghe et al, 1979b) or the long arms of No. 8 and No. 22 [t(8;22)(q24;q11)] (Berger et al, 1979b). Although the consistent change in the different Burkitt translocations appears to be the involvement of band 8q24, it is still too early to determine whether there are important biological differences in the behaviour of Burkitt cells when the variant translocations are present.

Non-Hodgkin lymphomas

Poorly differentiated lymphocytic lymphoma (PDL) Partial or complete cytogenetic studies are available on 38 patients with PDL. In 27 of these cases, analysis was performed on lymph nodes or effusions; peripheral blood was used in the remaining cases (Rowley and Fukuhara, 1980). All but two of the peripheral blood samples contained a chromosomally abnormal clone, and specimens that definitely contained malignant cells (i.e., lymph nodes of effusions) were found to have a chromosomally abnormal clone in every case but one. In more than half of the lymph nodes, 12 to 50% of the cells had a normal karyotype.

Patients with PDL often have very few dividing cells in their lymph nodes, and the banding patterns tend to be somewhat indistinct. Nevertheless, a 14q+ chromosome could be identified in 24 of the 35 chromosomally abnormal patients, and other abnormalities of No. 14

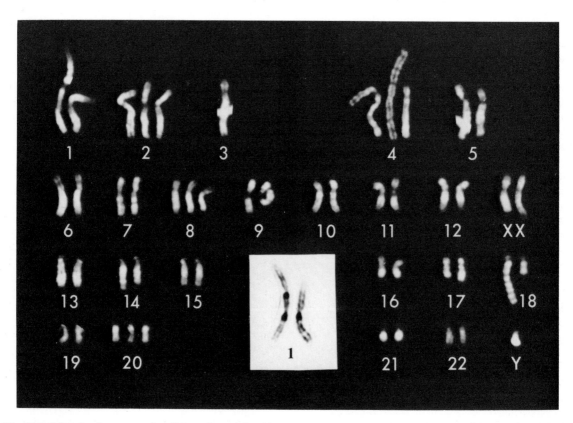

Fig. 77.7 Q-banding karyotype of a cell from the peripheral blood of a 59-year-old male patient in the leukemic phase of diffuse histiocytic lymphoma (the tumor was composed of large noncleaved cells); the patient's leukemic cells were IgMk. This cell has 50 chromosomes, with additional Nos. 2, 4, 8, 20, and an X, and with a missing No. 3. Chromosome No. 1 is involved in a complex rearrangement which includes duplication of all of the long arm. The first two No. 4 chromosomes have a series of repeating bands of unknown origin at the end of the short arm (4p+). The end of the first 18q (18q+) also has a series of repeating bands. The first No. 14 has an extra band which appears to be a translocation from the end of the third No. 8[t(8;14)(q24;q32)]. C-banding of No. 1 (inset) shows that the 1q+ marker represents a duplication of all of 1q. (Reproduced from Fukuhara et al, 1978, Blood 52:989).

Table 77.3 Chromosomes commonly affected in chronic leukaemia and lymphoma.[a]

Type of chromosome change	Chromosome number		
	Diffuse histiocytic lymphoma[b] (28 patients)	Poorly differentiated lymphocytic lymphoma (28 patients)	Chronic T-cell leukaemia and lymphoma (18 patients)
Gain	7, 8	3, 7	Infrequent
Loss	6, 15, 13	11	13, 17, 20, 22
Break in short arm	1, 3, 6, 8	1	1, 9
Break in long arm	1, 14, 3, 9	14, 11, 18, 8	14, 2, 9, 13, 18

[a] Reproduced from Rowley & Fukuhara (1980).
[b] Listed in order of descending frequency.

were seen in three additional patients. The donor chromosomes involved with No. 14 are listed in Table 77.2. Structural rearrangements of 11q and 18q were usually associated with translocation to No. 14. Finally, some abnormality of No. 1 (often leading to trisomy for 1q) was frequently observed in conjunction with a 14q marker.

Diffuse histiocytic lymphoma Banded chromosomal analyses are available on 32 patients with diffuse histiocytic lymphoma (Rowley & Fukuhara, 1980). Every patient had at least one chromosomally abnormal clone, and some had extremely complex karyotypic patterns (Fig. 77.7). In most cases, the tissue examined was lymph node or extra-nodal tumour tissue, although pleural or ascitic fluid or circulating leukaemic cells were used in some instances.

Based on the 28 patients on whom a reasonably complete analysis was accomplished, several generalizations appear valid. No patient had a gain of a No. 1; nor were gains of No. 6, No. 14, or the Y observed in any case. The single most common abnormality, seen in 15 patients, was a translocation to the end of the long arm of No. 14, usually at band 14q32. The donor chromosome could be identified in all 15 cases (Table 77.2).

T-cell lymphomas and related T-cell disorders

Although chromosomes from fewer than 20 patients in this category have been studied with banding, the results reveal interesting differences between the T-cell disorders and the lymphomas discussed above (Table 77.3).

Whereas gains and losses of chromosomes are not really characteristic of these disorders, five structural rearrangements should be noted. These include translocations and deletions, most often affecting the long arm of Nos. 2, 9, 13, and 18, in that order, in addition to the 14q+ abnormality. Nine of the 18 patients with T-cell malignancies had a structural rearrangement of No. 14, leading to a 14q+ chromosome (Table 77.2).

Multiple myeloma

Relatively few patients with multiple myeloma (MM) or

plasma cell leukaemia (PCL) have been studied with banding techniques. The normal karyotype observed in bone marrow cells from these patients may be related to the very low mitotic index of myeloma cells. In patients with abnormalities, the modal number tends to be hyperdiploid (47–55) and often includes many complex rearrangements (Rowley, 1981). A 14q+ marker chromosome has been reported in cells from six patients with MM and three patients with PCL (Gahrton et al, 1980b; Liang et al, 1979). Quite often, the 14q+ abnormality is associated with an abnormality of 1q. Gains of other chromosomes, especially Nos. 3, 5, 7, 9, and 11, also tend to occur together or in various combinations in these patients.

CONCLUSION

The occurrence of leukaemia and lymphoma in relatives of patients and in families with multiple cases suggests a genetic contribution to the multifactorial aetiology of these diseases. At present, however, the most compelling evidence for a genetic contribution comes from cytogenetic studies. Not only are individuals with certain constitutional aneuploidies or with inherited chromosome instability syndromes at an increased risk of malignancy (particularly of the lymphoreticular system), but consistent cytogenetic changes, including specific translocations, are now being detected in the malignant cells themselves.

As more genes are mapped to human chromosomes and as the breakpoints in the translocations are determined more precisely, it should become possible to determine the function of genes at these breakpoints. The genetic activity could be compared in cells with and without the translocations, and eventually such studies could indicate how chromosome changes provide selected cells in certain individuals with a growth advantage that results in malignancy.

REFERENCES

Alimena G, Brandt L, Dallapiccola B, Mitelman F, Nilsson P G 1979 Secondary chromosome changes in chronic myeloid leukaemia: Relation to treatment. Cancer Genetics and Cytogenetics 1: 79–85

Anderson D E 1975 Familial susceptibility. In: Fraumeni J F Jr (ed) Persons at high risk of cancer. Academic Press, New York

Autio K, Turunen O, Penttilä O, Erämaa E, de la Chapelle A, Schröder J 1979 Human chronic lymphocytic leukaemia. Karyotypes in different lymphocyte populations. Cancer Genetics and Cytogenetics 1: 147–155

Baikie A G, Buckton K E, Court Brown W M, Harnden D G 1961 Two cases of leukaemia and case of sex chromosome abnormality in same sibship. Lancet ii: 1003–1004

Barber R, Spiers P 1964 Oxford survey of childhood cancers: Progress report II. Monthly Bulletin of the Ministry of Health 23: 46–52

Benedict W F, Lange M, Greene J, Derencsenyi A, Alfi O S 1979 Correlation between prognosis and bone marrow chromosomal patterns in children with acute nonlymphocytic leukaemia: Similarities and differences compared to adults. Blood 54: 818–823

Berger R, Bernheim A, Brouet J-C, Daniel M T, Flandrin G 1979a t(8;14) Translocation in a Burkitt's type of lymphoblastic leukaemia (L3). British Journal of Haematology 43: 87–90

Berger R, Bernheim A, Weh H-J, Flandrin G, Daniel M T, Brouet J-C, Colbert N 1979b A new translocation in Burkitt's tumour cells. Human Genetics 53: 111–112

Bloomfield C D, Lindquist L L, Brunning R D, Yunis J J, Coccia P F 1978 The Philadelphia chromosome in acute leukaemia. Virchows Archiv B Cell Pathology 29: 81–92

Bloomfield C D, Peterson L C, Yunis J J, Brunning R D 1977 The Philadelphia chromosome (Ph¹) in adults presenting with acute leukaemia. A comparison of Ph¹ and Ph¹-patients. British Journal of Haematology 36: 347–358

Boveri T 1914 Zur Frage der Entstehung maligner Tumoren. Fischer, Jena

Brat S V 1979 Sister chromatid exchange and cell cycle in fibroblasts of Bloom's syndrome. Human Genetics 48: 73–79

Caspersson T, Gahrton G, Lindsten J , Zech L 1970 Identification of the Philadelphia chromosome as a number 22 by quinacrine mustard fluorescence analysis. Experimental Cell Research 63: 238–244

Chaganti R S K, Miller D R, Meyers P A, German J 1979 Cytogenetic evidence of the intrauterine origin of acute leukaemia in monozygotic twins. New England Journal of Medicine 300: 1032–1034

Chaganti R S K, Schonberg S, German J 1974 A manyfold increase in sister chromatid exchange in Bloom's syndrome lymphocytes. Proceedings of the National Academy of Sciences, USA 71: 4508–4512

Chessells J M, Janossy G, Lawler S D, Secker Walker L M 1974 The Ph¹ chromosome in childhood leukaemia. British Journal of Haematology 41: 25–4

Cimino M C, Rowley J D, Kinnealey A, Variakojis D, Golomb H M 1979 Banding studies of chromosomal abnormalities in patients with acute lymphocytic leukaemia. Cancer Research 29: 227–238

Clarkson B D, Boyse E A 1971 Possible explanation of the high concordance for acute leukaemia in monozygotic twins (letter to editor). Lancet i: 699–701

Cohen M M, Shaham M, Dagen J, Shmueli E, Kohn G 1975 Cytogenetic investigations in families with ataxia-telangiectasia. Cytogenetics and Cell Genetics 15: 338–356

Conen P E, Erkman B, Laski B 1966 Chromosome studies on a radiographer and her family:Report of one case of leukaemia and two cases of Down's syndrome. Archives of Internal Medicine 117: 125–132

Court Brown W M C 1964 Chromosomal abnormality and chronic lymphatic leukaemia. Lancet i: 986

Crossen P E 1975 Giemsa banding patterns in chronic lymphocytic leukaemia. Humangenetik 27: 151–156

Douglass E C,Magrath I T, Lee E C, Whang-Peng J 1980 Cytogenetic studies in non-African Burkitt lymphoma. Blood 55: 148–155

Drapkin R L, Gee T S, Dowling M D, Arlin Z, McKenzie S, Kempin S, Clarkson B 1978 Prophylactic heparin therapy in acute promyelocytic leukemia. Cancer 41: 2484–2490

Ebbin A J, Heath C W, Moldow R E, Lee J 1968 Down's syndrome and leukemia in a family. Journal of Pediatrics 73: 917–919

Esseltine D W, Vekemans M, Rudner M 1979 Is the (4:11) translocation associated with ALL, congenital leukemia or both? American Journal of Human Genetics 31: 92A

Finan J, Daniele R, Rowlands D, Nowell P 1978 Cytogenetics of chronic T cell leukemia, including two patients with a 14q+ translocation. Virchows Archiv B Cell Pathology 29: 121–127

First International Workshop on Chromosomes in Leukaemia 1978a Chromosomes in Ph¹-positive chronic granulocytic leukaemia. British Journal of Haematology 39: 305–309

First International Workshop on Chromosomes in Leukaemia 1978b Chromosomes in acute non-lymphocytic leukaemia. British Journal of Haematology 39: 311–316

Fitzgerald P H, Crossen P E, Adams A C, Sharman C V, Gunz F W 1966 Chromosome studies in familial leukaemia. Journal of Medical Genetics 3 96–100

Fitzgerald P H, Gunz F W 1964 Chromosomal instability and chronic lymphocytic leukemia. Lancet ii: 150

Fort S, Kanter R J, Phillips E A, Rai K R, Sawitsky A 1979 Chromosomal study of patients with chronic lymphocytic leukemia (CLL). Proceedings of the American Society of Clinical Oncology 20: 429

Fraumeni J F Jr (ed) 1975 Persons at High Risk of Cancer. Academic Press, New York

Friedberg E C, Ehmann U K, Williams J I 1979 Human diseases associated with defective DNA repair. Advances in Radiation Biology 8: 85–174

Gahrton G, Robèrt K-H, Friberg K, Zech L, Bird A G 1980a Extra chromosome 12 in chronic lymphocytic leukaemia. Lancet i: 146–147

Gahrton G, Zech L, Nillsson K, Lönnqvist B, Carlström A 1980b 2 Translocations, t(11;14) and t(1;6), in a patient with plasma cell leukaemia and 2 populations of plasma cells. Scandinavian Journal of Haematology 24: 42–46

Gahrton G, Zech L, Robèrt K-H, Bird A G 1979 Mitogenic stimulation of leukemia cells by Epstein-Barr virus. New England Journal of Medicine 301: 438

German J 1972 Genes which increase chromosomal instability in somatic cells and predispose to cancer. Progress in Medical Genetics 8: 61–101

Golomb H M, Vardiman J, Rowley J D 1976 Acute nonlymphocytic leukaemia in adults: Correlations with Q-banded chromosomes. Blood 48: 9–21

Golomb H M, Vardiman J W, Rowley J D, Testa J R, Mintz U 1978 Correlation of clinical findings with quinacrine-banded chromosomes in 90 adults with acute nonlymphocytic leukemia. New England Journal of Medicine 299: 613–619

Gorer F A, Vidabaek A 1949 Heredity in human leukemia and its relation to cancer (a review). Annals of Eugenics 14: 346–348

Gunz F W, Fitzgerald P H, Adams A 1962 An abnormal chromosome in chronic lymphocytic leukaemia. British Medical Journal 2: 1097–1099

Gunz F W, Veale A M O 1969 Leukemia in close relatives – accident or predisposition? Journal of the National Cancer Institute 42: 517–524

Hagemeijer A, Van Zanen G E, Smit E M E, Hahlen K 1979 Bone marrow karyotypes of children with nonlymphocytic leukemia. Pediatric Research 13: 1247–1254

Heath C W 1976 Hereditary factors in leukemia and lymphoma. In: Lynch H T (ed) Cancer genetics. C C Thomas, Springfield

Hecht F, McCaw B K 1977 Chromosome instability syndromes. In: Mulvihill J J, Miller R W, Fraumeni J F Jr (eds) Genetics of human cancer. Raven Press, New York

Holland W W, Doll R, Carter C O 1962 The mortality from leukemia and other cancers among patients with Down's syndrome (mongols) and among their parents. British Journal of Cancer 16: 178–186

Jackson E W, Turner J H, Klauber M R, Norris F D 1968 Down's syndrome: Variation of leukaemia occurrence in institutionalized populations. Journal of Chronic Diseases 21: 247–253

Juberg R C, Jones B 1970 The Christchurch chromosome (Gp-) mongolism, erythroleukemia and an inherited Gp-chromosome (Christchurch). New England Journal of Medicine 282: 292–297

Kakati S, Barcos M, Sandberg A A 1979 Chromosomes and causation of human cancer and leukemia. XXXVI. The 14q+ anomaly in an American Burkitt lymphoma and its value in the definition of lymphoproliferative disorders. Medical and Pediatric Oncology 6: 121–129

Kamada N, Okada K, Oguma N, Tanaka R, Mikami M, Uchino H 1976 C-G translocation in acute myelocytic leukemia with low neutrophil alkaline phosphatase activity. Cancer 37: 2380–2387

Kaneko Y, Rowley J D, Variakojis D, Chilcote R R, Moohr J W, Patel D 1981 Chromosome abnormalities in Down's syndrome patients with acute leukemia. Blood 58: 459–466

Kessous A, Corberand J, Robert A, Colombies P 1975 Caractères cytogénétiques des leucémies aiques de l'enfant. Aspects évolutifs à propos de 28 cas. Lyon Médical 233: 253–260

Klein G 1979 Lymphoma development in mice and humans: Diversity of initiation is followed by convergent cytogenetic evolution. Proceedings of the National Academy of Sciences, USA 76: 2442–2446

Knudson A G, Strong L C, Anderson D E 1973 Heredity and cancer in man. Progress in Medical Genetics 9: 113–158

Krivit W, Good R A 1957 Simultaneous occurrence of mongolism and leukemia. Report of a nationwide survey. American Journal of Diseases of Children 94: 289–293

Kurita S, Kamei Y, Ota K 1974 Genetic studies on familial leukemia. Cancer 34: 1048–1101

Levan A, Levan G, Mitelman F 1977 Chromosomes and cancer. Hereditas 86: 15–30

Liang W, Hopper J E, Rowley J D 1979 Karyotypic abnormalities and clinical aspects of patients with multiple myeloma and related paraproteinemic disorders. Cancer 44: 630–644

Lynch H T (ed) 1976 Cancer Genetics. C C Thomas, Springfield

MacMahon B, Levy M 1964 Prenatal origin of childhood leukemia: evidence from twins. New England Journal of Medicine 270: 1082–1085

Manolov G, Manolova Y 1972 Marker band in one chromosome 14 from Burkitt lymphomas. Nature 237: 33–34

Mark J 1977 Chromosomal abnormalities and their specificity in human neoplasms: An assessment of recent observations by banding techniques. Advances in Cancer Research 24: 165–222

Mark J, Dahlenfors R, Ekedahl C 1979 Recurrent chromosomal aberrations in non-Hodgkin and non-Burkitt lymphomas. Cancer Genetics and Cytogenetics 1: 39–56

Mayall B H, Carrano A V, Moore D H II, Rowley J D 1977 Qualification by DNA-based cytophotometry of the 9q+/22q- chromosomal translocation associated with chronic myelogenous leukemia. Cancer Research 37: 3590–3593

McCaw B K, Epstein A L, Kaplan H S, Hecht F 1977 Chromosome 14 translocation in African and North American Burkitt's lymphomas. International Journal of Cancer 19: 482–486

McCaw B K, Hecht F, Harnden D G, Teplitz R L 1975 Somatic rearrangement of chromosome 14 in human lymphocytes. Proceedings of the National Academy of Sciences L 72: 2071–2075

Meisner L F 1975 Cytogenetic analysis in leukemia. CRC Critical Reviews in Clinical Laboratory Sciences 6: 157–200

Miller O J, Breg W R, Schnickel R D, Tretter W 1961 A family with an XXXXY male, a leukaemic male, and two 21 trisomic mongloid females. Lancet ii: 78–79

Miller R W 1963 Down's syndrome (mongolism), other congenital malformations, and cancer among the sibs of leukemic children. New England Journal of Medicine 268: 393–401

Miller R W 1970 Neoplasia and Down's syndrome. Annals of the New York Academy of Sciences 171: 637–644

Miller R W 1971 Deaths from childhood leukaemia and solid tumors among twins and other sibs in the United States, 1960–67. Journal of the National Cancer Institute 46: 203–209

Mitelman F 1980 Cytogenetics of experimental neoplasms and non-random chromosome correlations in man. Clinics in Haematology 9: 195–219

Mitelman F, Anvret-Andersson M, Brandt L, Catovsky D, Klein G, Manolov G, Manolova Y, Mark-Vendel E, Nilsson P G 1979a Reciprocal 8;14 translocation in EBV-negative B-cell acute lymphocytic leukemia with Burkitt-type cells. International Journal of Cancer 24: 27–33

Mitelman F, Brandt L, Nilsson P G 1978 Relation among occupational exposure to potential mutagenic/carcinogenic agents, clinical findings, and bone marrow chromosomes in acute nonlymphocytic leukemia. Blood 52: 1229–1237

Mitelman F, Levan G 1978 Clustering of aberrations to specific chromosomes in human neoplasms. III. Incidence and geographic distribution of chromosome aberrations in 856 cases. Hereditas 89: 207–232

Mitelman F, Nilsson P G, Brandt L, Alimena G, Montuoro A, Dallapiccola B 1979b Chromosomes, leukaemia, and occupational exposure to leukaemogenic agents. Lancet ii: 1195–1196

Miyoshi I, Hiraki S, Kimura I, Miyamoto K, Sato J 1979 2/8 Translocation in a Japanese Burkitt lymphoma. Experientia 35: 742

Morse H, Hays T, Peakman D, Rose B, Robinson A 1979 Acute nonlymphocytic leukemia in childhood. Cancer 44: 164–170

Mulvihill J J, Miller R W, Fraumeni J F Jr (eds) 1977 Genetics of human cancer. Raven Press, New York

Nilsson P G, Brandt L, Mitelman F 1977 Prognostic implications of chromosome analysis in acute non-lymphocytic leukemia. Leukemia Research 1: 31–34

Nowell P C 1976 The clonal evolution of tumor cell populations Science 194: 23–28

Nowell P C, Hungerford D A 1960 A minute chromosome in human chronic granulocytic leukemia. Science 132: 1197

O'Riordan M L, Robinson J A, Buckton K E, Evans H J 1971 Distinguishing between the chromosomes involved in Down's syndrome (trisomy 21) and chronic myeloid leukemia (Ph^1) by fluorescence. Nature 230: 167–168

Oshimura M, Freeman A I, Sandberg A A 1977 Chromosomes and causation of human cancer and leukaemia. XXVI. Banding studies in acute lymphoblastic leukaemia (ALL). Cancer 40: 1161–1172

Prigogina E L, Fleischman E W, Puchkova G P, Kulagina O E, Majakova S A, Balakirev S A, Frenkel M A, Khvatova N V, Peterson I S 1979 Chromosomes in acute leukemia. Human Genetics 53: 5–16

Rosner F, Lee S L 1972 Down's syndrome and acute leukaemia: myeloblastic or lymphoblastic? Report of forty-three cases and review of the literature. American Journal of Medicine 53: 203–218

Roth D G, Cimino M C, Variakojis D, Golomb H M, Rowley J D 1979 B-cell acute lymphoblastic leukemia (ALL) with a 14q+ chromosome abnormality. Blood 53: 235–243

Rowley J D 1973 A new consistent chromosomal abnormality in chronic myelogenous leukaemia identified by quinacrine fluorescence and Giemsa staining. Nature 243: 290–293

Rowley J D 1974 Do human tumors show a chromosome pattern specific for each etiologic agent? Journal of the National Cancer Institute 52: 315–320

Rowley J D 1980a Ph^1 positive leukaemia, including chronic myelogenous leukaemia. Clinics in Haematology 9: 55–86

Rowley J D 1980b Chromosome abnormalities in acute lymphoblastic leukemia. Cancer Genetics and Cytogenetics 1: 263–271

Rowley J D 1980c Chromosome abnormalities in human leukemia. Annual Review of Genetics 14: 17–39

Rowley J D 1980d Chromosome abnormalities in cancer. Cancer Genetics and Cytogenetics 2: 175–198

Rowley J D 1982 Cytogenetic studies in hematologic disorders. Recent Advances in Hematology 3: 233–252

Rowley J D, Fukuhara S 1980 Chromosome studies in non-Hodgkin lymphomas. Seminars in Oncology 7: 255–266

Rowley J D, Golomb H M, Vardiman J W 1981 Nonrandom chromosome abnormalities in acute leukemia and dysmyelopoietic syndromes in patients with previously treated malignant disease. Blood 58: 759–767

Sakurai M, Hayata I, Sandberg A A 1976 Chromosomes and causation of human cancer and lukemia. XV Prognostic value of chromosomal findings in Ph^1-positive CML. Cancer Research 36: 313–318

Sakurai M, Sandberg A A 1976 Chromosomes and causation of human cancer and leukemia. XI Correlations of karyotypes with clinical features of acute myeloblastic leukemia. Cancer 37: 285–299

Sandberg A A 1979 Chromosomes in human cancer and leukemia. Elsevier North-Holland, New York.

Saxon A, Stevens R H, Golde D W 1979 Helper and suppressor T-lymphocyte leukemia in ataxia telangiectasia. New England Journal of Medicine 300: 700–704

Schroeder T M, German J 1974 Bloom's syndrome and Fanconi's anemia: demonstration of two distinctive patterns of chromosome disruption and rearrangement. Humangenetik 25: 299–306

Secker Walker L M, Lawler S D, Hardisty R M 1978 Prognostic implications of chromosomal findings in acute lymphoblastic leukaemia at diagnosis. British Medical Journal 2: 1529–1530

Second International Workshop on Chromosomes in Leukemia 1980 Cancer Genetics and Cytogenetics 2: 89–113

Sonta S, Sandberg A A 1977 Chromosomes and causation of human cancer and leukemia. XXIV Unusual and complex Ph^1 translocations and their clinical significance Blood 50: 691–697

Testa J R, Golomb H M, Rowley J D, Vardiman J W, Sweet D L 1978 Hypergranular promyelocytic leukemia (APL): cytogenetic and ultrastructural specificity. Blood 52: 272–280

Testa J R, Mintz U, Rowley J D, Vardiman J W, Golomb H M 1979 Evolution of karyotypes in acute nonlymphocytic leukemia. Cancer Research 39: 3619–3627

Testa J R, Rowley J D 1980a Chromosomes in leukaemia and lymphoma with special emphasis on methodology. In: Catovsky D (ed) The leukemic cell. Churchill Livingstone, Edinburgh p 184–202

Testa J R, Rowley J D 1980b Chromosomal banding patterns in patients with acute nonlymphocytic leukemia. Cancer Genetics and Cytogenetics 1: 239–247

Thompson M W, Bell R E, Little A S 1963 Familial 21-trisomic mongolism coexistent with leukemia. Canadian Medical Association Journal 88: 893–894

Van den Berghe H, David G, Broeckaert-Van Orshoven A, Louwagie A, Verwilghen R, Casteels-VanDaele M, Eggermont E, Eeckels R 1979a A new chromosome anomaly in acute lymphoblastic leukemia (ALL). Human Genetics 46: 173–180

Van den Berghe H, Parloir C, Gosseye S, Englebienne V, Cornu G, Sokal G 1979b Variant translocation in Burkitt lymphoma. Cancer Genetics and Cytogenetics 1: 9–14

Vidabaek A 1947 Heredity in human leukemia and its relation to cancer. Munksgaard, Copenhagen

Whang-Peng J, Canellos G P, Carbone P P, Tjio J H 1968 Clinical implications of cytogenetic variants in chronic myelocytic leukemia (CML). Blood 32: 755–766

Whang-Peng J, Knutsen T, Ziegler J, Leventhal B 1976 Cytogenetic studies in acute lymphocytic leukemia: special emphasis on long-term survival. Medical and Pediatric Oncology 2: 333–351

Zech L, Haglund U, Nilsson K, Klein G 1976 Characteristic chromosomal abnormalities in biopsies and lymphoid-cell lines from patients with Burkitt and non-Burkitt lymphomas. International Journal of Cancer 17: 47–56

Zuelzer W W, Cox D E 1969 Genetic aspects of leukemia. Seminars in Hematology 6: 228–249

Zuelzer W W, Inoue S, Thompson R I, Ottenbreit M J 1976 Long-term cytogenetic studies in acute leukemia of children; the nature of relapse. American Journal of ematology 1: 143–190

Immunodeficiency disorders

R. Hirschhorn and K. Hirschhorn

INTRODUCTION

The immune deficiency diseases are part of a spectrum of conditions involving defects in host defense against infections. Adequate host defense is dependent upon the interaction between phagocytic cells, immunocompetent cells and their products and the complement system. Diseases involving disorders of phagocytes and deficiencies of complement components will be discussed in subsequent chapters. Here we will concern ourselves with disorders of the immune system, including cellular and humoral immunity, both of which play a central role in our ability to resist infection. It is of course the occurrence of unusual types or frequency of infection which draws our attention to the possibility that a patient may be suffering from a host defense disorder.

The immune system as opposed to the other components of host defense is specific. Normal immunologic defenses are dependent upon memory of cells which recognise foreign antigens and are capable of appropriate responses, either by producing cytotoxic lymphocytes or releasing circulating antibodies specifically directed against the invading antigen. One other component of host defense which is specific involves the ability of lymphocytes to recognize infected cells, a process which is partly mediated by products of the major histocompatibility complex, another topic to be discussed in a subsequent chapter. Derangements of the immune system not only lead to deficient or abnormal responses to foreign antigens, such as invading organisms, but can also lead to abnormalities of another property of the immune system that of non-response to antigens of the host or recognition of self. This difficulty in appropriate recognition mechanisms leads in a number of immune deficiency diseases to a state of autoimmunity, either against specific antigens on cells of the host or against multiple organs. Therefore the discovery of autoimmune phenomena along with infection represents another clue leading to suspicion of the presence of an immune deficiency disease. Several reviews and monographs have appeared in the past few years (Ammann & Fudenberg, 1980; Asherson & Webster, 1980; Lawton & Cooper, 1980; Rosen, 1981; Waldman, Strober &Blaese, 1980) which contain numerous original references to matters described and discussed in this chapter, which we will not repeat in our bibliography.

Immunodeficiency disorders are usually classified as if they represent arrests at different stages of differentiation from a common stem cell along a pathway leading to two different major classes of immunologically com-

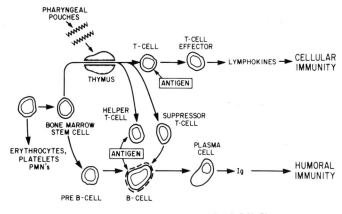

Fig. 78.1 Development of the immune system

petent cells (Fig. 78.1). This developmental approach, although not truly satisfactory, is currently the commonly used framework for diagnosis and classification. (World Health Organization Technical Report, 1978).

Several excellent text books exist which give detailed descriptions of the fields of basic and clinical immunology (Eisen, 1980; Sell, 1980; Roitt, 1980; Hood, Weissman & Wood, 1978; Fudenberg et al, 1980; Parker, 1980; Samter, 1978; Stiehm & Fulginiti, 1980). In order to lay a groundwork for our description of specific immunodeficiency disorders, we will briefly sketch some of the basic principles.

A pluripotent haematopoietic stem cell is thought to be the progenitor for both a lymphoid stem cell and a stem cell which gives rise to all of the other formed elements of the blood. The lymphoid stem cell can then further differentiate into two developmentally divergent but functionally interacting families of lymphocytes termed T and B cells. These two families of cells are respectively responsible for cellular and humoral immunity (Fig. 78.1).

CELLULAR IMMUNITY (T CELLS) (Table 78.1)

Under the influence of the thymus epithelium the lymphoid stem cell differentiates into cells expressing T cell characteristics, and which account for over 65% of peripheral blood lymphocytes in man. Further differentiation occurs following migration to peripheral tissues and is influenced by thymic humoral factors. This group of thymus dependent or 'T' cells can be recognized by their characteristic cell surface receptors. Differentiated

T cells in man carry receptors for sheep erythrocytes and can be identified, enumerated and separated by use of the rosettes which sheep erythrocytes form around these T cells. It is now apparent that this group of cells is not homogeneous, but contains several functionally and probably developmentally different classes of T cells which exert helper, suppressor and/or cytotoxic effects. More recently, monoclonal antibodies have been developed which have the potential to recognize either all T cells, the various different functionally distinct subsets of T cells, or T cell precursors. Several of these monoclonal antibodies are now commercially available and it can be expected that new insights will develop as such reagents are more widely used in the study of immunodeficient patients. Mature T cells also carry receptors for specific antigens. These receptors do not appear to be classical immunoglobulin but appear to share recognition sites for antigen with the appropriate antigen specific immunoglobulin.

T cells can be assessed functionally as well as enumerated and, in some immunodeficiency disorders, there is a dissociation of T cell function and number. In vivo, abnormalities of cellular immune function usually result in infections with intracellular organisms which are then not limited in course by the normal host defenses. Patients classically have moniliasis, pneumocystis carinii, generalized vaccinia and varicella, or other similar infections. Normal T cell function is also required for delayed type skin reactions to common 'recall' antigens such as candida, streptokinase-streptodonorase, tetanus and tuberculin. However, negative tests often occur in normal children under a year of age and skin testing with phytohaemagglutinin has therefore been utilized. De novo

Table 78.1

Lymphoid cells	Cell markers	In vitro functions	In vivo functions
T Cells (Cellular immunity)	1. Sheep erythrocyte ('E') rosettes 2. T cell specific antigens defined by monoclonal antibodies	1. Proliferation responses to soluble and cell surface antigens or polyclonal activators (e.g. PHA) 2. Mediator production 3. Cytotoxic responses (CML) 4. Regulatory functions	1. 80% of peripheral blood lymphocytes 2. Delayed type skin responses to antigens 3. Defense against intracellular fungi, parasites, viruses 4. Graft rejection 5. Graft vs. Host Disease (GVH)
B Cells (Humoral immunity)	1. C_3 receptors 2. E_c receptors 3. EBV receptors 4. Surface Ig 5. Intracellular Ig 6. B cell specific antigens	1. Immunoglobulin synthesis 2. Proliferation responses to EBV, some polyclonal activators and T cell factors	1. Serum immunoglobulin (IgG, IgA, IgM, IgE, IgD) 2. Specific antibodies 3. Defense against extracellular bacteria and viruses
Null Cells	1. No 'E' or surface Ig 2. Heterogeneous for C_3 and F_c receptors and I_a antigens	1. Precursors of T, B, myeloid and erythroid cells 2. Natural killer (NK) activity 3. Antibody dependent cellular cytotoxicity (ADCC)	1. ? Defense against tumour cells

sensitization with DNCB tests the ability both to mount and to recall a delayed hypersensitivity skin reaction. However, because of the intense reaction which occurs in normal individuals, this test is usually utilized only if in vitro tests reveal a profound defect of cellular immune function.

Initial assessment of cellular immune function can therefore be provided by determination of the peripheral lymphocyte count, enumeration of T cells, skin testing, routine chest X–ray in order to visualize the thymic shadow and a careful clinical history of types and frequencies of infections, as well as a family history.

In vitro, T cells respond to several different stimuli including 'polyclonal activators', specific antigens and allogeneic cells. As a result of interaction with these stimuli, lymphocytes increase their rates of synthesis of RNA, protein and DNA and then divide. This proliferative response is most commonly measured by determining the incorporation of radio-labelled thymidine into DNA, although mitotic rate can be used as a rough estimate. Virtually all T cells respond to a group of substances including plant lectins such as PHA, which are therefore termed 'polyclonal activators'. Only a subclass of 'antigen specific' T lymphocytes initially respond to antigens or foreign molecules. This 'antigen specific' response is only detected (under the standard in vitro conditions) if the donor of the lymphocytes has been previously exposed in vivo to the antigen. Finally, a subclass of T lymphocytes responds to alloantigens on cell surfaces, primarily to antigens coded for by the Ia like or 'D' region of the histocompatibility complex, and present on surfaces of B lymphocytes. This response to allogeneic determinants is termed the mixed lymphocyte reaction or MLR since lymphocytes from two different individuals are mixed to elicit the response. The MLR is usually measured in such a fashion that the response of cells from only one of the individuals is measured (one way MLR). It is now clear that many of these stimuli also activate T cells which can then either suppress or help the reaction of other T cells and modulate the reactions of B cells.

T cells function either directly by means of cell to cell contact or by releasing soluble mediators. Thus, activated T cells release a number of factors or 'lymphokines' which modulate the activity not only of other lymphoid cells but also of eosinophils, polymorphonuclear leucocytes and macrophages. The nature of these factors and their role in regulating the immune response is currently under active investigation. Immunodeficient patients may show a dissociation of ability to release soluble mediators and ability to respond to various stimuli. T lymphocytes when activated can also exhibit both nonspecific and specific cytotoxicity.

HUMORAL IMMUNITY (B CELLS) (Table 78.1)

The second major pathway of lymphoid development results in a terminally differentiated B cell secreting immunoglobulins (antibodies) which have recognition sites for specific antigens. Immunoglobulins are a group of related glycoproteins containing two 'heavy' polypeptide chains and two 'light' polypeptide chains (Fig. 78.2). The prototypic four chain molecule can be broken into two major fragments; an Fab portion consisting of the light chains linked to the N-terminal half of the heavy chains, and the Fc portion, consisting of the carboxy terminal half of the two heavy chains. The Fab portion contains the antigen binding site while the Fc

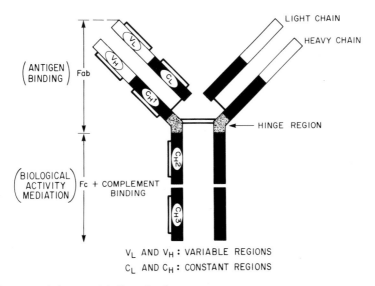

V_L AND V_H : VARIABLE REGIONS

C_L AND C_H : CONSTANT REGIONS

Fig. 78.2 Diagram of a prototypic immunoglobulin molecule

portion contains sites for activation of complement and for binding of immunoglobulin to diverse cell types via cell membrane Fc receptors. The area of the heavy chains which joins the Fc and Fab portions is the hinge region and the two heavy chains are joined at this site by several disulphide bonds. The Fab portion can be further subdivided into an N-terminal region which is variable in amino acid sequence in both the heavy and light chains and which determines antibody specificity, and a constant region (C_H1 and C_L) which is constant in amino acid sequence for a given class or subclass of heavy or light chains. There are five different types of heavy chains, gamma, alpha, mu, delta and epsilon, which differ from each other in the amino acid sequence of their constant regions. There are only two different classes of light chains, kappa and lambda, which differ from each other as to their constant regions. Both kappa and lambda light chains combine with all of the different classes of heavy chains, but a single immunoglobulin molecule contains only one class of light chain and one class of heavy chain. The combination of heavy and light chains results in five different classes of immunoglobulins in man: IgG, IgA, IgM, IgD and IgE. IgG is the most abundant serum immunoglobulin and is also the only immunoglobulin transferred across the placenta. IgA is the primary immunoglobulin in secretions, where it is associated as a dimer with a 'secretory component'. IgM is the next most abundant serum immunoglobulin, usually exists as a 17S pentamer and rises first after a primary response to antigenic challenge. Elevation of IgM in neonates usually indicates intrauterine infection. IgD concentrations in serum are minute but IgD is present on B cell surfaces. IgE is lowest in concentration in serum, and is responsible for immediate hypersensitivity or allergic reactions and release of mediators such as histamine from basophils and mast cells. Normal values of all the immunoglobulins vary with age and environment and diminished concentrations may reflect increased rates of degradation as well as decreased rates of synthesis.

Genetic polymorphisms have been described for the kappa light chain (Inv), for the gamma heavy chain (Gm), and for the alpha heavy chain (Am). Recent studies have indicated that the heavy chain for immunoglobulin of IgG, IgA and IgM and, by analogy, IgD and IgE are located on the fourteenth human chromosome (Croce et al, 1979; Smith et al, 1981). The gene for the kappa light chain has been mapped to chromosome two (McBride et al, 1982), and that for the lambda light chain to chromosome twenty two (Erickson et al, 1981). The molecular genetics of immunoglobulin synthesis has proven to be a complex process, so far unique for any gene product. In brief, the genes for the variable and hinge regions are combined with different constant regions by a series of translocations and deletions. As a result, the same variable region can be expressed by immunoglobulin molecules of several different classes. Several recent reviews have appeared on this rapidly moving subject (Davis, Kim & Hood, 1980; Maki et al, 1980).

The development of the terminally differentiated immunoglobulin secreting plasma cell from the primary stem cell occurs in several steps, probably beginning first in fetal liver and then in the bone marrow. The first stage in the differentiation of the stem cell is the appearance of small amounts of cytoplasmic immunoglobulin of the IgM class and possibly only of mu heavy chains. These cells subsequently develop surface immunoglobulin, initially of the IgM class, later of the IgD, IgG, and IgA classes. During this stage, B cells develop receptors for EBV virus, C3 complement components and the Fc portion of aggregated immunoglobulin. Indirect evidence from patients with immunodeficiency suggests that the development of EBV receptors occurs earliest and can be dissociated from the development of the complement receptors. By this stage of maturation, the B cell secretes as well as synthesizes immunoglobulins. The next stage of B cell differentiation is antigen specific, in that the B cells secrete antibodies which are specifically directed against an immunising antigen. In some disorders, there is a marked dissociation between the ability to synthesize immunoglobulins and that to synthesize specific antibodies in response to immunisation with antigens. It is also clear that T cell function is required for the synthesis of certain antibodies and that T cell function markedly modulates the ability of B cells both to synthesize immunoglobulins and specific antibodies.

Humoral immune function can be evaluated in vivo and in vitro. In vivo, severely defective humoral immunity is usually associated with recurrent pyogenic infections such as pneumococcal pneumonia, haemophilus influenza meningitis, otitis media, etc. With more prolonged defective humoral immunity (i.e. late onset and/or treated infantile agammaglobulinaemia), the effects of chronic pulmonary disease, diarrheal disorders, 'autoimmune phenomena' and infections with viruses which follow an unusual 'slow virus' type of course, are more prominent. In vivo assessment includes quantitative determination of serum IgG, IgM, IgA and IgE by radial immunodiffusion, and/or radioimmunoassay, isohaemagglutinins for evaluation of functional IgM, and if still available, Schick test. Specific antibodies are assessed both by reimmunising and/or actively immunising with a variety of protein and polysaccharide antigens (never as live agents) such as diptheria, tetanus, killed poliomyelitis vaccine, pneumococcal vaccine, etc. and determining the presence and/or the rise of specific antibody titer.

In vitro studies include enumeration of B cells by virtue of cell surface and intracytoplasmic immunoglobulins (complement and Fc receptors are also found on other cell types and are therefore less useful for initial screening). In vitro functional assays are performed by stimulating peripheral blood lymphocytes with B cell mitogens such as pokeweed mitogen, (although this mitogen is not totally B cell specific) and measuring rates of immunoglobulin synthesis.

OTHER LYMPHOID CELLS

The last class of lymphocytes are the so called null cells which derive their name from the fact that they bear neither the sheep E rosette receptor characteristic of T cells nor the immunoglobulins characteristic of B cells. This null cell population is truly a heterogeneous population and includes within it the so called natural killer (NK) cell. Studies of natural cytotoxicity or NK activity are currently an active area of research.

SPECIFIC INHERITED IMMUNODEFICIENCY DISORDERS (Table 78.2)

Combined cellular and humoral immune defects

Severe combined immunodeficiency disease
Severe combined immunodeficiency disease (SCID) is characterized by profound defects of both cellular and humoral immunity and is the most rapidly progressive and devastating of the primary immunodeficiency syndromes. This syndrome was originally called 'essential lymphocytophthisis', thymic alymphoplasia or Swiss type agammaglobulinemia, depending upon the parameters which could be measured at the time. Patients present within the first few months of life with recurrent, persistent infections due to bacterial, viral and fungal pathogens. Candida infection is almost universal and chronic pneumonitis due to infection with *pneumocystis carinii* or other organisms is extremely common. Chronic watery diarrhea, associated with various organisms was almost universal in the past. A morbilliform exanthematous rash or exfoliative dermatitis may develop, the latter usually following blood transfusion and probably representing *graft versus host disease* (GVH) due to transfusion of foreign lymphocytes. Chimaerism and GVH can also result from transplacental passage of maternal lymphocytes and in either case, the occurrence of GVH with attendant hepatosplenomegaly and eosinophilia can obscure the diagnosis of SCID. Only irradiated blood should be transfused. Immunisation with live viruses (e.g. polio or vaccinia) can have disastrous consequences and should not be performed. The course of SCID, even without iatrogenic complications, is rapidly progressive, associated with wasting and runting and, if untreated, is fatal by two years of age.

Virtually all parameters of cellular and humoral immunity (Table 78.1) are abnormal. Patients usually have absent tonsils, small or absent lymph nodes, absent thymic shadow, are lymphopenic and have markedly diminished numbers of T cells. Lymphopenia may wax and wane but in vitro responses are absent or reduced. Immunoglobulins are usually absent, although passively transferred maternal immunoglobulin of the IgG class can be present during the first six months of life. Gm typing can indicate if IgG is maternally derived. Failure of development of serum IgA and/or IgM (which do not cross the placenta) can often provide a sensitive marker for immunoglobulin abnormality early in life. B cells may be present. Pathologically, there is a lack of normal lymph node architecture and a small, dysplastic or fetal thymus.

The clinical picture of recently reported cases of SCID would appear to be slightly less severe at initial diagnosis (Hitzig &Kenny, 1978). This may reflect earlier diagnosis due to the development and wider availability of more sensitive and easily applied in vitro diagnostic tests for evaluation of both cellular immunity and quantitation of immunoglobulins. Additionally, development and widespread and vigorous use of effective antibacterial, antifungal and antiprotozoal agents may have altered the rapidity of the clinical course and immunologic attrition. For example, the incidence of diarrhea has declined from 80% in 1968 to only 47% in 1976. Lymphopenia was found in 90% of cases in 1968 compared to 50% in 1976, but in all cases response to PHA was absent or markedly diminished. Further immunologic attrition would appear to account for the fact that all untreated children, independent of their status at diagnosis, still die early in life.

It is now clear that some patients may initially have relatively normal amounts of immunoglobulins, albeit usually of restricted heterogeneity and that further immunologic attrition then occurs over time. Such patients, previously classified as Nezelof syndrome, are considered to represent part of the spectrum of SCID (see ADA deficiency as an example).

Autosomal recessive SCID and adenosine deaminase (ADA) deficiency
In 1972, Giblett and coworkers described two children who presented with autosomal recessive combined immunodeficiency, who both also had autosomal recessive inherited absence of the enzyme adenosine deaminase (ADA). This represented the first molecular defect defined in immunodeficiency disorders. (Reviewed in Ciba Foundation Symposium, 1979; Pollara et al, 1979; and Hirschhorn & Martin, 1978).

ADA deficiency has been estimated to account for SCID in 1/3 to 1/2 of families where the mode of inheritance is not clearly X–linked. In a small sample of definitely autosomal recessively inherited SCID (as defined by the occurrence of an affected female), the incidence of ADA deficiency has been found to be 57% with 95% confidence limits of 18–90%. Therefore a substantial proportion of autosomal recessive SCID appears to be due to deficiency of ADA. These estimates are consistent with the results of an informal survey of 130 patients with SCID (both autosomal recessive and X–linked) which revealed 22% with ADA deficiency. Approximately 80–90% of ADA deficient SCID patients are indistinguishable clinically as well as by in vitro tests of immune function from other patients with SCID. Normal numbers of lymphocytes and T lymphocytes as well as some degree of response to PHA may be found at birth and the diagnosis can most reliably be made at birth in a family at risk by determination of ADA activity in the red cells. The disease is progressive and any residual T cell function found at birth rapidly disappears. In 10–15% of the cases, onset of disease may occur later than 3–6

months. For example, one of the first reported patients, followed closely because of the prior death of a sib, was apparently immunocompetent and healthy until over two years of age. The outstanding feature in this late onset group is the persistence of immunoglobulins and even the presence of specific antibody. These patients were undoubtedly originally classified as having Nezelof syndrome. However, immunoglobulin levels eventually fall and in one case there was a preterminal monoclonal IgG. Unless treated, death has occurred by three years of age and usually earlier.

While genetic heterogeneity may contribute to the phenotypic diversity, this degree of differences in clinical manifestations has been found between sibs, probably indicating influence of environmental factors, although interaction with other genetic loci has not been ruled out.

Bony abnormalities, originally appreciated radiologi-

Table 78.2 Primary immunodeficiency disorders

	Mode of inheritance	
	X–linked	AR
1. *Combined humoral (B Cell) and cellular (T Cell) immune defects*		
Severe combined immunodeficiency (SCID)		+
Adenosine deaminase deficiency	–	+
Other SCID	+	+
With leukopaenia (reticular dysgenesis)	–	+
Cellular immunodeficiency with abnormal immunoglobulins (? Nezelof)	?	?
2. *Humoral (B Cell) immune defects*		
Infantile agammaglobulinaemia	+	(rare)
Immunodeficiency with hyper IgM	+	?
Common variable hyogammaglobulinaemia	?	?
Lymphoproliferative syndrome	+	?
Selective IgA deficiency	–	+ (? AD)
Selective IgM deficiency	?	?
Selective IgG subclass deficiency	–	+
Hyper IgE, eczema and recurrent infections	–	+ (? AD)
3. *Cellular (T Cell) immune defects*		
Purine nucleoside phosphorylase deficiency	–	+
Chronic mucocutaneous candidiasis (with or without endocrinopathy)	–	+
Nezelof syndrome	?	?
4. *Specific syndromes involving other organ systems with immunodeficiency as a significant manifestation*		
Wiskott Aldrich syndrome	+	–
Ataxia telangiectasia	–	+
Short limbed dwarfism with cartilage hair hypoplasia and cellular immunodeficiency		
with SCID	?	+
With antibody deficiency	–	+
Transcobalamin II deficiency	–	+
Multiple carboxylase deficiency	–	+
Chromosome 18 abnormalities		
Down syndrome		
5. *Metabolic disorders with suspected immunodeficiency*		
Orotic aciduria	–	+
Methylmalonic aciduria	–	+
Storage disorders	+	+

AR = autosomal recessive; AD = autosomal dominant; X-linked = X-linked recessive

cally and subsequently studied pathologically, occur frequently in patients with ADA deficient SCID. This bony abnormality (8 of 13 families) was evident on physical examination as prominence of the costochondral rib junctions, similar to a rachitic rosary. On X–ray, cupping and flaring of the costochondral junctions was seen as well as a dysplastic pelvis. However, these changes are not pathognomonic and similar radiologic changes can be observed in non-immunodeficient, severely malnourished patients as well as ADA-normal immunodeficient patients. Although the radiologic changes may not be specific, these bony alterations have served to alert physicians to the possibility of ADA-deficient SCID. Thymic pathology is also proposed to differ in the ADA deficient cases, with the retention of some Hassall's corpuscles suggesting secondary atrophy of a previously differentiated thymus. However, on a practical level, examination of thymic pathology in patients from seven kindreds with and without ADA deficiency did not allow for consistent correlation between the type of thymic pathology and the presence or absence of ADA deficiency.

Currently, numerous investigators are attempting to define the precise pathophysiologic mechanisms responsible for the relatively specific toxicity for the immune system. Whatever the mechanism, it is clear that affected children accumulate the substrates of the deficient enzyme, adenosine and deoxyadenosine, that they excrete massive amounts of deoxyadenosine in urine and that they accumulate massive amounts of the phosphorylated compound deoxy ATP in their cells. The most probable toxic metabolite is deoxy ATP, a potent allosteric inhibitor of ribonucleotide reductase and therefore of DNA synthesis. Other compounds, such as methylated adenine derivatives, have been found to accumulate, but their significance is speculative.

ADA deficiency without immunodeficiency. At least four individuals have been described who lack ADA in their erythrocytes and who are immunocompetent. Two such individuals have been found to have ADA in other cells, sufficient to prevent accumulation of toxic metabolites. In these two cases, an unstable enzyme appears to explain the lack of enzyme in erythrocytes but its presence in cells actively synthesizing new proteins.

Other forms of SCID with unusual characteristics

Dissociation of quantitative measures and function. Normal numbers of lymphocytes with markers characteristic of T and B cells, plasma cells and normal quantities of immunoglobulin have been reported in two male offspring of a consanguineous family. (Gelfand et al, 1979). However, all functional parameters (Table 78.1) were markedly abnormal. A defect in the mobility of Con A receptors was found in the patients' lymphoid cells. It can be expected that more cases of SCID with

dissociation of quantitative and functional parameters (with or without a Con A capping defect) will be described as the appropriate functional assays are applied more widely.

Bare lymphocyte syndrome. Five kindred have been described in which lymphocytes and platelets from affected children lack HLA A, B and C determinants as well as the associated subunit, beta$_2$-microglobulin (Touraine, 1981). These proteins are present in normal amounts on other cell types, suggesting a membrane defect limited to lymphocytes and platelets. The clinical picture has ranged from classical SCID, albeit with some retention of parameters of cellular and humoral immunity to a less rapidly progressive clinical picture and a less complete absence of HLA A, B and C antigens and beta$_2$-microglobulin. The inheritance appears to be autosomal recessive.

Reticular dysgenesis or SCID with granulocytopenia Six cases in five families have been reported of this rare disorder characterized by virtually complete loss of granulocytes and lymphocytes, a small thymus, but normal erythrocytes and platelets. In some cases, the diminution in lymphocyte and granulocyte numbers may initially be less profound and in one case, although response of cord blood lymphocytes to PHA was absent, the percentage of T lymphocytes was normal (Ownby et al, 1976). All reported patients died of infections by four months of age, which is not surprising in view of the deficit in two major host defense systems. The disorder appears to be autosomally recessively inherited. Prenatal diagnosis might in theory be feasible by examination of fetal peripheral blood obtained by fetoscopy. Attempts at bone marrow transplantation have not been reported.

Therapy

Complete immunologic reconstitution (as well as clearing of abnormal metabolites in ADA deficiency) can be obtained by bone marrow transplantation if a histocompatible sib (or other family member in a consanguineous family) is available (Bortin & Rimm, 1977). However, there is only a 1/4 chance for a normal sib to be histocompatible. Given a reasonable probability of two normal living sibs, the probability of finding a compatible sib donor is less than half (7/16). However, if the patient is the offspring of a first cousin marriage, not only will there be a higher probability of finding a compatible sib donor, but there is a small but significant chance (3/64) that one of the parents is compatible. In addition, the search for compatible donors in such consanguineous families should extend at least to aunts and uncles since even they have a reasonable although smaller chance of being compatible. These are important considerations because there is an increased rate of consanguinity in the parents of children with rare recessive disorders. GVH reactions can occur even when current 'typing' procedures predict a successful transplant. Currently, no equally effective alternative therapy is available. Therapy is generally supportive and includes early and vigorous use of antibiotics for infections, administration of gammaglobulin and attempts at replacement of thymic derived factors by administration of thymosin Fraction V or cultured thymic epithelial explants. Transplantation of fetal liver cells, which contain lymphoid cell precursors which presumably are too immature to be capable of mounting a GVH, has also been attempted with some reported success in rare patients. Isolation in a completely sterile environment has also been successful but is clearly impractical. In ADA deficient SCID, multiple partial exchange transfusions with normal irradiated packed erythrocytes (which contain both the deficient enzyme and transport sites for the accumulated substrates) has resulted in marked diminution of abnormal metabolites, increased growth rate and length of survival and partial restoration of immunologic function. However, it is now apparent that such therapy provides only temporary and/or partial amelioration in the hope that in the interim, more permanent therapy will become available.

Genetics

The syndrome of SCID is genetically heterogeneous. The incidence of SCID has been estimated as between 1/100 000 and 1/500 000 live births, but the diagnosis is often missed and this may be a gross under-estimate of the incidence of this disorder. Both X–linked and autosomal recessive modes of inheritance as well as 'sporadic' cases have been found. The ratio of affected males to females in the whole group is approximately 3:1, suggesting that half of all cases are X–linked and that a majority of families with a single affected child who is male will be carrying an X–linked gene for SCID. A more accurate estimate in a particular family can be calculated by the use of Bayesian mathematics. The *gene* frequency for the X–linked gene is $\frac{1}{2}$ the incidence of SCID in the population. The *gene* frequency of the autosomal recessive would be markedly greater (the square root of $\frac{1}{2}$ the population incidence), if all autosomal cases were caused by the same abnormal gene. Since, however, there are at least two, and probably more, different loci responsible for autosomal recessive SCID (see below), the combined frequencies of genes responsible for autosomal recessive SCID is even higher.

Based upon newborn screening, the incidence of complete ADA deficiency in the population would appear to be less than one in a million and the incidence of heterozygous carriers would then be less than one in 500. ADA deficient SCID can be diagnosed prenatally by assay of amniotic fluid fibroblasts for ADA activity. Other forms of SCID could in theory be diagnosed prenatally be testing in vitro responses of fetal blood lym-

phocytes obtained by fetoscopy to polyclonal activators and allogeneic cells (responses known to develop in the beginning of the second trimester). This approach has not as yet been tested in a pregnancey at risk. In X–linked SCID, females will be unaffected, but it must be emphasized that occurrence of multiple male affected children does not establish X–linkage. For example, even in a family with three affected males, there is approximately a 12.5% risk of autosomal recessive inheritance. Therefore, except in cases of clear, well documented X–linkage, all cases of SCID should be tested for ADA deficiency, since this is currently the only form of SCID which can be easily diagnosed prenatally.

Detection of heterozygous carriers of SCID is currently feasible only for ADA deficiency. Using quantitative determination of erythrocyte ADA, there is an approximately 10% overlap between carriers and normals. All living family members should be phenotyped for the normal genetic polymorphism of ADA (codominant expression of two common alleles) since anomalous inheritance of the polymorphism can demonstrate that a 'null' allele is segregating in the family. Based upon the gene frequency of the polymorphic forms of ADA, this approach can be diagnostic in approximately 30% of families if grandparents, uncles, aunts, etc. are tested.

Primary B cell deficiencies: humoral immune defects

Disorders of humoral immunity or antibody deficiency disorders can be of infantile or late onset, involve absence of all classes or only specific classes of immunoglobulins, with or without absence of B cells of different maturational stages. In rare cases, quantitatively normal but functionally inactive immunoglobulins can occur. The primary clinical manifestation in all of these disorders is recurrent, invasive, severe infection with common pyogenic bacteria such as *haemophilus influenza* and *streptococcus pneumoniae*. The infections usually respond to vigorous antibiotic therapy but recur. The response to most viral, fungal or mycobacterial infections is normal, reflecting the retention of normal T cell immunity. In the later onset form, diarrheal disorders, chronic pulmonary disease and autoimmune phenomena are more prominent features and variable degrees of cellular immune defects may become apparent.

Infantile agammaglobulinaemia

Infantile X–linked agammaglobulinaemia (Bruton disease) is the classical example of an isolated B cell defect (Rosen, 1980). The clinical course of these patients is such that they are usually healthy during the first six months of life, probably reflecting the presence of adequate amounts of placentally transferred maternal IgG. They then begin to suffer from multiple recurrent infections usually with pyogenic organisms, while infections with viruses and gram negative bacteria are not strikingly increased. The infections are most prominent at sites of initial contact with pathogens and include infections of the upper and lower respiratory tract and skin and eventually complications of sepsis such as meningitis. Although the use of antibiotics has lessened mortality from acute infections, without more specific therapy, these patients will go on to develop chronic pulmonary disease, bronchiectasis and respiratory failure. These children are more susceptible to infection with hepatitis virus and enteroviruses, particularly ECHO and poliomyelitis viruses. Paralytic polio can follow administration of live polio vaccine and a dermatomyositis-like syndrome apparently due to ECHO virus can evolve even in patients treated with gammaglobulin. These patients also often develop rheumatoid-like arthritis which improves with therapy. Haemolytic anaemia and asthma are also seen.

The diagnosis is made by demonstrating a severe deficiency of IgG, IgM and IgA by immunoelectrophoresis or quantitative determination of immunoglobulins. The diagnosis is often suggested by the presence of hypoplastic tonsils; lymph nodes may appear to be present, but biopsy reveals hyperplasia of reticular cells. As expected, B cells are lacking in over 90% of patients with X-linked agammaglobulinaemia although pre-B cells can be detected and isolated from bone marrow by special techniques. There may be some degree of intra-familial variation as to the completeness of absence of B cells. In rare cases of X-linked agammaglobulinaemia, B cells are present although these probably represent less mature B cells. T cell immunity is normal in affected children and childhood exanthems are handled normally. Standard therapy consists of 0.6 ml/kg immunoglobulin (100 mg/kg) every month by deep IM injection preceded by three loading doses, but a newly developed intravenous preparation may, after additional clinical testing, become the treatment of choice. Almost all cases of agammaglobulinaemia are X-linked in that there is no male to male transmission, the healthy sisters of affected patients have affected male children and maternal uncles are affected.

Infantile agammaglobulinaemia must be differentiated from transient hypogammaglublinaemia of infancy in which there is a prolongation of the normal physiologic decline in IgG. Normally, after birth, the total IgG initially falls precipitously, then slowly begins to rise after a nadir at 5–6 months of age, reflecting the catabolism of maternal IgG counterbalanced by the slow increase in the child's own synthesis of IgG. Simultaneously, IgA and IgM concentrations begin to increase. In transient hypogammaglobulinaemia, the expected rises can be delayed until 3 years of age. Sequential measurements demonstrating increases in IgA and IgM as well as determination of B cell numbers help to differentiate this temporary disorder from X-linked agammaglobulinaemia. When present, a family history of maternal male relatives or previous male sibs with persistant agammaglobulinaemia (IgG less than 200 mg percent, and virtually absent IgM, IgA, IgD and IgE) aids in diagnosis.

Genetics. Inheritance is that of a classical X-linked disorder. As in any lethal X-linked disorder, one third of patients should reflect new mutations and therefore a family history may not be obtained. The X-linkage indicates that the defect is not at the level of the structural genes for immunoglobulins which are located on autosomal chromosomes (number 14 for the heavy chains). No definite linkage to X-chromosome markers has been reported, although loose linkage to Xga is possible with low positive lod scores at a recombination fraction of 30 per cent (Race & Sanger, 1975). Prenatal diagnosis is not available other than that based on the 50% chance of males being affected and all females being unaffected. Absence of B cells in fetal blood might in theory be diagnostic, if a previously affected child is known to have lacked B cells at birth. Heterozygote detection for female carriers is not currently available.

There is a familial incidence of transient hypogammaglobulinaemia but the formal genetics of this undoubtedly heterogeneous disorder has not been delineated. There is a high incidence of transient hypogammaglobulinaemia in sibs of children with immunodeficiency disorders but definitive studies are lacking to demonstrate that the increased incidence does not simply reflect more frequent determinations of immunogloblins in these children. In a small population of patients with transient hypogammaglobulinaemia, we could not detect any heterozygotes for ADA deficiency, although transient hypogammaglobulinaemia has been observed in heterozygous sibs of ADA deficient patients. The bulk of transient hypogammaglobulinaemia would appear to be unassociated with a familial incidence of immunodeficiency.

Autosomal recessive infantile agammaglobulinaemia

Rare cases have been described of females affected with infantile agammaglobulinaemia, clinically indistinguishable from the X-linked form. They are unlikely to represent cases of an X-linked recessive mutant gene which is expressed in females because of extreme Lyonisation, since more than one affected female in a family has been reported, and patients have appeared in families without a history of the X-linked disorder.

X-linked agammaglobulinaemia and isolated growth hormone deficiency

A kindred with X-linked agammaglobulinaemia and isolated growth hormone deficiency has recently been reported (Fleisher et al, 1980).

Late onset or common variable hypogammaglobulinaemia

Common variable hypogammaglobulinaemia is essentially a wastebasket diagnosis and encompasses a majority of patients with humoral immune defects. This group of disorder has unfortunately been previously termed 'acquired agammaglobulinaemia'. This term should not be used in view of the common occurence of genetic disorders which are not phenotypically manifest until adult life and of genetic disorders such as alpha-1-antitrypsin deficiency which require as yet poorly defined environmental challenges to result in disease. This is a clinical entity characterized by late-onset panhypogammaglobulinaemia, although IgE production may be unaffected. A significant proportion of patients also have defects in some parameters of cell mediated immunity. Men and women are equally affected and the disorder can begin at any age. The clinical manifestations (Hermans, Diaz-Buxo & Stobo, 1976) include recurrent sinobronchopulmonary infections, chronic diarrhea with malabsorption, giardiasis and small bowel abnormalities including nodular lymphoid hyperplasia. In addition, other phenomena including pernicious anaemia, abnormalities of complement, cholelithiasis, thyroid abnormalities and neoplasia occur in a significant proportion of patients. Lymphadenopathy and splenomegaly due to reticular cell hyperplasia is common.

This group of disorders is also heterogeneous when examined at the cellular level. Patients may have no B cells as in the X–linked infantile syndrome but more often B cells are normal or even increased in number. B cells from a small subset of patients synthesize but do not secrete immunoglobulin in vitro. Some of these latter patients appear to be unable to glycosylate immunoglobulin normally and their B cells either lack or have markedly diminished EBV receptors (Schwaber et al, 1980). In some cases, increased T cell suppression of B cell function is found (Waldmann et al, 1976).

The possible role of heredity in this heterogeneous group is presently basically undefined. Several investigators have documented an increased incidence of serologic abnormalities or impairment of leucocyte function and autoimmunity in family members. Unfortunately, many of these studies do not have a carefully age matched control population. Familial constellations with manifestations among sibs ranging from agammaglobulinaemia to selective immunoglobulin deficiency have been described. Although some of these disorders may well represent primarily the effects of environmental factors, it is highly likely that further dissection and discovery of specific molecular defects will reveal a strong genetic component for these disorders.

Hyper IgM with hypogammaglobulinaemia
Hypogammaglobulinaemia with raised IgM is a group of disorders characterized by the presence of increased amounts of IgM and usually also IgD with a decrease in the other immunoglobulins. Clinically, patients show increased susceptibility to recurrent pyogenic infections, to autoimmune disease associated with IgM antibodies and to malignant lymphoproliferation of IgM producing B cells (Geha et al, 1979). B cells are normal in number but qualitatively abnormal in that they either spontaneously secrete or can be driven to secrete IgM in vitro but cannot be induced in vivo to secrete IgG. The disease is often seen as an X–linked form, but autosomal recessive, sporadic early or later onset forms have also been reported.

X–linked lymphoproliferative syndrome
The precise definition of this syndrome is currently evolving and it is not listed in the WHO classification. The relationship of the X–linked lymphoproliferative syndrome (Duncan Disease) to common variable hypogammaglobulinaemia and/or Hyper IgM is not clear. This syndrome could illustrate the marked variation in phenotype which can be expected in the immunodeficiency disorders because of the dependence upon interaction with environment for expression. An X–linked recessive lymphoproliferative syndrome has been described in several large kindreds (Purtillo et al, 1977). The phenotypes described in a single family are of two major types, a proliferative phenotype including fatal infectious mononucleosis, Burkitt's lymphoma or plasmacytoma and an aproliferative phenotype including late onset agammaglobulinaemia, agranulocytosis or aplastic anaemia. (Other abnormalities were described in a large kindred but may reflect some degree of earlier inbreeding, suggested by the marriages of three sisters to three brothers in the kindred.) What is clear is that there appears to be an X–linked recessive disorder which results in an inability to contain infection with EBV virus. Affected male children at some time in the course may develop hyper IgM, agammaglobulinaemia, aplastic anaemia or lymphoid malignancies.

Selective IgA deficiency
Selective IgA deficiency is the most commonly observed immunodeficiency with an incidence of 0.1–0.2% in normal blood donors. There is a 14 fold increase in incidence of IgA deficiency among the first degree relatives of these normal individuals. (Koistinen, 1976; Ammann & Hong, 1980). In most of such individuals, this deficiency is not associated with any disease. However, normal blood donors are by definition healthy adults and therefore individuals with an increases predisposition to infection beginning in childhood would not be included. A prospective study with matched controls beginning at an early age would be required to more critically determine the significance of IgA deficiency in the general population. Familial occurrence of IgA deficiency has been reported on numerous occasions, with patterns of inheritance consistent with both an autosomal dominant and

autosomal recessive mode of inheritance and associated with increased infections, primarily sinopulmonary in nature. Discordance of IgA deficiency in identical twins has been described, indicating a strong environmental component for the determination of serum IgA. A high incidence of IgA deficiency has also been reported in patients with recurrent infections, autoimmune disorders such as rheumatoid arthritis, systemic lupus erythematosus, malabsorption syndrome, sometimes with gluten sensitivity, childhood asthma and other atopic disease. The possible aetiologic relationship of IgA deficiency and the disease are difficult to evaluate since most studies involve correlating types of disease with IgA deficiency in a population referred because of frequent infections, atopy, etc.

IgA deficiency is also found in $\frac{1}{3}$ to $\frac{1}{2}$ of individuals with a wide variety of chromosome 18 abnormalities, is associated with ataxia telangiectasia (see below) and can presage development of hypogammaglobulinaemia. Clearly, the IgA deficiency associated with defects in either the short or long arm of chromosome 18 does not involve the structural gene for IgA which presumably would be on a different chromosome (chromosome 14). As a note of warning, IgA deficient individuals often have antibodies to IgA and can have a severe transfusion reaction when given normal whole blood or plasma.

Selective IgM deficiency

Selective IgM deficiency, in contrast to selective IgA deficiency, is rare. It has been reported in two patients with septicaemia, meningococcal meningitis, malabsorption, haemolytic anaemia and eczema. Familial aggregation has been noted and the deficiency has been described in sibs. A study in Great Britain reported fairly high frequency of isolated deficiency of IgM. Approximately 20% of subjects were asymptomatic while 60% had severe recurrent infections, often with bacteraemia. The condition was frequently familial and was four times more common in males than females (Hobbs, 1975).

Selective IgG subclass deficiency

Selective deficiency of specific IgG subclasses either due to regulatory or structural mutations could in theory lead to inability to cope with a limited spectrum of infectious agents. This hypothesis is based upon the observation that certain antibody activities occur largely within specific subclasses of IgG. Various abnormalities in subclass distribution and an apparent structural gene defect in a family have been reported in patients examined because of immunodeficiency (Yount et al, 1970). Here again, cause and effect relationships are unclear and possibly must await dissection at the level of the DNA. Alternatively, these variants may reflect primary imbalance of T cell subsets.

Hyper IgE and recurrent infections

The hyper IgE syndrome would appear to encompass at least two or more different syndromes which are often confused. The first is a rare syndrome described by Buckley (Buckley, 1980) characterized by recurrent staphylococcal abscesses, markedly elevated serum IgE, coarsened facies and a history of pruritic dermatitis. The severe recurrent staphylococal abscesses often begin in infancy and involve skin, lungs, joints and other sites, with virtually universal development of pneumatocoeles. The abscesses are tender and warm although systemic toxicity is less than expected. Infections with other bacterial and fungal agents can occur. All patients at some time have a pruritic dermatitis, but the distribution and characteristics of the lesion are said to be different from classical atopic dermatitis. Eosinophilia has been a consistent finding. A neutrophil or monocyte chemotactic defect is *not* a necessary part of this syndrome and is an inconstant finding. Variable abnormalities in cellular immunity are seen, manifested usually as skin test anergy and diminished proliferation in vitro to antigens and allogeneic cells.

Several patients have been described under the eponym of Job's syndrome. The original patients were fair skinned, red headed girls with eczema and recurrent 'cold' staphylococcal abscesses of the skin, subcutaneous tissue, lymph nodes, lung, liver and abdominal cavity. There were systemic signs of infection but little local inflammatory reaction. These patients were subsequently found to have hyper IgE and a chemotactic defect.

Additional patients have been described with neutrophil chemotactic defects, hyper IgE, severe weeping atopic dermatitis, cellulitis and recurrent staphylococcal abscesses. The exact relationship of the various syndromes remains to be elucidated.

Genetics. In the Buckley syndrome, both males and females have been affected with equal frequency and members of succeeding generations have also been affected, suggesting an autosomal dominant mode of inheritance with incomplete penetrance.

Cellular (T cell) immune defects

Thymic hypoplasia (DiGeorge syndrome)

Until recently, the DiGeorge syndrome (thymic hypoplasia) had been considered the classic prototypic example of an isolated T cell defect. The DiGeorge syndrome is usually a congenital sporadic disorder in which there are abnormalities of structures derived from the third and fourth pharyngeal pouches, including the thymus and parathyroids. The absence of the parathyroid glands often results in neonatal tetany. Patients have a characteristic facies with micrognathia, low set malformed 'pixie' ears, cleft palate, short philtrum of the lip and anti-mongoloid slant of the eyes. There are often associated abnormalities of the aortic arch (commonly truncus arteriosus communis) and the cardiac manifestations may overshadow the other features of this disorder. Although the thymic shadow is absent radiographically, some ectopic thymic tissue may be identified at autopsy. This variability in the degree of thymic hypoplasia presumably explains the variability in the extent of the T cell defect in different patients. Patients are not usually profoundly lymphopenic but cellular immune function is usually absent or markedly diminished with severely reduced to absent T cells as determined by cell surface markers and absence of response to mitogens or antigens. These patients classically have multiple candida and viral infections, while antibody function is usually normal. B cell percentages are elevated. These abnormalities can be explained by a lack of thymic factors needed to differentiate T cell precursors into mature mitogen and antigen responsive T cells. The immune defect appears to respond to implantation of fetal thymus. Therapy is difficult to evaluate critically since, in some patients, immune function gradually improves, presumably reflecting growth of thymic remnants.

Genetics. The incidence is not known, and less than 100 cases have been reported in the literature (Conley et al, 1979; Raatikka et al, 1981). The diagnosis is often made at autopsy, suggesting that the syndrome is often missed. Almost all cases have been solitary but three families with familial pharyngeal pouch syndrome have been reported. In these families, the findings were consistent with autosomal recessive inheritance.

Purine nucleoside phosphorylase deficiency

Genetic deficiency of purine nucleoside phosphorylase (PNP) results in an isolated defect of cellular immunity and is the second specific genetic molecular defect which results in immunodeficiency. The disorder was initially discovered in a five year old girl with a history of recurrent infections. At least nine children with PNP deficiency in six families have been found to date. (Ciba Foundation Symposium, 1979; Pollara et al, 1979; Hirschhorn & Martin, 1978.) It is apparent that all the patients have had severe T cell dysfunction as measured by marked reduction in T cell numbers, reduced response to mitogens and allogeneic cells and severe recurrent fungal and viral infections. The latter infections are often fatal. In marked contrast to ADA deficiency, humoral immunity has been quantitatively normal or increased as measured by normal numbers of B cells in the blood and of plasma cells in lymphoid tissue, normal to elevated immunoglobulin concentration in vivo and normal antibody production. Several patients have had abnormally excessive antibody production, usually with concurrent viral infections. These abnormalities have included Coombs positive haemolytic anaemia, positive ANA, rheumatoid factor and mono-

clonal gammopathy, all suggesting abnormalities in T suppressor function.

In several patients, the disease has shown a course of immunologic attrition. Clinical onset of disease has varied from six months to six years of age. Non-immunologic abnormalities have included anaemia in five patients (four of the six families). Three patients (two families) have had neurologic abnormalities of spastic tetraplegia or ataxia and tremor, reminiscent of the abnormalities seen in a few ADA deficient patients.

Purine nucleoside phosphorylase (PNP) reversibly catalyzes the phosphorylysis of the purine nucleosides guanosine, inosine, deoxyguanosine and deoxyinosine and is thus the next enzyme in the purine salvage pathway following adenosine deaminase. Although the equilibrium of the reaction in vitro favours nucleoside synthesis, in vivo the direction is towards the generation of the free purine base from the corresponding nucleoside. Patients with PNP deficiency therefore accumulate large amounts of all four nucleoside substrates (inosine, guanosine, deoxyinosine and deoxyguanosine) in their urine. Because the block is near the terminal portion of the major common pathway to uric acid, patients with complete PNP deficiency have low serum uric acid and excrete diminished amounts of uric acid. However, excretion of total purine precursors of uric acid is increased, indicating purine overproduction. Of the four substrates, only deoxyguanosine has been reported to be directly phosphorylated, without prior conversion to hypoxanthine or guanine, a reaction which is blocked in PNP deficiency. It is therefore not surprising that deoxy GTP is the major phosphorylated metabolite accumulated by PNP deficient children. Deoxy GTP like deoxy ATP is also an allosteric inhibitor of ribonucleotide reductase, albeit not as potent or all encompassing. It has been hypothesized that accumulation of deoxy GTP accounts for the lymphospecific and T cell specific effects of PNP deficiency. In vitro enzymatic and metabolic studies, similar to those described for deoxy ATP, also support this hypothesis.

PNP deficiency would appear to be a rarer disorder than ADA deficiency. It is inherited in an autosomal recessive mode, and obligate heterozygotes have usually been found to have half normal PNP activity in their red cells. The disorder is clearly genetically heterogeneous, with several different mutant alleles at the PNP locus. Thus, in one of the families (Toronto) the two affected brothers have detectable residual PNP activity but with an abnormal K_m. Correlated with the presence of residual enzyme activity, the two brothers are the oldest survivors, at over ten years of age and one of the brothers had the latest age of onset. The two brothers, who are products of a non-consanguineous mating, would appear to be doubly heterozygous for two different mutant PNP alleles. Thus, the father has an electrophoretically abnormal PNP which is also detectable with anti PNP antibodies as excess cross reacting material, while the mother has reduced enzyme and reduced CRM and no electrophoretic aberrations of the enzyme molecule. Another patient has been demonstrated to have yet another mutation, resulting in an electrophoretically altered enzyme but different from that seen in the brothers mentioned above.

Prenatal diagnosis has not yet been reported for PNP deficiency but should be feasible since amniotic fluid cells express PNP. Bone marrow transplantation has also not been attempted. Therapy has been supportive. Partial exchange transfusions, as in ADA deficiency have also been utilized, with marked metabolic clearing and some signs of clinical improvement. Complete immunologic reconstitution has not resulted.

Chronic mucocutaneous candidiasis
Chronic mucocutaneous candidiasis is a syndrome characterized by persistent Candida infection of the mucous membranes, scalp, skin and nails. It is often associated with an endocrinopathy. The defect appears to involve the cellular immune response only to Candida since susceptibility to other infectious agents is uncommon. Cutaneous anergy to Candida and often other antigens is observed. Following in vitro challenge with Candida, there is usually a diminished proliferative response and diminished release of the lymphokine MIF. Antibody to Candida as well as to other antigens is usually present. Other variable immunologic abnormalities have been described.

The syndrome can be classified into four types (Lehrer et al, 1978). The first form is early onset, severe disease in which associated endocrinopathy, usually hypothyroidism, is common and granulomas are seen. Survival past the third decade is unusual. The late onset type is the mildest and its only manifestations may be paranychia or involvement or of the buccal mucosa. These two forms are usually sporadic. The two familial forms of the syndrome essentially differ as to the presence or absence of endocrinopathies. The juvenile onset form is associated with polyendocrinopathies, most commonly hypoparathyroidism. The endocrine disorder can precede the candidiasis by several years. In other families, endocrinopathy rarely occurs. In both types inheritance is consistent with an autosomal recessive mode.

Specific syndromes involving other organ systems with immunodeficiency as a significant manifestation
Some of these disorders have conventionally not been listed as primary immunodeficiency diseases. However, as testing of immune function becomes more widespread, immunologic abnormalities are likely to be detected in a variety of syndromes (e.g. TC II deficiency).

We have therefore segregated immunodeficiencies which are associated with specific clinical syndromes, generally detected by virtue of their non-immunological manifestations.

Wiskott-Aldrich syndrome
The Wiskott-Aldrich syndrome is a rare X–linked recessive disorder characterized by thrombocytopenia, eczema and recurrent infections usually with polysaccharide containing pyogenic bacteria but also with other bacteria, viruses and fungi. Affected males have a median survival to 6 years and approximately 70% are dead by age 14 (Perry et al, 1980). The major cause of death is infection, commonly of the respiratory system, followed by bleeding, most often into the CNS. Lymphoid malignancies occur frequently (over 12 percent of patients). Thrombocytopenia is usually observed at birth and is often exacerbated during periods of infection.

Platelets are small in size, respond abnormally to aggregating agents and have a diminished half life. Splenectomy usually results in increase in platelet number and size, a normal half life of autologous platelets and a normal aggregating response to epinephrine (Lum et al, 1980). These recent observations suggest that the diminished half life, decreased size and abnormalities of aggregation may not be intrinsic defects but are alterations requiring splenic processing of abnormal platelets for expression. Following splenectomy, episodes of profound thrombocytopenia, possibly of an autoimmune nature, still occur. While splenectomy reduces the incidence of bleeding, there is an increased incidence of overwhelming sepsis which increases mortality unless antibiotics are administered prophylactically.

The eczema usually appears by one year of age and may be superinfected. The recurrent infections are associated with variable defects in humoral and cellular immunity. Immunoglobulins are both catabolised and synthesized more rapidly than normal and the most common resulting pattern of serum immunoglobulin is elevated serum IgA and IgE with low IgM. Serum isohaemagglutinins are absent or very low. Patients are unable to mount an antibody response to polysaccharide antigens (eg. pneumococcal vaccine) but can generate relatively normal antibody responses to protein antigens. B cells are normal but in vitro synthesis of Ig is variably abnormal, depending on the stimulant utilized. Cellular immunity can also be abnormal. Patients are generally anergic to skin test antigens including DNCB, and cells do not proliferate normally in vitro in response to antigens or allogeneic cells. However, proliferation response to polyclonal activators (non-specific mitogens), lymphocyte count and number of T cells are usually normal early in the course. Hepatosplenomegaly and autoimmune phenomena (eg. haemolytic anaemia) are seen.

Genetics

Wiskott-Aldrich syndrome has a crude incidence of approximately four per million male births. There is no widely accepted method for detection of heterozygous carriers. Although platelet abnormalities have been described in obligate heterozygotes, these observations are not consistent with reports that there is selection against platelets and lymphocytes expressing the X–chromosome which bears the Wiskott-Aldrich mutation (as detected by clonal expression in G6PD heterozygotes). A population of small platelets has reportedly not been detected in obligate carriers. Recombination between the G6PD locus and the Wiskott-Aldrich gene (Gealy et al, 1980), indicates that linkage between G6PD and Wiskott-Aldrich is not likely to provide accurate prenatal diagnosis.

Prenatal detection (other than the 50% risk for a male) is not currently feasible. It has not been determined if affected fetuses have small abnormally functioning platelets and/or thrombocytopenia in utero. Recently, several children have been successfully engrafted with histocompatible bone marrow with return of platelet function to normal. This manoeuver must be preceded by measures to extirpate the patient's own marrow, but it remains to be determined if such measures will result in a markedly increased incidence of malignancy in these patients who already have increased susceptibility to lymphoid malignancies.

Ataxia telangiectasia

Ataxia telangiectasia is characterized clinically by the occurrence of progressive cerebellar ataxia, ocular and cutaneous telangiectases, frequent and severe sinopulmonary infections, a very high incidence of neoplasia and variable abnormalities of both cellular and humoral immunity (McFarlin, Strober & Waldmann, 1972). More recent investigations at the molecular level indicate that this may be a genetically and clinically heterogeneous group of disorders.

The disease is usually first recognized as the child attempts to walk. The ataxia and dysarthria are progressive and additional neurologic abnormalities develop, including choreoathetosis, myoclonic jerks, nystagmus, and oculomotor apraxia. Increased infections become evident during the first year of life but are usually not prominent until 3–8 years of age. The telangiectases usually appear between 2 and 8 years of age. Progeric changes develop in the adult and include premature graying of the hair, early loss of subcutaneous tissue, sclerodermoid changes, vitiligo and cafe au lait spots.

The most prominent and consistent immunologic abnormality is absent or deficient serum and secretory IgA and serum IgE and the presence of a low molecular weight IgM. The latter may result in factitiously high IgM measurements by radial immunodiffusion. Autoantibodies are common. Diminished *in vitro* cellular immune responses are also common and the thymus often has a fetal-like histologic pattern. Endocrine abnormalities, involving several organs, are also frequent. Over half of the patients have hyperinsulinism, insulin resistance and hyperglycemia, due to a circulating factor (? anti-receptor antibody) that interferes with insulin binding. Many patients show hypogonadism with absent or hypoplastic ovaries in females. Hepatic abnormalities also occur and elevated alpha fetoprotein is common. Patients usually die before early adulthood as a result of the recurrent respiratory infections or a lymphoproliferative neoplasm.

Ataxia telangiectasia is one of the chromosome instability syndromes and patients' cells develop chromosome abnormalities at high frequency. The chromosome abnormalities typically involve the translocation of the long arm of chromosome 14 with the breakpoint at 14q12. In addition to showing an increased rate of 'spontaneous' chromosome rearrangements, cells from patients with ataxia telangiectasia are also more sensitive to ionizing radiation and radiomimetic chemicals. In vivo, patients react adversely to standard radiotherapy and may die in the course of treatment. Studies of gamma induced radiation repair suggest that there are two major complementation groups and a 'variant' group (Paterson, 1979).

Genetics. Ataxia telangiectasia has an incidence of approximately 25 per million and appears to be inherited as an autosomal recessive. The disorder occurs in higher frequency among Moroccan Jews. Obligate heterozygotes have been reported to be at increased risk for development of neoplasia. Definitive detection of heterozygotes is not available although autoimmunity and occulocutaneous telangiectases have been reported in some heterozygotes. Prenatal diagnosis has recently been reported in one case, based upon the ability of the amniotic fluid to induce chromosome aberrations in normal cells. Bone marrow transplantation, has been attempted, but there was no evidence for permanent successful engraftment.

Short limbed dwarfism (SLD) with immunodeficiency

Short limbed dwarfism is associated with at least three distinct forms of immunodeficiency and appears to encompass at least three different disorders (Ammann et al, 1974). McKusick (McKusick et al 1965) described the phenotype of 77 Amish children in 53 sibships affected with a form of short limbed dwarfism associated with cartilage hair hypoplasia. In addition to the cartilage and hair abnormalities, affected individuals typically could not fully extend their elbows, had hyperextensibility of fingers and wrists and often had a marked sternal deformity. The authors very astutely noted that two of the 77 died of chicken pox and at least three others had virulent varicella. They therefore suggested that increased susceptibility to viral infections, as well as intestinal abnormalities, could be part of the syndrome. Subsequent studies have indeed demonstrated in vitro-immune defects limited to cellular immune function. Although the in vitro defect is general, increased susceptibility to infection appears to be limited to vaccinia and varicella, while candida infections are notably absent. A similar disorder has been described in high frequency in the Finnish population (Virolainen et al, 1978). The Finnish group appears to have a very mild defect in cellular immunity and an increased susceptibility to viral infections has not been noted. However, the number of individuals examined was smaller (28). Chronic non-cyclic neutropenia has been described in a non-Amish affected girl (Lux et al, 1970) and congenital hypoplastic anaemia in an affected Amish boy (Harris et al, 1981).

The second form of SLD is much rarer and fewer than 10 patients have been described. The clinical course and prognosis are indistinguishable from severe combined immunodeficiency. Redundant skin folds, scaly skin and variably progressive hair loss can be seen. Aplastic anaemia has been reported in at least one case and we have seen an additional case with marked anaemia. The inheritance appears to be autosomal recessive. Because of the bony abnormalities, we have tested two of these children and found normal erythrocyte ADA. Prenatal diagnosis could conceivably be made by detection of bony abnormalities in utero. At least one patient has had a successful bone marrow transplant. The disorder is otherwise fatal.

The last form of SLD is rare and is associated only with defective humoral immunity and apparently without cartilage hair hypoplasia. The reported male and female sibs of gypsy extraction had a prominent nose, high forehead and large ears, but it is not clear if the facies are typical for the syndrome or for the family.

Inheritance in all three types is compatible with an autosomal recessive mode. The disorder is frequently misdiagnosed during infancy as achondroplasia, an autosomal dominant disorder, and thus may lead to inaccurate counseling. In the Amish group, the frequency is 1–2 per 1000 live births and the inheritance is compatible with an autosomal recessive mode. If, as suggested, there is reduced (70%) penetrance, the estimated gene frequency among the Amish is 0.05.

Transcobalamin II deficiency

Inherited deficiency of transcobalamin II (the vitamin B_{12} binding protein necessary for transport of vitamin B_{12} into cells) is characterized by infantile megaloblastic anaemia, leukopenia, thrombocytopenia, infections and failure to gain weight. In several cases of transcobalamin II deficiency, agammaglobulinaemia has been detected. The various abnormalities are correctable by pharmacologic doses of vitamin B_{12}. Interestingly, this deficiency appears to result in a block of clonal expansion and maturation of plasma cells, as well as of synthesis of antibodies, but not in the differentiation of antigen specific memory cells. Thus, following vitamin B_{12} therapy, an affected child synthesized specific antibodies to antigens with which he had been immunized several months previously during the unresponsive state (Hitzig, 1979).

This is a rare disorder and fewer than 5 families have been reported. Transcobalamin II is a genetically polymorphic protein and null alleles can thus be detected by anomalous inheritance of the polymorphic markers. Obligate heterozygotes have had half normal amounts of transcobalamin II and in at least one family an electrophoretically abnormal protein has been detected. Partial deficiency of transcobalamin II with only megaloblastic anemia as a manifestation also has been reported. Therapy is provided by administration of pharmacologic doses of vitamin B_{12}.

Biotin responsive multiple carboxylase deficiency

Two sibs have been reported with biotin responsive multiple carboxylase deficiency (Cowan et al, 1979) who in addition to seizures, alopecia and intermittent ataxia, also both had clinically significant candidiasis and an in vitro defective response to Candida antigen. The alopecia, organic aciduria and candidiasis cleared following therapy with biotin. However, the abnormal response to Candida remained and there were still several brief episodes of ataxia, suggesting that the biotin therapy was not totally effective. It remains to be determined if the organic acids which are accumulated in this disorder are toxic for immune function, or if biotin is also a cofactor for yet another enzyme crucial for immune function.

We have not attempted to cover all metabolic disorders in which patients have had multiple infections with unusual pathogens and/or died of varicella, vaccinia, etc. It is very likely that children with many of the inherited metabolic defects which have severe global manifestations will exhibit measurable abnormalities in immune function. Such abnormalities are likely to be less informative than, and should be differentiated from, the yet to be discovered additional metabolic defects which primarily result in abnormalities of the immune system. Investigations of the purine pathway have been fruitful to date and there are indeed several immunodeficiency syndromes where the association of bony abnormalities and neurologic abnormalities with immunodeficiency suggest that investigations of this pathway may still be rewarding. However, one must remember that the initial discovery of the importance of the purine pathway was serendipitous and totally unexpected, and unrelated metabolic pathways may subsequently be found to be important for normal immune function.

CONCLUSION

It should be clear from the descriptions above that, as in other genetic diseases, there is a great deal of heterogeneity in the immunodeficiency disorders. Such heterogeneity can be due to different alleles at the same locus or mutations at different loci resulting in similar phenotypes. Not only is there this expected genetic heterogeneity within each general phenotype, but due to the dependence of many of the symptoms upon chance exposure to environmental agents, there is superimposed a significant degree of non-genetic individual variation. In fact, a number of individuals demonstrating immunodeficiency, sometimes indistinguishable from the genetic diseases, develop their conditions as a result of such non-genetic problems as severe viral infections, malignancies or therapy with immunosuppressive and cytotoxic agents. Additionally, a number of inborn errors of metabolism, including storage diseases, urea cycle defects and organic and amino-acidurias, as well as several chromosomal disorders, such as those involving chromosome 18 as well as Down syndrome, demonstrate a variety of immunologic defects leading to increased susceptibility to infection. In great part, the difficulty of accurate classification, with a few notable exceptions, is due to our general lack of understanding of the fundamental molecular defects responsible for most of these conditions. In addition, the dependence of current classification systems upon the developmental model of stem cell, B cell or T cell defects, while initially highly useful, has become somewhat naive and therefore constricting.

The continuous advance in our understanding of interaction and interdependence of the components of the immune system with each other and with even more cells and molecules makes it clear that many modifications of the definitions of immunodeficiencies will come about. No doubt these discoveries, especially when they become understood on a molecular basis, will bring about the definition of many new defects associated with host defense problems.

One example of a fascinating puzzle to be solved is the role of genes on the X–chromosome, which seem to be responsible for so many defects involving hematopoietic cells. Among the diseases covered in this chapter are X–linked agammaglobulinaemia, the Wiskott-Aldrich syndrome, most of the hyper IgM states, a proportion of SCID and the X–linked lymphoproliferative syndrome. Other X–linked diseases involving bone marrow elements include agranulocytosis, a form of thrombocytopenia and chronic granulomatous disease. It may well be that a set of related genes on the X–chromosome determine the orderly differentiation from primitive stem cells to the various functional elements and that different mutations result in one or other of these abnormalities.

It is not only our hope but our sincere conviction that the increased application of modern biochemical and molecular methodology and thought will, over the next few years, lead to a clearer understanding of the genetics and fundamental defects of primary immunodeficiency. It is only with such understanding that more rational counseling and therapy can develop. As so often true in the past for other fields, a dissection of these genetic defects will inevitably help to take the field of clinical and cellular immunology from its current state of descriptive phenomenology into the realm of a proper science, such as is already becoming the case in our understanding of the immunoglobulins and antibody diversity.

REFERENCES

Ammann A J, Sutliff W, Millinchick E 1974 Antibody mediated immunodeficiency in short-limbed dwarfism. Journal of Pediatrics 84: 200–203

Ammann A J, Fudenberg H H 1980 Immunodeficiency diseases. In: Fudenberg H H, Stites D P, Caldwell J L, Wells J V (eds) Basic and clinical immunology, Lange, Los Altos, ch 29, p 409–442

Ammann A J, Hong R 1980 Disorders of the IgA system. In: Stiehm E R, Fulginiti V A (eds) Immunologic disorders in infants and children, W B Saunders, Philadelphia, ch 14, p 260–273

Asherson G L, Webster A D B 1980 Diagnosis and treatment of immunodeficiency diseases, Blackwell, Oxford, p 1–375

Baehner, R L 1980 Lymphocytes. In: Miller D R, Pearson H A (eds) Blood diseases in infancy and childhood, Mosby, St. Louis, ch 20, p 557–572

Bortin M M, Rimm A A 1977 Severe combined immunodeficiency disease – characterization of the disease and results of transplantation – report of the advisory committee of the international bone marrow transplant registry. Journal of the American Medical Association 238: 591–600

Buckley R H 1980 Disorders of the IgE system. In: Stiehm E R, Fulginiti V A (eds) Immunologic disorders in infants and children, W B Saunders, Philadelphia, ch 15, p 274–285

Ciba foundation symposium 68 1979 Enzyme defects and immune dysfunction, Excerpta Medica, Amsterdam, p 1–279

Conley M E, Beckwith J B, Mancer J F K, Tenckhoff L 1979 The spectrum of the DiGeorge syndrome. Journal of Pediatrics 94: 883–890

Cowan M J, Packman S, Wara D W, Ammann A J, Yoshimo M, Sweetman L, Nyhan W 1979 Multiple biotin-dependent carboxylase deficiencies associated with defects in T-cell and B-cell immunity. Lancet I: 115–118

Croce C M, Shander M, Martinis J, Cicurel L, D'Ancona G, Dolby T, Koprowski H 1979 Chromosomal location of the genes for human immunoglobulin heavy chains. Proceedings of the National Academy of Science, USA 76: 3416–3419

Davis M M, Kim S K, Hood L E 1980 DNA sequences mediating class switching in α-immunoglobulin. Science 209: 1353–1359

Eisen H N 1980 Immunology, Harper and Row, Hagerstown

Erickson J, Martiuis J, Croce C M 1981 Assignment of the genes for human λ immunoglobulin chains to chromosome 22. Nature 294: 173–175

Fleisher T A, White R M, Broder S, Nissley S P, Blaese R M, Mulvihill J J, Olive G, Waldmann T A 1980 X–linked hypogammaglobulinemia and isolated growth hormone deficiency. New England Journal of Medicine 302: 1429–1434

Fudenberg H H, Stites D P, Caldwell J L, Wells J V (eds) 1980 Basic and clinical immunology, Lange, Los Altos

Gealy W J, Dwyer J M, Harley J B 1980 Allelic exclusion of glucose-6-phosphate dehydrogenase in platelets and T lymphocytes from a Wiskott-Aldrich syndrome carrier. Lancet I: 63–65

Geha R S, Hyslop N, Alami S, Farah F, Schneeberger E E, Rosen F S 1979 Hyper immunoglobulin M immunodeficiency (dysgammaglobulinemia). Journal of Clinical Investigation 64: 385–391

Gelfand E W, Oliver J M, Shuurman R K, Matheson D S, Dosch H-M 1979 Abnormal lymphocyte capping in a patient with severe combined immunodeficiency disease. New England Journal of Medicine 301: 1245–1249

Giblett E R, Anderson J E, Cohen F, Pollara B, Meuwissen H J 1972 Adenosine deaminase deficiency in two patients with severely impaired cellular immunity. Lancet II: 1067–1069

Harris R E, Baehner R L, Gleiser S, Weaver D D, Hodes M E 1981 Cartilage-hair hypoplasia, defective T-cell function and Diamond-Blackfan anemia in an Amish child. American Journal of Medical Genetics 8: 291–297

Hermans P E, Diaz-Buxo J A, Stobo J D 1976 Idiopathic late-onset immunoglobulin deficiency. American Journal of Medicine 61: 221–237

Hirschhorn R, Martin D W Jr 1978 Enzyme defects in immunodeficiency disorders. In: Miescher P, Muller-Eberhard H (eds) Springer seminars in immunopathology, Springer-Verlag, p 299–321

Hitzig W H 1979 Immunodeficiency due to transcobalamin II deficiency. In: Ciba foundation symposium 68, enzyme defects and immune dysfunction, Excerpta Medica, Amsterdam

Hitzig W H, Kenny A B 1978 Inheritance, incidence and epidemiology of severe combined immunodeficiency syndromes. In: Japan medical research foundation (ed) Immunodeficiency. Its nature and etiological significance in human disease, University of Tokyo Press, Tokyo, p 257–270

Hobbs J R 1975 IgM deficiency. In: Bergsma D, Good R A, Finstad J (eds) Immunodeficiency in man and animals – birth defects: original article series, vol XI, 1, Sinauer Press, Sunderland, MA, p 112–117

Hood L E, Weissman I L, Wood W B 1978 Immunology, Benjamin Cummings, Menlo Park

Koistinen J 1976 Familial clustering of selective IgA deficiency. Vox Sangvinis 30: 181–190

Lawton A R III, Cooper M D 1980 Immune deficiency diseases. In: Isselbacher K J, Adams R D, Braunwald E, Petersdorf R G, Wilson J D (eds) Harrison's principles of internal medicine, 9th edn, McGraw Hill, New York, p 325–333

Lehrer R I, Stiehm E R, Fischer T J, Young L S 1978 Severe candidal infections: clinical perspective, immune defense mechanisms and current concepts of therapy. Annals of Internal Medicine 89: 91–106

Lum L G, Tubergen D G, Corash L, Blaese R M 1980 Splenectomy in the management of the thrombocytopenia of the Wiskott-Aldrich syndrome. New England Journal of Medicine 302: 892–896

Lux S E, Johnston R B Jr, August C S, Say B, Penchaszadeh V B, Rosen F S, McKusick V A 1970 Chronic neutropenia and abnormal cellular immunity in cartilage-hair hypoplasia. New England Journal of Medicine 282: 231–236

Maki R, Kearney J, Paige C, Tonegawa S 1980 Immunoglobulin gene rearrangements in immature B cells. Science 290: 1360–1365

McBride O W, Hieter P A, Hollis G F, Swan D, Otey M C, Leder P 1982 Chromosomal location of human kappa and lambda immunoglobulin light chain constant region genes. Journal of Experimental Medicine 155: 1480–1490

McFarlin D, Strober W, Waldmann T A 1972 Ataxia-telangiectasia. Medicine 51: 281–314

McKusick V A, Eldridge R, Hostetler J A, Ruangwit U, Egeland J A 1965 Dwarfism in the Amish II: cartilage hair hypoplasia. Bulletin of Johns Hopkins Hospital 116: 285–326

Ownby D R, Pizzo S, Blackmon L, Gall S A, Buckley R H 1976 Severe combined immunodeficiency with leukopenia (reticular dysgenesis): immunologic and histopathologic findings. Journal of Pediatrics 89: 382–387

Parker C W (ed) 1980 Clinical immunology, W B Saunders, Philadelphia

Paterson M C 1979 Environmental carcinogenesis and imperfect repair of damaged DNA in Homo Sapiens: causal relation revealed by rare hereditary disorders. In: Griffin A C, Shaw C R (eds) Carcinogens: identification and mechanisms of action, Raven Press, New York, p 251–276

Perry G S III, Spector B D, Schuman L M, Mandel, J S, Anderson, V E, McHugh R B, Hanson, M R, Fahlstrom S M, Krivit W, Kersey J H 1980 The Wiskott-Aldrich syndrome in the United States and Canada (1892–1979). Journal of Pediatrics 97: 72–78

Pollara B, Pickering R J, Meuwissen H J, Porter I H (eds) 1979 Inborn errors of specific immunity, Academic Press, New York, p 1–469

Purtilo D T, DeFlorio D, Hutt L M, Bhawan J, Yang J P S, Otto R, Edwards W 1977 Variable phenotypic expression of an X–linked recessive lymphoproliferative syndrome. New England Journal of Medicine 297: 1077–1081

Raatikka M, Rapola J, Tuuteri L, Louhimo I, Savilahti E 1981 Familial third and fourth pharyngeal pouch syndrome with Truncus Arteriosus: DiGeorge syndrome. Pediatrics, 67: 173–175

Race R R, Sanger R 1975 Blood groups in man, Blackwell Scientific, Oxford, p 606

Roitt I 1980 Essential immunology, Blackwell Scientific, Oxford

Rosen F S 1981 Primary immunodeficiencies and serum complement defects. In: Nathan D G, Oski F A (eds) Hematology of infancy and childhood, 2nd edn, vol II, Saunders, Philadelphia, ch 26, p 497–519

Rosen F S, Merler E 1978 Genetic defects in gamma globulin synthesis. In: Stanbury J B, Wyngaarden J B, Fredrickson D S (eds) The metabolic basis of inherited disease, 4th edn, McGraw-Hill, New York, p 1726–1737

Samter M (ed) 1978 Immunological diseases, Little Brown, USA

Schwaber J F, Klein G, Ernberg I, Rosen A, Lazarus H,

Rosen F S 1980 Deficiency of Epstein-Barr virus (EBV) receptors on B lymphocytes from certain patients with common varied agammaglobulinemia. Journal of Immunology 124: 2191–2196

Sell S 1980 Immunology, immunopathology and immunity, Harper and Row, Hagerstown

Shaham M 1981 Personal communication

Smith M, Krinsky A M, Arrendondo V F, Wang A-L, Hirschhorn K 1981 Confirmation of the assignment of genes for human immunoglobulin heavy chains to chromosome 14 by analyses of Ig synthesis by man-mouse hybridomas. European Journal of Immunology 11: 852–855

Stiehm E R, Fulginitti V A (eds) 1980 Immunologic disorders in infants and children, Saunders, Philadelphia

Touraine J L 1981 The bare lymphocyte syndrome: report on the registry. Lancet I: 319–321

Waldmann T A, Strober W, Blaese R M 1980 T and B cell immunodeficiency diseases. In: Parker C W (ed) Clinical immunology, W B Saunders, Philadelphia, ch 1, p 314–375

Waldmann T A, Broder S, Krakauer R, MacDermott R P, Durm M, Goldman C, Meade B 1976 The role of suppressor cells in the pathogenesis of common variable hypogammaglobulinemia and in the immunodeficiency associated with myeloma. Federation Proceedings 35: 2067–2072

Virolainen M, Savilahti E, Kaitila I, Perheentupa J 1978 Cellular and humoral immunity in cartilage hair hypoplasia. Pediatric Research 12: 961–966

World Health Organization 1978 Immunodeficiency; technical report series 630, Geneva

Yount W S, Hong R, Seligmann M, Good R A, Kunkel H G 1970 Imbalances of gamma globulin subgroups and gene defects in patients with primary hypogammaglobulinemia Journal of Clinical Investigation 49: 1957–1966.

79

Complement defects

F.S Rosen and C.A. Alper

INTRODUCTION

The complement system is a formidably complex system of interacting plasma proteins, strongly conserved in vertebrate evolution which functions as the principal effector system for antibody-mediated immune reactions. Three types of genetic variation in complement components have been discovered:

1. Polymorphism of individual components based on differences in electric charge. Such polymorphisms are well studied for C3, Factor B, and C6 where there are at least two high frequency alleles and also for C4, C2, C7, and C8 where the frequency of the second most common allele is less.

One of the more interesting results from this work is the discovery that the genes for Factor B, C2 and C4 are coded within HLA in close proximity to the HLA-B locus. The gene for C6 is closely linked to that for C7, but the locus for C6-C7, as well as those for C3, and C8 are so far unassigned (Alper).

2. Genes controlling the level of certain components of which the s gene in the mouse is the best known.

3. The isolated deficiencies which are dealt with elsewhere.

THE COMPLEMENT REACTION PATHWAYS

From a functional point of view the complement activation sequence occurs in two overlapping but distinct parts.

The first of these is a triggered enzyme cascade culminating in the cleavage and fixation of C3. This is, in quantitative terms, the major reaction of complement fixation and the fixation of C3 at complement fixation sites is probably the system's most important activity. Bound C3 reacts with the various receptors on phagocytic cells, platelets, erythrocytes (in primates) and certain lymphocytes. The retention of cells at complement fixation sites contributes largely to the phlogistic activity of the complement system.

The cleavage of C3 is brought about by two distinct pathways known for historical reasons as the 'classical' and 'alternative' pathways. It is possible to picture these as homologues of each other and this is shown in Figure 79.1. Here it can be seen that the C3 cleaving enzyme of the classical pathway C4b,2a is generated·from a complex between C4b and C2a in the presence of magnesium ions by proteolytic cleavage by C1. Similarly, in the alternative pathway, a complex C3b,Bb is formed between C3b and Factor B in the presence of magnesium ions cleaved by Factor D. There are sufficient physicochemical resemblances between C4b and C3b on the one hand, and C2 and Factor B on the other to suggest that the similarities at this level are not fanciful and that indeed one may be looking at the results of a duplicated enzyme system. The significant difference between the two pathways is that in the alternative pathway it is C3b itself which is the essential component of the C3 splitting enzyme, and this enables the alternative pathway to act as a positive feedback amplification loop for C3 activation no matter how C3 cleavage is originally produced. Thus,

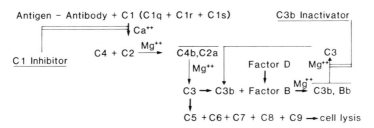

Fig. 79.1 Pathways of C3 cleavage.

this pathway can amplify not only immunologically-induced C3 activation, but also that produced by other enzymes as, for example, plasmin or leucocyte proteases, which may occur at inflammation sites even if this is not primarily of immunological origin. The initial activating steps of the alternative pathway are not fully understood. Properdin is now believed to act as a stabilizing factor for the alternative pathway C3 converting enzyme, C3bBb, rather than as an initiating factor. It seems probable that the alternative pathway may 'tick-over' continuously and that the triggering of the system by activators is a consequence of the stabilization of feedback enzyme. It has recently been suggested that C3b bound to activating particles may be more resistant to C3b inactivator which would be sufficient to account for the triggering role (Müller-Eberhard, 1975).

COMPLEMENT DEFECTS

Hereditary angioneurotic oedema

Hereditary angioneurotic oedema was recognized during the last century, but the molecular basis of the disease, a genetically determined deficiency of the C1 inhibitor, was not defined until 1963. The defect is transmitted as an autosomal dominant. The serum of most affected patients contains between 5 and 30% of the normal concentration of C1 inhibitor (Donaldson & Evans, 1963; Rosen et al, 1971).

Patients with this disease are prone to recurrent episodes of swelling. The oedema fluid accumulates rapidly in the affected part, which becomes tense but not discoloured; no itching, no pain, and no redness are associated with the oedema. Laryngeal oedema may be fatal because of airway obstruction and consequent pulmonary oedema. If the intestinal tract is involved, most often the jejunum, severe abdominal cramps and bilious vomiting ensue. Diarrhea, which is clear and watery in character occurs when the colon is affected. The attacks last 48–72 hours. Although they are often unheralded, attacks may occur subsequent to trauma, menses, excessive fatigue, and mental stress. Attacks of angioedema are infrequent in early childhood; the disease intensifies during adolescence and tends to subside in the sixth decade of life. In children especially, a mottling of the skin reminiscent of erythema marginatum may be frequently noticed and not necessarily be associated with attacks of angioedema.

The pathophysiology of hereditary angioneurotic oedema is directly related to the diminished activity of the C1 inhibitor in the plasma of affected persons. The latter leads to increased 'spontaneous' activation of C1 and attack on C4 and C2, the natural substrates of the C1, resulting in a marked lowering of the serum concentrations of these proteins, particularly during attacks. The

swelling that is the essential clinical feature of hereditary angioneurotic oedema appears to result from the action of the C2-kinin, a low molecular weight fragment of C2, modified by plasmin, on the postcapillary venule (Donaldson et al).

The autosomal dominant inheritance of hereditary angioneurotic oedema presents an interesting puzzle. Obviously, affected individuals are heterozygous for the abnormality. Despite this, their serum contains very little C1 inhibitor (average: 17 per cent of normal). Liver biopsy specimens can be shown to contain no hepatic parenchymal cells detectably engaged in synthesis of C1 inhibitor, whereas 3–5% of normal hepatic cells give positive fluorescence with a fluorescein-labeled antibody to C1 inhibitor.

In 15% of affected kindreds, sera of patients contain normal or elevated concentrations of an immunochemically cross-reacting (CRM+), nonfunctional protein. The CRM+, nonfunctional C1 inhibitors differ from kindred to kindred with respect to electrophoretic mobility, ability to bind to activated C1 esterase, and ability to inhibit the cleavage of certain synthetic esters by C1 esterase. However, all CRM+ C1 inhibitors fail to inhibit destruction of C4 by C1. The clinical expression of hereditary angioneurotic oedema is the same in CRM+ and CRM- patients, and the CRM+ proteins are inherited as autosomal dominant traits. No normal C1 inhibitor is detectable in serum from patients with CRM+ proteins.

Approximately 50% of patients with hereditary angioneurotic oedema will have a complete cessation of symptoms by taking a methyl-testosterone linguet daily. Recent studies with synthetic androgens have shown even more striking suppression of attacks and, remarkably, a rise in C1 inhibitor serum levels in deficient patients. In those patients with increased levels of dysfunctional protein, the latter have fallen in concentration with the appearance of normal C1 inhibitor. C4 and C2 levels in serum of patients under treatment have increased toward normal. Epsilon-aminocaproic acid and its analogue, tranexamic acid, are also effective as prophylactic therapy. It is now known that plasmin is required for the production of the C2-kinin, and this fact explains the efficacy of plasminogen inhibitors in the therapy of this disease. Although plasma infusions have been attempted in the therapy of acute attacks of angioedema, this procedure has no merit in light of present knowledge and may in fact be dangerous in that substrate for C1 is being infused along with inhibitor (Gelfand et al, 1976).

C3b inactivator deficiency

There are now six patients in four families known to have inherited deficiency of C3b inactivator. Three of the patients have had lifelong histories of severe infections with such organisms as *Diplococcus pneumoniae, Hemophilus influenzae, Neisseria meningitidis,* and β-haemolytic streptococci. The infections have included septicaemia, pneumonia, meningitis, and otitis media (Alper et al, 1970a; Alper et al, 1970b). The serum of all affected persons shows the same complement protein and functional abnormalities. The primary defect in each case is an absence, detected both immunochemically and functionally, of the C3b inactivator (Alper et al, 1972b). Because of this absence, there is spontaneous activation of the alternative pathway of complement activation with continuous conversion and consumption in vivo of C3 and Factor B. Native C3 concentration is about 5% of normal, and C3b is present in the patients' circulating plasma in moderately high concentration (20–25 mg/dl). No Factor B is detectable but the conversion products Bb and Ba are present in trace amounts. B added to the patients' serum is immediately cleaved. The classical pathway proteins C1, C4, and C2 are entirely normal in concentration, there is only a slight decrease in C5 concentration, and C6–9 are at normal levels. Almost all complement-mediated functions such as bactericidal activity for smooth gram-negative organisms, opsonization of pneumococci and endotoxin particles, haemolytic activity for antibody-sensitized sheep red cells, and the like are markedly diminished or absent in their serum. The functional abnormalities in vitro can be reversed only by the addition of C3b inactivator, C3, and B to the serum but not by any single protein. Partial normalization in vivo, on the other hand, can be achieved by the infusion of whole plasma or purified C3b inactivator. This partial normalization lasts for two weeks (Ziegler et al, 1975).

In family studies of C3b inactivator deficiency, heterozygotes are detected with 50% normal levels. These carriers have no abnormalities in C3 or B levels or in complement-mediated functions.

C1q deficiency

Two cases in the literature may represent inherited deficiency of C1q. One is of a 4 year old Asian boy with a lupus-like syndrome and glomerulonephritis. Absent haemolytic complement activity could be restored to this patient's serum by the addition of purified C1q. There was evidence for a structurally abnormal C1q in this patient's serum that was antigenically deficient, and of different charge, molecular weight, and subunit structure from normal C1q. This protein interacted with immune complexes, but this interaction did not result in activation of C1. The abnormal C1q was also found in several close, healthy relatives of the propositus. The second case was of a 10 year old boy with recurrent skin lesions, chronic infections, anti-smooth muscle antibody, circulating immune complexes, and anti-HB,Ag. This child died of sepsis and was found at autopsy to have had

mesangioproliferative glomerulonephritis (Berkel et al, 1979).

C1r deficiency

Seven patients in three families have inherited deficiency of C1r. All other components of complement are in normal concentration except for C1s, which is reduced to about half-normal. One patient at 16 y of age had a lupus-like syndrome with malar rash, arthralgia, and subacute focal membranous glomerulitis but negative lupus erythematosus (LE) cell test. His 24 year old sister had recurrent fever, arthralgia, and a malar rash. An unrelated 11 year old girl had chronic glomerulonephritis. The last two cases were of young adult siblings with severe discoid LE, recurrent fevers, and polyarthritis, one with antinuclear antibody, one without, but both with positive latex fixation tests. These two patients had two affected but healthy siblings. In all patients, C1r was absent by both immunochemical and functional assay of the serum. Obligatory heterozygotes sometimes had normal C1r levels, but not invariably (De Bracco et al, 1974).

C4 deficiency

The serum of an 18 year old girl with a lupus-like syndrome was found to be totally deficient in C4 by functional and immunochemical criteria. Although she had a typical malar rash and arthralgia, her LE cell test was negative. The serum of the patient's mother contained half-normal levels of C4. Other family members are possible heterozygotes (Hauptmann et al, 1974).

A second C4-deficient subject has been identified. This patient was a five year old boy with typical systemic lupus erythematosus (SLE). He had fever, myalgia, arthritis, and, more recently, nephrotic syndrome. Renal biopsy showed diffuse proliferative glomerulonephritis. He has since died with clear-cut severe SLE. As pointed out above, the identification of carriers for C4 deficiency of this sort is difficult if not impossible. By determining C4 haplotypes in the second family, it was possible to demonstrate that the proband had inherited a 'double deletion' haplotype *C4AQO C4BQO* (Ochs et al, 1977).

C2 deficiency

Inherited deficiency of C2 is probably the most common of genetic complement deficiency states (Klemperer et al, 1966). One healthy C2-deficient blood donor was found in a survey of 10 000 blood donors in Manchester, England. Glass and coworkers found 1.2% of random individuals to be heterozygous for C2 deficiency, in approximate keeping with the Manchester findings (Stratton, I., unpublished observations).

Many reports of individuals homozygous for C2 deficiency have appeared in the literature. The defect is transmitted as an autosomal recessive trait, but heterozygotes are usually detected by their half-normal serum

C2 concentration as determined by functional or immunochemical measurements.

The probands in the first four kindred discovered to have C2 deficiency and four homozygous affected siblings were all found to be healthy individuals. In fact, in two cases the discovery was made in immunologists whose blood was being used for routine haemolytic or immune adherence tests. Subsequently, four more kindreds were discovered because the probands presented with SLE. The probands in three further kindreds presented with Schönlein-Henoch purpura, and yet another, with polymyositis. These findings suggested the C2 deficiency may be associated with a high incidence of connective tissue disease. This subject is dealt with in more detail below.

Serum from homozygotes for C2 deficiency lacks certain complement-mediated functions: haemolytic activity, bactericidal activity, and immune adherence. The deficiency gene for C2 is an allele of the structural locus for this protein.

C3 deficiency

Hereditary deficiency of C3 was first detected in heterozygotes who had approximately 50% of the normal level of this protein (Alper et al, 1969). Affected persons were entirely healthy, although minor defects in complement-mediated functions could be detected in their serum. Serum haemolytic complement was variably slightly reduced, and the enhancement of phagocytosis of antibody-sensitized pneumococci was subnormal.

Analysis of the inheritance patterns of partial C3 deficiency revealed that affected persons had inherited a silent C3 gene, C3-, that produced no detectable protein. This gene was allelic to the common structural genes, and it has been shown that some C3 is produced in homozygous-deficient subjects. This C3 is normal in molecular weight, subunit composition, and surface charge (Alper et al, 1972a; Alper et al, 1976).

Subsequently, five unrelated patients homozygous for C3 deficiency have been identified. Four of them have had numerous episodes of infection by pyogenic bacteria, including pneumonia, septicemia, otitis media, and meningitis. The fifth patient was 3 years old with no history of severe infections who had an episode of fever, rash, and arthralgia, which suddenly terminated with the infusion of normal plasma. In two of the C3-deficient patients there was no leukocytosis or a blunted response in connection with systemic infection with gram-positive organisms. This may relate to a known role for C3, and specifically the C3e fragment, in leukocyte mobilization (Ballow et al, 1975; Davis et al, 1977).

Studies in vitro of serum from homozygous C3-deficient subjects have uniformly revealed marked depression or absence of most complement-mediated functions such as haemolytic activity for antibody-sensitized sheep red cells, chemotactic activity, opsonization of endotoxin particles, and bactericidal activity. Purified C3 corrected these abnormalities. In contrast to these severe deficits, immune adherence was near normal, consistent with the requirement only for the first two complement components, C1 and C4, for this function.

C5 deficiency

Inherited deficiency of the fifth component of complement has been studied in detail in at least three families. Most heterozygotes for the deficiency had about half-normal levels of C5 and inheritance is Mendelian. One of five homozygous deficient persons had SLE, two had disseminated gonococcal sepsis, and one had recurrent *N. meningitidis* meningitis.

Serum from deficient subjects showed decreased or absent total haemolytic complement, bactericidal activity, and chemotactic activity. Opsonization for endotoxin particles and a variety of microorganisms, including Baker's yeast, was entirely normal. The abnormalities in vitro in C5-deficient serum were corrected by the addition of purified C5 (Rosefeld et al, 1976; Snyderman et al, 1979).

C6 deficiency

Four patients homozygous for C6 deficiency have been studied in detail. All have had repeated episodes of neisserial sepsis involving either meningococcemia or gonococcemia. As with other complement component deficiencies, the gene for the deficiency state appears to be a null or blank allele at the structural locus for the protein, and severely deficient patients are homozygous for this blank allele.

The only defects in complement function detectable in C6-deficient serum in vitro are absent hemolytic and bactericidal activities. In particular, opsonization and chemotaxis induction are normal (Leddy et al 1974; Lim et al 1976).

C7 deficiency

There are at least seven unrelated individuals homozygous for C7 deficiency. C7 levels are undetectable to 10 per cent of normal in these sera. One patient had SLE and a second had renal disease with recurrent urinary tract infection, but most of the remaining patients have had recurrent neisserial infections (Wellek & Opferkuch, 1975).

Of all the complement-mediated functions tested, only haemolytic and bactericidal activities were reduced to absent in C7-deficient serum. Inheritance is autosomal recessive and carriers have about half-normal C7 concentrations.

A single family has been reported with a healthy proband whose serum had low but detectable levels of both C6 (1%) and C7 (8%). This combined defect was inherited as a single trait, reflecting the close linkage of the genetic loci for C6 and C7. The specific nature of this combined defect is unknown but is complicated since the small amount of C6 present is smaller in size than and antigenically deficient compared with normal C6.

C8 deficiency

Homozygous C8 deficiency has been reported in a number of individuals with a variety of clinical disorders, including lupus, xeroderma pigmentosum (which was clearly fortuitous) and several cases with severe neisserial infection. The homozygotes for C8 deficiency in these families had no detectable C8, heterozygotes often but not always had reduced C8 levels, and of the complement-mediated functions, only haemolytic and bactericidal activity were affected (Petersen et al, 1976; Matthews et al, 1980; Jasin, 1977).

There are, in addition to these families with straightforward C8 deficiency, four families with individuals who apparently have dysfunctional C8 molecules which are antigenically deficient compared with the normal molecule. No C8 function or total complement haemolytic activity was detected in the serum of the probands, some of whom had recurrent neisserial infections.

C9 deficiency

Two unrelated elderly healthy men were found to have no C9 in both functional and immunochemical tests. The only abnormalities of complement-mediated functions in these sera were slower haemolysis of antibody-sensitised sheep red blood cells and bacteriolysis than that produced by normal serum. Both haemolytic and bacteriocidal activity approached normal with longer incubation times (Lint et al, 1978).

BIOLOGICAL SIGNIFICANCE OF COMPLEMENT DEFICIENCY STATES IN HUMANS

In general, persons deficient in specific complement proteins have one or more kinds of disorders (if they have symptoms at all): 'allergic' vascular, increasing susceptibility to bacterial infections, and collagen vascular. These associations are dealt with separately (Lachmann & Rosen, 1978).

'Allergic' vascular manifestations

Persons with hereditary angioedema (C1 inhibitor deficiency) and C3b inactivator deficiency have clear-cut vascular permeability changes related to their basic genetic abnormalities. In both disorders there is unbridled activation of complement, either through the classical or the alternative pathway.

As mentioned above, the uninhibited action of C1 on C4 and C2 is attended by cleavage of these substrates, and the elaboration of a vasoactive peptide that has been isolated from patients' plasma and partly characterized. Recently, this material has been generated in vitro from mixtures of purified C1, C4, C2, and plasmin. With sufficient input of C2, C4 can be eliminated, providing further evidence for the earlier conclusion that the vasoactive peptide is derived from C2. The requirement for plasmin in the in vitro generation system is almost certainly important in vivo, because C1 inhibitor inhibits plasmin and synthetic inhibitors of plasminogen activation, such as ε-aminocaproic acid or tranexamic acid, can provide effective prophylaxis against attacks of angioedema in this disease. Although patients with hereditary angioedema have hyperhistaminuria, perhaps from some elaboration of C3a in vivo, they do not have urticaria.

In contrast, there is massive histaminuria in C3b inactivator deficiency, and the first patient to be described with this disorder had intermittent urticaria, particularly after a shower or when given normal plasma (and hence C3 as substrate). It is reasonable to attribute these abnormalities to the elaboration in vivo of large amounts of C3a from uninhibited alternative pathway activation with attendant C3 cleavage.

Increased susceptibility to infection

There appear to be two groups of complement-deficient patients with undue susceptibility to infection: those with deficits of C3 directly, or of C3 and Factor B secondary to C3b inactivator deficiency; and those with deficiencies of later-acting, or common pathway proteins, particularly C6 and C8. The organisms involved in C3-deficient patients are chiefly the pyogens: the streptococcus, the pneumococcus, the meningococcus and *H. influenzae*. These bacteria are much the same as those that afflict agammaglobulinaemics. Although severe deficits in most complement-mediated functions can be demonstrated in serum from these patients, it appears that a deficit in opsonization is central to their reduced host resistance. It is dangerous to be too simplistic, however, inasmuch as one C3-deficient subject had had no serious infections by the age of 4 years, and an 11 year old with C3b inactivator deficiency has also been infection free. Clearly, other factors, including environment, play their part in any specific instance.

Deficiency of the late-acting complement components, C5 through C8, is associated in a little over half the propositi with *N. meningitides* and *N. gonorrhoeae* systemic infections. There is some ascertainment bias in assessing the incidence of such infections in these subjects since the incidence in homozygous deficient sibs of index cases is only 14%. Of patients with recurrent meningococcal meningitis, it is estimated that about 10% have a deficiency of a late-acting complement component. The mechanism for this increased susceptibility is presumably a defective bactericidal capacity for *Neisseriae*.

Collagen vascular disease

There is a striking incidence of SLE, 'lupus-like' disease, and a variety of phenomena probably not the same, but all suspected of having an immunologic basis, among all patients with complement deficiencies, including hereditary angioedema. These associations are with deficiencies of late-acting components of complement as well as of early components. Because C2 deficiency is so common, most attention has been directed to this deficiency. Of 38 homozygous C2-deficient subjects, 23 have disease, chiefly of suspected immunologic type. Fourteen had systemic lupus erythematosus or discoid lupus erythematosus, and of these, the female/male ratio was 6:1, whereas the overall female/male ratio in the non-SLE C2-deficient subjects was nearly 1:1.

This association between lupus and C2 deficiency may have one or more of several explanations. The gene for C2 deficiency (and the structural lucus for C2) is on the sixth human chromosome, closely linked with the HLA regions. The C2 locus is very close to HLA-B and probably even closer to HLA-D. In other words, the genes at the C2 locus are inherited together with those for HLA with only minimal recombination. Furthermore, there is marked linkage disequilibrium between the C2 deficiency gene (*C2D*) and *HLA A10 B18*, and even more striking linkage disequilibrium between *C2D* and *HLA Dw2* and *Bf*s. Thus, among random, apparently unrelated individuals, *C2D* is found linked to specific nearby genes. This disequilibrium could be the result of selective pressure keeping them together or could result because the C2 deficiency mutation occurred fairly recently in human evolution. That the latter is the case is suggested by the fact that all the cases of C2 deficiency uncovered to date have been in white people. In contrast many of the homozygotes for deficiency of later-acting components, such as C5, C6, or C8 are in black people.

In any event, it is possible that an unusual immune response gene linked with *C2D* is somehow involved in an increased incidence of lupus in C2-deficient subjects. This possibility is enhanced by the evidence that lupus may result from viral infection. Further evidence for this hypothesis was obtained in a study of C2-deficient heterozygotes wherein it was found that although the incidence among normal individuals was 1.2%, the incidence in patients with lupus was significantly greater (two or three times).

Homozygous deficiency of complement proteins, particularly early-acting components, may predispose to lupus because of the deficiency per se. A possible mechanism is the requirement for complement in the solubilization of immune complexes. This would help explain the observed high incidence of lupus in C4 deficiency, hereditary angioedema, and Clr deficiency. Because the system only through C3 appears to participate in this function, it cannot be invoked to explain lupus in association with deficiencies of C5 and C8.

Finally, there is the problem of bias in the ascertainment and reporting of cases of complement deficiencies that favors a higher incidence of disease in general and collagen vascular disease in particular. Total haemolytic complement was measured initially only in specialised laboratories, so that it is not surprising that the first few cases of C2 deficiency were found among immunologists. As the test became a relatively common routine procedure, those tested tended to have or be suspected of having 'immunologic disease' and, in particular, lupus. The association may therefore reflect the incidence of these diseases in the tested population.

That there is a real association is suggested by the studies in heterozygous deficient subjects mentioned above. It is also suggested by a brief consideration of numbers. Assuming that the incidence of lupus (both systemic and discoid varieties) is between 1 and 0.1% of the general population in the United States and the incidence of homozygous C2 deficiency is 1 in 10 000, there are approximately 20 000 homozygous for C2 deficiency in the United States, of whom 20–200 would be expected to have lupus by chance alone. To have already identified 14 such subjects suggests that the number who have both C2 deficiency and lupus is much greater than the random association would predict. Thus, it appears likely that C4 and C2 deficiency (and perhaps other complement deficiencies) predispose to lupus, but the exact relationship and possible explanations need further exploration.

REFERENCES

Alper C A 1980 Complement and the MHC. In: Dorf M E (ed). The role of the major histocompatibility complex in immunobiology. Garland Press Publishing, Inc., New York, pp 173–220, 1981

Alper C A, Abramson N, Johnston R B Jr, Jandl J H, Rosen F S 1970a Increased susceptibility to infection associated with abnormalities of complement-mediated functions and of the third component of complement (C3). New England Journal of Medicine 282: 349–354

Alper C A, Abramson N, Johnston R B Jr, Jandl J H, Rosen F S 1970b Studies in vivo and in vitro on an abnormality in the metabolism of C3 in a patient with increased susceptibility to infection. Journal of Clinical Investigation 49: 1975–1985

Alper C A, Colten H R, Gear J S S, Rabson A R, Rosen F S 1976 Homozygous human C3 deficiency. The role of C3 in antibody production, Cls-induced vasopermeability, and cobra venom-induced passive hemolysis. Journal of Clinical Investigation 57: 222–229

Alper C A, Colten H R, Rosen F S, Rabson A R, Macnab G M, Gear J S S 1972a Homozygous deficiency of C3 in a patient with repeated infections. Lancet 2: 1179–1181

Alper C A, Propp R P, Klemperer M R, Rosen F S 1969 Inherited deficiency of the third component of human complement (C3) Journal of Clinical Investigation 48: 553–557

Alper C A, Rosen F S, Lachmann P J 1972b Inactivator of the third component of complement as an inhibitor in the properdin pathway. Proceedings of the National Academy of Sciences USA 69: 2910–2913

Ballow M, Shira J E, Harden L, Yang S Y, Day N K 1975 Complete absence of the third component of complement in man. Journal of Clinical Investigation 56: 703–710

Berkel A I, Loos M, Sanal O, Mauff G, Güngen G, Örs Ü, Ersay F, Yegin O 1979. Clinical and immunological studies in a case of selective complete Clq deficiency. Clinical and Experimental Immunology 38: 52–63

Davis A E III, Davis J S IV, Rabson A R, Osofsky S G, Colten H R, Rosen F S. Alper C A 1977 Homozygous C3 deficiency: Detection of C3 by radioimmunoassay. Clinical Immunology and Immunopathology 8: 543–550

De Bracco M M E, Windhorst D, Stroud R M, Moncada B 1974 The autosomal recessive mode of inheritance of Clr deficiency in a large Puerto Rican family. Clinical and Experimental Immunology 16: 183–188

Donaldson V H, Evans R R 1963 A biochemical abnormality in hereditary angioneurotic edema. Absence of serum inhibitor of Cl esterase. American Journal of Medicine 35: 35–45

Donaldson V H, Rosen F S, Bing D H 1977 Role of the second component of complement (C2) and plasmin in kinin release in hereditary angioneurotic edema (H.A.N.E.) plasma. Transactions of the Association of American Physicians 90: 174–183

Gelfand J A, Sherins R J, Alling D W, Frank M M 1976 Treatment of hereditary angioneurotic edema with Danazol. Reversal of clinical and biochemical abnormalities. New England Journal of Medicine 295: 1444–1448

Hauptmann G, Grosshans E, Heid E, Mayer S, Basset A 1974 Lupus erythemateux aigu avec deficit complet de la fraction C4 du complement. Nouveau Presse de Medicine 3: 881–882

Jasin H E 1977 Absence of the eighth component of complement in association with systemic lupus erythematosus-like disease. Journal of Clinical Investigation 60: 709–715

Klemperer M R, Woodworth H C, Rosen F S, Austen K F 1966 Hereditary deficiency of the second component of complement in man. Journal of Clinical Investigation 45: 880–890

Lachmann P J, Rosen F S 1978 Genetic defects of complement in man. Seminars in Immunopathology 1: 339–353

Leddy J P, Frank M M, Gaither T, Baum J, Klemperer M R 1974 Hereditary deficiency of the sixth component of complement in man. I. Immunochemical, biologic, and family studies. Journal of Clinical Investigation 53: 544–553

Lim D, Gewurz A, Lint T F, Ghaze M, Sepheri B, Gewurz H 1976 Absence of the sixth component of complement in a patient with repeated episodes of meningococcal meningitis. Journal of Pediatrics 89: 42–47

Lint T F, Zeitz H J, Scott D, Malkinson J R, Gewurz H 1978 Hereditary deficiency of the ninth component of complement (C) in man (abstract) Clinical Research 26: 714

Matthews N, Stark J M, Harper P S, Doran J, Jones D M 1980 Recurrent meningococcal infections associated with a functional deficiency of the C8 component of human complement. Clinical and Experimental Immunology 39: 53–59

Müller-Eberhard H J 1975 Complement. Annual Review of Biochemistry 44: 697–724

Ochs H D, Rosenfeld S I, Thomas E D, Giblett E R, Alper C A, Dupont B, Schaller J G, Gilliland B C, Hansen J A, Wedgwood R J 1977 Linkage between the gene (or genes) controlling synthesis of the fourth component of complement and the major histocompatibility complex. New England Journal of Medicine 296: 470–475

Petersen B H, Graham J A, Brooks G F 1976 Human deficiency of the eighth component of complement. The requirement of C8 for serum Neisseria gonorrhoeae bactericidal activity. Journal of Clinical Investigation 57: 283–290

Rosen F S, Alper C A, Pensky J, Klemperer M R, Donaldson V H 1971 Genetically determined heterogeneity of the Cl esterase inhibitor in patients with hereditary angioneurotic edema. Journal of Clinical Investigation. 50: 2143–2149

Rosenfeld S J, Kelly M E, Leddy J P 1976 Hereditary deficiency of the fifth component of complement in man. I. Clinical, immunochemical, and family studies. Journal of Clinical Investigation 57: 1626–1634

Snyderman R, Durack D J, McCarthy G A, Ward F E, Meadows L 1979 Deficiency of the fifth component of complement in human subjects. American Journal of Medicine 67: 638–645

Wellek B, Opferkuch W 1975 A case of deficiency of the seventh component of complement in man. Biological properties of a C7-deficient serum and description of a C7-inactivating principle. Clinical and Experimental Immunology 19: 223–235

Ziegler J B, Alper C A, Rosen F S, Lachmann P J, Sherington L 1975 Restoration by purified C3b inactivator of complement-mediated function in vivo in a patient with C3b inactivator deficiency. Journal of Clinical Investigation 55: 668–672

80

Disorders of leucocyte function

M.E. Miller

Over the past 15 years, the field of phagocytic disorders has attained major clinical and biological significance. Despite this relatively short period of time, much literature has accumulated on these disorders which are frequently hereditary.

HISTORICAL BACKGROUND

Two major observations, one basic and one clinical, set the foundation for current knowledge of this field. In the late 1800s, Elie Metchnikoff (1893) established that 'the essential and primary element in typical inflammation consists in a reaction of the phagocyte *against* a harmful agent.' Prior to this, it was believed that phagocytes were harmful to the host and that they contributed to the untoward consequences of bacterial infection. However, once Metchnikoff had established that phagocytes were helpful rather than harmful to the human host, he predicted that defects in phagocyte function might predispose the host to increased numbers and toxicity of infections with foreign microorganisms. The last 15 years of clinical recognition of phagocyte disorders have proven his hypothesis to be true.

Holmes and co-workers (1966) provided the first evidence of an inborn error of phagocyte function. They studied patients with chronic granulomatous disease (CGD), a disorder characterized by indolent, granulomatous type infections. The disease most frequently occurs in an X–linked pattern and usually proves fatal to afflicted males within the first decade of life.

In in vitro experiments, it was shown that polymorphonuclear leucocytes (PMNs) from the afflicted children were able to ingest bacteria normally but were unable to kill the ingested organisms. This was in sharp contrast to normal PMNs which effectively killed the same organisms intracellularly. Of additional interest was the observation that PMNs from the mothers (presumed carriers in an X–linked disorder) were intermediate in their killing capacity. Not only did these observations establish the first intrinsic defect of PMN function, but the intermediate bactericidal defect in maternal PMNs

was consistent with the Lyon hypothesis.

Baehner and Nathan (1968) demonstrated a primary metabolic abnormality in PMNs from CGD patients by utilizing a colorless dye – nitroblue tetrazolium (NBT) – which turns to blue formazan in the reduced state. It was shown that normal PMNs stimulated to ingest and kill bacteria reduced the dye, but similarly stimulated PMNs from the children with CGD were unable to reduce the dye. Again, maternal PMNs were found to be intermediate in dye reduction. This suggested a biochemical lesion under genetic control as the underlying basis for the bactericidal defect.

On a broader scale, the observation that dysfunction of one PMN activity, i.e. bactericidal mechanisms, could lead to a clinically recognizable syndrome suggested that other PMN functions such as movement and/or ingestion could also, if deficient, lead to recurrent infections. Further, the observation that one of these defects was genetically determined suggested that other disorders of PMN function might also have a hereditary basis.

Over the past 15 years, these hypotheses have been proven true. An entire spectrum of disorders of PMN, and more recently monocyte-macrophage (MNL) functions, have been recognized, many of which are genetically determined. In this chapter, we will summarize the current status of this exciting field. To grasp the subject better, it will be helpful first to review three basic mechanisms of normal phagocytic cells – movement, ingestion and bactericidal activities. This review is intended only to provide the reader with the necessary background to interpret the clinical findings. More comprehensive reviews of each function are cited in the appropriate sections.

BASIC PHAGOCYTIC ACTIVITIES

Polymorphonuclear leucocytes (PMNs)

Movement
Mobilization of phagocytic cells from the bone marrow and other storage sites of the body requires active move-

ment. The mechanisms by which phagocytes move have been the focus of extensive recent laboratory interest.

A major advance in the ability to study movement of PMNs was provided by the development of an in vitro filter assay by Stephen Boyden (1962). Prior to that time, it was commonly held that there was little, if any, biologic significance to the movement of phagocytic cells. In principle, the Boyden assay consists of measuring the migration of cells through a small-pored filter towards a chemotactically active gradient. Such a gradient can be generated by a variety of methods, but is usually derived by activation of complement following exposure of fresh serum to endotoxin or antigen-antibody complexes. Such activated sera contain a variety of chemotactically active materials, including C5a. Additional substances found to have chemotactic activity include: serum factors, coagulation-derived factors, bacterial metabolites, secretory products of sensitized lymphocytes and PMNs, denatured proteins, and synthetic chemotactic factors such as the N-formylmethionyl peptides (Gallin & Quie, 1978; Ackerman & Douglas, 1979). Also, lipoxygenases in a variety of mammalian cells transform arachidonic acid to stable mono-hydroxyeicosatetraenoic (HETE) products. Various endogenously produced HETE products are chemotactic for PMNs (Goetzl & Sun, 1979).

The precise mechanisms by which a PMN initiates and sustains movement following exposure to chemotactically active material are surrounded by controversy. A number of potentially important steps have, however, been identified.

Initially, a brief but rapid membrane depolarization occurs. This is coincident with calcium and/or sodium influx, and is followed by a prolonged hyperpolarization associated with increased potassium permeability (Gallin, et al, 1978).

Subsequent events include: increased levels of cyclic guanosine monophosphate (cGMP) (Hill, 1978); lysosomal enzyme release (Becker and Showell, 1974); increased glycolysis and hexosemonophosphate shunt activity (Goetzl and Austen, 1974); cell swelling (Becker, 1976); increased numbers of microtubules (Stossel, 1978); and probable activation of contractile proteins (Boxer, et al, 1974).

While considerable information on overall cell movement has been gained from filter, i.e. Boyden-type assays, such techniques yield little information on the process(es) of cell movement. In other words, cells are placed on one side of a filter and counted on the opposite side. How they got there, however, is anyone's guess. Such information is obviously critical if we are to understand and diagnose individual disorders of PMN movement.

Partial answers to these questions have been provided by the development of assays which permit observations of single and/or small numbers of cells during movement.

These include direct visualization (Wilkinson & Allan, 1978); the visual assay system of Zigmond (1978) in which cells are observed under phase microscopy on a bridge across which a gradient of chemotactic factor is established; deformability of PMNs by the technique of cell elastimetry (Miller & Myers, 1975); and cinemicrography and videotape analysis of PMNs subjected to a chemotactic gradient (Cheung & Miller, 1980). Such techniques have now been applied not only to normal PMNs but to PMNs from patients with various defects of movement. Since data so derived will be of significance in the following clinical discussion, the results will be briefly summarized.

(a) Deformability. Deformability is measured by the technique of cell elastimetry, which measures the amount of negative pressure required to aspirate a cell into a micropipette. In 1970, Lichtman utilized this technique in the study of human bone marrow granulocytes and found that less negative pressure was required for aspiration as cells matured. In other words, myeloblasts and promyelocytes were relatively resistant to deformation while myelocytes were more easily deformed. Mature PMNs were highly deformable, and it was postulated that increasing deformability of PMNs correlated with the ability of granulocytes to leave the bone marrow. Miller and Myers (1975) adapted the technique to the study of human peripheral blood PMNs and demonstrated a correlation between deformability and cell motility. Deformability of PMNs from patients with PMN movement disorders provides one means of demonstrating heterogeneity of the group (Miller, 1979).

(b) Visual assays. Several visual techniques have been applied to the study of motile PMNs. Early assays employed time-lapse photography and demonstrated that motile PMNs were able to turn in response to a chemotactic stimulus. Zigmond utilized an improved technique for studying the nature and mechanisms responsible for the turning (1978). Basically, the system consisted of a microscope slide with a bridge separated by a shallow well on either side. A chemotactic gradient could be established by placing a chemoattractant in one well and a suitable buffer in the other well. A suspension of PMNs was then deposited on the bridge and the cells observed microscopically. Cells appeared to orient or turn towards the chemotactic stimulus, and once oriented, retained their direction and moved towards the chemotactic stimulus. These observations led to a new terminology for PMN movement. Formerly, the term 'chemotaxis' was applied to the general phenomenon of PMNs moving towards a chemical gradient (as measured in a Boyden or filter type assay). The more current terminology, however, designates the turning or orientation phase as *chemotaxis*, and the increased rate of locomotion of motile cells as *chemokinesis* (Gallin and Quie, 1978). These new terms are important in understanding disorders of human PMN movement as some of the defects appear to be ones of abnormal chemotaxis and some of abnormal chemokinesis.

More recent studies have described the use of high speed cinemicrography and videotape analysis in the study of motile human PMNs (Cheung & Miller, 1980). Such studies suggest that the concept of PMNs turning towards the chemotactic stimulus may not be correct. Although human PMNs oriented towards a chemotactic gradient move steadily towards the gradient in terms of net activity, individual cells constantly oscillate and re-orient during the process. This is accomplished not by turning in any one direction, but rather by extending one or more pseudopodia from any area of the cell surface. A primary requirement of the PMN in order to move effectively is a highly deformable membrane (see above).

Phagocytosis

Ingestion of foreign substances of particulate nature (phagocytosis) or soluble nature (pinocytosis) involves two distinct phases – recognition and ingestion. The recognition phase involves specific receptors on the cell membrane. Several PMN membrane receptors which have been identified include a receptor for the Fc fragments of immunoglobulin molecules and receptors for several activation products of complement (C3b and C5a) (Henson, 1976). These receptros presumably play a significant role in increasing efficiency of the ingestion process by fixing opsonised particles to the cell surface.

Following adherence, particles are then actually ingested. This involves many of the same cellular functions and activities as in movement, and some investigators feel that the two activities are part of the same overall process. Ingestion involves the flow of cytoplasmic hyaline pseudopods around the phagocytosed particle (Stossel, 1975; Wilkinson, 1976). Formation of these pseudopods probably involves active participation of the actin-myosin filament system of the PMN (Stossel, 1975; Stossel & Hartwig, 1976). The pseudopods surround and fuse about the attached particle in forming a phagosome. The internalized phagosome is then merged with lysosomes and degranulation occurs with ultimate discharge of lysosomal contents into the phagosome, i.e. phagolysosome.

Bactericidal activity

An immense literature has accumulated on the characterization of bactericidal mechanisms of human PMNs. A comprehensive review of this topic is obviously outside the scope of this chapter, and we will, therefore, summarize those points which are relevant to the following clinical discussion.

A sophisticated array of biochemical processes are available to the human PMN in killing of ingested microorganisms. Bactericidal activity of human PMNs is associated with oxidative activity, although the precise

relationships are not yet known. Upon contact with the PMN membrance by a foreign particle, and coincident with ingestion and onset of killing, a sequence of metabolic events occurs. This is known as the 'respiratory burst' and includes increased oxygen consumption, oxidation of glucose via the hexosemonophosphate shunt, and the generation of hydrogen peroxide (Johnston, Jr. & Newman, 1977).

A group of potentially bactericidal products is generated during this process. The reaction is initiated by contact of the cell surface with a foreign particle or microbe. This presumably activates an enzyme upon, or closely related to the cell surface. Oxidases such as NADH, NADPH or glutathione peroxidase are particularly likely candidates. Activation of the oxidase(es) results in the transfer of a single electron to oxygen, thereby forming an unstable radical known as superoxide anion (O_2^-). Two superoxide radicals can form hydrogen peroxide (H_2O_2) when they spontaneously interact. The continuing reaction between H_2O_2 and O_2^- yields free hydroxyl radical (OH), a potent oxidizing agent. Transfer of energy from O_2^- to an unstable, excited species called singlet oxygen may result in a burst of energy which can be measured as emitted light in the chemiluminescence assay. Transfer of 'extra' electrons from superoxide anions may be responsible for NBT dye reduction.

Each of these oxidation products – superoxide anion, hydrogen peroxide, hydroxyl radicals and singlet oxygen – possess potent bactericidal activities. While the extent to which any one shares in normal PMN bactericidal activity has not yet been determined, it seems likely that some, if not all, are of clinical significance. Additional microbicidal activities result from the release of PMN lysosomal materials such as myeloperoxidase, lysozyme, phagocytin and other cationic proteins.

Monocytes and macrophages

These cells subserve many of the same functions as PMNs, including movement, ingestion and microbicidal activities. In addition, a major role in modulating the immune response has been demonstrated. The macrophage is involved in the enhancement of antibody responses and cell-mediated immunity, particularly towards T cell-dependent antigens. This topic is reviewed in detail elsewhere (Cohn, 1978; Karnovsky & Lazdins, 1978; North, 1978).

The importance of macrophages in the inflammatory response was first suggested by Metchnikoff (1893), who noted from his observations of tubercle bacilli that:

The polynuclear cells engulf the tubercle bacilli readily but perish after a short time, and then with the microbes they contain, are eaten up by various mononuclear phagocytes which may be classed together under the term of macrophages. These latter cells have a much greater power of resistance, and in some cases are even capable of destroying the tubercle bacilli.

The relationship between macrophages and the circulating monocytes has not been conclusively determined. It is generally believed, however, that blood monocytes evolve into macrophages (histiocytes) in various anatomic sites, including the peritoneal cavity, lung, bone marrow, spleen, lymph nodes, and liver. Increasing evidence suggests that subpopulations of macrophages from different and even the same tissues exist. For example, alveolar and peritoneal macrophages differ metabolically and functionally.

Mackaness (1962) immensely heightened interest in the role of the macrophage in the immune-inflammatory response when he demonstrated that macrophages which had been infected with the intracellular pathogen, *Listeria monocytogenes*, were able to significantly inhibit the growth and infectivity of other intracellular organisms (which normal macrophages cannot do).

Thus was born the concept of the 'activated macrophage' (Cohn, 1978; Karnovsky, 1978; North, 1978). These cells are larger and adhere and spread more on glass than normal macrophages. A number of functional and biochemical activities are enhanced in activated macrophages over those seen in normal macrophages. Phagocytosis of some (but not all) materials is increased. Glucose utilization through the hexosemonophosphate shunt is increased. Membrane enzymes such as adenylate cyclase, and cytoplasmic enzymes such as lactic dehydrogenase show increased activities. Increased numbers of lysosomes and enhanced release of lysosomal enzymes – e.g. collagenase – are also seen.

The functional consequences of these changes remain unclear. The major effects which have been noted in activated macrophages are enhanced bactericidal activities and increased tumour inhibition and killing. These two activities do not, however, consistently correlate. In other words, macrophages which have been 'activated' in enhanced killing may not always show increased tumoricidal activities, and vice versa.

It is not yet known whether all clinical disorders of phagocyte function involve both PMNs and MNLs, or whether there are entities which only involve one or the other cell line. To the extent that data is available, comparative studies will be noted in the following clinical discussion.

CLINICAL DISORDERS OF PHAGOCYTE FUNCTION

DISORDERS OF BACTERICIDAL FUNCTION

Chronic granulomatous disease
The CGD syndrome is characterized by recurrent, purulent infections of the skin, reticulo-endothelial organs and lungs, associated with an inability of the patient's phagocytes to kill intracellular, catalase positive, non-

Table 80.1 Signs and symptoms in 168 patients with chronic granulomatous disease (Johnston, Jr. and Newman, 1977)

Findings	Number of patients involved
Marked lymphadenopathy	137
Pneumonitis	134
Dermatitis	120
Hepatomegaly	114
Onset by one year	109
Suppuration of nodes	104
Splenomegaly	95
Hepatic-perihepatic abscess	69
Osteomyelitis	54
Onset with dermatitis	42
Onset with lymphadenitis	38
Facial periorificial dermatitis	35
Persistent diarrhea	34
Septicemia or meningitis	29
Perianal abscess	28
Conjunctivitis	27
Death from pneumonitis	26
Persistent rhinitis	26
Ulcerative stomatitis	26

hydrogen peroxide producing bacteria. Onset of symptoms usually occurs within the first year of life, although cases have been reported where the initial infections occurred as late as 12 years of age. Although common signs and symptoms may affect virtually any part of the body, suppurative, indolent lymphadenitis, pneumonitis, dermatitis, hepatomegaly, splenomegaly and osteomyelitis are particularly frequent findings. Table 80.1 summarizes the relative frequency of clinical findings in CGD. The dermatologic involvement may be in the form of low grade abcesses, or frequently as a perioral eczematoid lesion.

A unique group of bacteria is associated with CGD. This includes primarily catalase-positive, non-hydrogen peroxide producing organisms. As shown in Table 80.2, *Staphylococcus aureus* and enteric organisms predominate. Of additional significance is the relatively high frequency of the enteric organisms *Klebsiella-Aerobacter* and *Serratia Marcescens*. In many of the earlier case descriptions, post-mortem examinations yielded these organisms but those interpreting the findings tended to discard them as insignificant. Notably absent from the list of common pathogens in patients with CGD are *Hemophilus influenzae*, streptococci and pneumococci. This correlates with the ability of the patients' phagocytes to kill these catalase-negative, peroxide-producing organisms in vivo (Mandell & Hook, 1969; Johnston, Jr. & Newman, 1977). In addition to bacterial organisms, the fungi Aspergillus and Candida are relatively frequent pathogens.

An additional laboratory finding in CGD is an almost constant neutrophilia, even during periods when the patient does not appear to be acutely infected. As we

Table 80.2 Microorganisms cultured from blood, cerebrospinal fluid, or purulent foci (Johnston, Jr. Newman, 1977)

Organism	Number of patients involved*
Staphylococcus aureus	87
Klebsiella-Aerobacter organisms	29
E. coli	26
Serratia marcescens	16
Pseudomonas organisms	15
Staphylococcus albus	13
Aspergillus organisms	13
Candida albicans	12
Salmonella organisms	10
Proteus organisms	9
Streptococci	9
Nocardia organisms	4
Mycobacteria	4
Paracolobactrum organisms	4
Actinomyces organisms	2
Other enteric bacteria	9

* Refers to number of different patients from whom that organism was cultured.

shall later describe, this contrasts with the neutropenia of the patient with a chemotactic defect.

Laboratory diagnosis

Two procedures are generally performed in the confirmation of a diagnosis of CGD. The first is a screening technique which measures the ability of the patient's PMNs to reduce nitroblue tetrazolium dye (NBT). Reduction converts the colourless oxidized NBT to blue formazan, which can be measured qualitatively or spectrophotometrically (Johnston, Jr. & Baehner, 1971). Normal PMNs reduce NBT as a consequence of metabolic products generated during the bactericidal process. PMNs from patients with CGD fail, however, to reduce the dye. Decreased total dye reduction could result if all of the PMNs were working at diminished capacity or if two populations of PMNs – one normal and one defective – were present. This is important as the carrier state would more readily fit the Lyon hypothesis if two populations were present. Histochemical techniques (Ochs & Igo, 1973) have confirmed the presence of two populations.

Regardless of the results from an NBT test, specific diagnosis of CGD must be confirmed by an in vitro bactericidal assay (Holmes, Quie, et al, 1966). Ideally, this should be performed with isolates of the patient's infecting organism, but if not available, staphylococci or E. coli can be used.

Recent modifications of the chemiluminescence assay have increased its sensitivity and utility in the study of patients and carriers with CGD (Mills, et al, 1980). It

remains to be proven, however, that this relatively easy assay can be relied upon in lieu of a specific bactericidal test. Studies of monocytes from CGD patients have yielded essentially the same results as PMNs.

Mechanisms of CGD

The CGD syndrome reflects a number of related, yet specific, underlying molecular abnormalities. Until such molecular defects are precisely identified, however, separation of the cases into specific entities is not possible. Despite this limitation, much has been learned of the probable mechanisms. The basic molecular defect is deficient activity of an enzyme responsible for conversion of oxygen to bactericidal species. NADH oxidase, NADPH oxidase and glutathione peroxidase have each been proposed as the critical enzyme, but definitive proof for any one is lacking. Most investigators currently favour NADPH oxidase (Johnston, Jr. & Newman, 1977).

In the absence of oxidase activation, the events associated with the normal respiratory burst fail to occur. PMNs from patients with CGD fail to show a phagocytosis-associated increase in oxygen consumption, generation of superoxide and hydrogen peroxide. As a consequence, NBT reduction and chemiluminescence responses fail to occur. Decreased bactericidal activity presumably reflects the absence of these potent bactericidal oxidation products of normal PMN respiration.

Genetics of CGD

X–linked recessive inheritance has been established in the majority of males with CGD (Windhorst, Page, et al, 1968). In reported cases, a male:female ratio of 6:1 further supports this mode of inheritance as the most frequent (Johnston, Jr. & Newman, 1977). In familial studies, the use of the histochemical NBT test has supported X–linked transmission and provided confirmation of the Lyon hypothesis. In this test, over 90% (usually in excess of 98%) of PMNs from normal individuals will reduce the dye upon appropriate stimulation. Virtually none of the patients' PMNs will reduce the NBT. PMNs from the patients' mothers, sisters or female maternal relatives who are presumed carriers of the disease generally have a mixture of normal and abnormal PMNs (35 to 65% of PMNs will reduce the dye). If inactivation of one X–chromosome is, as required by the Lyon hypothesis, a completely random event, then one might expect to occasionally find a female carrier with wide deviation from 50% normal PMNs. Such has been reported by Repine, et al (1975) who found that PMNs from one sister of a boy with CGD had only 20% normal cells by NBT reduction.

In the absence of identified basic molecular defects in CGD, much controversy surrounds the question of other modes of inheritance. The two most widely cited occurrences are case reports of CGD in females (Baehner & Nathan, 1968; Quie et al, 1968; Azimi et al, 1968; Ochs & Igo, 1973; Wilson et al, 1974; Biggar et al, 1976; Carruthers & Greaves, 1976; McPhail et al, 1977; Clark & Klebanoff, 1978; Segal et al, 1978), and in boys without demonstrable leucocyte defects in either parent (Kontras & Bass, 1969; Dupree et al, 1972; Repine et al, 1975).

The mode of inheritance in females with CGD is unknown. Data yielded by the NBT and bactericidal assays has generally failed to demonstrate PMN defects in either parent. This inability to detect the carrier state in families of females with chronic granulomatous disease has been interpreted as suggesting a non-X-linked inheritance in these patients. Recently, however, Mills et al (1980) applied the luminol-dependent chemiluminescence assay to detect subtle abnormalities in PMN oxygen metabolism in females with CGD. PMNs from three of four CGD females showed extremely low chemiluminescence production. Their asymptomatic mothers' PMNs had intermediate values, and PMNs from the fathers were normal. PMNs from two affected males in these kinships also generated virtually no chemiluminescence. All unaffected males showed normal PMN chemiluminescence, but two of seven female relatives had intermediate values. PMNs in three of the families were also studied by NBT reduction. In each family, two populations of PMNs were demonstrated for the female patients and/or their mothers. The authors suggested that these findings support an X-linked inheritance in at least these families of females with CGD based upon (a) the wide phenotypic variability for clinical disease, (b) evidence of two; PMN populations in the patients or their mothers and (c) low but detectable chemiluminescence in PMNs from the affected females.

In reports of boys with CGD whose parents have lacked demonstrable PMN abnormalities, transmission by an autosomal recessive gene or, in some cases, the possibility of spontaneous mutation has been postulated. Study of these kindreds with senssitive assays such as the luminol enhanced chemiluminescence have not yet been reported but may help shed light on the problem.

Variants of CGD

Most reported 'variants' of CGD have provided relatively indirect evidence, such as apparent selectivity of bacterial strains to which the patient was susceptible or, the presence of PMN defects in addition to the bactericidal defect. Such case reports are difficult to interpret.

Several probable variants have, however, been reported. A brother and sister with clinical CGD were described, whose PMNs could ingest, but not kill, staphylococci (Van Der Meer et al, 1975; Weening et al, 1976). As expected, PMNs from either patient demonstrated defective oxygen consumption, O_2^- production, hexose monophosphate shunt activation and iodination of ingested particles upon in vitro ingestion of serum-opsonized zymosan or latex. Upon ingestion of latex particles heavily coated with IgG or IgG aggregates, however, the same PMNs demonstrated normal oxidative, 'respiratory burst' activities. It, thus, appeared that the patients' PMNs possessed normal oxidative metabolic activities, but had an abnormal trigger or activating mechanism. Six other patients (three boys and three girls) with CGD studied by the authors failed to demonstrate this finding.

Clark and Klebanoff (1978) described a brother and sister, ages 24 and 20, who had classical clinical and laboratory findings of CGD and also marked impairment in the chemotactic responses of their PMNs and in the level of chemotactic activities generated in their serums by activation of the complement system. Impaired leucocyte migration has not generally been found in patients with CGD. As noted by the authors, however,

It remains to be determined what the relationship between the leukocyte bactericidal and chemotactic defects is, what their relative contributions to increased susceptibility to infections are, and whether similar impairment of chemotaxis is present in other patients with chronic granulomatous disease.

Giblett et al (1971) observed that patients with the X-linked form of CGD carried the very rare null Kell blood group phenotype K_o, in which all antigenic products of the Kell locus are absent. Marsh and co-workers (1975, 1977) found K_o phenotypes in five boys with X-linked CGD, while 50 normal individuals possessed a Kell group antigen, designated K_x. In the brother and sister with CGD (presumably not X-linked) described by Clark and Klebanoff (178), both patients were K_x. Although these findings support an association between K_o phenotype and the X-linked form of CGD, more recent evidence suggests that the correlation is not always present.

Glucose-6-phosphate dehydrogenase (G6PD) deficiency

Patients with severe leucocyte G6PD deficiency (generally 5% or less of normal G6PD levels) have a clinical syndrome which mimics CGD, although infections are usually somewhat milder. Oxidative metabolic defects are also similar to CGD, with the exception that methylene blue stimulates glucose-C-1 oxidation by the PMNs of CGD patients, but not always of G6PD deficient subjects (Holmes et al, 1967). The actual existence of functionally significant intrinsic leucocyte G6PD deficiency has been questioned. An increased lability of G6PD in PMNs of CGD patients has been described (Bellanti et al, 1970) which may be due to a deficiency in a stabilizing factor (Erickson et al, 1972). It should be emphasized that the vast majority of subjects with erythrocyte G6PD deficiency have normal leucocyte G6PD activity (Marks et al, 1959; Klebanoff & Clark, 1978).

Clinical management

Specific therapy for CGD must await definite identification and replacement of primary molecular deficiencies. Despite this, significant improvements have occurred in management and long term prognosis. Prolonged antimicrobial therapy with an agent as specific as possible for the infecting organism is the treatment of choice. This means that the treating physician must be alert to the most subtle signs of infection in these compromised hosts and take seriously the results of appropriate cultures. In particular, organisms such as *Klebsiella aerobacter* or *Serratia marcescens* must be regarded as pathogens in patients with CGD.

Long term administration of sulphonamides has been utilized with some success. These agents may exert an effect upon intracellular PMN microbicidal mechanisms (Johnston, Jr. & Newman, 1977). Other reported therapeutic trials include bone marrow transplantation (Delmas et al, 1975) and repeated granulocyte transfusions (Quie, 1969; Raubitschek et al, 1973). These measures are of doubtful benefit.

Glutathione synthetase deficiency

Glutathione synthetase deficiency occurs in two forms – with or without associated 5-oxoprolinuria. GSD without 5-oxoprolinuria is usually limited in clinical findings to haemolytic anaemia and acidosis (Mohler et al, 1970). GSD with associated 5-oxoprolinuria may be of broader clinical significance with the additional findings of CNS dysfunction cataracts (at least in experimental animals), increased susceptibility to infections and PMN bactericidal defects (Spielberg et al, 1977; Boxer et al, 1979).

Mechanism of GSD

We will concentrate the discussion on GSD with 5-oxoprolinuria. The basic defect is presumed to result from negative effects of superoxide and hydrogen peroxide. Although, as previously discussed, these metabolites are important contributors to normal PMN bactericidal activities, they are also highly reactive waste products which must eventually be eliminated by the phagocyte. This elimination is accomplished by (a) superoxide dismutase which converts superoxide to hydrogen peroxide, and (b) catalase and the glutathione peroxidase-glutathione reductase system which convert hydrogen peroxide to water and molecular oxygen. In the absence of these enzymes, significant auto-oxidative damage occurs to the phagocytic cells (Oliver et al, 1976).

PMNs from a patient with GSD with 5-oxoprolinuria were studied for oxidant damage (Boxer et al, 1979). Compared with normal PMNs, GSD PMNs released 60% more hydrogen peroxide; iodinated 20–25% as many ingested particles; showed markedly decreased bactericidal activity towards ingested *S. aureus* 502A, and failed to assemble microtubules during phagocytosis.

Genetics of GSD

Genetic heterogeneity has been demonstrated in GSD. In GSD without 5-oxoprolinuria, Mohler et al (1970) demonstrated an autosomal recessive pattern. Erythrocytes from their patient (a 32 year old male) lacked glutathione synthetase, while erythrocytes from each of his parents and his four children had intermediate levels. Spielberg et al (1977) demonstrated that GSD without associated 5-oxoprolinuria resulted from an unstable mutant enzyme. Nucleated cells such as PMNs and fibroblasts maintained adequate levels of GS and glutathione, but erythrocytes did not.

GSD with 5-oxoprolinuria is also inherited as an autosomal recessive disorder (Spielberg et al, 1977). Almost undetectable levels of GS were found in cell lines from two patients, and intermediate levels in each of the parents studied. Unlike the erythrocyte defect, however, deficient GS activity was found in erythrocytes, PMNs and cultured skin fibroblasts. Further genetic heterogeneity was suggested by the finding of different enzyme kinetics for the mutant glutathione synthetases of the two patients studied. More studies will be necessary before concluding that different forms of GSD with oxoprolinuria exist.

Clinical management of GSD

Boxer et al (1979) reported successful treatment of a patient with GSD and 5-oxoprolinuria with alpha-tocopherol (vitamin E) therapy. The patient was placed on 400 IU of alpha-tocopherol per day for three months. Normalization of PMN defects occurred including improved microtubule assembly during phagocytosis. The mechanism of this response is unclear. Despite the improvement in PMN functions, glutathione levels remained at 25% normal levels. The authors suggested that vitamin E might have hastened the destruction of excess peroxide within the PMNs during phagocytosis.

Congenital myeloperoxidase deficiency

In congenital myeloperoxidase deficiency (*MPOD*), there is a complete absence of MPO from PMNs and MNLs. The eosinophil peroxidase differs in several respects from the PMN enzyme and is present in normal amounts (Archer et al, 1965; Desser et al, 1972). The clinical picture in hereditary MPOD is considerable less severe than that of CGD, and a number of the patients have been in reasonably good health (Klebanoff & Clark, 1978). In addition to occasional difficulty with the same spectrum of bacteria as encountered in CGD, several of these patients have encountered severe difficulty with *C. albicans* (Lehrer & Cline, 1969; Moosmann & Bojanovsky, 1975).

Mechanism of MPOD

Peroxidases do not exert direct antimicrobial activities,

but may catalyze the conversion of a substance from a weak to a strong antimicrobial agent. The mechanism of the MPO-mediated antimicrobial activity in human PMNs is complex. Hydrogen peroxide reacts with the iron of the heme prosthetic groups of MPO to form an enzyme-substrate complex or complexes with strong oxidative capacity. The oxidizable cofactors are presumably halides. The oxidation of a halide by MPO and hydrogen peroxide results in the formation of (a) strong antimicrobial agent(s) (iodine>bromine>chlorine) (Klebanoff & Clark, 1978).

Diagnosis of MPOD
MPOD is diagnosed by the complete absence of peroxidase-positive granules.in the cytoplasm of PMNs and MNLs. Eosinophils stain normally for peroxidase. A more accurate quantitative MPO assay from lysed PMNs has been described (Lehrer & Cline, 1969; Stehndahl & Lindgren, 1976; Rosen & Klebanoff, 1976).

Genetics of MPOD
Of the 12 reported cases, six were female and 12 were male. Three pairs of siblings were found within this relatively small group, suggesting a hereditary basis. In at least one family with MPOD, autosomal recessive inheritance has been proposed (Lehrer & Cline, 1969). Quantitative MPO assays of the patient's four sons each yielded MPO levels in their PMNs from 22–38% of the mean control value.

Chediak-Higashi syndrome
Chediak-Higashi Syndrome (CHS) is characterized by increased susceptibility to bacterial infections, oculocutaneous albinism, peripheral granulocytopaenia and giant azurophil lysosomes in PMNs (Blume & Wolff, 1972). The majority of patients succumb at an early age to recurrent pyogenic infections. PMNs from the affected patients have impaired chemotaxis, poor degranulation and kill bacteria inefficiently (Boxer et al, 1976). Occasionally, patients develop lymphoreticular infiltration in the liver, spleen, lymph nodes and bone marrow, which bear many similarities to malignant lymphoma. This pattern of CHS is known as the 'accelerated phase' (Kritzler et al, 1964). Animal models of CHS occur in mink, cattle, mice, killer whales and cats.

The upper and lower respiratory tract and the skin are among the most frequent sites of involvement. Pneumonitis, bronchitis, otitis, pharyngitis and sinusitis are also regularly encountered in CHS (Blume & Wolff, 1972). The causative agents in the CHS infections are the usual pyogenic bacteria.

Mechanism of CHS
An abnormality of microtubule assembly has been demonstrated in CHS (Boxer et al, 1976). Normal PMNs demonstrate aggregation, or 'capping' of the lectin, concanavalin A (con A) following treatment with colchicine. PMNs from patients with CHS, however, cap spontaneously upon con A treatment in the absence of colchicine (Boxer et al, 1976). This functional defect has been linked to abnormal levels of cyclic nucleotides in CHS PMNs, in turn leading to impaired function of cytoplasmic microtubules. Con A treatment of normal PMNs results in polymerization of cytoplasmic microtubules. This does not occur in CHS PMNs. Impaired lysosomal degranulation with consequent bactericidal deficiency may result from the generalized impairment of microtubule structural support.

Diagnosis of CHS
This is probably the easiest of the phagocyte disorders to diagnose. A history of recurrent pyogenic infections and at least some manifestations of partial oculocutaneous albinism are usually present. Additional findings such as lymphadenopathy, hepatosplenomegaly and neurologic dysfunction may be noted if the patient is in the accelerated phase. Confirmation of the diagnosis is made by examination of an ordinary Wright's stained peripheral blood smear. Up to 100% of the PMNs contain one or more 2–4µ azurophilic, peroxidase-positive cytoplasmic granules.

Genetics of CHS
This is a well established, simple autosomal recessive disorder. In the first reported family, the parents were consanguinous and four of the thirteen sibs were affected. Consanguinity has been reported in approximately half of the published cases (Blume & Wolff, 1972). Breeding experiments in various animal models of CHS have also demonstrated an autosomal pattern of inheritance in the various involved species. Detection of heterozygotes has had limited success, perhaps due to the paucity of homozygotes. Heterozygotes are usually healthy and lack albinoid features. Controversy exists over published reports of subtle PMN granule abnormalities (Klebanoff & Clark, 1978). Tanaka (1980) has reported a marked decrease in lysosomal enzymes of PMNs from patients with CHS.

Surprisingly, PMNs from heterozygous family members showed significantly elevated levels of different lysosomal enzymes. Tanaka suggested that CHS heterozygotes could, therefore, be detected by the altered PMN granule enzyme levels. Confirmation of this observation and explanation for the decreased levels in CHS patients and increased levels of different enzymes in the heterozygotes are necessary.

Clinical management of CHS
Treatment of CHS remains largely symptomatic, with vigorous treatment of infections with appropriate anti-

biotics. Although the accelerated phase has been treated with corticosteroids and chemotherapeutic agents such as vincristine, their success is questionable. Boxer et al (1976) exposed PMNs from patients with CHS to ascorbic acid, both in vitro and in vivo. Cyclic AMP levels were reduced to near normal, PMN functions were corrected and normal numbers of microtubules were restored. Improvement in clinical course of the patients, however, has not yet been conclusively demonstrated.

DISORDERS OF PHAGOCYTIC FUNCTION

No intrinsic, isolated abnormalities of PMN or MNL phagocytosis have been described. Boxer et al (1974) have described an 8 month old infant with pyogenic infections from birth whose PMNs were deficient in chemotaxis, bactericidal activity and phagocytosis. Cytoplasmic actin isolated from the patient's PMNs was quantitatively equal to that extracted from PMNs of a normal 8 month old. In vitro polymerization of the patient's actin was markedly decreased, however, in comparison to polymerization of the normal actin. No comment was made of the potential genetic implications.

Numerous phagocytic dysfunction syndromes resulting from deficiencies of various opsonins have been recognized. These have been extensively reviewed elsewhere (Miller, 1975; Johnston, Jr. & Stroud, 1977; Spitzer, 1977), and are also discussed in another chapter.

DISORDERS OF PHAGOCYTE MOVEMENT

Disorders of PMN and MNL movement constitute a large and important group of functional phagocyte deficiency states. As reviewed in the section of this chapter dealing with normal phagocyte movement, a number of mechanisms are involved and are, therefore, potential sites for clinically significant perturbations. To date, few of these disorders have been positively shown to be genetically determined. It should be stressed, however, that improvements in methodology of study of individual steps in PMN and MNL movement make it highly likely that some of these deficiencies will turn out to have a hereditary basis. In order to prepare the reader for these future developments, several general points should be stressed:

(a) Extensive heterogeneity exists among these disorders (Miller, 1975; Klebanoff & Clark, 1978). No single clinical or laboratory finding is consistently abnormal within this group of disorders. Assays such as the Boyden chamber reflect a number of individual steps in the overall movement process.

(b) Four basic types of movement defects have been recognized (Miller, 1975): (1) Intrinsic defects of only phagocyte movement; (2) Intrinsic defects of phagocyte movement with the addition of at least one other deficiency of phagocyte function such as phagocytosis or bactericidal activity; (3) Disorders of phagocyte movement secondary to deficiencies of humoral chemotactic agents, such as in primary disorders of the complement system; (4) Disorders of phagocyte movement secondary to the effects of a humoral inhibitor. Inhibitors may be directed either towards the phagocyte, or towards a humoral chemotactic factor which in turn results in deficient stimulation of phagocyte movement.

(c) At least one primary disorder of phagocyte movement appears to have a hereditary basis (Miller et al, 1973). Three children – a girl in one family a brother and sister in another family – presented with a symtom complex of congenital ichthyosis and *Trichophyton rubrum* infections. Movement of PMNs from each of the patients was abnormal in filter movement, but normal in undirected, or random movement (as measured in a capillary tube assay). On examination of PMNs from the two sets of parents, each of the fathers' PMNs showed an identical pattern of abnormalities in vitro. Upon further questioning, it was found that each father had been troubled intermittently throughout life by low-grade cutaneous fungal infections. These clinical and laboratory findings supported the suggestion of a familial chemotactic defect.

REFERENCES

Ackerman S K, Douglas S D 1979 Pepstatin A – a human leukocyte chemoattractant. Clinical Immunology and Immunopathology 14: 244–250

Archer G T, Air G, Jackas M, Morell D B 1965 Studies on rat eosinophil peroxidase. Biochemica et Biophysiica Acta (Amsterdam) 99: 96–101

Azimi P H, Bobenbender J G, Hintz R L, Kontras S B 1968 Chronic granulomatous disease in three female siblings. Journal of the American Medical Association 206: 2865–2870

Baehner R L, Nathan D G 1968 Quantitative nitro-blue tetrazolium test in chronic granulomatous disease. New England Journal of Medicine 278: 971–976

Becker E L 1976 Some interrelations among chemotaxis, lysosomal enzyme secretion and phagocytosis by neutrophils. In: Johansson S G O, Strandberg K, Uvnas B (eds) Molecular and Biological aspects of the acute allergic reaction, Plenum Publishing Corp., New York, pp 353–370

Becker E L, Showell H J 1974 The ability of chemotactic factors to induce lysosomal enzyme release. II. The mechanism of release. Journal of Immunology 112: 2055–2062

Bellanti J A, Cantz B E, Schlegel R J 1970 Accelerated decay of glucose-6-phosphate dehydrogenase activity in chronic granulomatous disease. Pediatric Research 4: 405–411

Biggar W D, Buron S, Holmes B 1976 Chronic granulomatous disease in an adult male: a proposed X–linked defect. Journal of Pediatrics 88: 63–70

Blume R S, Wolff S M 1972 The Chediak-Higashi syndrome: Studies in four patients and a review of the literature. Medicine 51: 247–280

Boxer L A, Hedley-Whyte E T, Stossel T P 1974 Neutrophil actin dysfunction and abnormal neutrophil behavior. New England Journal of Medicine 291: 1093–1099

Boxer L A, Oliver J M, Spielberg S P, Allen J M, Schulman J D 1979 Protection of granulocytes by vitamin E in glutathione synthetase deficiency. New England Journal of Medicine 301: 901–905

Boxer L A, Watanabe A M, Rister M, Besch H R Jr, Allen J, Baehner R L 1976 Correction of leukocyte function in Chediak-Higashi syndrome by ascorbate. New England Journal of Medicine 295: 1041–1045

Boyden S V 1962 The chemotactic effect of mixtures of antibody and antigen on polymorphonuclear leukocytes. Journal of Experimental Medicine 115: 453–466

Carruthers J A, Greaves M W 1976 Chronic granulomatous disease. British Journal of Dermatology (Supplement) 14: 72–74

Cheung A T W, Miller M E 1982 Movement of human polymorphonuclear leukocytes: a videotape analysis. Journal of Reticuloendothelial Society 31: 193–205

Clark R A, Klebanoff S J 1978 Chronic granulomatous disease. Studies of a family with impaired neutrophil chemotactic, metabolic and bactericidal function. American Journal of Medicine 65: 941–948

Cohn A A 1978 The activation of mononuclear phagocytes: Fact, fancy, and future. Journal of Immunology 121: 813–816

Delmas Y, Goudemand J, Ferriaux J P 1975 La granulomatose familiale chronique: Traitment per greffe de moelle (une observation). Nouvelle Presse Medicale 4: 2334

Desser R K, Himmelhoch S R, Evans W H, Januska M, Mage M, Shelton E 1972 Guinea pig heterophil and eosinophil peroxidase. Archives of Biochemistry 148: 452–465

Dupree E, Smith C W, Taylor-MacDougall N L 1972 Undetected carrier state in chronic granulomatous disease. Journal of Pediatrics 81: 770–774

Erickson R P, Stites D P, Fudenberg H H, Epstein C J 1972 Altered levels of glucose-6-phosphate dehydrogenase stabilizing factors in X–linked chronic granulomatous disease. Journal of Laboratory and Clinical Medicine 80: 644–653

Gallin J I, Gallin E K, Malech H L, Cramer E B 1978 Structural and ionic events during leukocyte chemotaxis. In: Gallin J I, Quie P G (eds) Leukocyte chemotaxis, Raven Press, New York, pp 123–141

Gallin J I, Quie P G (eds) 1978 Leukocyte chemotaxis: Methods, physiology, and clinical implications. Raven Press, New York

Giblett E R, Klebanoff S J, Pincus S H, Swanson J, Park B H, McCullough J 1971 Kell phenotypes in chronic granulomatous disease: A potential transfusion hazard. Lancet I: 1235–1236

Goetzl E J, Austen K F 1974 Stimulation of human neutrophil leukocyte aerobic glucose metabolism by purified chemotactic factors. Journal of Clinical Investigation 53: 591–599

Goetzl E J, Sun F F 1979 Generation of unique monohydroxyeicosatetraenoic acids from arachinoid acid by human neutrophils. Journal of Experimental Medicine 150: 406–411

Henson P M 1976 Membrane receptors on neutrophils. Immunology Communication 5: 757–775

Hill H R 1978 Cyclic nucleotides as modulators of leukocyte chemotaxis. In: Gallin J I, Quie P G (eds) Leukocyte chemotaxis. Raven Press, New York, pp 179–193

Holmes B, Page A R, Good R A 1967 Studies of the metabolic activity of leukocytes from patients with a genetic abnormality of phagocytic function. Journal of Clinical Investigation 46: 1422–1432

Holmes B, Quie P G, Windhorst D B, Good R A 1966 Fatal granulomatous disease of childhood: An inborn abnormality of phagocytic function. Lancet 1: 1225–1228

Johnston R B Jr, Baehner R L 1971 Chronic granulomatous disease: Correlation between pathogenesis and clinical findings. Pediatrics 48: 730–739

Johnston R B Jr, Newman S L 1977 Chronic granulomatous disease. Pediatric Clinics of North America 24: 365–376

Johnston R B Jr, Stroud R M 1977 Complement and host defense against infection. Journal of Pediatrics 90: 169–179

Karnovsky M L, Lazdins J K 1978 Biochemical criteria for activated macrophages Journal of Immunology 121: 809–813

Klebanoff S J, Clark R A 1978 The Neutrophil: Function and Clinical Disorders. North-Holland Publishing Company, New York

Kontras S B, Bass J C 1969 Chronic granulomatous disease. Lancet II: 646–647

Kritzler R A, Terner J Y, Lindenbaum J, Magidson J, Williams R, Preisig R, Phillips G B 1964 Chediak-Higashi syndrome. Cytologic and serum lipid observations in a case and family. American Journal of Medicine 36: 583–594

Lehrer R I, Cline M J 1969 Leukocyte myeloperoxidase deficiency and disseminated candidiasis: The role of myeloperoxidase in resistance to Candida infection. Journal of Clinical Investigation 48: 1478–1488

Lichtman M A 1970 Cellular deformability during maturation of the myeloblast: Possible role in marrow egress. New England Journal of Medicine 283: 493–498

Mackaness G B 1962 Cellular resistance to infection. Journal of Experimental Medicine 116: 381–406

Mandell G L, Hook E W 1969 Leukocyte bactericidal activity in chronic granulomatous disease: Correlation of bacterial hydrogen peroxide production and susceptibility to intracellular killing. Journal of Bacteriology 100: 531–532

Marks P A, Gross R T, Hurwitz R E 1959 Gene action in erythrocyte deficiency of glucose-6-phosphate dehydrogenase: Tissue enzyme levels. Nature (London) 183: 1266–1267

Marsh W L, 1977 The Kell blood group, K_x antigen, and chronic granulomatous disease. Mayo Clinic Proceedings 52: 150–152

Marsh W L, Uretskv S C. Douglas S D 1975 Antigens of the Kell blood group system on neutrophils and monocytes: Their relation to chronic granulomatous disease. Journal of Pediatrics 87: 1117–1120

McPhail L C, DeChatelet L R, Shirley P S, Wilfert C, Johnston R B Jr., McCall C E 1977 Deficiency of NADPH oxidase activity in chronic granulomatous disease. Journal of Pediatrics 90: 213–217

Metchnikoff E 1893 Lectures on the comparative pathology of inflammation. Kegan, Paul, Trench, Trubner & Co., Lindon

Miller M E 1975 Pathology of chemotaxis and random mobility. Seminars in Hematology 12: 59–82

Miller M E 1979 Cell elastimetry in the study of normal and abnormal movement of human neutrophils. Clinical Immunology and Inmunopathology 14: 502–510

Miller M E, Myers K A 1975 Cellular deformability of human peripheral blood polymorphonuclear leukocyte: Method of study, normal variation, and effects of physical and chemical alterations. Journal of the Reticuloendothelial Society 18: 337–345

Miller M E, Norman M E, Koblenzer P J, Schonauer T 1973 A new familial defect neutrophil movement. Journal of Laboratory and Clinical Medicine 82: 1–8

Mills E L, Rholl K S, Quie P G 1980 X–linked inheritance in females with chronic granulomatous disease. Journal of Clinical Investigation 66: 332–340

Mohler D N, Majerus P W, Minnich V, Hess C E, Garrick M D 1970 Glutathione synthetose deficiency as a cause of hereditary hemolytic disease. New England Journal of Medicine 283: 1253–1257

Moosmann K, Bojanovsky A 1975 Rezidivierende candidosis bei myeloperoxidase-mangel. Mschr. Kinderheilk 123: 408–409

North R J 1978 The concept of the activated macrophage. Journal of Immunology 121: 806–809

Ochs H D, Igo R P 1973 The NBT slide test: a simple screening method for detecting chronic granulomatous disease and female carriers. Journal of Pediatrics 83: 77–82

Olver J M, Albertini D F, Berlin R D 1976 Effects of Glutathione-oxidizing agents on microtubule assemble and microtubule-dependent surface properties of human neutrophils. Journal of Cell Biology 71: 921–932

Quie P G 1969 Chronic granulomatous disease of childhood. Advances in Pediatrics 16: 287–300

Quie P G, Kaplan E L, Page A R, Gruskay F L, Malawista S E 1968 Defective polymorphonuclear leukocyte function and chronic granulomatous disease in two female children. New England Journal of Medicine 289: 976–980

Raubitschek A A, Levin A S, Stites D P, Shaw E B, Fudenberg H H 1973 Normal granulocyte infusion therapy for aspergillosis in chronic granulomatous disease. Pediatrics 51: 230–233

Repine J E, Clawson C C, White J G, Holmes B 1975 Spectrum of function of neutrophils from carriers of sex–linked chronic granulomatous disease. Journal of Pediatrics 87: 901–907

Rosen H, Klebanoff S J 1976 Chemiluminescence and superoxide production by myeloperoxidase-deficient leukocytes. Journal of Clinical Investigation 58: 50–60

Schulman J D, Mudd S H, Schneider J A, Spielberg S P, Boxer L, Oliver J, Corash L, Sheetz M 1980 Genetic Disorders of Glutathione and sulfur amino-acid metabolism. Annals of Internal Medicine 93: 330–346

Segal A Q, Jones O T G, Webster D, Allison A C 1978 Absence of a newly described cytochrome b from neutrophils of patients with chronic granulomatous disease. Lancet II: 446–449

Spielberg S P, Kramer L I, Goodman S I, Butler J, Tietze F, Quinn P, Shulman J D 1977 5-Oxoprolinuria: Biochemical observations and case report. Journal of Pediatrics 91: 237–241

Spitzer R E 1977 The complement system. Pediatric Clinics of North America 24: 341–364

Stendahl O, Lindgren S 1976 Function of granulocytes with deficient myeloperoxidase-mediated iodination in a patient with generalized pustular psoriasis. Scandinavian Journal of Haematology 16: 144–153

Stossel T P 1975 Phagocytosis: Recognition and ingestion. Seminars in Hematology 12: 83–116

Stossel T P 1978 The mechanism of leukocyte locomotion. In: Gallin J I, Quie P G (eds) Leukocyte chemotaxis, Raven Press, New York, pp 143–160

Stossel T P, Hartwig J H 1976 Interaction of actin, myosin, and a new actin-binding protein of rabbit pulmonary macrophage. II. Role in cytoplasmic movement and phagocytosis. Journal of Cell Biology 68: 602–619

Tanaka T 1980 Chediak-Higashi syndrome: Abnormal lysosomal enzyme levels in granulocytes of patient and family members. Pediatric Research 14: 901–904

van der Meer J W M, van Zwet T L, van Furth R, Weemaes C M R 1975 New familial defect in microbicidal function of polymorphonuclear leucocytes. Lancet ii: 630–632

Weening R S, Roos D, Weemaes C M R, Homan-Müller J W T, vanSchaik M L J 1976 Defective initiation of the metabolic stimulation in phagocytizing granulocytes: A new congenital defect. Journal of Laboratory and Clinical Medicine 88: 757–768

81

The HLA system

R. Harris

INTRODUCTION

From an early stage it was appreciated that leucocyte antigens were relevant to human organ transplantation and this provided a major incentive for the investigation of HLA. It had been noted that antibodies directed against leucocytes appeared following the rejection of skin grafts and that the duration of skin graft survival was related to the degree of leucocyte antigen compatibility between the donor and the immunised recipient. Spurred on by the hope that these observations would facilitate organ transplantation, and by later findings associating HLA with a variety of diseases, a large number of HLA antigens were identified and found to be controlled by a single complex genetic system involving several closely linked loci. Four of these loci HLA-A, HLA-C, HLA-B and HLA-DR are defined by a serological test using carefully selected antisera obtained mainly from parous women. These antisera are reacted in the microlymphocytotoxic test with lymphocytes (enriched with B-lymphocytes in the case of DR) which are killed in the presence of complement and the appropriate HLA antigen. An additional locus, HLA-D, controls a series of alleles identified by the mixed lymphocyte response (MLR). For a general outline of HLA methodology the reader is referred to Dick and Kissmeyer-Nielson (1979).

Table 81.1 shows a recent listing of the antigens of the HLA system. The frequency of many of these antigens varies greatly between different human populations. The degree of polymorphism of HLA antigens is considerably greater than that of any other known human genetic system.

GENETICS OF HLA

Assignment of HLA to chromosome 6p (Lamm & Peterson, 1979; McKusick, 1978)

This assignment originated with family studies showing that the enzyme locus PGM3 and HLA were closely linked. PGM3 was then found to be syntenic with chromosome 6 in human-rodent hybrid cells. The location on the short arm of chromosome 6 and the relation of HLA to the centromere was suggested by studies of ovarian tumour material. Because of the large number of different HLA genotypes most families allow informative segregation studies and it is possible to relate particular HLA genotypes to cytogenetic markers or structural rearrangements of chromosome 6. By such studies it has been shown conclusively that HLA is located on the short arm of chromosome 6 in the 6p21 region.

Genetics of HLA and related loci

Complement components (Lachmann & Hobart, 1978)
In addition to HLA-A, -C, -B and -D (DR), two components of the classical complement pathway (C2 and C4) and one of the alternative pathways (Factor B, Bf) are controlled by the segment of chromosome which includes the structural genes for HLA. This segment, because of its involvement in transplant rejection, is known as the Major Histocompatibility Complex (MHC). Several electrophoretic variants of C2, C4 and Bf are known while recessive deficiency syndromes for C2 and C4 have been identified. Electrophoretic differences presumably represent amino-acid substitutions and thus it is believed that the structural genes for these complement components lie within the MHC. The red cell and serum blood groups Rogers (Rg^a) and Chido (Ch^a) have been shown to coincide with, respectively, C4F and C4S electrophoretic variants of C4 and are probably the products of separate but closely linked genes. Null alleles are believed to occur at each of the C4 loci but the genetics of C4 is complex and is in the process of being worked out. Bf and C2 are each at present believed to be controlled by a single genetic locus closely linked to HLA-B and -DR.

Other loci linked to HLA (Lamm & Peterson, 1979; McKusick, 1978)
Congenital adrenal hyperplasia due to 21-hydroxylase deficiency is closely linked to HLA-B (Dupont et al, 1980) and there is also strong evidence for linkage

Table 18.1 HLA nomenclature 1980 (modified from Tissue Antigens 1980 16: 113–117). Listing of recognised HLA specificities.

HLA-A	HLA-B	HLA-C	HLA-D	HLA-DR
HLA-A1	HLA-B5	HLA-Cw1	HLA-Dw1	HLA-DR1
HLA-A2	HLA-B7	HLA-Cw2	HLA-Dw2	HLA-DR2
HLA-A3	HLA-B8	HLA-Cw3	HLA-Dw3	HLA-DR3
HLA-A9	HLA-B12	HLA-Cw4	HLA-Dw4	HLA-DR4
HLA-A10	HLA-B13	HLA-Cw5	HLA-Dw5	HLA-DR5
HLA-A11	HLA-B14	HLA-Cw6	HLA-Dw6	HLA-DRw6
HLA-Aw19	HLA-B15	HLA-Cw7	HLA-Dw7	HLA-DR7
HLA-Aw 23 (9)	HLA-Bw16	HLA-Cw8	HLA-Dw8	HLA-DRw8
HLA-Aw24 (9)	HLA-B17		HLA-Dw9	HLA-DRw9
HLA-A25 (10)	HLA-B18		HLA-Dw10	HLA-DRw10
HLA-A26 (10)	HLA-Bw21		HLA-Dw11	
HLA-A28	HLA-Bw22		HLA-Dw12	
HLA-A29	HLA-B27			
HLA-Aw30	HLA-Bw35			
HLA-Aw31	HLA-B37			
HLA-Aw32	HLA-Bw38 (W16)			
HLA-Aw33	HLA-Bw39 (W16)			
HLA-Aw34	HLA-B40			
HLA-Aw36	HLA-Bw41			
HLA-Aw43	HLA-Bw42			
	HLA-Bw44 (12)			
	HLA-Bw45 (12)			
	HLA-Bw46			
	HLA-Bw47			
	HLA-Bw48			
	HLA-Bw49 (W21)			
	HLA-Bw50 (W21)			
	HLA-Bw51 (5)			
	HLA-Bw52 (5)			
	HLA-Bw53			
	HLA-Bw54 (W22)			
	HLA-Bw55 (W22)			
	HLA-Bw56 (W22)			
	HLA-Bw57 (17)			
	HLA-Bw58 (17)			
	HLA-Bw59			
	HLA-Bw60 (40)			
	HLA-Bw61 (40)			
	HLA-Bw62 (15)			
	HLA-Bw63 (15)			
	HLA-Bw4			
	HLA-Bw6			

HLA-A, -B, -C loci are defined by the microlymphocytotoxic test employing specific antisera and peripheral blood lymphocytes. HLA-DR uses a similar test but enriched with B-lymphocytes.
HLA-D involves the mixed lymphocyte response (MLR).
Although closely associated, especially in families, the antigens HLA-D and HLA-DR ('D-Related') are not identical.
Very few new determinants or blanks remain to be detected at the HLA-A and -B loci, while the genetic diversity of HLA-A, -B, -C and -DR is such that more than 300 million theoretical genotypes exist and more than 75% of Caucasians have four different HLA-A and -B antigens.
The letter 'w' (Workshop) denotes an antigen whose definition is still provisional. HLA-Bw4 and HLA-Bw6 are supertypic specifications including other HLA-B series antigens in two complex cross-reacting families. Recently supertypic specifications MB and MT have been identified in the HLA-DR series. A 'new' locus, SB, is being defined by the in vitro lymphocyte response. Broad specificities are given in parenthesis after named specificities: generally, broad specificities were discovered first, then new antisera were found which revealed that an original specificity could be 'split' into two or more discrete antigens.

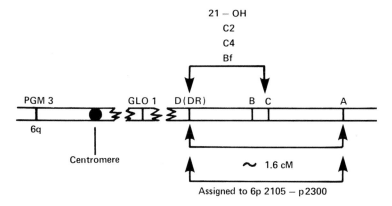

Fig. 81.1 The Major Histocompatibility Complex of man

D(DR) = HLA-D(DR) | PGM 3 = Phosphoglucomutase 3
B = HLA-B | GLO 1 = Glyoxalase 1
C = HLA-C | 21-OH = 21-Hydroxylase deficiency
A = HLA-A | C2,C4 = Complement components
| Bf = Properdin factor B

between HLA and major genes involved in haemochromatosis and olivopontocerebellar ataxia. Glyoxalase-1 (GLO) and phosphoglucomutase-3 (PGM3) are also within measurable distance of HLA. Other genetic loci strongly suspected of being linked to the MHC include immune response (Ir) genes, rag-weed sensitivity, neutrophil differentiation factor and asymmetrical atrial septal defect of the heart.

Figure 81.1 shows the genetic loci firmly assigned to the MHC. The map distance between HLA-A and HLA-D is approximately 1.6 centiMorgans.

Haplotypes and linkage disequilibrium (Hiller et al, 1978)

The number of different permutations of HLA antigens is enormous but it has been found that some combinations are much commoner than would be expected from a consideration of the population frequency of the individual antigens. For example, the antigens HLA-A1 and HLA-B8 are linked in the coupling phase on the same chromosome (constituting a haplotype) in European populations with greater frequency than expected. Figure 81.2 shows the segregation of HLA in a typical Caucasian family which illustrates the en-bloc transmission from generation to generation of intact haplotypes. Even if the population initially contains a non-random distribution of alleles in haplotypes, recombination should, within a predictable number of generations, randomise the linkage groups so that coupling and repulsion phases become equally frequent. The time required to achieve linkage *equilibrium* is conditioned by the closeness of the linkage but may be modified if some combinations have a selective advantage. The association between HLA

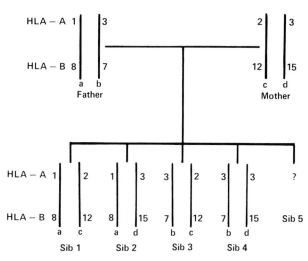

Fig. 81.2 Segregation of HLA haplotypes in a typical Caucasian family. One of the father's No. 6 chromosomes (a) is marked by HLA-A1, B8 and his other (b) by HLA-A3, B7. Similarly the mother's No. 6 chromosomes are marked by (c) HLA-A2, B12 and (d) HLA-A3 B15. a, b, c and d are referred to as haplotypes and each child inherits only one haplotype from each parent. Barring genetic recombination sib 5 must be HLA identical to one of his sibs. For clarity, only HLA-A and -B loci included.

and a variety of diseases (see below) is believed to depend upon linkage *disequilibrium*.

The chemistry of HLA (Kaufman et al, 1980; Stromiger et al, 1980)

HLA-A, -C and -B molecules (Class I) appear to have a similar basic structure which differs from HLA-D and

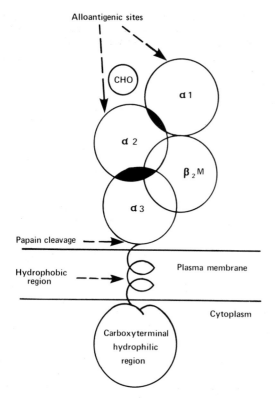

Fig. 81.3 Simplified diagramatic representation of HLA-B molecule (see text).

DR (Class II). Class I molecules consist of a polymorphic polypeptide heavy chain (mol. wt. = 45 000 daltons = 45 K) and an invariant polypeptide light chain, β2 microglobulin (mol. wt. = 12K). HLA-D antigens, Class II, have an invariant heavy chain (mol. wt. = 34K) and a polymorphic light chain (mol. wt. = 29K). Figure 81.3 illustrates the suggested configuration of an HLA-B molecule (Class I) which spans the cell membrane. Most of the molecule lies outside the cell with a small hydrophobic segment anchored in the cell membrane and the carboxy-terminal hydrophilic piece within the cytoplasm. The HLA molecule appears well placed to signal across the membrane by interactions within the cell between the hydrophilic piece and the actin of the cytoskeleton. The heavy chain is non-covalently bound outside the cell membrane to β2 microglobulin which, although not antigenically polymorphic itself, is essential if the HLA antigenicity of the heavy chain is to be expressed. The heavy chain can be divided into three domains one of which, α3, has amino-acid sequences which are highly conserved among HLA antigens and are partly homologous with both β2 microglobulin and Ig constant domains. The HLA antigenic determinants are probably in the α1 and α2 domains. There seems to be little inter-

nal homology between the domains suggesting that they have not evolved by duplication of a single gene. It is hoped that by preparing cloned cDNA copies it will be possible to probe genomic DNA so as to yield much information about the genetic structure of the human MHC.

HLA AND DISEASE (Bodmer, 1980a, b; Harris, 1981)

Genetic linkage

21-hydroxylase, C2 and C4 deficiencies are known to be due to genes that segregate with HLA-B in family studies. This constitutes genetic linkage and barring crossing-over during meiosis results in the inheritance by members of a family of the disease gene with the same HLA-B allele. However it is not necessarily the case that the disease gene will be inherited with the same HLA-B allele in different families. Linkage is with a *locus* and not with a particular allele at that locus. Evidence for genetic linkage is thus sought in families and not in populations.

Association

In contrast, associations between disease and individual HLA antigens are sought in groups of *unrelated* patients from the general population. The biological basis for association is not always clear but sometimes underlying genetic linkage can be shown to be responsible. A clear example of this is seen in the Caucasian population with the association between the rare HLA-Bw47 antigen and 21-hydroxylase deficiency in children (Klonda et al, 1978). This phenomenon is attributable to linkage disequilibrium (qv) between 21-hydroxylase deficiency and HLA-Bw47. Table 81.2 lists some of the very large number of diseases which have been found to occur with increased frequency in individuals of specific HLA types. The strongest known of these associations is still that between ankylosing spondylitis and HLA-B27 which is found in nearly all populations which have been studied. In Caucasians 90% or more patients with this disease are B27 positive compared with 5–10% amongst normal controls representing a Relative Risk (RR) compared to normal of about 90 times (Table 81.3). A young man who is B27 positive has a 20% risk of developing clinical disease at some stage in his life. The basis for this association is unknown, although recent work suggests that the B27 antigen may be related to cell surface receptors for pathogenic organisms or that there may be antigenic similarity ('molecular mimicry') between host and pathogen. Another category of association is represented by some autoimmune diseases, e.g. Graves disease which tends to occur more frequently in

Table 81.2 Some established HLA-associated disorders.

Rheumatology
Ankylosing spondylitis and related disorders
Rheumatoid arthritis

Neurology
*Olivopontocerebellar ataxia (one type)
Multiple sclerosis
Myasthenia gravis

Dermatology
Psoriasis
Discoid lupus erythematosus
Dermatitis herpetiformis
Behçet disease

Endocrinology
Juvenile insulin dependent diabetes mellitus
Graves disease
Sub-acute thyroiditis
Addison disease
Hypergonadotrophic hypogonadism
*21-Hydroxylase deficiency

Gastroenterology
Gluten-sensitive enteropathy
Pernicious anaemia
Chronic active hepatitis
*Haemochromatosis

Immunopathology
Atopy
*Complement deficiencies
Systemic lupus erythematosus
Sjögren disease

Malignant disease
Hodgkin disease
Acute lymphatic leukaemia
Acute myeloid leukaemia
Asiatic nasopharyngeal carcinoma

Occupational disease
Asbestosis

Drug reactions
Hydralazine lupus

* Known genetic linkage with HLA

Table 81.3 The association between HLA-B27 and ankylosing spondylitis in Caucasians. Findings from 21 studies reported to the Copenhagen HLA and Disease Registry, 1977.

967 patients	71–100% B27
7879 controls	3–12% B27
Relative risk*	90, p< 10^{-9}
Heterogeneity	p > 0.05

* Relative risk (RR) =

$$\frac{\text{B27-positive patients}}{\text{B27-positive controls}} \times \frac{\text{B27-negative controls}}{\text{B27-negative patients}}$$

great care if false associations are to be avoided and true ones are not to be missed (Svejgaard & Ryder, 1979).

Antigenic restriction (Doherty et al, 1976; Munro & Waldmann, 1978)
A particularly important series of interactions has been described between the products of several HLA loci and with the antigens of pathogens. In brief, lymphocytes are stimulated to divide by HLA-D antigens but the resulting cytotoxic 'T' cells capable of destroying virus infected target cells are 'restricted' to targets that bear both self HLA-A and HLA-B antigens and those of the infecting virus. Antigenic restriction of this type has been interpreted to mean that adjoining loci e.g. HLA-D and HLA-B within the MHC may function in concert. One may speculate that antigenic restriction of cell-cell interactions is involved in a wide range of developmental processes in ontogeny involving differentiation antigens, as well as in the mature immune system when pathogens provide the antigen. Some combinations (haplotypes) may then be more favourable than others and tend to be preserved, providing a basis of selection for maintaining linkage disequilibrium.

Table 81.4 summarises some of the possible explanations for HLA and disease associations.

PRACTICAL APPLICATIONS OF HLA

Clinical transplantation (Morris et al, 1978)
One in four is the probability that two sibs will be HLA identical (Figure 81.2) and it has been found that kidney grafts between such sibs are more likely to be successful than with any other donor category except identical twins. This provides the best evidence that HLA represents the Major Histocompatibility Complex. However it is in practice uncommon to have available a suitable HLA identical sib donor and most grafts have to come from unrelated cadavers. Attempts are made using a National or Continental pool of HLA data on prospective recipients to obtain HLA matches as near identical to

individuals who are HLA-DR3 positive. Linkage disequilibrium between HLA-DR genes and immune response (Ir) genes for high or low immune responsiveness, and responses to specific but generally unknown antigens, are believed to underlie autoimmune diseases. Other associations are known or strongly suspected to be due to linkage disequilibrium between HLA and disease genes. In this category there are 21-hydroxylase deficiency, C2 deficiency, haemochromatosis and one form of olivopontocerebellar ataxia. It is important to note that that disease associations have been found with antigens coded for by all the HLA loci, suggesting that susceptibility and/or resistance to a wide variety of diseases is regulated by genetic loci spread throughout the MHC.

The statistical analysis of disease associations requires

Table 81.4 Some explanations for HLA and disease associations.

1. True linkage	21-Hydroxylase deficiency and C2 deficiency: population associations depend upon *linkage disequilibrium* between deficiency genes and one or more HLA markers e.g. HLA-Bw47 and 21-hydroxylase deficiency.
2. Autoimmune diseases	Generally associated with HLA-D(DR) antigens and believed to represent linkage disequilibrium between HLA-D(DR) and immune response (Ir) genes (see 3 below)
3. Antigenic restriction and interaction between cells guided by products of different MHC loci	Cell-cell interaction in mature immune system (and perhaps in ontogeny too) depends upon collaboration between different cell types controlled by membrane antigenic products of the MHC. 45K molecules (HLA-A, -B, -C) guide cytotoxic T cells allowing them to destroy target cells which also bear viral antigens. 28K-32K molecules (HLA-D) guide T cells to activate macrophages and to become helper cells in amplifying immune responses. Disorders of these interactions will prove a fertile source of pathology.
4. Molecular mimicry	Postulated but not proven. Similarity between antigens of pathogens and HLA of host rendering pathogen 'immunologically invisible'.
5. Receptor for pathogens	HLA-B27 has been proposed as a component of a cell surface receptor for micro-organisms, leading by unknown pathogenesis to ankylosing spondylitis.
6. Functions of HLA molecules	HLA-A, -B and -C heavy chains are known to traverse cell membranes and may operate in regulating function of cell by influencing transport of substances across membrane or by signalling to cell interior events at the cell surface.

those of a cadaver donor as possible. The results of matching in this way have been disappointing and it is believed that the reason for this is that the 'real' transplant loci within MHC have not yet been identified. However, several important facts have emerged including the paradoxical need for previous blood transfusions to generate a protective immune response while subsequently, by a cross-match procedure, avoiding recipients who have damaging antibodies against the donor organ.

Recent studies, with the transfusion of white blood cells to treat resistant infections, platelets for thrombocytopenia and bone marrow transplants for bone marrow aplasia, appear to require good HLA matching for success and to avoid graft versus host reactions.

Genetic counselling and prenatal diagnosis

Using genetic linkage between disease genes and HLA
Three autosomal recessive deficiency syndromes (21-hydroxylase, C2 and C4) are very closely linked to HLA and genetic recombination is rare between HLA-B and these loci. HLA typing is very precise within a family and if the HLA genotype of an affected homozygote is known, normal homozygotes, heterozygotes and homozygotes for the mutant gene may be distinguished. This knowledge has been used for counselling and prenatal diagnosis in families in which 21-hydroxylase deficiency has occurred. However, prenatal diagnosis using HLA depends upon growing amniotic cells in vitro and when time is at a premium a more rapid method is required. 17-hydroxyprogesterone assay of amniotic fluid is used for the diagnosis of 21-hydroxylase deficiency but, in the future, extraction and identification of soluble HLA substances from the amniotic fluid itself may prove to be helpful.

Using associations between HLA and disease
In the absence of genetic linkage, HLA associations have at the moment only limited practical value as a tool for risk prediction in genetic counselling. However in the case of insulin dependent diabetes mellitus (IDDM) some use can be made of HLA (Svejgaard et al, 1980). The empirical risk of recurrence in a sib is approximately 5% but if the HLA genotypes are known from family studies, it can be shown that the risks of recurrence are about 12%, 4% and less than 1% for sibs who share 2, 1 and 0 haplotypes with the proband. In ankylosing spondylitis the son of an HLA-B27 positive father with ankylosing spondylitis is unlikely to develop the disease himself unless he too is B27 positive. Outside the family situation, HLA associations will become more valuable in risk prediction when the frequency of a disease amongst individuals who have the HLA marker is known or the true 'disease gene' within the MHC is identified. Further, when more is known about the relative penetrance of the MHC linked disease genes in populations and families it will be possible to use Bayes' method to modify a priori empirically derived risks for multifactorial conditions.

Population and epidemiological studies (Dausset & Colombani, 1973; Bodmer, 1980)
The extreme polymorphism of the HLA system and inter-population variability is of considerable importance

to population geneticists and epidemiologists. Use has been made of the polymorphism to estimate genetic distances between various populations to gain further insight into evolutionary mechanisms and the effects of migration.

Paternity studies

It is usually a simple matter to exclude paternity on the basis of HLA studies alone while with some of the rarer haplotypes, having a population frequency of 1 in 1000 or less, it may be possible positively to attribute paternity with a very small probability of error especially if other genetic markers are also taken into account. However the system has been insufficiently tested in Courts of Law and in some instances the existence of cross-reactions between antigens would allow for legal as well as serological imprecision.

SUMMARY AND CONCLUSIONS

The Major Histocompatibility Complex has been assigned to the short arm of chromosome 6 and codes for important cell surface molecules. These molecules provide a prodigous antigenic polymorphism and the basis for cell-cell interaction in ontogeny and in the mature immune system. The biochemical structure of the molecules is now firmly established. The MHC has a homologue in *all vertebrates* studied suggesting evolutionary conservation of a functionally important genetic complex. The role of tissue-matching in transplantation is still controversial. The feto-maternal relationship represents the adaptation of immunological polymorphisms on which natural selection has operated. The association of HLA antigens with a wide variety of diseases involves immunological and other mechanisms and promises to allow the function of these molecules to be worked out and will in its turn provide new insights into the pathogenesis of disease. The HLA polymorphism, its geographical polytypism and its association with disease provides a unique genetic system in man. Within the MHC, genes have been identified coding for four sets of serologically defined antigens, one set of antigens defined by lymphocyte response (MLR), three complement components, 21-hydroxylase deficiency and several other functions. It is likely that other loci remain to be discovered within the MHC and that existing ones are more complex than we now believe.

REFERENCES

Bodmer Julia G 1980 The HLA system: The HLA-DR antigens and HLA haplotypes in 24-populations. In: Population Structure and Genetic Disorders. Eriksson A W (ed) Academic Press, London

Bodmer W F 1980a Models and mechanisms for HLA and disease associations. Journal of Experimental Medicine 152: 353–357

Bodmer W F 1980b The HLA system and diseases: the Oliver Sharpey Lecture 1979. Journal of the Royal College of Physicians 14: No. 1, 43–50

Dausset J, Colombani J (eds) 1973 Histocompatibility testing 1972. Report of an International Workshop held at Evian, 23–27 May 1972, Munksgaard, Copenhagen

Dick H M, Kissmeyer-Nielson F (eds) 1979 Histocompatibility techniques. Elsevier/North Holland Biomedical Press Amsterdam, New York, Oxford

Doherty P C, Blanden R V, Zinkernagel R M 1976 Specificity of virus-immune effector T cells for H-2D or H-2K compatible interactions: Implications for H-antigen diversity. Transplantation Reviews 29: 89–124

Dupont B O, Pollack S, Levine S, O'Neill J, Hawkins B, New M I 1980 Congenital adrenal hyperplasia and HLA: Joint report from the Eighth International Histocompatibility Workshop, Los Angeles, In: Terasaki R I, (ed) Histocompatibility Testing. Munksgaard, Copenhagen

Harris R 1981 HLA antigens and disease susceptibility. Medicine, The monthly Add-on Journal: 5

Hiller C M, Bischoff A, Schmidt T, Bender K 1978 Analysis of the HLA – ABC linkage disequilibrium: decreasing strength of gametic association with increasing map distance. Human Genetics 41: 301–312

Kaufman J F, Andersen R L, Strominger J L 1980 HLA-DR antigens have polymorphic light chains and invariant heavy chains as assessed by lysine-containing tryptic peptide analysis. Journal of Experimental Medicine 152: 37–53

Klonda P T, Harris R, Price D A 1978 HLA and congenital adrenal hyperplasia. Lancet 2: 1046

Lachmann P J, Hobart M J 1978 Complement genetics in relation to HLA. British Medical Bulletin 34(3): 247–252

Lamm L U, Peterson G B 1979 The HLA genetic linkage group. Transplantation Proceedings XI(4): 1692–1698

McKusick V A 1978 Mendelian Inheritance in Man, 5th edn Johns Hopkins University Press, Baltimore & London

Morris P J, Batchelor J R, Festenstein H 1978 Matching for HLA transplantation. British Medical Bulletin 34(3): 259–262

Munro A, Waldmann H 1978 The major histocompatibility system and the immune response. British Medical Bulletin 34(3): 253–258

Strominger J L, Engelhard V H, et al 1980 Chemistry of HLA. In: Current topics in developmental biology, developmental immunology Vol 14. Academic Press, New York

Svejgaard A, Ryder L P 1979 Disease associations. In: Dick H M, Kissmeyer-Nielson (eds) Histocompatability techniques. Elsevier/North Holland Biomedical Press, Amsterdam, New York, Oxford

Svejgaard A, Platz P, Ryder L P 1981 Insulin dependent diabetes mellitus. Joint results of the 8th Workshop Study. In: Terasaki P I (ed) Histocompatibility Testing 1980 UCLA Tissue Typing Laboratory, Los Angeles

Genetic disorders of the pituitary gland

D.L. Rimoin

The pituitary gland is composed of two embryologically, morphologically and functionally distinct units – the *anterior pituitary* (adenophypophysis) and *posterior pituitary* (neurohypophysis). Disease processes usually involve only one of the units unless the disease affects both glands because of their anatomic proximity or because of hypothalamic involvement. Thus disorders of anterior and posterior pituitary function will be discussed separately in this chapter.

DISORDERS OF THE ANTERIOR PITUITARY

The anterior pituitary is derived from an epithelial invagination of the roof of the posterior pharynx, known as Rathke's pouch (Daughaday, 1974). This mass of cells migrates upwards towards the base of the brain to meet an out-pouching of the third ventricle – the future posterior pituitary. The pituitary gland comes to lie in a bony cavity of the sphenoid bone known as the sella turcica. It is separated from the brain superiorly by the diaphragma sella, an extension of the dura mater. The pituitary stalk, composed primarily of neurohypophyseal tissue surrounded by nerves and blood vessels, passes through the diaphragma sella, connecting the gland with the hypothalmus. It is this intimate vascular connection between the hypothalmus and pituitary which allows for the sensitive hypothalmic control of pituitary function. The anterior pituitary gland contains a number of distinct cell types responsible for the secretion of the seven or more pituitary hormones: growth hormone (hGH), thyrotropic hormone (TSH), adrenocorticotropic hormone (ACTH), luteinizing hormone (LH), follicle stimulating hormone (FSH), prolactin (Pr) and melanocyte stimulating hormone (MSH). The secretion of each of these pituitary hormones is under the direct control of the hypothalamus. This hypothalamic control of pituitary secretion is mediated by a variety of hypothalamic releasing hormones, which stimulate the secretion of the specific pituitary hormones (e.g. TRH stimulates TSH secretion) and hypothalamic inhibitory hormones, which inhibit the secretion of the specific pituitary hormones

(e.g. somatostatin which inhibits hGH secretion). It is the interplay between the specific releasing and inhibitory hormones that directly controls the secretion of each of the pituitary hormones. In turn, the secretion of the hypothalamic inhibitory and releasing hormones by the hypothalamus is modulated by a variety of humoral and central nervous system factors. The pituitary hormones, once released into the plasma, exert their effects on a variety of specific target organs, either a specific endocrine gland (e.g. thyroid, adrenal gland) or a variety of end organs. Growth hormone is unique in that it affects receptors in a variety of tissues including the liver; stimulation of the hepatic receptors results in the release of the somatomedins, a class of peptide hormones which stimulate growth and anabolism in a variety of other tissues. Because of the complexity of this hypothalamic-pituitary axis, a wide variety of pathogenetic mechanisms can operate at each level of the system, resulting in a widely heterogeneous group of disorders, with similar symptoms of pituitary insufficiency (Fig. 82.1).

Hereditary disorders of both pituitary hypofunction and hyperfunction have been described. Similar to genetic disorders of the other endocrine glands, diseases involving the hormonal deficiency states are much more common and better delineated than hereditary forms of hyperpituitarism. Pituitary deficiency disorders may involve a single tropic hormone (monotropic deficiency) or a combination of two or more pituitary hormones (multitropic hormone deficiency) and may result from disturbances in any part of the hypothalamic-hypophyseal-target organ complex (Rimoin & Horton, 1978 a & b). Theoretically, a syndrome of pituitary hormonal insufficiency might result from developmental degenerative or receptor lesions of the hypothalmus, deficiencies of the hypothalamic releasing hormones or their receptors, developmental or degenerative lesions of the pituitary gland, deficiencies or structural abnormalities of the pituitary hormones, or defects in target organ responsiveness to hormonal action. Each of these mechanisms has now been described in patients with pituitary insufficiency, resulting in the marked genetic heterogeneity that has been observed in pituitary dwarfism.

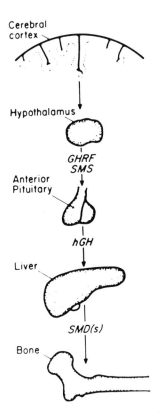

Fig. 82.1 Growth hormone axis. GHRF – Growth hormone releasing factor; SMS – somatostatin; hGH – human growth hormone; SMD(s) – somatomedin(s). Defects at each of the steps of the axis have now been described which result in proportionate dwarfism.

HEREDITARY FORMS OF GROWTH HORMONE DEFICIENCY

Proportionate dwarfism may result from a wide variety of endocrinologic, metabolic, nutritional, emotional, and genetic disorders. Pituitary deficiency has long been recognized as a cause of proportionate short stature and it is now apparent that pituitary dwarfism represents a heterogeneous group of disorders secondary to a variety of genetic and acquired defects in human growth hormone (hGH) secretion or action (Rimoin, 1976; Rimoin & Schimke, 1971). Indeed, defects at all levels of the hypothalamic - pituitary - somatomedin - chondroosseous end organ axis have now been described in proportionate dwarfs (Fig. 82.1). Delineation of the distinct disorder in each pituitary dwarf has obvious implications for genetic counselling; when growth hormone releasing factor becomes available, an exact diagnosis will also have great therapeutic significance.

The various types of pituitary dwarfism can be classified on the basis of (1) the level of the defect in the hypothalamic-pituitary axis; (2) whether it is a genetic or acquired disorder, and if genetic, on the mode of inheritance; (3) whether or not there is an obvious developmental or degenerative disease of the hypothalamus or pituitary; (4) whether the pituitary deficiency is monotropic (isolated growth hormone deficiency) or multitropic (panhypopituitary dwarfism); and (5) in those cases due to a defect in growth hormone action, as to whether somatomedin generation is normal or defective (Table 82.1).

Developmental anomalies and complex genetic syndromes associated with pituitary dwarfism

Although the pathogenesis of the growth hormone deficiency is unknown in most forms of pituitary dwarfism, a number of developmental anomalies of the hypothalamus and pituitary and complex genetic syndromes associated with degeneration of the hypothalamus or pituitary have been described which result in growth hormone deficiency with or without other tropic hormone deficiencies.

Table 82.1 Genetic forms of hGH deficiency and resistance

A. Developmental anomalies and complex genetic syndromes associated with pituitary dwarfism
 1. Congenital absence of the pituitary
 2. Familial pituitary dwarfism with abnormal sella turcica
 3. Familial hypopituitarism with large sella turcica
 4. Anencephaly
 5. Holoprosencaphaly
 6. Transsphenoidal encephalocele
 7. Septooptic dysplasia
 8. Simple cleft lip and palate associated with pituitary insufficiency
 9. Solitary maxillary central incisor syndrome
10. Histiocytosis X
11. Congenital hypothalamic hamartoblastoma, hypopituitarism, imperforate anus, postaxial polydactyly syndrome (Hall syndrome)
12. Rieger syndrome (iris-dental dysplasia)
13. Pituitary dwarfism associated with sensorineural deafness
14. Fanconi anaemia
15. Neurofibromatosis
16. Primary microcephaly
17. Gonadal dysgenesis

B. Genetic non syndromal forms of pituitary dwarfism
1. Familial panhypopituitary dwarfism (multitropic hormone deficiency)
   a. Sporadic
   b. Autosomal recessive
   c. X–linked recessive
2. Isolated human growth hormone deficiency (IGHD)
   a. Type I IGHD
   b. Type II IGHD
   c. Type A IGHD
   d. Biologically Inactive hGH
   e. X–linked Hypogammaglobulinemia and IGHD
3. Laron dwarfism
4. The African Pygmies
5. Pituitary dwarfism with somatomedin unresponsiveness

Congenital absence of the pituitary

Complete absence of the anterior pituitary gland results in severe neonatal adrenal insufficiency, hypothyroidism and hypoglycaemia, and if untreated, usually results in neonatal death (Steiner & Boggs 1965; Sadeghi-Nejad & Senior, 1974). This syndrome probably goes unrecognised in the majority of cases unless the adrenal insufficiency is diagnosed early and pituitary function is then studied or postmortem examination includes detailed examination of the pituitary fossa. The sella turcica is usually small and no trace of anterior pituitary tissue is found at autopsy. Posterior pituitary tissue may be present or absent. There is atrophy of the adrenals with absence of the fetal zone, presumably secondary to ACTH deficiency.

Clinical features include early lethargy, cyanosis, convulsions, circulatory collapse and hypoglycaemia. Neonatal jaundice has been documented in most patients and Herman et al (1975) have pointed out that hyperbilirubinaemia may be associated with most forms of neonatal hypopituitarism (Moncrieff et al, 1972). The thyroid and gonads may be hypoplastic and the penis is usually minute. Survival past the neonatal period will result in severe dwarfism, hypogonadism, and cretinism, but early total hormone replacement therapy should result in complete phenotypic reversal.

This disorder has been described in at least 3 sets of sibs and there is an increased prevalence of consanguinity, suggesting autosomal recessive inheritance (Steiner & Boggs, 1965; Sadeghi-Nejad & Senior, 1974; Willard, 1973). The adrenal atrophy leads to a deficiency in maternal urinary oestriol excretion and thus, urinary oestriol levels may provide a means of prenatal diagnosis, as might studies of fetal thyroid function.

Lovinger et al (1975) have described a syndrome of congenital hypopituitarism with severe hypoglycaemia and microphallus which resembles congenital absence of the pituitary clinically. Plasma prolactin was normal or elevated and there was a TSH rise following TRH administration, indicative of hypothalamic defect. All of these cases were sporadic. Thus for genetic counselling purposes, these 2 syndromes must be distinguished.

Hypoplasia or ectopia of the pituitary gland has also been described with pituitary insufficiency (Mosier, 1957; Ehrlich, 1957). It is impossible to state whether these latter disorders are simply less complete forms of pituitary agenesis or secondary to distinct pathogenetic mechanisms.

Familial pituitary dwarfism with abnormal sella turcica

Ferrier and Stone (1969) described 2 sisters who had severe growth failure, hypoglycaemia, and mental retardation, and manifested evidence of relative growth hormone, thyrotropin and ACTH deficiency. These individuals differed from the usual form of hereditary panhypopituitary dwarfism in that both had a very small sella turcica located in a morphologically abnormal sphenoid bone. They postulated that the association of panhypopituitary dwarfism, mental retardation and abnormal sella turcica may represent a distinct syndrome inherited as an autosomal recessive trait. Two sisters with a similar syndrome of panhypopituitarism with a poorly developed sella turcica were recently described by Sipponen et al (1978). On autopsy, no pituitary gland could be found in one child and a rudimentary, partly ectopic pituitary in the other. Thus there is some question as to whether this represents a distinct syndrome or is simply a less severe form of congenital absence of the pituitary.

Familial hypopituitarism with large sella turcica

Parks et al (1978) have described three sibs from a non-consanguinous mating who had short stature, growth hormone deficiency and thyrotropin deficiency. Skull X-rays demonstrated abnormally large sella turcicas (3.7–5.9 standard deviations above age specific means). Computed tomography and pneumoencephalography showed full sellae without suprasellar extension and a normal ventricular system ruling out the 'empty sella syndrome'. ACTH reserve and prolactin appeared normal. The $18\frac{1}{2}$ year old sister had lack of pubertal development and the 10 year old brother had extremely small testes, suggesting gonadotropin deficiency. Although their gonadotropin levels were normal for skeletal age, the latter was markedly retarded and true gonadotropin deficiency is likely. The authors postulate that this syndrome is secondary to a pituitary tumour or a regulatory defect, but elucidation of the pathogenesis will probably require direct visualization of pituitary tissue. This probably represents a distinct syndrome inherited as an autosomal recessive trait. It must be differentiated from the empty sella syndrome, which has been described in sibs, associated with short stature, unusual facies, spinal anomalies and delayed sexual maturation (Merle et al 1979).

Anencephaly

Anencephaly is associated with the complete absence of a normal hypothalamus, absence or severe hypoplasia of the posterior pituitary and a variable degree of anterior pituitary hypoplasia (Naeye & Blanc, 1971; Angevine, 1938). These infants have hypoplastic adrenals and often die from adrenal insufficiency. Plasma hGH levels have been found to vary from low normal to deficient in anencephalics (Hayek et al, 1973; Grunt & Reynolds, 1970). Basal thyrotropin levels were low, and plasma prolactin levels normal. Hayek et al (1973) found that the intravenous insulin tolerance test failed to evoke elevations in plasma growth hormone in anencephalics. Administration of lysine-vasopressin caused an active growth hormone release, however, and there was a large increase in serum thyrotropin concentration following administration of thyrotropin releasing hormone. Thus, the anterior pituitary appears to be capable of releasing growth hormone and thyrotropin when directly stimulated, but anterior pituitary function mediated by hypothalamic releasing hormones appears to be totally deficient. The normal prolactin values presumably reflect the absence of the hypothalamic prolactin inhibitory hormone, the major factor controlling prolactin secretion from the pituitary. These endocrinologic data are supported by the morphologic observation of thyrotropin, gonadotropin, and somatotropin secreting cells in the pituitary of these infants.

It is of interest that while anencephalics, who lack a hypothalamus, usually have some basal growth hormone secretion, albeit lower than normal, some individuals with idiopathic hypopituitarism have essentially no basal growth hormone secretion. One might postulate that in the anencephalic, there is an absence of both growth hormone releasing factor and growth hormone inhibitory hormone (somatostatin), while in the idiopathic hypopituitary dwarf secondary to a hypothalamic defect, there may be an isolated deficiency of growth hormone releasing factor, with normal somatostatin secretion completely blocking growth hormone secretion from the pituitary.

Holoprosencephaly

The holoprosencephalies form a spectrum of developmental anomalies associated with impaired midline cleavage of the embryonic forebrain, aplasia of the olfactory bulbs and tracts and midline dysplasia of the face, ranging from cyclopia to cleft lip and palate with hypotelorism. Anomalies of the pituitary gland have been described in all forms of holoprosencephaly, ranging from malformation of the gland to its complete absence (Edmonds, 1950; Haworth et al, 1961; Gorlin et al, 1968). In individuals with absence of the pituitary, the adrenals are also hypoplastic and there may or may not be thyroid hypoplasia as well. Hypoplastic or aplastic pancreas, testes and ovaries have also been described (Cohen et al, 1971). ACTH deficiency and vasopressin-sensitive diabetes insipidus have been documented (Hintz et al, 1968). All degrees of insufficiency may occur in the holoprosencephalies and the degree of pituitary dysfunction appears to be unrelated to the severity of the facial deformity. The pituitary insufficiency is presumably secondary to a developmental anomaly of the hypothalamus. Romshe and Sotos (1973) have described growth hormone deficiency in a sib of 2 sisters with classic holoprosencephaly. This dwarfed brother had normal facies other than for mild hypotelorism. The holoprosencephalies are a genetically heterogeneous group of disorders associated with trisomy 13, deletion of the short arm of chromosome 18, simple autosomal recessive inheritance and a variety of unusual chromosomal anomalies (Rimoin & Schimke, 1971).

Transsphenoidal encephalocele

A number of cases of transsphenoidal encephalocele associated with variable degrees of hypothalamic-pituitary dysfunction have been reported (Ellyin et al, 1980; Lieblich et al, 1978). In transsphenoidal encephalocele, a defect exists in the sphenoid bone, and the encephalocele usually extends into the epipharynx. Associated features include an epipharyngeal or nasopharyngeal mass, hypertelorism, midfacial or midline craniocerebral anomalies and optic nerve abnormalities. The facies are characterized by a broad nasal root, increased interpupillary distance and a wide bitemporal diameter. A wide variety of pituitary hormonal deficiences have been reported in these patients, indicating hGH, TSH, ACTH, LH, FSH, Prolactin and ADH deficiencies. In individual patients, pituitary function has ranged from normal to a single hormonal deficiency to multitropic hormone deficiencies (Ellyen et al, 1980; Lieblich et al, 1978; Yagnik et al, 1973). In one proband autopsied, degeneration of the hypothalamus and agenesis of the supraoptic nuclei were found (Pollock et al, 1968). Duplication of the pituitary and agenesis of the corpus collosum have also been described (Bale & Reye, 1976). Diagnosis of this syndrome is important, as iatrogenic hypopituitarism has been described following extirpation of a nasopharyngeal mass containing anterior and posterior pituitary tissue, whose sphenoidal defect was not recognized postoperatively (Weber et al, 1977). Although the majority of cases of transsphenoidal encephalocele are sporadic, 2 sibs with transsphenoidal pituitary herniation, midfacial anomalies and multitropic hormonal deficiencies, who were the offspring of a consanguinous mating, have been described, suggestive of autosomal recessive inheritance (Ellyin et al, 1980).

Septooptic dysplasia

The association of hypoplasia of the optic discs with absence of the septum pellucidum was described by de Morsier in 1956. In 1970, Hoyt et al described 9 dwarfed children with this developmental anomaly in whom they documented growth hormone deficiency, with or without other tropic hormone deficiencies. Septooptic dysplasia is a rare malformation of anterior midline structures of the brain, including agenesis of the septum pellucidum, primitive optic ventricle and hypoplasia of the chiasm, optic nerves and infundibulum. Severely affected neonates may present with hypotonia, seizures, hypoglycaemia and prolonged jaundice progressing to a young infant with defective vision, behavioural delay, hypotonia and seizures (Patel et al, 1975; Harris and Haas, 1972). In midly affected cases, the children may simply present with proportionate short stature and pendular nystagmus, with or without amblyopia. Ophthalmologic examination reveals bilateral hypoplasia of the optic nerves, with small optic discs and irregular field defects. On pneumencephalography, or computed tomography, absence of the septum pellucidum is usually found, but it has now been documented that agenesis of the septum pellucidum is inconstant and not essential for diagnosis (Patel et al, 1975; Manelfe & Rochicciolo, 1979). Intelligence may be normal or mild to moderately subnormal. The sella turcica and suprasellar cisterns have been normal. The pituitary insufficiency, which may vary from isolated growth hormone deficiency to panhypopituitarism is probably secondary to a diencephalic malformation resulting in deficiency of one or more of the hypothalamic releasing hormones (Benoit-Gonin, et al, 1978; Toublanc et al, 1976). Diabetes insipidus is found in nearly one half of the cases. One case of septo-optic dysplasia with sexual precocity has been described. Autopsy has shown absence of the posterior pituitary and diffuse lesions of the hypothalmus, optic nerves, corpus callosum and olfactory tract (Patel, et al, 1975). This syndrome should be considered in any child with pituitary dwarfism who has nystagmus or abnormalities of the optic disc. All of the cases described to date with septooptic dysplasia and growth retardation have been sporadic, with no evidence of ocular anomalies or dwarfism in their parents or sibs. The relationship of this syndrome to the holoprosencephaly syndromes has been questioned.

Simple cleft lip and palate associated with pituitary insufficiency

Functional pituitary insufficiency has been described in a number of individials with cleft lip and palate who did not have other facial or neurologic abnormalities (Frances et al, 1966; Laron et al, 1969; Rudman et al, 1979). Pituitary insufficiency may vary from complete panhypopituitarism associated with congenital aplasia of the pituitary to isolated growth hormone deficiency. Rudman et al (1978) studied 200 children with isolated clefts and found 4% with hGH deficiency: 40 times higher than the frequency in children without clefts. Short children with cleft lip and palate and growth retardation should thus be subjected to a complete pituitary evaluation. One can speculate that this disorder is simply the mild end of the spectrum of the holoprosencephaly-septooptic dysplasia range of hypothalamic anomalies associated with pituitary insufficiency.

Solitary maxillary central incisor

Rappaport et al (1977) have described seven patients with a single maxillary central incisor in both deciduous and permanent dentition and short stature. Five of the patients had documented hGH deficiency and the two who were treated had good growth response to growth hormone therapy. No other pituitary hormone deficiencies were found. All had normal skull radiographs except for one patient with a 'small J-shaped sella'. They had normal facies or only mild midline facial anomalies and there was no evidence of hypothalamic or optic defects. All of the cases were sporadic, although Lowry (1974) has observed a solitary maxillary central incisor in the normal sized mother of a child with holoprosencephaly and median cleft lip. The aetiology and pathogenesis of this syndrome are unknown.

Histiocytosis X (Letterer-Siwe disease, Hand-Schuller-Christian disease, eosinophilic granuloma)

Histiocytosis X is characterized by foamy histiocyte infiltration in many areas of the body, including the hypothalamus. It is now been well documented that when the histiocytic infiltration involves the hypothalamus, prepubertal growth retardation associated with growth hormone deficiency and diabetes insipidus frequently occur (Latorre et al, 1974; Braunstein and Kohler, 1972). Delayed puberty and hypogonadism are also frequent accompaniments of this syndrome. Autopsy reports in adults with histiocytosis X suggest that the pituitary insufficiency is secondary to hypothalamic destruction. Diabetes insipidus and growth hormone deficiency frequently occur together, but either endocrine abnormality may exist alone. In contrast to a previous suggestion of hGH unresponsiveness, Braunstein et al (1975) have documented a significant increment in growth rate in response to growth hormone therapy in these individuals.

Congenital hypothalamic hamartoblastoma, hypopituitarism, imperforate anus, postaxial polydactyly syndrome (Hall syndrome)

Hall et al (1980) have described a neonatally lethal malformation syndrome consisting of hypothalamic hamartoblastoma, hypopituitarism, postaxial polydactyly and imperforate anus. Variable features include laryngeal cleft, abnormal lung lobulation, renal agenesis and/or renal dysplasia, short 4th metacarpals, nail dysplasia, multiple buccal frenula, hypoadrenalism, microphallus, congenital heart defect and intrauterine growth retardation. The hypothalamic tumour was apparent on the inferior surface of the cerebrum and extended from the optic chiasma to the interpeduncular fossa (Claren et al, 1980). The tumour replaced the hypothalamus and other nuclei which originate in the embryonic hypothalamic plate. It was principally composed of cells resembling primitive undifferentiated germinal cells. The olfactory bulbs and tracts were short and thick suggesting a relationship to the holoprosencephaly syndromes. An anterior pituitary gland was absent in all cases. The posterior pituitary was absent in the majority. The adrenal hypoplasia, small thyroid and microphallus are presumably secondary to pituitary insufficiency. All patients were sporadic and there was no consanguinity; thus the aetiology of the syndrome is not known.

Rieger syndrome (iris-dental dysplasia)
The Rieger syndrome is an autosomal dominant disorder associated with malformation of the iris, with pupillary anomalies and hypoplasia of the teeth, with or without maxillary hypoplasia (Feingold et al, 1969). Sadeghi-Nejad and Senior (1974b) reported a large family in which 3 and possibly 5 individuals had both Rieger syndrome and isolated growth hormone deficiency. Sibs of the proband had Rieger syndrome with normal pituitary function, but a deficiency of growth hormone was not present in any member of the family who did not have Rieger syndrome. Affected individuals had insulin hypersensitivity, but normal plasma insulin responses to arginine and glucose. One subject who was treated with growth hormone exhibited substantial enhancement of his rate of growth. It is postulated that the basic pathogenetic mechanism in this autosomal dominant disorder is maldevelopment of the neural crest resulting in ocular, dental and hypothalamic abnormalities.

Primary empty sella with normal pituitary function has also been reported in association with dominantly inherited Rieger syndrome in multiple members of a large kindred (Kleinmann et al, 1981). Gorlin et al, (1975) has described an apparently distinct syndrome in two brothers, consisting of Rieger anomaly, growth retardation, normal pituitary function, joint hypermobility, inguinal hernia, delayed dentition, and megalocornea. Definition of this syndrome must await the recognition of other similarly affected patients.

Pituitary dwarfism associated with sensorineural deafness
Winklemann et al (1972) described 2 sisters, offspring of a nonconsanguineous mating, who had pituitary dwarfism, primary amenorrhea and sensorineural deafness. Deficiency of human growth hormone and gonadotropins was documented, and thyroid and adrenal function were normal. It was postulated that the combination of sensorineural deafness with pituitary insufficiency could represent a simple autosomal recessive trait. Further families with this combination of abnormalities will have to be described before it can be accepted as a distinct syndrome.

Fanconi anaemia
The Fanconi syndrome is an autosomal recessive disorder characterized by chronic pancytopenia with bone marrow hypoplasia, abnormal pigmentation, upper limb malformations, kidney anomalies, growth retardation, small genitalia and increased frequency of chromosomal breaks in cultured lymphocytes. Nilsson (1960) found that 38 of 68 published cases of Fanconi anaemia had

stunted growth and 24 had genital anomalies. In 1965, Cussen reported a child with Fanconi anaemia who appeared to be a pituitary dwarf and pointed out that small pituitary glands, adrenocortical atrophy and atrophic testis have been described in this syndrome. A number of investigators have now documented hGH deficiency in patients with Fanconi anaemia, in most of whom other endocrine function was normal (Pochedly et al, 1971; Clark & Weldon, 1975; Zachman et al, 1972; Costin et al, 1972). Administration of hGH resulted in excellent short-term and long-term responses in most of these patients but Gleadhill et al (1975) were unable to find evidence of growth acceleration in response to long-term hGH treatment in their patients. In view of the intrauterine growth retardation commonly associated with this syndrome, it appears that both cellular factors and growth hormone deficiency probably contribute to their short stature.

Neurofibromatosis
A variety of endocrine disturbances have been reported in patients with neurofibromatosis (Saxena, 1970). The most common associated endocrine disorder in children is sexual precocity, while pheochromocytoma is the most common in adults. Marked growth retardation unrelated to skeletal anomalies, has also been reported. Andler et al (1979) have documented a variety of pituitary dysfunctions in affected children including hGH deficiency, both diminished and elevated TSH response to TRH and hyperprolactinaemia. All of their patients with neurofibromatosis and pituitary dysfunction had a suprasellar tumour.

Primary microcephaly
Since somatic growth is impaired in most microcephalic children, Dacou-Voutetakis et al (1974) studied pituitary function in 5 children with primary microcephaly. In many of these children, growth hormone levels were deficient both in the basal state and following insulin-induced hypoglycaemia, while thyroid function was normal. There was no correlation between the degree of microcephaly and the presence or absence of growth hormone deficiency. Thus, a wide variety of central nervous system defects appear to be associated with pituitary insufficiency, presumably secondary to hypothalamic abnormalities.

Gonadal dysgenesis
Although growth hormone secretion has been reported to be normal or paradoxically increased following glucose in most patients with gonadal dysgenesis, pituitary insufficiency has now been reported in several patients. Faggiono et al (1975) described two women with X0/XX mosaicism who showed absent hGH response to arginine and insulin induced hypoglycaemia, low levels of gono-

dotropins and limited ACTH reserve. In addition, Kauli et al (1979) have described a girl with XY gonadal dysgenesis who was deficient in both growth hormone and gonadotropin secretion. Although the most likely explanation for these cases is chance association, a hypothalamic disturbance in gonadal dysgenesis has been postulated.

Genetic non syndromal forms of pituitary dwarfism

Hereditary forms of pituitary insufficiency unassociated with apparent anatomical defects of the CNS, hypothalamus or pituitary represent a genetically heterogeneous group of disorders. These disorders can be primarily classified into: (1) multitropic pituitary hormone deficiency (panhypopituitarism) and, (2) isolated growth hormone deficiency. Each of these disorders, in turn, is heterogeneous and must be distinguished from the various genetic forms of growth hormone unresponsiveness.

Familial panhypopituitary dwarfism (multitropic hormone deficiency)

Panhypopituitary dwarfism is associated with hGH deficiency and a deficiency of one or more of the other pituitary tropic hormones. Although the great majority of cases of panhypopituitary dwarfism are sporadic, at least 2 distinct genetic types of the disease have been described (Rimoin, 1976). Numerous kindreds with multiple affected family members have been described, the majority of which have occurred in inbred communities. The occurrence of affected sibs of both sexes, the high frequency of consanguinity and a segregation ratio of close to 25% in familial cases indicates that one form of panhypopituitary dwarfism is inherited as an autosomal recessive trait (Rimoin et al, 1968) (Fig. 82.2). Schimke et al (1971) and Phelan et al (1971) have reported pedigrees in which panhypopituitary dwarfism appears to be inherited as an X-linked recessive trait, and review of the older reported pedigrees reveals several families with only male sibs affected, compatible with either autosomal or X-linked recessive inheritance. Thus, there appear to be at least 2 distinct forms of hereditary panhypopituitary dwarfism, one inherited as an autosomal recessive and one as an X–linked recessive trait. Unfortunately, there are no clinical or endocrinologic differences between the 2 genetic disorders and the more common acquired disease, and thus in a sporadic case or in a family in which only male sibs are affected, accurate genetic counselling is impossible.

The clinical features of hereditary panhypopituitary dwarfism are identical to those of the nongenetic forms of the disease and are dependent upon which of the tropic hormones are deficient. The most frequently associated hormonal deficiency is that of gonadotropin, followed in order of frequency by ACTH and TSH deficiency. Deficiency of hGH results in proportionate dwarfism,

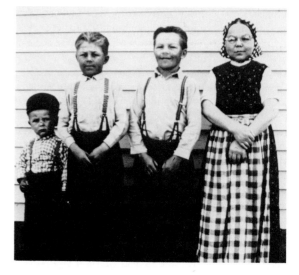

Fig. 82.2 Autosomal recessive multitropic pituitary hormone deficiency. Three affected Hutterite sibs on the right and their cousin on the left.

increased subcutaneous adipose tissue and characteristic high-pitched voice and wrinkled skin. Gonadotropin deficiency results in sexual immaturity with primary amenorrhea and lack of secondary sexual characteristics in the female and small testes and phallus and lack of beard in the male. TSH deficiency, when it occurs, does not often result in severe thyroid deficiency, but in certain instances definite signs of hypothyroidism can occur with myxedematous facies, slow reflexes, hypometabolism and epiphyseal dysplasia. ACTH deficiency may contribute to severe hypoglycaemia in infancy and childhood. There is both inter- and intrafamilial variability in the associated hormonal deficiencies; in certain families one individual may lack all of the tropic hormones, whereas another may lack only hGH and gonadotropin. In families with multitropic deficiencies, however, at least both hGH and gonadotropin deficiency occur in all affected members, there being no familial crossovers between panhypopituitary dwarfism and isolated hGH deficiency yet reported.

In hereditary panhypopituitary dwarfism, it would be difficult to visualize a metabolic defect or structural gene mutation resulting in the deficiency of 2 or more tropic hormones which lack a common subunit; thus, it is quite likely that a structural, degenerative, or secretory defect in the pituitary or hypothalamus exists in these disorders. Studies with TRH and LHRH in panhypopituitary dwarfs have demonstrated that the basic defect in the majority of cases lies in the hypothalamus, rather than in the pituitary, since TRH and LHRH administration resulted in TSH and LH secretion, respectively, in approximately two thirds of the patients (Medeiros-Neto et al, 1973; Costom et al, 1971; Folley et al, 1972). In those patients with a positive response to the hypothalamic releasing hormone, the pituitary is capable of synthesizing and secreting the tropic hormone, indicating that the basic defect lies in the hypothalamus. In the minority of cases who do not respond to TRH or LHRH a defect located in the pituitary itself would be more likely.

Isolated human growth deficiency (IGHD)

An isolated deficiency of hGH with otherwise normal pituitary function has now been well established as a cause of proportionate dwarfism with normal sexual development (Rimoin, 1976; Rimoin & Schimke, 1971; Goodman et al, 1968). It is likely that the majority of cases previously described under the designation of 'sexual ateliotic dwarfism' had an isolated deficiency of hGH. Although the majority of cases of hGH deficiency have a fairly typical physical appearance and characteristic metabolic abnormalities, it is now apparent that on the basis of clinical, genetic, and metabolic variability, IGHD is a heterogeneous group of disorders.

1. Type I IGHD. The most common form of IGHD, which has been called Type I, is inherited as an autosomal recessive trait and is associated with proportionate dwarfism, increased subcutaneous fat, typical pinched facies with high forehead, wrinkled skin and high-pitched voice (Rimoin, 1976; Rimoin & Schimke, 1971; Royer et al, 1970; Donaldson et al, 1980) (Fig. 82.3). They may have spontaneous hypoglycaemic episodes in infancy, but spontaneous hypoglycaemia is not a problem after early childhood, although they maintain hypersensitivy to exogenous insulin into adulthood. As adults, abnormal glucose tolerance associated with insulinopenia is a characteristic feature, both of which quickly revert to normal following hGH therapy. Puberty occurs spontaneously, but is frequently delayed to the late teens or early twenties. Puberty frequently appears abruptly during the first few months of hGH therapy. Thus, in the prepubertal individual, IGHD cannot be clinically distinguished from a combined deficiency of hGH and gonadotropins until at least the early twenties. LHRH stimulation studies may well prove to be valuable in distinguishing between these 2 disorders.

Since the structure of growth hormone releasing hormone is not yet known, it is presently impossible to utilize releasing factor stimulation studies in IGHD to pinpoint the pathogenetic defect. Autopsy studies in 3 cases of IGHD Type I have all revealed the presence of typical somatotropic cells in the pituitary, and in the one case assayed, the presence of significant amounts of immunoreactive growth hormone (Hewer, 1944; Rimoin & Schechter, 1973; Merimee et al, 1975). Though the relative number of somatotropic cells in the pituitary differed between the 3 cases studied, they clearly demonstrate the pituitary's capability of synthesizing growth

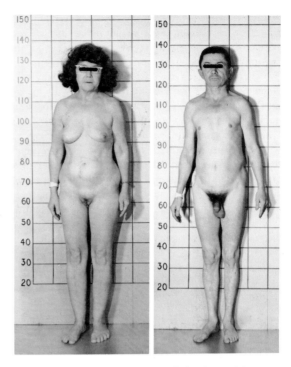

Fig. 82.3 Autosomal recessive type 1 isolated growth hormone deficiency in two sibs who are the offspring of a consaguineous meeting.

hormone. Thus, the defect in these patients would appear to be a deficiency of growth hormone releasing factor or a defect in the releasing factor receptor of the somatotropic cell.

2. Type II IGHD. Merimee et al (1969) described a distinct form of hGH deficiency, apparently inherited as an autosomal dominant trait, which they called Type II IGHD. These individuals did not have the wrinkled skin or characteristic voice seen in other pituitary dwarfs. They had glucose intolerance, but an increased rather than decreased insulin response to both glucose ingestion and arginine infusion. Furthermore, they were relatively resistant to exogenous insulin and to the metabolic effects of exogenous hGH. It is now quite clear that there is further heterogeneity in the IGHD syndromes than a simple division into Type I and Type II, as previously suggested, since there have been families reported with apparent dominant inheritance who have the metabolic features of the recessive form of the disease. For example, Poskitt and Rayner (1974) have described 2 families with a father and son with IGHD, suggestive of autosomal dominant inheritance. These individuals had wrinkled skin, spontaneous hypoglycaemia of infancy, hyperresponsiveness to exogenous insulin and a marked increase in growth velocity following hGH therapy, all features of the 'recessive' form of the disease. Sheikholislam and Stempfel (1972) have described a family in which a father and 4 of his 7 children had IGHD, again suggestive of autosomal dominant inheritance. These individuals had the typical features of IGHD Type I with high-pitched voice, infantile facies, delayed onset of puberty and marked growth acceleration following hGH therapy, but they had glucose intolerance with relative hyperinsulinism, which increased even further following hGH administration. On the other hand, Bierich (1973) described 2 sibs with normal insulin sensitivity, but plasma hyperinsulinism in response to an intravenous glucose load. Unfortunately, they did not mention whether or not a parent was affected, so it is impossible to state whether the syndrome is dominantly or recessively inherited in this family. It is thus apparent that the heterogeneity of the IGHD syndromes is much more complex than the original Type I and II classification, involving more than 2 disorders which differ in their mode of inheritance and metabolic features.

3. Type A IGHD. Illig (1970) described a type of growth hormone deficiency, called Type A, which was felt to be distinct from Type I, on the basis of the appearance of high concentrations of hGH antibodies following hGH therapy. This syndrome is also inherited as an autosomal recessive trait and results in shortness at birth and even more severe dwarfism and exaggerated pinched facies than the more common forms of hGH deficiency. Nitrogen retention following exogenous hGH is greater as well. The major distinguishing feature, however, is that during hGH therapy they develop hGH antibodies in high concentration, which suppress the growth promoting effects of hGH. The authors postulated that these children have a hereditary complete deficiency of hGH, which is effective before birth and which causes a lack of immune tolerance to homologous hGH.

Phillips et al (1981) have recently studied the growth hormone genes in Illig's original family using restriction endonuclease techniques. All affected children in this family were found to be homozygous for a 7.5 kilobase deletion in their growth hormone gene, whereas their parents and two thirds of their unaffected sibs appeared to be heterozygous for the deletion. Thus type A IGHD appears to be the result of a deletion in the hGH gene resulting in the congenital absence of normal hGH and a lack of immunotolerance to homologous hGH. This would explain their total absence of immunoreactive plasma hGH and their high antibody titers following hGH administration. In contrast to the patients with the Type A syndrome, patients with Type I and II IGHD had normal restriction patterns in their hGH genes. This would support the anatomic data suggesting that Type I IGHD is the result of a hypothalamic rather than a primary hGH defect.

4. Pituitary dwarfism with biologically inactive hGH. Kowarski et al (1978) and Hayek et al (1978) have described patients with the clinical features of isolated growth hormone deficiency who achieved normal plasma immunoactive growth hormone levels following stimulation, but low levels of somatomedin. Following hGH administration, however, they generated normal somatomedin levels and had a significant increase in their growth rates. TSH and ACTH secretion were normal. In view of their clinical syndrome of isolated growth hormone deficiency, normal plasma hGH, low basal somatomedin levels and their normal response to exogenous hGH, they appear to secrete a biologically inert growth hormone. Since their endogenous growth hormone reacted normally in the immunossay, this appears to represent a CRM (cross-reactive-material) positive mutation.

5. X-linked hypogammaglobulinaenia and isolated growth hormone deficiency. Fleisher et al (1980) described a kindred in which two brothers and their two maternal uncles had a syndrome consisting of hypogammaglobulinaenia and isolated hGH deficiency. They had proportionate short stature, retarded bone age in childhood, delayed onset of puberty, lack of plasma hGH response to insulin-arginine stimulation, low bio and immunoassayable somatomedin and normal TSH, ACTH, FSH and LH secretion. Recurrent sinopulmonary infections were a problem in two patients, which were abated by parenteral gamma globulin therapy. Three of the patients had panhypogammaglobulinaemia and absence of circulating B cells, whereas the other patient had normal serum IgA and IgM levels and decreased levels of circulating B cells. All had an absence of specific in vitro antibody production after antigenic stimulation and a failure of in vitro immunoglobulin production. Two of the patients had normal appearing tonsils. T cell function and number was normal. Thus these patients appear to have a distinct X-linked recessive syndrome consisting of isolated hGH deficiency and hypogammaglobulinaemia.

Laron dwarfism

Laron et al (1966) described a syndrome with the clinical features of pituitary dwarfism, associated with high plasma concentrations of immunoreactive hGH (Fig. 82.4). Although their patients were all oriental Jews, this autosomal recessive syndrome has since been described in numerous other ethnic groups (Van Gemund et al, 1969; Najjer et al, 1971; Van den Brant et al, 1974). These individuals have the clinical appearance of patients with IGHD to an exaggerated extent, with severe growth retardation, severly pinches facies, high-pitched voices and small male genitalia (Laron, 1974). Males have delayed puberty. Birthweight is normal but birth length may be retarded. Motor development may be delayed and some are mildly retarded. Teething and fontanel closure are delayed. Their hands and feet are small and like pituitary dwarfs, they are

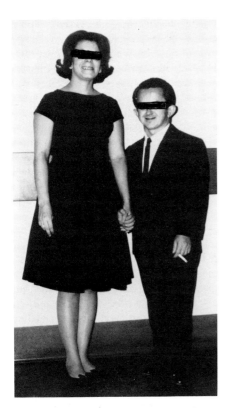

Fig. 82.4 A woman with isolated growth hormone deficiency and her husband with Laron dwarfism.

obese and their body proportions are childlike. They may have spontaneous hypoglycaemic episodes in infancy and usually have insulinopenia in response to glucose and arginine. ACTH, TSH, gonadotropin and vasopressin secretion are normal. Fasting plasma hGH concentrations are usually elevated, but may fluctuate from normal levels to over 100 ng/ml in the same patient. There is further elevation of plasma immunoreactive growth hormone concentration following insulin induced hypoglycaemia and arginine infusion. Plasma somatomedin levels are low, and unlike hGH deficient patients, do not respond to hGH administration (Laron et al, 1971). Furthermore, they are relatively unresponsive to metabolic and growth promoting effects of growth hormone. Laron et al (1966) first postulated that this disorder was due to the synthesis of a structurally altered hGH molecule which was immunologically active but biologically inert. Several groups of investigators, however, have been unable to distinguish between plasma hGH of Laron dwarfs and normal individuals on the basis of serial immunoassay dilutions, electrofocusing and molecular size distribution (Van den Brandt et al, 1974; Eshet et al, 1973; Bala & Beck, 1973; Eldes et al, 1973; Pierson et al, 1978). Furthermore, substantial quantities of receptor active hGH have been found in their sera by a hepatic radioreceptor assay (Jacobs et al, 1976). Golde et al (1980) have directly demonstrated specific cellular resistance to hGH in Laron dwarfs, utilizing an in vitro erythyroid progenitor technique. Thus, the pathogenetic mechanism in Laron dwarfism appears to involve a defect in somatomedin generation, which may be secondary to a universal defect in growth hormone receptors.

The African Pygmies
Peripheral unresponsiveness to human growth hormone administration, in the presence of normal concentrations of immunoreactive plasma hGH and normal bioassayable somatomedin activity, has been documented in the African Pygmies (Rimoin et al, 1969; Merimee et al, 1972). This population, who inhabit the rain forests of equatorial Africa, resemble pituitary dwarfs in size and skeletal proportions, but do not have the truncal obesity, peculiar facies and wrinkled skin of pituitary dwarfism. Following insulin induced hypoglycaemia and arginine infusion, plasma hGH levels are normal, but like Type I IGHD, they are insulinopenic and hypersensitive to the effects of exogenous insulin. They are completely unresponsive to the lipolytic, insulinotropic and nitrogen retaining properties of hGH and their small size is presumably secondary to a similar unresponsiveness to the growth promoting properties of the molecule. Their immediate responses to hGH, however, are normal. Unlike Laron dwarfs, who are unable to generate somatomedin, the African Pygmies may well have a defect in somatomedin receptors. Although no well-documented cases of peripheral unresponsiveness to hGH with normal plasma hGH and somatomedin activity have been described in other ethnic groups, it is possible that somatomedin resistance may be a relatively common cause of short stature in the population at large. Merimee et al (1981) have recently reported a deficiency of insulin-like growth factor I in these pygmies.

Pituitary dwarfism with somatomedin unresponsiveness
Lanes et al (1980) have described an adolescent male with proportionate dwarfism, normal plasma hGH response to stimulation and elevated somatomedin by bioassay, radioreceptor assay and radioimmunoassay. Bone age was clinically retarded, but by age 15 years his sexual development was well established. Twenty-four hour growth hormone secretion was normal, as were his ACTH, TSH and gonadotropin functions. In view of his elevated somatomedin and clinical hypopituitarism, peripheral unresponsiveness to somatomedin, at either the receptor or postreceptor level was postulated.

Isolated deficiencies of TSH, ACTH, LH and FSH
Isolated deficiencies of each of these pituitary hormones have been reported. Since the clinical symptoms produced are the result of the target organ hormonal defi-

ciency (eg hypothyroidism, hypoadrenalism or hypogonadism), they will be discussed in the appropriate endocrine organ chapters (Thyroid-Chapter 83; Adrenal-Chapter 86 and Gonadal disorders-Chapter 87).

DISORDERS OF PITUITARY HYPERSECRETION AND/OR NEOPLASIA

Genetic disorders of pituitary hyperfunction are far less common than those of pituitary insufficiency. Furthermore, except in instances of multiple endocrine adrenomatosis or in patients who have a positive family history of pituitary hyperfunction, it is impossible to denote which of the sporadic cases have a genetic form of pituitary disease. The most common form of hereditary pituitary neoplasia is the multiple endocrine adenomatosis syndrome, Type I (Chapter 98). Although multiple cases of familial acromegaly and of the amenorrhea-galactorrhea syndrome have been described in certain kindreds with no evidence of other endocrine involvement, these disorders may well represent limited forms of the multiple endocrine adenomatosis syndrome.

Acromegaly
Hypersecretion of human growth hormone by a pituitary neoplasm leads to the classic syndromes of acromegaly and gigantism, depending upon the age of onset of the disorder. The clinical features and diagnostic criteria of acromegaly have been well reviewed in the endocrinological literature and will not be discussed here (Daughaday, 1981). The diagnosis can be readily made on the basis of high fasting plasma concentrations of human growth hormone, which usually do not suppress following oral glucose ingestion.

Although the majority of cases of acromegaly are sporadic, many families have been reported in which multiple members are said to be affected (Koch & Tiwisima, 1959; Rimoin & Schimke, 1971). This literature must be regarded with caution, however, as very few of the familial cases have been anatomically confirmed or had high hGH levels documented by radioimmunoassay. Indeed, a number of the families described in the literature as hereditary acromegaly represent instead, cases of pachydermoperiostosis, a dominantly inherited disorder (Rimoin & Schimke, 1971). In other reports of familial acromegaly, the affected relatives are said to be 'acromegaloid' rather than acromegalic; that is, they are of tall stature but have no evidence of pituitary dysfunction (Lehmann, 1964). Another syndrome that might be confused with acromegaly is cerebral gigantism, in which increased growth rate occurs from infancy but no abnormalities in hGH secretion are found (Hook & Reynolds, 1967). In spite of these reservations, pathologic and radiographic documentation of pituitary adenomas have

been described in successive generations in several families, strongly suggesting autosomal dominant inheritance. Two cousins from a highly inbred family have also been described with 'acromegaly,' suggesting autosomal recessive inheritance (Leva, 1915). Objective evidence for the disease was obtained in only one of these cousins, however; thus the presence of a recessive form of the disorder must be interpreted with caution. It would be of great value to study hGH secretion in the 'acromegaloid' relatives of documented acromegalic cases to see if minor abnormalities of hGH secretion do exist. Many of the familial cases of acromegaly may represent partial expression of the multiple endocrine adenomatosis syndrome.

Familial amenorrhea-galactorrhea syndrome (Chiari-Frommel syndrome, Forbes-Albright syndrome)
The association of secondary amenorrhea and galactorrhea is generally thought to occur in two distinct syndromes – the Forbes-Albright syndrome, in which amenorrhea and galactorrhea are accompanied by a pituitary tumour, with or without prior pregnancy; and the Chiari-Frommel syndrome, in which the amenorrhea and galactorrhea commence following pregnancy, unassociated with a pituitary neoplasm (Young et al, 1967). This distinction may be artificial, however, as the pituitary adenomata may be too small to recognize; progression from the benign Chiari-Frommel syndrome to the neoplastic Forbes-Albright syndrome has been documented. Linquette and associates (1967) have described a family in which both mother and daughter developed amenorrhea and galactorrhea associated with pituitary adenomas. The mother first developed the clinical signs of this syndrome following a pregnancy, whereas the daughter was never pregnant and amenorrhea ensued following emotional trauma. Both patients had a large sella turcica radiographically and were found on craniotomy to have pituitary adenomas. Histologically, the tumours resembled chromophobe adenomas, but there was fine eosinophillic granulation on tetrachrome staining, indicative of prolactin secreting cells. The amenorrhea-glactorrhea syndrome has also been described as a part of the multiple endocrine adenomatosis (MEA) I syndrome, associated with gastric ulcers, islet cell adenomas, and hyperparathyroidism. It is impossible to state whether or not the family reported by Linquette represents a distinct entity or whether both mother and daughter had partial forms of the MEA syndrome. In any case, the pituitary adenomata in this syndrome, like most other hereditary tumours, are inherited as dominant traits.

Multiple endocrine adenomatosis Type I (MEA Type I, Wermer syndrome)
Multiple endocrine adenomatosis is a familial disorder characterized by multiple tumours or hyperplasia of the

endocrine glands and a high incidence of multifocal, unremitting peptic ulcer disease (Zollinger-Ellison syndrome) (See Chapters 84 and 98).

Ballard and associates (1964) reviewed eighty-five cases of the MEA syndrome, of which fifty-five had pituitary involvement. The clinical manifestations of pituitary disease are dependent upon the predominating cell type. Chromophobe adenoma was the most common lesion and resulted in symptoms of pituitary insufficiency, especially hypogonadism and/or headache and visual disturbances secondary to mechanical pressure. Acromegaly, which was present in fifteen of the fifty-five cases, was associated with eosinophilic adenoma and did not differ clinically from acquired cases of this disease. Pituitary involvement has been found without other apparent endocrine disease in certain patients whose relatives have the full-blown syndrome, but it may occur in combination with any or all of the other manifestations of the disorder. On histopathological examination, the pituitary may show simple hyperplasia, benign adenoma, or invasive neoplasm.

LeBriggs and Powell (1969) described a woman with the MEA syndrome who developed the amenorrhea-galactorrhea syndrome following parturition. Although there was no clinical evidence of a pituitary neoplasm, pituitary gonadotropins were absent in the urine and she may well have had a small prolactin secreting adenoma. It is impossible to state whether or not the familial cases of 'pure' amenorrhea-galactorrhea syndrome and acromegaly are all part of the MEA syndrome or whether they represent distinct entities. In any patient with a pituitary neoplasm, however, an effort should be made to rule out involvement of the other endocrine organs, in both the patient and his close relatives.

The MEA I syndrome is inherited as an autosomal dominant trait, with marked intrafamilial variability.

POSTERIOR PITUITARY

The posterior pituitary gland (neurohypophysis), which is derived from an invagination of the hypothalamus, is embryologically and functionally distinct from the anterior pituitary. The primary function of the neurohypophysis is the storage and secretion of two octapeptide hormones: antidiuretic hormone (ADH, vasopressin) and oxytocin. These hormones are synthesized by neurones in the supraoptic and paraventricular nuclei of the hypothalamus. They are bound to a carrier protein (neurophysin) and transported down the neuronal axons (supraopticoneurohypophyseal tracts) to the posterior pituitary, in vesicular form. The hormones are stored in the posterior pituitary and released into the circulation following appropriate stimuli (Leaf & Coggins, 1974).

GENETIC DISORDERS OF VASOPRESSIN DEFICIENCY

Hereditary vasopressin-sensitive diabetes insipidus is a syndrome characterized by polyuria, polydipsia, and dehydration secondary to a deficiency of antidiuretic hormone. This syndrome is characterized by acute thirst, especially for cold water, enormous daily urinary output (3000 to 15 000 ml per day), and persistent nocturia. If water is withheld, the patient rapidly loses weight and develops hypertonic dehydration. A variety of acquired lesions of the hypothalamus, such as neoplasia, basilar skull fractures, granulomatous diseases, vascular lesions, meningitis, and encephalitis can result in ADH deficiency (Leaf and Loggins, 1974). In approximately 50% of the cases of diabetes insipidus, however, no obvious primary lesion can be found and the disease is termed 'idiopathic'. It is quite likely that many of the idiopathic cases of diabetes insipidus represent sporadic cases of the genetic form of the disease.

In 1841, Lacombe was the first to document a familial form of diabetes insipidus; he described excessive thirst and polyuria in five males and three females in two generations of a family. Numerous other families with multiple affected members have since been described (Blotner, 1942; Walker and Rance, 1954). Both males and females have been affected in successive generations, and male-to-male transmission has been documented on numerous occasions, indicating that vasopressin-sensitive diabetes insipidus can be inherited as an autosomal dominant trait. The signs and symptoms of this autosomal dominant disorder are quite similar to those of the acquired forms of diabetes insipidus. There is, however, a great deal of intrafamilial variability in the clinical severity and age of onset of the disease. Pender and Fraser (1953) reported a large family in which urinary output varied from 3 to 4 quarts per day to 15 to 20 quarts per day among affected relatives. Some, but not all, affected individuals have an increase in fluid requirements during febrile episodes, exercise, or pregnancy. In most cases the onset of the disease occurs in infancy, but in several well-studied families, symptoms did not occur until late childhood in certain members (Martin, 1959). In many of the affected families, the condition is regarded as an unpleasant family habit, rather than a disease. Other than for drinking enormous quantities of water, the disease did not impair health or well being.

If all forms of hereditary diabetes insipidus were inherited as an autosomal dominant trait, one would expect an equal number of affected males and females. A deficiency of female affected individuals was noted by several authors who assembled previously reported kindreds with this disease (Martin, 1959). Forssman (1945) has documented an X–linked recessive form of vasopressin-sensitive diabetes insipidus in several families and suggested that the previously reported unequal sex ratio was caused by inclusion of families with the X–linked form of the disease. He described several large kindreds in which a number of males were affected with vasopressin-sensitive diabetes insipidus, the disease apparently being transmitted through females, who were either completely unaffected or only minimally affected. Thus both autosomal dominant and X–linked recessive varieties of vasopressin-sensitive diabetes insipidus exist, but affected males of either type are clinically indistinguishable.

Hereditary vasopressin-sensitive diabetes insipidus is caused by a marked deficiency of vasopressin. In all reported autopsy studies of individuals with the hereditary or sporadic idiopathic forms of the disease, a severe reduction in the number of neurosecretory neurons in both the supraoptic and paraventricular nuclei of the hypothalamus was found (Gaup, 1941; Green et al, 1967). There is associated gliosis, and in the paraventricular nucleus, the small to medium-sized neurons may be normal or reduced in number. The posterior pituitary gland has been found to be normal in size or small in these cases, but no neurosecretory material was observed on special staining. Thus the vasopressin deficiency appears to be secondary to aplasia or degeneration of the neurosecretory neurons of the hypothalamus. Although these individuals appear to have no neurosecretory neurons in their hypothalamic nuclei and have all of the signs and symptoms of ADH deficiency, oxytocin secretion appears to be normal. Several females with the dominantly inherited form of vasopressin-sensitive diabetes, including one in whom a marked deficiency of neurosecretory cells was documented, have undergone normal pregnancies and deliveries and have successfully nursed their children. Thus they appear to secrete oxytocin, despite the deficiency of neurosecretory neurons. Although a small number of secretory cells remain in the paraventricular nuclei of these patients, Green and associates (1967) suggested that oxytocin might also be produced by cells located outside of these areas. Several patients with diabetes insipidus have been reported, however, who have had difficulty in expelling the fetus and placenta during labour, suggesting that oxytocin deficiency might also exist (Rimoin & Schimke, 1971).

Diabetes insipidus of the vasopressin-sensitive variety has been reported to be an autosomal recessive trait in the Battleboro strain of rat (Valtin, 1969). Although these animals have an absolute deficiency of antidiuretic hormone in their hypothalamic and posterior pituitaries, unlike the human disease, there is hypertrophy of the hypothalamo-pituitary system. The neurons in the supraoptic nucleus are extremely well developed. Similar, but less marked changes, are seen in the paraventricular nuclei, and the posterior lobe of the pituitary is three to four times heavier than normal. Heterozygous animals have a reduced concentration of vasopressin in the hypothalamus and pituitary and have deficient secretion and release of the hormone. Thus it appears as if the basic defect in the autosomal recessive variety of diabetes insipidus in the rat is decreased synthesis of active hormone with compensatory hypertrophy of the secretory neurons. The differences in the genetics and pathogenesis of diabetes insipidus between the human and rat support the general rule of recessive inheritance of peptide hormone deficiency syndromes. In the rat, the basic defect appears to be in the synthesis of the peptide hormone and the disease is inherited as an autosomal recessive trait. In man, the disease is inherited as an autosomal dominant trait, but the primary defect appears to involve a degenerative or developmental disorder of the hypothalamus, rather than a primary defect in peptide synthesis. It would be of great interest to study the hypothalamus in the X–linked recessive variety of the human disease.

Vasopressin deficiency associated with complex genetic syndromes

A variety of developmental malformations may result in both anterior and posterior pituitary deficiency. See previous discussion of congenital absence of pituitary, anencephaly, holoprosencephaly, transphenoidal encephaloeocle, septooptic dysplasia and histiocytosis X (see index for page numbers.)

The diabetes mellitus-optic atrophy, diabetes insipidus-deafness syndrome (DIDMOAD syndrome, Wolfram syndrome)

This autosomal recessive syndrome consists of diabetes mellitus, optic atrophy, diabetes insipidus and neurosensory deafness. Well over 100 cases have now been reported and it has been estimated that the frequency of this syndrome among patients with juvenile onset diabetes is approximately 1/150 (Gunn et al, 1976.) The optic atrophy is of the primary variety and is characterized by white discs and, in some instances, peripheral retinal pigmentation as well. The diabetes mellitus is of the severe juvenile onset variety and frequently precedes the other symptoms. Bilateral neurosensory deafness has more recently been considered to be an integral component of this syndrome; it begins as a high frequency hearing loss and may remain quite mild. Indeed, in many affected patients, the hearing loss was not suspected until audiograms were performed.

A number of other associated abnormalities have been described in certain families, including ataxia, autonomic dysfunction with a neurogenic bladder, sideroblastic anaemia, and hyperalaninuria (Jarnerot, 1973). In view of the progression with time of simple optic atrophy and diabetes mellitus to the full-blown syndrome with neurosensory hearing loss, atonic bladder and ataxia in the original family described by Wolfram (Wolfram, 1938; Turnbridge and Paley, 1956), it is quite likely that all of these anomalies are the result of a single pleiotropic mutant gene and represent one distinct syndrome.

Vasopressin sensitive diabetes insipidus occurs in over one-third of the patients with this syndrome (Bretz et al, 1970). Although the association of diabetes insipidus with diabetes mellitus and optic atrophy had been considered to represent a distinct autosomal recessive syndrome, several families have now been reported in which several members have the full blown syndrome whereas others have the diabetes mellitus and optic atrophy, without the diabetes insipidus (Gossain et al, 1975; Richardson & Hamilton, 1977). Thus it is clear that the diabetes insipidus is simply another pleiotropic effect of a single mutant gene. ADH deficiency has been documented in affected patients (Richardson & Hamilton, 1977). Post mortem examination of two sibs with this syndrome revealed degeneration of the hypothalamic nuclei, more severe in the paraventricular than supraoptic nuclei, and atrophy of the posterior lobe of the pituitary, adrenal cortex, pons and substantia nigra (Carson et al, 1972). Fraser and Gunn (1977) have performed a segregation analysis on 21 families from the literature and found that the data were entirely consistent with autosomal recessive inheritance, with widespread variability in expression. They also postulate that heterozygotes have an increased probability of developing juvenile diabetes mellitus. Although this syndrome is characterized by typical insulin dependent diabetes, it does not appear to be linked to the HLA locus (Stanley et al, 1979).

PERIPHERAL RESISTANCE TO VASOPRESSIN (NEPHROGENIC DIABETES INSIPIDUS)

Nephrogenic diabetes insipidus is an inherited disorder characterized by polyuria, polydipsia, and hyposthenuria, resistant to vasopressin (Rimoin & Schimke, 1971). There is renal unresponsiveness to vasopressin, biologically active antidiuretic hormone has been found to be present in the serum and urine of affected individuals and there is deficient cyclic AMP excretion in the urine following ADH administration.

These individuals have severe polyuria and polydipsia. A concentrating defect has been demonstrated within six days of birth. Polyuria and polydipsia, however, may be overlooked in the early days of life. Several patients have been described who have an absence of thirst. The infants are usually irritable, eager to suck, and vomit milk soon after ingestion. They show a distinct preference for water over milk in early life. They often have constipation, unexplained fever, and failure to gain weight. Episodes of hypernatremic dehydration may

result in seizures and death. Mental retardation was first thought to be one of the inherited features of the disease, but it is now known to result from the acute episodes of severe hypertonic dehydration in infancy (Hillman et al, 1958). These children are constantly preoccupied with drinking, ingest a hypocaloric diet, and have little opportunity for prolonged sleep. It is this preoccupation with drinking which is thought to result in the hypocaloric dwarfism and retardation of mental and emotional development. A large urinary volume and an effort to avoid urinary frequency and enuresis may result in distention and trabeculation of the bladder, with dilated ureters and calyces, which can mimic lower urinary tract obstruction. Chronic renal insufficiency may occur in late childhood. The renal lesion appears to be limited to vasopressin resistance, but associated generalized aminoaciduria and cysthioninuria have been occasionally described (Perry et al, 1967).

Nephrogenic diabetes insipidus must be differentiated from the various forms of vasopressin-sensitive diabetes insipidus, as well as from a number of other renal lesions that result in an inability to reabsorb adequate amounts of filtered water. These renal disorders include glomerulonephritis, chronic pyelonephritis, obstructive uropathy, multiple myeloma, amyloidosis, hypokalaemic and hypercalcaemic nephropathy, and unilateral renal artery occlusion (Leaf & Coggins, 1974). Several complex genetic disorders also result in the syndrome of vasopressin-resistant diabetes insipidus such as sickle cell anaemia, hereditary renal retinal dysplasia, juvenile nephronophthisis, and medullary cystic disease. The diagnosis of nephrogenic diabetes insipidus can be made only after excluding other renal and nonrenal involvement.

The majority of families described with nephrogenic diabetes insipidus suggests X–linked recessive inheritance. Forssman (1945) described families with both nephrogenic and vasopressin-sensitive diabetes insipidus in which X–linked inheritance was almost certain. Waring and associates (1945), in their original description of the disease, also suggested X–linked recessive inheritance. Dancis and associates (1948) were the first to describe a severely affected female with this disorder and challenged the X–linked hypothesis. This hypothesis has also been challenged by other authors (Robinson & Kaplan, 1960). The only reports of male-to-male transmission in this disease, however, were by Cannon (1955) in a large Mormon pedigree. He suggested autosomal dominant inheritance with incomplete penetrance in females on the basis of this pedigree, but in none of the six instances of male-to-male transmission were the patients examined and the disease documented. Crawford and Bode (1969) have illustrated the unreliability of a family history for diagnostic purposes in this disease. They studied one large pedigree extending over nine generations in which male-to-male transmission was suggested by history in six instances. In three of these males, concentrating ability was shown to be normal and in the remaining three, consanguinity of the parents was documented. Thus, no well-documented exception to the X–linked recessive hypothesis has been reported. The X–linked recessive hypothesis is further supported by the finding that the great majority of heterozygous females manifest partial concentrating defects and are unable to excrete urine with a specific gravity greater than 1.018 (Crawford & Bode, 1969). Discrimination by this test, however, is not perfect, as obligate heterozygotes have been reported who have normal concentrating capabilities (Feigen et al, 1970). The variable symptomatology in carrier females is probably due to 'Lyonization.' One affected female with this disorder has been reported in whom administration of chlorothiazide failed to alter urinary volume (Feigen et al, 1970). Administration of chlorothiazide to affected males will result in moderate water conservation, and in nonaffected individuals and some carrier females it results in diuresis. The failure to alter urinary volume in this affected female could also be the result of mosaicism of the renal tubular epithelium, as explained by the Lyon hypothesis. One further piece of evidence for the X–linked recessive hypothesis is the observation of a severely affected girl who was found to have a deletion of one X-chromosome (Bode & Crawford, 1969). There is absence of close linkage between the gene for nephrogenic diabetes insipidus and the Xg blood group (Bode & Miettinen, 1970).

Bode and Crawford (1969) have traced a large number of kindreds with this disorder to a group of Ulster Scotsmen who settled in Nova Scotia. These settlers arrived in Halifax in 1761 aboard the ship Hopewell, and the authors postulate that most, if not all, of the persons with nephrogenic diabetes insipidus in this country originated from these original settlers. At least three families with X–linked nephrogenic diabetes insipidus have been described in Blacks, and there has been a report of this disease in a large family of Samoan descent (Rimoin & Schimke, 1971). Thus, although the great majority of patients with this disorder originally may have inherited their mutant gene from a common ancestor, the infrequent occurrence of new mutations is quite likely.

REFERENCES

Andler W, Roosen K, Kohns U, Stolecke H 1979 Endokrine Storungen bei Kindern mit Neurofibromatose von Recklinghausen. Monatsschrift für Kinderheilkunde 127: 135

Angevine D M 1938 Pathologic anatomy of hypophysis and adrenals in anencephaly. Archives of Pathology 26: 507

Bala R M, Beck J C 1973 Fractionation studies on plasma of normals and patients with Laron dwarfism and hypopituitary gigantism. Canadian Journal of Physiology and Pharmacology 51: 845

Bale P M, Reye R D K 1976 Epignathus, double pituitary and agenesis of corpus callosum. Journal of Pathology 120: 161

Ballard H S, Frame B, Hartsock R J 1964 Familial multiple endocrine adenomapeptic ulcer complex. Medicine 43: 481

Benoit-Gonin J J, David M, Feit J P, Bourgeois J, Chopard A, Kopp N, Jeune M 1978 La dysplasie septo-optique avec deficit en hormone antidiuetique et insuffisance surrenal centrale. Nouvelle Press Medecine 37: 3327

Bierich J R 1973 On the aetiology of hypopituitary dwarfism. 'Proceedings of the International Congress of Endocrinology.' Excerpta Medica, Amsterdam p 408

Blotner H 1942 The inheritance of diabetes insipidus. American Journal of Medical Science 204: 261

Bode H H, Crawford J D 1969 Nephrogenic diabetes insipidus in North America-the Hopewell hypothesis, New England Journal of Medicine 280: 750

Bode H E, Miettinen O S 1970 Nephrogenic diabetes insipidus: absence of close linkage with Xg, American Journal of Human Genetics 22: 221

Braunstein G D, Kohler P P 1972 Pituitary function in Hand-Schuller-Christian disease: Evidence for deficient growth-hormone release in patients with short stature. New England Journal of Medicine 286: 1225

Braunstein G D, Raiti S, Hansen J W, Kohler P O 1975 Response of growth-retarded patients with Hand-Schuller-Christian disease to growth hormone therapy. New England Journal of Medicine 292: 332

Bretz G W, Baghdassarin A, Graher J D, Zacherle B J, Norum R A, Blizzard R M 1970 Coexistence of diabetes mellitus and insipidus and optic atrophy in two male siblings. American Journal of Medicine 48: 398

Cannon J F 1955 Diabetes insipidus: clinical and experimental studies with consideration of genetic relationship. Archives of Internal Medicine 96: 215

Carson M J, Slager U T, Steinberg R M 1972 Occurrence of diabetes insipidus, simultaneous and optic atrophy in a brother and sister. American Journal of Diseases of Children 131: 1382

Clarke W L, Weldon V V 1975 Growth hormone deficiency and Fanconi anaemia. Journal of Pediatrics 86: 814

Clarren S K, Alvord E C, Hall J G 1980 Congenital hypothalamic hamartoblastoma, hypopituitarism imperforate anus and postaxial polydactyly – a new syndrome? Part II. American Journal of Medical Genetics 7: 75

Cohen M M, Jirasek J E, Guzman R T, Gorlin R J, Peterson M Q 1971 Holoprosencephaly and facial dysmorphia. Birth Defects: Original Article Series 7(7): 125

Costin G, Kogut M D, Hyman C B, Ortega J 1972 Fanconi's anaemia associated with isolated growth hormone (GH) deficiency. Clinical Research 20: 253

Costom B H, Grumbach M M, Kaplan S L 1971 Effect of thyrotropin-releasing factor on serum thyroid stimulating hormone. Journal of Clinical Investigation 50: 2219

Crawford J D, Bode H H 1975 Disorders of the posterior pituitary in children. In Gardner L I, editor: Endocrine and Genetic Diseases of Childhood, Philadelphia, W B Saunders Co. p 126

Cussen L J 1965 Primary hypopituitary dwarfism with

Fanconi's hypoplastic anaemia syndrome, renal hypertension and phycomycosis: Report of a case. Medical Journal of Australia 2: 367

Dacou-Voutetakis C, Karpathios Th, Logothetis N et al 1974 Defective growth hormone secretion in primary microcephaly. Journal of Pediatrics 85: 498

Dancis J, Birmingham J R, Leslie S H 1948 Congenital diabetes insipidus resistant to treatment with pitressin. American Journal of Diseases of Children 75: 316

Daughaday W H 1981 The adenohypophysis. In Williams R H, editor: Textbook of Endocrinology, 6, ed, Saunders, Philadelphia. p. 73

de Morsier G 1968 Etudes sur les dysraphies cranio-encephaliques. III. Agenesie du septum lucidum avec malformation du tractus optique: La dysplasie septo-optique. Schweizer Archiv für Neurologie, Neurochirurgie und Psychiatrie 77: 267

Donaldson M D C, Tucker S M, Grant D B 1980 Recessively inherited growth hormone deficiency in a family from Iraq. Journal of Medical Genetics 17: 288

Edmonds H W 1950 Pituitary, adrenal and thyroid in cyclopia. Archives of Pathology 50: 727

Ehrlich R M 1957 Ectopic and hypoplastic pituitary with adrenal hypoplasia. Journal of Pediatrics 51: 377

Elders M J, Garland J T, Daughaday W A, Fisher D A, Whitney J E, Hughes E R 1973 Laron's dwarfism: studies on the nature of the defect. Journal of Pediatrics 83: 253

Ellyin F, Khatir A H and Singh S P 1980 Hypothalamic – pituitary functions in patients with transsphenoidal encephalocoele and midfacial anomalies. Journal of Clinical Endocrinology 51: 854

Eshet R, Laron Z, Brown M and Arnon R 1973 Immunoreactive properties of the plasma hGH from patients with the syndrome of familial dwarfism and high plasma IR-hGH. Journal of Clinical Endocrinology and Metabolism 37: 819

Faggiano M, Lombardi G, Carella C and Criscoulo T 1975 Two cases of the chromatin positive variety of ovarian dysgenesis (XO/XX mosaicism) associated with hGH deficiency and marginal impairment of other hypothalamic-pituitary functions. Clinical Genetics 8: 324

Feigin R D, Rimoin D L and Kaufman R L 1970 Nephrogenic diabetes insipdus in a Negro kindred. American Journal of Diseases of Children 120: 64

Feingold M, Shiere F, Fogels H R, Donaldson D 1969 Rieger's syndrome. Pediatrics 44: 564

Ferrier P E, Stone E F 1969 Familial pituitary dwarfism associated with an abnormal sella turcica. Pediatrics 43: 858

Fleisher T A, White R M, Broder S, Nissley S P, Blaese R M, Mulvihill J J, Olive G, Waldmann T A 1980 X–linked hypogammaglobulinemia and isolated growth hormone deficiency. New England Journal of Medicine 302: 1429

Folley T P, Owings J, Hayford J T, Blizzard R M 1972 Serum thyrotropin responses to synthetic thyrotropin-releasing hormone in normal children and hypopituitary patients. Journal of Clinical Investigation 51: 431

Forssman H 1945 On hereditary diabetes insipidus. With special reference to a sex-linked form. Acta Medica Scandanavica 121: 1

Frances J M, Knorr D, Martinez R, Neuhauser G 1966 Hypophysarer Zwergwuchs bei Lippen-Kiefer-Spalte. Helvetica Paediatrica Acta 21: 315

Fraser F C, Gunn T 1977. Diabetes mellitus, diabetes insipidus, and optic atrophy. An autosomal recessive syndrome? Journal of Medical Genetics 14: 190

Gaupp R 1941 Ueber den Diabetes Insipidus, Zentralblatt für die gesamte Neurologie und Psychiatrie 171: 514

Gleadhill V, Bridges J M, Hadden D R 1975 Franconi's aplastic anaemia with short stature. Absence of response to human growth hormone. Archives of Disease In Childhood 50: 318

Golde D W, Bersch N, Kaplan S, Rimoin D L, Li C H 1980 Peripheral unresponsiveness to human growth hormone in Laron dwarfism. New England Journal of Medicine 303: 1156

Goodman H D, Grumbach M M, Kaplan S L 1968 Growth and growth hormone, II. Comparison of isolated growth hormone deficiency and multiple pituitary hormone deficiencies in 35 patients with idiopathic hypopituitary dwarfism. New England Journal of Medicine 278: 57

Gorlin R, Yunis J, Anderson V 1968 Short arm deletion of chromosome 18 in cebocephaly. American Journal of Diseases of Children 115: 473

Gorlin R J, Cervenka J, Moller K, Horrobin M, Witkop C J 1975 A selected miscellany. Birth Defects original article series XI(2): 39

Gossain V V, Sugawara M, Hagen G A 1975 Co-existent diabetes mellitus and diabetes insipidus, a familial disease Journal of Clinical Endocrinology and Metabolism 41: 1020

Green J R, Buchan G C, Alvard E J, Jr, Savonson A G 1967 Hereditary and idiopathic types of diabetes insipidus. Brain 90: 707

Grunt J A, Reynolds D W 1970 Insulin, blood sugar and growth hormone levels in anencephalic infant before and after intravenous administration of glucose. Journal of Pediatrics 76: 112

Gunn T, Bortolussi R, Little J M, Andermann F, Fraser F C, Belmonte M M 1976 Juvenile diabetes, optic atrophy, sensory nerve deafness, and diabetes insipidus – a syndrome. Journal of Pediatrics 89: 565

Hall J G, Pallister P D, Clarren S K, Beckwith J B, Wiglesworth F W, Fraser F C, Cho S, Benke P J, Reed S D 1980 Congenital hypothalamic hamartoblastoma, hypopituitarism, imperforate anus and postaxial polydactyly – a new syndrome? Part 1. American Journal of Medical Genetics 7: 47

Harris R J, Haas L 1972 Septo-optic dysplasia with growth hormone deficiency (de Morsier syndrome). Archives of Disease in Childhood 47: 973

Haworth J C, Medovy H, Lewis A J 1961 Cebocephaly with endocrine dysgenesis. Journal of Pediatrics 59: 726

Hayek A, Driscoll S G, Warshaw J B 1973 Endocrine studies in anencephaly. Journal of Clinical Investigation 52: 636

Hayek A, Peake G T, Greenberg R E 1978 A new syndrome of short stature due to biologically inactive growth hormone. Pediatric Research 12: 413

Herman S P, Baggenstoss A H, Cloutier M D 1975 Liver dysfunction and histologic abnormalities in neonatal hypopituitarism. Journal of Pediatrics 87: 892

Hewer T F 1944 Ateliotic dwarfism with normal sexual function: A result of hypopituitarism. Journal of Endocrinology 3: 397

Hillman D A, Neyzi O, Porter P, Cushman A, Talbot N B 1958 Renal (vasopressin resistant) diabetes insipidus: definition of the effects of a homeostatic limitation in capacity to conserve water on the physical, intellectual and emotional development of a child. Pediatrics 21: 430

Hintz R L, Menking M, Sotos J T 1968 Familial holoprosencephaly with endocrine dysgenesis. Journal of Pediatrics 72: 81

Hook E B, Reynolds J W 1967 Cerebral gigantism: endocrinological and clinical observations of six patients including a congenital giant, concordant monozygotic twins and a child who achieved adult gigantic size. Journal of Pediatrics 70: 900

Hoyt W F, Kaplan S L, Grumbach M M et al: Septo-optic dysplasia with pituitary dwarfism. Lancet 1: 893

Illig R 1970 Growth hormone antibodies in patients treated with different preparations of human growth hormone (HGH). Journal of Clinical Endocrinology 31: 679

Jacobs L S, Sneid D S, Garland J T, Laron Z, Daughaday W A 1976 Receptoractive growth hormone in Laron dwarfism. Journal of Clinical Endocrinology 42: 403

Jarnerot G 1973 Diabetes mellitus with optic atrophy-thalassemia-like sideroblastic anemia and weak isoagglutinins – a new genetic syndrome. Acta Medica Scandanavica 193: 359

Kauli R, Pertzelan A, Prager-Lewin R, Maimon Z, Ovadia J, Laron Z 1979 XY gonadal dysgenesis associated with hGH and gonadotrophin deficiencies. Clinical Genetics 15: 369

Kleinmann R E, Kazarian E L, Raptopoulos V, Braverman L E 1981 Primary empty sella and Rieger's anomaly of the anterior chamber of the eye. New England Journal of Medicine 304: 90

Koch G, Tiwisina T 1959 Beitrag Zur Erblichkeit der Akromegalie und der Hyperostosis Generalisata mit Pachydermie. Arzneimittel-Forschung 13: 489

Kowarski A A, Schneider J, Ben-Galim E, Weldon V V, Daughaday W H 1978 Growth failure with normal serum RIA-GH and low somatomedin activity: somatomedin restoration and growth acceleration after exogenous GH. Journal of Clinical Endocrinology 47: 461

Lacombe L U 1841 De la polydipsia. L'experience. 7: 309

Lanes R, Plotnick L P, Spencer E M, Daughaday W A, Kowarski A A 1980 Dwarfism associated with normal serum growth hormone and increased bioassayable, receptorassayable, and immunoassayable somatomedin. Journal of Clinical Endocrinology 50: 485

Laron Z 1974 Syndrome of familial dwarfism and high plasma immunoreactive growth hormone. Israel Journal of Medical Science 10: 1247

Laron Z, Pertzelan A, Karp M 1966 Pituitary dwarfism with high serum concentration of human growth hormone – A new inborn error in metabolism? Israel Journal of Medical Science 2: 152

Laron Z, Pertzelan A, Karp M, Kowaldo-Silbergeld A, Daughaday W H 1971 Administration of growth hormone to patients with familial dwarfism with high plasma immunoreactive growth hormone. Journal of Clinical Endocrinology 33: 332

Laron Z, Taube E, Kaplan I 1969 Pituitary growth hormone insufficiency associated with cleft lip and palate. An embryonal developmental defect. Helvetica Paediatrica Acta 24: 576

Latorre H, Kenney F M, Lahey M E, Drash A 1974 Short stature and growth hormone deficiency in histiocytosis X. Journal of Pediatrics 85: 813

Leaf A, Coggins C H 1974 The Neurohypoplysis: In: William RH (ed) Textbook of Endocrinology. 5th edition, Saunders, Philadelphia

Le Briggs R, and Powell J R 1969 Chiari-Frommel syndrome as a part of the Zollinger-Ellison multiple endocrine adenomatosis complex. California Medicine 111: 92

Lehmann V W 1964 Krankheiten der Drusen mit innerer Sekretion. In Becker P E, editor: Humangenetick, Stuttgart, Verlang

Leva J 1915 Uber familiare Akromegalie. Medicine Klinik 11: 1266

Lieblich J M, Rosen S W, Guyda H, Reardan J, Schaaf M 1978 The syndrome of basal encephalocoele and hypothalamic – pituitary dysfunction. Annals of Internal Medicine 89: 910

Linquette M, Herlant M, Laine E, Fossati P, Dupont-Lecompte M 1967 Adenome a prolactine chez une jeune fille dont la mére etait porteuse adénome hypophysaire avec aménorrhée. Annals of Endocrinology (Paris) 28: 773

Lovinger R D, Kaplan S L, Grumbach M M 1975 Congenital hypopituitarism associated with neonatal hypoglycaemia. Journal of Pediatrics 87: 1171

Lowry R B 1974 Holoprosencephaly. American Journal of Diseases of Chidlren 128: 887

Manelfe C, Rochicciolo P 1979 CT of septo-optic dysplasia. Amerian Journal of Roentgenology 133: 1157

Martin F I R 1959 Familial diabetes insipidus. Quarterly Journal of Medicine 28: 573

Medeiros-Neto G A, Toledo S P A, Pupo A A et al 1973 Characterization of the LH response to luteinizing hormone-releasing hormone (LG-RH) in isolated and multiple tropic hormone deficiencies. Journal of Clinical Endocrinology and Metabolism 37: 972

Merimee T J, Zapf J, Froesch E R 1981 Dwarfism in the pygmy. An isolated deficiency of insulin-like growth factor I. New England Journal of Medicine 305: 965

Merimee T J, Ostrow P, Aisner S C 1975 Clinical and pathological studies in a growth hormone-deficient dwarf. Johns Hopkins Medical Journal 136: 150

Merimee T J, Rimoin D L, Hall J D, McKusick V A 1969 A metabolic and hormonal basis for classifying ateliotic dwarfs. Lancet 1: 963

Merimee T J, Rimoin D L, Penetti E, Cavalli Sforza L L 1972 Growth retardation in the African pygmy. Journal of Clinical Investigation 51: 395

Merle P, Georget A M, Goumy P, Jarlot D 1979 Primary empty sella turcica in children. Pediatric Radiology 8: 209

Moncrieff M W, Hill D S, Archer J, Arthur L J H 1972 Congenital absence of pituitary gland and adrenal hypoplasia. Archives of Diseases in Childhood 47: 136

Mosier H D 1957 Hypoplasia of the pituitary and adrenal cortex: Report of occurrence in twin siblings and autopsy findings. Journal of Pediatrics 51: 377

Naeye R L, Blanc W A 1971 Organ and body growth in anencephaly. Archives of Pathology 91: 140

Najjar S S, Khachadurian A K, Ilbawi M N, Blizzard R M 1971 Dwarfism with elevated levels of plasma growth hormone. New England Journal of Medicine 284: 809

Nilsson L R 1960 Chronic pancytopenia with multiple congenital abnormalities. Acta Paediatrica 49: 518

Parks J S, Tenore A, Bongiovanni A M, Kirkland R T 1978 Familial hypopituitarism with large sella turcica. New England Journal of Medicine 298: 698

Patel H, Tze J W, Crichton J U et al 1975 Optic nerve hypoplasia with hypopituitarism. American Journal of Diseases of Children 129: 175

Pender C B, Fraser F C 1953 Dominant inheritance of diabetes insipidus. Pediatrics 11: 246

Perry T L, Robinson G C, Teasdale J M, Hansen S 1967 Cystathioninuria, nephrogenic diabetes insipidus and anemia. New England Journal of Medicine 276: 721

Phelan P D, Connelly J, Martin F I R, Wettenhall H N B 1971 X–linked recessive hypopituitarism. In: The Endocrine System, Birth Defects: Original Article Series Vol VII, no. 6. Williams and Wilkins, Baltimore for The National Foundation – March of Dimes, 1971, Part X p 21.

Phillips J A, Hjelle B L, Seeburg, P H, Zachmann M, 1981 Molecular basis of familial isolated growth hormone deficiency. Proceedings of the National Academy of Sciences USA 78: 6372.

Pierson M, Malaprade D, Fortier G, Belleville F, Lasbennes A, Wuilbreq L 1978 Le nanisme familial de type Laron, deficit genetique primaire en somatomedine. Archives Francais Pediatrics 35: 151

Pochedly C, Collip P J, Wolman S R et al 1971 Fanconi's anemia with growth hormone deficiency. Journal of Pediatrics 79: 93

Pollock J A, Newton T H and Hoyt W 1968 Transphenoidal and transethmoidal encephaloceles. Radiology 90: 442

Poskitt E M E, Rayner P H W 1974 Isolated growth hormone deficiency. Two families with autosomal dominant inheritance. Archives of Disease in Childhood 49: 55

Rappaport E B, Ulstrom R A, Gorlin R J, Lucky A W, Colle E, Miser J 1977 Solitary maxillary central incisor and short stature. Journal of Pediatrics 91: 924

Richardson J E, Hamilton W 1977 Diabetes insipidus, diabetes mellitus, optic atrophy and deafness. Archives of Disease in Childhood 52: 796

Rimoin D L 1976 Hereditary forms of growth hormone deficiency and resistance. Birth Defects: Original Article Series 12(6): 15

Rimoin D L, Horton W A 1978a Short Stature, Part I. Journal of Pediatrics 92: 523

Rimoin D L, Horton W A 1978 Short Stature, Part II. Journal of Pediatrics 92: 697

Rimoin D L, Merimee T J, Rabinowitz D, McKusick V A 1968 Genetic aspects of clinical endocrinology. 24: 365

Rimoin D L, Merimee T J, Rabinowitz D et al 1969 Peripheral subresponsiveness to human growth hormone in the African pygmies. New England Journal of Medicine 281: 1383

Rimoin D L, Schechter J E 1973 Histological and ultrastructural studies in isolated growth hormone deficiency. Journal of Clinical Endocrinology and Metabolism 37: 725

Rimoin D L, Schimke R M 1971 Genetic Disorders of the Endocrine Glands. C V Mosby Company, St Louis

Robinson M C, Kalan S A 1960 Inheritance of vasopressin resistant ('nephrogenic') diabetes insipidus. American Journal of Diseases of Children 99: 164

Romshe C A, Sotos J F 1973 Hypothalamic – pituitary dysfunction in siblings of patients with holoprosencephaly. Journal of Pediatrics 83: 1088

Royer P, Rappaport R, Gabilan J C, Canet J, Bonnici F 1970 Manifestations hypoglycemiques initials dans une forme familiale de defaut isole en somathormone. Annales de Pediatrie 17: 828

Rudman D, Davis G T, Priest J H, Patterson J H, Kutner M H, Heymsfield S B, Bethel R A 1978 Prevalence of growth hormone deficiency with cleft lip or palate. Journal of Pediatrics 93: 378

Sadeghi-Nejad A and Senior B 1974a A familial syndrome of isolated 'aplasia' of the anterior pituitary. Journal of Pediatrics 84: 79

Sadeghi-Nejad A, Senior B 1974b Autosomal dominant transmission of isolated growth hormone deficiency in iris-dental dysplasis (Rieger's syndrome). Journal of Pediatrics 85: 644

Saxena K M 1970 Endocrine manifestations of neurofibromatosis in children. American Journal of Diseases of Children 120: 265

Schimke R N, Spaulding J J and Hollowell J G 1971 X–linked congenital panhypopituitarism. In: Bergsma D

(ed) The Endocrine System, Birth Defects: Original Article Series 7(6): 21. Baltimore: Williams and Wilkins, Baltimore for The National Foundation – March of Dimes, 1971, Part X

Sheikholislam B M and Stempfel R S 1972 Hereditary isolated somatotropin deficiency: Effects of human growth hormone administration. Pediatrics 49: 362

Sipponen P, Simila S, Collan Y, Autere T, Herva R 1978 Familial syndrome with panhypopituitarism, hypoplasia of the hypophysis, and poorly developed sella turcica. Archives of Disease in Childhood 53: 664

Stanley C A, Spielman R S, Zmijewski C M and Baker L 1979 Wolfram syndrome not HLA linked. New England Journal of Medicine 301: 1398

Steiner M M, Boggs J D 1965 Absence of pituitary gland, hypothyroidism, hypoadrenalism and hypogonadism in a 17-year-old dwarf. Journal of Clinical Endocrinology and Metabolism 25: 1591

Toublanc J E, Chaussain J L, Lejeune D, dePaillerets F, Job J C 1976 Hypopituitarisme avec hypoplasie des nerfs optiques. Archives Francais Pediatrie 33: 67

Turnbridge R E, Paley R G 1956 Primary optic atrophy in diabetes mellitus. Diabetes 2: 295

Valtin H 1969 Hereditary diabetes insipidus-lessons learned from animal models. Excerpta Medicine International Congress 184: 321

Van den Brande J L, Du Caju M V L, Visser H K A et al 1974 Primary somatomedin deficiency. Archives of Disease in Childhood 49: 297

Van Gemund J J, de Angulo M S L, Van Gelderen H H 1969 Familial prenatal dwarfism with elevated serum immunoreactive growth hormone levels and end-organ unresponsiveness. Maandsch. Kindergeneesk. 37: 372

Walker N F, Rance C P 1954 Inheritance of diabetes insipidus. American Journal of Human Genetics 6: 354

Waring A J, Kajdi L, and Tappan V 1945 A congenital defect of water metabolism. American Journal of Diseases of Children 69: 323

Weber F T, Donnelly W H and Bejar R L 1977 Hypopituitarism following extirpation of a pharyngeal pituitary. American Journal of Diseases of Children 131: 525

Willard D 1973 Primary pituitary dysgenesis. Journal of Pediatrics 73: 586

Winkelmann W, Solbach H G, Wiegelmann W et al 1972 Hypothalamo-hypophysarer Minderwuchs mit Innenohrschwerhorigkeit bei zwei Schwestern. Internist (Berlin) 13: 52

Wolfram D J 1938 Diabetes mellitus and simple optic atrophy among siblings: report of four cases. Proc. staff meet. Mayo Clinic 13: 715

Yagnik R, Reber R M, Katz R, Root R 1973 Anterior pituitary function in a neonate with craniofacial dysraphia. Journal of Pediatrics 83: 1090

Young R L, Bradley E M, Goldzieher J W, Myers P W, Lecocq F R 1967 Spectrum of nonpuerperal galactorrhea: report of two cases evolving through the various syndromes. Journal of Clinical Endocrinology 27: 461

Zachman lM, Illig R, Prader A 1972 Fanconi's anemia with isolated growth hormone deficiency. Journal of Pediatrics 80: 159

83

Thyroid disorders

D.A. Fisher

INTRODUCTION

The mammalian thyroid gland, a derivative of the primitive gut, evolved from an iodine-concentrating gland in lower vertebrates to an endocrine gland capable of storing and secreting iodothyronines in higher vertebrate species (Van Wyk & Fisher, 1977). The active iodothyronines, tetraiodothyronine (thyroxine or T4) and 3,5,3'-triiodothyronine (T3) are amino acids bearing, respectively, four and three iodine atoms per molecule. They are synthesized within the thyroid gland follicular cells from tyrosine and iodine substrates. Efficient synthesis requires an optimal dietary iodine intake and appropriate pituitary thyroid stimulating hormone (TSH) stimulation (Ingbar and Woeber, 1974). TSH synthesis and secretion by the anterior pituitary thyrotroph cell is, in turn, stimulated by hypothalamic thyrotropin releasing factor (TRF or TRH) and inhibited by circulating thyroid hormone via a classic endocrine negative feedback control system. TSH is secreted directly into blood where, via thyroid perfusion, it has access to TSH receptors on the thyroid follicular cell. TSH binding to plasma membrane receptors activates a membrane bound adenyl cyclase-cyclic AMP second messenger system and stimulates iodine uptake and organification, thyroglobulin degradation and thyroid hormone secretion. T4 (and to a lesser extent T3), like TSH, is secreted directly into peripheral blood, but unlike TSH, T4 is stored in plasma and in extracellular fluids tightly bound to one of three carrier protein species, thyroxine-binding globulin (TBG), thyroxine-binding prealbumin (TBPA), or albumin. The saturation of thyroid-hormone binding protein sites on TBG is regulated by the pituitary TSH negative feedback control system to adjust circulating free (or unbound) T4 concentrations within narrow limits (Van Wyk & Fisher, 1977: Ingbar & Woeber, 1974).

Circulating free T4 diffuses into peripheral tissue cells where it is enzymatically monodeiodinated to a triiodothyronine. A beta ring monodeiodinase converts T4 to T3, an analogue with 3 to 4 times the metabolic potency of T4. An alpha ring monodeiodinase converts T4 to reverse T3 (rT3), an inactive iodothyronine analogue (Chopra et al, 1979. The triiodothyronines then diffuse back into circulating blood where they, too, are bound to TBG, although less avidly than T4 is bound. The control of T4 to T3 conversion, and the regulation of production of active triiodothyronine is not well understood. T4 beta ring monodeiodinase activity and T4 to T3 conversion are minimal in the fetus so that fetal serum T3 levels are low; alpha ring monodeiodination does occur and fetal serum rT3 levels are elevated. T4 to T3 conversion and serum T3 levels increase markedly after birth. After birth, a variety of circumstances are known to inhibit T4 to T3 conversion, including undernutrition, starvation, severe illness, adrenal corticosteroids, propylthiouracil, propranalol, and some iodine-containing radiographic contrast agents.

Thyroid hormone effects on tissue are mediated via binding to specific nuclear, chromosomal, nonhistone protein in thyroid responsive tissues (Oppenheimer et al, 1976). These receptors have a predominant affinity for T3; T4 binds with only one tenth the affinity of T3. It is possible that T4 may bind directly to nuclear chromosomal receptors and mediate thyroid hormone action, but the most active hormone at the tissue level is T3. The thyroid gland can secrete T3, but the normal secretion ratio of T4/T3 approximates 15 to 20/1; after birth, as indicated, most of the circulating T3 is derived from tissue conversion from T4. The metabolic effects of thyroid hormone are largely mediated by T3 from three sources: (1) circulating T3 derived from T4 in tissues and released into blood; (2) circulating T3 secreted by the thyroid gland; and (3) intracellular T3 derived directly from intracellular monodeiodination of T4.

Optimal thyroid function and tissue metabolism are dependent on integrity of the entire hypothalamic-pituitary-thyroid tissue axis; and a variety of congenital anomalies, environmental factors, and inborn defects are known to alter thyroid function parameters in the newborn; some may result in congenital hypothyroidism (Fisher, 1980). These defects may occur at four levels, the hypothalamus, the pituitary, the thyroid gland, or the peripheral tissue levels. A listing of possible abnormalities is shown in Table 83.1.

Table 83.1 Congenital disorders of thyroid function

I Hypothalamus
  A. Hypothalamic dysplasia
  B. TRH deficiency

II Pituitary gland
  A. Pituitary aplasia or hypoplasia
  B. TSH deficiency

III Thyroid gland
  A. Dysgenesis
    Agenesis, hypoplasia or ectopy
  B. Dyshormonogenesis
    (1) Iodide concentrating defect
    (2) Organification defects
    (3) Iodotyrosine deiodinase deficiency
    (4) Defects in thyroglobulin synthesis
  C. TSH unresponsiveness
  D. Goitrogen exposure in utero
  E. Abnormal thyroid stimulator (neonatal Graves disease)

IV Peripheral thyroid metabolism
  A. Disorders of thyroid hormone transport
    (1) Abnormalities of TBG concentration
    (2) Abnormalities of TBPA or TBPA-like protein
    (3) Analbuminaemia
  B. Decreased tissue response to thyroid hormones
  C. Hyperthyroidism (neonatal Graves disease)

HYPOTHALAMIC-PITUITARY HYPOTHYROIDISM

Hypothalamic-pituitary disorders associated with hypothalamic-pituitary anomalies and with panhypopituitarism are reviewed in another Chapter.

Familial isolated TSH deficiency

Miyae and colleagues (1971) first reported familial isolated TSH deficiency in 1971 (3a). Two sisters aged 12 and 14 years with nongoitrous cretinism were described. Both had low serum T4 and TSH concentrations and were markedly retarded with IQ values of 28 and 49. Pituitary growth hormone, ACTH and gonadotropin secretion were intact. The thyroid gland responded to exogenous TSH but there was no TSH response to TRH. The sisters were products of a consangiuneous marriage. One other sib was retarded and died at age 3 years. Later studies indicated detectable levels of circulating TRH, normal prolactin responses to TRH (Miyai et al, 1976), normal LH and FSH responses to gonadotropin releasing hormone (GnRH), normal GH responses to insulin hypoglycaemia and normal urinary 17 OHCS responses to metyrapone (normal ACTH reserve). These patients appear to have an inherited isolated defect in pituitary capacity of synthesize or release TSH. An abnormal TSH is a less likely possibility because of the absence of TSH-like immunoreactivity in serum.

THYROID DYSGENESIS

The major cause for congenital hypothyroidism in nonendemic areas is thyroid dysgenesis due to abnormal thyroid gland embryogenesis. The aetiology of thyroid dysgenesis is not clear; a variety of mechanisms presumably are represented including single gene defects and familial autoimmune factors (Fisher, 1980; Stanbury et al, 1979). The majority of cases, however, represent sporadic nonfamilial embryologic defects. A high risk population has not been identified. There is a marked female predominance in reported series (female to male ratio is 5:2), and a seasonal variation with a summer predominance has been reported from Japan (Miyai et al, 1979). Thyroid aplasia or hypoplasia as well as thyroid ectopia have been described. Ectopic tissue may occur at the base of the tongue or in the midline along the line of descent of the thyroid gland during embryogenesis. The relative prevalence of thyroid aplasia, thyroid ectopy, and thyroid hypoplasia may vary geographically; preliminary estimates for North America are 40%, 25% and 25%, respectively, of the total cases of thyroid dysgenesis (Fisher et al, 1979).

Although in the usual case only one affected infant occurs in a sibship, familial instances have been reported, and nongoitrous hypothyroidism has been reported both in identical and non-identical twins (Greiger et al, 1966). The mechanism is not clear.

GOITROUS HYPOTHYROIDISM (FAMILIAL GOITER)

Patients with inborn defects in thyroid metabolism often are referred to as having goitrous hypothyroidism or familial goiter (Stanbury, 1978; Stanbury et al, 1979). The events in thyroid hormone synthesis and release by thyroid follicular cells and the sites of identified or postulated defects in patients with goitrous hypothyroidism are illustrated in Fig. 83.1. These defects include (1) absence or malfunction of the cell membrane mechanism for trapping and transporting iodide from blood. (2) absence or inefficiency of the mechanisms for oxidizing iodide and 'organifying' or covalently binding the iodide to tyrosine, possibly including an inefficient 'coupling' of iodotyrosines to form thyroid hormones, (3) absent or defective enzymes for deiodinating iodotyrosines released into thyroid follicular cell cytoplasm in the process of thyroglobulin hydrolysis and thyroid hormone release, and (4) abnormalities in thyroglobulin synthesis, storage, or release. All appear to be transmitted as autosomal recessive traits, and all may be associated with congenital hypothyroidism.

Except for the familial incidence and tendency for affected individuals to develop large goiters, the clinical manifestations of congenital hypothyroidism due to a

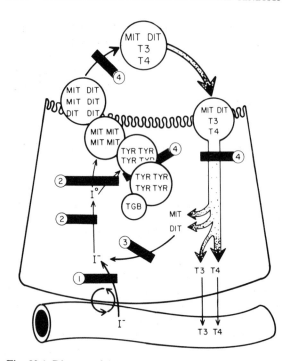

Fig. 83.1 Diagram of the pathways of thyroid hormone synthesis and release by the thyroid follicular cell. Iodine is transported across the plasma membrane, and oxidized to a reactive state. Thyroglobulin (TBG) is synthesized by the cell and transported to the apical cell membrane where the incorporated tyrosine residues react with the reactive iodine first to form monoiodotyrosine (MIT) and then diiodotyrosine (DIT). The iodinated tyrosine (TYR) residues spatially oriented for coupling combine to form the iodothyronines: DIT + DIT = T4 and MIT + DIT = T3. TBG stored in colloid reenters the cell via endocytosis and is digested under the influence of lysosomal enzymes to release the iodotyrosines as well as T4 and T3. The MIT and DIT are deiodinated and the release iodine reutilized. The T3 and T4 are secreted. Numbers indicate sites of possible abnormality. See text for details. (Reproduced with permission from Pediatrics in Review 2: 70, 1980. © American Academy of Pediatrics 1980)

biochemical defect are similar to those arising from an embryologic error in development. Thyroid enlargement may appear at birth but in many patients the goiter is delayed for months or years and may be absent altogether. Presumably, similar but less severe errors in synthesis may produce goiters that first make their appearance in later childhood or adulthood; such patients may remain euthyroid or may develop only mild hypothyroidism.

Failure to concentrate iodide

The transport of iodide across the thyroid follicular cell membrane from plasma to cytosol is the first step in thyroid hormone biosynthesis (DeGroot & Stanbury, 1975; Stanbury, 1978). Under normal circumstances the thyroid cell membrane iodide pump generates a thyroid/serum

(T/S ratio) concentration gradient in excess of 20–30; this gradient can reach several hundredfold when the thyroid gland is stimulated by a low-iodine diet, by thyroid stimulating hormone (TSH), by a variety of thyroid-stimulating immunoglobulins in Graves disease, or by drugs that impair the efficiency of hormone synthesis. Other tissues such as the salivary glands, gastric mucosa, mammary glands, ciliary body, choroid plexus, and placenta also are capable of concentrating iodide against a gradient. However, these tissues are not capable of organifying inorganic iodide.

TSH stimulates iodide transport through a sequence of increased cyclic AMP formation and RNA and protein synthesis. Certain anions that are themselves accumulated by the thyroid are capable of competitively inhibiting iodide transport. These, in order of increasing potency, include bromide (Br^-), nitrite (NO_2^-), thiocyanate (SCN^-), selenacyanate ($SeCN^-$), fluoroborate, (BF_4^-), and perchlorate (ClO_4^-). Thiocyanate and perchlorate have been utilized clinically to block iodide transport.

Several patients have been described with hyperplastic thyroid glands but only minimal uptake of radioactive iodide at 24 hours (Feldman et al, 1958; Gilboa et al, 1963; Wolff et al, 1964; Stanbury, 1978). The thyroid glands in these patients are enlarged twofold to fourfold, and the patients usually are hypothyroid cretins. Other iodine-concentrating tissues (salivary glands, gastric mucosa) also fail to concentrate iodide from the circulation. Lugol solution ameliorates the hypothyroidism by increasing the serum iodide to high levels and increasing the intrathyroidal inorganic iodide concentration via diffusion. The molecular defect in this disorder is not known.

Several patients have been reported with a partial defect in iodide trapping also manifest in thyroid salivary and gastric tissues (Papadopoulos et al, 1970; Medeiros-Neto et al, 1972). Thyroid radioiodine uptake was decreased but not absent in these patients and did not respond to TSH. The salivary/plasma ratio of radioiodine also was reduced but not entirely absent. Nonetheless the patients were hypothyroid with mental retardation.

Peroxidase system defects (organification defects)

Normally, iodide concentrated by the thyroid follicular cell is rapidly oxidized and bound in organic form (organified); less than 1% of the total thyroidal iodine is present as inorganic iodide (Ingbar & Woeber, 1974; Stanbury, 1978). Organification of iodide involves two processes: oxidation of iodide and iodination of thyroglobulin-bound tyrosine. First, iodide is oxidized to an active intermediate (perhaps I° or I^+) followed by iodination of thyroglobulin-bound tyrosyl residues to form the iodotyrosines MIT and DIT. These processes are very rapid; the half-time of incorporation of iodide into protein approximates 2 minutes. Two DIT residues are 'coupled' to form T4 and MIT and DIT couple to form T3. The coupling reaction however is relatively slow. Both tyrosyl iodination and 'coupling' are catalyzed by a thyroid peroxidase enzyme system. Thyroid peroxidase is a membrane-bound haem protein that requires peroxide and an acceptor, which in the normal thyroid gland is thyroglobulin, but can be albumin or other proteins or peptides. The hydrogen peroxide may be provided by one or more of several flavoprotein enzyme systems.

Deficient thyroid peroxidase

The first of the iodide organification defects described by Stanbury was attributed to an absence or deficiency of the peroxidase enzyme(s) necessary to oxidize thyroidal iodide to iodine (Stanbury & Hedge, 1950). Patients with the defect presented as goitrous cretins. The administration of thiocyanate or perchlorate to a patient with such a defect within 2 hours after administration of a test dose or radioiodine is followed by a precipitous fall in thyroid radioactivity. This 'perchlorate (or thiocyanate) discharge' indicates an organification defect assuming the patient has no other reason for defective iodination, such as antithyroid drugs, high iodine intake, Hashimoto's thyroiditis. The diagnosis of the specific defect is confirmed by measuring low or absent levels of thyroid peroxidase activity in thyroid tissue obtained at the time of biopsy (Stanbury & Hedge, 1950; Valenta et al, 1973; Pommier et al, 1974; Hagen et al, 1971; Niepomniszcze et al, 1973, Mederios-Neto, 1980).

Abnormal thyroid peroxidase

More recently, two patients have been described who were euthyroid or mildly hypothyroid but manifested goiter and partial discharge of radioiodine following perchlorate administration. In these patients the thyroid gland was found to contain no peroxidase activity, but such activity could be restored by adding haematin, the noncovalently bound prosthetic group of the peroxidase (Niepomniiszcze et al, 1972; 1975). This suggests an abnormal peroxidase apoenzyme deficient in binding to its haem moiety.

Deficient H_2O_2 generation

An adult woman presenting with euthyroidism and a non-toxic goiter in association with a positive perchlorate discharge was reported by Kusakabe in 1975. In vitro iodination in thyroid homogenates was reduced in tissue obtained from thyroidectomy. However, iodination capacity was restored by addition of riboflavin, FMN, oxidized cytochrome b_2, cytochrome C, NADH or NADPH. Microsomal NADH-cytochrome b_2 reductase activity was low and restored by addition to flavine-adenine dinucleotide (FAD); FAD, 250 mg/day, admin-

istered prior to thyroidectomy decreased goiter size, serum TSH and thyroid radioiodine uptake whereas treatment with riboflavin, a precursor of FAD, was without effect. A defect in thyroid H_2O_2 generation was postulated due to a defect in biosynthesis of FAD from riboflavin.

Pendred syndrome

A large group of patients with familial goiter and congenital eighth nerve deafness have been described. These patients are referred to as having Pendred syndrome; Pendred in 1896 described two sisters with deafness and goiter living in a nonendemic goiter area (Pendred, 1896). Subsequently many such patients have been described (Stanbury, 1978; Fraser, 1969; Fraser et al, 1960; Medeiros-Neto, 1980; Nilsson et al, 1964). The prevalence is estimated to be 1.5 to 3 cases per 100 000 school children (DeGroot & Stanbury, 1975; Nilsson et al, 1964). The syndrome includes high tone or complete congenital deafness, goiter of variable degree appearing in middle or late childhood and euthyroidism or mild hypothyroidism. Perhaps a third of patients have the complete syndrome; others present without hearing loss or with mild goiter (Medeiros-Neto, 1980). Most patients have a positive perchlorate discharge test, but atypical patients without an abnormal perchlorate discharge have been described (Cave & Dunn, 1975; Medeiros-Neto, 1980). The biochemical defect in these patients is not clear; thyroid peroxidase activity is normal (Burrow et al, 1973; Cave & Dunn, 1975; Ljunggren et al, 1973). The cause of deafness is not known, a cochlear defect due to hypothyroidism in utero and a defect common to the thyroid and cochlea have been postulated. If the former, a variety of thyroid defects could produce the same phenotype.

Coupling defect

An abnormality of the thyroid peroxidase system can lead to an apparent inability of the thyroid to couple iodotyrosines to form thyroid hormones (Stanbury, 1978). It now seems clear that 'coupling' of iodotyrosines also is catalyzed by thyroid peroxidase. Pommier et al (1974) have reported a patient with a euthyroid familial goiter, a positive perchlorate discharge test, and a high level of thyroid peroxidase activity. After solubilization, thyroid peroxidase enzyme activity was found to be abnormal; it catalyzed iodide peroxidation similarly to a control hog peroxidase but catalyzed hormone synthesis 3 to 6 times less efficiently than the hog peroxidase. A structural defect in the thyroid peroxidase was postulated; the defective enzyme showed little iodide peroxidation activity, but retained 'coupling' activity (Pommier et al, 1974).

Iodotyrosine deiodinase defect

Deficiency of the iodotyrosine dehalogenase enzyme can produce an hereditary defect causing either congenital hypothyroidism or a less severe form of familial goiter. Failure to deiodinate thyroid MIT and DIT as they are released from thyroglobulin leads to severe iodine wastage, since these non-deiodinated iodotyrosines diffuse out of the thyroid and are excreted in urine. As a result the iodine is lost rather than being recycled within the thyroid gland. Iodotyrosine deiodinases are present in both thyroid cells and in peripheral tissues, and abnormalities involving both deiodinase systems have been described.

The patients originally described were cretinous and hypothyroid with goiters presenting at birth or shortly thereafter (Stanbury, 1978). Detailed studies of three patients by Stanbury and colleagues (Stanbury et al, 1956) showed early rapid thyroid radioiodine uptake and rapid spontaneous discharge; by 48 hours most of the thyroidal radioiodine had been discharged. After administration of a test dose of radioiodine, the serum of these patients contained high concentrations of labeled iodotyrosines. Moreover, these patients excreted essentially all of an intravenous dose of labeled iodotyrosine directly into urine, whereas normal subjects excrete the label almost entirely as free iodide. Thyroid tissue, when examined, also failed to deiodinate labeled diiodotyrosine to iodide. Administration of thyroid hormone or iodide induced remission (Stanbury, 1978).

Kusakabe and Miyake (1963; 1964) have reported patients with euthyroid goiter and partial defects in deiodination of iodotyrosine (a) in both thyroid and peripheral tissues, (b) in peripheral tissues only, or (c) in thyroid tissue only. Three sibs with goiter and mild hypothyroidism and selective thyroidal iodotyrosine deiodinase deficiency also were reported by Ismail-Beigi and Rahimifar (1977).

Defects in thyroglobulin synthesis

Thyroglobulin is an essential substrate for organification and is the major protein component of thyroid colloid. It is an iodinated glycoprotein with a molecular weight approximating 650 000 daltons and a sedimentation coefficient of 19.7 (19S). It is composed of two 12S subunits, each of which is composed of two to four peptide chains (Stanbury et al, 1979). The iodine content of thyroglobulin depends on dietary iodine intake. MIT, DIT, T3 and T4 (and to a lesser extent rT3) are present within the protein molecule as iodoaminoacyl residues that can be cleaved by proteolytic enzymes. The tyrosine residues, which are the iodine acceptors of thyroglobulin, comprise about 3% of the weight of the protein, and about two-thirds of these residues are spatially oriented to be susceptible to iodination.

Thyroglobulin synthetic defects probably comprise a spectrum of related abnormalities. Coupling of iodotyrosines is a complex chemical transformation that requires the presence of normal thyroglobulin. A number of possible defects may lead to similar functional abnormalities, so that the defects are difficult to distinguish. A coupling defect could be caused by absent or abnormal thyroglobulin. In this instance alternative protein substrates for the organification reactions would result in release of increased quantities of iodoalbumin or other iodoproteins. An abnormal perchlorate discharge also might occur, as well as abnormal ratios of iodotyrosines to iodothyronines within the gland. A structural abnormality of thyroglobulin could be so minimal that only the spatial orientation of the tyrosyl residues is altered or the postulated receptor for the peroxidase enzyme could be altered.

Impaired thyroglobulin synthesis

A number of patients have been described with findings suggestive of impaired thyroglobulin synthesis. These patients present with familial congenital hypothyroidism of variable degree associated with goiter and circulating non-thyroglobulin iodoprotein. The latter is detected as butanol insoluble iodoprotein or radioiodoprotein. Some have a positive perchlorate discharge test (Lissitzky et al, 1973; Desai et al, 1974; Savoie et al, 1973; Bernal & Abregon; 1974). Interestingly these patients tend to excrete abnormal quantities of iodohistidine, presumably as a degradation product of the iodinated iodoalbumin (Savoie et al, 1973).

Thyroglobulin transport defect

Lissitzky and colleagues in 1975 reported two brothers with an apparent defect in thyroglobulin transport as well as synthesis. The boys presented with congenital goiter and hypothyroidism, circulating non-thyroxine iodoprotein, and decreased thyroidal thyroglobulin. Further evaluation revealed partially immunoreactive carbohydrate deficient thyroglobulin associated with intracytoplasmic membranes. The immunoreactive thyroglobulin chains were synthesized and discharged into the intracisternal cisternae, but not into the colloid spaces.

Structurally abnormal thyroglobulin

Kusakabe (1972) reported a woman with a euthyroid goiter and positive thiocyanate discharge with normal thyroid peroxidase, catalase, transaminase and protease and a normal thyroglobulin content. However, assessment of absorbance as a function of pH and susceptibility to iodination or acetylation suggested that two thirds of the tyrosyl residues were buried within the molecule, and Kusakabe postulated an abnormal stereostructure of the thyroglobulin in this patient.

TSH UNRESPONSIVENESS

The thyroid follicular cell response to TSH involves a series of coordinated steps including TSH binding to a receptor in the plasma membrane, activation of adenyl cyclase, synthesis of cyclic AMP, activation of protein kinase(s), phosphorylation of receptor protein(s), and stimulation of the several intracellular events of thyroid hormone synthesis and release. A defect at one of several sites could, therefore, lead to an abnormality in thyroid responsiveness to TSH.

To date only a few such patients have been reported. The first, reported by Stanbury et al (1968) was an 8 year old male with severe growth and mental retardation. His parents were consanguineous and his thyroid was not enlarged in spite of the fact that his serum TSH level was markedly increased. Thyroid slices in vitro failed to respond to TSH.

Codaccioni et al (1980) reported a 12 year old boy with a history of congenital hypothyroidism diagnosed at 18 months. The boy's grandparents were first cousins, but there was no family history of thyroid disease. His serum thyroxine was low and TSH markedly increased. Thyroid radioiodine uptake increased significantly in response to dibutyryl cAMP but not in response to TSH. The thyroid follicles, histologically, were devoid of colloid. Studies of thyroid TSH receptors on thyroid membrane preparations showed normal TSH receptor binding and normal flouride-stimulated TSH receptor-adenylate cyclase system activity. TSH stimulation of the TSH receptor-adenylate cyclase system was markedly reduced suggesting a TSH receptor-adenylate cyclase coupling abnormality (Codaccioni et al, 1980). Medeiros-Neto et al (1979) reported a 19 year old hypothyroid male without thyroid development, with increased serum levels of bioactive TSH and normal radioactive iodine uptake unresponsive to TSH. The thyroid gland contained no thyroglobulin and there was no increase in cyclic AMP levels in thyroid series in response to TSH. Impaired generation of cyclic AMP was postulated. Job and colleagues in 1969 reported an infant with hypothyroidism and a normal radioiodine uptake unresponsive to TSH. The child did not have a goiter and in vitro studies were not conducted.

DECREASED PERIPHERAL RESPONSIVENESS TO THYROID HORMONES

Refetoff and associates in 1967 first described a familial syndrome in 3 siblings with deaf-mutism, stippled epiphyses, retarded skeletal age, goiter, and greatly elevated levels of serum free T4 and free T3, but normal plasma TSH concentrations. Growth rate, metabolic rate, and intelligence were normal. Kinetic studies indicated that the thyroid glands were secreting about five times the normal amount of T4 daily. Administration of 1000 μg/day of T4 or 375 μg/day of T3 produced little or no metabolic effects. As the patients matured, the plasma T4 tended to return to normal levels, the epiphyses closed, and the goiters disappeared (Refetoff et al, 1967; 1972b). Recent studies of the youngest affected sib show a normal TSH response to TRH despite 3 fold elevated serum free T4 and free T3 levels (Refetoff et al, 1980). Administration of T3 produced paradoxical enhancement of the TSH response to TRH whereas administration of glucocorticoid produced a normal suppression of the TSH and prolactin responses to TRH. These results indicate that the pituitary shares the TSH resistance. A nuclear T3 receptor with low affinity has been identified in the circulating lymphocytes of one sibling suggesting a defect at the level of nuclear receptors (Bernal et al, 1978).

Several other patients have been described with variable degrees of thyroid hormone unresponsiveness and goiter (Bode et al, 1973; Elewaut et al, 1976; Lamberg et al, 1978; Seif et al, 1978; Schneider et al, 1975). Both single (Bode et al, 1973; Seif et al, 1978; Schneider et al, 1975) and familial cases (Elewaut et al, 1976; Lamberg et al, 1978) were included. The family of Refetoff et al (1967; 1972b) manifest consanguinity and presumed autosomal recessive inheritance. The families reported by Elewaut et al (1976) and Lamberg et al (1978), in contrast, seemed most consistent with a dominant inheritance pattern.

DISORDERS OF THYROID HORMONE TRANSPORT

Several presumably genetic abnormalities of iodothyronine-binding serum proteins have been described. These include (1) absent TBG, (2) decreased (low) TBG, (3) excess TBG, (4) increased TBPA, (5) an increased TBPA-like protein and (6) analbuminemia.

TBG deficiency

Tanaka and Starr in 1959 first reported TBG deficiency in a euthyroid male. Since that time many reports of a familial TBG deficiency syndrome have appeared (Stanbury et al, 1979; Robbins, 1973). The disorder seems to be transmitted as an X–linked trait; serum TBG levels measured either by immunoassay or T4 binding capacity are very low in affected males and approximately half normal in carrier females. Serum T4 levels vary similarly, but affected subjects are euthyroid with normal serum free T4 concentrations, normal serum TSH levels and normal serum TSH responses to exogenous TRH. Male to male transmission has not been observed and there is invariable transmission of the trait from affected males to female offspring (Stanbury et al, 1979). An abnormality in hepatic TBG synthesis rate has been postulated on the basis of TBG production rate measurements; variations in TBG production rates have been shown to correlate highly with variations in TBG concentrations (Refetoff et al, 1976).

The prevalence of very low TBG levels is not entirely clear. Stanbury et al (1979) comment that at least 14 families have been reported. However, preliminary results from the provincial newborn thyroid screening program in Quebec indicate a prevalence of 1 in 14 000 newborn infants (Dussault et al, 1977); this prevalence estimate may include infants with low TBG as well as TBG deficiency.

Low TBG

A second disorder has been described characterized by diminished but not absent TBG. A number of families have been reported (Stanbury et al, 1979; Refetoff et al, 1976; 1972b; Bode et al, 1973; Levy et al, 1971). Careful studies indicate that in these families, as in those with very low serum TBG levels, serum free T4 and TSH levels are normal. The TBG levels were diminished in affected males and there is a tendency to decreased concentrations in carrier females. However, the carrier state in females is sometimes difficult to identify because of overlap with affected males or normals; Bode et al (1973) were able to more definitively characterize the genotype of 15 of 16 females tested by utilizing the product of the T4 concentration and the T4 binding capacity of TBG. This abnormality also seems to be transmitted as an X−linked trait (Refetoff et al, 1972a; Bode et al, 1973). More recently TBG levels have been assessed directly by radioimmunoassay (Levy et al, 1971). Kinetic studies using purified TBG in these patients have shown that the total daily degradation rate of TBG is proportional to the serum concentration of the protein indicating that the abnormality, like the absent TBG abnormality, is due to altered TBG production (Refetoff et al, 1976).

High TBG

Subjects with increased levels of TBG have increased total serum T4 concentrations with normal free T4 and TSH levels; thus they are euthyroid (Robbins 1973; Refetoff et al, 1976). Studies in these subjects as in those with low TBG concentrations have shown correlation between TBG production rates and serum levels suggesting that the mechanism for the high TBG concentrations is increased production, presumably by the liver (Refetoff et al, 1976). TBG levels are increased up to 4.5 times normal in affected individuals (Stanbury et al, 1979) and carrier females have serum concentrations intermediate between normal values and the high levels in affected males (Stanbury et al, 1979; Robbins, 1973). Early reports suggested a dominant mode of inheritance (Beierwaltes et al, 1961; Florsheim et al, 1962), but subsequent studies and review of the earlier data are compatible with an X−linked mode of inheritance (Stanbury et al, 1979; Robbins, 1973; Refetoff et al, 1972a). Refetoff

and colleagues (1972a) have proposed that the several TBG concentration abnormalities reflect mutations at a single X-linked gene locus involved in the control of TBG synthesis.

High TBPA

Moses et al (1980) reported a 52 year old euthyroid male with an elevated serum T4 not corrected by the use of a free T4 index, but with normal free T4, normal total serum T3 and TSH concentrations and normal TSH and T3 responses to TRH. Serum TBG and albumin levels were normal, but the serum TBPA concentration measured by radioimmunoelectrophoresis was 2.5–3.0 times above the level in a normal human serum pool. Moreover 70% of the serum T4 was selectively removed by an anti-TBPA immunoglobulin affinity column. One of the subject's three children had a similar abnormality, but the mode of inheritance was not clearly defined (Moses et al, 1980).

Increased TBPA-like protein

Several groups of investigators have reported euthyroid subjects with increased serum T4 concentrations not corrected by the use of the free T4 index correction and with normal free T4, total serum T3 and TSH levels (Lee et al, 1979; Hennemann et al, 1979; Barlow et al, 1980). Thus, thyroid function parameters in these subjects resemble those in the patients with high TBPA reported by Moses et al (1980). These subjects have not been studied using affinity column absorption or TBPA radioimmunoassay, but the abnormal T4 binding protein does not seem to be TBPA. It migrates with albumin by conventional polyacrylamide electrophoresis (Lee et al, 1979; Henneman et al, 1979), and the patients of Barlow et al (1980) had normal TBPA levels on the basis of saturation-binding studies in vitro (Barlow et al, 1980). The abnormal TBPA-like protein seems to be transmitted as an autosomal dominant trait. There is male to male transmission and an affected to unaffected ratio of one or greater in first degree relatives (Barlow et al, 1980).

Analbuminaemia

Analbuminaemia is a rare autosomal recessive trait associated with serum albumin concentrations less than 100 mg/ml. Serum albumin levels in heterozygotes are within the normal range (Stanbury et al, 1979; Bennhold et al, 1954–55; Bennhold and Kallee, 1959). There is little clinical disability. Since albumin normally binds a significant proportion of circulating thyroid hormones, the distribution of T4 and T3 binding to serum proteins in these patients is abnormal (Hollander et al, 1968). In association with essentially absent iodothyronine binding to albumin, both serum TBG and T4 binding prealbumin (TBPA) binding capacities are increased, perhaps due to increased levels of these binding proteins (Hollander et al, 1971). After long term infusion of albumin, TBG and TBPA binding return to normal. Free T4 and free T3 concentrations are normal and the patients are euthyroid.

FAMILIAL GRAVES DISEASE AND HASHIMOTO THYROIDITIS

Graves disease and Hashimoto thyroiditis now are recognized to be autoimmune thyroid disorders associated with circulating autoantibodies to thyroid and other tissues as well as cell mediated immunity directed against one or more thyroid antigens (Kidd et al, 1980). Graves disease comprises a constellation of hyperthyroidism, opthalmopathy and dermopathy; Hashimoto thyroiditis usually is characterized by progressive lymphoid infiltrate of the thyroid gland with a gradual progression to hypothyroidism. The hyperthyroidism in Graves disease is believed to be due to the production by sensitized lymphocytes of one or more circulating thyroid stimulating immunoglobulins. Hashimoto thyroiditis is thought to be caused by progressive destruction of thyroid follicular cells by sensitized lymphocytes.

The familial incidence of Graves disease and Hashimoto thyroiditis are well documented. Both disorders tend to aggregate in families and both occur in the same family (Kidd et al, 1980; Friedman & Fialkow, 1978). In a recent study nearly half of first order relatives of patients with Graves disease or Hashimoto thyroiditis were found to have some evidence of thyroid autoimmunity with or without evidence of thyroid dysfunction (Chopra et al, 1977). In another report, 36% of children of parents with Graves disease had one or more physical, functional or autoimmune markers of thyroid dysfunction as compared to 24% of control children (Carey et al, 1980). During a 3 year follow-up of these children of Graves disease patients, one child out of 129 developed thyrotoxicosis, one developed Hashimoto thyroiditis and one each manifested vitiligo and exopthalmos (Carey et al, 1980).

Age specific incidence rates for Graves disease and Hashimoto thyroiditis show an increasing rate of onset through the fifth decade and a decline thereafter (Volpe, 1978; Volpe et al, 1973). This has been interpreted as suggesting the existence of a subpopulation of subjects with genetic predisposition who develop thyroid autoimmune disease with increasing exposure to some environmental factor(s). Ultimately the unaffected portion of the subpopulation becomes so small that age specific incidence rates for the entire population fall with increasing age (Kidd et al, 1980; Volpe, 1978; Volpe et al, 1973). A genetic predisposition to thyroid autoimmunity also is suggested by observations in twins. There is an approximately 50% concordance for Graves disease in monozygotic twins as contrasted with a 5% concordance rate in fraternal twins (Kidd et al, 1980; Volpe, 1978). Moreover there are several reports of monozygotic twin pairs in which one twin manifested Graves disease and the other Hashimoto thyroiditis (Jayson et al, 1967; Chertov et al, 1973).

Graves disease may occur in the newborn, usually as a result of transplacental passage of maternal thyroid stimulating immunoglobulins (Van Wyk & Fisher, 1977; Smallridge et al, 1978). In this instance neonatal Graves disease is transient, abating as the maternal thyroid stimulator degrades in the newborn. There are, however, a group of newborns with more prolonged or recurrent disease (Hollingsworth & Mabry, 1972). These patients usually are born into families with a high prevalence of Graves disease and may represent familial hyperthyroidism with fetal-neonatal onset.

The mechanism of thyroid autoimmunity in Graves disease and Hashimoto thyroiditis remains unclear. Recent studies have documented an increased incidence of HLA-B8 and HLA-DRW3 transplantation antigens in caucasian patients with Graves disease, HLA-BW35 antigen in Japanese patients and HLA B46 in Chinese patients with the disorder (Kidd et al, 1980; Friedman & Fialkow, 1978; Grume et al, 1974; Chan et al, 1978; Allannic et al, 1980; Farid et al, 1980). An increased risk for Hashimoto thyroiditis in subjects with an HLA DW3 haplotype has been reported (Moens & Farid, 1978) but not confirmed (Kidd et al, 1980). These studies suggest that the relative risk of thyroid autoimmune disease, particularly Graves disease, probably is the result of an abnormal response conditioned by an unidentified antigen stimulus governed by immune response gene(s) located in close linkage disequilibrium with the HLA marker gene on chromosome No. 6. Volpe and colleagues have proposed that Graves hyperthyroidism, Graves exophthalmos and Hashimoto thyroiditis are related organ-specific autoimmune disorders mediated by inherited defect(s) in immunoregulation, possibly a specific defect(s) in suppressor T lymphocyte function (Volpe, 1978; Kidd et al, 1980). The mode of transmission is not clear (Kidd et al, 1980; Friedman & Fialkow, 1978; Chopra et al, 1977; Carey et al, 1980) and polygenic inheritance is a possibility.

MULTIPLE ENDOCRINE DEFICIENCY DISEASE

Many case reports have connected Hashimoto (lymphocytic) thyroiditis with other diseases suspected to include immune features. An increased incidence of Hashimoto disease or hypothyroidism has been documented in patients with multiple endocrine deficiency syndromes involving the thyroid gland, the adrenal glands, the gonads, the parathyroid glands, and the pancreas (Irvine,

1968; Blizzard et al, 1966, 1967; Faber et al, 1979; Carpenter et al, 1964; Edmonds et al, 1973; Spinner et al, 1968; Winter & Green, 1976). There also have been reports of an association between diabetes mellitus and hyperthyroidism (Hung et al, 1978). In addition many such patients have gastric mucosal involvement, vitiligo and/or moniliasis. The syndromes involve deficiency of glandular or tissue function associated with the presence of organ-specific antibodies (Blizzard et al, 1966, 1967; Spinner et al, 1968). Thus, syndromes in which Hashimoto thyroiditis occurs in association with idiopathic Addison disease, idiopathic hypoparathyroidism, hypogonadism, diabetes mellitus, pernicious anemia and/or moniliasis are believed to result from an autoimmune process. Perhaps the most common clinical entity is Schmidt syndrome, the combination of Hashimoto thyroiditis, adrenal insufficiency, and more recently, diabetes mellitus; deficiency syndromes involving any two of the three glands are being more frequently recognized. The familial nature of the syndromes (Spinner et al, 1968) suggests a genetic predisposition and a degree of homogeneity. However, genetic heterogeneity has been invoked to explain the wide of variety of manifestations, differences among families and varying age of onset.

THYROID DISEASE AND CHROMOSOMAL DISORDERS

Hashimoto (lymphocytic) thyroiditis has been reported with increased frequency in patients with Turner syndrome. Down syndrome and Klinefelter syndrome (Sparkes et al, 1978; Williams et al, 1964; Pai et al, 1977; Fialkow et al, 1971; Vallotton & Forbes, 1967). Patients with Noonan syndrome who have phenotypic features of Turner syndrome without a chromosomal disorder also have been reported (Vesterhus & Aarskog, 1973). Thus, there is no specific chromosomal disorder associated with lymphocytic thyroiditis or with the production of thyroid autoantibodies. Families of these patients also have an increased incidence of thyroid autoantibodies as well as thyroid autoimmune disease, so that the association may be coincidental.

MEDULLARY THYROID CARCINOMA

In addition to thyroid hormone secreting cells within the thyroid gland, there are parafollicular 'C' cells which secrete calcitonin. These cells usually lie between the follicular cells and the basement membrane and form small nests of cells in an apparent interfollicular location. Hazard et al in 1959, recognized that medullary carcinoma

of the thyroid is a tumour derived from the 'C' cells and is a separate entity from other thyroid tumours (Hazard et al, 1959; Williams, 1979). Since that time medullary carcinoma has been reported as a feature of a variety of genetically conditioned syndromes. An association between familial pheochromocytoma and medullary thyroid carcinoma has been reported (Williams, 1979; Sipple, 1961; Schimke and Hartmann, 1965). Medullary carcinoma also can be inherited alone (Block et al, 1967) or in association with multiple mucosal neuromas, pheochromocytomas, ganglioneuromas of the intestinal tract and other anomalies (Williams, 1979; Williams and Pollock, 1966; Nankin et al, 1970; Melvin et al, 1972). It is of interest that parathyroid hyperplasia or clinical hyperparathyroidism with hypercalcemia may occur in any patient with medullary thyroid carcinoma (Williams, 1979; Melvin et al, 1972). Moreover, elevated serum levels of parathyroid hormone are commonly seen (Williams, 1979; Melvin et al, 1972). The mechanism is not clear.

These three familial syndromes account for some 20% of all cases of medullary thyroid carcinoma (Williams, 1979). All three are separately heritable and appear to be transmitted as autosomal dominant traits with high penetrance (Williams, 1979). The combination of medullary carcinoma and pheochromocytoma has been referred to as Sipple syndrome. The term multiple endocrine neoplasia (MEN) also has been utilized. MEN IIa and IIB or MEN II and MEN III have been terms utilized to designate the combination syndromes without and with mucosal neuromata, respectively. Williams (1979) proposes utilizing the term MEN II for the several syndromes of genetically conditioned medullary carcinoma with the qualifying terms 'with neuromas' or 'without pheochromocytomas'.

The medullary carcinomas found in these syndromes often are bilateral and may appear during childhood or later; the average age of presentation ranges from 19–36 years (Williams, 1979). The pheochromocytomas are usually bilateral and may be multiple. Either medullary thyroid carcinoma or pheochromocytomas may be the presenting abnormality. There is suggestive evidence that the incidence of malignancy is greater in these syndromes than with sporadic pheochromocytomas (Williams, 1979). In MEN IIb, the mucosal neuromata occur in the eyelid, lip and tongue.

Medullated nerves sometimes are visible in the cornea (Williams, 1979; Melvin et al, 1972). The ganglioneuromas of the gastrointestinal tract involve enlargement of Auerbach's plexus and may extend from the esphagus to the rectum. These patients also may manifest a marfanoid habitus, muscular weakness, pes cavus, and a high arched palate, as well as other less frequent anomalies (Williams, 1979; Melvin et al, 1972).

REFERENCES

Allannic H, Fouchet R, Lorey Y, Heim J, Gueguen M, Leguerrier A M and Genetet B 1980 HLA and Graves disease: an association with HLA DRW 3. Journal of Clinical Endocrinology and Metabolism 51: 863

Barlow J W, Topliss D J, White E L, Hurley D M, Funder J W and Stockigt J R 1980 Familial euthyroid thyroxine excess due to increase prealbumin-like binding in plasma. In: Stockigt J R and Nagataki S (eds) Thyroid Research VIII, Australian Academy of Science, Canberra p 509–512.

Beierwaltes W H, Carr E A Jr and Hunter R L 1961 Hereditary increase in the thyroxine binding in the serum alpha globulin. Transactions of the Association of American Physicians 74: 170

Bennhold H and Kallee E 1959 Comparative studies of the half-life of I[131]-labeled albumins and nonradioactive human serum albumin in a case of analbuminemia. Journal of Clinical Investigation 38: 863

Bennhold H, Peters H and Roth E 1954–55 Ueber einen fall von kompletter analbuminaemie ohne wesentliche klinische krankheitszeichen. Verhandlungen der Deutschen Gesellschaft für innere medizin 4: 72

Bernal J and Abregon M J 1974 Thyroglobulin-like antigens in a goiter with impaired thyroglobulin synthesis. Journal of Clinical Endocrinology and Metabolism 39: 592

Bernal J, Refetoff S and DeGroot L J 1978 Abnormalities of triiodothyronine binding to lymphocyte and fibroblast nuclei from a patient with peripheral resistance to thyroid hormone action. Journal of Clinical Endocrinology and Metabolism 47: 1266

Blizzard R M, Chee D and Davis W 1966 The incidence of parathyroid and other antibodies in the sera of patients with idiopathic hypoparathyroidism. Clinical and Experimental Immunology 1: 119

Blizzard R M, Chee D and Davis W 1967 The incidence of adrenal and other antibodies in the sera of patients with idiopathic adrenal insufficiency (Addison's disease). Journal of Experimental Immunology 2: 119

Block M A, Horn R C Jr. Miller J M, Barrett J L and Brush B E 1967 Familial medullary carcinoma of the thyroid. Annals of Surgery 166: 403

Bode H H, Danon M and Weintraub B D 1973 Partial target organ resistance to thyroid hormone. Journal of Clinical Investigation 52: 776

Bode H H, Rothman K J and Danon M 1973 Linkage of thyroxine binding globulin deficiency to other X–chromosome loci. Journal of Clinical Endocrinology and Metabolism 37: 25

Burrow G N, Spaulding S W, Alexander N M and Bower B F 1973 normal peroxidase activity in Pendred's syndrome. Journal of Clinical Endocrinology and Metabolism 36: 522

Carey C, Skosey C, Pinnamaneni K M, Barsano C P and DeGroot L J 1980 Thyroid abnormalities in children of parents who have Graves' disease: possible pre-Graves' disease. Metabolism 29: 369

Carpenter C C J, Solomon N, Silverberg S G, Bledsoe T, Northcutt R C, Klinenberg J R, Bennett L I Jr and Harvey A M 1964 Schmidt's syndrome (thyroid and adrenal insufficiency): a review of the literature and a report of fifteen new cases including ten instances of coexistant diabetes mellitus. Medicine 43: 153

Cave W T Jr and Dunn J T 1975 Studies on the thyroidal defect in an atypical form of Pendred's syndrome. Journal of Clinical Endocrinology and Metabolism 41: 590

Chan S H, Yeo P P B, Lui K F, Wee G B, Woo K T, Pin L and Cheak J S 1978 HLA and thyrotoxicosis (Graves disease) in Chinese. Tissue Antigens 12: 109

Chertov B S, Fidler W J and Fariss B L 1973 Graves disease and Hashimoto's thyroiditis in monozygotic twins. Acta Endocrinologica 72: 18

Chopra I J, Solomon D H, Chopra U, Wy S Y and Fisher D A 1979 Pathways of metabolism of thyroid hormones. Recent Progress in Hormone Research 34: 556

Chopra I J, Solomon D H, Chopra U, Yoshihara E, Terasaki P I and Smith F 1977 Abnormalities in thyroid function in relatives of patients with Graves' disease and Hashimoto's thyroiditis: Lack of correlation with inheritance of HLA-B8. Journal of Clinical Endocrinology and Metabolism 45: 45

Codaccioni J L, Carayon P, Michel-Becket M, Foucault F, Lefort G and Pierron H 1980 Congenital hypothyroidism associated with thyrotropin unresponsiveness and thyroid cell membrane alterations. Journal of Clinical Endocrinology and Metabolism 50: 932

DeGroot L J and Stanbury J B 1975 Hereditary defects in hormone synthesis, transport or action. In: DeGroot L J and Stanbury J B (eds) The thyroid and its diseases, John Wiley and Sons, New York, p 538–571

DeLange F, Beckers C, Hofer R 1979 Screening for congenital hypothyroidism in Europe. Acta Endocrinol Suppl 223, 90: 1

Desai K B, Mehta M N. Patel M C, Sharma S M, Ramana L and Ganatra R D 1974 Familial goitre with absence of thyroglobulin and synthesis of thyroid hormones from thyroidal albumin. Journal of Endocrinology 60: 389

Dussault J H, Letarte J, Guyda H and Laberge C 1977 Serum thyroid hormone and TSH concentrations in newborn infants with congenital absence of thyroxine-binding globulin. Journal of Pediatrics 90: 264

Edmonds M, Lamki L, Killinger D W and Volpe R 1973 Autoimmune thyroiditis, adrenalitis and oophoritis. American Journal of Medicine 54: 782

Elewaut A. Mussche M and Vermeulen A 1976 Familial partial target organ resistance to thyroid hormones. Journal of Clinical Endocrinology and Metabolism 43: 575

Faber J, Colin D, Kirkegaard C, Christy M, Siersback-Nielsen K, Friis T and Nerup J 1979 Subclinical hypothyroidism in Addison's disease. Acta Endocrinologica 91: 674

Farid N R, Moens H, Larsen B, Payne R, Saltman K, Fifield F and Ingram D W 1980 HLA haptotypes in familial Graves disease. Tissue Antigens 15: 492

Federman D, Robbins J and Rall J E 1958 Some observations on cretinism and its treatment. New England Journal of Medicine 259: 610

Fialkow P J, Thuline H C, Hecht F and Bryant J 1971 Familial predisposition to thyroid disease in Down's syndrome: controlled immunoclinical studies. American Journal of Human Genetics 23: 67

Fisher D A 1980 Hypothyroidism in childhood. Pediatrics in Review 2: 67

Fisher D A, Dussault J H, Foley T P Jr, Klein A H, LaFranchi S, Larsen P R, Mitchell M L, Murphey W H and Walfish P G 1979 Screening for congenital hypothyroidism: results of screening 1 million North American infants. Journal of Pediatrics 94: 700

Florsheim W II, Dowling J T, Meister L and Bodfish R E 1962 Familial elevation of serum thyroxine-binding capacity. Journal of Clinical Endocrinology and Metabolism 22: 735

Fraser G R 1969 The genetics of thyroid disease. In: Steinberg A G and Bearn A G (eds) Progress in medical genetics, Vol VI Grune and Stratton, New York, p 89–115

Fraser G R, Morgans M E, Trotter W R 1960 The syndrome of sporadic goiter and congenital deafness. Quarterly Journal of Medicine 53: 279

Friedman J M and Fialkow P J 1978 The genetics of Graves' disease. Journal of Clinical Endocrinology and Metabolism 7: 47

Gilboa Y, Ber A, Lewitus Z and Hasenfratz J 1963 Goitrous myxedema due to iodide trapping defect. Archives of Internal Medicine 112: 110

Grieg W R, Henderson A S, Boyle J A, McGirr E M and Hutchison J H 1966 Thyroid dysgenesis in two pairs of monozygotic twins and in a mother and child. Journal of Clinical Endocrinology and Metabolism 26: 1309

Grumet F C, Payne R O, Konishi J, Kriss J P 1974 HLA antigens as marker for disease susceptibility and autoimmunity in Graves disease. Journal of Clinical Endocrinology and Metabolism 39: 115

Hagen G A, Niepomniszcze H, Haibach H, Bigazzi M, Hati R, Rapoport B, Jiminez C, DeGroot L J and Frawley T F 1971 Peroxidase deficiency in familial goiter with iodide organification defect. New England Journal of Medicine 285: 1394

Hazard J B, Hawk W A and Crile G Jr 1959 Medullary (solid) carcinoma of the thyroid – a clinicopathologic entity. Journal of Clinical Endocrinology and Metabolism 19: 152

Henneman G, Docter R, Krenning E P, Box G, Otten M and Visser T J 1979 Raised total thyroxine and free thyroxine index but normal free thyroxine. Lancet 1: 639

Hollander C S, Bernstein G and Oppenheimer J H 1968 Abnormalities of thyroxine binding in analbuminemia. Journal of Clinical Endocrinology and Metabolism 28: 1069

Hung W, August G P and Glasgow A M 1978 Hyperthyroidism in juvenile diabetes mellitus. Pediatrics 61: 583

Ingbar S H and Woeber K A 1974 The thyroid gland. In: Williams R H (ed) Textbook of endocrinology, 5th edn. W B Saunders Co, Philadelphia p 95–227

Irvine W J 1968 Clinical and immunological associations in adrenal disorders. Proceedings of the Royal Society of Medicine 61: 271

Ismail-Beigi F and Rahimifar M 1977 A variant of iodotyrosine dehalogenase deficiency. Journal of Clinical Endocrinology and Metabolism 44: 499

Jayson M I V, Doniach D, Benhamour-Glynn N 1967 Thyrotoxicosis and Hashimoto goitre in a pair of monozygotic twins with long acting thyroid stimulator. Lancet 2: 15

Job J C, Canlorbe P, Thomassin N, et al 1969 L'hypothyroidie infantile a debut precoce avec glande en place, fixation faible de radio-iode et default de response a la thyreostimuliue. Annales d'endocrinologie (Paris) 80: 696

Kidd A, Okita N, Row V V and Volpe R 1980 Immunologic aspects of Graves' and Hashimoto's diseases. Metabolism 29: 80

Kusakabe T 1972 A goitrous subject with structural abnormality of thyroglobulin. Journal of Clinical Endocrinology and Metabolsim 35: 785

Kusakabe T 1975 Deficient cytochrome b5 reductase activity in nontoxic goiter with iodide organification defect. Metabolism 24: 1103

Kusakabe T and Miyake T 1963 Defective deiodination of I[131]-labeled 1-diiodotyrosine in patients with simple goiter. Journal of Clinical Endocrinology and Metabolism 23: 132

Kusakabe T and Miyake T 1964 Thyroidal deiodination defect in three sisters with simple goiter. Journal of Clinical Endocrinology and Metabolism 24: 456

Lamberg B A, Rosengard S, Liewendahl K, Saarinen P and Evered D C 1978 Familial partial peripheral resistance to thyroid hormones. Acta Endocrinologica 87: 303

Lee W N P, Golden M P, Van Herle A J, Lippe B M and Kaplan S A 1979 Inherited abnormal thyroid hormone-binding protein causing selective increase in total serum thyroxine. Journal of Clinical Endocrinology and Metabolism 49: 292

Levy R P, Marshall J S and Velayo N L 1971 Radioimmunoassay of human thyroxine binding globulin. Journal of Clinical Endocrinology and Metabolism 32: 372

Lissitzky S, Bismuth J, Jaquet P, Castay M, Michel-Bechet M, Koutras D A, Pharmakiotis A D, Maschos A, Psarras A and Malamos B 1973 Congenital goiter with impaired thyroglobulin synthesis. Journal of Clinical Endocrinology and Metabolism 36: 17

Lissitzky S, Torresani J, Burrow G N, Bouchilloux S and Chabaud O 1975 Defective thyroglobulin export as a cause of congenital goiter. Clinical Endocrinology 4: 363

Ljunggren J G, Lindstrtom H and Hjern B 1973 The concentration of peroxidase in normal and adenomatous human thyroid tissue with special reference to patients with Pendred's syndrome. Acta Endocrinologica 72: 272

Medeiros-Neto G A, Bloise W and Ulhoa Cintra A G 1972 Partial defect of iodide trapping mechanism in two siblings with congenital goiter and hypothyroidism. Journal of Clinical Endocrinology and Metabolism 35: 370

Medeiros-Neto G A, Knobel M, Bronstein M D, Simonetti J, Filho F F and Mattar E 1979 Impaired cyclic-AMP response to thyrotropin in congenital hypothyroidism with thyroglobulin deficiency. Acta Endocrinologica 92: 62

Medeiros-Neto G A 1980 Inherited disorders of intrathyroidal metabolism, in Thyroid Research VIII, Stockigt JR and Nogataki S, Eds, Australian Acad Sci, Canberra, pp. 101–108

Melvin K E W, Tashjian A H Jr and Miller H H 1972 Studies in familial (medullary) thyroid carcinoma. Recent Progress in Hormone Research 28: 399

Miyai K, Azukizawa M and Kumahara Y 1971 Familial isolated thyrotropin deficiency with cretinism. New England Journal of Medicine 285: 1043

Miyai K, Ichihara K, Amino N 1979 Seasonality of birth in sporadic cretinism. Early Human Development 3: 85

Miyai K, Azukizawa M, Onishi T, Hashimoto T, Sawazaki N, Nishi K and Kumahara Y 1976 Familial isolated thyrotropin deficiency. In: James V H T (ed) Excerpta Medica International Congress Series No 403, Endocrinology, p 345–349

Moens H and Farid N R 1978 Hashimoto's thyroiditis is associated with HLA DRW3. New England Journal of Medicine 299: 133

Moses A A C, Lawlor J F, Haddow J E and Jackson I M D 1980 A new syndrome of familial euthyroid hyperthyroxinemia: elevated thyroxine caused by increased immunoreactive thyroid-binding prealbumin (TBPA). Prog 56th Meeting of Americal Thyroid Association, p

Nankin H, Hydovitz J and Sapira J 1970 Normal chromosomes in mucosal neuroma variant of medullary thyroid carcinoma syndrome. Journal of Medical Genetics 7: 374

Niepomniszcze H, DeGroot L J and Hagen G A 1972 Abnormal thyroid peroxidase causing iodide organification defect. Journal of Clinical Endocrinology and Metabolism 34: 607

Neipomniszcze H, Castells S, DeGroot L J, Refetoff S, Kim O S, Rapoport B and Hati R 1973 Peroxidase defect in congenital goiter with complete organification block. Journal of Clinical Endocrinology and Metabolism 36: 347

Niepomniszcze H, Rosenbloom A L, DeGroot L J, Shimaoka K, Refetoff S and Yamamoto K 1975 Differentiation of two abnormalities in thyroid peroxidase causing organification defect and goitrous hypothyroidism. Metabolism 24: 57

Nilsson L R, Borgfors N, Gamstrop I, Holst H E and Liden G 1964 Nonendemic goitre and deafness. Acta Paediatrica 53: 117

Oppenheimer J H, Schwartz H L, Surks M I, Koerner D and Dillman W H 1976 Nuclear receptors and the initiation of thyroid hormone action. Recent Progress in Hormone Research 32: 529

Pai G S, Leach D C, Weiss L, Wolf C and Van Dyke D L 1977 Thyroid abnormalities in 20 children with Turner's syndrome. Journal of Paediatrics 91: 267

Papadopoulos S N, Vagenakis A G, Maschos A, Koutras D A, Matsaniotis N and Malamos B 1970 A case of a partial defect of the iodide trapping mechanism. Journal of Clinical Endocrinology and Metabolism 30: 302

Pendred V 1896 Deaf-mutism and goitre. Lancet 2: 532

Pommier J, Tourniaire J, Deme D, Chalendar P, Bornet H and Nunez J 1974 A defective thyroid peroxidase solubilized from a familial goiter with iodine organification defect. Journal of Clinical Endocrinology and Metabolism 39: 69

Refetoff S, DeGroot L J and Barsano C P 1980 Defective thyroid hormone feedback regulation in the syndrome of peripheral resistance to thyroid hormone. Journal of Clinical Endocrinology and Metabolism 51: 41

Refetoff S, DeWind L T and DeGroot L J 1967 Familial syndrome combining deaf-mutism, stippled epiphyses, goiter and abnormally high PBI: possible target organ refractoriness to thyroid hormone. Journal of Clinical Endocrinology and Metabolism 27: 279

Refetoff S, Robin N I and Alper C A 1972a Study of four new kindreds with inherited thyroxine binding globulin abnormalities. Journal of Clinical Investigation 51: 848

Refetoff S, DeGroot L J, Bernard B, DeWind L T 1972b Studies of a sibship with apparent hereditary resistance to the intracellular action of thyroid hormone. Metabolism 21: 723

Robbins J 1973 Inherited variations in thyroxine transport. Mount Sinai Journal of Medicine NY 40: 511

Savoie J C, Massin J P and Savoie F 1973 Studies on mono and diiodohistidine. II congenital goitrous hypothyroidism with thyroglobulin defect and iodohistidine-rich iodoalbumin production. Journal of Clinical Investigation 52· 116

Schimke R N and Hartmann W H 1965 Familial amyloid producing medullary thyroid carcinoma and pheochromocytoma. Annals of Internal Medicine 63: 1027

Schneider G, Keiser H R and Bardin C W 1975 Peripheral resistance to thyroxine: a cause of short stature in a boy without goiter. Clinical Endocrinology 4: 111

Seif F J, Sherbaum W and Klinger W 1978 Syndrome of elevated thyroid hormone and TSH blood levels: a case report. Acta Endocrinologica 87 Suppl 215: 81–88

Sipple J H 1961 The association of pheochromocytoma with carcinoma of the thyroid gland. American Journal of Medicine 31: 163

Smallridge R C, Wartofsky L, Chopra I J, Morinelli P V, Broughton R E, Dimond R C and Burman K D 1978 Neonatal thyrotoxicosis: alterations in serum concentrations of LATS- protector, T4, T3, reverse T3 and 3,3'T2. Journal of Pediatrics 93: 118

Sparkes R S and Motulsky A G 1963 Hashimoto's disease in Turner's syndrome with isochromosome X. Lancet 1: 947

Spinner M W, Blizzard R M and Childs B 1968 Clinical and genetic heterogeneity in idiopathic Addison's disease and hypoparathyroidism. Journal of Clinical Endocrinology and Metabolism 28: 795

Stanbury J B 1978 Familial goiter. In: Stanbury J B, Wyngaarden J B and Fredrickson D S (eds) The metabolic basis of inherited disease, 4th edn. McGraw Hill, New York, p 206–239

Stanbury J B and Hedge A M 1950 A study of a family of goitrous cretins. Journal of Clinical Endocrinology and Metabolism 10: 1471

Stanbury J B, Aiginger P and Harbison M D 1979 Familial goiter and related disorders. In: DeGroot L J, Cahill G F Jr, Martini L, Nelson D H, Odell W D, Potts J T Jr, Steinberger E and Winegrad A I (eds) Endocrinology, Grune and Stratton, New York p 523–539

Stanbury J B, Meijer J W A and Kassenaar A A H 1956 The metabolism of iodotyrosines I The fate of mono and diiodotyrosine in certain patients with familial goiter. Journal of Clinical Endocrinology and Metabolism 16: 735

Stanbury J B, Rocmans P, Buhler U K and Ochi Y 1968 Congenital hypothyroidism with impaired thyroid response to thyrotropin. New England Journal of Medicine 279: 1132

Tanaka S and Starr P 1959 A euthyroid man without thyroxine binding globulin. Journal of Clinical Endocrinology and Metabolism 19: 485

Valenta L J, Bode H, Vickery A L, Caulfield J B and Maloof F 1973 Lack of thyroid peroxidase activity as the cause of congenital goitrous hypothyroidism. Journal of Clinical Endocrinology and Metabolism 36: 830

Vallotton M B and Forbes A P 1967 Autoimmunity in gonadal dysgenesis and Klinefelter's syndrome. Lancet 1: 648

Van Wyk J J, and Fisher D A 1977 The thyroid. In: Rudolph A, Barnett H L, and Einhorn A H (eds) Pediatrics 16, 16th edn. Appleton-Century-Crofts, New York p 1663–1692

Vesterhus P and Aarskog D 1973 Noonan's syndrome and autoimmune thyroiditis. Journal of Pediatrics 83: 237

Volpe R 1978 The genetics and immunology of Graves and Hashimoto's diseases. In: Rose N, Bigazzi P E and Warner N L (eds) Genetic control of autoimmune disease, Elsevier/North Holland, New York, p 43–56

Volpe R, Clarke P V and Row V V 1973 Relationship of age-specific incidence rates to immunologic aspects of Hashimoto's thyroiditis. Canadian Medical Association Journal 109: 898

Williams E D 1979 Medullary carcinoma of the thyroid. In: DeGroot L J, Cahill G F Jr, Martini L, Nelson D H, Odell W D, Potts J T Jr, Steinberger E and Winegrad A I (eds) Endocrinology, Grune and Stratton, New York, p 777–792

Williams E D and Pollock D J 1966 Multiple mucosal neuromata with endocrine tumours: a syndrome allied to von Recklinghausen's disease. Journal of Pathology and Bacteriology 91: 71

Williams E D, Engel E and Forbes A P 1964 Thyroiditis and gonadal dysgenesis. New England Journal of Medicine 270: 805

Winter R J and Green O C 1976 Carbohyte homeostasis in chronic lymphocytic thyroiditis: increased incidence of diabetes mellitus. Journal of Pediatrics 89: 401

Wolff J, Thompson R H and Robbins J 1964 Congenital goitrous cretinism due to absence of iodide-concentrating ability. Journal of Clinical Endocrinology and Metabolism 24: 699

84

Parathyroid disorders

C. E. Jackson

INTRODUCTION

This chapter is concerned with the genetic aspects of clinical disorders of the parathyroid glands. The topics will be discussed under the main headings of primary hyperparathyroidism, primary hypoparathyroidism, (or hormone deficiency) and pseudohypoparathyroidism (or end organ unresponsiveness). Genetic factors are important in each of these 3 heterogeneous conditions to a variable extent. Knowledge of parathyroid conditions has considerable practical importance not only in genetic counselling but also in their treatment potential.

PRIMARY HYPERPARATHYROIDISM

Clinical description and pathogenesis

Primary hyperparathyroidism is a generalised disorder of calcium and phosphate metabolism resulting from an increased production of parathyroid hormone (PTH) by the parathyroid glands without identifiable cause. In secondary hyperparathyroidism, the increased PTH production is most often secondary to chronic renal disease or intestinal malabsorption with the exact mechanism of the parathyroid hyperplasia being not well understood. Primary hyperparathyroidism was initially recognized most frequently by the development of severe bone disease, osteitis fibrosa cystica. Later the association of nephrolithiasis and kidney stones led to the diagnosis of this entity. Since the reports of the detection of hyperparathyroidism by elevated serum calcium determinations on routine analysis (Boonstra & Jackson, 1962) and the advent of the almost universal clinical use of multiphasic biochemical screening procedures, this condition has become recognized with increasing frequency. It is estimated that 1 per 800–1000 patients seen in a general medical clinic will have this condition (Boonstra & Jackson, 1965–1971). The disease is no longer thought of as being one of just 'bones and stones' but one also of 'abdominal groans and psychic moans with fatigue overtones' or at times almost completely asymptomatic and evident only by an elevated serum calcium value obtained

as a routine screening procedure. Primary hyperparathyroidism is generally related to the presence of an adenoma of one of the 4 parathyroid glands in the neck (Fig. 84.1). However, some cases (about 15–20%) are related to an adenoma of more than one gland or to diffuse hyperplasia of all glands. The pathologic differentiation of adenoma from hyperplasia is difficult if not impossible.

Glucose-6-phosphate-dehydrogenase studies of parathyroid 'adenomas' have disclosed that those studied are of multicellular origin as one would expect of hyperplastic lesions (Fialkow et al, 1977). Although these findings would not have been unexpected in hereditary hyperparathyroidism, multicellular origin in sporadic cases suggests that unknown factors are stimulating many cells in the parathyroid glands to become hyperplastic instead of some neoplastic change occurring as a mutation originating in one cell only. Thorough family studies of patients with primary hyperparathyroidism have revealed that 1/6–1/8 of the cases have other family members affected with hyperparathyroidism alone or manifestations of the hereditary multiple endocrine neoplasia syndromes (Jackson et al, 1977).

Natural history and complications

The natural history of primary hyperparathyroidism is quite variable, at times being asymptomatic into old age and at other times causing symptoms in early adulthood (or in infancy as in familial neonatal hyperparathyroidism). The symptoms may involve different organ systems such as the bones, gastrointestinal tract, kidneys or central nervous system and are thought to generally represent the effect of hypercalcaemia on those particular systems. The age of onset is usually considerably earlier in the hereditary syndromes associated wity hyperparathyroidism than in the cases of sporadic primary hyperparathyroidism. Rarely is hyperparathyroidism detected by symptomatic bone disease at the present time. Nephrolithiasis and kidney stones often lead to the diagnosis as do the gastrointestinal complications of ulcer, pancreatitis or nonspecific nausea and vomiting. The complications of other organ involvement associated with the hereditary multiple endocrine neoplasia syndromes will be discussed under those topics.

Differential diagnosis

The differential diagnosis of primary hyperparathyroidism from other conditions causing hypercalcaemia has become increasingly important with the frequent detection of hypercalcaemia in biochemical screening programmes. Non-parathyroid hypercalcaemia occurs with vitamin D intoxication, the milk-alkali syndrome, sarcoidosis and hyperthyroidism. However, the most frequent and often the most difficult differential diagnosis lies between primary hyperparathyroidism and the hypercalcaemia of malignancy either related to multiple myeloma, bony metastases or the ectopic production of substances which elevate the serum calcium (Stewart et al, 1980). This differentiation requires a thorough study of the patient for tumours of those organs (lungs, kidneys, ovaries or breasts) which are most likely to cause hypercalcaemia. Another important differential diagnosis is the determination of the type of genetic disease present in those 1/6–1/8 of all cases of hyperparathyroidism which represent hereditary conditions. It is felt that studies of the relatives of patients with hypercalcaemia can contribute greatly to the establishment of the correct diagnosis. The finding of another relative with hypercalcaemia provides evidence for primary hyperparathyroidism being the correct diagnosis if hereditary hypocalciuric hypercalcaemia is excluded by calcium:creatinine clearance studies. The finding of a hypercalcaemic relative also requires investigation of the patient for manifestations of the multiple endocrine neoplasia (MEN) syndromes. The important conditions are pancreatic islet cell adenoma or carcinoma causing hyperinsulinism; or more commonly, the Zollinger-Elli-son syndrome with peptic ulceration and pituitary tumours of the MEN 1 syndrome; or rarely, the pheochromocytoma or medullary thyroid carcinoma of the MEN 2 syndrome.

Therapy

The treatment of primary hyperparathyroidism is still by surgery with the excision of all hyperfunctioning parathyroid tissue by a competent neck surgeon. Those patients with hereditary hyperparathyroidism, whether from hereditary hyperparathyroidism alone or associated with MEN 1 or 2, are much more likely to have multiple parathyroid gland involvement or generalised hyperplasia of all parathyroid glands which may require subtotal (usually 3–1/2 gland removal) parathyroidectomy. It is the policy of some surgeons (Block et al 1975) however, to do a selective parathyroidectomy in MEN-2 removing only those glands which are enlarged. In hereditary hyperparathyroidism, Jackson and Boonstra (1967) found the frequency of multiple parathyroid gland involvement to be 40% with selective parathyroid excision being carried out in these cases. Some surgeons have advocated subtotal parathyroidectomy in all cases with

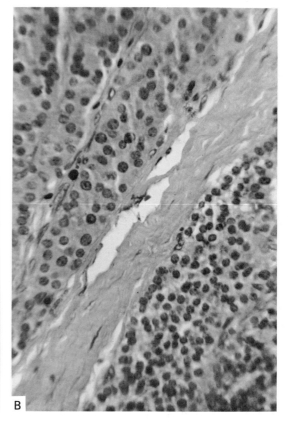

Fig. 84.1 Extremely large parathyroid adenoma from patient with multiple endocrine neoplasia type 1. (A) Gross appearance (B) Microscopic appearance (H & E stain) showing hyperplasia of two different cell types.

the hereditary types of hyperparathyroidism and Wells et al (1976) have recommended total parathyroidectomy and autotransplantation of parathyroid tissue into forearm muscle in patients with parathyroid hyperplasia. Clearly the apparent increasing prevalence of hyperparathyroidism (what has been termed the epidemic of hyperparathyroidism) suggests the need for effective medical treatment which would preclude surgery although the prospects for this possibility are bleak at present.

The heterogeneity of hereditary conditions causing hyperparathyroidism

Several hereditary entities are known at the present time to cause hyperparathyroidism. These include neonatal primary hyperparathyroidism, hereditary hyperparathyroidism, multiple endocrine neoplasia (MEN) type 1, and multiple endocrine neoplasia type 2 (or 2a) — (Table 84.1). Each of these is a distinct entity and will be discussed separately. Although not truly hereditary hyperparathyroidism, hereditary hypocalciuric hypercalcaemia will be included in this discussion because it is associated with parathyroid hyperplasia and is an important condition to be differentiated from the various entities causing hereditary hyperparathyroidism.

Hereditary hypocalciuric hypercalcaemia
This entity was described by Marx et al (1977) in a report of family studies of patients with parathyroid hyperplasia. They found a high failure rate in parathyroid exploration in two kindreds with a syndrome which they termed familial hypocalciuric hypercalcaemia (FHH). The name was derived from the fact that this appeared to be an autosomal dominant condition of high penetrance of the hypercalcaemia with the hypocalciuria being the distinctive characteristic. They emphasized that this condition could be distinguished from primary hyperparathyroidism by the low ratio of urinary calcium clearance to creatinine clearance and that this distinction was important not only because of the benign nature of the condition but also because of the high failure rate of parathyroid surgery for correcting the hypercalcaemia. In a subsequent article Marx et al (1980b) have emphasized that this condition was of sufficient prevalence to account for 9% of a large group of patients referred after unsuccessful parathyroidectomy. Following the description of this entity by Marx's group (1977, 1980b) we have reinvestigated a large family which we reported earlier as hereditary hyperparathyroidism (Jackson & Boonstra, 1967). This family had 19 members (Fig. 84.2) with hypercalcaemia in an autosomal dominant type of inheritance pattern with failure to correct the hypercalcaemia in 3 members having surgery (2, 3–1/4 and 3–1/2 parathyroid glands removed). It was recognized (Jackson & Boonstra, 1966) that this condition was a separate entity from hereditary hyperparathyroidism but it was not until

Table 84.1 Heterogeneity of hereditary conditions causing hyperparathyroidism

	Mode of inheritance	Age of onset	Pathology	Main ass'd conditions	Surgical treatment
Hereditary hypocalciuric hypercalcaemia	Autosomal dominant	Birth	Parathyroid hyperplasia	None	Not true hyperparathyroidism – surgery not indicated
Neonatal hyperparathyroidism	Autosomal recessive	Birth	Parathyroid hyperplasia	None	Early surgery with subtotal parathyroidectomy
Hereditary hyperparathyroidism	Autosomal dominant	About puberty	Parathyroid hyperplasia, single or multiple adenomas	None	Selective parathyroidectomy
Multiple endocrine neoplasia type 1	Autosomal dominant	About puberty	Generally parathyroid hyperplasia	Pancreatic islet cell adenoma or carcinoma; pituitary tumours	Subtotal parathyroidectomy. Surgery for pancreatic neoplasm may be the first treatment with total gastrectomy
Multiple endocrine neoplasia type 2 (or 2a)	Autosomal dominant	Childhood	Parathyroid hyperplasia	Pheochromocytomas; medullary thyroid carcinoma	Pheochromocytoma removal first. Total thyroidectomy and selective parathyroidectomy
Multiple endocrine neoplasia type 2b (or 3)	Autosomal dominant	Childhood	Parathyroids generally *not* affected	Mucosal neuromas, pheochromocytoma; medullary thyroid carcinoma	Pheochromocytoma removal first. Total thyroidectomy

WAL KINDRED

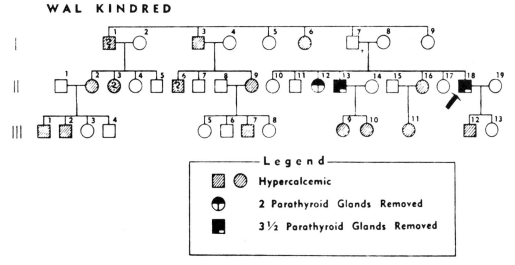

Fig. 84.2 Pedigree of family with hereditary hypocalciuric hypercalcaemia originally reported by Jackson & Boonstra (1967) as hereditary hyperparathyroidism.

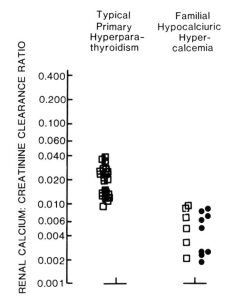

Fig. 84.3 Calcium: creatinine clearance ratios in primary hyperparathyroidism and hypocalciuric hypercalcemia from Marx et al (1980a) indicated by the open squares and from individuals in Figure 84.2 indicated by closed circles.

the work of Marx et al (1977) that the distinguishing characteristics became evident. Further studies have revealed calcium:creatinine clearance ratios in this family consistent with the diagnosis of this entity (Fig. 84.3). The findings in this family (Jackson & Kleerekoper, 1981) have re-emphasized the benign nature of this condition – one member is living at 82 having been asymptomatic his entire life, with several known affected members having died in their 70's without ever having had symptoms.

This condition is characterized by the presence of hypercalcaemia in the neonatal period and throughout childhood, which contrasts with hereditary hyperparathyroidism or the hyperparathyroidism associated with the multiple endocrine neoplasia syndromes in which hypercalcaemia generally does not occur until late childhood and mostly after the age of puberty. The early age of hypercalcaemia therefore would most resemble that occurring with neonatal primary hyperparathyroidism from which it should be distinguished. Marx et al (1980a) state that the principle differences appear to be the higher degree of hypercalcaemia seen in the reported cases of neonatal primary hyperparathyroidism and its apparent autosomal recessive mode versus the autosomal dominant mode of inheritance of FHH.

Familial hypocalciuric hypercalcaemia should probably have been termed hereditary hypocalciuric hypercalcaemia since the hereditary nature has been established. Heath and Purnell (1980) have chosen to use the term 'familial benign hypercalcaemia' because of the priority in the literature, with this term being used in the 1972 description of the entity by Foley et al. It should actually not be listed under the heading of primary hyperparathyroidism since it is not associated with an increased production of parathyroid hormone. The entity deserves much emphasis because of the prognostic and treatment implications apparent in its diagnosis and differentiation from true hereditary primary hyperparathyroidism. It has been emphasized that the families of hypercalcaemic patients should be studied prior to surgery since the finding of an affected relative tends to support the diagnosis and provides further incentive to the surgeon to investigate all parathyroid glands because of the greater likelihood of multiple involvement. (It is at this time also that maximum cooperation can be obtained from family members for such studies). The differentiation of the entity of FHH from primary hyperparathyroidism provides an important additional reason for thoroughly studying the families of all patients with hypercalcaemia prior to surgery.

Neonatal primary hyperparathyroidism

Hypercalcaemia in the neonatal period is extremely rare. It may be related to familial hypocalciuric hypercalcaemia (FHH) or to neonatal primary hyperparathyroidism. In the former condition, surgery is not indicated but in the latter the disease is very serious and often fatal without surgery (Goldbloom et al 1972, Marx et al 1980b) making the differential diagnosis crucial. The hereditary cases of neonatal primary hyperparathyroidism appear to be autosomal recessively inherited, although 2 families with 2 generations affected have been reported as reviewed by Thompson et al (1978). Besides the necessity to differentiate this condition from FHH, it is important to differentiate it from the hypercalcaemia seen in infants of hypoparathyroid mothers and from a syndrome known as idiopathic hypercalcaemia of infancy, in each of which surgery is not indicated. Here again the study of the parents and other family members is sometimes critical in the differential diagnosis.

Hereditary hyperparathyroidism

Hereditary hyperparathyroidism without features of the multiple endocrine neoplasia syndromes may occur as a separate dominantly inherited entity. It has been postulated however (Jackson & Boonstra, 1967) that most cases thought to be this entity are part of the multiple endocrine neoplasia type 1 syndrome in which the family has not been followed long enough or thoroughly enough to note the other endocrine involvement. Figure 84.4 shows the affected members in the pedigree of the family of hereditary hyperparathyroidism first observed in association with pancreatitis by Jackson (1958). Most affected members were found by performing serum calcium tests on asymptomatic members of the family. It was the finding of these cases of hyperparathyroidism in this family which led to the performance of serum calcium screening (Boonstra & Jackson, 1965; 1965; 1971) which has become routine almost throughout the world and which has led to the recognition of the remarkably high prevalence of a disease previously thought to be somewhat rare.

Study of the families of all cases of hyperparathyroidism has disclosed that 12–18% of all cases have other family members affected, (Jackson & Boonstra, 1967; Boonstra & Jackson, 1971; Jackson et al, 1977) some

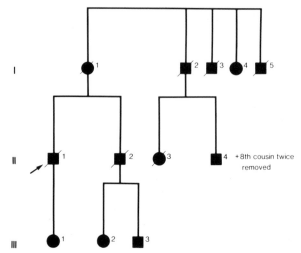

Fig. 84.4 Pedigree indicating only the affected individuals with hyperparathyroidism in the family reported by Jackson (1958).

with hyperparathyroidism alone and others with other associated endocrine tumours. Hereditary hyperparathyroidism has the same spectrum of manifestation as does sporadic or non-hereditary hyperparathyroidism. However, the age of onset tends to be much earlier, even excluding those cases found by family studies. It may be that affected individuals have an increased risk of parathyroid carcinoma as is discussed under familial parathyroid carcinoma (Jackson et al, 1980).

Multiple endocrine neoplasia type 1 (MEN-1)

The term multiple endocrine neoplasia was emphasized by Steiner et al (1968) for these syndromes rather than the previously used term of multiple endocrine adenomatosis (MEA) originally proposed by Wermer (1954). The change in terminology has a solid basis since the lesions are known to be neoplastic with carcinoma occurring frequently and not just adenomas. Ptak and Kirsner (1970) emphasized that 50% of the pancreatic islet cell lesions of the Zollinger-Ellison syndrome are malignant. Reports of parathyroid carcinoma occurring in hereditary hyperparathyroidism and MEN-1 are reviewed later in this chapter. In the autosomal dominantly inherited type 1 syndrome, the parathyroid glands are involved most frequently (Ballard et al, 1964) with pancreatic islet cell and pituitary gland involvement also frequent (88%, 81% and 65% respectively of 85 cases). Thorough study of the families of patients with hereditary hyperparathyroidism has disclosed that often affected members have other endocrine involvement (Jackson & Boonstra, 1967; Boey et al, 1975; Jackson et al, 1977). Pancreatic islet cell manifestations may involve tumours producing gastrin (Zollinger-Ellison syndrome) insulin (insulinomas) or glucagon (glucagonomas). The literature reports of the MEN-1 syndrome are voluminous and will not be reviewed in detail here. They generally reveal an autosomal dominant type of inheritance with variable expressivity which sometimes appears to represent decreased penetrance.

Although the MEN syndromes have been generally thought to be distinct clinical and genetic entities with parathyroid tumours being shared by each (Schimke & Hartmann, 1965), overlap situations have been reported. Pheochromocytomas are reported to occur in the same patients and the same families with pancreatic islet cell neoplasms (Carney et al, 1980). The overlap families reviewed and others (including one with glucagonomas, medullary thyroid cancer and pheochromocytoma reported by Boden & Owen, 1977) suggest that a mechanism may be present resulting in a wider spectrum of endocrine involvement than was originally anticipated (Table 84.2). It is probable that in the future other hereditary endocrine neoplasia syndromes will be identified which may be separable from those recognized at present. These may be separated from each other by clinical findings, genetic linkage investigations or chromosomal studies.

Multiple endocrine neoplasia type 2 (MEN-2)
Although the syndrome of medullary thyroid carcinoma with pheochromocytoma was identified earlier by Sipple (1961), Steiner et al (1968), in reporting a large kindred,

originated the term multiple endocrine neoplasia type 2. This has appropriately come to be the accepted terminology for the autosomal dominant syndrome which also includes parathyroid gland involvement.

The 1970 report by Tashjian et al on radioimmunoassay for calcitonin in patients with medullary thyroid cancer has provided the tool not only for the early detection of this cancer in families but also for a greater understanding of the mechanisms of neoplasia. The value of calcitonin assay for detection of medullary thyroid cancer has been established in many other studies (Wells et al, 1975; Jackson et al, 1973; Sizemore et al, 1977; Gagel et al, 1975; Samaan et al, 1973; Keiser et al, 1973 and many others). The provocative test used initially was a 4 hour calcium infusion. Pentagastrin (Hennessy et al, 1974) has largely replaced the 4 hour calcium infusion as the stimulating agent because of convenience (requiring only a rapid injection and measurements of calcitonin at 2, 5 & 10 minutes) and generally increased sensitivity (Fig. 84.5) Wells et al (1978) have utilized the combination of calcium infusion (2 mg/kg) and pentagastrin (0.5 mcg/kg) to obtain what they feel to be the optimum stimulus to create the most sensitive test. Silva et al (1979) have advocated the assay of urine for calcitonin to improve the early diagnosis of medullary thyroid carcinoma. The utilization of calcitonin radioimmunoassay in such studies for the early detection of medullary thyroid cancer in families has provided one of the best examples of the practical application of genetic studies.

Table 84.2 Endocrine neoplasia overlap

Gland involvement	Adrenal cortex	Pituitary	Pancreas	Parathyroid	Medullary thyroid cancer	(Pheochyromocytoma) Adrenal Medulla	Mucosal neuroma
Typical MEN-1		+	+	+	+		
Typical MEN-2 or 2a				+	+	+	
Typical MEN-2b or 3					+	+	+
Boden & Owen (1977)			+		+	+	
Cameron & Spiro (1978)			+		+		
Heikkinen & Åkerblom (1977)			+	+		+	
Block et al (1980)			+		+		
			+		+		
			+		+		
Carney et al (1980)			+			+	
Alberts et al (1980)	+		+	+		+	
Janson et al (1978)		+	+			+	
						+	
Hansen et al (1976)	+			+	+		
Tateishi et al (1978)			+			+	

Other combinations have been reported in association with von Hippel-Lindau disease

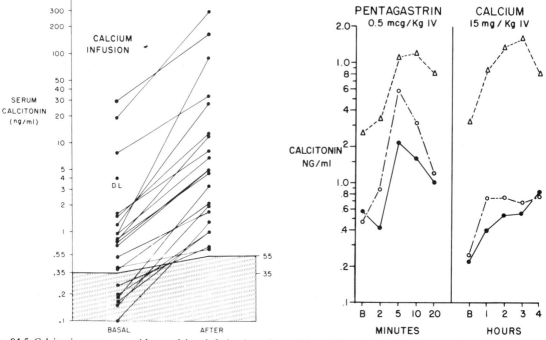

Fig. 84.5 Calcitonin responses to 4 hour calcium infusion in patients with medullary thyroid carcinoma and comparison of results in 3 patients between a 1-1/2 minute pentagastrin infusion and 4 hour calcium infusion.

SMI KINDRED

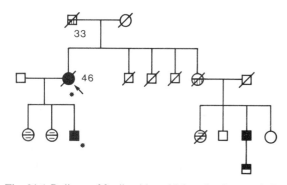

Fig. 84.6 Pedigree of family with multiple endocrine neoplasia (MEN) type 2 with medullary thyroid cancer, pheochromocytoma and parathyroid tumours. The 46 year old woman in generation II also had Cushing's syndrome secondary to ACTH production by the thyroid cancer.

■	●	Medullary thyroid carcinoma
◨	◐	Pheochromocytoma
◫	◒	Negative calcitonin test
◨	◔	Negative catecholamines
⊞	⊕	Probable pheochromocytoma
*		Parathyroid adenoma

Parathyroid gland involvement in this syndrome is quite variable from family to family and also within families. Within the group of the families with MEN-2 studied at Henry Ford Hospital, some have been noted (Block et al, 1980) to have the entire spectrum of med-

ullary thyroid cancer, pheochromocytoma and parathyroid tumours (Fig. 84.6) whereas others have had medullary thyroid cancer and parathyroid tumours (Fig. 84.7) and others only the medullary thyroid cancers. The treatment of patients with this syndrome involves a thorough study of the patients for their particular gland involvement. If a pheochromocytoma can be identified as being present, surgery for this serious and potentially fatal condition should be performed first. Because of the high frequency of bilateral and multicentric involvement and because of the presence of adrenal medullary hyperplasia in these hereditary cases (Carney et al, 1976; DeLellis et al, 1976) bilateral adrenalectomy should be performed. Unfortunately urinary and plasma catecholamine determinations do not permit as early a diagnosis as is possible in medullary thyroid carcinoma with provocative calcitonin testing. Computerized tomographic and isotope scans of the adrenal will probably come to be helpful in patients with suspected pheochromocytomas. Generally patients with this syndrome have their thyroid condition detected and treated and need to be followed periodically for the development of pheochromocytomas. They also need to be followed periodically by the sensitive provocative calcitonin procedures in order to detect recurrences of medullary thyroid carcinoma. Block et al (1978) have suggested a conservative approach in those patients with elevated calcitonin levels, but no palpable nodes, postoperative to total thyroidectomy.

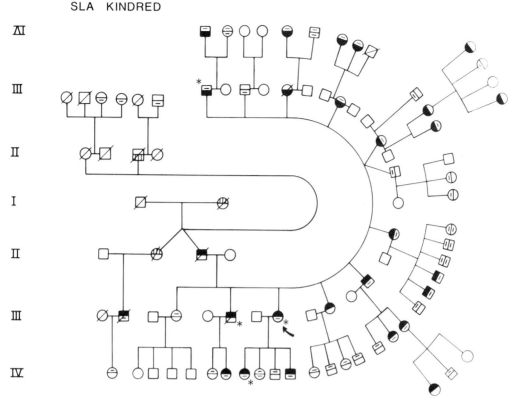

Fig. 84.7 Pedigree showing 5 generations of a family affected with MEN-2 with medullary thyroid cancer and parathyroid tumours without pheochromocytomas being present in any member (key as in Figure 84.6).

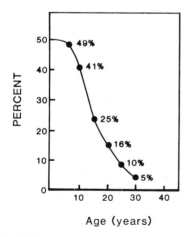

Fig. 84.8 Probability of subsequently developing the autosomal dominantly inherited medullary carcinoma of the thyroid (MCT) for individuals who have a negative stimulated calcitonin (CT) procedure at the stated age even though they have a 50% risk at birth (based on data of Gagel et al, 1982).

For the medullary thyroid cancer, total thyroidectomy is advised along with neck lymphatic node dissection as indicated. For the parathyroid involvement some surgeons have advocated subtotal parathyroidectomy whereas others (Block et al, 1975) have advocated selective parathyroidectomy of any enlarged parathyroid glands.

The following of young patients at risk of inheriting medullary thyroid carcinoma has permitted the construction of curves which have proven useful in genetic counselling of this autosomal dominant condition. The curve provided from data on 38 patients whose provocative calcitonin tests had converted from negative to positive is illustrated in Figure 84.8 (Gagel et al 1982). For example, an individual in the 50% risk category at birth and a normal calcitonin level following either pentagastrin or calcium infusion at age 25 has only a 10% chance of subsequently developing this tumour.

Approximately 25% of all medullary thyroid cancers are hereditary (Block et al, 1980). Comparisons of the clinical and pathologic characteristics have provided evidence for distinctive differences important not only in prognosis but also in therapy (Table 84.3). These findings are also of potential significance in the aetiology of cancer. Reports in 1973 of the new entity of C-cell hyperplasia of the thyroid (Jackson et al and Wolfe et al) postulated this condition to be the expression of the initial genetic mutation in Knudson's (1971) two mutational event theory on the initiation of cancer. Ages of

Table 84.3 Comparison of hereditary and sporadic medullary thyroid carcinoma (from Block et al 1980)

	Hereditary	*Sporadic*
Others in family	Yes, autosomal dominant pattern	No
Pathology	Bilateral, associated C-cell hyperplasia	Unilateral, no C-cell hyperplasia
Other endocrine involvement	Adrenal medulla & parathyroid glands as part of MEN-2 syndrome	Not part of MEN-2
Age of onset of palpable lesions	Average 36 years	Average 50 years
Curability by surgery based on calcitonin assay	Almost 100% of non-palpable tumours detected by calcitonin studies within families; 17% of palpable tumours	45% (all palpable)
Average life expectancy	Age about 50 (average for palpable tumours)	Age about 66

onset curves for palpable hereditary medullary thyroid cancer (MCT) (Fig. 84.9) when compared with those sporadic MCT are similar to those obtained by Knudson with retinoblastoma and what is predictable on a one-hit occurrence for the hereditary tumours and two-hit occurrence for the sporadic type (Jackson et al, 1979). Data from Gagel et al (1982) (Fig. 84.9) on the age of detectability of hereditary cases by provocative calcitonin testing (38 cases with conversion from negative to positive tests) also provide evidence for this theory.

C-cell hyperplasia (CCH) has been observed (Jackson et al, 1979) peripheral to the cancers invariably in the thyroid glands of patients with the hereditary type but not in those of patients with the sporadic type. This is predictable if CCH is actually the manifestation of the first or genetic mutation in Knudson's theory. This finding also has practical value in enabling the pathologist to indicate which patients are most likely to have the hereditary type of tumour so that more concentrated studies can be performed on the families of such patients. G6PD studies showing the clonal origin of medullary thyroid cancer by Baylin et al (1976 & 1978) also provide evidence for the concept that these cancers occur as a change in a cell genetically predisposed by the first mutation to

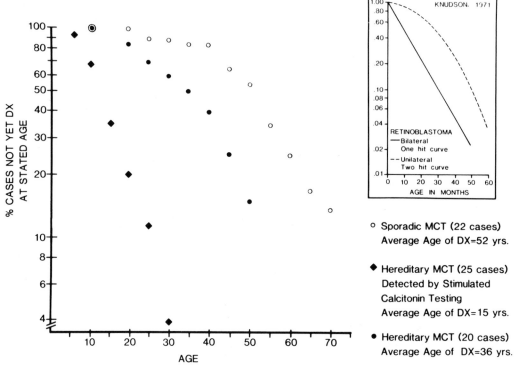

Fig. 84.9 Comparison of the proportion of cases of medullary cancer of the thyroid not yet detected at various ages for palpable sporadic cases and palpable hereditary cases (from Jackson et al, 1979) and nonpalpable hereditary cases detected in family studies by calcitonin testing (Gagel et al, 1982).

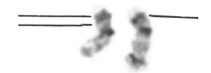

Fig. 84.10 Homologous number 20 chromosomes from patient with MEN-2 showing suggestive deletion in short arm of one of the pair (Van Dyke et al, 1981).

cancer formation. In the 1978 paper by Baylin et al, tumours of one origin in one thyroid lobe were reported with tumours of another origin in the other lobe suggesting that the second mutation had occurred in different cells predisposed by prior mutations.

Two tumours, retinoblastoma (Yunis & Ramsey, 1978) and Wilm's tumours (Francke et al, 1979) have forms associated with specific chromosomal deletions. Using the prometaphase culture techniques of Yunis et al (1978), Van Dyke, Jackson and Babu (1981) reported a deletion in the short arm of number 20 chromosome in members of several kindreds with MEN-2 (Fig. 84.10). If the deletion in MEN-2 can be confirmed in other laboratories, it should be valuable in providing the diagnosis even earlier than has been possible by calcitonin testing and eventually lead to prenatal diagnosis. Of more importance is the theoretical significance of finding a visible chromosome deletion in a condition for which the manifestation (C-cell hyperplasia) of the mendelian dominantly inherited mutation is known. Knudson (1980) has suggested that cancer may develop when a heterozygous cell becomes homozygously defective by a mutation at a specific chromosomal site, resulting in a loss of growth control of a particular cell type. One could postulate in the MEN-2 Syndrome that the chromosomal deletion results in C-cell hyperplasia (described by Wolfe et al, 1973), the adrenal medullary hyperplasia (described by DeLellis et al, 1976 and Carney et al, 1976) and also parathyroid hyperplasia. If a second mutagenic event occurs at the allelic site on the homologous chromosome of one of the cells in these endocrine tissues, that cell becomes a malignant cell with all the potential associated with such cells. The multiple endocrine neoplasia syndrome may be providing a better understanding of the pathogenesis of malignancy than has been previously possible.

The syndrome of mucosal neuromas, medullary thyroid carcinoma and pheochromocytoma was recognized as a separate syndrome by Schimke et al (1968) and Gorlin et al (1968). It has been termed MEN-2b by the Mayo Clinic group (Chong et al 1975) and MEN-3 by Khairi et al (1975). In this distinct entity, which also includes the marfanoid habitus, parathyroid involvement is rarely observed. The inheritance is autosomal dominant with the condition apparently more frequently resulting from mutation.

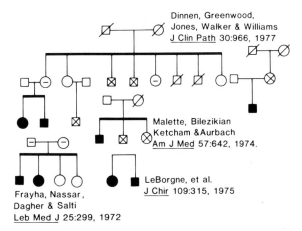

Fig. 84.11 Pedigrees from the literature showing 8 cases of parathyroid cancer within 5 families with hereditary hyperparathyroidism.
■ ● Parathyroid carcinoma
⊠ ⊗ Hyperparathyroidism

Familial parathyroid carcinoma

Parathyroid carcinoma is a rare disease, considered on the basis of autopsy findings to represent about 3–4% of all cases of primary hyperparathyroidism (Schantz & Castleman, 1973). The increasingly frequent detection of hyperparathyroidism by automated chemical screening probably indicates that 3–4% is likely an overestimate. Eight cases of parathyroid carcinoma have been reported in 5 families with hereditary hyperparathyroidism (Fig. 84.11). The ages of onset of the parathyroid cancers in these families is considerably younger than that of apparently sporadic cases reported (Table 84.4). The presence of this many cases of the rarely occurring parathyroid cancer in families with hereditary hyperpar-

Table 84.4 Comparison of ages of onset of sporadic and hereditary parathyroid cancer

	Cases	Average age
Parathyroid carcinoma		
Schantz & Castleman (MGH) 1973	64	44.3
Van Heerden et al (Mayo) 1979	14	50.6
	78	45.3
Hereditary cases		
Leborgne et al 1975	1	35
	1	38
Frayha et al 1972	1	25
	1	33
Mallette et al 1974	1	51
Dinnen et al 1977	1	33
(2 Families)	1	35
	1	32
	8	35.2

athyroidism suggests that those individuals with hereditary parathyroid tumours are at greater risk of malignancy. Glucose-6-phosphate dehydrogenase studies have revealed findings compatible with multiple cell origin in one case of hereditary hyperparathyroidism (Jackson et al, 1980). This finding is compatible with the parathyroid hyperplasia of this hereditary condition being a manifestation of the genetic event in the two mutational event theory on the initiation of cancer of Knudson (1971). The ages of onset of the 8 cases of parathyroid cancer reported in hereditary hyperparathyroidism are also compatible with this theory.

Genetic counselling

Genetic counselling in hyperparathyroidism clearly is dependent on the establishment of the correct diagnosis of the aetiology of the particular entity involved. Although most conditions are inherited as autosomal dominant diseases, the age of onset is variable as are the ramifications and the seriousness of the various conditions. Prenatal diagnosis is not possible at present in any of the conditions. Establishment of the specific diagnosis and the providing of risk figures will allow recommendations to be given to the individuals as to the procedures available for the early diagnosis and treatment possible in most of the entities.

PRIMARY HYPOPARATHYROIDISM

Primary hypoparathyroidism is caused by a group of heterogeneous conditions associated with a deficiency of parathyroid hormone production. These are characterized by hypocalcaemia and consequent neuromuscular symptoms. As in hyperparathyroidism, hypoparathyroidism is important clinically because it is generally related to conditions for which adequate and effective treatment is available making the need for recognition of the condition critical to the health of the individuals. Excellent classifications of hypoparathyroid disease states have been presented by Bronsky in 1970 and by Nusynowitz et al in 1976. The latter authors separated these into two major categories – hormonopenic hypoparathyroidism and hormonoplethoric hypoparathyroidism. The hormonoplethoric states will be discussed in this chapter under the heading of pseudohypoparathyroidism (or hormone resistance states). An excellent discussion of the genetic disorders of parathyroid hormone deficiency is found in Rimoin & Schimke's book (1971) on genetic disorders of the endocrine glands.

Hypoparathyroidism is most commonly non-genetic and surgically acquired (with the excision of parathyroids or damage to the glands or their blood supply with thyroid or parathyroid surgery). Rarely hypoparathyroidism may occur following ^{131}I therapy for hyperthyroidism.

Neonatal hypoparathyroidism may occur due to maternal hyperparathyroidism and subsequent suppression of the fetal parathyroid glands by maternal hypercalcaemia. This is usually transient although it may be associated with convulsions. Hypocalcaemia may also occur secondary to hypomagnesemia which may occur neonatally (Friedmann et al, 1967) and as a hereditary condition (Stromme et al, 1969) – these cases would be expected to respond to magnesium therapy but not to calcium alone.

Hypoparathyroidism can occur neonatally as a part of the third and fourth branchial arch syndrome reported by DiGeorge (1965). This condition is associated with congenital aplasia of the parathyroid glands and thymus. The patients with this syndrome have a characteristic appearance with low set ears. It is apparently sporadic although Steele et al (1972) have reported a girl, her maternal half brother and possibly their mother as being affected by a condition resembling this syndrome. Idiopathic hypoparathyroidism has been reported as an X–linked recessive trait (Peden, 1960) with the distribution of cases within other families suggesting autosomal recessive and autosomal dominant transmission as discussed in Rimoin & Schimke's book (1971).

Hypoparathyroidism occurs in association with adrenal cortical insufficiency (Addison disease) in a group of conditions which are clinically and genetically heterogeneous (Spinner et al 1968). Hypoparathyroidism and Addison disease in association with moniliasis has been termed autoimmune polyglandular syndrome type I (Neufeld et al, 1980), the inheritance pattern of which seems to be most consistent with that of an autosomal recessive condition. This syndrome should be distinguished from Schmidt syndrome in which Addison disease is associated with autoimmune thyroid disease. Knowledge of the variable characteristics of these syndromes will allow physicians to screen the individuals and members of their families for other associated diseases.

Therapy

Therapy for hypoparathyroidism (and also for pseudohypoparathyroidism) involves the correction of the hypocalcaemia with oral calcium supplementation and with the addition of a proper dose of vitamin D or one of its more potent analogues or metabolites with attention also being directed toward any associated conditions.

PSEUDOHYPOPARATHYROIDISM(or end-organ unresponsiveness)

Pseudohypoparathyroidism (PHP) is a heterogeneous group of disorders characterized by end-organ unresponsiveness to parathyroid hormone. They may occur with

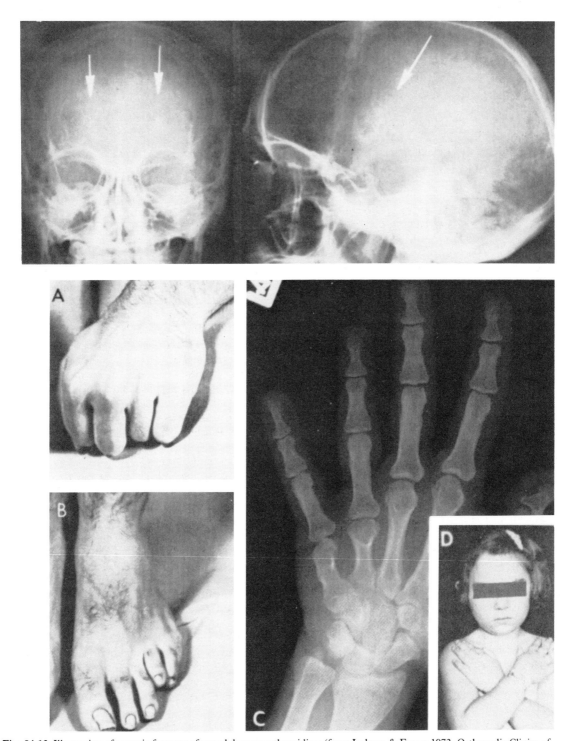

Fig. 84.12 Illustration of somatic features of pseudohypoparathyroidism (from Jackson & Frame 1972, Orthopedic Clinics of North America). Shortened metacarpal bones are illustrated in (A) & (C) and the shortened metatarsals are shown in (B). The rounded face in a girl who has short stature is shown in (D). Basal ganglia calcification seen on skull X–ray is shown on the top illustration.

or without the typical skeletal or somatic abnormalities of Albright's osteodystrophy. Fuller Albright et al (1942) described patients with the clinical picture of hypoparathyroidism in whom the cause was a lack of response to parathyroid hormone, instead of being related to insufficient hormone production. The biochemical findings are hypocalcaemia, hyperphosphataemia and elevated parathyroid hormone levels.

PHP has been classified into 2 types: PHP type 1 with no increase in urinary cyclic AMP (cAMP) levels after parathyroid extract (PTE) infusion and PHP type 2 with an increase in cAMP after PTE (Drezner et al, 1973). The clinical picture is one of convulsions and tetany and other evidence of neuromuscular irritability similar to that seen in patients with primary or post-surgical hypoparathyroidism. Additionally, some patients with PHP show characteristic somatic abnormalities of short stature and shortened fingers and toes (Fig. 84.12). Some patients with PHP are mentally retarded. The diagnosis of PHP depends on demonstrating resistance to PTH by the lack of increase in urinary excretion of phosphate following PTH administration. The serum parathyroid hormone level is elevated in PHP accounting for the term hormonoplethoric type of hypoparathyroidism used by Nusynowitz et al (1976). Farfel et al (1980) described a generalized deficiency of the N protein component of adenyl cyclase in some patients with PHP type 1, which was measurable at about 50% of normal levels in erythrocyte membranes. Erythrocytes of PHP type II contained normal levels of this receptor-cyclase coupling protein, as would be expected, since the defect in this condition is associated with a decreased urinary cAMP response to PTH, but is related to a defect in response to cAMP itself. They described the classic PHP-1 phenotype (with the brachydactyly and short stature and the deficiency of erythrocyte N protein) as following a pattern suggestive of an autosomal dominant mode of inheritance. Farfel et al (1980) reported some families in which PHP-1 not associated with abnormalities of N protein. Another family reported by this group (Bourne et al 1981) have the erythrocyte defect in a pattern of affected individuals suggesting autosomal recessive inheritance.

The application of the knowledge of a deficiency of erythrocyte N protein to the study of families should make it possible to elucidate the genetic mechanisms in particular kindreds and the delineation of specific types of PHP-1. It should also allow the early detection and treatment of some cases. It will be very important to determine which types are associated with mental retardation and whether or not such early detection and treatment will prevent the mental retardation which is so troublesomely and unpredictably associated with pseudohypoparathyroidism.

Pseudo-pseudohypoparathyroidism (PPHP) is a condition described by Albright et al (1952) to indicate those patients who have the skeletal or somatic defects of pseudohypoparathyroidism (Fig. 84.12) with normal calcium values (a false PHP). Cases in which PPHP and PHP exist in the same individuals at different stages (Palubinskas & Davies, 1959) and PPHP and PHP exist in different members of the same families (Mann et al, 1962; Williams et al, 1977) suggest that these conditions may represent variable expression of one genetic disease entity.

Genetics

Pseudohypoparathyroidism has in the past been considered to be inherited by an X–linked mechanism as discussed in McKusick's catalogues (1978). The problems of attributing PHP to this genetic mechanism are discussed by McKusick. These problems are especially evident as the result of an increasing appreciation of the variability in the biochemical defects in a syndrome in which the heterogeneity is so evident.

Genetic counselling

Genetic counselling in pseudohypoparathyroidism is extremely difficult and will continue to be so until we have a more firm biochemical understanding of the heterogeneous entities which comprise this condition. The mental retardation associated at times is a great concern to the counsellor even in those families in which it has not been evident in known affected individuals. At present genetic counselling in PHP must be individualized and must depend on thorough pedigree taking within the family of that individual and the delineation of the manifestations in those affected within that kindred. This requires the utilization in those family studies of all the biochemical parameters available at the time. In the many instances in which the cases appear to be sporadic or to be a part of only a limited number of affected individuals in a kindred, the genetic counsellor must express to the patients and their families the difficulties of providing accurate predictions of risk in the state of knowledge of the condition at that particular time.

REFERENCES

Alberts W M, McMeekin J O, George, J M 1980 Mixed multiple endocrine neoplasia syndromes. JAMA 244: 1236–1237
Albright F, Burnett C H, Smith P H, Parson, W 1942 Pseudohypoparathyroidism, an example of 'Seabright-Bantam Syndrome.' Endocrinology 30: 922–932
Albright F, Forbes A P, Henneman P H 1952 Pseudo-pseudo hypoparathyroidism. Transactions of the Association of American Physicians 65: 337–350

Ballard H S, Frame B, Hartsock R J 1964 Familial multiple endocrine adenoma – peptic ulcer complex. Medicine (Baltimore) 43: 481–515

Baylin S B, Gann, D S Hsu, S H 1976 Clonal origin of inherited medullary thyroid carcinoma and pheochromocytoma. Science 193: 321–323

Baylin S B, Hsu S H, Gann D S, Smallridge R C, Wells S A Jr 1978 Inherited medullary thyroid carcinoma: a final monoclonal mutation in one of multiple clones of susceptible cells. Science 199: 429–431

Block M A, Jackson C E, Tashjian A H Jr 1975 Management of parathyroid glands in surgery for medullary thyroid carcinoma. Archives of Surgery 110: 617–624

Block M A, Jackson C E, Tashjian A H Jr 1978 Management of occult medullary thyroid carcinoma: evidenced only by serum calcitonin elevations after apparently adequate neck operations. Archives of Surgery 113: 368–372

Block M A, Jackson C E, Greenawald K A, Yott J B, Tashjian A H Jr 1980 Clinical characteristics distinguishing hereditary from sporadic medullary thyroid carcinoma. Archives of Surgery 115: 142–148

Boden G, Owen O E 1977 Familial hyperglucagonemia – an autosomal dominant disorder. New England Journal of Medicine 296: 534–538

Boey J H, Cooke T J C, Gilbert J M, Sweeney E C, Taylor S 1975 Occurrence of other endocrine tumours in primary hyperparathyroidism. Lancet 2: 781–784

Boonstra C E, Jackson C E 1962 The clinical value of routine serum calcium analysis. Annals of Internal Medicine 57: 963–969

Boonstra C E, Jackson C E 1965 Hyperparathyroidism detected by routine serum calcium analysis: prevalence in a clinic population. Annals of Internal Medicine 63: 468–474

Boonstra C E, Jackson C E 1971 Serum calcium survey for hyperparathyroidism: results in 50 000 clinic patients. American Journal of Clinical Pathology 55: 523–526

Bourne H R, Farfel Z, Brickman A S 1981 Pseudo-hypoparathyroidism: an inherited disorder of adenylate cyclase. In: Advances in Cyclic Nucleotide Research Research 14: 43–49

Bronsky D 1970 Hyperparathyroidism with Albright's osteodystrophy: Case report and a proposed new classification of parathyroid disease. Journal of Clinical Endocrinology and Metabolism 31: 271–276

Cameron D, Spiro H M 1978 Zollinger-Ellison Syndrome with multiple endocrine adenomatosis type II. New England Journal of Medicine 299: 152–153

Carney J A, Sizemore G W, Sheps S G 1976 Adrenal medullary disease in multiple endocrine neoplasia, type 2: pheochromocytoma and its precursors. American Journal of Clinical Pathology 66: 279–290

Carney J A, Go V L W, Gordon H, Northcutt R C, Pearse A G E, Sheps S 1980 Familial pheochromocytoma and islet cell tumor of the pancreas. American Journal of Medicine 68: 515–521

Chong G C, Beahrs O H, Sizemore G W, Woolner L H 1975 Medullary carcinoma of the thyroid gland. Cancer 35: 695–704

DeLellis R A, Wolfe H G, Gagel R F 1976 Adrenal medullary hyperplasia: a morphometric analysis in patients with familial medullary thyroid carcinoma. American Journal of Pathology 83: 177–196

DiGeorge A M 1965 Discussions on a new concept of the cellular basis of immunity. Journal of Pediatrics 67: 907–908

Dinnen J S, Greenwood R H, Jones J H, Walker D A, Williams E D 1977 Parathyroid carcinoma in familial hyperparathyroidism. Journal of Clinical Pathology 30: 966–975

Drezner M, Neelon F A, Lebovitz H E 1973 Pseudohypoparathyroidism type II: a possible defect in the reception of the cyclic AMP signal. New England Journal of Medicine 289: 1056–1060

Farfel Z, Brickman A S, Kaslow H R, Brothers V M, Bourne H R 1980 Defect of receptor – cyclase coupling protein in pseudohypoparathyroidism. New England Journal of Medicine 303: 237–242

Fialkow P J, Jackson C E, Block M A, Greenawald K A 1977 Multicellular origin of parathyroid adenomas. New England Journal of Medicine 297: 696–698

Foley T P Jr, Harrison H C, Arnaud C D, Harrison H E 1972 Familial benign hypercalcemia. Journal of Pediatrics 81: 1060–1067

Francke U, Holmes L B, Atkins L 1979 Aniridia – Wilm's tumor association: evidence for specific deletion of 11 p13. Cytogenetics and Cell Genetics 24: 183–192

Frayha R A, Nassar V H, Dagher F, Salti I S 1972 Familial parathyroid carcinoma. Lebanese Medical Journal 25: 299–309

Friedman M, Hatcher G, Watson I 1967 Primary hypomagnesemia with secondary hypocalcemia in an infant. Lancet 1: 703–705

Gagel R F, Melvin K E W, Tashjian A H Jr, Miller H H, Feldman Z T, Wolfe H J, DeLellis R A, Cervi-Skinner S, Reichlin S 1975 Natural history of the familial medullary thyroid carcinoma – pheochromocytoma syndrome and the identification of preneoplastic stages by screening studies, a five year report. Transactions of the Association of American Physicians 88: 177–191

Gagel R F, Jackson C E, Block M A, Feldman Z T, Reichlin S, Hamilton B P, Tashjian A H Jr 1982 Age-related risk of development of hereditary medullary thyroid carcinoma. Journal of Pediatrics 101: 941–946

Goldbloom R B, Gillis D A, Prasad M 1972 Hereditary parathyroid hyperplasia: a surgical emergency of early infancy. Pediatrics 49: 514–523

Gorlin R J, Sedano H O, Vickers R A, Cervenka J 1968 Multiple mucosal neuromas, pheochromocytoma and medullary carcinoma of the thyroid – a syndrome. Cancer 22: 293–299

Hansen O P, Hansen M, Hansen H H, Rose B 1976 Multiple endocrine adenomatosis of mixed type. Acta Medica Scandinavica 200: 327–331

Heath H, Purnell D C 1980 Urinary cyclic 3',5' adenosine monophosphate responses to exogenous and endogenous parathyroid hormone in familial benign hypercalcemia and primary hyperparathyroidism. Journal of Laboratory and Clinical Medicine 96: 974–984

Heikkinen E S, Akerblom H K 1977 Diagnostic and operative problems in multiple pheochromocytomas. Journal of Pediatric Surgery 12: 157–163

Hennessy J F, Wells S A Jr, Ontjes D A, Cooper C W 1974 A comparison of pentagastrin injection and calcium infusion as provocative agents for the detection of medullary carcinoma of the thyroid. Journal of Clinical Endocrinology and Metabolism 39: 487–500

Jackson C E 1958 Hereditary hyperparathyroidism associated with recurrent pancreatitis. Annals of Internal Medicine 49: 829–836

Jackson C E, Boonstra C E 1966 Hereditary hypercalcemia and parathyroid hyperplasia without definite hyperparathyroidism. Journal of Laboratory and Clinical Medicine 68: 883

Jackson C E, Boonstra C E 1967 The relationship of

hereditary hyperparathyroidism to multiple endocrine adenomatosis. American Journal of Medicine 43: 727–734

Jackson C E, Frame B 1972 Diagnosis and management of parathyroid disorders. Orthopedic Clinics of North America 3: 699–712

Jackson C E, Kleerekoper M 1981 Hereditary hypocalciuric hypercalcemia is benign in 15 year followup. Clinical Research 29: 409A

Jackson C E, Tashjian A H Jr, Block M A 1973 Detection of medullary thyroid cancer by calcitonin assay in families. Annals of Internal Medicine 78: 845–852

Jackson, C E, Frame B, Block M A 1977 Prevalence of endocrine neoplasia syndromes in genetic studies of parathyroid tumors. In: Mulvihill J J, Miller R W, Fraumini J F Jr (ed) Genetics of Human Cancer, Raven Press, New York, p 205–208

Jackson C E, Block M A, Greenawald K A, Tashjian A H Jr 1979 The two-mutational-event theory in medullary thyroid cancer. American Journal of Human Genetics 31: 704–710

Jackson C E, Block M A, Greenawald K A, Fialkow P J 1980 Multiple cell origin of hyperparathyroidism. Clinical Research 28: 788A

Janson K L, Roberts J A, Varela M 1978 Multiple endocrine adenomatosis: in support of the common origin theories. Journal of Urolology 119: 161–165

Keiser H R, Beaven M A, Doppman J, Wells S Jr, Buja L M 1973 Sipple's syndrome: medullary thyroid carcinoma, pheochromocytoma, and parathyroid disease. Annals of Internal Medicine 78: 561–579

Khairi M R A, Dexter R N, Burzynski N J, Johnston C C Jr 1975 Mucosal neuroma, pheochromocytoma and medullary thyroid carcinoma: multiple endocrine neoplasia type 3. Medicine (Baltimore) 54: 89–112

Knudson A G Jr 1971 Mutation and cancer: statistical study of retinoblastoma. Proceedings of the National Academy of Sciences USA 68: 820–823

Knudson A G Jr 1980 Genetics and Cancer. American Journal of Medicine 69: 1–3

Leborgne J, Le Neel J-C, Buzelin F, Malvy P 1975 Cancer familial des parathyroides. Journal de Chirurgie (Paris) 109: 315–326

Mallette L E, Bilezikian J P, Ketcham A S, Aurbach, G D 1974 Parathyroid carcinoma in familial hyperparathyroidism. American Journal of Medicine 57: 642–648

Mann J B, Alteman S, Hill A G 1962 Albright's hereditary osteodystrophy comprising pseudohypoparathyroidism and pseudo-pseudohypoparathyroidism with report of two cases representing the complete syndrome occurring in successive generations. Annals of Internal Medicine 56: 315–342

Marx S J, Spiegel A M, Brown E M, Aurbach G D 1977 Family studies in patients with primary parathyroid hyperplasia. American Journal of Medicine 62: 698–706

Marx S J, Spiegel A M, Brown E M, Gardner D G, Downs R W, Attie M, Aurbach G D 1980a Familial hypocalciuric hypercalcemia. In: DeLuca H F & Anast C C (eds) Pediatric Diseases Related to Calcium, Elsevier North Holland, New York p 413–431

Marx S J, Stock J L, Attie M F, Downs R W Jr, Gardner D G, Brown E M, Spiegel A M, Doppman J L, Brennan M F 1980b Familial hypocalciuric hypercalcemia: recognition among patients referred after unsuccessful parathyroid exploration. Annals of Internal Medicine 92: 351–356

McKusick V A 1978 Mendelian inheritance in man: catalogs of autosomal dominant, autosomal recessive and X–linked

phenotypes. Fifth edn. The Johns Hopkins University Press, Baltimore p 710

Neufeld M, Maclaren N, Blizzard R 1980 Autoimmune polyglandular syndromes. Pediatric Annals 9: 154–162

Nusynowitz M L, Frame B, Kolb F O 1976 The spectrum of the hypoparathyroid states: a classification based on physiologic principles. Medicine (Baltimore) 55: 105–119

Palubinskas A J, Davies H 1959 Calcification of the basal ganglia of the brain. American Journal of Roentgenology 82: 806–822

Peden V H 1960 True idiopathic hypo-parathyroidism as a sex–linked recessive trait. American Journal of Human Genetics 12: 323–337

Ptak T, Kirsner J B 1970 The Zollinger-Ellison Syndrome, polyendocrine adenomatosis and other endocrine associations with peptic ulcer. Advances in Internal Medicine 16: 213–242

Rimoin D L, Schimke R N 1971 Genetic disorders of the endocrine glands. C V Mosby, St Louis p 79–112

Samaan N A, Hill C S Jr, Beceiro J R, Schultz P N 1973 Immunoreactive calcitonin in medullary carcinoma of the thyroid and in maternal and cord serum. Journal of Laboratory and Clinical Medicine 81: 671–681

Schantz A, Castleman B 1973 Parathyroid carcinoma: a study of 70 cases. Cancer 31: 600–605

Schimke R N, Hartmann W H 1965 Familial amyloid-producing medullary thyroid carcinoma and pheochromocytoma: a distinct genetic entity. Annals of Internal Medicine 63: 1027–1039

Schimke R N, Hartmann W H, Prout T E, Rimoin D L 1968 Syndrome of bilateral pheochromocytoma, medullary thyroid carcinoma and multiple neuromas. New England Journal of Medicine 279: 1–7

Silva O L, Snider R H, Moore C F, Becker K L 1979 Urine calcitonin as a test for medullary thyroid cancer: a new screening procedure. Annals of Surgery 189: 269–274

Sipple J H 1961 The association of pheochromocytoma with carcinoma of the thyroid gland. American Journal of Medicine 31: 163–166

Sizemore G W, Carney J A, Heath H 1977 Epidemiology of medullary carcinoma of the thyroid gland: a 5 year experience (1971–1976) Surgical Clinics of North America 57: 633–645

Spinner M W, Blizzard R M, Childs B 1968 Clinical and genetic heterogeneity in idiopathic Addison's disease and hypoparathyroidism. Journal of Clinical Endocrinology and Metabolism. 28: 795–804

Steele R W, Limas C, Thurman G B, Schuelein M, Bauer H, Bellanti J A 1972 Familial thymic aplasia. New England Journal of Medicine 287: 787–791

Steiner A L, Goodman A D, Powers S R 1968 Study of a kindred with pheochromocytoma, medullary thyroid carcinoma, hyperparathyroidism and Cushing's disease: multiple endocrine neoplasia type 2. Medicine (Baltimore) 47: 371–409

Stewart A F, Horst R, Deftos L J, Cadman E C, Lang R, Broadus A E 1980 Biochemical evaluation of patients with cancer-associated hypercalcemia: evidence for humoral and nonhumoral groups. New England Journal of Medicine 303: 1377–1383

Stromme J H, Nesbakken R, Normann T, Skyorten F, Skyberg D, Johannessen B 1969 Familial hypomagnesemia. Acta Paediatrica Scandinavica 58: 433–444

Tashjian A H Jr, Howland B G, Melvin K E W 1970 Immunoassay of human calcitonin. Clinical measurement, relation to serum calcium and studies in patients with medullary carcinoma. New England Journal of Medicine 283: 890–895

Tateishi R, Wada A, Ishigura S, Ehara M, Sakamoto H, Miki T, Mori Y, Matsui Y, Ishikawa O 1978 Coexistence of bilateral pheochromocytoma and pancreatic islet cell tumor: report of a case and review of the literature. Cancer 42: 2928–2934

Thompson N W, Carpenter L C, Kessler D L, Nishiyama R H 1978 Hereditary neonatal hyperparathyroidism. Archives of Surgery 113: 100–103

Van Dyke D L, Jackson C E, Babu V R 1981 Prometaphase chromosomes in cancer families: multiple endocrine neoplasia 2 syndrome and neurofibromatosis. Clinical Research 29: 37A

Van Heerden J A, Weiland L H, ReMine W H, Walls J T, Purnell D C 1979 Cancer of the parathyroid glands. Archives of Surgery 114: 475–480

Wells S A Jr, Ontjes D A, Cooper C W, Hennessy J F, Ellis G J, McPherson H T, Sabiston D C 1975 The early diagnosis of medullary carcinoma of the thyroid gland in patients with multiple endocrine neoplasia type II. Annals of Surgery 182: 362–370

Wells S A Jr, Ellis G J, Gunnells J C, Schneider A B,

Sherwood L M 1976 Parathyroid autotransplantation in primary parathyroid hyperplasia. New England Journal of Medicine 295: 57–62

Wells S A Jr, Baylin S B, Linehan W M, Farrell R E, Cox E B, Cooper C W 1978 Provocative agents and the diagnosis of medullary carcinoma of the thyroid gland. Annals of Surgery 188: 139–141

Wermer P 1954 Genetic aspects of adenomatosis of the endocrine glands. American Journal of Medicine 16: 363–371

Williams A J, Wilkinson J L, Taylor W H 1977 Pseudohypoparathyroidism: variable manifestations within a family. Archives of Disease in Childhood 52: 798–800

Wolfe H J, Melvin K E W, Cervi-Skinner S J, Al Saadi A A, Juliar J F, Jackson C E, Tashjian A H Jr 1973 C-cell hyperplasia preceding medullary thyroid carcinoma. New England Journal of Medicine 289: 437–441

Yunis J J, Ramsay N 1978 Retinoblastoma and sub band deletion of chromosome 13. American Journal of Diseases of Children 132: 161–163

Yunis J J, Sawyer J R, Ball D W 1978 The characterization of high-resolution G-banded chromosomes of man. Chromosoma (Berlin) 67: 293–307

85

Diabetes mellitus

J. I. Rotter and D. L. Rimoin

INTRODUCTION

Diabetes mellitus is a diagnostic term for a group of disorders characterized by abnormalities in glucose homeostasis, or more simply, 'too much sugar' in the blood and/or urine (West, 1978; Cahill, 1979a). Its manifestations can range from asymptomatic glucose intolerance (i.e. higher than normal blood glucose levels to an administered glucose load) to an acute medical emergency (diabetic ketoacidosis) to chronic complications such as nephropathy, neuropathy, retinopathy, or accelerated atherosclerosis. It is among the most common of chronic disorders, affecting up to 5–10% of the adult population of the Western world. Its prevalence varies over the globe, with certain populations at extremely high risk, such as certain American Indian tribes and the inhabitants of Micronesia and Polynesia (West, 1978; Zimmet, 1979; Knowler et al, 1981).

It has been clearly established in recent years that diabetes mellitus is a genetically heterogeneous group of disorders that share glucose intolerance in common (Creutzfeldt et al, 1976; Rotter et al, 1978; Fajans et al, 1978; Friedman & Fialkow, 1980; Rotter & Rimoin, 1981a, b). (Heterogeneity implies that different genetic and/or environmental aetiologic factors can result in similar phenotypes). The concept of genetic heterogeneity has significantly altered the genetic analysis of this common disorder. It is now apparent that diabetes and glucose intolerance are not diagnostic terms, but like anaemia, are simply symptom complexes or laboratory abnormalities respectively, which can result from a number of distinct aetiologic factors. Diabetes mellitus is currently classified into 'idiopathic diabetes mellitus' and 'diabetes or glucose intolerance associated with genetic syndromes and other conditions' (National Diabetes Data Group, 1979). The majority of cases of diabetes mellitus currently are placed into the idiopathic category, and the exact prevalence of the latter category is unknown. The 'idiopathic' category is subdivided into two major groups – an insulin dependent type (IDDM) (often referred to as juvenile onset) and a non-insulin dependent type (NIDDM) (often referred to as maturity

onset). This separation is based on family, twin, metabolic, immunologic, and HLA association studies, to be reviewed below. There is now evidence that even these major categories can be further subdivided. This subclassification is of major importance, because it is only through the delineation of this heterogeneity that distinct disease entities will be identified. To be meaningful, pathophysiological studies, genetic analysis, epidemiologic prospective studies, delineation of risk factors, and creation of risks tables for genetic counselling, must be performed on each of the specific disease entities constituting the diabetic phenotype.

DIFFICULTIES IN GENETIC STUDIES AND ANALYSIS

For many years the genetics of diabetes mellitus was one of the most confused topics in medicine. Although familial aggregation of diabetes has been apparent for years, and classic twin studies indicated that a large component of this familial aggregation is due to genetic factors, there has been little agreement as to the specific nature of the genetic factors involved (Rimoin & Schimke, 1971; Rotter & Rimoin, 1981a). All possible modes of inheritance have been proposed for diabetes and proponents for most of these hypotheses exist today. Indeed, they are probably all correct, at least for specific types of the diabetic syndrome. Why has there been such confusion?

The geneticist is confronted with a number of obstacles in his attempts to unravel this problem, including differences in the definition of affected individuals, modification of the expression of the diabetic genotype by environmental factors, and variability in the age of onset of the disease. One of the major sources of confusion in the study of diabetes mellitus has been, and often still is, the definition of an 'affected' individual. Some investigators will call an individual diabetic only if he has clinical symptoms of the disease, while others will accept a mildly abnormal glucose tolerance test. There is still some argument as to whether diabetes mellitus, or at least some forms, are a distinct disease or simply the tail end of a normal distribution of blood sugar concentrations.

Another problem in the definition of affected individuals is the marked clinical variability of diabetes. The phenotypic expression of the diabetic genotype appears to be modified by a variety of environmental factors, including diet, obesity, infection, and physical activity, as well as sex and parity. Obese adult diabetics may lose all signs of the disorder, clinical as well as chemical, if their weight returns to normal. Because of the marked variability in the age of onset of the disease, at any given time only a fraction of those individuals possessing the diabetic genotype may be recognized. Therefore, it is impossible to say at any given point in time whether a clinically unaffected individual carries the mutant genotype. Thus, longitudinal studies may be required to detect affected family members with clinical disease.

The high prevalence of the disease in the population presents additional difficulties for the geneticist. Is a relative affected because he has the same genotype, shares the same environment, or has a chance occurrence of a common disorder? The diabetic syndromes are sufficiently common that different forms of them may occasionally occur in the same family by chance alone.

The most important impediment to genetic analysis is the lack of knowledge concerning the basic defect(s) in each of the disorders leading to diabetes. Because of this there is no certain method for detecting all individuals with the mutant genotype prior to its clinical manifestation, that is, individuals who possess the diabetic genotype but have no signs of abnormal carbohydrate metabolism.

Nevertheless, with all these obstacles, major strides have been made in the last several years in the search for delineating the genetic basis of the diabetic syndromes. This progress has come through increasing recognition of the potential genetic heterogeneity of diabetes, and its delineation by a variety of lines of evidence.

EARLY GENETIC STUDIES

To provide a background, the earlier observations regarding the genetics of diabetes will be briefly reviewed.

Familial aggregation of diabetes
Clinical heterogeneity and the importance of genetic factors have long been recognized in diabetes. For example, the Hindu physicians Charaka and Sushruta, over 2000 years ago, commented on 'honey urine' of two causes – genetic, i.e., passed from one generation to another in 'the seed', and environmental, i.e., injudicious diet; and also the existence of two types of disease, one associated with emaciation, dehydration, polyuria and lassitude,

and the other associated with stout build, gluttony, obesity, and sleepiness (Simpson, 1976; Cahill, 1979a).

Many authors have shown that diabetics have an 'increased family history' of the disease (Rimoin & Schimke, 1971). In most reports the frequency of diabetics with positive family histories of the disease ranges from 25 to 50%. Since the frequency of non-diabetic individuals with a positive family history of diabetes has usually been found to be below 15%, this family history information has been used to support the hypothesis that diabetes mellitus is a hereditary disorder. These types of data, however, are not very powerful. A more accurate method of assessing familial aggregation is by comparing the prevalence of the disorder among specific relatives of an affected individual to that found among similar relatives of a control group. Pincus and White (1933) were the first to use this method in the study of diabetes when they statistically established the increased prevalence of the disease among the relatives of diabetics. These findings have since been confirmed by many other investigators (Table 85.1). Using more sensitive markers of the diabetic genotype, such as oral, intravenous, and cortisone-induced glucose tolerance tests, the prevalence of affected individuals among the relatives of diabetics is even higher (usually ranging between 10 and 30% of the parents, sibs, or close relatives, as compared to a prevalence of 1 to 6% of the relatives of nondiabetic individuals). Thus the prevalence of both clinical diabetes and abnormal glucose tolerance is significantly greater among the close relatives of diabetics than among similar relatives of nondiabetic individuals.

Early twin studies
Familial aggregation of a trait may be caused by either genetic or environmental factors. Twin studies represent one approach to resolving this question. The frequency of concordance (both members of the twin pair affected) of monozygotic (identical) twins is compared with that of dizygotic (fraternal) twins. Monozygotic twins share all genes, and thus theoretically should be concordant for disorders with pure genetic aetiology. Dizygotic twins share only half their genes and are no more alike genetically than any pair of siblings.

Twin studies have confirmed the importance of genetic factors in the aetiology of diabetes (Table 85.2). Using clinical diabetes as the critera for affected, most investigators have found the concordance rate for monozygotic twins to vary from 45 to 96% and that for dizygotic twins to range between 3 and 37%. With NIDDM, when glucose tolerance tests are performed in the 'non-diabetic' monozygotic co-twins, the concordance rate is usually above 70%. Thus the concordance of diabetes mellitus in monozygotic twins is significantly greater than for dizygotic twins. Furthermore, the concordance for older monozygotic twins approaches 100% and concordance

Table 85.1 Prevalence of diabetes and glucose intolerance among the relatives of diabetic and control patients

Author	Relatives studied	Criteria	Percent affected [†] Diabetic	control
Keen & Track (1968)*	Parents	Clinical	4.0-9.7	1.1-2.9
Working Party College of Practitioners (1965)*	Parents	Clinical	4.2-9.2	1.5-3.1
Levit and Pessikova (1934)	Parents	Clinical	4.3	
Simpson (1964)	Parents	Clinical	4.8	
Harris (1950)	Parents	Clinical	5.0	
Thompson & Watson (1952)	Parents	Clinical	7.1	
Pincus & White (1933)	Parents	Clinical	8.3	2.0
Bartels (1953)	Parents	Clinical	9.0	
Hunter & McKay (1967)**	Parents	IV GTT	24.0	
Braunsteiner et al (1966)	Parents	IV GTT	76.0	
Working Party College of Practitioners (1965)	Sibs	Clinical	2.4-4.8	0.2-2.1
Keen and Track (1968)*	Sibs	Clinical	3.3-3.5	0.5-0.8
Levit & Pessikova (1934)	Sibs	Clinical	3.6	
Harris (1950)	Sibs	Clinical	4.3	
Pincus & White (1933)	Sibs	Clinical	5.9	0.6
Thompson & Watson (1952)	Sibs	Clinical	9.0	
Kobberling (1969)**	Sibs	Clinical	10.9	
Bartels (1953)**	Sibs	Clinical	11.7	
Burkeholder et al (1957)**	Sibs	Oral GTT	18.0	
Sisk (1968)**	Sibs	Oral GTT	23.0	
Pickens (1964)**	Sibs	Oral GTT	29.0	
Kobberling et al (1969)	Sibs	Oral GTT	38.9	
Hanhart (1951)	Close relatives	Clinical	5.3	1.2
Lambert et al (1961)	Relatives	Oral GTT	6.0	3.0
Notelovitz (1969)	Close relatives	Oral GTT	12.3	6.0
Jakobson & Nikkila (1969)	Close relatives	Oral GTT	13.7	
Joslin et al (1959)	Close relatives	Random Sugar	14.0	2.0
Conn & Fajans (1961)	Close relatives	Oral GTT	18.0	<1
Joslin et al (1959)	Close relatives	Oral GTT	25.0	2.0
Lambert et al (1961)	Relatives	Cortisone GTT	23.0	6.0
Conn & Fajans (1961)	Close relatives	Cortisone GTT	26.0	4.0

* Depending on age of proband.
[†] Figures rounded off to one decimal place.
** Probands are all juvenile diabetics.

increases with more sensitive markers for the diabetic genotype (Pyke, 1979; Barnett et al, 1981a, b). Since concordance is not complete among younger monozygotic twins or when clinical criteria alone are used, it is obvious that environmental factors are important for the phenotypic expression of the diabetic genotype.

THE HETEROGENEITY HYPOTHESIS – EARLY EVIDENCE

Although the evidence derived from studies of familial aggregation and twins leaves no doubt as to the importance of genetic factors in the aetiology of diabetes, there had been little agreement as to the nature of the genetic factors involved. During the past several decades every possible mode of genetic transmission has been proposed, objections to all of them have been raised, and even today there are proponents of each of these hypotheses. This confusion could, in a large part, be explained by genetic heterogeneity. Indeed the evidence marshalled for the concept of heterogeneity within diabetes is now overwhelming (Creutzfeldt et al, 1976; Rotter et al, 1978; Fajans et al, 1978; Friedman & Fialkow, 1980; Rotter & Rimoin 1981a, b). In 1966, the hypothesis of genetic heterogeneity was proposed based on several lines of evidence (Rimoin, 1967). Indirect evidence included: (1) to the existence of distinct, mostly rare genetic disorders, now numbering some 45, that have glucose intolerance as one of their features; (2) genetic heterogeneity in diabetic animal models; (3) ethnic variability in prevalence and clinical features; (4) clinical variability between the thin ketosis prone, insulin dependent juvenile onset diabetic versus the obese, nonketotic insulin resistant adult onset diabetic; and (5) physiologic variability – the demonstration of decreased plasma insulin in juvenile versus the relative hyperinsulinism of maturity onset diabetics. In addition,

Table 85.2 Concordance of diabetes and glucose intolerance in twins

Author	Criteria	Age of patients	Per cent concordant monozygotic	dizygotic
White (1965)	Clinical		48.0	3.0
Werner (1936)	Clinical		75.0	10.0
Lemser (In Mimura & Miyao, 1962)	Clinical		85.5	29.2
Verschuer (In Mimura & Miyao, 1962)	Clinical		84.0	37.0
Steiner (1936)	Clinical		96.6	9.1
Harvald & Hauge (1963, 1965)	Clinical		47.0	9.5
Harvald & Hauge (1963, 1965)	Clinical	> 70 years	73.0	32.0
Harvald & Hauge (1963)	GTT		57.0	9.0
Gottlieb & Root (1968)	Clinical	<40 years	10.0	3.1
Gottlieb & Root (1968)	Clinical	>40 years	70.0	3.5
Gottlieb & Root (1968)	GTT		14.0	35.0
Then Berg (1939)	GTT		65.0	22.0
Then Berg (1939)	GTT	>43 years	100.0	39.0
Pyke & Taylor (1967)	GTT		78.0	
Cerasi & Luft (1967)	Glucose infusion		92.0	
Mimura & Miyao (1962)	Combined data		80.5	28.0
Tattersall & Pyke (1972)	Clinical & GTT (96 pairs)	<40 years	52.5	
		>40 years	91.9	
Pyke & Nelson (1976)	Clinical & GTT (106 pairs)	<40 years	50.0	
		>40 years	92.9	
Pyke (1978)	Clinical & GTT (150 pairs)	<45 years	50.9	
		>45 years	88.6	
Pyke (1979)	Clinical & GTT (185 pairs)	Insulin dependent	55.3	
		Noninsulin dependent[†]	88.6	
Barnett et al (1981a)	Clinical & GTT (200 pairs)	Insulin dependent	54.4	
		Noninsulin dependent[†]	90.6	

[†] In the NIDDM discordant pairs, the index twin has been ascertained only within the last 5 years)

some direct evidence for heterogeneity came from clinical genetic studies which suggested that juvenile and adult onset diabetes differ genetically (Simpson, 1976; Rotter et al, 1978).

Genetic syndromes associated with glucose intolerance

There are some 45 distinct genetic disorders associated with glucose intolerance, and in some cases, clinical diabetes (see Table 85.3) (Rimoin & Schimke, 1971; Rimoin, 1976; Rotter & Rimoin, 1981a; Rimoin & Rotter, 1982). Although individually rare, these syndromes demonstrate that mutations at different loci can produce glucose intolerance. Furthermore, they illustrate the wide variety of pathogenetic mechanisms which can result in glucose intolerance. The pathogenetic mechanisms range from absolute insulin deficiency due to pancreatic degeneration, in such disorders as hereditary relapsing pancreatitis, cystic fibrosis, and polyendocrine deficiency disease; to relative insulinopaenia in the growth hormone deficiency syndromes; to inhibition of insulin secretion in the hereditary pheochromocytoma syndromes associated with elevated catecholamines; to various deficits in the interaction of insulin and its receptor in the non-ketotic insulin resistant states such as

myotonic dystrophy and the lipoatrophic diabetes syndromes; to relative insulin resistance in the hereditary syndromes associated with obesity. Even within these individual categories, further division can be made, either by mechanism or by genetic criteria. For example, the lipoatrophic syndromes – characterized by the total or partial absence of adipose tissue, hyperlipidaemia, insulin resistance, nonketotic diabetes mellitus, increased basal metabolic rate, and hepatomegaly – can be further subdivided into a recessive, several dominant, and nongenetic forms (Kobberling, 1976b; Rotter & Rimoin, 1982). There are a variety of syndromes which are characterized by marked insulin resistance. The pathophysiology of the resistance in many of these disorders has recently been defined by studies of the insulin receptor and its interactions (Flier et al, 1979; Rimoin and Rotter, 1982). Even within what is currently felt to be one genetic entity, multiple endocrine adenoma type I, an autosomal dominant disorder characterized by pituitary, parathyroid, and pancreatic adenomas, a variety of different hormonal mechanisms can result in insulin antagonism; e.g. eosinophilic adenomas of the pituitary may secrete growth hormone, adenomas of the adrenal gland can secrete cortisol, and nonbeta islet cells of the pancreas can produce glucagon. Each of the hormones indi-

Table 85.3 Genetic syndromes associated with glucose intolerance and diabetes mellitus

Syndromes	Types of DM	Associated clinical findings	Pattern of inheritance
Syndromes associated with pancreatic degeneration			
Congenital absence of the pancreas	IDDM (Congenital)	IUGR, poor adipose and muscle, malabsorption, dehydration	? AR
Congenital absence of the islets of Langerhans	IDDM (Congenital)	IUGR, dehydration	? AR or XR
Hereditary relapsing pancreatitis	IGT → IDDM	Abdominal pain, chronic pancreatitis	AD
Cystic fibrosis	IGT → IDDM	Malabsorption, chronic respiratory disease	AR
Polyendocrine deficiency disease (Schmidt syndrome)	IDDM	Autoimmune endocrine disease: hypothyroidism, hypoadrenalism	?AR, AD
IgA deficiency, malabsorption and diabetes	IDDM	IgA deficiency, malabsorption	?AD
Haemochromatosis	NIDDM	Hepatic, pancreatic, skin, cardiac, and endocrine complications of iron storage	AR
Thalassaemia	IGT → NIDDM	Anaemia, iron overload	AR
Alpha-1-antitrypsin deficiency	IGT	Emphysema, cirrhosis	AR
Hereditary endocrine disorders with glucose intolerance			
Isolated growth hormone deficiency	NIDDM	Proportionate dwarfism	AR, AD
Hereditary panhypopituitary dwarfism	NIDDM	Proportionate dwarfism, hypogonadism ± TSH & ACTH deficiency	AR, XR
Laron dwarfism	NIDDM	Proportionate dwarfism	AR
Pheochromocytoma	IGT	Hypertension, tremor, paroxysmal sweating	AD
Multiple endocrine adenomatosis I syndrome	IGT	Pituitary (acromegaly), parathyroid (renal stones), pancreatic adenomas (peptic ulcer)	AD
Inborn errors of metabolism with glucose intolerance			
Glycogen storage disease type I (von Gierke's disease)	IGT	Hepatomegaly, early hypoglycemia	AR
Acute intermittent porphyria	IGT	Paroxysmal abdominal pain, hypertension	AD
Hyperlipidaemias	NIDDM	Hyperlipidemia, coronary artery disease	AD
Fanconi syndrome-hypophosphataemia	NIDDM	Renal tubular dysfunction, metabolic bone disease	AR
Thiamine responsive megaloblastic anaemia	IDDM, IGT	Megaloblastic anemia, deafness	?AR
Syndromes with non-ketotic insulin resistant early onset diabetes mellitus			
Ataxia telangiectasia	Insulin resistant (IGT → NIDDM)	Ataxia, telangiectasia, IgA deficiency	AR
Myotonic dystrophy	Insulin resistant (IGT → NIDDM)	Myotonia, cataracts, balding, testicular atrophy	AD
Lipoatrophic diabetes syndromes	Insulin resistant (NIDDM)	Lipoatrophy, hyperlipidenia acanthosis nigricans	AD, AR
Leprechaunism	Insulin resistant (NIDDM)	Unusual facies, hirsutism, clitoromegaly, mental retardation, growth retardation	AR
Insulin resistance and acanthosis nigricans syndromes	Insulin resistant (NIDDM)	Acanthosis nigricans A-ovarian dysfunction B-autoimmune disease	?
Mendenhall syndrome	Insulin resistant	Unusual facies, hyperpigmentation, enlarged genitalia, pineal hypoplasia	AR

Table 85.3 (cont'd)

Syndromes	Types of DM	Associated clinical findings	Pattern of inheritance
Hereditary neuromuscular disorders associated with glucose intolerance			
Muscular dystrophies	IGT → NIDDM	Muscular dystrophy	AD, AR, XR
Late onset proximal	IGT → NIDDM	Myopathy, cataracts	?AR
Huntington's chorea	IGT → NIDDM	Chorea, demenitia	AD
Machado disease	NIDDM	Ataxia	AD
Herrman syndrome	NIDDM	Photomyoclonus, deafness, nephropathy, dementia	AD
Diabetes mellitus-optic atrophy – diabetes insipidus-deafness syndrome (Wolfram syndrome)	IDDM	Optic atrophy, diabetes insipidus, deafness, neurologic symptoms	AR
Friedrich's ataxia	IDDM or NIDDM	Spinocerebellar degeneration	AR
Alstrom syndrome	NIDDM	Retinitis pigmentosa, deafness, obesity	AR
Laurence-Moon-Biedl syndrome	NIDDM	Retinitis pigmentosa, polydactyly, obesity, hypogonadism, mental retardation	AR
Pseudo-Refsum syndrome	NIDDM	Muscle atrophy, ataxia, retinitis pigmentosa	?AD
Progeroid syndromes associated with glucose intolerance			
Cockayne syndrome	IGT	Dwarfism, progeria, MR, deafness, blindness	AR
Werner syndrome	NIDDM	Premature ageing, cataracts, arteriosclerosis	AR
Syndromes with glucose intolerance secondary to obesity			
Prader-Willi syndrome	NIDDM	Obesity, short stature, acromicria, MR	? deletion chromosome 15
Achondroplastic dwarfism	IGT	Disproportionate dwarfism	AD
Miscellaneous syndromes associated with glucose intolerance			
Steroid induced ocular hypertension	IGT	Steroid induced ocular hypertension	AD
Epiphyseal dysplasia and infantile onset diabetes mellitus	IDDM (congenital)	Epiphyseal dysplasia, tooth and skin defects	AR
Progressive cone dystrophy, degenerative liver disease, endocrine dysfunction, and hearing defect	MODY	Color blindness, liver disease, deafness, hypogonadism	AR
Cytogenetic disorders associated with glucose intolerance			
Down syndrome	IGT	MR, short stature, typical facies	Trisomy 21
Klinefelter syndrome	IGT → NIDDM	Hypogonadism, tall stature, MR	47,XXY
Turner syndrome	IGT → NIDDM	Short stature, gonadal dysgenesis, web neck	45,XO

Abbreviations
IDDM – Insulin dependent diabetes mellitus (type I)
NIDDM – Noninsulin dependent diabetes mellitus (type II)
IGT – Impaired glucose tolerance
AR – Autosomal recessive
AD – Autosomal dominant
XR – X–linked recessive
IUGR – Intrauterine growth retardation
MR – Mental retardation
MODY – Maturity onset type diabetes of the young

vidually is an insulin antagonist and their excess can lead to marked glucose intolerance. Thus, each of these 45 different genetic diseases are capable of resulting in carbohydrate intolerance through a variety of different pathogenetic mechanisms. These rare syndromes clearly suggest that similar heterogeneity, both genetic and pathogenetic, may exist in 'idiopathic' diabetes mellitus.

Genetic heterogeneity in animal models

Genetic heterogeneity for glucose intolerance has been well documented in the rodent (Herberg & Coleman, 1977; Coleman, 1982). A number of distinct single gene mutants have been found to result in glucose intolerance, which are due to mutations at different unlinked loci. In addition, a number of polygenic forms of glucose intolerance have been described in the rodent. Coleman's studies have not only documented clear genetic heterogeneity for glucose intolerance in the mouse, but have also shown that the phenotypic expression of the mutant gene influenced by the total genotype of the animal (Herberg & Coleman, 1977). The *db* mutant, which produces severe hyperglycaemia with islet cell atrophy in the homozygous state, was first described in the C57BL/KsJ strain of mouse. The *ob* mutant, which produces a mild form of maturity onset diabetes, with obesity and islet cell hyperplasia in the homozygous state, was first described in a different strain of mouse (C57BL/6). When the *db* mutant, however, was introduced into the C57BL/6 strain of mouse, they developed a maturity onset type of diabetes that was much like that of the *ob* mouse; in contrast, when the *ob* mutant was introduced into the KsJ strain, they developed a severe juvenile onset type of diabetes. Thus, the overall genetic constitution of the individual can clearly influence the phenotypic expression of the mutant diabetogenic gene. Similarly, differences in the genetic background of humans could result in differences in clinical expression of diabetes in different ethnic groups.

Ethnic variability

Marked ethnic variability in the prevalence and clinical features of diabetes mellitus has also been well documented (Rimoin, 1969; Rimoin & Schimke, 1971; West, 1978). Variability in the prevalence and pattern of disease among ethnic groups can be secondary to both genetic and environmental modifying factors, but may also indicate the presence of heterogeneity. Epidemiological surveys have revealed significant differences in the prevalence of diabetes among different populations (West, 1978). There appears to be a general correlation between overnutrition and the prevalence of diabetes. In certain populations, such as the Kurdish and Yemenite Jews in Israel, the prevalence of diabetes has markedly increased following their migration to Israel and a subsequent change in diet (Cohen, 1961). Similar increases in diabetes prevalence has occurred in the Micronesian population with changes in diet, activity, and migration (Zimmet et al 1981) and in the intensively studied Pima Indians of the American Southwest (Knowler et al, 1981).

Nevertheless, there are clear differences in the clinical phenotype of diabetes between different ethnic groups that do not appear to be totally the result of environmental differences (Rimoin, 1969; West, 1978). For example, there are different ethnic groups with low fat-high carbohydrate diets, some of which have common vascular complications and rare ketosis, whereas in other ethnic groups with similar diets, ketosis is the usual presenting symptom and vascular complications are rare (Rimoin & Schimke, 1971). There are even types of diabetes frequent in tropical countries – namely type J and pancreatic diabetes, that do not appear to occur in temperate zones (West, 1978).

INSULIN DEPENDENT (JUVENILE TYPE, IDDM) VS NON-INSULIN DEPENDENT (MATURITY TYPE, NIDDM) – HETEROGENEITY CONFIRMED

Heterogeneity within the more common forms of diabetes, unassociated with complex genetic syndromes, has been considered for years because of the clear clinical and physiological distinction between the thin, ketosis prone, insulin dependent juvenile onset diabetic versus the obese, non-ketotic, non-insulin dependent adult onset diabetic. A number of family studies clearly indicated that juvenile and adult onset diabetes appear to be separate disorders genetically (Cammidge, 1928, 1934; Harris, 1949, 1950; Simpson, 1962, 1964, 1968; Working Party, 1965; Degnbol & Green, 1978; Kobberling, 1969; Lestradet, 1972; MacDonald, 1974). This distinction remains when the diabetics are categorized as to insulin dependence, i.e., the insulin dependent and non-insulin dependent types also segregate independently (Irvine et al, 1977b; Cudworth, 1978).

The extensive monozygotic twin studies by Pyke and his coworkers in England strongly supported the separation of juvenile insulin dependent and maturity non-insulin dependent diabetes (Pyke, 1979). In contrast to the usual twin studies, where one compares concordance rates among monozygotic vs dizygotic twin pairs, Pyke and coauthors examined only monozygotic twins looking for differences between the concordant and discordant pairs. Of 106 monozygotic twin pairs studied, 71 were concordant and 35 discordant (Tattersall and Pyke, 1972). When the pairs were classified according to age of onset, however, only 50% of the pairs, in whom the age of onset of diabetes in the index twin was below age 40, were concordant, as opposed to 100% of those in whom the index twin developed diabetes after age 50. Of the discordant pairs, most have remained discordant for more than 10 years and showed no trend toward increasing concordance with time. Pyke and coworkers have now studied 200 twin pairs with similar results (Barnett et al, 1981a). Thus, among twin pairs with maturity onset type of non-insulin dependent diabetes, concordance approached 100%; whereas in those twin pairs with insulin dependent juvenile type diabetes, concordance was only approximately 50%. This would suggest that there are a large group of individuals with juvenile onset diabetes in whom, although the predisposition to diabetes can be genetically determined, non-genetic factors are of major importance.

The study of the insulin response to a glucose load provided early physiologic evidence for heterogeneity in diabetes. The absolute insulinopenic response of juvenile onset diabetics and the relative hyperinsulinaemic response of maturity onset diabetes parallels therapeutic observations of the absolute insulin requirement of the juvenile (insulin dependent) in contrast to the ability to manage most adult cases with oral hypoglycemics and/or diet (insulin independent). This, plus the immunologic and HLA observations mentioned below, led the recent international NIH working group to use insulin dependence, rather than age of onset, as a basis of classification (National Diabetes Data Group, 1979).

Immunologic studies have also supported this separation into insulin dependent and non-insulin dependent diabetic types (Irvine, 1980; Cahill & McDevitt, 1981). The first evidence was indirect, in that only insulin dependent diabetes was found to be clinically associated with Addison disease, certain thyroid disorders, and pernicious anemia, and with increased antibodies to the thyroid, gastric mucosa, intrinsic factor, and the adrenal gland (Irvine, 1977). Direct evidence for an autoimmune role in the pathogenesis of insulin dependent diabetes came from the discovery of organ specific cell mediated immunity to pancreatic islets, and then the eventual successful demonstration of antibodies to the islet cells of the pancreas (Bottazzo et al, 1974; MacCuish et al, 1974). While these antibodies were first detected only in insulin dependent diabetics with coexistent autoimmune endocrine disease, it soon became apparent that they were common (60 to 80%) in newly diagnosed juvenile diabetics. Islet cell antibody studies supported the differentiation of insulin dependent from non-insulin dependent diabetes, as antibodies were present in 30–40% of former group, as opposed to 5 to 8% of the latter. Of interest, the majority of the insulin independent, yet antibody positive, patients appeared to become insulin dependent with time. They also have flat insulin responses to a glucose load. This has suggested that aetiologically they belong in the insulin dependent category (that is they are just in an intermediate state in the

development of insulin dependence) (Irvine et al, 1977a). These immunologic studies have thus both separated disorders (juvenile vs adult) and combined others (insulin dependent and non-insulin dependent yet antibody positive).

The clear and consistent association of juvenile insulin dependent, but not maturity onset insulin independent diabetes, with HLA antigens B8 and B15, has been a major argument for aetiologic differences between these disorders (Nerup et al, 1977; Cudworth, 1978; Rotter & Rimoin, 1981a). These associations appear to be even stronger for antigens Dw3 and Dw4 of the HLA D locus. These HLA alleles are believed to serve as markers for closely linked, but as yet untypeable, 'diabetogenic' genes which may be immune response genes that are directly responsible for the individual's susceptibility to IDDM (see below).

The family, twin, metabolic, immune and HLA studies clearly indicate that juvenile onset insulin dependent and maturity onset non-insulin dependent diabetes are genetically distinct (Table 85.4). The NIH National Diabetes Data Group (1979) sponsored International Workgroup on the Classification of Diabetes considered that this division between insulin dependent type and noninsulin dependent type diabetes is firmly established. Therefore, in its classification, it divided diabetes into an 'insulin-dependent type', IDDM (that is, insulin dependence regardless of age of onset, therefore including the classical juvenile diabetes) and a 'non-insulin-dependent type', NIDDM (classical maturity onset insulin independent diabetes, regardless of age of onset).

A few cautions are in order. First, just because we are able to separate the bulk of patients and families into insulin dependent and non-insulin dependent types does not mean this phenotypic distinction is absolute. There is at least some evidence that families of either type have more of the other type than do the general population (Cahill, 1979b; Gottlieb, 1980). Part of this may be attributed to the insulin independent phase of the insulin dependent type (the frequency of which is not yet defined) (Irvine et al, 1977a). But this observation may also hint at as yet indelineated further heterogeneity. Second, it is appropriate to point out that age of onset is still a helpful criterion in describing the diabetic phenotype. While the distinction on the basis of insulin dependence versus independence has the greatest support, the use of age of onset as an additional, not substitute, clinical criterion has delineated further heterogeneity. Tattersall and Fajans have described a distinct form of non-insulin dependent diabetes which they have called 'maturity onset diabetes of the young' (MODY) (Tattersall, 1974; Tattersall & Fajans, 1975) (to be discussed below). The recent delineation of this entity clearly demonstrates that age of onset is a useful clinical criterion. Similarly, there is tentative evidence

Table 85.4 Separation of IDDM from NIDDM

Other nomenclature	IDDM Type I (juvenile onset type)	NIDDM Type II (maturity onset type)
1. Clinical	Thin Ketosis prone Insulin required for survival Onset predominantly in childhood and early adulthood	Obese Ketosis resistant Often treatable by diet or drugs Onset predominantly after 40
2. Family studies	Increased prevalence of juvenile or Type I	Increased prevalence of maturity or Type II
3. Twin studies	<50% concordance in monozygotic twins	Close to 100% concordance in monozygolic twins
4. Insulin response to a glucose blood	Flat	Variable
5. Associated with other autoimmune endocrine diseases and antibodies	Yes	No
6. Islet cell antibodies and pancreatic cell mediated immunity	Yes	No
7. HLA associations	Yes	No

that age of onset may still be a helpful additional classification criterion in the insulin dependent type. Initial reports have suggested that B15 and Dw4 were increased principally in younger insulin dependent diabetes, while B8 and Dw3 were increased more prominently in older IDDM patients, thus suggesting heterogeneity within IDDM (Svejgaard & Ryder, 1979; Svejgaard et al, 1980).

GENETICS AND HETEROGENEITY OF INSULIN DEPENDENT DIABETES MELLITUS (IDDM)

Difficulties in genetic analysis

The aforementioned family, twin, metabolic, and immunologic studies all helped separate IDDM from NIDDM. The discovery of HLA antigen associations with juvenile type insulin dependent diabetes mellitus, or IDDM, provided some of the stronger evidence separating this disorder, or group of disorders, from maturity type non-insulin dependent diabetes, as well as adding to the evidence for an immunologic pathogenesis. It was hoped that the use of these disease marker associations in appropriate studies might clarify the genetics of IDDM. While these associations have provided a useful tool to further investigate the genetics and pathogenesis of IDDM, the genetics of this group of disorders remains an area of great controversy, with many different modes of inheritance being proposed (Rotter, 1981). There are several major difficulties that confound any attempt to analyze the genetics of IDDM. These include the reduced penetrance of the disorder, the confounding of linkage and association, and the heterogeneity within the disorder.

First is the problem of the reduced penetrance of the IDDM diabetic genotype. When the mode of inheritance

is unclear, the only estimate we have for this is identical twin concordance data. The largest twin data set is that of the British diabetic twin study, which reports concordance for IDDM of some 50% (Pyke, 1979). However it is clear that this sample is a biased one, with only a fraction of the twins in the British isles identified, and thus a presumed bias toward concordant pairs (Pyke, 1978). Reports from less biased but much smaller samples report concordances of 20% (Gottlieb and Root, 1968; Cahill, 1979b). What this basically means is that what is inherited in IDDM is disease susceptibility, and other factors, presumably environmental, convert susceptibility into clinical disease. This view is supported both by the observations that the onset of IDDM clusters in families (Gamble, 1980); and the epidemiologic, experimental animal, and clinical evidence for viral infections as a supervening factor in at least some cases (Craighead, 1978; Rayfield & Seto, 1981).

The second problem is that genes genes in the HLA region appear both to be associated with IDDM in the population at large, and in families. The former observation connotes association, the latter linkage. Association and linkage are usually felt to be entirely distinct. The principal goal of disease association studies is to study the prevalence of a disorder among individuals with different well defined genetic traits, such as blood groups or serum enzyme polymorphisms. If the given disease occurs more commonly with a particular allele of a well defined genetic locus (e.g., increased duodenal ulcer among blood group O individuals) there is a positive association; then the genetically determined trait is usually considered to be of importance in the pathogenesis of the disorder in question (Rotter & Rimoin, 1979; 1981c). In most instances, linkage is an entirely different phenomenon from association. Linkage refers to the position for the gene locus on the chromosome map. If two genes are linked, they tend to accompany one another through meiosis and therefore vertically down a pedigree. But because of crossing over or recombination, specific alleles at the linked loci are not associated throughout a population. Association usually implies that there is some relationship between the two factors which are associated and does not imply linkage. For example, the association between blood group O and duodenal ulcer does not imply any linkage between the ABO locus and duodenal ulcer gene. Thus, linkage is usually a phenomenon within families and not across populations, whereas association is a phenomenon in the population, and not necessarily in families. Most mathematical techniques for linkage detection include a necessary assumption that there is no population association between the disease (phenotype) under study and the genetic marker alleles. However, the genetics of the HLA region (also known as the major histocompatibility complex, or MHC, located on chromosome 6) violate the cardinal rule of separation between linkage and association, because alleles at its own loci are in linkage disequilibrium. The HLA region has at least four well defined loci – three serologically defined (now known as loci A, B, and C) and one defined by the mixed lymphocyte reaction (MLC) (D locus) (Bodmer, 1978). A fifth locus, called the B lymphocyte alloantigen locus, Ia or Dr locus, which is also serologically defined and may be the serologic analogue of the D locus, is currently being characterized. A number of other genes, most notably several components of the complement sequence, have also been localized to this region of the human genome. Each of these loci has several alleles or antigens. All of these genes are located close to one another on chromosome 6; they are linked. Yet certain pairs of HLA antigens are also found in the population together in greater frequency than would be expected from multiplying their individual frequencies; i.e. they are associated. Since they are both linked and associated, this is known as linkage disequilibrium. The most popular explanation for linkage disequilibrium is that selective forces exist that tend to select for certain advantageous combinations of antigens. One of the major speculations regarding the aetiology of various autoimmune diseases is that we are seeing today the residual of the selective advantage of these antigen associations against the infectious diseases that our species was exposed to in the past (McMichael & McDevitt, 1977; Svejgaard et al, 1975).

A large number of studies have consistently found an increased frequency of HLA antigens B8 and B15, and D3 (DR3) and D4 (DR4) among IDDM patients. These population associations, initially reported by Singal and Blajchman (1973), Nerup et al (1974), and Cudworth & Woodrow (1975a), are now well established. In addition, studies within families have revealed that sibs who are both affected with IDDM share both HLA haplotypes more often than is expected by chance alone. (A haplotype is the set of alleles at the 4 closely linked HLA loci, A, B, C, and D, on one chromosome 6. Each individual inherits two haplotypes, one from each parent) If there were no linkage – association between the HLA region and IDDM, affected pairs of siblings would be expected to share 2 haplotypes (HLA identical) one haplotype (HLA haploidentical) and O haplotypes) (HLA nonidentical) in a ratio of 25% to 50% to 25%. Instead a number of reports indicate that pairs of diabetic siblings share 2 haplotypes approximately 55–60% of the time, share one haplotype approximately 40%, and in only a few cases share zero haplotypes (Cudworth & Woodrow, 1975b; Barbosa et al, 1977; Spielman et al, 1980; Walker & Cudworth, 1980; Svejgaard et al, 1980). This is between the 100% and 0% for two and one shared haplotypes that would be expected for simple autosomal recessive inheritance (for rare disorders) and the 50% and 50% expected for a rare autosomal dominant.

Most investigators have concluded that these data are most easily explained by a susceptibility locus (or loci) closely linked (probably within) the HLA complex. Certain alleles at the susceptibility locus (or loci) would then predispose to IDDM. These alleles are presumed to be in linkage disequilibrium with the respective HLA B and D alleles since there is such a great deal of linkage disequilibrium within the HLA complex. It should be pointed out that this is not the only possible explanation. An alternative is that the HLA alleles themselves predispose to IDDM (presumably the HLA D alleles, since they have the highest population association). Since not all IDDM diabetics have these alleles, and these alleles are frequent in the general nondiabetic population, presumably additional genes at other loci would be required, a model that implicates two or more loci. Such an alternative model can explain much of the population and family observations in HLA associated diseases in general (Clerget–Darpoux & Bonaiti–Pellie, 1980; Hodge & Spence, 1981).

Heterogeneity within insulin dependent diabetes (IDDM)

Possibly the greatest problem in any attempt to determine the mode of inheritance of IDDM is the increasing evidence for heterogeneity within this type of diabetes. Thus any attempt to determine a single mode of inheritance might very well be trying to combine different disorders with different patterns of inheritance. The evidence for heterogeneity within insulin dependent diabetes has been developing for some time. It could be inferred when the first detailed argument for heterogeneity within all of diabetes was proposed, since frank insulin dependent diabetes was a component of certain defined genetic syndromes, such as the optic atrophy-diabetes mellitus syndrome and a syndrome with epiphyseal dysplasia and infantile onset diabetes (Rimoin 1967, 1976; Rotter & Rimoin, 1981a; Rimoin & Rotter, 1982). More direct evidence came from immunologic studies which suggested that there were forms of insulin dependent diabetes associated with autoimmunity and those which were not, and that this occurred on a familial basis (Nissley et al, 1973; Fialkow et al, 1975; Bottazo et al, 1978). On the basis of the additive risk of B8 and B15, the Danish group suggested the possibility that more than one gene in the HLA complex affected the susceptibility to insulin dependent diabetes (Svejgaard et al, 1975; Svejgaard & Ryder, 1981). Subsequently Bottazo and Doniach (1976) and Irvine (1977) proposed that insulin dependent diabetes can be subdivided into autoimmune and viral-induced types, with an intermediate group in the Irvine classification. The autoimmune type would be characterized by pancreatic islet cell antibodies, which may occur years before the onset of clinical diabetes and persist for years after its onset, by the presence of other associated autoimmune endocrinopathies and antibodies, by an onset at any age, and by a higher incidence in females. In contrast, the hypothesized viral induced type would have transient islet cell antibodies at the onset of disease which disappear within the next year, would not be associated with autoimmunity, would tend to have an age of onset less than 30 (but may occur later) and have an equal sex incidence. During the same period, Rotter and Rimoin (1978), on the basis of an analysis of published immunologic and metabolic studies, proposed further heterogeneity among the juvenile insulin dependent form of diabetes based on differential immunologic correlations with different HLA phenotypes, and postulated that the HLA B8-Dw3, and

the B15-Dw4 associated forms of diabetes are distinct diseases – B8-Dw3, an autoimmune form, and B15-Dw4, an insulin antibody responder type.

The accumulated evidence strongly suggests that genetic heterogeneity exists even within the typical insulin dependent juvenile onset type of diabetes (see Table 85.5). It appears that there are at least two clearly distinct forms of juvenile onset diabetes, one of which is associated with HLA B8 and the other with B15 (Rotter and Rimoin, 1978, 1981a; Rotter, 1981). B8 could be replaced by Dw3 and B15 by Dw4 without any change in concept or conclusion. The HLA-B8 form of the disease (autoimmune form) is characterized by an increased prevalence of the Dw3 allele of the HLA D locus, an increased persistence of pancreatic islet cell antibodies and antipancreatic cell mediated immunity, and lack of antibody response to exogenous insulin. This form apparently has onset throughout life and probably accounts for a significant fraction of older onset IDDM, which in the older age groups may present for a significant period as treatable without insulin, but in whom the presence of islet cell antibodies presages eventual insulin dependence (Irvine et al, 1979). Since such cases have an increased frequency of B8, it would appear they belong to the general group of IDDM patients. The second form of juvenile onset insulin dependent diabetes is associated with HLA B15 and is less well characterized. It is associated with the Cw3 allele of the HLA C locus and Dw4 of the D locus, is not associated with autoimmune disease or islet cell antibodies, and it is accompanied by an increased antibody response to exogenous insulin. This disorder also appears to have an earlier age of onset that the B8-Dw3 type. Irvine et al (1978b) have shown a direct relationship between persistent islet anti-

Table 85.5 Heterogeneity within insulin-dependent diabetes mellitus (For references, see Rotter, 1981)

Evidence	B8	B15	B18	B8(Dw3)/B15(Dw4) Combined form
Relative risk for diabetes				
Linkage disequilibrium	D3, Dr3, A1	Cw3, D4, Dr4	BfF1, D3, Dr3	↑ occurrence in MZ twins
Insulin antibodies	Nonresponder (no antibodies)	High responder (produce antibodies)		↑ risk to siblings ↑ occurrence in familial cases
Islet cell antibodies	Persistent	Transient		
Antipancreatic cell-mediated immunity	Increased	Not increased		
Thyroid autoimmunity in IDDM	Yes	Less frequent		
Associated with other autoimmune endocrine diseases	Yes	No		
IgA deficiency in IDDM	Increased	Not increased		
Isolated pedigrees	Autoimmune disorder	Defect in insulin release		
Age of onset	Any age	Younger age	?Younger age	Youngest
Levels of C-peptide			Highest	Lowest

bodies and lower insulin antibody levels, thus directly confirming the differential immunologic features of the two forms.

Not all investigators conclude that these observations indicate genetic heterogeneity. For example, Rubinstein et al (1981) and Curie – Cohen (1981) argue that this phenotypic heterogeneity only reflects other linked (in disequilibrium) immune reactivity in the HLA complex, that may not have anything to do with diabetes pathogenesis per se. However, the ability of mathematical models based on these heterogeneity arguments to make accurate population predictions (see below) would seem to be additional evidence in their favour.

There is reasonably good evidence for even further heterogeneity with insulin dependent diabetes. There appears to exist a third form, the compound B8-Dw3/B15-Dw4 heterozygote (Rotter & Rimoin, 1979; Rotter, 1981). This form is characterized by an increased relative risk. Evidence hints that it may also have an increased prevalence among concordant twins, an increased prevalence among familial cases, and an increased risk to sibs for diabetes (Cudworth, 1978; Christy et al, 1979; Nerup et al, 1976). In addition, this group may have the earliest age of onset and greater islet cell damage, as indicated by the lowest levels of measureable C-peptide (Ludvigsson et al, 1977). To further complicate matters, it appears that the recently described Bf-F1 IDDM association identifies a third diabetogenic haplotype, one that carries Bf-F1, HLA B18 and Dw3 (Raum et al, 1979; Bertrams, 1982). In addition, besides the positive HLA associations mentioned, negative associations have also been noted. For example, there is a decreased frequency of HLA antigen B7 (Ludwig et al, 1976) and a marked decrease, to the point of almost complete absence, of the D2 and Dr2 alleles in IDDM patients (Ilonen et al, 1978; Nerup et al, 1978).

Mode(s) of inheritance

There currently exists an ongoing lively debate regarding the mode of inheritance of IDDM. Based on population studies of HLA antigens and family studies of HLA haplotypes, susceptibility to IDDM has been variously proposed to be inherited in a single autosomal dominant fashion, as a single autosomal recessive, as some recessive and some dominant forms, in an intermediate gene dosage mode, in a heterogeneous three allele or two HLA loci model, and as a two locus disorder (Table 85.6). The reasons for much of this confusion-the reduced penetrance, confounding of linkage and association, and heterogeneity-have been reviewed above.

Autosomal dominant inheritance has been proposed several times, most recently by MacDonald (1980), who demonstrated that such a model was consistent with US Black-Caucasian differences in the frequency of IDDM.

However, in terms of family data, a simple dominant model is consistent with no more than 50% of affected sib pairs sharing HLA haplotypes in common (Thomson & Bodmer, 1977). Since a clear excess, 55–60%, of affected sib pairs is observed, the simple dominant model can be rejected (Svejgaard et al, 1980). The autosomal recessive model can explain the sib pair haplotype data alone, but to do so would require a gene frequency for the diabetes susceptibility allele of 0.2 to 0.3 or higher (Rubinstein et al, 1981). This would necessitate the population prevalence of the disease to be some ten or more fold higher than actually observed (Christy et al, 1979). Thus, unless one invokes radically different penetrances for familial and nonfamilial cases, the simple recessive model can be rejected. The gene dosage model of Spielman et al (1980), by invoking a higher penetrance for an individual with two doses of the susceptibility allele, can resolve both the prevalence and sib pair data. However, neither the gene dosage model, nor its simpler extremes (dominant or recessive) can account for the consistent excess of DR3/DR4 heterozygotes observed (Svejgaard et al, 1980; Rotter, 1981). This persistent observation appears central to the population genetics of IDDM. Thus the simple gene dosage model must be rejected as well.

The accumulated evidence for heterogeneity, plus the observations regarding the compound form, make the simple autosomal recessive and autosomal dominant hypotheses increasingly less tenable. A more restricted hypothesis would be that at least some forms of juvenile diabetes are due to inheritance of recessive or dominant susceptibility. Barbosa et al (1980a) ascertained their patients in order to select two sets of families: those with horizontal and those with vertical aggregation. For the purpose of linkage analysis, they then assume recessive inheritance for the first set and dominant for the second (Barbosa et al, 1977; 1978a; 1980a). However, without further phenotypic distinctions, it is not clear whether these different aggregation patterns truly reflect different modes of inheritance.

For the most part these models ignore the increasingly documented heterogeneity within IDDM. Formal genetic analyses which fail to take this heterogeneity into account and treat IDDM as one entity probably suffer from the same defect as did earlier genetic analyses which failed to distinguish insulin dependent from noninsulin dependent diabetes. Other genetic models besides simple autosomal dominant or recessive must be developed to take this heterogeneity into account. For example, Hodge et al (1980) have recently developed a three allele model for a diabetic susceptibility locus tightly linked to the HLA complex which incorporates the immunogenetic heterogeneity observed within IDDM.

Hodge, Rotter, and Lange (1980) postulated a susceptibility locus S for insulin dependent diabetes tightly

Table 85.6 Proposed modes of inheritance of IDDM susceptibility*

Mode of inheritance	Comments	Problems	Proposers and suggesters
Autosomal dominant	1. Fits racial admixture and prevalence of IDDM in U.S. Blacks	1. Does not explain excess sharing of 2 haplotypes in sibships 2. Does not explain heterogeneity	Svejgaard et al, 1975; Spielman et al, 1979; MacDonald, 1980
Autosomal recessive	1. Explains excess of 2 shared haplotypes	1. High estimate for gene frequency (implausible, but not impossible) 2. Requires different penetrances in familial cases and the population at large 3. Does not explain U.S. Black-Caucasian incidence differences 4. Does not explain heterogeneity	Thomson & Bodmer, 1977; Rubinstein et al, 1977; 1981
Some autosomal recessive, some autosomal dominant	1. Uses observed familial aggregation pattern, and assumes mode of inheritance	1. Without further phenotypic differences, different inheritance not demonstrable 2. Both sets of families have high incidence of HLA associated alleles 3. Does not explain immunologic heterogeneity	Barbosa et al, 1977; 1978a; 1980a
Intermediate, gene dosage model	1. One dose of the gene is sufficient, but 2nd dose increases susceptibility 2. Explains excess of shared haplotypes	1. Does not explain heterogeneity	Spielman et al, 1980
Two different susceptibility alleles (and/or two HLA linked loci)	1. Different immunologic forms of IDDM differentially associated with B8-Drw3, & B15-Drw4, and a compound form 2. Accounts for immunologic differences 3. Predicts autoimmunity in U.S. Blacks less frequent than in U.S. Whites	1. Too many parameters, can't be fully tested on existing data sets (i.e. some parameters such as tight linkage must be assumed)	Svejgaard et al, 1975; Bottazzo & Doniach, 1976; Rotter & Rimoin, 1978; 1979; Cudworth & Festenstein, 1978; Irvine et al, 1978a;b; Hodge et al, 1980; Rotter & Hodge, 1980
Two unlinked loci	1. Unlinked genes interacting with HLA alleles, or HLA linked alleles 2. Evidence for additional non-HLA linked genes in other B8 associated disorders-coeliac disease, Graves disease, chronic active hepatitis	1. Again, too many parameters, can't be tested without additional assumptions 2. Does not explain heterogeneity unless incorporate different HLA linked alleles	Thomson, 1980; Rotter, 1981; Clerget-Darpoux et al, 1981

* These are propositions made in the 'HLA era'.

linked to the HLA complex with 3 alleles: S_1, S_2, and s. S_1 and S_2 would be the diabetogenic alleles for Forms 1 and 2, respectively, while s is a normal nondiabetic allele. Genotypes S_1s and $S_1 S_1$ were presumed to be at risk (with penetrance ϕ_1) for the autoimmune B8 associated form of the disease (Form 1); S_2S_2 and S_2s were presumed to be at risk (with penetrance ϕ_2) for Form 2, characterized by antibodies to exogenous insulin and associated with B15; S_1S_2 was presumed to be at risk (with penetrance ϕ_3) for Form 3, the compound form, which would share the features of both 1 and 2. The normal allelic state ss would not be susceptible to insulin dependent diabetes. This model therefore takes into account the differential immunologic and HLA associations, and the greatly increased relative risk for the B8/B15 (Dw3/Dw4) heterozygotes. Hodge et al (1980) incorporated the population prevalence of the disease, the HLA relative risks, the concordance rates for sibs and monozygotic twins, and the percentages of HLA haplotypes shared in common by affected sib pairs. They then were able to solve for the penetrances of the various forms, and the gene frequencies of the three susceptibility alleles. One solution set which provided a particular good fit to the observations gave gene frequencies of 0.111, 0.006, 0.883 for S_1, S_2 and little s, respectively, and penetrances $\phi_1 = 0.001$, $\phi_2 = 0.107$, $\phi_3 = 0.436$. The predicted relative proportions of the three forms among all juvenile diabetics in the Caucasian population were 10%, 60% and 30% for Forms 1, 2 and 3 respectively, a prediction consistent with various reported immunologic studies. It should be noted that the reason Form 3 is so frequent among diabetics, even though the underlying gentotype frequency is rare compared to the other two forms, is because of its high disease penetrance. This model also predicts, due to the higher penetrance of Form 3, that the distribution of the forms of the disease will differ among affected individuals and families with multiple members affected. That is, of all affected individuals, approximately 30% will have Form 3, but in contrast almost 50% of all affected sib pairs will have Form 3.

There were several predictions and conclusions from this modelling. First, it demonstrates that other models, besides dominant and recessive, can account for the population and HLA observations. Second, in a sense, this model has both dominant and recessive features. Since only one diabetogenic allele is required for susceptibility, genetic transmission mimics dominant inheritance on a population basis. However the familial forms often involve two alleles, and therefore can mimic recessive inheritance within families.

This heterogeneity model can also account for the racial differences commented upon by MacDonald (1980). In addition, the heterogeneity model makes certain predictions regarding racial differences that would not follow from either simple dominant or recessive susceptibility or the more general one-locus, two-allele gene dosage model. Given the racial differences and gene admixture proposed by MacDonald (1980), the heterogeneity model predicts that the relative incidence of the autoimmune form of the disease would be proportionately less among U.S. Black IDDM patients than among U.S. White IDDM patients (Rotter & Hodge, 1980). This prediction has received direct support from the studies of Maclaren and coworkers who have found the prevalence of islet cell antibodies and adrenal antibodies to be less in U.S. Black IDDM patients than U.S. IDDM Whites (Neufeld et al, 1980; Riley et al, 1980). The frequency of pancreatic autoimmunity observed in U.S. Whites was twice that observed in U.S. Blacks, precisely what was predicted by the heterogeneity model (Rotter & Hodge, 1980; Neufeld et al, 1980).

To make an already complicated area even more complex, there are theoretical grounds for considering two independent genetic loci as predisposing to IDDM. The evidence is suggestive but growing. First the association of B8-Dw3 is not only with IDDM, but with a host of autoimmune disorders such as Graves disease, Addison disease, coeliac disease, chronic active hepatitis, and others (McMichael & McDevitt, 1977). What then provides the specificity? Either a specific disease predisposing gene for each different disease must be in linkage disequilibrium with the B8-Dw3 haplotype, or the B8-Dw3 haplotype provides some general predisposition to autoimmune disease. Direct evidence for a second non-HLA linked B cell alloantigen that more specifically predisposes to coeliac disease has been provided by Peña, Strober and coworkers (Pēna et al, 1978; Strober, 1980). Population genetic analysis also supports a two locus model for coeliac disease (Greenberg & Rotter, 1981). Equally suggestive is the data regarding Graves disease and chronic active hepatitis, where besides the HLA B8-Dw3 association, an association with alleles at the Gm locus (IgG heavy chain allotypes) has also been identified (Farid et al, 1978; Whittingham et al, 1981). In an analogous fashion we should consider investigating a second locus for IDDM. Specifically if insulin antibodies have any pathogenetic role in IDDM, then Gm locus alleles (or as always, closely linked genes) may be important, as an association between the antibody response to exogeneous insulin and certain Gm allotypes has recently been observed by Nakao et al (1981). Another suggestive piece of evidence is the report by Gorsuch et al (1980) that IDDM and the thyrogastric autoimmunity segregate independently in IDDM families. A population genetic analysis has been reported to be consistent with a two locus model for IDDM (Thomson, 1980), though the analysis did not take into account the heterogeneity reviewed above. Possibly the most direct evidence for a second locus has just been reported, specifically tentative linkage of IDDM with a second linkage marker, this one not located close to HLA on chromosome 6, the Kidd blood group (Hodge et al, 1981).

Probably the major difficulty in fully resolving the genetics of IDDM remains the problem of identifying those who carry the predisposing diabetic genotype yet do not manifest the disorder, i.e. those individuals who are not fully penetrant. When we don't know the pattern of inheritance, the only estimate of penetrance available is that from identical twin data. Since estimates of monozygotic twin concordance range from 20 to 50%, this means the majority of individuals in the population with the IDDM genetic predisposition are clinically normal. This will continue to confound and bedevil all attempts at rigorous genetic analysis. We must work toward identifying the IDDM genotype in the absence of full blown clinical disease. In this regard, the recent work of Barbosa et al (1980b) is noteworthy. They have demonstrated subtle abnormalities of glucose and insulin levels in HLA identical siblings as opposed to HLA non-identical siblings of IDDM diabetics. Even more significant was a high incidence of intense immune fluorescent staining of albumin in the skeletal muscle extracellular membrane in the HLA-identical siblings, those at highest risk, than in non-identical sibs, who were comparable to controls. Such biological advances provide the hope of eventually identifying those individuals who are genetically susceptible, thus resolving not only the genetics, but providing an invaluable tool in studying the natural history, pathogenesis, preventive measures, and providing genetic counselling as well.

HETEROGENEITY WITHIN NON-INSULIN DEPENDENT DIABETES MELLITUS (NIDDM)

The monozygotic twin studies reviewed above demonstrate almost complete concordance in NIDDM identical twins (Barnett et al, 1981a; 1981b). Yet the familial aggregation of either clinical disease or glucose levels is not consistent with a single mode of inheritance (Friedman & Fialkow, 1980; Rotter & Rimoin, 1981a). Again, genetic heterogeneity would seem the most likely explanation. In addition, population studies have shown a marked increase in the frequency of NIDDM when primitive populations migrate to more urban and affluent environments (Cohen, 1961; Zimmet et al, 1981), demonstrating that environmental factors are important as well. The identical twin data suggest that, in the urbanized western world, the environment is sufficiently constant that what determines the onset of clinical disease is primarily the genetic susceptibility.

Clinical genetic studies have indeed suggested heterogeneity within NIDDM. Kobberling (1971) divided his adult onset probands into low, moderate, and markedly overweight categories. He found a significantly higher frequency of affected sibs in the light proband category (38%) and a significantly lower frequency in the heavy proband category (10%). While Kobberling (1976a) commented that one explanation for these findings could be an additive gene model, with obesity as an additional risk factor, this could also be explained by different monogenic forms with different susceptibilities, i.e., different dependence on exogenous predisposing factors. Irvine et al (1977b) also suggested a differences between the non-obese and obese insulin independent propositi, in that they observed a different clinical range of diabetes in the relatives of the non-obese and obese probands.

Fajans (1976) and coworkers have demonstrated metabolic heterogeneity in non-obese latent diabetes. They were able to divide their patients with latent diabetes into two broad groups, one who had an insulinopenic form of glucose intolerance, in contrast to those with high levels of plasma immunoreactive insulin. The high responders and low responders remained consistent and distinct following many years of follow-up suggesting that they represented different metabolic disorders. Fajans suggests that in the under-responder category, the lack of insulin is one of the principal determinants of

abnormal glucose tolerance. On the other hand, in the over-responder category, the hyperinsulinaemia is secondary to other factors which cause glucose intolerance. This could be insulin resistance due to insulin receptor or postreceptor abnormalities, or the production of an abnormal insulin with diminished biologic activity. The former seems the most common occurrence. However, one NIDDM patient with significant hyperinsulinaemia has been discovered whose glucose intolerance appears to be due to secretion of a biologically abnormal insulin (Given et al, 1980).

The best delineated heterogeneity within non-insulin dependent diabetes is the distinct form of diabetes described by Tattersall and Fajans which they have called 'maturity onset diabetes of the young' (MODY) (Tattersall, 1974; Tattersall & Fajans, 1975; Fajans et al 1978; Fajans, 1982) and which Pyke and colleagues refer to as 'Mason type' diabetes (Pyke, 1979). This group of patients have an early age of onset but have few symptoms, no ketonuria, and can be controlled without insulin, with little progression in severity of carbohydrate intolerance over 20 years or more. These 'maturity onset diabetics of young people' (MODY patients) are clearly phenotypically different from the classical juvenile onset diabetic (JOD). Physiologic studies of these patients supports this phenotypic differentiation, as they have insulin response to glucose loads much more characteristic of maturity onset diabetes. Genetic studies provided further evidence that this is a separate entity. Of the MODY propositi, 85% had a diabetic parent, usually with a similar phenotype, 53% of sibs tested had diabetes, and 46% of the families showed three generations of direct vertical transmission of the trait, suggesting autosomal dominant inheritance. In contrast, only 11% of JOD parents were diabetic, 8 of 74 sibs were diabetic, six with similar JOD phenotype, and only 6% of the families showed three-generation transmission. Thus the MODY patients clearly have a distinct dominantly inherited syndrome, distinct from IDDM and from most NIDDM patients. The delineation of this disorder most clearly demonstrates the need to carefully dissect out the phenotypic differences among diabetics before genetic analysis is possible. If these MODY patients had been classified by either age of onset or by diabetic phenotype (insulin independence) alone, they would have been lumped together with 'classic' JOD's or the non-insulin dependent type of the current NIH classification respectively, and their distinctive pattern of inheritance would have been obscured.

Fajans has provided evidence for clinical, metabolic, and genetic heterogeneity even within MODY (Fajans et al, 1978; Fajans, 1982). While several authors have commented on the rarity of vascular complications in MODY (Tattersall, 1974; Barbosa et al, 1978b) a number of Fajan's patients have had frequent vascular complications, a difference that may well occur on a familial basis (Fajans et al, 1978; Fajans, 1982). Fajans also reports that his MODY patients differ in their insulin response to a glucose load, with both hypoinsulinemic and hyperinsulinemic responses, and that there is familial aggregation of the level of insulin response (Fajans, 1982) It is of interest that some of the hypoinsulinemic patients haveprogressed to require insulin to control hyperglycaemia. In contrast, Barbosa et al (1978b) in a study of two MODY families, found both hypoinsulinaemic and hyperinsulinaemic affected individuals in the same family.

A potentially exciting development regarding the genetics of MODY (or 'Mason type') diabetes in particular, and non-insulin dependent diabetes in general, was the description by Leslie and Pyke of chlorpropamide primed alcohol induced flushing, or CPAF, as a purported preclinical marker of MODY type diabetes (Leslie & Pyke, 1978; Pyke & Leslie, 1978; Pyke, 1979). After observing that diabetic members of the original Mason family, who were being treated with chlorpropamide, experienced facial flushing after alcohol, Drs. Leslie and Pyke studied their MODY families and found that most of the diabetics in these families flushed after alcohol (after being primed 12 hours earlier with a tablet of chlorpropamide) and that most of the nondiabetics in these families did not. They proposed that CPAF is a dominantly inherited trait, as in their hands the CPAF positive individuals had a CPAF positive parent, approximately 50% of their sibs and offspring had CPAF, and the trait was demonstrable through three generations in two families (Leslie & Pyke, 1978). Leslie and Pyke (1978) also demonstrated that many non-insulin dependent diabetics who would not be recognized as MODY type (that is they had an adult age of onset) also were CPAF positive. They also observed that CPAF negative patients have both a higher incidence and greater severity of complications than CPAF positive patients (Leslie et al, 1979b). Leslie, Pyke and Stubbs (1979a) also have suggested that an increased sensitivity to enkephalins (the endogeneous opiates) is the cause of CPAF, as the flushing is reproduced in these patients with enkephalin analogues, and is blocked by the specific opiate antagonist naloxone. This has led Pyke to hypothesize that the pathogenesis of CPAF positive non-insulin dependent diabetes is centrally mediated, analogous to the piqure diabetes of Claude Bernard (Pyke, 1979). However, other groups of investigators have failed to confirm an association of either NIDDM or MODY type diabetes with the CPAF trait. They observed no increase of CPAF in NIDDM patients compared to IDDM patients or controls (Kobberling et al, 1980; Dreyer et al, 1980; de Silva et al, 1981). Entire MODY pedigrees have been reported where no one flushed (Kobberling et al, 1980), and other MODY families have been observed to have CPAF positive and negative patients in the same kindred (Fajans, 1982). Thus, it is not clear that CPAF predisposes to

diabetes. It is possible that the high incidence of CPAF positivity in the London series of diabetes may be related to specific use of chlorpropamide in that clinic. While CPAF negativity may indeed be associated with diabetic complications, this may reflect effect rather than cause, analogous to an early form of autonomic neuropathy. Genetic factors may still be important, as the CPAF positive patients did have a stronger family history of diabetes, but the genetic relationship is not as clearcut as originally proposed.

Two recent observations may add to the knowledge regarding the genetics of NIDDM. Bottazzo and coworkers have recently observed antibodies to specific endocrine cells of the gut, namely GIP (glucose insulinotropic peptide) cells, in 15–20% of NIDDM patients (Mirakian et al, 1980; Bottazzo et al, 1982). This hormone plays a role in the modulation of insulin secretion. It is conceivable that these antibodies are identifying an autoimmune form of NIDDM, due to destruction of the gut endocrine influences on glucose homeostasis. Of interest, some IDDM patients were also found to have these anti-GIP cell antibodies (Botazzo et al, 1982). This would be one possible explanation for the overlap of NIDDM and IDDM seen in some families.

The most recent development regarding NIDDM is the report of an association with a DNA restriction polymorphism of the insulin gene. Owerbach et al (1981) localized the insulin gene to the short arm of chromosome 11, using nucleic acid hybridization techniques applied to mouse-human somatic cell hybrids. Extending this work, Owerbach and Nerup (1981) examined restriction fragment length polymorphisms of the insulin gene in NIDDM and IDDM patients, and found a positive population association between NIDDM and a certain insulin gene polymorphism. If confirmed, this would be analogous to the HLA associations with IDDM, and could be used in population and family studies to clarify the genetics of NIDDM.

CLASSIFICATION, COUNSELLING, AND CONCLUSIONS

Heterogeneity within both the insulin dependent and non-insulin dependent types appears extensive. A classification of the heterogeneous entities within these 'idiopathic' types is given in Table 85.7.

An important question arises from the population genetic viewpoint. These diabetic disorders, whose susceptibility appears to be primarily genetically determined, are deleterious, and thus reproductive fitness should be impaired. How then did these genes become so frequent? As regards IDDM, a disorder in which autoimmunity and immune response genes seem implicated, a possible role in the resistance to infectious agents seen likely. As regards NIDDM, a possible explanation

Table 85.7 Heterogeneity within 'idiopathic' diabetes mellitus, genetic-aetiologic classifications (Overlapping features that may yield separate classifications)

I. Insulin dependent type
A. *By HLA association*
  1. B8-Dw3-autoimmune type
  2. B15-Dw4-Cw3-insulin antibody responder
  3. B18-BfF$_1$-Dw3
  4. B8/B15(Dw3/Dw4) compound
  5. ? Non HLA associated
B. *By islet cell antibodies*
  1. Positive
    a) Transient
    b) Persistent
  2. Negative
C. *Proposed pathogenesis*
  1. Autoimmune-clinical and serologic associations
  2. Viral-mumps, rubella, coxsackie
  3. Mixed
  4. Other mechanisms

II. Non-insulin dependent type
A. *By obesity*
  1. Non-obese
  2. Obese
B. *By age of onset*
  1. MODY
  2. MOD
C. *By chlorpropamide – alcohol flushing*
  1. CPAF positive
  2. CPAF negative
D. *Other mechanisms*
  1. Abnormal insulin
  2. Antibody to GIP cells

is the concept of a 'thrifty' genotype, first proposed by Neel (1962). Neel proposed that the diabetic genotypic somehow allowed more efficient utilization of foodstuffs by the body in periods of famine to which primitive man was often exposed. Such a 'thrifty' gene would therefore have a selective survival advantage and would tend to increase in frequency. However, in the modern western world, with its continuous abundance of calories, such a gene would lead to diabetes and obesity. Neel's hypothesis has recently received support by observations in both man and animals. The extremely high frequency of diabetes and obesity in populations such as the Pima Indians (Knowler et al, 1981) and Pacific Islanders (Zimmet, 1979), and its apparent increase with modernization and urbanization, are entirely consistent with the thrifty genotype hypothesis. Direct support comes from studies by Coleman (1979) who has shown that heterozygotes for rodent diabetes-obesity genes exhibit a much better ability to survive fasting than normal rodents.

The heterogeneity that has so far been discovered among typical diabetes mellitus probably represents just the tip of the iceberg. But even this currently demonstrable heterogeneity has immediate relevance to current research efforts into the pathogenesis and therapy of the diabetic state. Various agents, e.g. viruses, have been proposed as the inciting or promoting factors for diabetes in individuals with the appropriate genetic predisposition (Craighead, 1978; Rayfield and Seto, 1981). The susceptibility to a given agent may very well depend on the heterogeneity elucidated by these studies. The long-standing debate on the efficacy of tight vs loose control in preventing vascular complications might very well be answered when this heterogeneity is taken into account in appropriately designed studies – ie., there may be forms of diabetes where control is vital, and others where it is less so, subgroups with inexorable complications, and others complication free (Barbosa, 1980; Rimoin & Rotter, 1981). A variety of conflicting observations regarding HLA types and complications have been reported, and so any relation to specific HLA types must be considered tentative at best (Rimoin & Rotter, 1981). The observation by Leslie et al (1979) that CPAF negative non-insulin dependent patients had a much higher incidence of retinopathy than CPAF positive patients, and the different frequency of a positive family history between these groups, does suggest at least some genetic determination of diabetic complications. Thus, delineation of genetic heterogeneity and the search for genetic markers should have profound implications not only for understanding the genetics and aetiology of diabetes, but also for its vascular complications. Only when each of the many disorders resulting in diabetes mellitus and/or glucose intolerance are delineated will specific prognostication and therapy be possible for all diabetic patients.

Given these recent advances in our knowledge of the genetics and heterogeneity of the diabetic syndrome, what is the genetic counselling we can provide at his time to our diabetic patients? First, as in all genetic counselling, an accurate diagnosis must be made. On clinical grounds one can distinguish between juvenile insulin-dependent type diabetes, maturity-onset non-insulin-dependent type diabetes, and maturity-onset diabetes of the young. In distinguishing between these phenotypes, one already has important counselling information. As discussed above, in a given family the increased risk for diabetes over the general population is only for that specific type of diabetes that has already occurred in the family, not for all diabetes. Thus, if the index case presenting for counselling is a juvenile insulin-dependent diabetic, the increased risk for that patient's relatives is for insulin dependent diabetes. If the index case is a non-insulin-dependent diabetic, the increased risk for the patient's relatives is, for the most part, for non-insulin dependent diabetes only. Associated abnormalities or diseases may suggest the rare genetic syndromes that include diabetes – each of which has its own risk of recurrence (see Table 85.3).

Once we have accurately characterized the clinical phenotype of the patient, how do we then proceed? At this stage, we must fall back for the most part on observed empirical recurrence risks, i.e., data concerning the actually observed recurrence of these disorders in a large number of families. Even these empiric recurrence risks have limitations, since for the most part they have been reported only from Caucasian populations. Even with the reservation that these empirical risks can be safely applied only to the populations from which they were derived, the most reassuring aspect of the data is the overall low absolute risk for the development of clinical diabetes in first degree relatives, especially for insulin-dependent diabetes (Table 85.8). If a child has juvenile insulin-dependent diabetes, published studies report an average risk to his sibs of 5 to 10%. If a parent has juvenile-onset diabetes, the risk for the offspring of overt diabetes during the first decade of life is generally reported as 1 to 2% or less. For non-insulin-dependent diabetes, the empiric recurrence risk to first degree relatives is of the order of 5–10% for clinical diabetes, and 15–25% for an abnormal glucose tolerance test (Rotter & Rimoin, 1981a). Since maturity-onset diabetes of the young (MODY) appears to be an autosomal dominant disorder, the offspring and sibs of such patients would be at a 50% risk. But though the numerical risk of recurrence is relatively high in the disorder, the lower burden of this type of diabetes must be made clear to the family, since this type of diabetes appears to be milder, with fewer complications.

Certain studies would indicate that subgroups at higher risk can theoretically be identified. Thus the HLA haplotype studies discussed earlier indicate that within an IDDM sibship, sibs can be classified into those who share two haplotypes with the diabetic proband and who have a higher risk for IDDM than the general sib empirical risks, sibs who share one haplotype with the proband and have approximately the same risk as the overall empirical risk, and sibs who share no haplotypes with the proband and have a decreased recurrence risk. Similarly there have been reports of islet cell antibody positivity in ostensibly normal sibs of an IDDM diabetic who have gone on to frank insulin dependent diabetes. More recently Bottazzo et al (1980, 1982) have claimed the delineation of a more specific islet cell antibody with complement fixing properties, and suggest that this may particularly identify relatives at risk. As regards non-insulin-dependent diabetes, the trait of chlorpropamide alcohol induced flushing may be a preclinical marker of some forms of the MODY or Mason type NIDDM. If confirmed by others, this could identify those individuals at risk in younger generations who have not yet manifested the diabetes. However, for the most part these tools currently remain in the realm of research, rather than providing clinical tools. Advances have been so rapid that any recommendations made here should be considered working guidelines, subject to revision as new knowledge becomes available. In the near future we should be able to utilize many of these markers and our increasing knowledge of the genetic heterogeneity of diabetes to aid in counselling diabetic patients and their families.

Table 85.8 Empiric recurrence risks for juvenile insulin dependent diabetes

Reference	Proband	Risk to sibs %	Risk to offspring %	Comments
1. Harris (1950)	<30	4.1		Interview
			1.4	Predicted by age 40
2. Working Party, College of Practitioners (1965)	<30	4.8		Interview
3. Simpson (1962)	<20	5.7	.9	Interview
4. Simpson (1968)	<20	2.4	1.8	Mailed questionnaire
	<40	3.4	1.1	
5. Kobberling (1969)	<25	10.9±3.9		Predicted by age 25
6. Darlow et al (1973)	<25	4.7–7.6		Predicted by age 25
		5.2–12.6		Predicted by age 45
7. Tattersall & Fajans (1975)	<25	11		Interview and GTT
8. Nerup et al (1976)	juvenile	9.7		HLA typed
9. Degnbol & Green (1978)	<20	6.2±1.3	5.4±2.9*	Questionnaire interview – predicted by age 35
10. West et al (1979)	<17	4.1%		Medical record review
11. Gottlieb (1980)	<20	4.5%	3.1%	Mailed questionnaire of proband and relatives
12. Gamble (1980)	<16	5.6%		Observed by age 16, mailed questionnaire of families
13. Koberling & Bruggeboes (1980)	insulin treated since dianosis		2.4%	Medical questionnaire, includes both parents affected
			1.5%	Only mother affected

* Actual observed recurrence 2.8%

REFERENCES

Barbosa J, King R, Noreen H, Yunis E J 1977 The histocompatibility (HLA) system in juvenile insulin dependent diabetic multiplex kindreds. Journal of Clinical Investigation 60: 989–998

Barbosa J, Chern M M, Noreen H, Anderson V E 1978a Analysis of linkage between the major histocompatibility system and juvenile insulin dependent diabetes in multiplex families, reanalysis of data. Journal of Clinical Investigation 62: 492–495

Barbosa J, Ramsay R, Goetz F C 1978b Plasma glucose, insulin, glucagon, and growth hormone in kindreds with maturity-onset type of hyperglycemia in young people. Annals of Internal Medicine 88: 595–601

Barbosa J 1980 Nature and nurture: the genetics of diabetic microangiopathy. In: Podolsky S and Viswanathan M, (eds) Secondary Diabetes, The Spectrum of the Diabetic Syndromes, Raven Press, New York, p 67–74

Barbosa J, Chern M M, Anderson V E, Noreen H, Johnson S, Reinsmoen N, McCarty R, King R, Greenberg L 1980a Linkage analysis between the major histocompatibility system and insulin-dependent diabetes in families with patients in two consecutive generations. Journal of Clinical Investigation 65: 592–601

Barbosa J, Cohen R A, Chavers B, Michael A F, Steffes M, Hoogwerf B, Szalapski E, Mauer M 1980b Muscle extracellular membrane immunofluorescence and HLA as possible markers of prediabetes. Lancet ii: 330–333

Barnett A H, Eff C, Leslie R D G, Pyke D A 1981a Diabetes in identical twins. A study of 200 pairs. Diabetologia 20: 87–93

Barnett A H, Spiliopoulos A J, Pyke D A, Stubbs W A, Burrin J, Alberti K G M M 1981b Metabolic studies in unaffected co-twins of non-insulin-dependent diabetics. British Medical Journal ii: 1656–1658

Bartels E D 1953 Endocrine disorders. In: Sorbsy A (ed) Clinical Genetics, 2nd ed., C V Mosby Company, St Louis

Bertrams J 1982 Non HLA markers for type I diabetes on chromosome 6. In: Kobberling J and Tattersall R (eds) Genetics of Diabetes Mellitus, Academic Press, London, pp 91–98

Bodmer W F 1978 The HLA system: Introduction. British Medical Bulletin 34: 213–216

Bottazzo G F, Florin-Christensen A, Doniach D 1974 Islet-cell antibodies in diabetes mellitus with autoimmune polyendocrine deficiencies. Lancet ii: 1279–1282

Bottazzo G F and Doniach D 1976 Pancreatic autoimmunity and HLA antigens. Lancet ii: 800

Bottazzo G F, Mann J I, Thorogood M, Baum J D, Doniach D 1978 Autoimmunity in juvenile diabetics and their families. British Medical Journal ii: 165–168

Bottazzo G F, Dean B M, Gorsuch A N, Cudworth A G, Doniach D 1980 Complement-fixing islet-cell antibodies in type-I diabetes, possible monitors of active beta-cell damage. Lancet i: 668–672

Bottazzo G F, Mirakian R, Dean B M, McNally J M, Doniach D 1982 How immunology helps to define heterogeneity in diabetes mellitus. In: Kobberling J and Tattersall R (eds) Genetics of Diabetes Mellitus, Academic Press, London, pp 79–90

Braunsteiner H, Hansen W, Jung A, Sailer S 1966 Latent diabetes in parents of juvenile diabetics. German Medical Monthly 11: 227–232

Burkeholder J N, Pickens J M, Womack W N 1967 Oral glucose tolerance test in siblings of children with diabetes mellitus. Diabetes 16: 156–160

Cahill C F Jr 1979a Diabetes mellitus. In: Beeson P B,

McDermott W, Wyngaarden J B (eds) Cecil Textbook of Medicine, W B Saunders, Philadelphia, p 1969–1989

Cahill C F Jr 1979b Current concepts of diabetic complications with emphasis on hereditary factors: a brief review. In: Sing C F and Skolnick M H (eds) Genetic Analysis of Common Diseases: Applications to Predictive Factors in Coronary Heart Disease, Alan R Liss, New York, pp. 113–129

Cahill G F Jr, McDevitt H O 1981 Insulin dependent diabetes mellitus: The initial lesion. New England Journal of Medicine 304: 1454–1464

Cammidge P J 1928 Diabetes mellitus and heredity. British Medical Journal ii: 738–741

Cammidge P J 1934 Heredity as a factor in the aetiology of diabetes mellitus. Lancet i: 393–395

Cerasi F, Luft R 1967. Insulin response to glucose infusion in diabetic and nondiabetic monozygotic twin pairs, Genetic control of insulin response? Acta Endocrinologia 55: 330–345, 1967

Christy M, Green A, Christau B, Kromann H, Nerup J, Platz P, Thomsen M, Ryder L P, Svejgaard A 1979 Studies of the HLA system and insulin dependent diabetes mellitus. Diabetes Care 2: 209–214

Clerget-Darpoux F and Bonaiti-Pellie C 1980 Epistasis effect: an alternative to the hypothesis of linkage disequilibrium in HLA associated diseases. Annals of Human Genetics 44: 195–204

Clerget-Darpoux F, Bonaiti-Pellie C, Deschamps I, Hors J, Feingold N 1981 Juvenile insulin-dependent diabetes: a possible susceptibility gene in interaction with HLA. Annals of Human Genetics 45: 199–206

Cohen A M 1961 Prevalence of diabetes among different ethnic Jewish groups in Israel. Metabolism 10:50–58.

Coleman D L 1979 Obesity genes: beneficial effects in heterozygous mice. Science 203: 663–644

Coleman D L 1982 The genetics of diabetes in rodents. In: Kobberling J and Tattersall R (eds) Genetics of Diabetes Mellitus, Academic Press, London pp 183–193

Conn J W and Fajans S S 1961 The prediabetic state. American Journal of Medicine 31: 839–850

Craighead J E 1978 Current views on the etiology of insulin-dependent diabetes mellitus. New England Journal of Medicine 299: 1439–1445

Creutzfeldt W, Kobberling J, Neel J V (eds) 1976 The Genetics of Diabetes Mellitus, Springer-Verlag, Berlin

Cudworth A G and Woodrow J C 1975a HLA system and diabetes mellitus. Diabetes 24: 345–349

Cudworth A G and Woodrow J C 1975b Evidence for HLA linked genes in juvenile diabetes mellitus. British Medical Journal ii: 133–135

Cudworth A G 1978 Type I diabetes mellitus. Diabetologia 14: 281–291

Cudworth A G and Festenstein H 1978 HLA genetic heterogeneity in diabetes mellitus. British Medical Bulletin 34: 285–290

Curie-Cohen M 1981 HLA antigens and susceptibility to juvenile diabetes: do additive relative risks imply genetic heterogeneity? Tissue Antigens 17: 136–148

Darlow J M and Smith C 1973 A statistical and genetical study of diabetes. III. Empiric risks to relatives. Annals of Human Genetics 37: 157–174

Degnbol B and Green A 1978 Diabetes mellitus among first- and second-degree relatives of early onset diabetics. Annals of Human Genetics 42: 25–34

DeSilva N E, Tunbridge W M G, Alberti K G M M 1981 Low incidence of chlorpropamide-alcohol flushing in diet-treated, non-insulin-dependent diabetes. Lancet i: 128–131

Dreyer M, Kuhnau J, Rudiger H W 1980 Chlorpropamide-alcohol flushing is not useful for individual genetic counseling of diabetic patients. Clinical Genetics 18: 189–190

Fajans S S 1976 The natural history of idiopathic diabetes mellitus. Heterogeneity in insulin responses in latent diabetes. In: Creutzfeldt W, Kobberling J, Neel J V (eds) The Genetics of Diabetes Mellitus, Springer-Verlag, Berlin, p 64–78

Fajans S S, Cloutier M C, Crowther R L 1978 Clinical and etiologic heterogeneity of idiopathic diabetes mellitus. Diabetes 27: 1112–1125

Fajans S S 1982 Heterogeneity between various families with noninsulin dependent diabetes of the MODY type, In: Kobberling J and Tattersall R (eds) Genetics of Diabetes Mellitus, Academic Press, London, pp 251–260

Farid N R, Newton R M, Noel E P, Barnard J M, Marshall W H 1978 The operation of immunological networks in Graves' disease. Tissue Antigens 12: 205–211

Fialkow P J, Zavala C, Nielsen R 1975 Thyroid autoimmunity: increased frequency in relatives of insulin dependent diabetes patients. Annals of Internal Medicine 83: 170–176

Flier J S, Kahn C R and Roth J 1979 Receptors, antireceptor antibodies and mechanisms of insulin resistance. New England Journal of Medicine 300: 413–419

Friedman J M and Fialkow P J 1980 The genetics of diabetes mellitus, In: Steinberg A G, Bearn A G, Motulsky A G, Childs B (eds) Progress in Medical Genetics Vol IV, W.B. Saunders, Philadelphia, p 199–232

Gamble D R 1980 An epidemiological study of childhood diabetes affecting two or more siblings. Diabetologia 19: 341–344

Given B D, Mako M E, Tager H S, Baldwin D, Markese J, Rubenstein A H, Olefsky J, Kobayashai M, Kolterman O, Poucher R 1980 Diabetes due to secretion of an abnormal insulin. New England Journal of Medicine 302: 129–135

Gorsuch A N, Dean B M, Bottazzo G F, Lister J, Cudworth A G 1980 Evidence that type I diabetes and thyrogastric autoimmunity have different genetic determinants. British Medical Journal i: 145–147

Gottlieb M S and Root H F 1968 Diabetes mellitus in twins. Diabetes 17: 693–704

Gottlieb M S 1980 Diabetes in offspring and siblings of juvenile and maturity-onset-type diabetics. Journal of Chronic Diseases 33: 331–339

Greenberg D A and Rotter J I 1981 Two locus models for gluten sensitve enteropathy: population genetic considerations. American Journal of Medical Genetics 8: 205–214

Hanhart E 1951 Zur Vererbung des diabetes mellitus. Schweiz Med Wchnschr 81: 1127–1131

Harris H 1949 The incidence of parental consanguinity in diabetes mellitus. Annals of Eugenics 14: 293–300

Harris H 1950 The familial distribution of diabetes mellitus: a study of the relatives of 1241 diabetic propositi. Annals of Eugenics 15: 95–110

Harvald B and Hauge M 1963 Selection in diabetes in modern society. Acta Medica Scandinavica 173: 459–465

Harvald B and Hauge M 1965 Heredity factors elucidated by twin studies. In: Neel J V, Shaw M W, Schull W J (eds) Genetics and the Epidemiology of Chronic Diseases, Public Health Service Publication No 1163, p 61–76

Herberg L and Coleman D L 1977 Laboratory animals exhibiting obesity and diabetes syndromes. Metabolism 26: 59–99

Hodge S E, Rotter J I and Lange K L 1980 A three allele model for heterogeneity of juvenile onset dependent diabetes. Annals of Human Genetics 43: 399–412

Hodge S E and Spence M A 1981 Some epistatic two-locus models of disease II: The confounding of linkage and

association. American Journal of Human Genetics 33: 396–406

Hodge S E, Anderson C E, Neiswanger K, Field L L, Spence M A, Sparkes R S, Sparkes M C, Crist M, Terasaki P I, Rimoin D L, Rotter J I 1981 Close linkage between IDDM and the Kidd blood group, Lancet ii: 893–895

Hunter S and McKay E 1967 Intravenous glucose tolerance test in parents of diabetic children. Lancet i: 1017–1019

Ilonen J, Herva E, Tiilikainen A, Akerblom H K, Koivukangas T, Kouvalainen K 1978 HLA-Dw2 as a marker of resistance against juvenile diabetes mellitus. Tissue Antigens 11: 144–146

Irvine W J 1977 Classification of idiopathic diabetes. Lancet i: 638–642

Irvine W J, Gray R S, McCallum C J, Duncan L J P 1977a Clinical and pathogenic significance of pancreatic islet cell antibodies in diabetics treated with oral hypoglycaemic agents. Lancet i: 1025–1027

Irvine W J, Toft A D, Holton D E, Prescott R J, Clarke B F, Duncan L J P 1977b Familial studies of type I and type II idiopathic diabetes mellitus. Lancet ii: 325–328

Irvine W J, Mario U D, Feek C M, Gray R S, Ting A, Morris P J, Duncan L J P 1978a Autoimmunity and HLA antigens in insulin dependent (type 1) diabetes. Journal of Clinical and Laboratory immunology 1: 107–110

Irvine W J, Mario U D, Feek C M, Ting A, Morris P J, Gray R S, Duncan L J P 1978b Insulin antibodies in relation to islet cell antibodies and HLA antigens in insulin dependent (type 1) diabetes. Journal of Clinical and Laboratory Immunology 1: 111–114

Irvine W J, Sawen J S A, Prescott R J, Duncan L J P 1979 The value of islet cell antibody in predicting secondary failure of oral hypoglycaemic agent therapy in diabetes mellitus. Journal of Clinical and Laboratory Immunology 2: 23–26

Irvine W J (ed) 1980 Immunology of Diabetes, Teviot, Edinburgh

Jakobson T and Nikkila E A 1969 Serum lipid levels and response of plasma insulin to the oral administration of glucose in first degree relatives of diabetic patients. Diabetologia 5: 427

Joslin E P, Root F H, White P, Marble A 1959 In: The Treatment of Diabetes Mellitus, ed 10, Lea and Febiger, Philadelphia, p 47–98

Keen H and Track N S 1968 Age of onset and inheritance of diabetes: the importance of examining relatives. Diabetologia 4: 317–321

Kobberling J 1969 Utersuchungen zur Genetik des Diabetes Mellitus. Eine Geeignete Methode zur Durchfuhrung von Alterskorrekturen. Diabetologia 5: 392–396

Kobberling J, Appels A, Kobberling G, Creutzfeldt W 1969 Glucose tolerance test; 727 first degree relatives of maturity-onset diabetics. German Medical Monthly 14: 290–294

Kobberling J 1971 Studies on the genetic heterogeneity of diabetes mellitus. Diabetologia 7: 46–49

Kobberling J 1976a Genetic heterogeneities within idiopathic diabetes. In: Creutzfeldt W, Kobberling J, Neel J V (eds) The Genetics of Diabetes Mellitus, Springer-Verlag, Berlin, p 79–87

Kobberling J 1976b Genetic syndromes associated with lipatrophic diabetes, In: Creutzfeldt W, Kobberling J, Neel J V (eds) The Genetics of Diabetes Mellitus, Springer-Verlag, Berlin, p 147–154

Kobberling, J and Bruggeboes B 1980 Prevalence of diabetes among children of insulin-dependent diabetic mothers. Diabetologia 18: 459–462

Kobberling J, Bengsch N, Bruggeboes B, Schwarch H, Tillil H, Weber M 1980 The chlorpropamide alcohol flush, Lack of specificity for familial non-insulin dependent diabetes. Diabetologia 19: 359–363

Knowler W C, Pettitt D J, Savage P J, Bennett P H 1981 Diabetes incidence in Pima Indians: Contributions of obesity and parental diabetes. American Journal of Epidemiology 113: 144–156

Lambert T H, Johnson R B, Geoffrey P R 1961 Glucose and cortisone-glucose tolerance in normal and prediabetic humans. Annals of Internal Medicine 54: 916–923

Leslie R D G and Pyke D A 1978 Chlorpropamide-alcohol flushing: a dominantly inherited trait associated with diabetes. British Medical Journal ii: 1519–1520

Leslie R D G, Pyke D A, Stubbs W A 1979a Sensitivity to enkephalin as a cause of non-insulin dependent diabetes. Lancet i: 341–343

Leslie R D G, Barnett A H, Pyke D A 1979b Chlorpropamide alcohol flushing and diabetic retinopathy. Lancet i: 997–999

Lestradet H, Battistelli J, Ledoux M 1972 L'heredite dans le diabete infantile. Le Diabete 2: 17–21

Levit S G and Pessikova L N 1934 The genetics of diabetes mellitus. Proc Maxim Gorky Medico Biol Institute 3: 132–147

Ludvigsson J, Safwenberg K, Heding L G 1977 HLA-types, C-peptide and insulin antibodies in juvenile diabetes. Diabetologia 13: 13–17

Ludwig H, Schernthaner G, Mayr W R 1976 Is HLA-B7 a marker associated with a protective gene in juvenile-onset diabetes mellitus? New England Journal of Medicine 294: 1066

MacCuish A C, Barnes E W, Irvine W J, Duncan L J P 1974 Antibodies to pancreatic islet cells in insulin-dependent diabetics with coexistent autoimmune disease. Lancet ii: 1529–1531

MacDonald M J 1974 Equal incidence of adult-onset diabetes among ancestors of juvenile diabetics and non diabetics. Diabetologia 10: 767–773

MacDonald M J 1980 Hypothesis: The frequencies of juvenile diabetes in American Blacks and Caucasians are consistent with dominant inheritance. Diabetes 29: 110–114

McMichael A and McDevitt H 1977 The association between the HLA system and disease. In: Steinberg A G, Bearn A G, Motulsky A G and Child B (eds) Progress in Medical Genetics, Vol II, W B Saunders, Philadelphia, p 39–100

Mimura G and Miyao S 1962 Heredity and constitutions of diabetes mellitus. Bull Res Inst Diathetic Med Kumamoto Univ 12: 1–82

Mirakian R, Bottazzo G F, Doniach D 1980 Auto-antibodies to duodenal gastric-inhibitory-peptide (GIP) cells and to secretin (S) cells in patients with coeliac disease, tropical sprue and maturity-onset diabetes. Clinical and Experimental Immunology 41: 33–42

Nakao Y, Matsumoto H, Miyazaki T, Mizuno N, Arima N, Wakisaka A, Okimoto K, Akazawa Y, Tsuji K, Fujita T 1981 IgG heavy-chain (Gm) allotypes and immune response to insulin in insulin-requiring diabetes mellitus. New England Journal of Medicine 304: 407–409

National Diabetes Data Group International Workgroup 1979 Classification of diabetes mellitus and other categories of glucose intolerance. Diabetes 28: 1039–1057

Neel J V 1962 Diabetes mellitus, a "thrifty" genotype rendered detrimental by "progress?". American Journal of Human Genetics 14: 353–362

Nerup J, Platz P, Ortved-Anderson O, Christy M, Lyngsoe J, Poulsen J E, Ryder L P, Staub-Nielsen L, Thomsen M, Svejgaard A 1974 HLA antigens and diabetes mellitus. Lancet ii: 864–866

Nerup J, Platz P, Ortved-Anderson O, Christy M, Egeberg J,

Lyngsoe J E, Poulsen J E, Ryder L P, Thomsen M, Svejgaard A 1976 HLA, autoimmunity and insulin-dependent diabetes mellitus. In: Creutzfeldt W, Kobberling J, Neel J V (eds) The Genetics of Diabetes Mellitus, Springer-Verlag, Berlin, p 106–114

Nerup J, Cathelineau C, Seignalet J, Thomsen M 1977 HLA and endocrine diseases. In: Dausset J and Svejgaard A (eds) HLA and Disease, Munksgaard, Copenhagen, p 149–161

Nerup J, Platz P, Ryder L P, Thomsen M, Svejgaard A 1978 HLA, islet cell antibodies, and types of diabetes mellitus. Diabetes 27: (supplement) 247–250

Neufeld M, Maclaren N K, Riley W J, Lezotte D, McLaughlin J V, Silverstein J, Rosenbloom A L 1980 Islet cell and other organ-specific antibodies in U.S. Caucasians and Blacks with insulin-dependent diabetes mellitus. Diabetes 29: 589–592

Nissley P S, Drash A L, Blizzard R M, Sperling M, Childs B 1973 Comparison of juvenile diabetes with positive and negative organ specific antibody titers; evidence for genetic heterogeneity. Diabetes 22: 63–65

Notelovitz M 1969 Genetics and the Natal Indian diabetic. South African Medical Journal 43: 1245–1247

Owerbach D, Bell G I, Rutter W J, Brown J A, Shows T B 1981 The insulin gene is located on the short arm of chromosome 11 in humans. Diabetes 30: 267–270

Owerbach D and Nerup J 1981 Restriction fragment length polymorphism of the insulin gene in diabetic individuals. Diabetologia, 21: 311

Peña A S, Mann D L, Hague N E, Heck J A, Van Leeuwen A, Van Rood J J, Strober W 1978 Genetic basis of gluten-sensitive enteropathy. Gastroenterology 75: 230–235

Pickens J M 1964 The prediabetic state in siblings of known juvenile diabetic children. 51st Ross Conference on Pediatric Research, p 64–68

Pincus G and White P 1933 On the inheritance of diabetes mellitus, I. An analysis of 675 family histories. American Journal of Medical Science 186: 1–14

Pyke D A and Taylor K W 1967 Glucose tolerance and serum insulin in unaffected identical twin of diabetics. British Medical Journal ii: 21–24

Pyke D A, Nelson P G 1976 Diabetes mellitus in identical twins. In: Creutzfeldt W, Kobberling J, Neel J V (eds) The Genetics of Diabetes Mellitus, Springer-Verlag, Berlin, p 194–205

Pyke D A 1978 Twin studies in diabetes. In: Nance W E, Allen G and Parisi P (eds) Twin Research, Part C, Clinical Studies, Alan R Liss, New York, p 1–12

Pyke D A and Leslie R D G 1978 Chlorpropamide-alcohol flushing: a definition of its relation to non-insulin dependent diabetes. British Medical Journal ii: 1521–1522

Pyke D A 1979 Diabetes: the genetic connections. Diabetologia 17: 333–343

Raum D, Alper C A, Stein R, Gabbay K H 1979 Genetic marker for insulin-dependent diabetes mellitus. Lancet i: 1208–1210

Rayfield E J and Seto Y 1981 Etiology: viruses. In: Brownlee M (ed) Handbook of Diabetes Mellitus, Garland STPM Press, Vol 1: 95–120

Riley W J, Maclaren N K, Neufeld M 1980 Adrenal autoantibodies and Addison disease in insulin-dependent diabetes mellitus. Journal of Pediatrics 97: 191–195

Rimoin D L 1967 Genetics of diabetes mellitus. Diabetes 16: 346–351

Rimoin D L 1969 Ethnic variability in glucose tolerance and insulin secretion. Archives of Internal Medicine 124: 695–700

Rimoin D L and Schimke R N 1971 Endocrine pancreas. In: Genetic Disorders of the Endocrine Glands, C V Mosby, St Louis, p 150–216

Rimoin D L 1976 Genetic syndromes associated with glucose intolerance. In: Creutzfeldt W, Kobberling J, Neel J V (eds) The Genetics of Diabetes Mellitus, Springer-Verlag, Berlin, p 43–63

Rimoin D L and Rotter J I 1981 Genetic heterogeneity in diabetes mellitus and diabetic microangiopathy. Hormone and Metabolic Research, Supplement ii: 63–72

Rimoin D L and Rotter J I 1982 Genetic syndromes associated with diabetes mellitus and glucose intolerance. In: Kobberling J and Tatterall R (eds) Genetics of Diabetes Mellitus, Academic Press, London, pp 149–181

Rotter J I and Rimoin D L 1978 Heterogeneity in diabetes mellitus – update 1978: Evidence for further genetic heterogeneity within juvenile onset insulin dependent diabetes mellitus. Diabetes 27: 599–608

Rotter J I, Rimoin D L, Samloff I M 1978 Genetic heterogeneity in diabetes mellitus and peptic ulcer. In: Morton N E and Chung C S (eds) Genetic Epidemiology, Academic Press, New York, p 381–414

Rotter J I and Rimoin D L 1979 Diabetes mellitus: the search for genetic markers. Diabetes Care 2: 215–226

Rotter J I and Hodge S E 1980 Racial differences in diabetes are consistent with more than one mode of inheritance. Diabetes 29: 115–118

Rotter J I 1981 The modes of inheritance of insulin dependent diabetes, American Journal of Human Genetics, 33: 835–851

Rotter J I and Rimoin D L 1981a Etiology-genetics. In: Brownlee M (ed) Handbook of Diabetes Mellitus. Garland STPM Press, New York Vol 1: 3–93

Rotter J I and Rimoin D L 1981b The genetics of the glucose intolerance disorders. American Journal of Medicine 70: 116–126

Rotter J I and Rimoin D L 1981c The genetics of insulin dependent diabetes. In: Martin J M, Ehrlich R M, Holland F J (eds) Etiology and Pathogenesis of Insulin Dependent Diabetes Mellitus, Raven Press, New York, p 37–59

Rubinstein P, Suciu-Foca N, Nicholson F 1977 Genetics of juvenile diabetes mellitus, a recessive gene closely linked to HLA D and with 50 percent penetrance. New England Journal of Medicine 297: 1036–1040

Rubinstein P, Ginsberg-Fellner F, Falk C 1981 Genetics of type I diabetes mellitus: a single, recessive predisposition gene mapping between HLA-B and GLO. American Journal of Human Genetics, 33: 865–882

Simpson N E 1962 The genetics of diabetes: a study of 233 families of juvenile diabetics. Annals of Human Genetics 26: 1–12

Simpson N E 1964 Multifactorial inheritance: a possible hypothesis for diabetes. Diabetes 13: 462–471

Simpson N E 1968 Diabetes in the families of diabetics. Canadian Medical Association Journal 98: 427–432

Simpson N E 1976 A review of family data. In: Creutzfeldt W, Kobberling J, Neel J V (eds) The Genetics of Diabetes Mellitus, Springer-Verlag, Berlin, p 12–26

Singal D P, Blajchman M A 1973 Histocompatibility (HL-A) antigens, lymphocytotoxic antibodies and tissue antibodies in patients with diabetes mellitus. Diabetes 22: 429–432

Sisk C W 1968 Application of a one hour glucose-tolerance test to genetic studies of diabetes in children. Lancet i: 262–266

Spielman R S, Baker L, Zmijewski C M 1979 Inheritance of susceptibility to juvenile-onset diabetes. In: Sing C F and Skolnick M H (eds) Genetic Analysis of Common Diseases: Applications to Predictive Factors in Coronary Heart Disease, Alan R Liss, New York, p. 567–585

Spielman R S, Baker L, Zmijewski C M 1980 Gene dosage and susceptibility to insulin dependent diabetes. Annals of Human Genetics 44: 135–150

Steiner F 1936 Untersuchungen zur Frage der Erblichkeit des diabetes mellitus. Deutches Archiv für Klinische Medezin 178: 497–510

Strober W 1980 Genetic factors in gluten-sensitive enteropathy. In: Rotter J I, Samloff I M, Rimoin D L (eds) The Genetics and Heterogeneity of Common Gastrointestinal Disorders, Academic Press, San Francisco and New York, p 243–259

Svejgaard A, Platz P, Ryder L P, Staub-Nielsen L, Thomsen M 1975 HLA and disease associations – a survey. Transplantation Reviews 22: 3–34

Svejgaard A and Ryder L P 1979 HLA markers and disease. In: Sing C F and Skolnick M (eds) Genetic Analysis of Common Diseases: Applications to Predictive Factors in Coronary Heart Disease Alan R Liss, New York, p 523–543

Svejgaard A, Platz P, Ryder L P 1980 Insulin dependent diabetes mellitus, In: Terasaki P I (ed) Histocompatibility Testing 1980, UCLA Tissue Typing Laboratory, Los Angeles, p 638–656

Svejgaard A and Ryder L P 1981 HLA genotype distribution and genetic models of insulin-dependent diabetes mellitus. Annals of Human Genetics 45: 293–298

Tattersall R B and Pyke D A 1972 Diabetes in identical twins. Lancet ii: 1120–1124

Tattersall R B 1974 Mild familial diabetes with dominant inheritance. Quarterly Journal of Medicine 43: 339–357

Tattersall R B and Fajans S S 1975 A difference between the inheritance of classical juvenile onset and maturity onset type diabetes of young people. Diabetes 24: 44–53

Then Berg H 1939 The genetic aspect of diabetes mellitus. J A M A 112: 1091

Thompson M W and Watson E M 1952 The inheritance of diabetes mellitus: an analysis of the family histories of 1,631 diabetics. Diabetes 1: 268–275

Thomson G and Bodmer W 1977 The genetic analysis of HLA and disease associations. In: Dausset J and Svejgaard A (eds) HLA and Disease, Munksgaard, Copenhagen, p 84–93

Thomson G 1980 A two locus model for juvenile diabetes. Annals of Human Genetics 43: 383–398

Walker A and Cudworth A G 1980 Type I (insulin-dependent) diabetic multiplex families, mode of genetic transmission. Diabetes 29: 1036–1039

Werner N 1936 Blutzuckerregulation und Erbanlage. Deutches Archiv Für Klinische Medezin 178: 308

West K M 1978 Epidemiology of Diabetes and its Vascular Lesions, Elsevier, New York

West R, Belmonte M M, Colle E, Crepeau P, Wilkins P, Poirier R 1979 Epidemiologic survey of juvenile-onset diabetes in Montreal. Diabetes 28: 690–693

White P 1965 The inheritance of diabetes. Medical Clinics of North America 49: 857–863

Whittingham S, Mathews J D, Schanfield M S, Tait B D, Mackay I R 1981 Interaction of HLA and Gm in autoimmune chronic active hepatitis. Clin Exp Immunol 43: 80–86

Working Party, College of General Practitioners 1965 Family history of diabetes. British Medical Journal i: 960–962

Zimmet P 1979 Epidemiology of diabetes and its macrovascular manifestations in Pacific populations, the medical effects of social progress, Diabetes Care 2: 144–153

Zimmet P, Faaiuso S, Ainuu J, Whitehouse S, Milne B, DeBoer W 1981 The prevalence of diabetes in the rural and urban Polynesian population of Western Samoa. Diabetes 30: 45–51

86

Congenital adrenal hyperplasia

M.I. New, K. Grumbach, L.S. Levine

INTRODUCTION

Congenital adrenal hyperplasia (CAH) is a family of inherited disorders of adrenal steroidogenesis. Each disorder results from a deficiency of one of the several enzymes necessary for normal steroid synthesis.

Since the earliest documented case of CAH in 1865 by the Neapolitan anatomist De Crecchio (1865), numerous investigators have unravelled the mechanisms of adrenal steroid synthesis and the associated enzyme defects responsible for the adrenogenital syndrome.

PATHOPHYSIOLOGY

Biochemistry of steroidogenesis

The adrenal gland synthesizes three main classes of hormones: mineralocorticoids, glucocorticoids, and sex steroids. Figure 86.1 presents a simplified scheme of the adrenal synthesis of these steroids from the cholesterol precursor molecule. Each hydroxylation step is indicated and the newly added hydroxyl group is circled.

Defects in the enzymes necessary for steroidogenesis produce clinically recognizable syndromes that depend upon the specific hormones that are deficient and those that are produced in excess.

The most common form of CAH results from a defect of the 21-hydroxylation enzyme. This defect selectively impairs aldosterone and cortisol synthesis while sparing the androgen pathway. A deficiency of the 11β-hydroxylase enzyme similarly blocks cortisol but not androgen synthesis. Disorders of adrenal steroidogenesis have also been described in association with deficiencies of the enzymes 3β-hydroxysteroid dehydrogenase (3β-HSD), 17α-hydroxylase, cholesterol desmolase, 18-hydroxylase, 18-dehydrogenase, and 17β-hydroxysteroid dehydrogenase.

A summary of the clinical and biochemical features of these disorders is presented in Table 86.1.

Adrenal steroid regulation

The pituitary regulates adrenal steroidogenesis via adrenocorticotropic hormone (ACTH). ACTH acts on the adrenals to increase the conversion of cholesterol to pregnenolone. The central nervous system controls the secretion of ACTH, its diurnal variation, and its increase in stress via corticotropin-releasing factor (Ganong, 1963; Guillemin & Schally, 1963). The hypothalamic-pituitary-adrenal feedback is mediated through the circulating level of plasma cortisol such that any condition which decreases cortisol secretion will result in increased ACTH secretion. In those forms of CAH in which an enzyme deficiency causes impaired cortisol synthesis, there is excessive ACTH secretion and hyperplasia of the adrenal cortex (Fig. 86.2).

Reference to Figure 86.1 indicates the pathophysiology of adrenal hyperplasia in the case of 21-hydroxylase deficiency. An enzymatic deficiency of 21-hydroxylase results in decreased cortisol (F) synthesis, which in turn induces increased ACTH secretion. Consequent to the increased ACTH secretion, there is overproduction of cortisol precursors (viz. 17-hydroxyprogesterone) and sex steroids (viz. testosterone), the biosynthesis of which do not require 21-hydroxylation.

The excess of adrenal androgen is responsible for the virilization characteristic of CAH due to 21-hydroxylase deficiency.

Reference to Figure 86.1 indicates that an enzymatic deficiency of 11β-hydroxylase also results in decreased cortisol synthesis, as in 21-hydroxylase deficiency. The decreased cortisol synthesis induces increased ACTH secretion, with the resultant overproduction of cortisol precursors and sex steroids. Thus, 11β-hydroxylase deficiency CAH shares the clinical feature of virilization with the 21-hydroxylase disorder.

An additional finding in many, but not all, patients with 11β-hydroxylase deficiency CAH is hypertension. The hypertension is thought to be the result of the excess production of the aldosterone precursor deoxycorticosterone (DOC), itself a mineralocorticoid with salt-retaining activity.

In addition to the hypothalamic-pituitary regulation of adrenal steroidogenesis, the renin-angiotensin system exerts a primary influence on the adrenal secretion of aldosterone. In brief, the renin-angiotensin system is

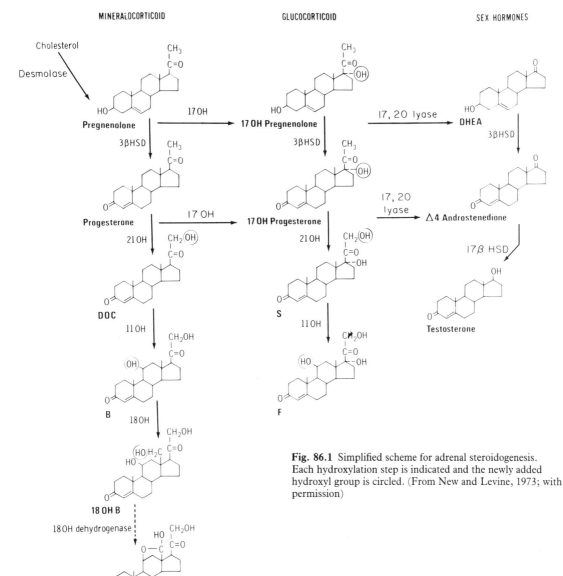

Fig. 86.1 Simplified scheme for adrenal steroidogenesis. Each hydroxylation step is indicated and the newly added hydroxyl group is circled. (From New and Levine, 1973; with permission)

responsive to the state of electrolyte balance (Fig. 86.3). The justaglomerular apparatus produces renin, an enzyme which reacts with an α_2 globulin known as renin substrate to release angiotensin I. Angiotensin I is then enzymatically converted to angiotensin II, a potent stimulator of aldosterone secretion (Laragh et al, 1971).

The fact that the pituitary and the renin-angiotensin system act as two distinct and largely independent regulators of adrenal steroidogenesis has prompted the theory that the adrenal zona fasciculata and zona glomerulosa function as two separate glands (New & Seaman, 1970). According to this proposal, ACTH stimu-

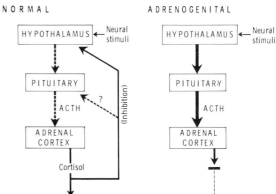

Fig. 86.2 The regulation of cortisol secretion in normal subjects and in patients with congenital adrenal hyperplasia. (From New and Levine, 1973; with permission)

Table 86.1 Clinical and laboratory features of various forms of adrenal disorders of steroidogenesis

Clinical features					
Newborn with sexual ambiguity					
Female	Male	Salt wasting	Hypertension	Postnatal virilization	Enzyme deficiency
					21-Hydroxylase
+	0	0	0	+	– not salt wasting
+	0	+	0	+	– salt wasting
+	0	+	0	+	11β-Hydroxylase
+	0	0	+	+	11β-Hydroxylase
+	+	+	0	0	3β-HSD[b]
0	+	0	+	0	17α-Hydroxylase
0	+	+	0	0	Cholesterol desmolase
0	0	+	0	0	18-Hydroxylase
					18-Dehydrogenase of 18 hydroxycorticosterone
0	0	+	0	0	(Methyloxidase Type II)
?	+	–	–	+[c]	17β-Hydroxysteroid[f] dehydrogenase

nl = normal

[a] Mostly THS

[b] The values presented apply to the infant and very young child

[c] Mostly △5–17 ketosteroids

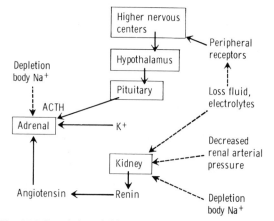

Fig. 86.3 Regulation of aldosterone secretion (From New and Peterson, 1966; with permission)

lates the fasciculata to secrete sex steroids, glucocorticoids, and the weak mineralocorticoid precursors of aldosterone such as corticosterone. The fasciculata lacks, however, the enzyme necessary to complete the terminal step of aldosterone synthesis. In contrast, the glomerulosa secretes aldosterone but not cortisol or testosterone under the stimulation of the renin-angiotensin system; ACTH exerts only a transient influence on glomerulosa aldosterone synthesis.

An extension of this theory is that an enzymatic deficiency may occur in the fasciculata, but not in the glomerulosa. Several reports have suggested that this is the case for the genetic defect of 11β-hydroxylation (Zach-

mann et al, 1971; Sizonenko et al, 1972; Tan et al, 1978; Gregory & Gardner, 1976). Recent extensive studies in four patients with 11β-hydroxylase deficiency (Levine et al, 1980a) have confirmed that this enzyme defect occurs only in the fasciculata.

Additional evidence supporting the concept that the adrenal fasciculata and glomerulosa function as two separate glands has been gained from the recent study of patients with 21-hydroxylase deficiency.

In CAH due to 21-hydroxylase deficiency, two different clinical syndromes are recognized: the simple virilizing and the salt wasting forms. In both forms, there is defective 21-hydroxylation of the 17-hydroxysteroids leading to the elevation of 17-hydroxyprogesterone (17-OHP) and diminished production of cortisol (Bongiovanni & Eberlein, 1958). The salt wasting form, however, evidences a deficiency of mineralocorticoid activity in addition to the virilization caused by excess androgen secretion. The exact nature of the 21-hydroxylase enzyme defect in the 17-desoxy (mineralocorticoid) pathway in both the salt wasting and simple virilizing forms of CAH remains controversial, though it is widely accepted that aldosterone synthesis is more deficient in salt wasters than in simple virilizers. The hypotheses proposed to explain the different syndromes are based either on a 'one-enzyme' or a 'two-enzyme' defect. However, neither in vivo nor in vitro studies have been conclusive and results compatible with both theories have been reported (New et al, 1981b).

The 'one-enzyme' theory attributes the difference between salt wasting and simple virilizing CAH to a dif-

Laboratory findings								
Urinary excretion				Circulating hormones				
17-KS	17-OH	P'triol	Aldo	17-OHP	△4	DHEA	Testosterone	Renin
↑↑	nl or ↓	↑↑	nl	↑↑	↑↑	nl or ↑ (DHEA/△4 ↓)	↑	nl or ↑
↑↑	↓	↑↑	↓	↑↑	↑↑	nl or ↑	↑	↑↑
↑↑ [c]	↑↑ [a]	↑	↓		↑↑	↑	↑	↓↓
↑	↓↓	↑	↓	nl or ↑	nl or ↑	↑↑↑	↓ or nl	↑
↓↓	↓↓	↓↓	↓↓	↓	↓	↓	↓	↓
nl	nl	nl	↓↓	nl	nl	nl	nl	↑
nl	↑ [d]	nl	↓↓	nl	nl	nl	nl	↑
nl ↑	nl	nl	nl	nl	↑↑	nl or ↑	nl or ↓ (△4/T ↑↑)	nl

[d] Largely 18-hydroxy THA, which gives a Porter-Silber reaction
[e] Only in males at puberty
[f] This defect may occur only in the gonad

ferent degree of enzymatic deficiency, the most severe deficiency leading to salt wasting. The 'two-enzyme' theory postulates that the simple virilizers have an enzymatic deficiency in the 17-hydroxy (glucocorticoid) pathway, whereas the salt wasters have a deficiency in both the 17-hydroxy and 17-desoxy pathway of adrenal steroidogenesis. This theory is supported by normal or even elevated aldosterone secretion or excretion in simple virilizers in contrast to the impaired aldosterone production in salt wasters (New et al, 1981b).

Recent studies from our laboratory have suggested a new hypothesis to explain the differences in salt wasting and simple virilizing adrenal hyperplasia (New et al, 1981b). This hypothesis states: (a) in both simple virilizers and salt wasters, there is a fasciculata defect of 21-hydroxylation in both the 17-hydroxy and 17-desoxy pathways, and (b) in the salt waster there is a defect in 21-hydroxylation in the glomerulosa as well, while in the simple virilizer, the glomerulosa is spared this defect. This hypothesis is schematically presented in Figure 86.4.

A new study verifies this hypothesis. Kuhnle et al (1980, 1981) found that both normal subjects and simple virilizers, but not salt wasters, demonstrated a rise in serum and urinary aldosterone and 18-hydroxycorticosterone when the glomerulosa was stimulated with a low sodium intake while the zona fasciculata was suppressed by dexamethasone. These results indicate the absence of a 21-hydroxylase deficiency in the zona glomerulosa of the simple virilizer and show that in both normal subjects and in the simple virilizers, the zona glomerulosa can increase aldosterone secretion in response to renin stimulation independent of precursor hormones of the zona fasciculata.

These data support the hypothesis that there is a 21-hydroxylation defect in the zona fasciculata of simple virilizers and salt wasters whereas the zona glomerulosa is defective in salt wasters and not in simple virilizers (Fig. 86.4). In addition, the data indicate that there is one enzyme involved in the 21-hydroxylation of the 17-hydroxy and 17-desoxy pathways of adrenal steroidogenesis in the zona fasciculata. These findings are consistent with the reports of an enzymatic deficiency only in the fasciculata, sparing the glomerulosa, in CAH due to 11β-hydroxylase deficiency (Sizonenko et al 1972; Levine et al 1980a).

These findings further suggest the possibility of separate genetic loci for the regulation of 21-hydroxylation in the zona fasciculata and the zona glomerulosa. Studies of genetic recombination, discussed below, are also suggestive of the possibility that more than one locus on the sixth chromosome code for 21-hydroxylation. However, the hormonal data suggest that within the fasciculata, only one genetic locus seems to regulate the 21-hydroxylase enzyme activity in both the 17-hydroxy and 17-desoxy pathways.

CLINICAL ASPECTS

Ambiguous genitalia at birth

The most prominent clinical feature of both 21-hydroxylase and 11β-hydroxylase deficiency CAH is virilization

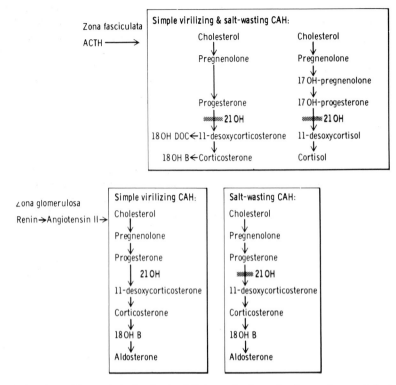

Fig. 86.4 Pathway of adrenal steroidogenesis in the simple virilizing and salt wasting forms of congenital adrenal hyperplasia.

of the external genitalia of the genetic female presenting at birth. In order to understand the pathophysiology of CAH, it is necessary to discuss normal sexual differentiation briefly.

According to the hypothesis developed by Jost (1966), normal differentiation of male genitalia is dependent on two functions of the fetal testis:

1. secretion of the fetal androgen, perhaps testosterone, to cause stimulation of the Wolffian ducts and differentiation of male external genitalia. When differentiation is complete, the urethra opens at the tip of the penis. In the male, the source of androgen is the fetal testis, but any source of androgen can cause masculinization of external genitalia, e.g. adrenal androgen during the first trimester of pregnancy.

2. secretion of a non-steroidal substance (Josso, 1972) which inhibits Mullerian development such that normal males are born without a uterus.

Since the fetal ovary secretes neither testosterone nor the inhibiting factor necessary to inhibit Mullerian structures, the normal female is born without male differentiation of external genitalia (i.e., with female external genitalia), and without Mullerian repression (i.e., with a uterus and fallopian tubes). This is shown schematically in Figure 86.5.

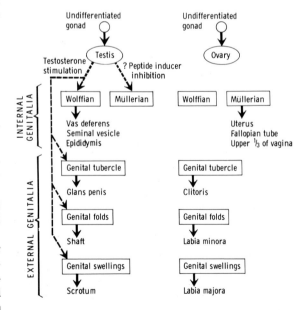

Fig. 86.5 Fetal sex differentiation. (From New and Levine, 1973; with permission)

Thus, in the above scheme, the ovary does not play a determining role in sex differentiation.

Female fetuses exposed to either high levels of androgen consequent to CAH, an androgen producing tumor in the mother, or administration of androgens to the mother, manifest virilization of the external genitalia but normal internal genitalia (Federman, 1968).

Since adrenocortical function begins in the third month of gestation, in cases of 21-hydroxylase or 11β-hydroxylase deficiency the fetus is exposed at the critical time of sexual differentiation to the oversecreted adrenal androgens. In the case of a female fetus, the excessive adrenal androgen masculinizes the external genitalia and female pseudohermaphroditism results. In rare cases the masculinization is so profound that the urethra is penile (Wilkins, 1962). The internal female genitalia (i.e., uterus and fallopian tubes) are normal, however, since the female fetus does not possess testes to secrete Mullerian inhibitor. The female genital abnormalities are present only in the androgen-responsive external genitalia.

Males with disorders of 21-hydroxylase or 11β-hydroxylase do not manifest genital abnormalities at birth.

Postnatal virilization

The result of continued excess adrenal androgen secretion in untreated virilizing CAH is progressive penile or clitoral enlargement; advanced bone age and transient tall stature followed by ultimate short stature due to premature epiphyseal closure; early appearance of facial, axillary, and pubic hair; and acne. As mentioned above, in cases of 11β-hydroxylase deficiency, hypertension is frequently an additional symptom.

Further complications arise at puberty in untreated patients with CAH. The female fails to develop breasts, remains amenorrheic, and develops a male habitus. In the male, the testes generally remain small and fail to develop and function. Without appropriate therapy adults may be expected to be sterile.

Treatment

Sex assignment at birth
The newborn infant with ambiguous genitalia presents a complex problem. The decision as to sex assignment at birth has obvious life-long implications. Furthermore, the correct decision cannot be based solely on the anatomical appearance of the external genitalia.

For example, a highly virilized genetic female with CAH due to a 21-hydroxylase defect may be born with extremely masculine appearing genitalia, e.g. a penile-like clitoris and complete labioscrotal fusion. Yet a male sex assignment would be in error in this case because of the female genetic sex and the normal female internal genitalia. A male sex assignment in the case of female pseudohermaphroditism due to 21-hydroxylase deficiency would be particularly tragic since with proper treatment the infant could become a reproductive female capable of full sexual and gender role activity.

The specific enzymatic defects causing the clinically observed CAH can be distinguished by hormonal testing. In patients with 21-hydroxylase deficiency, there is excessive excretion of pregnanetriol, the metabolite of 17-hydroxyprogesterone (Bongiovanni, 1953; Bongiovanni et al, 1954), and urinary 17-ketosteroids, which result from the metabolism of dehydroepiandrosterone (DHEA), △4-androstenedione, and testosterone. Laboratory diagnostic tests include the measurement of increased levels of 17-ketosteroids and pregnanetriol in urine. More recently, techniques have permitted the measurement of accumulated precursors in the blood, as well as the measurement of the secretion of adrenal corticoids (Korth-Schutz et al, 1978; Pang et al, 1979).

In patients with 11β-hydroxylase deficiency, elevated serum and urinary concentrations of DOC and androgens are found. Serum levels of 11-deoxycortisol (Compound S) and urinary excretion of Compound S metabolites, including 17-hydroxysteroids, are also elevated (New & Levine 1973; Levine et al, 1980a).

An exciting new development in the laboratory diagnosis of 21-hydroxylase deficiency has been the application of a microfilter paper method for 17α-hydroxyprogesterone radioimmunoassay as a rapid screening test for CAH in newborns (Pang et al 1977). This convenient test requires only 20 μl of blood to provide a reliable diagnostic measurement of serum 17-hydroxyprogesterone (Fig. 86.6).

Once a sex assignment has been made based on a reliable diagnosis of the underlying endocrine disorder, appropriate surgical measures may be taken to repair the ambiguous external genitalia. In cases of female pseudohermaphroditism due to 21- or 11β-hydroxylase deficiency, the aim of surgical repair should be to remove the redundant erectile tissue, preserve the sexually sensitive glans clitoris, and provide an exteriorized vagina that will function adequately for menstruation and intromission (Mininberg et al, 1979). In these patients, normal puberty, fertility, and childbearing are possible when there is early therapeutic intervention.

Endocrine therapy
The aim of therapy is to provide replacement of the deficient hormones. In the case of the most common 21-hydroxylase form of CAH, this means replacing cortisol, both to replace the deficiency in secretion and to suppress ACTH overproduction. Proper replacement will prevent excessive stimulation of the androgen pathway, thus averting further virilization and allowing normal growth and a normal onset of puberty.

Although salt retaining steroids in addition to glucocorticoids have been used in the treatment of the salt wasting form of 21-hydroxylase deficiency, it has not

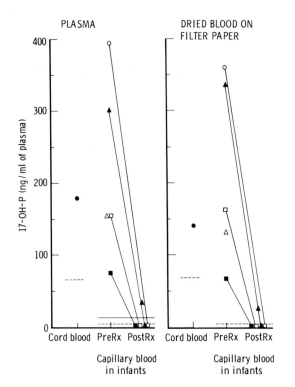

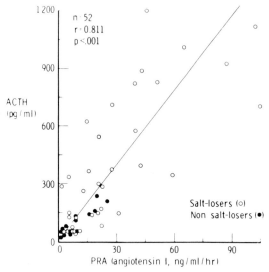

Fig. 86.7 Correlation between ACTH and plasma renin activity (PRA) levels in patients with CAH treated with constant replacement doses of glucocorticoids equivalent to 25 mg/m²/day of hydrocortisone. Patients were studied during different states of sodium balance. (From Rösler et al, 1977; with permission)

Fig. 86.6 17α-OH-progesterone concentrations in cord and capillary blood samples in infants with CAH. Ages of infants at diagnosis were as follows: ● = cord blood, △ = 2 days □ = 4 days, ■ = 7 days, ▲ = 2 weeks, ○ = 4 weeks. Samples on treatment were taken from five days to one month after treatment was begun. The dashed line indicates upper limit of normal infants. The solid line indicates upper limit of pooled plasma in sick infants. Plasma samples were pipetted quantitatively and assayed. Cord blood samples were also quantitatively pipetted onto filter paper. Capillary samples were directly applied to filter paper without quantitation and a 3 mm disc punched out for analysis.

been customary to treat non-salt wasting patients with salt retaining steroids, despite the recognition that plasma renin activity (PRA) is elevated in the non-salt wasting form as well as in the salt wasting form (Dillon & Ryness, 1975; Bartter, 1977; Strickland & Kotchen, 1972; Godard et al, 1968). However, in a clinical study, Rösler et al (1977) have demonstrated that the addition of salt retaining hormone to glucocorticoid therapy in patients with elevated PRA does in fact improve the hormonal control of the disease. Rösler showed that the PRA was closely correlated to the ACTH level (Fig. 86.7). Thus, when PRA was normalized by the addition of 9α-fludrocortisone acetate administration (9FF), the ACTH level fell and excessive androgen stimulation by ACTH decreased (Fig. 86.8). The addition of salt retaining steroids to the therapeutic regimen often made possible a decrease in the glucocorticoid

dose. Normalization of PRA also resulted in improved statural growth (New et al, 1981a) (Fig. 86.9).

In the past, urinary 17-ketosteroids and pregnanetriol excretion have been the biochemical monitors of hormonal control. Since the advent of radioimmunoassay, it has been possible to establish normal serum androgen concentrations for children of various ages (Korth-Schutz et al, 1976). Recent studies have indicated that the serum 17-hydroxyprogesterone and △4-androstenedione levels provide a sensitive index of biochemical control. The serum testosterone is useful in females and prepubertal males but not in newborn or pubertal males (Korth-Schutz et al, 1978).

The combined determinations of PRA, 17-hydroxyprogesterone, and serum androgens and the clinical assessment of growth and pubertal status must all be considered in adjusting the dose of glucocorticoid and salt retaining steroid. In our clinic, we employ hydrocortisone and 9α-fluorocortisone acetate modalities. This approach to therapy has been confirmed by Winter (1980). Measurement of PRA can be used to monitor efficacy of treatment not only in 21-hydroxylase deficiency but also in the other salt losing forms of CAH (cholesterol desmolase, 3β-HSD). PRA is also useful as a therapeutic index in those forms of CAH with mineralocorticoid excess and suppressed PRA (11β-hydroxylase and 17-hydroxylase). In the former, the PRA is elevated in poor control whereas in the latter it is suppressed (Fig. 86.10).

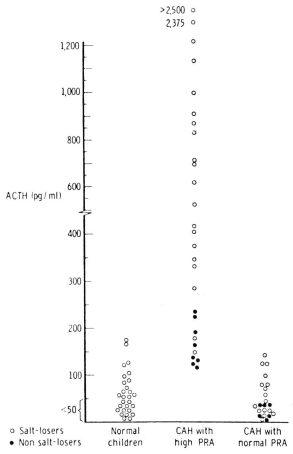

Fig. 86.8 ACTH levels in normal children and in seven patients with CAH treated with constant replacement doses of glucocorticoids equivalent to 25 mg/m²/day of hydrocortisone. Samples were drawn between 0800 and 0900 h. Levels of plasma renin activity (PRA) were high during the ad lib, normal and low sodium diets. Normal PRA levels were achieved by sodium repletion with a high sodium diet and/or additional 9α-fludrocortisone acetate. (From Rösler et al, 1977; with permission)

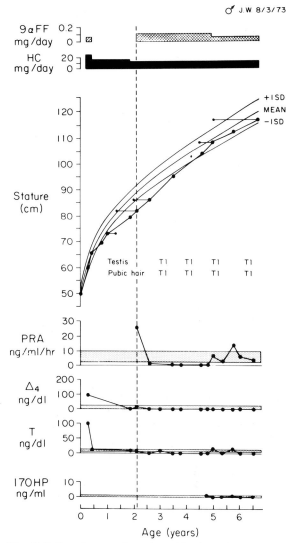

Fig. 86.9 Growth curve of a patient with salt wasting congenital adrenal hyperplasia before and after therapeutic control of plasma renin activity. Note that with renin suppression, hydrocortisone dose could be lowered, growth improved and androgen suppression was maintained despite the decrease in hydrocortisone dose. (From New et al, 1981b; with permission)

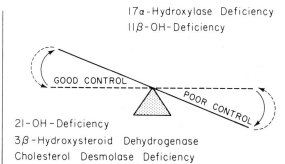

Fig. 86.10 The pivotal role of monitoring plasma renin activity in therapy of various forms of congenital adrenal hyperplasia. In poor control, renin is elevated in 21-hydroxylase deficiency, 3β-hydroxysteroid deficiency and cholesterol desmolase deficiency and decreases with proper mineralocorticoid treatment. In contrast in 17α-hydroxylase deficiency and 11β-hydroxylase deficiency, renin is suppressed in poor control and rises with proper treatment. (From New et al, 1981b, with permission)

GENETICS

Population studies

Several surveys have established that the 21-hydroxylase deficiency is transmitted as an autosomal recessive trait (Prader, 1958; Wilkins, 1962; Childs et al, 1956). Males and females are equally at risk (Baulieu et al, 1967). With few exceptions (Rosenbloom & Smith, 1966b), the severity of the 21-hydroxylase deficiency, which parallels the degree of salt wasting, is consistent within one family.

In Europe and the USA recent estimates of the incidence have been between 1:5000 and 1:15,000. In Alaska the incidence in Yupik Eskimos is unusually high, while the low incidence reported in Maryland may be due to inadequate case ascertainment (Table 86.2).

The gene frequency is estimated as one in 50 and one in 100 in different populations (Müller et al, 1979). The salt wasting variety occurs in about 30–80% of patients with 21-hydroxylase deficiency (Cohen, 1969; Rimoin & Schimke, 1971). A very high incidence of the salt wasting variety has been found among the Yupiks (Hirschfeld & Fleshman, 1969).

The 11β-hydroxylase deficiency is also transmitted as an autosomal recessive trait, but it is rarer than the 21-hydroxylase deficiency.

HLA linkage

In 1977, close genetic linkage between HLA and CAH due to 21-hydroxylase deficiency was first described (Dupont et al, 1977). In this initial study, HLA genotyping of parents and children in six families with more than one child affected with CAH due to 21-hydroxylase deficiency was performed. In five of these families, all of the affected offspring were HLA identical and different from their unaffected sibs.

Subsequently, studies of 34 unrelated families with a total of 48 patients were reported from New York and Zurich (Levine et al, 1978). The findings of this study are exemplified by the two typical pedigrees shown in Figure 86.11. As can be observed in Figure 86.11A, the three affected sibs are HLA identical. In Figure 86.11B, the unaffected sibs are all HLA different from their affected sister. Both HLA haplotypes of the patient are therefore presumed to be linked to the gene for 21-hydroxylase deficiency. Thus any member of the family who shares one HLA haplotype with the patient should also carry the gene for the enzyme defect.

In Figure 86.11B, the corresponding HLA haplotype presumed to carry the genetic enzyme defect is represented by an asterisk.

Thus each parent has transmitted one HLA haplotype carrying the gene for 21-hydroxylase deficiency to the patient. The brother and the sister having one haplotype linked to the gene for CAH are presumed heterozygotes, as is each parent who transmitted that haplotype. The sib sharing neither haplotype with the patient is presumed to not carry the gene for the 21-hydroxylase deficiency.

Thus, the HLA genotype can be a marker for the CAH genotype in a family with an index case.

Further international studies of the genetic linkage between HLA and CAH have provided a more detailed genetic mapping of the 21-hydroxylase deficiency gene within the HLA complex. The studies from twenty-five laboratories were recently summarized in the report from the Eighth International Histocompatibility Workshop (Dupont et al, 1980); the findings are presented in Table 86.3.

These findings complement earlier studies (Murtaza et al, 1978; Zappacosta et al, 1978; Grosse-Wilde et al, 1979) which clearly indicate that the 21-hydroxylase deficiency gene segregates with the HLA-B locus and can be separated by genetic recombination from the HLA-A and glyoxalase I (GLO) loci. These findings support the initial conclusion (Dupont et al, 1977; Levine et al, 1978) that both the salt wasting and non-salt wasting forms of 21-hydroxylase deficiency are in very close genetic linkage with HLA-B; that is, that the gene for 21-hydroxylation is located close to the locus for the HLA-B determinants.

Table 86.2 Estimated incidence of CAH (21-hydroxylase deficiency)

Reference	Population	Patient/live births
Childs et al (1956)	Maryland, USA	1:67 000
Prader (1958)	Zurich, Switzerland	1:5041
Hubble (1966)	Birmingham, England	1:7255
Rosenbloom and Smith (1966a)	Wisconsin, USA	1:15 000
Hirshfeld and	Alaska, USA	1:700★
Fleshman	Yupik Eskimo, USA	1:245
Qazi and Thompson (1972)	Toronto, Canada	1:13 000★
Mauthe et al (1977)	Munich, Germany	1:9831
Muller et al (1979)	Tirol, Austria	1:8991
Werder et al (1980)	All of Switzerland	1:15 472

★ Incidence was corrected for both variants of salt waster and non-salt waster

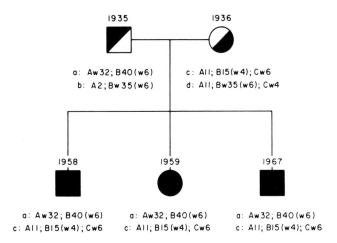

A.   FAMILY Zurich 7 (21-Hydroxylase Deficiency)

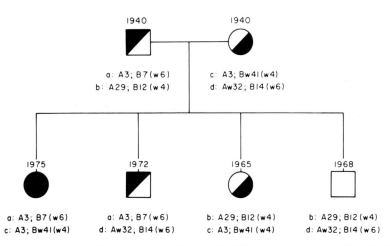

B.   FAMILY N.Y. 16 (21-Hydroxylase Deficiency)

Fig. 86.11 Pedigrees for two families with 21-hydroxylase deficiency. The HLA haplotypes for the HLA-A, HLA-B, and HLA-C alleles are given in each family. The paternal haplotypes are labeled a and b, and the maternal haplotypes c and d. The parents are obligate heterozygous carriers for the 21-hydroxylase deficiency gene (denoted by the half-black symbols). The affected children are denoted by black symbols. In (A) three affected siblings are HLA genotypically identical. In (B) one affected child is HLA genotypically different from the three unaffected siblings. One sibling who carries the parental a and d haplotypes is presumed to be a heterozygous carrier for 21-hydroxylase deficiency because he shares the a haplotype with the patient. Another sibling has the parental b and c haplotypes and shares the c haplotype with the patient, and should be a carrier of the 21-hydroxylase deficiency gene. The child with the b and d haplotypes should be normal for the gene. (From Levine et al, 1978; with permission)

The findings relative to the HLA-D/DR locus are less consistent. In one study of HLA-B:D/DR recombination, the 21-hydroxylase deficiency gene was reported to segregate with the HLA-B locus and separate from the HLA-D/DR gene (Pucholt et al, 1979); this suggests that the 21-hydroxylase gene lies *between* the HLA-B and HLA-D/DR loci. Two other studies, however, have reported rare cases of HLA-D/DR:GLO recombination in which the 21-hydroxylase deficiency gene segregated with the GLO locus and not with the HLA loci (Betuel et al, 1980; Klouda et al, 1980). These latter studies indicate that the 21-hydroxylase gene lies *below* the HLA-D/DR site relative to the centromere, between the HLA-D/DR and GLO loci. These seemingly inconsist-

Table 86.3 21-Hydroxylase deficiency: HLA recombinants

Recombination		21-OH-DEF gene	Reference
HLA	A : B	segregate with HLA-B	Dupont et al 1977
			Levine et al 1978
	A : B	segregate with HLA-B	Gelsthorpe et al 1980★
	A : B	segreate with HLA-B	Couillin et al 1980★
	A : C	segregate with HLA-C	Price et al 1978
	A : Bf	segregate with Bf or HLA-B	Weitkamp et al 1978
	or		
	A : B		
	C : B	segregate with HLA-B	Kastelan et al 1980★
	C : B	segregrate with HLA-B	Betuel et al 1980★
	B : D/DR	segregate with HLA-B	Pucholt et al 1979
	DR : GLO	segregate with DR in two families	Levine et al 1978
	DR : GLO	segregate with DR	Couillin et al 1980★
	DR : GLO	segregate with DR in two families	Manderville et al 1980★
	DR : GLO	segregate with DR in four families	Kastelan et al 1980★
	DR : GLO	segregate with DR	Mayer et al 1980★
	DR : GLO	segregate with GLO	Klouda et al 1980
	DR : GLO	segregate with DR in three families	Hansen et al 1980★
	HLA-A,B,C,DR/D id. sibs discordant for 21-OH-Def	21-OH-DEF outside HLA-D	Betuel et al 1980★

★ Denotes families reported only as part of the Eighth International Histocompatibility Workshop (Dupont et al., 1980)

ent findings suggest the possibility that there may be two separate but closely linked genetic loci which code for 21-hydroxylation. This possibility is particularly noteworthy in view of our earlier suggestion that two separate genetic loci may regulate 21-hydroxylase activity in the adrenal zona fasciculata and zona glomerulosa.

Statistical methods of genetic analysis have more formally demonstrated close genetic linkage between the 21-hydroxylase deficiency gene and HLA. Using LOD Score and recombination frequency (θ) indexes, studies have consistently reported high 21-hydroxylase gene linkage probability with the HLA-B locus and low probabilities with the HLA-A and GLO loci (Grosse-Wilde et al, 1978; Levine et al, 1978; Dupont et al, 1980). The statistical probabilities can be translated into a chromosomal distance scalar, indicating that the deficiency gene is very near the HLA-B locus, five to ten centimorgans from the GLO locus.

The loci mapped on chromosome number six within the HLA linkage group are shown in Figure 86.12.

The discovery of HLA linkage to the 21-hydroxylase deficiency gene has been applied to great advantage to the practice of clinical endocrinology. Prior to this discovery, it was difficult to distinguish CAH heterozygosity solely on the basis of hormonal testing. It is now possible to predict by HLA genotyping which sibs of a patient with CAH are heterozygote carriers for the enzyme deficiency and which sibs can be presumed to be genetically unaffected. Figure 86.11 demonstrates how HLA genotyping can be applied to heterozygosity prediction.

Hormonal studies can then verify the genetic prediction. In family studies, the response of 17-hydroxypro-

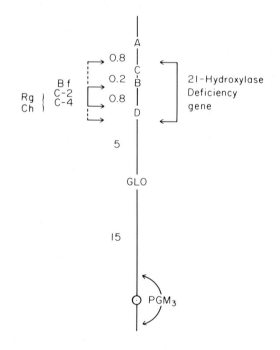

Fig. 86.12 HLA linkage group on chromosome 6. The recombinant fractions for the known linkages between A:C, C:B, B:D, B:GLO and GLO:PGM₃ are shown. The position of the genes for factor B (*Bf*), complement C-2 and complement C-4 and Rodgers (*Rg*) and Chido (*Ch*) blood groups is also indicated. The 21-hydroxylase deficiency gene can be mapped between HLA-A and Glyoxalase I (*GLO*). The most likely position of the 21-hydroxylase deficiency gene is very close to HLA-B. (From Levine et al, 1978; with permission)

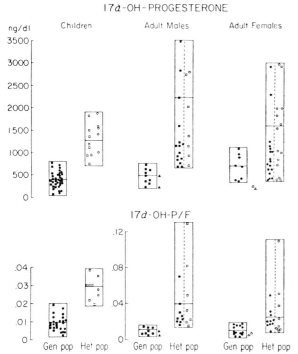

Fig. 86.13 Stimulated 17-OHP level and the stimulated 17-OHP to F ratio in prepubertal and early pubertal children, postpubertal males, and postmenarchal females. Gen. pop: general population (■, male, ●, female, ▲ homozygous normal brother of a patient with CAH, based on HLA typing). Het. pop.: heterozygous population (■, father, ●, mother, □, heterozygous brothers or heterozygous male family members, based on HLA typing; ○, heterozygous sisters or heterozygous female family members, based on HLA typing; △, homozygous normal sister, based on HLA typing). The bar represents the range; the heavy horizontal line represents the mean. (From Lorenzen et al, 1980; with permission)

gesterone (17-OHP) to ACTH stimulation was higher in family members who were predicted to be heterozygotes than in family members predicted to be genetically unaffected by HLA genotyping (Fig. 86.13). No other hormonal measurement was as useful in discriminating heterozygotes from normals (Lorenzen et al 1979, 1980).

The HLA genotyping of amniotic cells has been applied to the prenatal diagnosis of CAH. HLA genotyping, in combination with hormonal testing of amniotic fluid, can predict CAH in cases of a fetus at risk (Pollack et al, 1979) (Fig. 86.14).

Our HLA linkage studies have also led us to uncover a new and cryptic form of 21-hydroxylase deficiency in family members of patients with classical CAH. In the course of HLA genotyping and hormonal testing of families, we encountered a conflict between the HLA and hormonal predictions of CAH genotype in the sister of an index case who was predicted by HLA genotyping to be unaffected (Lorenzen et al, 1979) (Fig. 86.15). ACTH tests indicated that her stimulated 17-OHP level was within the heterozygote range (Fig. 86.16). This conflict between the HLA prediction and the hormonal findings was resolved when it was discovered that the father was an asymptomatic patient with mild 21-hydroxylase deficiency. Thus the genotype of the pedigree was revised to indicate that both the father's haplotypes were linked to a 21-hydroxylase deficiency gene (Fig. 86.15). One was transmitted to the index case and the other to the unaffected sib who responded appropriately to hormonal testing as a heterozygote. It was surprising to find that the father was a patient with 21-hydroxylase deficiency without the hallmarks commonly accompanying this disorder.

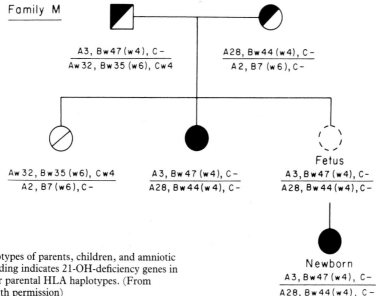

Fig. 86.14 HLA genotypes of parents, children, and amniotic cells in family M. Shading indicates 21-OH-deficiency genes in linkage with particular parental HLA haplotypes. (From Pollack et al, 1979, with permission)

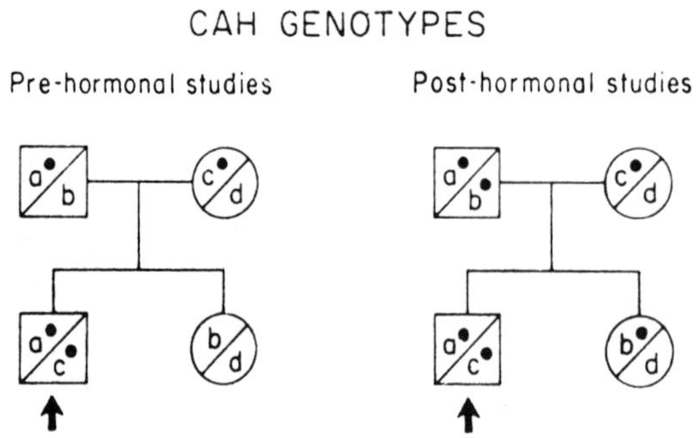

CAH GENOTYPES

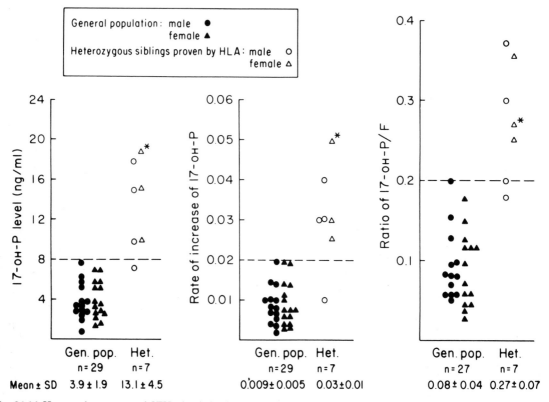

Fig. 86.15 Revision of interpretation of CAH genotyping before and after hormonal studies which revealed the father to be a patient with 21-hydroxylase deficiency.
a, b, c, and d represent HLA haplotypes.
a• and c• represent the HLA haplotypes linked with gene for CAH in the affected child (↑).
Hormonal studies revealed the father to be affected and thus the b haplotype was also linked with the gene for CAH. This resulted in reassignment of the sister as a heterozygote (b•/d).
(From Lorenzen et al, 1979; with permission)

We have now studied 120 families and have found eight pedigrees in which family members of an index case have a mild but asymptomatic 21-hydroxylase deficiency which we have called cryptic 21-hydroxylase deficiency. Within each generation the family members with cryptic 21-hydroxylase deficiency were HLA identical (Figures 86.17 & 86.18). Each shared one HLA haplotype with the index case with classical CAH and would have been predicted before hormonal testing to be heterozygote carriers. These family members are genetic compounds, having 21-hydroxylase deficiency as a result of two recessive genetic defects: a severe 21-hydroxylase deficiency gene present in the index case, and a mild 21-hydroxylase deficiency gene. Thus, the CAH genotype in the family members with cryptic 21-hydroxylase deficiency was $21\text{-}OH^{CAH}/21\text{-}OH^{CRYPTIC}$.

LOD Score analysis has established close genetic linkage between HLA and the 21-hydroxylase^{CRYPTIC} gene (Levine et al, 1980b).

These cryptic family members have no clinical signs or symptoms suggestive of 21-hydroxylase deficiency (e.g., virilization), although their biochemical profile indicates that they do have a mild 21-hydroxylase deficiency. The

Fig. 86.16 Hormonal response to ACTH stimulation in prepubertal and early pubertal children (Tanner I-III). Gen. pop.: general population; Het: assumed to be heterozygous for CAH according to HLA genotyping; (---): upper range in general population; △*: offspring of a probably affected father and heterozygous mother for CAH. (From Lorenzen et al, 1979; with permission)

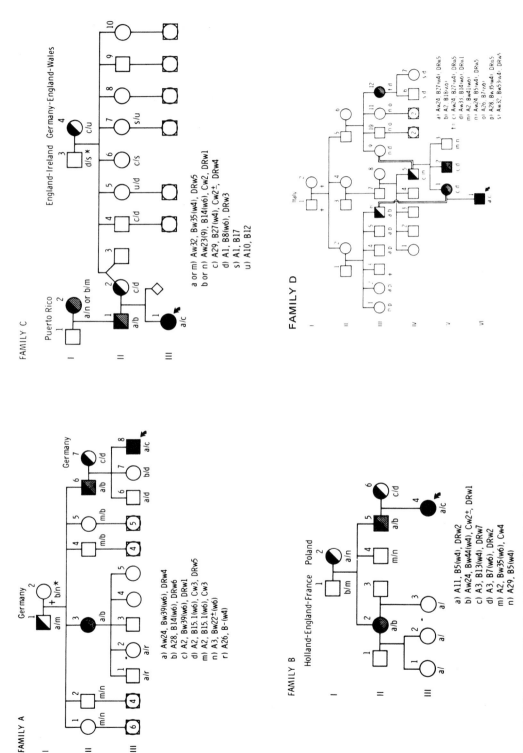

Fig. 86.17 Pedigrees of families A–D. The HLA haplotypes from the HLA-A, HLA-B, HLA-C, and HLA-D/DR are indicated for each family tested. The index case with CAH is assigned the haplotypes a/c. ✱ indicates haplotypes a/c. ✱ indicates haplotypes deduced from offspring. ● indicates obligate heterozygous carriers of the severe deficiency gene for CAH. ● ◨ indicates family members with cryptic 21-hydroxylase deficiency, having both a severe and a mild deficiency gene. ▢ indicates offspring, number if known. (From Levine et al, 1980b; with permission)

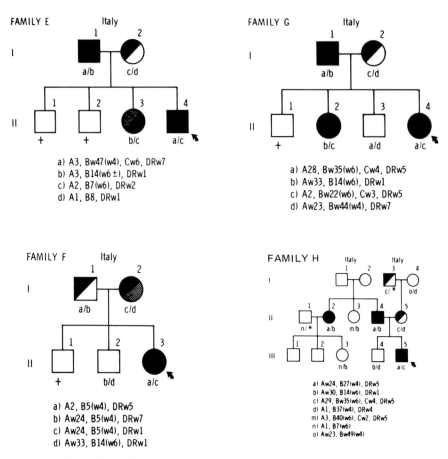

a) A3, Bw47(w4), Cw6, DRw7
b) A3, B14(w6±), DRw1
c) A2, B7(w6), DRw2
d) A1, B8, DRw1

a) A28, Bw35(w6), Cw4, DRw5
b) Aw33, B14(w6), DRw1
c) A2, Bw22(w6), Cw3, DRw5
d) Aw23, Bw44(w4), DRw7

a) A2, B5(w4), DRw5
b) Aw24, B5(w4), DRw7
c) Aw24, B5(w4), DRw1
d) Aw33, B14(w6), DRw1

a) Aw24, B27(w4), DRw5
b) Aw30, B14(w6), DRw1
c) A29, Bw35(w6), Cw4, DRw5
d) A1, B37(w4), DRw4
m) A3, B40(w6), Cw2, DRw5
n) A1, B7(w6)
o) Aw23, Bw49(w4)

Fig. 87.18 Pedigrees of families E-H. See Figure 86.17 for symbols. (From Levine et al, 1980b; with permission)

biochemical profile in these patients is best described by a nomogram relating the baseline and ACTH stimulable levels of 17-OHP, $\triangle$4-androstenedione ($\triangle$4), dehydroepiandrosterone (DHEA), the ratio of DHEA/$\triangle$4, and testosterone. Figure 86.19 demonstrates that 17-OHP levels in patients with classical CAH ($21\text{-}OH^{CAH}/21\text{-}OH^{CAH}$), cryptic 21-hydroxylase deficiency ($21\text{-}OH^{CAH}/21\text{-}OH^{CRYPTIC}$), and heterozygotes ($21\text{-}OH^{CAH}/21\text{-}OH^{NORMAL}$ or $21\text{-}OH^{CRYPTIC}/21\text{-}OH^{NORMAL}$ for these disorders aggregate into groups which are easily distinguished.

The groups are distributed on a regression line in the following descending order: classical adrenal hyperplasia, cryptic 21-hydroxylase deficiency, heterozygotes for the classical and cryptic 21-hydroxylase deficiencies, and subjects genetically unaffected (by HLA). The general population which was not HLA genotyped is at the lower end, but some fall in the heterozygote group suggesting that they may be carrying the gene for 21-hydroxylase deficiency. A similar distribution of groups along a regression line is observed for $\triangle$4 and testosterone in females (Figures 86.20 & 86.21).

Although the DHEA values (Fig. 86.22) do not aggregate in groups, the ratio of DHEA/$\triangle$4 aggregates in reverse order from that of 17-OHP (Fig. 86.23). The mean testosterone level in males with classical CAH was lower than that of heterozygotes (Fig. 86.24).

These nomograms provide a sensitive and powerful tool by which to assign the 21-hydroxylase deficiency genotype, i.e. patients whose hormonal values fall on a regression line within a defined group are assigned to that group.

Based on these nomograms, the genotype for 21-hydroxylase deficiency in the members of families A-H (Figs. 86.17 & 86.18) can now be refined (Figs. 86.25 & 86.26). In Figures 86.25 and 86.26, the family members who are heterozygous for the cryptic 21-hydroxylase deficiency and the classical 21-hydroxylase deficiency are shown.

HLA and hormonal studies in families of patients with late onset adrenal hyperplasia (21-hydroxylase deficiency) have also been reported. Late onset or 'acquired' adrenal hyperplasia is a puzzling syndrome in which virilization and menstrual disturbances associated with

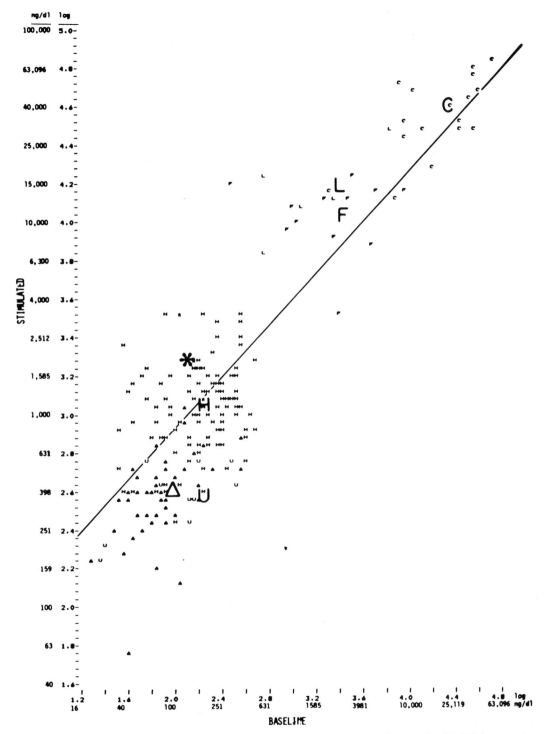

Fig. 86.19 Nomogram relating baseline to ACTH stimulated serum 17-hydroxyprogesterone concentration. Values for the log$_{10}$ and the antilog are indicated. The mean for each group is indicated by a large symbol.

C = Classical CAH patients off treatment
F = Cryptic 21-hydroxylase deficiency patients
★ = Heterozygotes for cryptic 21-hydroxylase deficiency
H = Heterozygotes for classical CAH

U = Family members predicted by HLA genotyping to be genetically unaffected
△ = General population
L = Patients with late onset 21-hydroxylase deficiency

The values for each group aggregate in descending order along the regression line. Note that the heterozygotes for the cryptic 21-hydroxylase defect are in the same range as the heterozygotes for the classical 21-hydroxylase defect. (From New et al, 1981b; with permission)

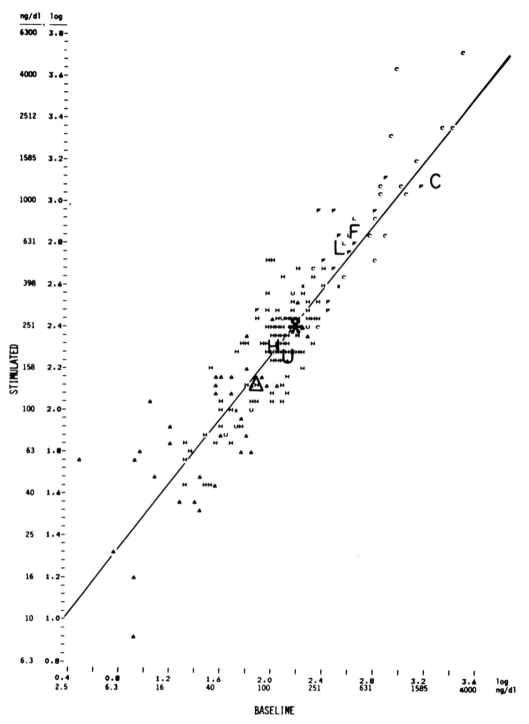

Fig. 86.20 Nomogram relating baseline to the ACTH stimulated △4 androstenedione concentration. Values for the $\log_{10}$ and the antilog are indicated. The mean for each group is indicated by a large symbol.

C   = Classical CAH patients off treatment
F   = Cryptic 21-hydroxylase deficiency patients
★   = Heterozygotes for cryptic 21-hydroxylase deficiency
H   = Heterozygotes for classical CAH
U   = Family members predicted by HLA genotyping to be genetically unaffected

△   = General population
L   = Patients with late onset 21-hydroxylase deficiency
The values for each group aggregate in descending order along the regression line. Note that the values for the asymptomatic patients with cryptic 21-hydroxylase deficiency are in the same range as the symptomatic virilized females with late onset 21-hydroxylase deficiency. (From New et al, 1981b, with permission)

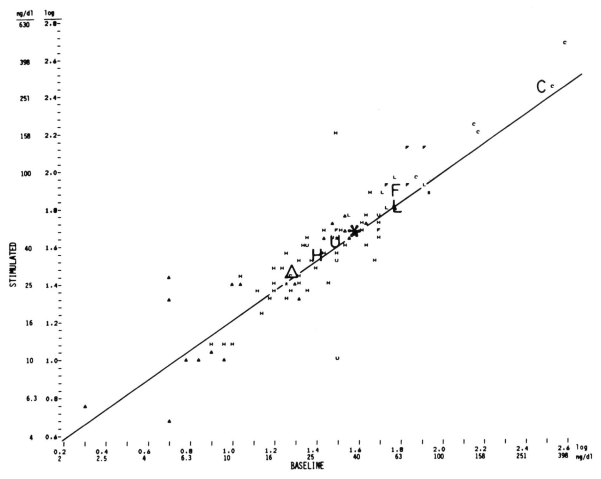

Fig. 86.21 Nomogram relating baseline to ACTH stimulated serum testosterone concentration in females. Values for the $\log_{10}$ and the antilog are indicated. The mean for each group is indicated by a large symbol.

C = Classical CAH patients off treatment
F = Cryptic 21-hydroxylase deficiency patients
★ = Heterozygotes for cryptic 21-hydroxylase deficiency
H = Heterozygotes for classical CAH
U = Family members predicted by HLA genotyping to be genetically unaffected

△ = General population
L = Patients with late onset 21-hydroxylase deficiency

The values for each group aggregate in descending order along the regression line. Note that the values for the asymptomatic females with cryptic 21-hydroxylase deficiency are in the same range as the symptomatic virilized females with late onset 21-hydroxylase deficiency. (From New et al, 1981b, with permission)

endocrinological features consistent with CAH due to 21-hydroxylase deficiency present in later childhood or early adulthood (Newmark et al, 1977). The late presentation of a biochemical enzyme defect has raised the question as to whether this is the same inherited disorder as CAH with delayed presentation or is an 'acquired' disorder distinct from CAH.

Although our first genetic study indicated that the late onset form was not linked to HLA (New et al, 1979), subsequent reports from other laboratories as well as our own have indicated that late onset 21-hydroxylase deficiency may indeed be linked to HLA (Blankstein et al, 1980; Laron et al, 1980). It is therefore likely that 21-

hydroxylase deficiency CAH and late onset 21-hydroxylase deficiency may be allelic forms of the same inherited disorder.

In cases of 11β-hydroxylase deficiency CAH, studies have found no significant linkage between the 11β-hydroxylase deficiency gene and HLA (Dupont et al, 1980).

An important consideration of genetic studies is the distinction between linkage, which we have described between HLA-B and the CAH gene, and genetic disequilibrium, which is the occurrence of alleles of two closely linked loci together at a higher frequency than would be expected. In CAH and cryptic 21-hydroxylase

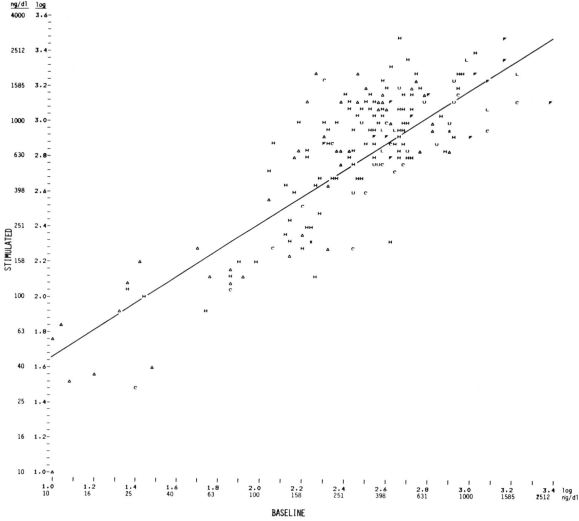

Fig. 86.22 Nomogram relating baseline to ACTH stimulated serum dehydroepiandrosterone concentration. Values for the $\log_{10}$ and the antilog are indicated. Note that the serum dehydroepiandrosterone concentration does not aggregate according to group.

C = Classical CAH patients off treatment
F = Cryptic 21-hydroxylase deficiency patients

★ = Heterozygotes for cryptic 21-hydroxylase deficiency
H = Heterozygotes for classical CAH
U = Family members predicted by HLA genotyping to be genetically unaffected
△ = General population
L = Patients with late onset 21-hydroxylase deficiency
(From New et al 1981b with permission)

deficiency both linkage and genetic linkage disequilibrium have been demonstrated.

The most significant association for classical 21-hydroxylase deficiency has been found for Bw47, where the combined relative risk is 15.4 (Dupont et al, 1980). Slight increases have also been reported for Bw51, Bw53, Bw60, and DR7. A review of the Bw47 positive haplotypes in patients with 21-hydroxylase deficiency reveals that this antigen frequently occurs on one particular haplotype: A3; Cw6; Bw47; BfF; DR7. Although the gene frequency for Bw47 in different Caucasian populations is always very low (<0.005), international studies have

found that Bw47 appears with remarkable frequency among 21-hydroxylase CAH patients; in one particular region of England, the Bw47 frequency among CAH patients is nearly 50%. Several studies have also demonstrated that A1, B8, and DRw3 are consistently decreased among 21-hydroxylase deficient patients (Klouda et al, 1978; Levine et al, 1978; Grosse-Wilde et al, 1979; Pollack et al, 1979).

Genetic linkage disequilibrium with HLA-B14 and DR1 has been detected in cryptic 21-hydroxylase deficiency (Dupont et al, 1980) and late onset adrenal hyperplasia (Blankstein et al, 1980; Laron et al, 1980).

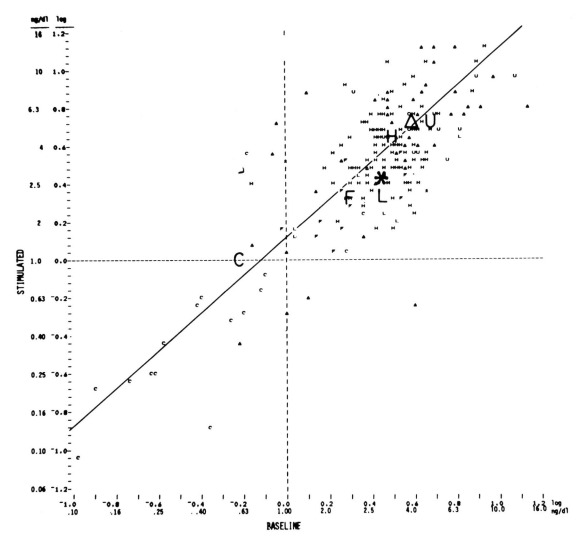

Fig. 86.23 Nomogram relating baseline to ACTH stimulated ratio of serum dehydroepiandrosterone/△4 androstenedione concentrations. Values for the log$_{10}$ and the antilog are indicated. The mean for each group is indicated by a large symbol.

  C = Classical CAH patients off treatment
  F = Cryptic 21-hydroxylase deficiency patients
  * = Heterozygotes for cryptic 21-hydroxylase deficiency
  H = Heterozygotes for classical CAH

  U = Family members predicted by HLA genotyping to be genetically unaffected
  △ = General population
  L = Patients with late onset 21-hydroxylase deficiency

The values for each group aggregate in descending order along the regression line. Note that the ratio of DHEA/△4 is lower in patients with classical congenital adrenal hyperplasia and that this group is easily distinguished from other groups by the ratio. (From New et al 1981b, with permission)

Allelic variants

In 1973, McKusick listed congenital adrenal hyperplasia due to 21-hydroxylase deficiency among the disorders in which the phenotypic diversity might be attributed to allelic series (McKusick, 1973). McKusick noted that genetic compounds were an additional source of phenotypic diversity. Although the phenotypic variants of salt wasting and simple virilizing CAH have long been recognized, the new phenotypic variant of cryptic 21-

hydroxylase deficiency has only recently been described (Levine et al, 1980b).

We propose that there are allelic variants at the 21-hydroxylase locus which produce different degrees of 21-hydroxylase deficiency resulting in the phenotypic diversity of classical, cryptic, and late onset 21-hydroxylase deficiency. Further, we suggest that the cryptic form of 21-hydroxylase deficiency represents a genetic compound of the classical (or more severe) 21-

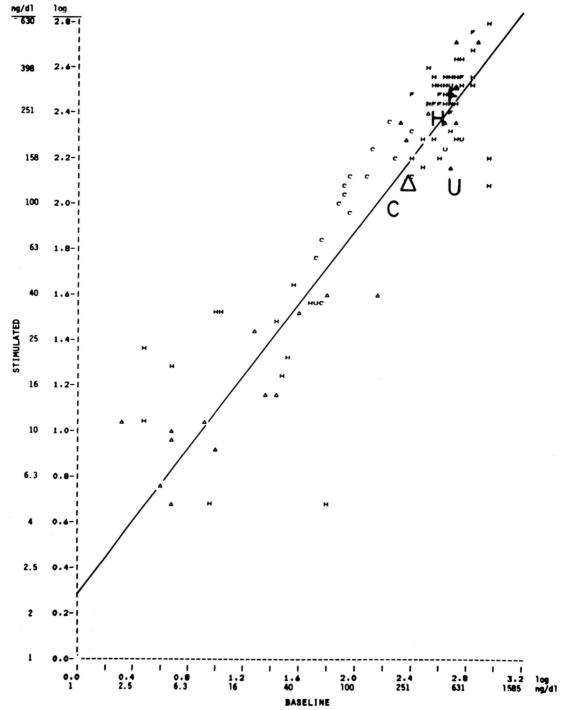

Fig. 86.24 Nomogram relating baseline to the ACTH stimulated serum testosterone concentration in males. Values for the log$_{10}$ and the antilog are indicated. The mean for each group is indicated by a large symbol.

C   = Classical CAH patients off treatment
F   = Cryptic 21-hydroxylase deficiency patients
*   = Heterozygotes for cryptic 21-hydroxylase deficiency
H   = Heterozygotes for classical CAH

U   = Family members predicted by HLA genotyping to be genetically unaffected
△   = General population
L   = Patients with the late onset 21-hydroxylase deficiency
Note that in males the serum testosterone does not distinguish the groups as well as in females. (From New et al 1981b, with permission)

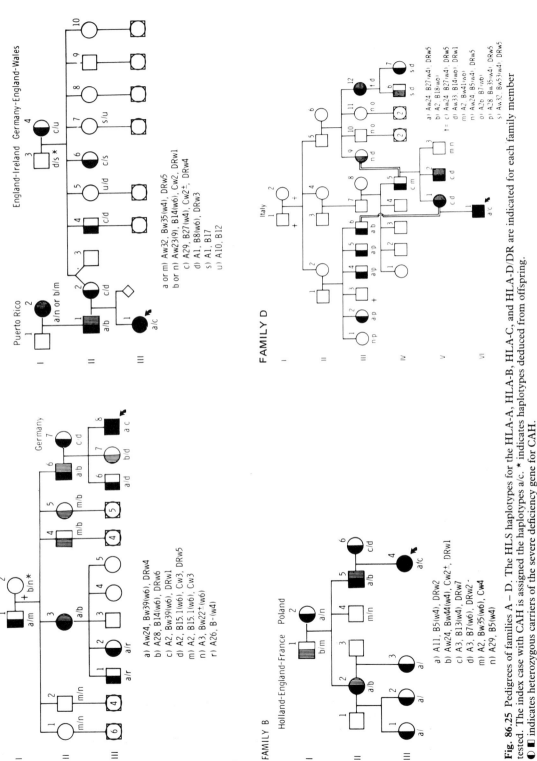

Fig. 86.25 Pedigrees of families A – D. The HLS haplotypes for the HLA-A, HLA-B, HLA-C, and HLA-D/DR are indicated for each family member tested. The index case with CAH is assigned the haplotypes a/c. * indicates haplotypes deduced from offspring.

● ■ indicates heterozygous carriers of the severe deficiency gene for CAH.
◐ ◧ indicates family members with cryptic 21-hydroxylase deficiency, having both a severe and a mild deficiency gene.
◍ ▤ indicates heterozygous carriers of the cryptic 21-hydroxylase deficiency gene.
▱ indicates offspring. (From New et al 1981b, with permission) number if known.

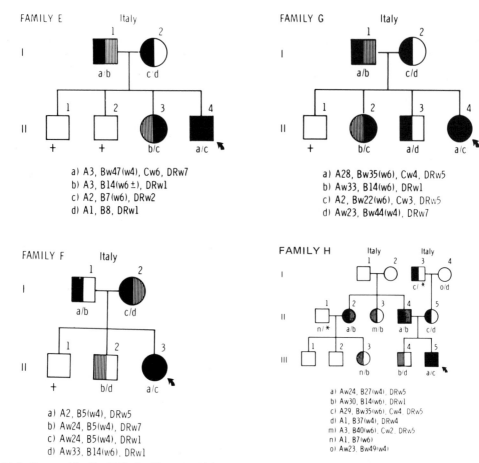

FAMILY E Italy

a) A3, Bw47(w4), Cw6, DRw7
b) A3, B14(w6 ±), DRw1
c) A2, B7(w6), DRw2
d) A1, B8, DRw1

FAMILY G Italy

a) A28, Bw35(w6), Cw4, DRw5
b) Aw33, B14(w6), DRw1
c) A2, Bw22(w6), Cw3, DRw5
d) Aw23, Bw44(w4), DRw7

FAMILY F Italy

a) A2, B5(w4), DRw5
b) Aw24, B5(w4), DRw7
c) Aw24, B5(w4), DRw1
d) Aw33, B14(w6), DRw1

FAMILY H Italy Italy

a) Aw24, B27(w4), DRw5
b) Aw30, B14(w6), DRw1
c) A29, Bw35(w6), Cw4, DRw5
d) A1, B37(w4), DRw4
m) A3, B40(w6), Cw2, DRw5
n) A1, B7(w6)
o) Aw23, Bw49(w4)

Fig. 86.26 Pedigrees of families E-H. See Figure 86.25 for symbols.

hydroxylase deficiency gene and the less severe cryptic 21-hydroxylase deficiency gene. This postulate awaits proof by complementation studies. Ultimate proof may be obtained by sequencing the gene by recombinant DNA techniques and demonstrating the site of genetic mutation for each allelic variant.

One may anticipate that a similar degree of genetic heterogeneity is likely to be found in the other inherited enzyme defects of steroidogenesis. Thus the phenotypic variability already recognized in 11β-hydroxylase and 17β-hydroxysteroid dehydrogenase deficiencies may be other examples of genetic heterogeneity.

SUMMARY

Disorders of steroidogenesis transmitted by an autosomal recessive gene have been investigated by hormonal and immunogenetic techniques.

Genetic linkage between the genes for HLA and steroid 21-hydroxylase has been demonstrated by family studies indicating that the gene for 21-hydroxylase is on the sixth chromosome close to the HLA-B locus. Various phenotypic forms of 21-hydroxylase deficiency have been described which may represent allelic variants at the 21-hydroxylase locus. Genetic linkage disequilibrium between HLA-Bw47 and the severe 21-hydroxylase deficiency has been demonstrated. The cryptic and late onset 21-hydroxylase defects appear to be in nonrandom gametic association with HLA-B14 and DR1. Hormonal tests have confirmed the prediction of heterozygosity by HLA genotyping.

Further hormonal and immunogenetic studies should prove helpful in elucidating the biological basis for the variable expression of these disorders of adrenal steroidogenesis.

REFERENCES

Bartter F C 1977 Adrenogenital syndromes from physiology to chemistry (1950–1975). In: Lee P A, Plotnick L P, Kowarski A A, Migeon C J (eds) Congenital Adrenal Hyperplasia, University Park Press, Baltimore, p 9–18

Baulieu E E, Peillon F, Migeon C J 1967 Adrenogenital syndrome. In: Eisenstein AB (ed) The Adrenal Cortex, Little, Brown and Co., Boston, p 553

Betuel H, Fauchet R, Gebuhrer L, Freidel C, Bouhallier O 1980 Informative families for the location of the congenital adrenal hyperplasia gene. Eighth International Histocompatibility Workshop Newsletter 20: 89

Blankstein J, Faiman C, Reyes F I, Schroeder M L, Winter J S D 1980 Adult-onset familial adrenal 21-hydroxylase deficiency. American Journal of Medicine 68: 441

Bongiovanni A M 1953 Detection of pregnanediol and pregnanetriol in urine of patients with adrenal hyperplasia: suppression with cortisone; preliminary report. Bulletin of the Johns Hopkins Hospital 92: 244

Bongiovanni A M, Eberlein W R 1958 Adrenogenital syndrome: uncomplicated and hypertensive forms. Pediatrics 21: 661

Bongiovanni A M, Eberlein W R, Cara J 1954 Studies on metabolism of adrenal steroids in adrenogenital syndrome. Journal of Clinical Endocrinology and Metabolism 14: 409

Childs B, Grumbach M M, van Wyk J J 1956 Virilizing adrenal hyperplasia: a genetic and hormonal study. Journal of Clinical Investigation 35: 213

Cohen J M 1969 Salt-losing congenital adrenal hyperplasia. Pediatrics 44: 621

De Crecchio L 1865 Sopra un caso di apparenze virile in una donna. Morgagni 7: 1951

Dillon M J, Ryness J 1975 Plasma renin activity and aldosterone concentrations in children: results in salt-wasting states. Archives of Disease in Childhood 50: 330

Dupont B, Oberfield S E, Smithwick E M, Lee T D, Levine L S 1977 Close genetic linkage between HLA and congenital adrenal hyperplasia (21-hydroxylase deficiency). Lancet 2: 1309

Dupont B, Pollack M S, Levine L S, O'Neill G J, Hawkins B R, New M I 1980 Congenital adrenal hyperplasia. In: Terasaki P I (ed) Histocompatibility Testing 1980, UCLA Tissue Typing Laboratory, Los Angeles, p. 693

Federman D D 1968 Abnormal Sexual Development. W B Saunders, Philadelphia p. 129

Ganong W F 1963 The central nervous system and the synthesis and release of adrenocorticotrophic hormone. In: Nalbandov A V (ed) Advances in Neuroendocrinology, University of Illinois Press, Urbana, p 92

Godard C, Riondel A M, Veyrat R, Megevand A, Muller A F 1968 Plasma renin activity and aldosterone in congenital adrenal hyperplasia. Pediatrics 41: 883

Gregory T, Gardner L I 1976 Hypertensive virilizing adrenal hyperplasia with minimal impairment of synthetic route to cortisol. Journal of Clinical Endocrinology and Metabolism 43: 769

Grosse-Wilde H J, Weil J, Albert E, Scholz S, Bidlingmaier F, Knorr D 1978 Linkage studies between HLA-A, B, D alleles and congenital adrenal hyperplasia (CAH). Pediatric Research 12: 1088

Grosse-Wilde H, Weil J, Albert E, Scholz S, Bidlingmaier F, Sippel W G, Knorr D 1979 Genetic linkage studies between congenital adrenal hyperplasia and the HLA blood group system. Immunogenetics 8: 41

Guillemin R, Schally A V 1963 Recent advances in the chemistry of neuroendocrine mediators originating in the central nervous system. In: Nalbandov A V (ed) Advances in Neuroendocrinology, University of Illinois Press, Urbana, Illinois p 314

Hirschfeld A J, Fleshman J K 1969 An unusually high incidence of salt-losing congenital adrenal hyperplasia in the Alaskan Eskimo. Journal of Pediatrics 75: 492

Hubble D 1966 Congenital adrenal hyperplasia. In: Holt K S, Raine D N (eds) Basic Concepts of Inborn Errors and Defects of Steroid Biosynthesis. Proceedings of the third Symposium of the Society for the Study of Inborn Errors of Metabolism, Churchill Livingstone, Edinburgh, p 68

Josso N 1972 Permeability of membranes to the Mullerian-inhibiting substance synthesized by the human fetal testis in vitro: a clue to its biochemical nature. Journal of Clinical Endocrinology and Metabolism 34: 265

Jost A 1966 Steroids and sex differentiation of the mammalian foetus. Excerpta Medical Internal Congress Service 132: 74

Klouda P T, Harris R, Price D A 1978 HLA and congenital adrenal hyperplasia. Lancet 2: 1046

Klouda P T, Harris R, Price D A 1980 Linkage and association between HLA and 21-hydroxylase deficiency. Journal of Medical Genetics 17: 337 1980

Korth-Schutz S, Levine L S, New M I 1976 Serum androgens in normal prepubertal and pubertal children and in children with precocious adrenarche. Journal of Clinical Endocrinology and Metabolism 42: 117

Korth-Schutz S, Virdis R, Saenger P, Chow D M, Levine L S, New M I 1978 Serum androgens as a continuing index of adequacy of treatment of congenital adrenal hyperplasia. Journal of Clinical Endocrinology and Metabolism 46: 452

Kuhnle U, Chow D, Levine L S, New M I 1980 The activity of the 21-hydroxylase (21-OH) enzyme in the glomerulosa and fasciculata of the adrenal cortex in congenital adrenal hyperplasia (CAH). Pediatric Research 14: 480/325

Kuhnle U, Chow D, Rapaport R, Pang S, Levine L S, New M I 1981 The activity of the 21-hydroxylase (21-OH) enzyme in the glomerulosa and fasciculata of the adrenal cortex in congenital adrenal hyperplasia (CAH). Journal of Clinical Endocrinology and Metabolism 52: 534

Laragh J H 1971 Aldosteronism in man: factors controlling secretion of the hormone. In: Christy N P (ed) The Human Adrenal Cortex, Harper and Row, New York p 483

Laron Z, Pollack M S, Zamir R, Roitman A, Dickerman Z, Levine L S, Lorenzen F, O'Neill G J, Pang S, New M I, Dupont B 1980 Late onset 21-hydroxylase deficiency and HLA in the Ashkenazi population: A new allele at the 21-hydroxylase locus. Human Immunology 1: 55

Levine L S, Zachmann M, New M I, Prader A, Pollack M S, O'Neill G J, Yang S Y, Oberfield S E, Dupont B 1978 Genetic mapping of the 21-hydroxylase deficiency gene within the HLA linkage group. New England Journal of Medicine 299: 911

Levine L S, Rauh W, Gottesdiener K, Chow D, Gunczler P, Rapaport R, Pang S, Schneider B, New M I 1980a New studies of the 11β-hydroxylase and 18-hydroxylase enzymes in the hypertensive form of congenital adrenal hyperplasia. Journal of Clinical Endocrinology and Metabolism 50: 258

Levine L S, Dupont B, Lorenzen F, Pang S, Pollack M, Oberfield S, Kohn B, Lerner A, Cacciari E, Mantero F, Cassio A, Scaroni C, Chiumello G, Rondanini G F, Gargantini L, Giovannelli G, Virdis R, Bartolotta E, Migliori C, Pintor C, Tato L, Barboni F, New M I 1980b Cryptic

21-hydroxylase deficiency in families of patients with classical congenital adrenal hyperplasia. Journal of Clinical Endocrinology and Metabolism 51: 1316

Lorenzen F, Pang S, New M I, Dupont B, Pollack M, Chow D, Levine L S 1979 Hormonal phenotype and HLA-genotype in families of patients with congenital adrenal hyperplasia (21-hydroxylase deficiency). Pediatric Research 13: 1356

Lorenzen F, Pang S, New M I, Pollack M, Oberfield S E, Dupont B, Chow D, Schneider B, Levine L S 1980 Studies of the C-21 and C-19 steroids and HLA genotyping in siblings and parents of patients with congenital adrenal hyperplasia due to 21-hydroxylase deficiency. Journal of Clinical Endocrinology and Metabolism 50: 572

Mauthe I, Lapse Knorr D 1977 The frequency of congenital adrenal hyperplasia in Munich. Klinische Paediatic 189: 172

McKusick V A 1973 Phenotypic diversity of human diseases resulting from allelic series. American Journal of Human Genetics 25: 446

Mininberg D T, Levine L S, New M I 1979 Current concepts in congenital adrenal hyperplasia. Investigative Urology 17: 169

Müller W, Prader M, Kofler J, Glatzl J, Geir W 1979 Frequency of congenital adrenal hyperplasia. Päediatrie und Paedologie 14: 151

Murtaza L M, Hughes I A, Sibert S R, Balfour I C 1978 HLA and congenital adrenal hyperplasia. Lancet 2: 524

New M I, Levine L S 1973 Congenital adrenal hyperplasia. In: Harris H, Hirschhorn K K (eds) Advances in Human Genetics, Plenum Press, New York, p 251

New M I, Peterson R E 1966 Disorders of aldosterone secretion in childhood. Pediatric Clinics of North America 13: 43

New M I, Seaman M P 1970 Secretion rates of cortisol and aldosterone precursors in various forms of congenital adrenal hyperplasia. Journal of Clinical Endocrinology and Metabolism 30: 361

New M I, Lorenzen F, Pang S, Gunczler P, Dupont B, Pollack M S, Levine L S 1979 'Acquired' adrenal hyperplasia with 21-hydroxylase deficiency is not the same genetic disorder as congenital adrenal hyperplasia. Journal of Clinical Endocrinology and Metabolism 48: 356

New M I, Dupont B, Levine L S 1981a HLA and adrenal disease. In: Farid N (ed) HLA in Endocrine and Metabolic Disorders. Academic Press p 177–208

New M I, Dupont B, Pang S, Pollack M, Levine L S 1981b An update of Congenital adrenal hyperplasia. In: Recent Progress in Hormone Research 37: 105

Newmark S, Dluhy R G, Williams G H, Pochi P, Rose L I 1977 Partial 11 and 21 hydroxylase deficiencies in hirsute women. American Journal of Obstetrics and Gynecology 127: 594

Pang S, Hotchkiss J, Drash A L, Levine L S, New M I 1977 Microfilter paper method for 17-α-hydroxyprogesterone radioimmunoassay: its application for rapid screening for congenital adrenal hyperplasia. Journal of Clinical Endocrinology and Metabolism 45: 1003

Pang S, Levine L S, Chow D, Faiman C, New M I 1979 Serum androgen concentrations in neonates and young

infants with congenital adrenal hyperplasia due to 21-hydroxylase deficiency. Clinical Endocrinology 11: 575

Pollack M S, Levine L S, Pang S, Owens R P, Nitowsky H M, Maurer D, New M I, Duchon M, Merkatz I R, Sachs G, Dupont B 1979 Prenatal diagnosis of congenital adrenal hyperplasia (21-hydroxylase deficiency) by HLA typing. Lancet 1: 1107

Prader A 1958 Die Häufigkeit des kongenitalen adrenogenitalen syndroms. Helvetica Paediatrica Acta 13: 426

Price D A, Klouda P T, Harris R 1978 HLA and congenital adrenal hyperplasia linkage confirmed. Lancet 1: 930

Pucholt V, Fitzsimmons J S, Reynolds M A, Gelsthorpe K 1979 Location of the gene for 21-hydroxylase deficiency. Pediatric Research 13: 1186

Qazi Q H, Thompson M W 1972 Incidence of salt-losing form of congenital virilizing adrenal hyperplasia. Archives of Diseases in Childhood 47: 302

Rimoin D L, Schimke R N 1971 Genetic Disorders of the Endocrine Glands. Mosby, St Louis

Rosenbloom A L, Smith D W 1966a Congenital adrenal hyperplasia. Lancet 1: 660

Rosenbloom A L, Smith D W 1966b Varying expression for salt losing in related patients with congenital adrenal hyperplasia. Pediatrics 38: 215

Rösler A, Levine L S, Schneider B, Novogroder M, New M I 1977 The interrelationship of sodium balance, plasma renin activity and ACTH in congenital adrenal hyperplasia. Journal of Clinical Endocrinology and Metabolism 45: 500

Sizonenko P-C, Riondel A M, Kohlberg I J, Paunier L 1972 11β-hydroxylase deficiency: steroid response to sodium restriction and ACTH stimulation. Journal of Clinical Endocrinology and Metabolism 35: 281

Strickland A L, Kotchen T A 1972 A study of the renin-aldosterone system in congenital adrenal hyperplasia. Journal of Pediatrics 81: 962

Tan S Y, Noth R H, Mulrow P J 1978 Deoxycorticosterone and 17-ketosteroids; elevated levels in adult hypertensive patients. JAMA 240: 123

Weitkamp L R, Bryson M, Bacon G E 1978 HLA and congenital adrenal hyperplasia linkage confirmed. Lancet 1: 931

Werder E A, Siebenmann R E, Knorr-Murset G, Zimmermann A, Sizonenko P C, Theintz P, Girard J, Zachmann M, Prader A 1980 The incidence of congenital adrenal hyperplasia in Switzerland: a survery of patients born in 1960 to 1974. Helvetica Paediatrica Acta 35: 5

Wilkins L 1962 Adrenal disorders. II. Congenital virilizing adrenal hyperplasia. Archives of Diseases in Childhood 37: 231

Winter J S D 1980 Current approaches to the treatment of congenital adrenal hyperplasia. Journal of Pediatrics 97: 81

Zachmann M, Völlmin J A, New M I, Curtius H-C, Prader A 1971 Congenital adrenal hyperplasia due to deficiency of 11β-hydroxylation of 17α-hydroxylated steroids. Journal of Clinical Endocrinology and Metabolism. 33: 501

Zappacosta S, De Felice M, Minozzi M, Lombardi G, Valentino R, Vancote G 1978 HLA and congenital adrenal hyperplasia. Lancet 2: 524

87

Disorders of gonads and internal reproductive ducts

J. L. Simpson

Genetic advances have greatly facilitated not only the understanding but also the delineation of disorders of sexual differentiation.

In this chapter we shall delineate some of the most common disorders of gonadal differentiation that result from mutant genes, emphasizing diagnosis and aetiology. Abnormalities involving sex chromosomes are reviewed elsewhere in this volume and will be considered only briefly here. Both genetic and cytogenetic disorders have been discussed by the author in greater detail elsewhere (Simpson, 1976; Simpson, 1978a, 1978b), publications that this review inevitably reflects.

H-Y ANTIGEN AND REPRODUCTIVE EMBRYOLOGY

If an X chromosome-bearing ovum is fertilized by an X-bearing sperm, a 46,XX female zygote results. If a normal X chromosome-bearing ovum is fertilized by a Y-bearing sperm, a 46,XY male zygote results. The major determinant(s) responsible for testicular differentiation are localized to the centromeric region on the Y, probably on the short arm (Simpson, 1976). The manner by which the testicular determinant(s) acts is not totally understood, but it appears that a cell surface antigen, H-Y antigen, is integrally involved in testicular differentiation (Wachtel, 1977, 1979; Wachtel & Ohno, 1979). Both circumstantial as well as direct evidence suggests that H-Y antigen can direct testicular differentiation. The following circumstantial data, referenced elsewhere (Wachtel & Ohno, 1979; Simpson, 1980) are consistent with this hypothesis: (1) H-Y is evolutionarily conservative, being present in all species tested in that sex containing the heterogametic sex chromosome (Y or W); (2) at least one locus for H-Y is near or identical to the locus for the testicular determinant(s); (3) YY males have twice the H-Y titer of XY males; (4) H-Y is present in XY humans and mice with androgen insensitivity, indicating that H-Y is not merely induced by androgens; (5) H-Y on XY cells continues to be expressed after transfer to a female host; (6) H-Y is present in approximately 50% of mouse blastocysts, a stage prior to organ differentiation and, hence, prior to testicular differentiation; (7) most sex-reversed 46,XX true hermaphrodites have H-Y antigen; (8) XY female lemmings are H-Y negative; and (9) H-Y antigen is present in the testicular but not the ovarian portion of ovotestes (Winters et al, 1979). In general, H-Y has thus been detected in individuals with testes, but not in those lacking testes.

Direct evidence also exists. Reaggregation of neonatal mouse or rat testes disassociated by Moscona-type disruption produces tubular-like (male) structures (Ohno et al, 1978; Zenzes et al, 1978a). However, H-Y antisera causes testicular cells to reaggregate into follicle-like (female) fashion. Moreover, H-Y antigen recovered from cultured Sertoli cells directs disassociated ovarian tissue into tubular-like structures (Zenzes et al, 1978b).

Although clearly an attractive hypothesis, testicular differentiation cannot yet be ascribed solely to H-Y antigen. In addition to major problems in assay reproducibility, much contradictory data remain to be explained. For example, most patients with XY gonadal dysgenesis are H-Y positive (Wolf, 1979), as are 45,X and 46,X, i(Xq) (Wolf et al, 1980; Wolf, 1981). Conversely, presence of ovaries in an XY phenotypic female who had an additional band on Yp was observed and explained by hypothesizing that the band suppressed expression of H-Y (Bernstein et al, 1980). Clearly, many facets of the H-Y story remain to be elucidated, not the least of which is the nature of H-Y receptors. That 45,X individuals are H-Y positive indicates that H-Y is not the gene product of the Y–linked testicular determinant. The structural locus for H-Y could be on an autosome or on the X chromosome possibly activated by a Y–linked regulatory locus corresponding to the testicular determinant.

After having differentiated from the indifferent gonad, the developing testes secrete two hormones (Fig. 87.1). Fetal Leydig cells produce an androgen, probably testosterone, which stabilizes the Wolffian ducts and permits differentiation of vasa deferentia, epididymides and seminal vesicles. After conversion by 5α-reductase to dihydrotestosterone, the external genitalia are virilized.

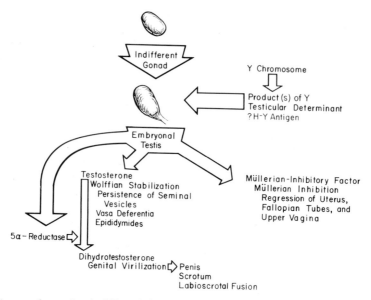

Fig. 87.1 Schematic diagram of normal male differentiation. From Simpson (1980).

These actions can be mimicked by the administration of testosterone to female or castrated male embryos, as demonstrated clinically by teratogenic forms of female pseudohermaphroditism. Fetal Sertoli cells produce a second hormone, a non-steroid hormone of high molecular weight that diffuses locally to cause regression of Mullerian derivatives (uterus and Fallopian tubes). The action of this hormone cannot be duplicated by any known compound. In the absence of these two hormones the external genitalia develop along female lines, the Mullerian ducts develop into a uterus and Fallopian tubes, and the Wolffian ducts regress. These changes thus occur in 46,XX embryos and in castrated 46,XY embryos.

In the absence of a Y–chromosome, or more specifically in the absence of H-Y antigen, the indifferent gonad develops into an ovary. This appears to occur in both 46,XX and in 45,X embryos. If two intact X–chromosomes are not present, most ovarian follicles degenerate by the time of birth.

MALE PSEUDOHERMAPHRODITISM

Male pseudohermaphrodites are individuals with a Y–chromosome whose external genitalia fail to develop as expected for normal males. Some authors apply the appellation only to those whose external genitalia are ambiguous enough to confuse the choice of sex rearing; however, applying the term more liberally seems more useful clinically. Three related disorders are also discussed in this chapter: persistence of Mullerian derivatives in males, anorchia, and the syndrome of rudimentary

testes. Cytogenetic forms (45,X/46,XY) will be discussed briefly in order to contrast their phenotype with those of genetic forms.

Cytogenetic forms

45,X/46,XY

Individuals with both a 45,X cell line and at least one line containing a Y–chromosome may manifest a variety of phenotypes, ranging from almost normal males with cryptorchidism or penile hypospadias to females indistinguishable from those with the 45,X Turner syndrome. The different phenotypes presumably reflect different tissue distributions of the various cell lines; however, this assumption is unproved. Not infrequently a structurally abnormal Y–chromosome is present, especially mitotically unstable (e.g. dicentric forms). Clinically, 45,X/46,XY individuals may be grouped into one of three categories, namely individuals with (a) unambiguous female external genitalia, (b) ambiguous external genitalia, i.e., the sex of rearing is in doubt, or (c) almost normal male external genitalia.

Female external genitalia. These individuals may have the Turner stigmata and thus be clinically indistinguishable from 45,X individuals. These 45,X/46,XY individuals are usually normal in stature and show no somatic anomalies. As in any type of gonadal dysgenesis, the external genitalia, vagina, and Mullerian derivatives remain unstimulated because of the lack of sex steroids. Breasts fail to develop, and little pubic or axillary hair develop. In fact, if breast development occurs in a 45,X/46,XY individual, one should suspect an oestrogen-secreting tumour, namely a gonadoblastoma or dysgerminoma.

Although the streak gonads of 45,X/46,XY individuals are usually histologically indistinguishable from the streak gonads of individuals with 45,X gonadal dysgenesis, gonadoblastomas or dysgerminomas develop in about 15–20% of 45,X/46,XY individuals, sometimes in the first or second decade.

Ambiguous genitalia. The terms asymmetric or mixed gonadal dysgenesis are applied to individuals who have one streak gonad and one dysgenetic testis. Individuals with mixed gonadal dysgenesis usually have ambiguous external genitalia and a 45,X/46,XY complement, but occasionally only 45,X or only 46,XY cells can be demonstrated. Many investigators believe that the phenotype is almost always associated with 45,X/46,XY mosaicism, apparent nonmosaic cases merely reflecting inability to sample appropriate tissues.

An important diagnostic observation is that 45,X/46,XY individuals with ambiguous external genitalia usually have Mullerian derivatives (e.g., a uterus). Presence of a uterus is thus diagnostically helpful because a uterus is absent in almost all genetic forms of male pseudohermaphroditism (see below). If an individual has ambiguous external genitalia, bilateral testes, and a uterus, it is therefore reasonable to infer that such a person has 45,X/46,XY mosaicism, regardless of whether both lines can be demonstrated cytogenetically. Occasionally the uterus is rudimentary, or a Fallopian tube may fail to develop ipsilateral to a testis.

Almost normal male genitalia. Occasionally 45,X/46,XY mosaicism is detected in individuals with almost normal male external genitalia. A uterus is less likely to be present than in 45,X/46,XY individuals with ambiguous or female external genitalia. 45,X/46,XY individuals with almost normal male external genitalia also probably do not develop neoplasia as often as 45,X/46,XY individuals with female or frankly ambiguous genitalia. In my opinion, gonadal extirpation is not necessary if a male sex-of-rearing is chosen and if gonads can be palpated within the scrotum for periodic examination.

45,X/47,XYY; 45,X/46,XY/47,XYY

These complements are rarer than 45,X/46,XY, but they are probably associated with the same phenotypic spectrum. Of particular interest is one family in which two and possibly three sibs with 45,X/46,XY/47,XYY mosaicism were products of a second cousin marriage (Hsu et al, 1970). This suggests recessive factors influencing non-disjunction.

Genetic forms

Hypospadias without other defects
In hypospadias the external urinary meatus terminates on the ventral aspect of the penis, proximal to its usual site at the tip of the glans penis. Hypospadias can be classified according to the site of the urethral meatus: glans penis, penile shaft, penoscrotal junction, or perineum. Sometimes testicular hypoplasia coexists, especially in penoscrotal or perineal hypospadias; however, more often testicular volume is normal.

Multiple affected sibs and affected individuals in several generations have been reported to have uncomplicated hypospadias. After the birth of one affected child the recurrence risk for subsequent male progeny is about 6–10%. These risks are higher than those usually associated with multifactorial/polygenic traits, suggesting genetic heterogeneity. In fact, hypospadias is sometimes only one of several components of a multiple malformation pattern, as in the X–linked recessive syndrome characterized by hypospadias and hypertelorism. Presence of other anomalies should, therefore, be excluded before offering the above recurrence risks.

Persistence of Mullerian derivatives in otherwise normal males
Occasionally, the uterus and Fallopian tubes (Mullerian derivatives) persist in ostensibly normal males. The external genitalia, Wolffian (mesonephric) derivatives and testes develop as expected; virilization occurs at puberty. However, the frequency of associated infertility is quite high, and about 5% of reported individuals have had a seminoma or other germ cell tumour. The disorder is sometimes ascertained because the uterus and Fallopian tubes produce inguinal hernias, hence the appellation uterine hernia inguinalis. Failure of Mullerian duct regression could theoretically result either from end-organ (uterus) insensitivity to the Mullerian inhibitory factor (MIF) or from failure of fetal Sertoli cells to synthesize or secrete MIF. In several families multiple affected sibs or monozygotic twins have been reported and in one family maternal half-sibs were affected (Sloan & Walsh, 1976). Thus, this disorder is probably inherited as an X–linked recessive trait.

Disorders with multiple malformation patterns
Genital ambiguity may occur in individuals with multiple malformation patterns, as tabulated elsewhere (Simpson, 1976).

Enzyme deficiencies in testosterone biosynthetic pathways
An enzyme deficiency should be suspected if secretion of testosterone or its metabolites is decreased. Deficiencies of 21- or 11β-hydroxylation, the most common causes of female pseudohermaphroditism, do not cause male pseudohermaphroditism. Indeed, androgen secretion is increased. However, males with 21-hydroxylase deficiency may lose sodium, whereas those with 11β-hydroxylase deficiency may retain sodium and develop hypervolemia and hypertension. Thus, newborn male infants whose sibs had 21- or 11β-hydroxylase deficien-

cies should be screened for electrolyte disturbances. Male pseudohermaphroditism may result from deficiencies of 17α-hydroxylase, 3β-ol-dehydrogenase, and the enzymes required to convert cholesterol to pregnenolone (congenital adrenal lipoid hyperplasia).

Congenital adrenal lipoid hyperplasia. These male pseudohermaphrodites have ambiguous or female-like external genitalia, severe salt wasting and adrenals characterized by foamy appearing cells filled with cholesterol (Prader and Gurtner, 1955). The accumulation of cholesterol indicates that this compound cannot be conversed to pregnenolone (Fig. 87.2). The specific enzyme deficient in this disorder is not known; however, any of the three enzymes required to convert cholesterol to pregnenalone could be deficient – 20α-hydroxylase, 20,22-desmolase, 22α-hydroxylase.

3β-ol-dehydrogenase deficiency. Deficiency of 3β-ol-dehydrogenase results in decreased synthesis of both androgens and estrogens (Fig. 87.2) The major androgen produced is dehydroepiandrosterone, a weaker androgen than testosterone. Diagnosis is usually made on the basis of elevated 16-hydroxy pregnenolone. 3β-ol-dehydrogenase deficiency is often associated with severe salt wasting because of the decreased levels of aldosterone and cortisol, but many older children with less severe defects are now being recognized (Bongiovanni, 1979). The incompletely developed external genitalia of affected males are similar to the external genitalia of most other male pseudohermaphrodites: small phallus, urethra that opens proximally on the penis, and incomplete labioscrotal fusion. The testes and Wolffian ducts differentiate normally.

17α-hydroxylase deficiency Males with deficiency of 17α-hydroxylase usually show ambiguous external genitalia, normal Wolffian duct development, and normal testicular differentiation. Some severely affected males show female external genitalia (Heremans et al, 1976). Unlike females deficient for 17α-hydroxylase, males usually have normal blood pressure (Simpson, 1978a). Autosomal recessive inheritance seems likely for this disorder.

Deficiency of 17,20-desmolase. Zachman et al (1972) reported a family in which three members apparently had 17,20-desmolase deficiency. This is the only family in which multiple members have been affected. Two maternal first cousins had genital ambiguity, bilateral testes, and no Mullerian derivatives; a maternal 'aunt' was said to have abnormal external genitalia and bilateral testes. Both cousins showed low plasma testosterone and low dehydroepiandrosterone (DHEA) but normal urinary excretion of pregnanediol, pregnanetriol, and 17-hydroxycorticoids. Incubation of testicular tissue revealed that testosterone could be synthesized from androstenedione or dehydroepiandrosterone, excluding 17-ketosteroid reductase and suggesting deficiency of 17, 20-desmolase. The disorder could be inherited in either an autosomal recessive or X–linked recessive fashion.

Deficiency of 17-ketosteroid reductase. Unable to convert dehydroepiandrosterone to testosterone, these males lack 17-ketosteroid reductase (Fig. 87.2). Plasma testosterone is usually decreased; androstenedione and dehydroepiandrosterone are increased. Affected males show ambiguous external genitalia, bilateral testes, and no Mullerian derivatives. Breast development may or may not be present, apparently depending upon the estrogen/testosterone ratio (Imperato-McGinley et al, 1979). Greater puberal

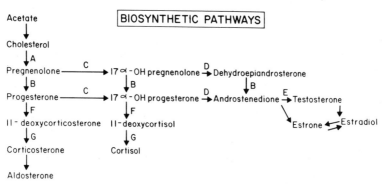

Fig. 87.2 Summary of important adrenal and gonadal biosynthetic pathways. Letters designate enzymes required for the appropriate conversions. From Simpson (1976).

A = 20-hydroxylase, 22R-hydroxylase, and 20, 22-desmolase
B = 3β-ol-dehydrogenase
C = 17α-hydroxylase
D = 17, 20-desmolase
E = 17-ketosteroid reductase
F = 21-hydroxylase
G = 11β-hydroxylase

virilization may occur in these male pseudohermaphrodites than in some of the other enzyme deficiencies, as illustrated by a report of an affected individual who underwent female-to-male sex role change after puberty (Imperato-McGinley et al, 1979). The disorder is either autosomal recessive or X–linked recessive.

Complete androgen insensitivity (testicular feminization)
In androgen insensitivity (testicular feminization) 46,XY individuals have bilateral testes, female external genitalia, a blindly-ending vagina, and no Mullerian derivatives. Affected individuals undergo breast development and pubertal feminization. Despite pubertal feminization, some individuals with androgen insensitivity have clitoral enlargement and labioscrotal fusion; to these patients the term incomplete androgen insensitivity (incomplete testicular feminization) has been applied. Both complete and incomplete androgen insensitivity are inherited in X–linked recessive fashion. However, not only are the two disorders clearly genetically distinct, but heterogeneity probably exists in each. Studies performed on cloned fibroblasts from mothers of affected males show that only half the maternal cells are androgen-responsive, as expected for X–linked genes (Meyer et al, 1975).

Clinical features of individuals with complete androgen sensitivity are well-known. These phenotypic females may be quite attractive and have excellent breast development, but probably most affected patients are similar in appearance to unaffected females. Breasts contain normal ductal and glandular tissue, but often the areolae are pale and poorly developed. Statural growth and body proportions are usually normal. Occasionally the arms and legs are disproportionately long, and the hands and feet disproportionately large. Pubic and axillary hair are usually sparse, but scalp hair normal. The vagina terminates blindly and is shorter than usual, presumably because Mullerian ducts fail to contribute to formation of the vagina. Occasionally the vagina is only 1–2 cm long or represented merely by a dimple. Neither a uterus nor Fallopian tubes are ordinarily present, although occasionally one detects fibromuscular remnants or rudimentary Fallopian tubes of presumptive Mullerian origin. The absence of Mullerian derivatives is not unexpected because the Mullerian-inhibitory factor secreted by the fetal testes is not an androgen; therefore, Mullerian regression occurs, as in normal males. Testes are usually normal in size, and may be located in the abdomen, inguinal canal, or labia, i.e., anywhere along the path of embryonic testicular descent. Testes located in the inguinal canal may produce inguinal hernias, and half of all individuals with testicular feminization develop inguinal hernias. It is therefore desirable to determine cytogenetic status of prepubertal girls with inguinal hernias, although most will be 46,XX.

The frequency of gonadal neoplasia is increased, but the precise extent is uncertain. In a frequently cited publication, Morris and Mahesh (1963) tabulated that 22% of reported patients had neoplasia, but because of various biases the actual risk is probably no greater than 5% (Simpson & Photopulos, 1976). Most investigators agree that the risk of neoplasia is low prior to age 25–30 years. Thus, it is probably preferable to leave the testes in situ until after pubertal feminization, thereafter performing orchiectomy inasmuch as risk of neoplasia increases with age. In postpubertal patients benign tubular adenomas (Pick adenomas) are especially common, probably as result of increased secretion of LH.

The pathogenesis of complete androgen insensitivity clearly involves end-organ insensitivity to androgens. Plasma testosterone is normal, and patients neither virilize nor retain nitrogen after administration of androgen (testosterone or dehydrotestosterone). In addition, presence of hyperplastic Leydig cells and elevated LH suggests abnormal gonadal-hypothalamic feed back. Although most cases result from an abnormality in the amount of the cytosol receptor for androgens (receptor negative), other mechanisms must be invoked for cases in which cytosol receptors appear normal (receptor positive) (Amrhein et al, 1976). Kaufman et al (1979) observed 4 receptor positive and 9 receptor negative cases among 13 clinically indistinguishable cases. Possible explanations for receptor positive cases include abnormalities of the receptor(s) that binds the hormonal/receptor complex to DNA to initiate transcription, or abnormalities at a later step involving the protein presumably necessary to exert androgen influence on cells.

Incomplete androgen sensitivity and the Reifenstein syndrome
At puberty certain individuals feminize (show breast development) because of androgen insensitivity, yet their external genitalia are characterized by phallic enlargement and partial labioscrotal fusion. Such individuals are said to have incomplete androgen insensitivity (incomplete testicular feminization). Both incomplete and complete androgen insensitivity share the following features: bilateral testes with similar histologic features, no Mullerian derivatives, pubertal breast development, lack of pubertal virilization, normal male plasma testosterone levels, normal response to HCG and ACTH, and failure to retain nitrogen following testosterone administration. The number of cytosol androgen receptors appears reduced (Griffin et al, 1976).

An epididymis and one or both vasa deferentia are usually present. The disorder is inherited in X–linked recessive fashion.

A disorder related to if not identical with incomplete androgen insensitivity is the Reifenstein syndrome. Most patients reported to have this X–linked recessive trait differ in no important respect from those with incomplete testicular feminization. Traditionally, however, the appellation Reifenstein syndrome was applied to males with phallic development more nearly normal than in incomplete androgen insensitivity, no vagina-like perineal orifice, and lack of pubertal virilization (Bowen et al, 1965). Logically, decreased virilization in the Reifenstein syndrome appeared to result not from androgen insensitivity, but from inadequate testosterone secretion.

In contrast to the usual trend toward genetic heterogeneity, it appears that the traditional distinctions between Reifenstein syndrome and incomplete androgen insensitivity (incomplete testicular feminization) may not be valid. Specifically, males with small testes and elevated gonadotropin levels may show partial androgen insensitivity (Amrhein et al, 1977). The Reifenstein syndrome and incomplete androgen insensitivity may thus merely represent different spectrums of a single X–linked recessive disorder (Wilson et al, 1974).

Irrespective, the clinical significance of the incomplete androgen insensitivity states is that they must be excluded before a male sex or rearing is assigned. Presence of androgen receptors and demonstration of a response to exogenous androgen (irrespective of receptor status) exclude these disorders.

5α-reductase deficiency (pseudovaginal perineoscrotal hypospadias)

For some 20 years it has been recognized that some genetic males show ambiguous external genitalia at birth, but otherwise develop like normal males. At puberty they undergo virilization–phallic enlargement, increased facial hair, muscular hypertrophy, voice deepening, and no breast development. The external genitalia consist of a phallus that resembles a clitoris more than a penis, a perineal urethral orifice, and usually a separate blindly ending perineal orifice that resembles a vagina (psuedovagina) (Fig. 87.3). Testes are relatively normal in size and secrete normal amounts of testosterone. In 1971–1972 colleagues and I showed conclusively that this trait, then called pseudovaginal perineoscrotal hypospadias (PPSH) was inherited in autosomal recessive fashion (Simpson et al, 1971c; Opitz et al, 1972). Other investigators later showed that the PPSH phenotype could result from deficiency of 5α-reductase (Imperato-McGinley et al, 1974; Walsh et al, 1974; Peterson et al, 1977; Fisher et al, 1978). The enzyme 5α-reductase converts testosterone to dihydrotestosterone, the androgen active within cells. That intracellular 5α-reductase deficiency results in PPSH is consistent with embryological findings showing that virilization of the external genitalia during embryogenesis requires dihydrotestosterone, whereas Wolffian differentiation requires only testosterone. 5α-reductase deficiency is also an autosomal reces-

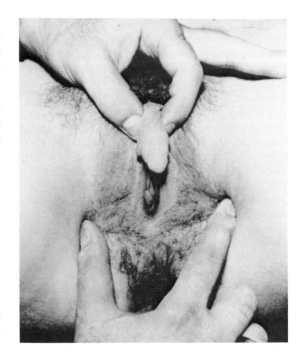

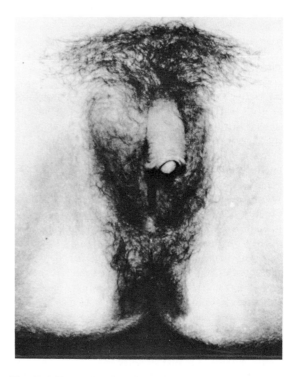

Fig. 87.3 External genitalia of one of three 46,XY sibs with the pseudovaginal perineoscrotal hypospadias (PPSH) phenotype. Many if not all individuals with this phenotype have deficiencies of 5α-reductase. From Opitz et al (1972).

sive trait, further substantiating that the PPSH phenotype may result from 5α-reductase deficiency.

The diagnosis is perhaps made most easily on the basis of elevated testosterone: dihydrotestosterone ratio after HCG stimulation (Pinsky, 1978). 5α-reductase (5α-R) is also present in cultured fibroblasts, in fibroblast homogenates and tissue homogenates. Levels are highest in genital tissue, for which reason most investigators prefer to assay cells derived from genital tissue (e.g., foreskin). There is also great variability in 5α-R activity among control genital strains, with near overlap between controls and patients clearly deficient for the enzyme (as shown by hormonal studies). Thus, presence of 5α-R in cultured genital fibroblasts usually excludes 5α-R deficiency; however, absence of 5α-R does not necessarily confirm the clinical diagnosis, especially if genital tissues were not studied. In addition to diagnostic pitfalls, there is evidence for genetic heterogeneity in 5α-R deficiency, based upon enzyme kinetics (Leshin et al, 1978).

Syndrome of rudimentary testes

Bergada et al (1962) reported four unrelated males who, despite well-formed testes less than 1 cm in greatest diameter, had small penises. These testes consisted of a few Leydig cells, small tubules containing Sertoli cells, and an occasional spermatogonium. Wolffian derivatives were present; Mullerian derivatives were absent. Relatively few individuals with the rudimentary testes syndrome have been described; however, Najjar et al (1974) described five affected sibs.

The pathogenesis is unclear, for it seems unlikely that such small testes could be responsible for normal male development. Perhaps the testes were initially normal during embryogenesis, only later decreasing in size. The aetiology might be analogous to anorchia (see below) yet with retention of some testicular tissue.

Agonadia

In agonadia the gonads are absent, the external genitalia abnormal, and all but rudimentary Mullerian or Wolffian derivatives absent. External genitalia usually consist of a phallus about the size of a clitoris, underdeveloped labia majora, and nearly complete fusion of the labioscrotal folds. A persistent urogenital sinus is often present. By definition, gonads cannot be detected. Likewise, neither normal Mullerian derivatives nor normal Wolffian derivatives are present, although structures resembling rudimentary structures may be present along the lateral pelvic wall. Somatic anomalies are common – craniofacial anomalies, vertebral anomalies, dermatoglyphic anomalies and possibly mental retardation (Sarto & Opitz, 1973). About 20 cases have been tabulated by Simpson (1978a) and Coulam (1979). Any pathogenic explanation for agonadia must take into account not only the absence of gonads, but also abnormal external geni-

talia and lack of normal internal ducts. At least two explanations seem reasonable: (1) fetal testes functioned sufficiently long to inhibit Mullerian development, yet not sufficiently long to complete male differentiation, or (2) the entire gonadal, ductal, and genital systems developed abnormally, as result of either defective anlage, defective connective tissue, or action of a teratogen. The frequent coexistence of somatic anomalies favors the existence of a teratogen or the existence of defective connective tissue. In one and possibly two kindreds affected sibs have been reported; thus, genetic factors should be considered. H-Y antigen is present (Schulte, 1979), suggesting that pathogenesis need not involve an abnormality of this system.

Although agonadia most often occurs in 46,XY individuals, 46,XX individuals may show the same phenotype (Duck et al, 1975).

Leydig cell agenesis

Four 46,XY patients have had complete absence of Leydig cells (Brown et al, 1970; Lee et al, 1981). They showed female external genitalia, no uterus and bilateral testes devoid of Leydig cells, and elevated LH levels. Interestingly, epididymes and vasa deferentia were present.

TRUE HERMAPHRODITISM

True hermaphrodites possess both ovarian and testicular tissue. They may have separate ovary and separate testis, or more often, one or more ovotestes. The disorder is clearly heterogeneous. Most true hermaphrodites have a 46,XX chromosomal complement; however, others have 46,XX/46,XY, 46,XX/47,XXY, 46,XY, or other complements (Simpson, 1978b). There are suggestions that phenotype depends upon karyotype, (Simpson, 1978b; Van Niekerk & Retief, 1981) but in this review we shall generalize about the phenotype of all true hermaphrodites.

Phenotype

About two-thirds of true hermaphrodites are raised as males, although their external genitalia may be frankly ambiguous or predominantly female. Paradoxically, breast development usually occurs at puberty despite male external genitalia, whereas virilization does not.

Gonadal tissue may be located in the ovarian, inguinal, or labioscrotal region. The greater the proportion of testicular tissue in an ovotestis, the greater the likelihood of gonadal descent. In 80% of ovotestes the testicular and ovarian components exist in end-to-end fashion (Van Niekerk, 1974); thus, ovotestes can usually be detected by inspection or possibly by palpation because testicular tissue is softer and darker than ovarian tissue. A testis

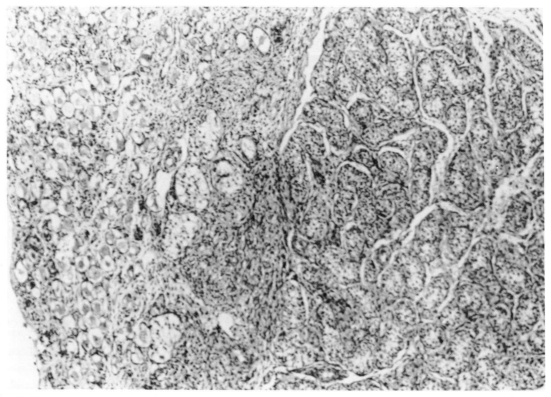

Fig. 87.4 Photomicrograph of the left ovotestis of patient No. 2 of Van Neikerk (1974). The patient had a 46,XX complement. Numerous primordial follicles are present in the smaller left portion; infantile testicular tissue is present on the right.

or an ovotestis is more likely to be present on the right than the left. Spermatozoa are rarely present; however, apparently normal oocytes are often present, even in ovotestes (Fig. 87.4). A uterus is usually present, often bicornuate or unicornuate. The absence of a uterine horn usually indicates an ipsilateral testis or ovotestis. The fimbriated end of the Fallopian tube may be occluded ipsilateral to an ovotestis, and squamous metaplasia of the endocervix may occur. Most true hermaphrodites with a uterus menstruate, and four 46,XX true hermaphrodites have become pregnant (Tegenkamp et al, 1979).

The diagnosis is usually made only after excluding the more common forms of male and female pseudohermaphroditism. A male sex-of-rearing is possible if genital status permits reconstruction and if the inappropriate (i.e., ovarian in male sex-of-rearing) tissue is extirpated. A few gonadal tumours have been observed, as has carcinoma of the breast.

Aetiology

The aetiology of true hermaphroditism is uncertain, but heterogeneous. 46,XX/46,XY cases may result from chimerism. (Chimerism is the presence or two or more cell lines, each derived from different zygotes, in a single individual.) In one survey by the author, 6 of 28 reported 46,XX/46,XY cases had been verified to be chimeras (Simpson, 1978b). However, experimental production of XX/XY mouse chimeras usually does not result in true hermaphroditism, nor do 46,XX/46,XY humans always have true hermaphroditism. 46,XX/47,XXY cases, which may result from either chimerism or mitotic nondisjunction, also have been reported.

A few 46,XX true hermaphrodites doubtless result from undetected chimerism; however, for various reasons undetected chimerism cannot easily explain all 46,XX true hermaphrodites. The presence of testicular tissue in 46,XX individuals is ostensibly perplexing because testicular determinants are localized to the Y–chromosome, specifically the short arm. Possible explanations for the presence of testes in individuals who ostensibly lack a Y include (1) translocation of testicular determinant(s) from the Y to an X, (2) translocation of testicular determinant(s) from the Y to an autosome, (3) undetected mosaicism or chimerism, and (4) sex-reversal genes. The first or possibly the second hypothesis is probably the likely explanation inasmuch as H-Y antigen is present in almost all 46,XX true hermaphrodites

(Wachtel & Ohno, 1979). Especially impressive are observations of H-Y antigen in each of two 46, XXX true hermaphrodite sibs (Fraccaro et al, 1979).

46,XX MALES (SEX-REVERSAL)

46,XX (sex-reversed) males are phenotypic males with bilateral testes. However, their chromosomal complement is that of a female (De La Chapelle, 1972; 1981).

Phenotype

Affected patients have small testes and signs of androgen deficiency, but otherwise have a normal male appearance. Facial and body hair are decreased, and pubic hair may be distributed in the pattern characteristic of females. About one-third have gynecomastia. The penis and scrotum are small but usually well differentiated, and Wolffian derivatives are normal. In one survey 9% of 46,XX males had hypospadias, but almost by definition the sex of rearing is not in doubt (De La Chapelle, 1972). Seminiferous tubules are decreased in number and in size, peritubular and interstitial fibrosis is present, Leydig cells are hyperplastic, and spermatogonia usually cannot be detected. Occasionally immature spermatogonia are detected, and sometimes the ejaculate contains spermatozoa.

Aetiology

In 46,XX males, as in 46,XX true hermaphrodites, testes develop contrary to expectations that a Y–chromosome is required for testicular differentation. As noted in the section on True hermaphroditism, several explanations have been proposed. Because all tested 46,XX males have been H-Y antigen positive (Wachtel, 1979), X-Y or Y-autosome translocation seems likely. Familial aggregates of 46,XX males alone, or either 46,XX males and 46,XX true hermaphrodites, have also been reported. Such families suggest sex-reversal genes, but in only one of the families studied were affected males H-Y positive (De La Chapelle et al, 1978). This could be explained by Y-X or Y-autosome translocation of portions of H-Y genes that are present in multiple copies; in females the translocated portion might be too small to confer maleness but large enough to behave in recessive sex-reversal fashion if a spouse were heterozygous for a similar mutant.

GENETIC FORMS OF GONADAL DYSGENESIS

Gonadal dysgenesis is usually associated with monosomy for the X–chromosome (45,X) or structural abnormalities of sex chromosomes, as reviewed previously by this author (Simpson, 1976) and elsewhere in this volume.

Occasionally individuals with apparently normal male (46,XY) or female (46,XX) chromosomal complements have gonadal dysgenesis. These disorders form the basis of this section.

XX gonadal dysgenesis

Gonadal dysgenesis histologically similar to that detected in individuals with an abnormal sex chromosome complement is known to occur in 46,XX individuals in whom mosaicism is reasonably excluded (XX gonadal dysgenesis) (Simpson, 1971a, 1979). Many well documented cases have been reported, and the trait does not appear unusually rare.

The external genitalia and the streak gonads of affected patients are indistinguishable from those of individuals who have gonadal dysgenesis and an abnormal chromosomal complement. Likewise, the endocrine findings (elevated gonadotropins) and the lack of secondary sexual development do not differ from those of other individuals with streak gonads. Most individuals with XX gonadal dysgenesis are normal in stature (mean height 165 cm) and somatic features of the Turner stigmata are usually absent.

In a number of families more than one member had XX gonadal dysgenesis, and in several families parents were consanguinous. Available data thus indicate autosomal recessive inheritance (Simpson, 1979). Of interest with respect to heterogeneity is one family in which one affected sib had streak gonads, whereas another had primary amenorrhea and extreme ovarian hypoplasia (a few ova were detected) (Boczkowski, 1970). Our group has also studied two affected sibs, one of whom showed not typical elongated streaks but rather small rounded gonads devoid of ova. These families suggest the mutant allele can exert a more variable effect than previously supposed, and therefore perhaps be more common than ordinarily expected. It could even explain sibships in which multiple members have had premature ovarian failure.

Both XX gonadal dysgenesis and neurosensory deafness have affected sibs in several families, as reviewed by Pallister and Opitz (1979). Although other explanations are possible, the most likely explanation for the association indicates existence of a pleiotropic gene different from the gene producing XX gonadal dysgenesis without deafness.

Finally, gonadal dysgenesis in 46,XX individuals may also result from nongenetic causes – e.g., infectious processes (e.g., mumps), infiltrative disorders (e.g., tuberculosis, tumours), autoimmunity.

XY gonadal dysgenesis

Individuals with apparently normal male (46,XY) chromosomal complements may also have gonadal dysgenesis (XY gonadal dysgenesis). Some authors apply the

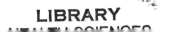

eponym Swyer syndrome. Almost all individuals with XY gonadal dysgenesis have been normal in stature, and somatic anomalies are usually absent. An estimated 20–30% of reported XY gonadal dysgenesis patients have had a dysgerminoma or gonadoblastoma (Simpson & Photopulos, 1976). Often the neoplasia arises in the first or second decade. Because of the relatively high probability of undergoing neoplastic transformation, gonads should therefore be extirpated from any patient with XY gonadal dysgenesis. The uterus and Fallopian tubes need not necessarily be removed, although often it is technically easier to remove these organs than to extirpate only the streaks.

The trait segregates in the fashion expected of an X–linked recessive or male-limited autosomal dominant gene (Simpson, 1971a, 1979 Simpson et al., 1981). Perhaps surprisingly, most affected patients are H-Y antigen positive (Wolf, 1979). Further studies are investigating the possibility that H-Y positive patients are at greater risk for neoplasia than are H-Y negative patients. Genetic heterogeneity clearly exists (Simpson et al, 1981) as shown also by the newly recognized association of camptomelic dwarfism and XY gonadal dysgenesis (Bricarelli et al, 1981; Puck et al, 1981.)

ANOMALIES LIMITED TO INTERNAL GENITAL DUCTS (MULLERIAN OR WOLFFIAN DERIVATIVES)

Many different developmental abnormalities affect the internal genital ducts. In this section only the most common disorders are mentioned.

Transverse vaginal septa

Transverse vaginal septa may occur at several locations, may be complete or incomplete. The septa are usually about 1 cm thick and located near the junction of the upper third and lower two-thirds of the vagina; however, they may be present in the middle or lower third of the vagina. If no perforation is present, mucus and menstrual fluid lack eggress; thus, hydrocolpos or hydrometrocolpos may develop. Other pelvic organs are usually normal, although occasionally the uterus is bicornuate.

Vaginal septa probably result from failure of the urogenital sinus derivatives and the Mullerian duct derivatives to fuse or to canalize. An autosomal recessive gene is responsible for some cases, at least in the Amish (McKusick et al, 1968). Cases with coexisting polydactyly may or may not be aetiologically distinct.

Longitudinal septa

Longitudinal vaginal septa (sagital or coronal) rarely produce clinical problems. They probably result from abnormal mesodermal proliferation or persisting epithelium. Occasionally such septa impede the second stage of labour. Heritable tendencies do not appear paramount in aetiology. However, Edwards and Gale (1972) reported an autosomal dominant syndrome characterized by a longitudinal vaginal septum, hand anomalies, and possible bladder neck anomaly. In addition a longitudinal septum may exist in Mullerian fusion defect (see below) of the most extreme type.

Vaginal atresia

In vaginal atresia the urogenital sinus fails to contribute the caudal portion of the vagina. The lower 20–40% of the vagina is therefore replaced by 2–3 cm of fibrous tissue, superior to which exist well differentiated upper vagina, cervix, uterine corpus, and Fallopian tubes. Vaginal atresia, a condition distinct from both transverse vaginal septa and Mullerian aplasia (see below) accounts for only 10–20% of patients who present clinically with 'absence of the vagina'. Familial aggregates of vaginal atresia have not been reported, and in general few data are available.

Winter et al (1968) described four sibs with an apparent autosomal recessive syndrome characterized by vaginal atresia, renal hypoplasia or agenesis, and middle ear anomalies (malformed incus, fixation of the malleus and incus). Another malformation syndrome in which vaginal atresia occurs is the Fraser (1962) syndrome, characterized by cryptophthalamos and resulting blindness.

Mullerian aplasia

Aplasia of the Mullerian ducts leads to absence of the uterine corpus, absence of the uterine cervix, and absence of the upper portion of the vagina. A vagina only 1–2 cm in depth is likely derived exclusively from invagination of the urogenital sinus. Despite primary amenorrhea, secondary sexual development is normal. Some investigators apply the appellation Rokitansky-Kustner-Hauser syndrome if rudimentary bands persist. The only disorder that ordinarily needs to be considered in the differential diagnosis is complete androgen insensitivity (complete testicular feminization). The latter can be excluded on the basis of chromosomal studies and gonadal composition. In addition, pubertal patients with Mullerian aplasia show pubic hair, whereas those with testicular feminization usually do not.

Renal anomalies are associated with Mullerian aplasia more frequently than expected by chance. The most frequent renal anomalies are pelvic kidney, renal ectopia, and unilateral renal aplasia. Vertebral anomalies are also relatively common. Excretory urography and vertebral roentgenograms are thus obligatory in the evaluation of patients with Mullerian aplasia.

Sibs with Mullerian aplasia have been reported on several occasions (Sarto & Simpson, 1978). Most observations are consistent with polygenic or multifactorial inheritance (Carson et al, 1982), despite Shokeir's (1978) report of several kindreds in which the trait appears to be inherited in sexlimited (female) autosomal dominant fashion.

Incomplete Mullerian fusion

During embryogenesis the Mullerian ducts are originally paired organs. Subsequently fusion and canalization produces the upper vagina, uterus and Fallopian tubes. Failure of fusion results in two hemiuteri, each associated with no more than one Fallopian tube. By contrast, in true Mullerian duplication, each hemiuterus has two tubes. (Thus, the common practice of applying the term 'double uterus' to incomplete Mullerian fusion constitutes a misnomer.) Sometimes one Mullerian duct fails to contribute to the definitive uterus, leading to a single rudimentary horn. Incomplete Mullerian fusion may be associated with second and early third trimester fetal losses. Surgical reconstruction may be helpful.

Several familial aggregates of incomplete Mullerian fusion have been reported, including multiple affected sibs as well as an affected mother and her daughter (Sarto & Simpson, 1978). Only one formal genetic study has been conducted. Both the low (3%) recurrence risk observed in female sibs (Elias et al, 1982) and the occasional reports of familial aggregates are consistent with polygenic or multifactorial inheritance. Incomplete Mullerian fusion may also be one component of a genetically determined malformation syndrome, e.g., the Meckel syndrome, the Fraser syndrome, and the Rudiger syndrome. One especially interesting syndrome is the 'hand-foot-uterus' syndrome, an autosomal dominant disorder in which affected females have a bicornuate uterus and characteristic malformations of the hands and feet.

Wolffian aplasia

Absence of Wolffian deriviates (Wolffian aplasia) may or may not be associated with absence of upper urinary tract. Complete agenesis of both the Wolffian duct derivatives and the upper urinary tract implies total failure of the mesonephric development. Agenesis of Wolffian derivatives alone implies resorption of Wolffian elements after the Wolffian duct has reached the cloaca. Even if absence of Wolffian derivatives is accompanied by upper urinary tract anomalies, the gonads are only rarely involved. More frequently the upper urinary tract is normal in individuals who lack an epididymis, ductus deferens, and seminal vesicle, or who lack only the ductus epididymis and proximal portion of the ductus deferens. If the defect is bilateral, affected patients are infertile. If the defect is unilateral, patients are usually asymptomatic. Absence of the ductus deferens has been observed in four sibs; none had cystic fibrosis, a disorder in which absence of the ductus deferens is common.

Failure of fusion of epididymis and testis

Another relatively common defect involves failure of fusion of (a) the rete cords of the testis and (b) the mesonephric tubules that form the ductuli efferentia (Simpson, 1976). Spermatozoa cannot exist from the testis and, if bilateral, infertility results. One or both testes may fail to descend.

These fusion anomalies are not nearly so rare as one might expect from the relative paucity of reports in the literature. Surveys indicate that fusion defects of this type occur in about 1% of cyrptorchid and in about 1% of azoospermic men. No genetic data are available.

SELECTED MISCELLANEOUS DISORDERS

Germinal cell aplasia (Sertoli-cell only syndrome; Del Castillo syndrome)

Del Castillo et al (1947) described several normally virilized yet sterile males. Their seminiferous tubules lacked spermatogonia and their testes were slightly smaller than average. However, Leydig cell function was normal; thus, secondary sexual development was normal. In germinal cell aplasia FSH is elevated but LH is normal. Tubular hyalinization and sclerosis usually do not occur. Occasionally a few spermatozoa are present, but affected individuals are usually sterile. Despite infertility, androgens are unnecessary because secondary sexual development is normal.

Anorchia

Males (46,XY) with anorchia have unambiguous male external genitalia, normal Wolffian derivatives, no Mullerian derivatives, and no detectable testes. Somatic abnormalities are rarely present. Despite absence of testes, the phallus is well differentiated. Pathogenesis presumably involves atrophy of fetal testes after 12–16 weeks gestation, by which time genital virilization has occurred. Vasa deferentia terminate blindly, often in association with the spermatic vessels. Unilateral anorchia is not extraordinarily rare, but bilateral anorchia is relatively rare. The diagnosis should be applied only if testicular tissue is detected in neither the scrotum, the inguinal canal or the entire path along which the testes descended during embryogenesis. Splenic-gonadal fusion can also occur, mimicking the disorder (Finkbeiner et al, 1977).

Heritable tendencies exist, but the occurrence of monozygotic twins discordant for anorchia suggests that genetic factors are not paramount in all cases (Simpson et al, 1971b). However, a heritable tendency toward in utero torsion of the testicular artery could exist, explaining occasional familial aggregates.

Normofunctional testicular hyperplasia with mental retardation

An X–linked syndrome characterized by macroorchidism and mental retardation exists (Cantu et al, 1978). Virilization is normal. Cytogenetic studies have indicated that this disorder corresponds to X–linked recessive mental retardation associated with 'the fragile X' chromosome (Howard-Peebles & Stoddard, 1979; Gerald, 1980).

'Rudimentary ovary syndrome' and unilateral streak ovary syndrome

The 'rudimentary ovary syndrome' is a poorly defined entity of unknown etiology said to be characterized by ovaries containing decreased numbers of follicles. Anatomically analogous to the rudimentary testes syndrome, the 'rudimentary ovary syndrome' is certainly heterogeneous and probably not be a true entity. Many cases have been associated with sex chromosomal abnormalities, particularly 45,X/46,XX mosaicism. Similar statements apply also to individuals said to have the unilateral streak ovary syndrome.

Polycystic ovarian disease (Stein-Leventhal syndrome)

Polycystic ovarian disease is a common gynecologic disorder characterized by obesity, oligomenorrhea, and virilization (hirsuitism). Clinicians appreciate the great variability shown by individuals with this disorder, frequently the cause of infertility. The LH/FSH ratio is increased, androstenedione is elevated and peripheral conversion of androstenedione to estrone is increased. Autosomal dominant or even X–linked dominant inheritance has been proposed (Cohen et al, 1975) consistent with the variable expressivity. Polycystic ovaries have been observed in patients with X–chromosomal abnormalities, but the relationship between these phenomena is uncertain. A further example of heterogeneity among females with polycystic ovarian disease are observations that this phenotype may be associated with adult-onset 21-hydroxylase deficiencies.

Mutant genes affecting meiosis

In plants and lower mammals meiosis is known to be under genetic control, and similar mechanisms presumably exist in humans. Mutation involving such genes could deleteriously after reproduction. Data are limited, but in some families mutant genes appearing to interfere with meiosis led to infertility (Changanti et al, 1980). Further studies of male and female meiosis should uncover further evidence for the role of meiotic mutants in infertility. This topic is considered elsewhere in this volume by Chandley.

REFERENCES

Amrhein J A, Meyer W J, Jones H W, Migeon C J 1976 Androgen insensitivity in man. Evidence for genetic heterogeneity. Proceedings National Academy of Science USA 73: 891

Amrhein J A, Klingensmith G J, Walsh P C, McKusick V A, Migeon C J 1977 Partial androgen insensitivity. The Reifenstein syndrome revisited. New England Journal of Medicine 297: 350

Bergada C, Cleveland W W, Jones H W, Wilkins L 1962 Variants of embryonic testicular dysgenesis: Bilateral anorchia and the syndrome of rudimentary testes. Acta Endocrinology 40: 521

Bernstein R, Koo G E, Wachtel S S 1980 Abnormality of the X–chromosome in human 46,XY female siblings with dysgenetic ovaries. Science 207: 768

Boczkowski K 1970 Pure gonadal dysgenesis and ovarian dysplasia in sisters. American Journal of Obstetrics and Gynecology 106: 626

Bongiovanni A M 1979 Further studies of congenital adrenal hyperplasia due to 3β-hydroxysteroid dehydrogenase deficiency. In: Vallet H L, Porter I H (eds) Genetic Mechanism of Sexual Development, Academic Press, New York. p 189

Bowen P, Lee C S N, Migeon C J, Kaplan N M, Whalley P J, McKusick V A, et al 1965 Hereditary male pseudohermaphriditism with hypogonadism, hypospadias, and gynecomastia (Reifenstein's syndrome). Annals Internal Medicine 62: 252

Bricarelli F D, Fraccaro M, Lindsten J, Miller U, Baggio P,

Carbone L D L et al 1981 Sex-reversed XY females with campomelic dysplasia are H-Y negative. Human Genetics 57: 15

Brown D M, Markland C, Dehner L P 1976 Leydig cell hypoplasia: A cause of male pseudohermaphroditism. Journal of Clinical Endocrinology and Metabolism 46: 1

Cantu J M, Scaglia H E, Gonzalez-Diddi M, Hernandex-Jawregui P, Morato T, Moreno M E, et al 1978 Inherited congenital nomofunctional testicular hyperplasia and mental deficiency. Human Genetics 41: 331

Carson S A, Simpson J L, Elias S, Sarto G E, Gerbie A B, Malinak L R, Buttram V C Jr 1982 Genetics of Mullerian aplasia. Fertility and Sterility 37: 306

Chaganti R S K, Jhanwar S C, Ehrenbard L T, Kourides I A, Williams J J 1980 Genetically determined asynapsis, spermatogenic degeneration and infertility in man. American Journal of Human Genetics 32: 833

Cohen B N, Givens J R, Wiser W L, Wilroy R S, Summitt R L, Coleman S A, et al 1975 Polycystic ovarian disease, maturation arrest of spermatogenesis and Klinefelter's syndrome in siblings of a family with familial hirsuitism. Fertility and Sterility 26: 1228

Coulam C B 1979 Testicular regression syndrome. Obstetrics and Gynecology 53: 45

De La Chapelle A 1972 Analytical review: Nature and origin of males with XX sex chromosomes. American Journal of Human Genetics 24: 71

De La Chapelle A 1981 The etiology of maleness in XX men. Human Genetics 58: 105

De La Chapelle A, Koo G C, Wachtel S S 1978 Recessive sex-determining genes in human XX male syndrome. Cell 15: 837

Del Castillo E B, Trabucco A, De La Balze R A 1947 Syndrome produced by absence of the germinal epithelium without impairment of the Sertoli or Leydig cells. Journal Clinical Endocrinology 7: 493

Duck S C, Sekhon G S, Wilbois R, Pagliara A S, Weldon V V 1975 Pseudohermaphroditism with testes and a 46,XX karyotype. Journal of Pediatrics 87: 58

Edwards J A, Gale R P 1972 Camptobrachydactyly: A new autosomal dominant trait with two probably homozygotes. American Journal of Human Genetics 24: 464

Elias S, Carson S A, Simpson J L, Verp M S, Sarto G E, Malinak L R Jr 1982 Genetic studies in incomplete Mullerian fusion (septate and bicornuate uteri) Fertility and Sterility 37: 305

Finkbeiner A E, DeRiddle P A, Ryden S E 1977 Splenic-gonadal fusion and adrenal cortical rest associated with bilateral cryptorchidism. Urology 10: 337

Fisher L K, Kogut M D, Moore R J, Goebelsmann U, Weitzman J J, Isaacs H, et al 1978 Clinical endocrinological, and enzymatic characterization of two patients with 5α-reductase deficiency: Evidence that a single enzyme is responsible for the 5α-reduction of cortisol and testosterone. Journal Clinical Endocrinology and Metabolism 47: 653

Fraccaro M, Tiepolo L, Zuffardi O, Chiumello G, DiNatale B, Gargantini L, et al 1979 Familial XX true hermaphroditism and the H-Y antigen. Human Genetics 48: 45

Fraser G K 1962 Our genetical 'load'. A review of some aspects of genetic malformations. Annals of Human Genetics 25: 387

Gerald P S 1980 X–linked mental retardation and an X–chromosome marker. New England Journal of Medicine 303: 696

Griffin J E, Punyashthiti K, Wilson 1976 Dihydrotestosterone binding by cultured human fibroblasts. Comparison of cells from control subjects and from patients with hereditary pseudohermaphroditism due to androgen resistance. Journal of Clinical Investigation 57: 1342

Heremans G F P, Moolenaar A J, Van Gelderen H M 1976 Female phenotype in a male child due to 17α-hydroxylase deficiency. Archives Diseases of Childhood 51: 721

Howard-Peebles P N, Stoddard G R 1979 X–linked mental retardation with macroorchidism and marker X–chromosome. Human Genetics 50: 247

Hsu L Y F, Hirschhorn K, Goldstein A, Barcinski M A 1970 Familial chromosomal mosaicism, genetic aspects. Annals of Human Genetics 33: 343

Imperato-McGinley J, Guerrero L, Gautier T, Peterson R E 1974 Steroid 5α-reductase deficiency in man: An inherited form of male pseudohermaphroditism. Science 186: 1213

Imperato-McGinley J, Peterson R E, Stoller R, Goodwin W E 1979 Male pseudohermaphroditism secondary to 17α-hydroxysteroid dehydrogenase deficiency: Gender role with puberty. Journal of Clinical Endocrinology and Metabolism 49: 391

Jones H W, Rary J M, Cummings D 1979 The role of the H-Y antigen in human sexual development. Johns Hopkins Medical Journal 145: 33

Kaufman M, Pinsky, L, Baird P A, Mc Gillivray B C 1979 Complete androgen insensitivity with a normal amount of 5α-dihydrotestosterone-binding activity in labium majis skin fibroblasts. American Journal of Medical Genetics 4: 401

Lee P A, Rock J A, Brown T R, Fichman K M, Migeon C J,

Jones H W Jr 1981 Leydig cell hypofunction resulting in male pseudohermaphroditism. Fertility and Sterility 37: 675

Leshin M, Griffin J E, Wilson J D 1978 Hereditary male pseudohermaphroditism associated with unstable form of 5α-reductase. Journal of Clinical Investigation 62: 685

McKusick V A, Weibaecher R G, Gragg G W 1968 Recessive inheritance of a congenital malformation syndrome. Journal American Medical Association 204: 113

Meyer W J, Migeon B R, Migeon C J 1975 Locus on human X–chromosome for dihydrotestosterone receptor and androgen insensitivity. Proceedings of National Academy of Science USA 72: 1469

Morris J M, Mahesh V B 1963 Further observations on the syndrome, 'testicular feminization'. American Journal of Obstetrics and Gynecology 87: 731

Najjar S S, Takla R J, Nassar V H 1974 The syndrome of rudimentary testes: Occurrence in five siblings. Pediatrics 84: 119

Ohno S, Nagai Y, Ciccarese S 1978 Testicular cells lysostripped of H-Y antigen organize ovarian follicle like aggregates. Cytogenetics Cell Genetics 20: 315

Opitz J M, Simpson J L, Sarto G E, Summitt R L, New M, German J 1972 Pseudovaginal perineoscrotal hypospadias. Clinical Genetics 3: 1

Pallister P D, Opitz J M 1979 The Perrault syndrome: Autosomal recessive ovarian dysgenesis with facultative, non-sex-limited sensorineural deafness. American Journal of Medical Genetics 4: 239

Peterson R E, Imperato-McGinley J, Gautier T, Sturla E 1977 Male pseudohermaphroditism due to steroid 5α-reductase deficiency. American Journal of Medicine 62: 170

Pinsky L 1978 The nosology of male pseudohermaphrotidism. Birth Defects, Original Article Series 14(6c): 73

Prader A, Gurtner N P 1955 Das syndrome des pseudohermaphroditismus masculinus bei kongenitaler nebennierenrinden-hyperplasie ohne androgenüberproduktion (adrenaler pseudohermaphroditismus masculinus) Helvetica Pediatrics Acta 10: 397

Puck S M, Haseltine F P, Francke U 1981 Absence of H-Y antigen in an XY female with campomelic dysplasia. Human Genetics 57: 23

Sarto G E, Opitz J M 1973 The XY gonadal agenesis syndrome. Journal of Medical Genetics 10: 288

Sarto G E, Simpson J L 1978 Abnormalities of the Mullerian and Wolffian duct systems. Birth Defects, Original Article Series 14(6c): 37

Schimke R N 1979 XY sex-reversal campomelia-possibly and X–linked disorder? Clinical Genetics 16: 62

Schulte M J 1979 Positive H-Y antigen testing in a case of XY gonadal absence syndrome. Clinical Genetics 16: 438

Shokeir M H K 1978 Aplasia of the Mullerian system: Evidence for probable sex-limited autosomal dominant inheritance. Birth Defects, Original Article Series 14(6c): 147

Simpson J L, Christakos A C, Horwith M, Silverman F S 1971a Gonadal dysgenesis in individuals with apparently normal chromosomal complements: Tabulation of cases and compilation of genetic data. Birth Defects, Original Article Series 7(6): 215

Simpson J L, Horwith M, Morillo-Cucci G, McGovern J H, Levine M I, German J 1971b Bilateral anorchia: Discordance in monozygotic twins. Birth Defects, Original Article Series 7(6): 196

Simpson J L, New M, Peterson R E, German J 1971c Pseudovaginal perineoscrotal hypospadias (PPSH) in sibs. Birth Defects, Original Article Series 7(6): 140

Simpson J L 1976 Disorders of Sexual Differentiation. Etiology and Clinical Delineation. Academic Press, New York

Simpson J L, Photopulos G 1976 The relationship of neoplasia to disorders of abnormal sexual differentiation. Birth Defects, Original Article Series 12(1): 15

Simpson J L 1978a Male pseudohermaphroditism: Genetics and clinical delineation. Human Genetics 44: 1

Simpson J L 1978b True hermaphroditism in humans: Etiology and phenotypic considerations. Birth Defects, Original Article Series 14(6c): 9

Simpson J L 1979 Gonadal dysgenesis and sex chromosome abnormalities: Phenotypic-karyotypic correlations. In: Vallet H L, Porter I H (eds) Genetic Mechanisms of Sexual Development, Academic Press, New York. p 365

Simpson J L 1980 Genetics of human reproduction. In: Hafez E S (ed) Human Reproduction, 2nd edition Harper & Row, Hagerstorm. p 395

Simpson J L, Blagowidow N, Martin A O 1981 XY gonadal dysgenesis: Genetic heterogeneity based upon clinical observations, H-Y antigen status and segregation analysis. Human Genetics 58: 9

Sloan W R, Walsh P C 1976 Familial persistent Mullerian duct syndrome. Journal of Urology 115: 459

Tegenkamp T R, Brazzell J W, Tegenkamp I, Labadi F 1979 Pregnancy without benefit of reconstructive surgery in a bisexually active true hermaphrodite. American Journal of Obstetrics and Gynecology 135: 427

Van Niekerk W A 1974 True Hermaphroditism. Harper & Row, New York

Van Niekerk W A, Retief A E 1981 The gonads of human true hermaphrodites. Human Genetics 58: 117

Wachtel S S 1977 H-Y antigen and the genetics of sex determination. Science 198: 797

Wachtel S S 1979 The genetics of intersexuality: Clinical and theoretic perspectives. Obstetrics and Gynecology 54: 671

Wachtel S S, Ohno S 1979 The immunogenetics of sexual development. Progress in Medocal Genetics 3: 109

Walsh P C, Madden J D, Harrod M J, Goldstein J L, MacDonald P C, Wilson J D 1974 Familial incomplete male pseudohermaphroditism, type 2. New England Journal of Medicine 291: 944

Wilson J D, Harrod M J, Goldstein J L, Hemsell D L, MacDonald P C 1974 Familial incomplete male pseudohermaphroditism, type 1. New England Journal of Medicine 290: 1097

Winter J S D, Kohn G, Mellman W J, and Wágner S 1968 A familial syndrome of renal, genital and middle ear anomalies. Journal of Pediatrics 71: 88

Winters J J, Wachtel S S, White B J, Koo G C, Javadpour N, Loriaux D L, et al 1979 H-Y antigen mosaicism in the gonad of a 46,XX true hermaphrodite. New England Journal of Medicine 300: 745

Wolf U 1979 XY gonadal dysgenesis and the H-Y antigen. Report on 12 cases. Human Genetics 47: 269

Wolf U 1981 Genetic aspects of H-Y antigen. Human Genetics 58: 25

Wolf U, Fraccaro M, Mayerova A, Hecht T, Zuffardi O, Hameister H. 1980. Turner syndrome patients are H-Y positive. Human Genetics 54: 315

Zachmann M, Vollmin J A, Hamilton W, Prader A 1972 Steroid 17,20-desmolase deficiency: A new cause of male pseudohermaphroditism. Clinical Endocrinology 1: 369

Zenzes M T, Wolf U, Gunther E 1978a Studies on the function of H-Y antigen: Dissociation and reorganization experiments on rat gonadal cells. Cytogenetics Cell Genetics 20: 365

Zenzes M T, Wolf W, Engel W 1978b Organization in vitro of ovarian cells into testicular structures. Human Genetics 44: 333

Disorders of amino acid metabolism

C. R. Scott

DISORDERS OF PHENYLALANINE
METABOLISM (Table 88.1)

The hyperphenylalaninaemias

The chemist, Følling, first recognized the existence of a disorder of phenylalanine metabolism in 1934 (Følling, 1934). He found the metabolites phenylpyruvic acid and phenylacetic acid in the urine of mentally retarded patients who were in a Norwegian institution for the retarded. This condition would eventually be called *phenylketonuria* and be a cornerstone of research in clinical and biochemical genetics. It is now recognized that several genetic entities can cause an elevation of blood phenylalanine and mimic the clinical phenotype of phenylketonuria. All interfere with the conversion of phenylalanine to tyrosine by reducing the activity of phenylalanine hydroxylase. They each cause an elevation of phenylalanine concentration in the blood and are referred to as the hyperphenylalaninaemias.

Phenylalanine hydroxylase reaction
Phenylalanine is hydroxylated to tyrosine by the enzyme

phenylalanine hydroxylase. The reaction requires molecular oxygen and tetrahydrobiopterin as the active cofactor (Kaufman, 1963; Kaufman, 1971). The tetrahydrobiopterin is generated from dihydrobiopterin by the enzyme *dihydrofolate reductase.* The dihydrobiopterin is normally synthesized de novo in man (Fig. 88.1).

The products of the phenylalanine hydroxylase reaction are tyrosine and an oxidized biopterin, quinonoid-XH_2. The quinonoid-XH_2 may be regenerated to tetrahydrobiopterine by *dihydropteridine reductase* for conservation and reutilization. In humans the conversion of phenylalanine to tyrosine occurs primarily, if not entirely, in the soluable fraction of the liver.

Classic phenylketonuria

Classic phenylketonuria is caused by a genetic deficiency of phenylalanine hydroxylase. This was first documented by Jervis in 1953 and subsequently by Mitoma et al (1957), Wallace et al (1957), and Kaufman (1958). Friedman et al (1973) and Kaufman (1976) have shown by immunological methods that the apoenzyme is structurally altered in classical phenylketonuria.

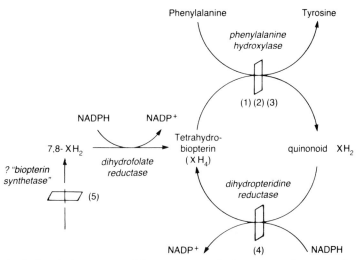

Fig. 88.1 The phenylalanine hydroxylating system and the reactions required to generate the active cofactor, tetrahydrobiopterine. The known genetic defects are phenylketonuria (1), benign hyperphenylalaninaemia (2), transient hyperphenylalaninaemia (3), dihydropteridine reductase deficiency (4), and a defect in biopterin synthesis (5).

Patients affected with classic phenylketonuria will develop mental retardation, eczema, hypopigmentation and neurological symptoms if untreated. Knox (1972) has reviewed the intellectual results of untreated children and adults with phenylketonuria and concluded that the majority would have an IQ at or below 20. Only 4% or less would have an IQ above 60. In screening approximately 250 000 blood samples submitted to the Massachusetts State Health Laboratory for syphilis testing, Levy et al (1970) found only three persons with an elevated blood phenylalanine; each was retarded. Thus, normal intelligence is rarely achieved in persons with phenylketonuria who remain untreated.

The characteristic 'mousey' odour that is present in untreated persons with phenylketonuria is from the excretion of phenylacetic acid. The hypopigmentation is related to the competitive inhibition of *tyrosine hydroxylase* by the increased concentration of phenylalanine. The inhibition of tyrosine hydroxylase activity prevents the conversion of tyrosine to DOPA and the subsequent formation of melanin. Thus, affected individuals have been described as having blue eyes, blonde hair and pale skin.

The neurological symptoms include the findings of hypertonicity, irritability, agitated behavior, tremors, hyperactivity and occasionally seizures. The exact mechanism that causes the neurological abnormalities and the development of mental retardation is unknown but is believed to be related to interference in the functioning of metabolic pathways within the nervous system by phenylalanine and its accumulated by-products (Knox, 1972).

Diagnosis

In most Western countries, newborns are being screened for phenylketonuria by the measurement of blood phenylalanine during the newborn period. The blood phenylalanine concentration may be near the normal range at birth but promptly rises within three to seven days of age. Patients with classic phenylketonuria will demonstrate a persistent elevation of phenylalanine in their blood of > 16 mg % while receiving a normal dietary intake of protein. Their plasma tyrosine will be in the normal range and O-OH-phenylacetic acid and phenylpyruvic acid may be detectable in the urine if the phenylalanine concentration has been consistently elevated for one to two weeks. Holtzman (1974a, b) has demonstrated that female infants may have a slower rise in plasma phenylalanine than males and that screening performed prior to 72 hours of age may not be epidemiologically efficient.

The majority of infants with an elevated blood phenylalanine detected through a screening programme do not have classic phenylketonuria, but rather, have one of the other forms of hyperphenylalaninaemia which is usually benign and does not require therapy.

Genetics

Genetic heterogeneity exists for the causes of persistent hyperphenylalaninaemia. These vary from the benign neonatal hyperphenylalaninaemia caused by a temporary derangement in tyrosine metabolism to the known defects of phenylalanine hydroxylase.

Classic PKU is inherited in an autosomal recessive manner and occurs in approximately 1:10 000 births in populations of Western European origin. In these populations, the gene for PKU can be considered a polymorphism since q approaches 0.01 and the heterozygote frequency is 0.02 ($2pq$). The chromosomal location of the gene coding for the apoenzyme of phenylalanine hydroxylase is unknown.

A considerable variation in gene frequency exists depending upon ethnic origin. The gene is most common in Ireland, Scotland, Belgium and West Germany, with estimated gene frequencies of $q = 0.012$ to 0.014 (Rosenberg, 1980) to populations in which PKU may be considered rare (Blacks, Asians and American Indians).

Heterozygote detection is feasible for classic PKU. The most reliable method utilizes only a single blood sample analyzed for phenylalanine and tyrosine by ion-exchange chromatography. If descriminate analysis is applied to the resulting values, reliable heterozygote detection can be achieved (Perry et al, 1967; Rosenblatt and Scriver, 1968). Less reliable are phenylalanine loading studies by either oral or intravenous administration. No studies have documented the ability to accurately identify heterozygotes from the general population.

The prenatal detection of PKU has not been documented. Since the enzyme is not active in cells derived from amniotic fluid, a direct assay is not feasible. Similarly, affected fetuses probably do not excrete increased quantities of phenylalanine products that would allow the detection of abnormal metabolites in amniotic fluid.

Maternal phenylketonuria

It has been recognized that children born to mothers with PKU have a high risk of having mental retardation or congenital defects. At least 90% of offspring will be affected with microephaly, mental and growth retardation, or congenital heart or vascular problems (Hsia, 1970; Howell & Stevenson, 1971; Lenke & Levy, 1980). These intrauterine effects on development are believed to be a direct consequences of the elevated maternal phenylalanine on the developing fetus.

Attempts to reduce the serum phenylalanine during pregnancy by the use of a low phenylalanine diet have resulted in confusing information. Some authors have reported successful outcomes of pregnancies (Arthur &

Hulme, 1970) but most attempts have been unsuccessful (Huntley & Stevenson, 1969; Busk & Dukes, 1975; unpublished data).

Women with PKU should be counselled of the 90% risk of having a damaged fetus with or without dietary intervention during pregnancy.

Therapy of phenylketonuria

Dietary therapy has been shown to be effective in preventing mental retardation in patients with PKU. In long-term studies in the United Kingdom, Canada and the United States, the restriction of dietary phenylalanine within 30 to 90 days of birth and continuing for six to eight years has resulted in intelligence comparable to normal sibs (Hudson et al, 1970; Hanley et al, 1971; Smith & Wolff, 1974; Dobson et al, 1976).

It is currently advised that a restriction of dietary phenylalanine should continue throughout childhood and probably through adulthood for affected patients. The diet should be managed by a competent team consisting of a nutritionist, a physician and a person with skills in social work to assure dietary compliance. It has been established that blood levels of 2 to 12 mg per 100 ml of phenylalanine are satisfactory for achieving normal development in patients with PKU.

Atypical phenylketonuria with dihydropteridine reductase deficiency

Several children have been identified with a deficiency of dihydropteridine reductase as a cause for their elevated blood phenylalanine (Bartholome et al, 1975; Kaufman et al, 1975). Such children are believed to be rare and account for no more than 1% of patients with phenylketonuria. Unfortunately, they lose intellectual function even though their blood phenylalanine values can be adequately managed by diet.

The deficiency of the reductase prevents the recycling of the quinonoid-XH_2 to the tetrahydrobiopterin, the active form of the cofactor necessary for the phenylalanine hydroxase reaction (Fig. 88.1). The reductase is also necessary for the formation of 5-hydroxytryptophane and DOPA from tryptophane and tyrosine, respectively. These two products are the precursors of the neurotransmittors serotonin and norepinephrin. It is presumed that the mental deficiency is a consequence of the lack of formation of these necessary compounds.

The enzyme deficiency is inherited as an autosomal recessive condition. Preliminary reports indicate the enzyme can be measured in peripheral leukocytes and cultured fibroblasts and that heterozygotes have less than normal activity (Firgaira et al, 1979).

Serotonin and 5-hydroxytryptophane have been given to affected children in an attempt to replace these deficient compounds. Tentative reports have been encouraging (Danks et al, 1978).

Transient phenylketonuria

Occasional infants are diagnosed as having phenylketonuria during infancy who eventually 'outgrow' their disorder. They have been referred to as 'transient phenylketonuria'. The mechanism of how this occurs is poorly understood. It is believed they have a partial deficiency of phenylalanine hydroxylase (Justice et al, 1967).

Hyperphenylalaninaemia, benign

A large number of infants are detected with elevated levels of phenylalanine, but with values below the level seen in children with 'classic phenylketonuria'. Their plasma phenylalanine values are usually between 4 and 10 mg % on a normal diet. They require no dietary intervention and do not develop neurological sequelae.

Table 88.1 Disorders of phenylalanine metabolism — the hyperphenylalaninaemias

Disorder	Enzyme deficiency	Inheritance pattern	Heterozygote detection	Prenatal diagnosis
Phenylketonuria (PKU)	Phenylalanine hydroxylase (1.14.16.1) ? chromosome 1	AR	Yes	No
Benign hyperphenylalaninaemia	Phenylalanine hydroxylase (1.14.16.1)	AR	?	No
Transient hyperphenylalaninaemia	Phenylalanine hydroxylase (?) (1.14.16.1)	AR?	No	No
Dihydropteridine reductase deficiency	Dihydropteridine reductase (1.6.99.7) ? chromosome 4	AR	?	Possible
Biopterin synthesis deficiency	'Biopterin synthetase' defect (?)	AR?	—	—

The information contained in this table and subsequent tables was obtained from several sources, the most helpful being Erbe (1977) and Scriver (1977).

Sibs may be affected, lending credence to the genetic nature of the condition. A partial deficiency of phenylalanine hydroxylase has been measured in a few cases (Justice et al, 1967; Kang et al, 1970).

DISORDERS OF TYROSINE METABOLISM
(Table 88.2)

The majority of the available tyrosine in humans is formed from the oxidation of phenylalanine. Tyrosine is essential for the composition of protein, the synthesis of thyroid hormones, the formation of pigment and the production of neurotransmitters. Tyrosine is normally degraded through a series of oxidative steps to form acetic and fumeric acid (Fig. 88.2). Enzyme deficiencies within the catabolic pathway may cause an accumulation of tyrosine or a tyrosine product. The only common disorder of tyrosine metabolism is *neonatal tyrosinaemia*, a problem of delayed developmental synthesis of a normal enzyme. The other known disorders are genetically determined and rare.

Neonatal tyrosinaemia
It is estimated that 30% of premature infants and 10% of full term infants develop neonatal tyrosinaemia (Avery et al, 1967). Gestational age rather than birth weight is the most consistent predisposing factor. Neonatal tyrosinaemia, per se, is not believed to be associated with significant clinical symptomatology or to cause developmental problems (Avery et al, 1967; Partington et al, 1968). Menkes and co-workers (1972) have suggested

however, that small infants with tyrosine values greater than 1 mM may be at risk for mild mental retardation.

The cause of the observed tyrosinaemia in immature infants has been shown to be an impairment in the activity of *p-hydroxyphenylpyruvic acid (pHPPA) oxidase*. Kretchmer and co-workers (1956) showed that the development of adequate enzyme activity in the liver tissue of infants was related to gestational age. Thus, young infants may have insufficient pHPPA oxidase to metabolize the pHPPA formed from tyrosine. The enzyme pHPPA oxidase is synthesized more efficiently after birth, may be stabilized by ascorbic acid, and is inhibited by its substrate pHPPA. Each of these factors are used to assist in the clinical management of infants who may demonstrate tyrosinaemia. Lowering the dietary protein to 2 gm/kg/day will decrease the formation of pHPPA from tyrosine, and administering 100 mg/day of ascorbic acid will stabilize those enzyme molecules that have been synthesized. Most infants with neonatal tyrosinaemia will promptly lower their plasma tyrosine concentration to the normal range (< 0.1 mM) with these two manoeuvres.

Neonatal tyrosinaemia is not believed to occur as the result of an abnormal allele. However, genetic factors may influence its incidence, since it is common in the Arctic Eskimo with a frequency of 12% in term births (Clow et al, 1972).

Hereditary tyrosinaemia
Hereditary tyrosinaemia has two clinical forms; an 'acute' infantile form associated with liver failure and early death, and a more 'chronic' form leading to growth

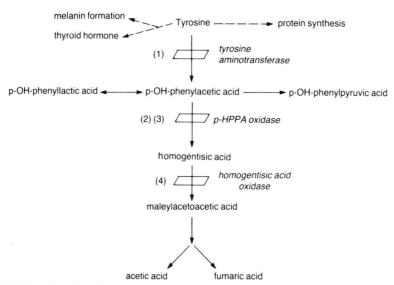

Fig. 88.2 The metabolic fate of tyrosine. The known defects in tyrosine metabolism include hypertyrosinaemia (1), neonatal tyrosinaemia (2), hereditary tyrosinaemia (3), and alkaptonuria (4).

Table 88.2 Disorders of tyrosine metabolism — the hypertyrosinaemias

Disorder	Enzyme deficiency	Inheritance pattern	Heterozygote detection	Prenatal diagnosis
Neonatal tyrosinaemia	p-OH-phenylpyruvic acid oxidase (1.13.11.27)	Not inherited		
Hereditary tyrosinaemia	p-OH-phenylpyruvic acid oxidase (?) (1.13.11.27)	AR	No	Yes
Tyrosinaemia	Tyrosine aminotransferase (cytoplasm) (2.6.1.5)	AR?		
Tyrosinosis	Tyrosine aminotransferase (mitochondrial) (?)			
Alkaptonuria	Homogentisic acid oxidase	AR	No	No

failure, nodular cirrhosis of the liver, and nephropathy. Both forms may be associated with hypoglycaemia and hyperplasia of the islets of Langerhans. Patients with the chronic form may also develop hypophosphataemic rickets from their kidney disease and are at high risk for hepatic carcinoma (Gentz et al, 1965; Scriver & Davis, 1967).

The observed biochemical abnormalities include the massive excretion of tyrosine, pHPPA and pHPLA. There is an increased concentration of tyrosine and methionine in the plasma. Serum α-fetoprotein has been noted to be increased during the postnatal period and has been recommended to be used as a screening assay for the condition (Belanger et al, 1973).

The primary enzymatic defect in hereditary tyrosinaemia is believed to be a deficiency of pHPPA oxidase (La Du, 1967; Toniguchi and Gjessing, 1965). However, there is evidence to suggest that deficiency of the oxidase could be secondary to inhibition by other metabolic derangements. Gaul and associates (1970) have specifically implicated defects in the catabolism of methionine.

Restriction of dietary intake for phenylalanine and tyrosine has been beneficial for affected patients (Partington et al, 1967; Aronsson et al, 1968). During the acute stage of the illness, methionine restriction has also been of value. Detailed instructions for the synthetic diet and its appropriate use have been published (Hill et al, 1970).

Hereditary tyrosinaemia is inherited as an autosomal recessive condition. Both forms of the disease have been documented to occur in the same sibship (Partington et al, 1967). The condition has been recognized in many ethnic groups. A particularly high incidence exists in a French Canadian isolate where the heterozygote frequency has been estimated to be 1 in 14 persons (Bergeron et al, 1974). Neither heterozygote detection nor prenatal diagnosis has been reported for the disorder.

Hypertyrosinaemia

A few patients have been reported with a markedly elevated concentration of tyrosine in their blood (> 1 mM) and painful hyperkeratosis of palmar and plantar surfaces. They have associated corneal ulcers and may have mental retardation. They do not have the hepatic or renal problems seen in hereditary tyrosinaemia (Goldsmith et al, 1973; Wadman et al, 1971).

Patients with hypertyrosinaemia excrete large quantities of pHPPA in their urine and smaller amounts of pHPLA, pHPAA and p-tyramine. They are unresponsive to ascorbic acid therapy.

The enzymatic defect has been shown to be a deficiency of the *cytosol* form of *hepatic tyrosine aminotransferase*. The mitochondrial form of this enzyme has normal activity (Fellman et al, 1972).

Dietary restriction of phenylalanine and tyrosine lowers the plasma tyrosine value in affected patients and decreases the urinary excretion of the tyrosyl products. Clinical improvement of the keratosis and corneal ulcers occurs with dietary therapy.

The disorder is probably inherited as an autosomal recessive condition. No information is available on heterozygote detection or prenatal diagnosis.

Tyrosinosis

A single patient was reported by Grace Medes in 1932 with a condition she called 'tyrosinosis'. Excretion data of tyrosyl products in the urine led her to suggest this patient had a defect in pHPPA oxidase (Medes, 1932). Subsequently, it was considered that the data was most consistent with a defect in tyrosine transaminase (La Du and Gjessing, 1978). The precise defect remains undetermined. Additional information is not available to offer any genetic conclusions about the condition.

DISORDERS OF GLYCINE METABOLISM (Table 88.3)

Glycine is the smallest and the most ubiquitous of the naturally occuring amino acids. It accounts for approx-

Table 88.3 Disorder of glycine metabolism

Disorder	Enzyme deficiency	Inheritance pattern	Heterozygote detection	Prenatal diagnosis
Non-ketotic hyperglycinaemia	Glycine cleavage reaction	AR	No	Yes
Sarcosinaemia	Sarcosine dehydrogenase (1.5.3.1)	AR	Possible	No
Hyperoxaluria				
Type I	2-oxo-glutarate: glyoxylate carboligase (soluable)	AR	No	
Type II	D-glyceric acid dehydrogenase	?		

imately 25% of the composition of many proteins, interacts in a multitude of biological reactions and can be synthesized from many pathways. It is not an essential amino acid.

The major source of nondietary glycine is from serine. Serine is converted to glycine by the enzyme *serine hydroxymethyltransferase* and uses tetrahydrofolate as a cofactor. The reaction favours the formation of glycine.

The hyperglycinaemias

The disorders of metabolism causing hyperglycinaemia have been divided into 'ketotic' and 'non-ketotic' categories. Those infants recognized to have hyperglycinaemia associated with metabolic acidosis and ketonuria, were originally labled 'ketotic hyperglycinaemia' (Childs et al, 1961). It subsequently was determined that children with 'ketotic hyperglycinaemia' had a disorder of propionate, methylmalonate, or isoleucine metabolism. The mechanism by which the elevated glycine concentration occurs remains unexplained but may be related to the accumulation of organic acids which interfere with the interconversion of glycine and serine (Hillman &

Otto, 1974). This group of 'ketotic' disease is summarized in the discussion of the disorders of branch chained amino acids.

Non-ketotic hyperglycinaemia

Non-ketotic hyperglycinaemia presents as a severe neurological disease of infants. The affected infants are often normal appearing at birth but quickly develop lethargy, listlessness, poor feeding and commonly, seizures. They remain neurologically damaged with no significant intellectual development for the remainder of their life. Most die from infections before two years of age.

The biochemical abnormality in non-ketotic hyperglycinaemia has been shown to be a defect in the conversion of glycine to serine. Glycine reacts with tetrahydrofolate to form methylene-tetrahydrofolate plus CO_2 and ammonia. The formed methylene-tetrahydrofolate reacts with another glycine molecule to form serine and regenerates tetrahydrofolate (Fig. 88.3). Tissue from patients with non-ketotic hyperglycinaemia have been shown to be unable to cleave the C_1 carbon of the glycine molecule to form CO_2 in the presence of tetrahydrofolate. This is

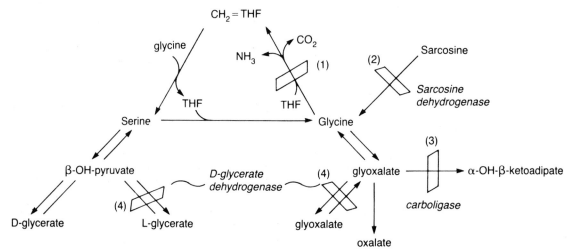

Fig. 88.3 Abbreviated pathway for some of the metabolic reactions related to glycine. The known genetic defects involve non-ketotic hyperglycinaemia (1), sarcosinaemia (2), type I oxalosis (3), and type II oxalosis (4).

believed to be the primary genetic defect (Ando, 1968; DeGroot et al, 1970; Tada et al, 1969).

Patients with this defect accumulate a 10 to 20 fold increase in plasma glycine and excrete massive quantities of glycine in the urine. The glycine concentration in the cerebal spinal fluid is markedly elevated and may be used as a diagnostic indicator of non-ketotic hyperglycinaemia.

Patients with non-ketotic hyperglycinaemia may be diagnosed on the basis of an elevated concentration of plasma glycine, the large excretion of glycine in the urine, a significant elevation of glycine in the spinal fluid, and the absence of metabolic acidosis associated with propionate or methylmalonate excretion.

No effective treatment is available. Low protein diets, sodium benzoate and folic acid have not been shown to be effective. Strichnine has been shown to improve muscle tone but no improvement in intellectual function has occured in affected infants.

Non-ketotic hyperglycinaemia is inherited as an autosomal recessive condition. Males and females are equally affected, there is an increased incidence of consanguinity among parents, and the disorder occurs in sibs. Heterozygote detection is not available. Prenatal diagnosis has been achieved in this disorder by quantitating amino acid concentrations is amniotic fluid at 17 weeks gestation. An elevated glycine/serine ratio was documented in an affected fetus (Garcia-Castro et al, 1982).

Sarcosinaemia

Sarcosine is an intermediate in one carbon metabolism and is a precursor of glycine. Sarcosine (N-methylglycine) is formed by the oxidative demethylation of N-dimethylglycine, and sarcosine undergoes further demethylation to form glycine. The enzyme responsible for this latter reaction is *sarcosine dehydrogenase.*

A genetic deficiency of sarcosine dehydrogenase allows for the accumulation of sarcosine in the plasma and the excretion of large quantities of sarcosine in the urine. Although originally suspected of being causally related to children with mental retardation, it is currently believed that sarcosinaemia is a benign condition, unrelated to clinical symptomatology (Gerritsen & Waisman, 1966; Scott et al, 1970).

Sarcosinaemia is inherited as an autosomal recessive condition. Heterozygote detection using oral loading studies of sarcosine is possible but unreliable. Prenatal diagnosis is not feasible since the enzyme is not expressed in cultured amniotic fluid cells.

Hyperoxaluria

Hyperoxaluria, type I
Two rare metabolic errors may result in primary hyperoxaluria. Hyperoxaluria type I, typically occurs in young children who have symptoms of renal colic and who develop calcium oxylate nephrolithiasis. The affected children may develop growth retardation, uraemia, and often succumb before the age of 20 years. A few patients have been reported who did not have symptoms in childhood and who did not develop symptoms until the third or fourth decade. Patients with hyperoxaluria type I excrete increased quantities of both oxalic acid and L-glyoxylic acid.

The primary defect in type I hyperoxaluria is a deficiency of *2-oxo-glutarate: glyoxylate carboligase (soluble)* (Koch et al, 1967). Urinary glyoxylate excretion has been consistently elevated in patients with the disorder. The excretion of glycolic acid is variable.

Type I hyperoxaluria is inherited as an autosomal recessive condition. It has been reported in sibs, identical twins and from consanguinous matings. The detection of heterozygotes is not reliable. Prenatal diagnosis has not been reported.

Hyperoxaluria, type II
A second rare form of hyperoxaluria has been reported to occur in children. The children suffer from L-glyceric aciduria and develop nephrocalcinosis, urolithiasis, and the consequences of renal disease with growth failure and uraemia.

Patients with type II hyperoxaluria excrete large amounts of oxylate and D-glyceric acid in the urine. Unfortunately this latter compound cannot be routinely measured.

Affected patients have been shown to lack activity for the enzyme *D-glyceric acid dehydrogenase* when assayed in peripheral leucocytes. (Williams & Smith, 1968).

Hyperoxaluria type II is probably inherited as an autosomal recessive condition, but confusion exists over its exact mode of inheritance. Shepard et al (1960) reported hyperoxaluria in at least two generations, and Williams and Smith (1968) have found decreased enzyme activity in the mothers of three patients but not in their fathers. Information on heterozygote detection will need to await clarification of the inheritance pattern.

DISORDERS OF SULPHUR AMINO ACIDS (Table 88.4)

Methionine and cysteine are the two sulphur containing amino acids that are incorporated into protein. Methionine is an essential amino acid and through a series of transulphuration reactions may be converted to cysteine. Methionine also serves as a primary methyl donor for the synthesis of some neurotransmitters. The metabolism of the sulphur amino acids is outlined in Figure 88.4.

Methionine forms S-adenosyl-L-methionine when cat-

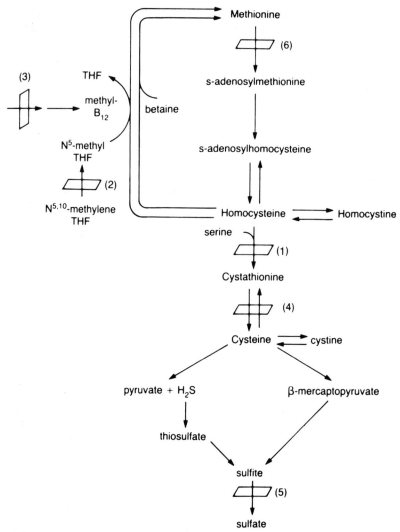

Fig. 88.4 Abbreviated diagram of the transsulphuration pathway. The known genetic defects are those that cause homocystinuria from a deficiency of *cystathionine-β-synthase* (1), $N^{5,10}$-*methylene-tetrahydrofolate reductase* (2), or deficient synthesis of methyl-B_{12} (3). Other defects in the pathway are cystathioninuria (4), *sulphite oxidase* deficiency (5), and hypermethioninaemia from *methionine adenosyl transferase* deficiency (6).

alyzed by *methionine-adenosyltransferase*. S-adenosyl-methionine is a major methyl donor in mammalian metabolism. S-adenosylhomocysteine is formed from S-adenosylmethionine, and is used by a number of methyl donor reactions. S-adenosylhomocysteine is cleaved to form homocysteine and adenosine.

Homocysteine plays a central role in the transulphur-ation pathway. It undergoes three important enzymatic conversions. Two of the reactions allow homocysteine to be resynthesized to methionine. *Betaine-homocysteineme-thyltransferase* uses betaine as a methyl donor to re-synthesize methionine; and the enzyme N^5-*methyltetrahydrofolate: homocysteinemethyltransferase* uses the N^5-methyl form of folic acid as a methyl donor

to recycle homocysteine to methionine. The latter reac-tion requires methyl-B_{12} as a cofactor.

Homocysteine may also be converted to cystathionine by the enzyme *cystathionine-β-synthase*. This step requires pyridoxylphoshate as a cofactor. Cystathionine under-goes further cleavage to form the amino acid cystathion-ine by the action of *γ-cystathionase*. This enzyme also requires pyridoxylphosphate as a cofactor.

Cysteine undergoes a number of reactions. It can be utilized for protein synthesis, formation of glutathione, participation in the formation of coenzyme A, or may be further oxidized to form inorganic sulphate.

The major inborn error of metabolism involving sul-phur amino acids has to do with the various defects which cause an accumulation of homocystine. They have been called 'homocystinuria'. There are three known enzymatic defects resulting in homocystinuria, the most common being a deficiency of *cystathionine-β-synthase*.

Cystathionine-β-synthase deficiency
A genetic deficiency of cystathionine-β-synthase prevents the conversion of homocysteine to cystathionine. Affected patients were originally confused with the Marfan syndrome because of a similar clinical phenotype. They tended to be tall, have light complexions, some degree of arachnodactyly and a significant number had mental retardation. Not all patients, however, fit this clinical description. Patients with homocystinuria do tend to be tall but the most consistent abnormality is ectopia lentis. This develops early in childhood and may be associated with progressive myopia, glaucoma and a propensity to retinal detachment. X–ray evidence of osteoporosis is present by late childhood. Mental retardation effects at least 50% of patients.

The major life threatening symptom is the predilection towards vascular thrombosis. It has been suggested that the thrombotic episodes may be one of the predisposing factors in the development of mental retardation.

Most patients with homocystinuria probably have a shortened life expectancy due to significant thrombotic episodes beginning in early adulthood. A number of patients have been documented to die in their 20's and 30's from vascular accidents.

Diagnosis
Patients with homocystinuria can be diagnosed by the presence of large amounts of homocystine in the urine. The urinary cyanide-nitroprusside test is quite sensitive for the detection of homocystine in urine. Definitive identification can be accomplished by chromatography. Plasma values of homocystine and methionine are elevated. Homocystine values are typically in the range of 0.2 mM and methionine is commonly 2 mM. The documentation of the elevated methionine concentration in plasma is necessary for the presumptive diagnosis of cystathionine-β-synthase deficiency in the absence of a direct enzymatic assay.

The finding of homocystinuria and the documentation of homocystinaemia does not confirm the diagnosis of cystathionine-β-synthase deficiency. It must be distinguished from the other defects which may cause homocystinuria: a deficiency of N^5-methyltetrahydrofolate-homocysteine methyltransferase, or a defect in cobalamin metabolism with a deficiency of methylcobalamin.

Therapy
Therapeutic interventions may be effective in assisting patients with the synthase defect. If the patients are responsive to pyridoxine, an appropriate daily oral dose

of pyridoxine can lower homocystine concentrations (50 to 500 mg/day). Decreasing the homocystine concentration is believed to protect the patients from developing many of their clinical symptoms (Brenton & Cusworth, 1971; Mudd et al, 1970).

A low methionine diet has been used to prevent the accumulation of homocystine. It has been documented that a low protein and low methionine diet can decrease the homocystine and methionine concentration in the plasma of affected patients (Perry, 1971; Komrower & Sardhawalla, 1971). Additional time is still needed to confirm the benefit of a long-term diet deficient in methionine to prevent the complications of homocystinuria. The use of agents aimed at preventing platelet mediated vascular injury have been advocated. The use of dipyridamole (100 mg daily) combined with aspirin (1 gm daily) has been recommended to prevent the thrombotic catastrophies which present such a major threat to the older patients with homocystinuria (Harker et al, 1976).

Genetics
Cystathionine-β-synthase deficiency is inherited as an autosomal recessive condition with an incidence of approximately 1:200 000 live births (Mudd & Levy, 1978).

Two forms of cystathionase-β-synthase deficiency are known to exist. Approximately 50% of the patients are believed to have a defect in the apoenzyme while the remainder are believed to have a defect that involves the binding site of the enzyme for its cofactor, pyridoxylphosphate. The latter group are defined by a lowering of their plasma homocystine concentration when large doses of pyridoxine are administered. Doses in the range of 50 to 500 mg/day will often reduce plasma homocystine concentrations to undetectable levels. This group of patients has been called 'pyridoxine responsive'.

In addition to the response that patients have to pyridoxine, there is additional clinical and biochemical evidence for genetic heterogeneity; considerable interfamilial variation exists in the clinical expression of the disorder; intrafamilial response to pyridoxine is always consistent; the mutant synthase enzyme isolated from affected patients has shown variability in its thermal stability; and the residual enzyme activity varies between patients (Mudd et al, 1964; Kim and Rosenberg, 1974; Fowler et al, 1978; and Fleisher et al, 1978).

Difficulty exists for the detection of heterozygotes for the synthase defect. Although assays for the enzyme in both cultured fibroblasts and stimulated peripheral lymphocytes have been shown to be below control values, a consistent and clean separation of heterozygotes from normal persons remains difficult (Mudd & Levy, 1978). Sardharwalla et al (1974) have reported a promising loading study using L-methionine under carefully controlled circumstances and the measurement of homocystine and other sulphydryl compounds in the urine as a means of distinguishing heterozygotes from normal persons.

Prenatal diagnosis for homocystinuria has not been achieved. There is evidence, however, that the enzyme activity is expressed in cultured amniotic fluid cells, and this information has been used to correctly predict an unaffected fetus (Fleisher et al, 1974).

Three other genetic conditions have been associated with the excretion of homocystine in the urine. A decrease in the activity of $N^{5,10}$-methylene-tetrahydrofolate reductase, a defect in the conversion of vitamin B_{12} to its active cofactors, and a genetic abnormality in th e absorption of vitamin B_{12}, have each been associated with homocystinuria.

$N^{5,10}$-methylene-tetrahydrofolate reductase deficiency

A small number of children have been reported with a deficiency of $N^{5,10}$-methylene-tetrahydrofolate reductase (Freeman et al, 1975). This enzyme catalyzes the conversion of $N^{5,10}$-methylene-tetrahydrofolate to N^5-methyltetrahydrofolate. The synthesized N^5-methyltetrahydrofolate is the active cofactor necessary for the conversion of homocysteine to L-methionine. Patients deficient in the synthesis of N^5-methyltetrahydrofolate accumulate homocysteine and have low plasma methionine values.

Affected patients have been reported with symptoms of mental retardation, acute psychosis, muscle weakness, ataxia and spastic paraperesis. Most have shown a significant improvement in clinical symptoms when supplemented with folate (15 mg/day).

The enzyme deficiency is most likely inherited as an autosomal recessive condition. Both males and females have been affected. In one family, reduced activity of the reductase was documented in the parents and a sib (Narisawa et al, 1977). Prenatal diagnosis has not been reported.

Deficiency of cobalamin reductase

Methyl-B_{12} is the active cofactor for the conversion of homocysteine to L-methionine by the enzyme N^5-methyltetrahydrofolate: homocysteine methyltransferase. Several children have been documented with an inability to synthesize methyl-B_{12} with the consequence of developing homocystinaemia, hypomethioninaemia and neurological symptoms. Some patients have died during infancy with failure to thrive while others have had milder clinical symptoms associated with megaloblastic anaemia and progressive neurological deterioration.

The primary defect is believed to be the failure to actively convert vitamin B_{12} to hydroxycobalamin (for review see Rosenberg, 1978). Hydroxycobalamin is a necessary precursor for methyl-B_{12} or adenosyl-B_{12}. The failure to synthesize methyl-B_{12} leads to the accumulation of homocysteine, and the failure to synthesize methyl-B_{12}

interferes with the conversion of methylmalonate to succinate. These patients are identified by the presence of methylmalonic acid and homocystine in the urine.

Heterozygotes have not been identified and prenatal diagnosis has not been reported.

Malabsorption of vitamin B_{12}

Two children have been reported with an inherited form of vitamin B_{12} malabsorption. These children excreted homocystine, methylmalonic acid and cystathionine in their urines (Hollowell et al, 1969). The children responded to vitamin B_{12} therapy. No genetic information is available.

Cystathioninuria

γ-cystathionase cleaves L-cystathionine to cysteine and α-ketobutarate. This reaction is necessary to complete the transfer of the sulphur atom from methionine to cysteine. Deficiency of γ-cystathionase activity causes a massive excretion of cystathionine in the urine. Although the original patients reported with cystathioninuria had symptoms of mental retardation, subsequent reports have indicated the condition is most likely benign and not associated with neurological symptoms (Scott et al, 1967): Frimpter reported less than 10% activity for γ-cystathionase in liver tissue from two affected patients (Frimpter et al, 1963).

Cystathioninuria is inherited as an autosomal recessive condition. Male and female siblings have been reported, and small amounts of cystathionine can be detected in the urines of obligate heterozygotes. At least two different genetic defects cause a deficiency of γ-cystathionase. This is based on the clinical observation that the majority of patients respond biochemically to parental and oral pyridoxine supplements. Other patients, in separate families, do not respond biochemically to pyridoxine.

Since cystathioninuria is a benign condition, pyridoxine therapy is not necessarily indicated in detected individuals. Similarly, prenatal diagnosis would not normally be indicated. Heterozygotes excrete detectable quantities of cystathionine in their urine.

Sulphite oxidase deficiency

Two families have been reported with a deficiency of sulphite oxidase (Mudd et al, 1967; Shih et al, 1977). Infants in both families had severe neurological abnormalities which were present at birth and persisted until they died in early childhood. The infants had the unusual finding of having ectopia lentis, similar to that which is seen in homocystinuria. The urine of affected infants contained greatly increased quantities of S-sulpho-L-cysteine, sulphite and thiosulphate. No sulphate was detectable in the urine. An absence of sulphite oxidase was shown to exist in postmortem samples from liver, kidney, brain.

Table 88.4 Disorders of sulphur amino acids

Disorder	Enzyme deficiency	Inheritance pattern	Heterozygote detection	Prenatal diagnosis
Hypermethioninaemia	Methionine adenosyl-transferase (2.5.1.6)	AR?		
The homocystinurias Homocystinuria (B_6 non-responsive)	Cystathionine β-synthase (4.2.1.22)	AR	Difficult	Possible
Homocystinuria (B_6 responsive)	Cystathionine β-synthase (4.2.1.22)	AR	Difficult	Possible
Homocystinuria (with folate deficiency)	$N^{5,10}$-methylene-tetrahydrofolate reductase (1.1.1.68)	AR	Probable	
Homocystinuria (with methylmalonic aciduria) 'cbl C'	Synthesis of methyl-B_{12} and adenosyl-B_{12} (? cobalamin reductase)	AR		Possible
'cbl D'	(Same as above, but less severe deficiency)	AR?		Possible
Cystathioninaemia (B_6 responsive)	γ-cystathionase (4.4.1.1)	AR	Yes	?
Cystathioninaemia (B_6 non-responsive)	γ-cystathionase (4.4.1.1.)	AR	Yes	?
Sulphite Oxidase Deficiency	Sulphite oxidase	AR?	?	

Sulphite oxidase deficiency most likely is an autosomal recessive condition. Intermediate levels of the enzyme could be detected in cultured fibroblasts from the parents of the child reported by Shih et al (1977). Prenatal diagnosis has not been reported.

DISORDERS OF THE BRANCHED CHAIN AMINO ACIDS (Table 88.5)

The amino acids leucine, isoleucine and valine each contain a methyl group which branches from the main aliphatic carbon chain. Because of this structure they are designated 'branched chain amino acids'. If the amino acids are not used for protein synthesis, they undergo a series of irreversible oxidation steps to form organic acids that eventually enter the tricarboxylic acid cycle.

There are nine categories of diseases within the oxidative pathway of the branch chain amino acids. The defects have traditionally been divided into disorders in which the primary metabolite which accumulates in body fluids is either an amino acid or an organic acid. The disorders which result in an accumulation of amino acids are (1) maple syrup urine disease, (2) hypervalinaemia and (3) leucine-isoleucinaemia. The disorders of organic acid accumulation include (1) isovaleric acidaemia, (2) methylmalonic acidaemia, (3) propionic acidaemia, (4) β-methylcrotonic aciduria, (5) α-methylacetoacetic aciduria and (6) β-hydroxy-β-methylglutaric aciduria. For reviews of the organic acidurias, see Rosenberg (1980), Rosenberg and Tanaka (1977) and Goodman (1980). Extensive heterogeneity has been recognized for propionic aciduria and methylmalonic aciduria and is succintly summarized in Table 88.5.

Maple syrup urine disease (MSUD)

Patients who inherit a deficiency of the branched chain α-keto acid dehydrogenase will develop symptoms of maple syrup urine disease. The enzyme is responsible for the oxidative decarboxylation of the α-keto acids formed by the deamination of the branched chain amino acids. The enzyme is a large multicomplex molecule similar to pyruvate dehydrogenase and α-ketoglutarate dehydrogenase. It is known to consist of three separate apoenzymes; a decarboxylase, a lipoate reductase transacylase and a lipoamide oxidoreductase (Connelly et al, 1968; Reed & Cox, 1966). The complexity of the enzyme system allows for the potential of many mutational events to effect the activity of the reaction.

A deficiency of the dehydrogenase prevents the further oxidation of the α-keto acids that are formed from their respective amino acids. Thus, patients accumulate α-ketoisocaproic acid, α-keto-β-methylcaproic acid and α-ketoisovaleric acid. These α-keto acids may be reaminated by transamination to again form branched chain

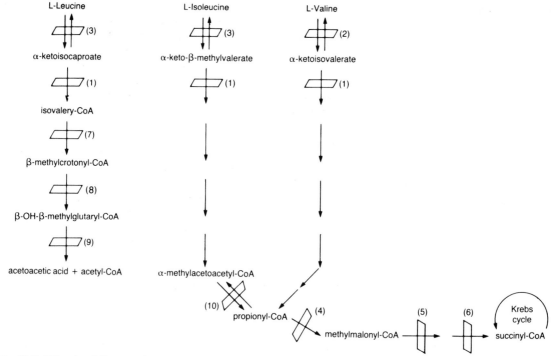

Fig. 88.5 Abbreviated diagram of the metabolism of the branched chain amino acids. The known enzyme defects are maple syrup urine disease (1), hypervalinaemia (2), leucine-isoleucinaemia (3), propionic acidaemia (4), methylmalonic acidaemia (5) and (6), isovaleric acidaemia (7), β-methylcrotonyl glycinaemia (8), β-OH-β-methylglutaric acidaemia (9) and α-methyl acetoacetic aciduria (10).

amino acids. Thus, patients with a dehydrogenase deficiency accumulate both α-keto acids and leucine, isoleucine and valine.

Affected infants with the 'classical' form of MSUD have symptoms of acidosis, lethargy and seizures soon after birth. They may have severe hypoglycaemia. If they survive the immediate newborn period, signs of brain damage are usually present. The characteristic odour of 'maple syrup' can usually be detected in the urine or on the skin of the infant (Dancis & Levitz, 1978).

There probably exists a continual spectrum of clinical heterogeneity for MSUD varying from the severe 'classical' form to the 'mild' form of the illness. The degree of severity would be related to the residual enzyme activity of the dehydrogenase that exists at physiological concentrations of the substrates. Thus, patients with an 'intermediate' form and a 'mild' form of the disorder have been described (Morris et al, 1966; Dancis et al, 1967; Shulman et al, 1970).

Infants with acidosis and neurological symptoms can be rapidly diagnosed as having MSUD. They will usually have the characteristic odour of maple syrup, their urine will react with ferric chloride to give a gray-blue colour, and with 2,4, dinitrophenylhydrazine to give a heavy

yellow precipitate. An excess quantity of leucine, isoleucine and valine can be detected in urine and plasma.

A variant of MSUD called 'thiamine – responsive form' has been described by Scriver et al (1971) in a girl who was diagnosed at 11 months of age. This patient had 25% of normal decarboxylase activity in cultured cells at physiological concentration of substrate. Her elevated plasma concentrations of the branched chain amino acids responded dramatically to 10 mg/day of thiamine with improvement in her clinical course.

In the 'classic form' of MSUD, therapeutic intervention has not been very rewarding. The majority of patients have either died as infants or have intellectual impairment in spite of special diets. Diets which limit the available source of leucine, isoleucine and valine have been used and are successful in lowering the plasma concentration of the amino acids (Snyderman et al, 1964; Committee Report, 1976). Management remains, however, difficult and expensive. Better results can be expected from those patients with milder defects of the dehydrogenase complex and less severe clinical symptomatology.

MSUD is inherited as an autosomal recessive trait. It is rare with an incidence no greater than 1 in 100 000 live births. Heterozygote detection is difficult to reliably ascertain (Langenbeck et al, 1975). The dehydrogenase reaction is expressed in cultured amniotic fluid cells and prenatal diagnosis can be reliably performed.

Hypervalinaemia

Valine undergoes deamination to form α-ketoisovaleric acid via a transaminase reaction (Fig. 88.5). An infant from Japan has been reported to be missing this enzymatic step and to accumulate only valine in the plasma (Wada et al, 1963; Dancis et al, 1967).

The child was detected because of developmental delay and symptoms of vomiting and lethargy. The infant did respond to a low valine diet.

The mode of inheritance remains unclear and an abnormality in valine metabolism could not be detected in the parents.

Hyperleucine – isoleucinemia

A single family with two sibs has been reported with a deficiency of the enzyme which deaminates leucine and isolecine to their respective α-keto acids (Fig. 88.5). The children had severe mental deficiency, seizures, deafness and retinal degeneration (Jeune et al, 1970). The defect was detected because of the presence of hyperprolinemia, type II.

The defect is likely an autosomal recessive condition, but an abnormality in leucine or isoleucine deamination could not be demonstrated in the parents.

Accumulation of organic acids from disorders of branched chain amino acid oxidation

The decarboxylation of the α-keto acids of leucine, isoleucine and valine is an irreversible reaction. Any metabolic block distal to this reaction will result in the accumulation of organic acids without an increase in concentration of a branched chain amino acid.

All of the organic acidaemias share a similar clinical presentation; an infant or young child with repeated bouts of metabolic acidosis associated with lethargy, vomiting and neurological depression. There may be a characteristic odour or hyperammonaemia depending upon the genetic defect. The two most common disorders are propionic acidaemia and methylmalonic acidaemia. The others are rare, even by genetic standards.

Diagnosis is dependent upon identification of the specific organic acid or one of its metabolites by gas chromatography (Goodman, 1980).

Propionic acidaemia

Propionyl-CoA is formed as an eventual oxidative product of valine and isoleucine. It then is converted to succinyl-CoA, via methylmalonyl-CoA, and enters the Kreb Cycle (for review see Rosenberg, 1978).

Patients with propionic acidaemia have a genetic deficiency of propionyl-CoA decarboxylase and are unable to convert propionyl-CoA to D-methylmalonyl-CoA. Affected patients have recurrent episodes of ketoacidosis during infancy associated with neutropenia, thrombocytopenia and hyperammonaemia. Hyperglycinaemia has been a common feature during periods of acidosis. The recognition of the hyperglycinaemia originally led to this entity being called 'ketotic hyperglycinaemia' (Child et al, 1961).

Defects of the propionic decarboxylase reaction are inherited as autosomal recessive traits. Genetic heterogeneity has been documented for the apoenzyme. Two complimentation groups have been identified through the use of somatic cell hybrids. The complimentation groups have been labeled *pcc A* and *pcc C* and presumably involve different polypeptide subunits of the apoenzyme (Gravel et al, 1977; Wolf & Rosenberg et al, 1978).

A third defect involving the decarboxylase reaction exists and is responsive to biotin therapy. It has been designated *bio*. Patients with the *bio* type defect also have decreased activity of 3-methylcrotonyl-CoA carboxylase and pyruvate carboxylase. Presumably this mutation effects the binding of biotin to the carboxylase molecule and prevents the formation of an active holoenzyme (Sweetman et al, 1979).

Heterozygote detection by measurement of propionyl-CoA decarboxylase in leukocytes or cultured fibroblasts has been achieved but is difficult (Wolf & Rosenberg, 1978). Reliability varies between the *pcc A* and *pcc C* complimentation groups. Heterozygote detection for the *bio* subgroup has not been achieved.

Infants with propionic acidaemia may respond to a low protein diet (1 gm/kg/day of protein) and careful management of febrile episodes. Chronic bicarbonate therapy may be useful. Those infants with the *bio* mutation will respond to oral biotin (10 mg/day).

Prenatal diagnosis of propionic acidaemia has been achieved by measuring the decarboxylase reaction in cultured amniotic fluid cells.

Methylmalonic acidaemia

D-methylmalonyl-CoA is formed by the decarboxylation of propionyl-CoA (Fig. 88.5). The D-methylmalonyl-CoA is then enzymatically rearranged to L-methylmalonyl-CoA by *D-methylmalonyl-CoA racemase*. The L-isomer of methylmalonate is converted to succinyl-CoA by the enzyme *L-methylmalonyl-CoA mutase* and requires adenosyl-B_{12} as a cofactor. Genetic defects of the racemase apoenzyme, the mutase apoenzyme, and the synthesis of adenosyl-B_{12} have been confirmed to cause methylmalonic aciduria (Morrow et al, 1969; Kang et al, 1978; Mahoney et al, 1975. For review see Rosenberg, 1978). Three distinct defects in the synthesis of adenosyl-

Table 88.5 Disorders of the branched chain amino acids

Disorder	Enzyme deficiency	Inheritance pattern	Heterozygote detection	Prenatal diagnosis
Branched chain ketoaciduria *(maple syrup urine disease)* Classic form	Branched chain α-ketoacid dehydrogenase	AR	Difficult	Yes
Intermediate and mild forms	Less severe deficiency of BCK dehydrogenase	AR	Difficult	Yes
Thiamine responsive form	Thiamine binding/stabalization/ activiation of BCK dehydrogenase	AR?		
Hypervalinaemia	Valine aminotransferase (2.6.1.42)	AR?		
Leucine-isoleucinaemia	Leucine-isoleucine aminotransferase (2.6.1.42)	AR?		
Propionic acidaemia 'pcc A'	Propionyl-CoA decarboxylase holocarboxylase (4.1.1.41)	AR	Possible	Yes
'pcc C'	(same enzyme)	AR	No	Yes
'bio'	Biotin binding/stabalization/ activiation of propionyl-CoA decarboxylase	AR	No	?
Methylmalonic aciduria Racemase	D-methylmalonyl-CoA racemase (5.1.99.1)	AR		Possible
Mutase	L-methylmalonyl-CoA mutase (5.4.99.2)	AR	Yes	Yes
'cbl A'	Synthesis of adenosyl-B_{12}	AR		Yes
'cbl B'	Synthesis of adenosyl-B_{12} (? ATP: Cob (I) alamin adenosyltransferase)	AR	Yes	Yes
Methylmalonic aciduria with homocystinuria 'cbl C'	Synthesis of adenosyl-B_{12} and methyl-B_{12} (? cobalamin reducatase)	AR		Possible
'cbl D'	(Same as above, but less severe deficiency)	AR?		Possible
Isovaleric acidaemia	Isovaleryl-CoA dehydrogenase	AR		Yes
β-methylcrotonylglycinaemia	(i) 3-methylcrotonyl carboxylase ii) 'Bio' defect of propionic acidaemia	AR?		
β-hydroxy-β-methylglutaric acidaemia	Hydroxymethylglutaryl-CoA lyase	AR		
Glutaric acidaemia, type I	Glutaryl-CoA dehydrogenase	AR		Yes
Glutaric acidaemia, type II	?	AR?		
Ptyroglutamic acidaemia	Glutathione synthetase	AR?		
α-methyl-β-hydroxybutyric acidaemia	β-ketothiolase	AR?		

B_{12} are known: two which interfere with the synthesis of adenosyl-B_{12} only, and one that prevents the formation of both methyl-B_{12} and adenosyl-B_{12} (Table 88.5).

Patients with either the mutase or the racemase defect may respond to a diet low in protein. Depending upon the severity of the enzyme deficiency, dietary protein may vary between 1–2 gm/kg/day (Nyhan et al, 1973). Those children with a defect in the synthesis of adenosyl-B_{12} usually respond to pharmacological doses of vitamin B_{12} (Hsia et al, 1970).

Methylmalonate may be detected in the urine of an affected child by a screening test (Giorgio & Luhby,

1969) or by using gas chromatography (Goodman, 1980). Methylmalonate is not detectable in the urine of unaffected children. Confirmatory enzyme assays may be performed on peripheral leucocytes or cultured fibroblasts.

Pedigree data and complimentation studies using heterokaryons (Gravel et al, 1975) are compatible with an autosomal recessive mode of inheritance for each form of methylmalonic aciduria. No evidence exists for either a dominant or X–linked variety of the disorder. Heterozygote detection has not been reliable by assaying for methylmalonate in urine or by propionate oxidation in lymphocytes or cultured fibroblasts.

Prenatal diagnosis is feasible for each of the genetic types of methylmalonic aciduria using cultured amniotic fluid cells (Morrow et al, 1970; Gompertz et al, 1974). In a vitamin responsive form of MMA prenatal therapy using vitamin B_{12} was instituted to the pregnant mother (Ampola et al, 1975).

Methylmalonic aciduria with homocystinuria
A rare form of methylmalonic aciduria with homocystinuria, cystathioninuria and hypomethioninaemia has been recognized. These patients are unable to synthesize either adenosyl-B_{12} or methyl-B_{12} from orally ingested vitamin B_{12} (Levy et al, 1970). Rosenbery and co-workers (1975) demonstrated that cells from the affected patients were unable to retain the cobalamin they took up and form the active vitamin B_{12} cofactors. They called this genetic defect 'cbl C'.

Methyl-B_{12} is a required cofactor for *homocysteine methyl-transferase*, an enzyme which transfers the methyl group from homocysteine to methionine (Fig. 88.5). Low activity of this enzyme accounts for the accumulation of homocysteine and cystathionine and the hypomethioninaemia.

The disorder has caused severe neurological damage and death in children. It is inherited as an autosomal recessive condition. Heterozygote detection has not been reported and prenatal diagnosis has not been attempted.

Other genetic disorders that cause organic acid accumulation in children are quite rare. In most cases, only a few patients have been identified. Each is probably inherited as an autosomal recessive condition with little information available on heterozygote detection or heterogeneity (for review see Goodman, 1980). These rare organic acidaemias are listed in Table 88.5.

DISORDERS OF HISTIDINE METABOLISM
(Table 88.6)

Histidine is an essential amino acid for human infants and probably for adults. The amino acid is necessary for protein synthesis and can be decarboxylated to form histamine. The major pathway of histamine metabolism, however, is to be degraded to eventually yield glutamic

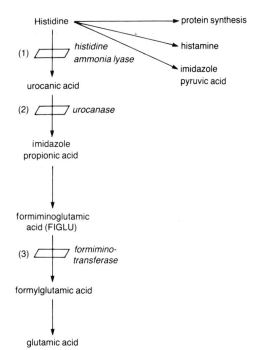

Fig. 88.6 The major metabolic reactions of histidine metabolism. The enzymatic blocks are for histidinaemia (1), urocanic aciduria (2), and formiminoglutamic aciduria (3).

acid (Fig. 88.6). A minor pathway allows histidine to undergo transamination with the formation of imidazole pyruvic acid.

Histidinaemia
Patients with histidinaemia are unable to adequately convert histidine to uroconic acid. The enzyme responsible for this reaction is *histidine ammonia lyase*, and it has been documented to be deficient in affected patients (La Du et al, 1963; Zannoni & La Du, 1963). Histidine is markedly increased in the urine, blood and CSF. The elevated blood histidine levels (> 0.5 mM) cause an increased formation of imidazole pyruvic acid which is excreted in the urine. This compound reacts with ferric chloride solution to yield a green colour, similar to that observed in phenylketonuria. Histidine ammonia lyase may be assayed in stratum corneum or in liver tissue.

The diagnosis of histidinaemia is typically dependent upon the documentation of histidinuria, histidinaemia and a deficiency of enzyme activity in the stratum corneum.

A consistent clinical picture for patients with histidinaemia has not evolved. Although the original patients had mental retardation (Woody et al, 1965; Ghadimi & Partington, 1967), this feature may have been unduly stressed because of ascertainment bias. Delayed speech development and defects in auditory perception have been present in some probands. When histidinaemic pro-

Table 88.6 Disorders of histidine metabolism

Disorder	Enzyme deficiency	Inheritance pattern	Heterozygote detection	Prenatal diagnosis
Histidinaemia	Histidine ammonia lyase (4.3.1.3)	AR	Possible	No
Urocanic aciduria	Urocanse	?		
Formiminoglutamic aciduria	Formiminotransferase	AR?		

bands are detected prospectively, it has been found to be a benign condition (Levy et al, 1974).

Histidinaemia is inherited as an autosomal recessive trait. It has an incidence of 1:15 000 in live born infants (Levy et al, 1972). Evidence for heterogeneity exists from variation in the expression of histidine ammonia lyase between liver and stratum corneum. The majority of patients are lacking this enzyme in both tissues, but at least one pedigree had activity of the enzyme in the stratum corneum (Woody et al, 1965).

Heterozygotes cannot reliably be detected by fasting histidine concentrations in blood or by enzyme activity from skin samples. The most consistent test for discriminating heterozygotes from normals within a pedigree is the measurement of urinary FIGLU following an L-histidine load (Rosenblatt et al, 1970).

Prenatal diagnosis has not been reported. The documentation of an affected fetus is unlikely since the enzyme is not expressed in cultured amniotic fluid cells.

Urocanic aciduria

Only a single family has been reported with urocanic aciduria from a deficiency of urocanase. Insufficient data exists to reach any conclusions concerning the clinical symptomatology or genetic transmission of the disorder.

Formiminoglutamic (FIGLU) aciduria

A small number of patients have been documented to excrete a marked excess of FIGLU and to have a deficiency of *formiminotransferase*. Some patients have had symptoms of profound mental retardation while others have been normal. The relationship of this enzyme deficiency to neurological symptoms remains unclear.

The pedigree information is consistent with an autosomal recessive trait. No information is available concerning the reliability of heterozygote detection or prenatal diagnosis.

DISORDERS OF LYSINE METABOLISM (Table 88.7)

Those patients that manifest an increased lysine concentration in plasma represent a confusing group of disorders. In most of the families reported, the primary

biochemical defect has not been clearly delineated and the relationship of the elevated blood lysine concentration to mental retardation or clinical symptoms remains unclear. These problems lend considerable difficulty in offering precise information concerning the genetic inheritance of the disorders.

Columbo and co-workers (1964) described a child with hyperlysinaemia associated with hyperammonaemia. Liver activity from this child showed a 75 per cent reduction in activity of *L-lysine dehydrogenase*, the enzyme which converts lysine to α-keto-epsilon-amino-caproic acid (Burgi et al, 1966).

Ghadimi et al (1965) have reported hyperlysinaemia associated with mental retardation. These patients excreted homoarginine and homocitrulline in addition to the lysine. The primary metabolic block was not defined.

Woody et al (1966) reported several family members with elevated lysine concentrations. The proband was mentally retarded but siblings with hyperlysinaemia were normal. An absence of *lysine-ketoglutarate reductase* activity in fibroblast extracts was documented by Dancis et al (1969). This finding and the observation that the parents were consanguineous, suggests that the en-

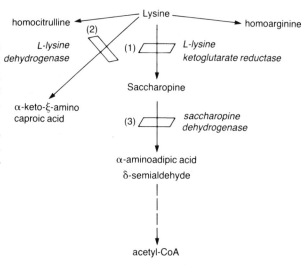

Fig. 88.7 Initial steps in the metabolism of lysine. The defects implicated in hyperlysinaemia are indicated at (1) and (2), and the presumptive defect in saccharopinuria is at (3).

Table 88.7 Disorders of lysine metabolism

Disorder	Enzyme deficiency	Inheritance pattern	Heterozygote detection	Prenatal diagnosis
Hyperlysinaemia	Lysine-ketoglutarate reductase (1.5.1.8)	AR		
	L-lysine dehydrogenase	AR?		
Saccharopinuria	Saccharopine dehydrogenase (1.5.1.10)	AR?		
Hydroxylysinaemia	Unknown	AR?		

zyme deficiency is inherited as an autosomal recessive condition.

Carson and co-workers (1968) identified a young adult with increased concentrations of lysine and saccharopine in plasma who also excreted homocitrulline and α-aminoadipic acid in urine. The enzymatic defect was not defined.

A number of patients have been described with elevations of hydroxylysine in the plasma and the excretion of increased quantities of hydroxylysine in urine (Goodman et al, 1972). Although all the patients have been mentally retarded, it is unclear whether the mental retardation is caused by the biochemical defect. The precise biochemical defect was not elucidated.

DISORDERS OF PROLINE AND HYDROXYPROLINE (Table 88.8)

Proline and hydroxyproline are nonessential amino acids. Proline is synthesized from glutamic acid and hydroxyproline is formed by the oxidation of proline which has been incorporated into peptide linkages.

Proline is synthesized through the intermediary of Δ'-pyrroline-5-carboxylic acid (PC) by the reduction of glutamic acid. PC is further reduced by Δ' -pyrroline-5-carboxylic reductase to form proline. The catabolism of proline is exactly the reverse of its chemical synthesis, but is performed by different enzymes. *Proline oxidase* converts proline to PC, and *PC dehydrogenase* will further oxidize PC to glutamic acid (Fig. 8).

Genetic deficiencies of proline oxidase and PC dehydrogenase exist which cause type I and type II hyperprolinaemmia, respectively. A deficiency of 'hydroxyproline oxidase' is believed responsible for hydroxyprolinaemia.

Hyperprolinaemia type I

Patients with type I hyperprolinaemia have increased plasma concentrations of proline (~ 1mM) and excrete proline, hydroxyproline and glycine in the urine (Scriver & Efron, 1978). Although the original reports suggested an association between the hyperprolinaemia and kidney

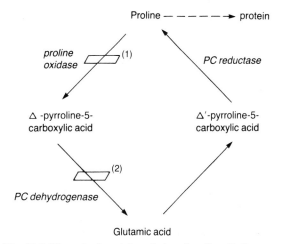

Fig. 88.8 Biosynthesis and degradation of proline. Proline oxidase deficiency (1) and PC dehydrogenase deficiency (2) cause type I and type II hyperprolinaemia, respectively.

disease, deafness and neurological disorders (Schafer et al, 1962), it is now believed that hyperprolinaemia is a benign clinical condition. A deficiency of proline oxidase has been documented in liver biopsy specimens from affected persons (Efron, 1965; Scriver & Efron, 1978).

Proline oxidase deficiency is inherited as an autosomal recessive condition, Heterozygotes for the condition may or may not have plasma proline values above the normal range. This feature of type I hyperprolinaemia tends to confuse the interpretation of the inheritance pattern in some pedigress (Scriver & Efron, 1978).

A mouse model exists for type I hyperprolinaemia with proline oxidase deficiency. It has been labeled PRO/Re, has similar residual enzyme activity as the human patients, and has no apparent developmental sequelae for the mouse.

Hyperprolinaemia, type II

Persons with type II hyperprolinaemia have greatly elevated concentrations of proline in their plasma (1.5 mM–3.0 mM) and excrete substantial quantities of proline, hydroxyproline, glycine and Δ'-pyrroline-5-carboxylic acid (PC). The concentration of plasma proline is

Table 88.8 Disorders of proline and hydroxyproline

Disorder	Enzyme deficiency	Inheritance pattern	Heterozygote detection	Prenatal diagnosis
Prolinaemia, Type I	Proline oxidase (1.5.1.2.)	AR	Possibly	
Prolinaemia, Type II	$\triangle'$-pyrroline-5-carboxylic acid dehydrogenase (1.5.1.12)	AR		
Hyperhydroxyprolinaemia	Hydroxyproline oxidase (?) (1.1.1.104)	AR		

greater than that observed in type I hyperprolinaemia. Cultured fibroblasts from a patient with type II hyperprolinaemia were documented to have no detectable activity of Δ'-pyrrole-5-carboxylate dehydrogenase (Valle et al, 1974). This condition has not been consistently associated with clinical symptoms and is believed to be benign.

Type II hyperprolinaemia is inherited as an autosomal recessive trait. Heterozygotes have normal plasma proline concentrations and have not been documented to excrete an increased quantity of PC. Intermediate enzyme values for PC dehydrogenase activity have not been reported.

Hyperhydroxyprolinaemia

Hyperhydroxyprolinaemia is a very rare disorder characterized by a markedly elevated concentration of hydroxyproline in the plasma. Although originally detected in a child with mental retardation, persons subsequently identified have been clinically normal. It is now considered to be a harmless trait. Although free hydroxyproline is found in the urine of affected persons, the concentration rarely reaches levels which would interfere with the imino-glycine transport system. Thus, an increased excretion of proline and glycine is not usually observed.

By inference from loading studies using oral hydroxyproline it has been deduced that the enzyme block is between hydroxyproline and Δ'-pyrroline-3-hydroxy-5-carboxylic acid (Efron et al, 1965; Pelkonen and Kivirikko, 1970). This enzymatic step is catalyzed by hydroxyproline oxidase an enzyme distinct from proline oxidase.

Pedigree data is consistent with the disorder being an autosomal recessive trait (Efron et al, 1965; Rama Rao, et al, 1974). A homozygous female has had normal children (Pelkonen & Kivirikko, 1970).

DISORDERS OF THE UREA CYCLE AND OF ORNITHINE (Table 88.9)

The urea cycle is the only known metabolic pathway for the removal of ammonia (Fig. 88.9). The primary site of ammonia removal is the liver with only a small amount of urea being formed in brain and other tissues.

Ammonia is formed as the breakdown product of protein or amino acids and must be converted to urea and excreted in the urine. Failure to convert ammonia to urea results in hyperammonaemia and the development of neurological suppression. Five enzymes have classically been considered part of the urea cycle and for each there is known to exist a disorder caused by a genetic deficiency of the enzyme. Each enzyme deficiency is associated with hyperammonaemia and significant neurological symptoms.

Carbamyl phosphate synthetase deficiency (CPS-I)

CPS-I is the first enzyme in the urea cycle and forms carbamyl phosphate from ammonia, ATP and carbon dioxide. The enzyme is mitochondrial bound and requires magnesium and acetylglutamine as cofactors.

Infants who are lacking CPS-I activity develop symptoms of severe ammonia toxicity during the first week of life. Vomiting, lethargy, comma, seizures and respiratory distress are the usual symptoms. Blood ammonia values are usually 1000 μg/dl or greater (normal: <150 μg/dl). These infants typically die during the first weeks of life. CPS-I activity in liver tissue has been documented to be <1% of normal (Gelehrter & Snodgrass, 1974).

A few infants may have clinical symptoms of episodic vomiting, lethargy and delayed intellectual development. Blood ammonia values are moderately elevated to the range of 600 μg/dl. Residual CPS-I activity in liver tissue has been reported to be 5–15% of normal (Shih, 1978). These infants may be aided by a restricted protein diet of 1.0 to 1.5 gm/kg/day.

The diagnosis of CPS-I can only be confirmed by direct enzyme assay of CPS-I from liver tissue. The diagnosis can be infered to exist by exclusion of the other disorders of the urea cycle and other genetic disorders which interfere with CPS-I activity (propionic acidaemia and methylmalonic acidaemia).

CPS-I deficiency is inherited as an autosomal recessive trait. Reliable heterozygote testing is not available. Prenatal diagnosis is not feasible since the enzyme is not expressed in cultured amniotic fluid cells.

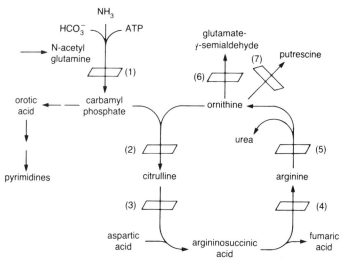

Fig. 88.9 Abbreviate pathway for the urea cycle and the degradation of ornithine. The known genetic conditions which interfere with this pathway are carbamyl phosphate synthetase – I deficiency (1), ornithine tanscarbamylase deficiency (2), citrullinaemia (3), argininosuccinic aciduria (4), and argininaemia (5). Two defects of ornithine metabolism include gyrate atrophy of the retina from ornithine aminotransferase (6), and hyperornithinaemia from a suspected defect in ornithine decarboxylase (7).

Ornithine transcarbamylase deficiency

Ornithine transcarbamylase (OTC) is the second enzyme in the urea cycle. The enzyme condenses carbamyl phosphate and ornithine to form citrulline. OTC is mitochondrial bound (Fig. 88.9).

Male infants with OTC deficiency have a lethal course during the perinatal period (Shih, 1978). The affected infants develop vomiting, lethargy and coma with associated respiratory distress (Campbell et al, 1973). Blood ammonia values are usually >1000 μg/dl. Increased concentration of glutamine may be present in plasma and urine.

Females may have a less severe deficiency of OTC and milder symptoms. Such females may demonstrate significant hyperammonaemia (400–800 μg/dl) with symptoms of vomiting, lethargy and mental retardation. Some females may only have such mild symptoms as aversion to high protein foods. OTC deficiency in females is one cause of 'cyclic vomiting'.

Patients with OTC deficiency excrete an excess of orotic acid in their urine. This occurs because the accumulation of carbamyl phosphate is shunted to pyrimidine metabolism via CPS-II (Fig. 88.9). CPS-II is a different enzyme to CPS-I, it is located in the cytoplasm and requires glutamate as a cofactor. The increased excretion of orotic acid may be used as an aid in the diagnosis of OTC deficiency.

OTC is primarily limited to liver tissue and is not detectable in cultured fibroblasts or leucocytes. In affected males, the enzyme is virtually absent with less than 1 per cent of normal activity. In symptomatic females, the enzyme activity has been shown to vary from 10 per cent to 40% of normal.

The allele for OTC has been shown to be X–linked by pedigree data (Scott et al, 1972; Campbell et al, 1973; Short et al, 1973) and by the demonstration of two populations of hepatocytes in female carriers (Ricciuti et al, 1976). The X–linkage of OTC explains the severe form of the disease in males and the variable expression of the disorder in females. OTC is also linked to the X–chromosome in the mouse (DeMars et al, 1976).

Allelic heterogeneity for OTC deficiency has been documented by biochemical and immunological studies of the mutant enzyme. Abnormal kinetic properties have been found for pH, affinity for ornithine, and affinity for carbamylphosphate (for review see Cathelineau et al, 1974).

Heterozygote detection in some females may be successful by either an ammonia tolerance test or by quantitating orotic acid in urine. Both have been shown to be abnormal in some carriers.

Therapy for males with OTC deficiency has been uniformly unsuccessful. Low protein diets, keto acid analogues, and standard medical means to lower blood ammonia have not prevented affected males from dying. For symptomatic females, the most effective therapy has been protein restriction. Most infants can grow satisfactorily on a diet containing 1 gm/kg/day of protein of high biological value.

Citrullinuria

Citrulline and aspartate condense to form argininosuccinic acid. This reaction is catalyzed by the enzyme *argininosuccinic acid (ASA) synthetase* (Fig. 88.9). A deficiency of ASA synthetase allows the accumulation of citrulline and a failure of processing ammonia to urea.

Patients with a deficiency of *ASA synthetase* may have a heterogenous clinical course. Some newborns have a severe and fulminant course with vomiting, lethargy, seizures and death associated with severe hyperammonaemia (Van der Zee et al, 1971). Others may present later in childhood with developmental delay, and some have been found to have a benign clinical course (Wick et al, 1973). This clinical heterogeneity is believed to be related to the degree of the enzyme deficiency which exists under physiological conditions.

ASA synthetase deficiency has been documented in patients with citrullinaemia. Activity has been found to be less than 5% in liver or cultured skin fibroblasts (Mohyuddin et al, 1967; Tedesco & Mellman 1967). Heterogeneity of the enzyme deficiency has been shown by alterations in the Km for both citrulline and aspartate and by variation in Vmax of the residual activity (Kennaway et al, 1975; Walser et al, 1977; Shih, 1978).

The diagnosis of citrullinaemia is not difficult. Affected children excrete massive amounts of citrulline in the urine and have a 10 to 20 fold increase of citrulline in blood. Enzyme confirmation of ASA deficiency can be performed on cultured skin fibroblasts.

The most effective approach to therapy has been a protein restricted diet (1 gm/kg/day) supplemented with 1 to 2 gm/day of arginine. In severely affected infants, peritoneal dialysis or hemodialysis may be necessary to decrease the blood ammonia prior to instituting diet therapy. The nitrogen free analogues of essential amino acids have been used for treatment but have not proven to be of great benefit (Thoene et al, 1973).

Citrullinaemia is inherited as an autosomal recessive trait. Heterozygote detection is not considered reliable, but Buist et al (1974) did document decreased ASA synthetase activity in cultured fibroblasts from three presumed heterozygotes. Prenatal diagnosis is possible on cultured amniotic fluid cells (Jacoby et al, 1980).

Argininosuccinic acidura

Argininosuccinic acid (ASA) is cleaved into two smaller molecules, arginine and fumarate by the enzyme argininosuccinase. The enzyme is active in liver, brain and kidney. A deficiency of the lyase causes an accumulation of ASA in CSF and plasma and a major excretion of ASA in the urine.

Infants who have a genetic absence of the lyase may have profound symptoms of lethargy and coma associated with hyperammonaemia. These severly symptomatic children often die during the newborn period (Carton et al, 1969). Many affected children, however, may have less severe symptoms and only be detected in childhood with mild mental retardation and a voluntary aversion to protein (Shih, 1978). Of clinical interest is the observation that some children develop trichorrhexis nodosa, a nodular condition of the hair which causes it to be friable.

Confirmation of ASA in symptomatic children is quite easy. They excrete large quantities of ASA in their urine which is readily detectable by any amino acid chromatography system.

Successful therapy is aimed at reducing the intake of protein to decrease the formation of ammonia. The diet may be supplemented with 1–2 gm/day of arginine to stimulate the conversion of ammonia to ASA.

Table 88.9 Disorders of the urea cycle and of ornithine

Disorder	Enzyme deficiency	Inheritance pattern	Heterozygote detection	Prenatal diagnosis
The hyperammonaemias				
Type I (severe and mild forms)	Carbamyl phosphate synthetase I (2.7.2.2)	AR	No	No
Type II	Ornithine transcarbamylase (2.1.3.3)	XL	Yes	No
Citrullinaemia (severe and mild forms)	Argininosuccinic acid synthetase (6.3.4.5) chromosome 9	AR	Unreliable	Yes
Argininosuccinic aciduria (severe and mild forms)	Argininosuccinic acid lyase (4.3.2.1) chromosome 7	AR	Yes	Yes
Argininaemia	Arginase (3.5.3.1)	AR	Possible	Possible by arginase activity in fetal RBC
The hyperornithinaemias				
Hyperornithinaemia with gyrate atrophy	Ornithine aminotransferase (2.7.2.2.)	AR	Yes	Possible
Hyperornithinaemia with mental retardation	Ornithine decarboxylase? (4.1.1.17)	AR?		

Argininosuccinic aciduria is inherited as an autosomal recessive trait. The enzyme has been shown to be absent in liver, fibroblasts and red cells of affected children. One report found the enzyme absent in liver, but present in brain and kidney (Glick et al, 1976). Heterozygotes may be detected by the presence of small amounts of ASA in their urine and Tomlinson et al (1964) have reported that ASA lyase activity in red cells from parents of affected children is less than normal. Prenatal diagnosis can be performed by using cultured cells from amniotic fluid.

Argininaemia

The urea cycle is completed by the cleavage of arginine by arginase to form ornithine and urea. Arginase is the most active of the urea cycle enzymes in hepatic tissue. The enzyme is present in liver, kidney, brain and red cells. Arginase is not expressed in leucocytes or cultured skin fibroblasts.

An absence of arginase activity has been reported to cause mental retardation, seizures and a progressive spastic diplegia (Terheggen et al, 1969; Cederbaum et al, 1977).

The diagnosis of argininaemia can be determined by the presence of excess arginine excretion in the urine and the presence of elevated arginine in the plasma. The pattern of urinary amino acid excretion may be confused with cystinuria. The increased arginine excretion competes with the renal tubular uptake sites for diabasic amino acids and cystine. This competition causes an increased renal loss of lysine, ornithine and cystine.

A low protein diet may assist in lowering blood ammonia and arginine values. Snyderman et al (1977) have used a synthetic protein diet consisting of essential amino acids with some success.

Arginase deficiency is inherited as an autosomal recessive condition. Parents of affected children have been noted to have less than normal arginase activity in their red cells. Prenatal diagnosis would be feasible if fetal red cells were available. The enzyme is not expressed in cultured amniotic fluid cells.

Hyperornithinaemia with gyrate atrophy (ornithine amino transferase deficiency)

Gyrate atrophy of the retina associated with a 10–20 fold elevation of plasma ornithine was described in the Finnish population in 1973 (Simell & Takki, 1973). The disorder appears to effect only the vision with no associated problems in intellectual development. Visual loss begins to occur during the second decade and is slowly progressive. The retinal atrophy begins in the periphery with loss of the pigment epithelium. The fundal picture is characterized by sharply defined margins of choroidal atrophy which slowly progress toward the posterior pole of the eye.

A deficiency of ornithine aminotransferase in affected patients has been documented in cultured fibroblasts (Trijbels et al, 1977; O'Donnell et al, 1977). Although no biochemical evidence exists for heterogeneity, clinical studies suggest that some patients may respond to pyridoxal phosphate by lowering their plasma ornithine concentration. One study reports are improvement in vision following a restriction of dietary ornithine (Kaiser-Kupfer et al, 1980).

The disorder is inherited as an autosomal recessive trait. The majority of reported patients have been of Finnish origin although patients of other ethnic groups have been identified. Heterozygotes have been noted to have an abnormal response to ornithine loading (Takki & Simell, 1974) and to have less than normal enzyme activity in cultured cells (Valle et al, 1977; O'Donnell et al, 1977). Prenatal diagnosis is feasible since the enzyme is expressed in cultured cells.

BIBLIOGRAPHY

Ampola M G, Mahoney M J, Nakamura E, Tanaka K 1975 Prenatal therapy of a patient with vitamin B₁₂-responsive methylmalonic aciduria. New England Journal of medicine 283: 313–317.

Ando T, Nyhan W L, Gerritsen T, Gong L, Heiner D C, Bray P F 1968 Metabolism of glycine in the nonketotic form of hyperglycinemia. Pediatric Research 2: 254–263.

Aronsson S, Engleson G, Jagenburg R, Palmgren B 1968 Long term dietary treatment of tyrosinosis. Journal of Pediatrics 72: 620–627.

Arthur L J, Hulme J D 1970 Intelligent, small for dates baby born to oligophrenic phenylketonuric mother after low phenylalanine diet during pregnancy. Pediatrics 46: 235–239.

Avery M E, Clow C L, Menkes J H, Ramos A, Scriver C R, Stern L, Wasserman B P 1967 Transient tyrosinemia of the newborn: dietary and clinical aspects. Pediatrics 39: 378–384.

Bartholome K, Byrd D J, Kaufman S, Milstien S 1977 Atypical phenylketonuria with normal phenylalanine hydroxylase and dihydropteridine reductase activity in vitro. Pediatrics 59: 757–761.

Belanger L, Belanger M, Prive L, Larochelle J, Tremblay M, Aubin G 1973 Tyrosinemie hereditaire et alpha-1-foetoproteine, 1. Interet clinique de l'alpha-foeto-proteine dans la tyrosinemie hereditaire. Pathologie et Biologie 21: 449–455.

Bergeron P, Laberge C, Grenier A 1974 Hereditary tyrosinemia in the province of Quebec: prevalence at birth and geographic distribution. Clinical Genetics 5: 157–162.

Brenton D P, Cusworth D C (ed) 1971 The response of patients with cystathionine synthase deficiency to pyridoxine. In: Inherited disorders of sulphur metabolism, N A Carson and D N Raine, London, Livingstone, p 264–274.

Buist N R M, Kennaway N G, Hepburn C A, Strandholm

J J, Ramberg D A 1974 Citrullinemia: investigation and treatment over a four year period. Journal of Pediatrics 85: 208–214.

Burgi W, Richterich R, Colombo J P 1966 L-Lysine dehydrogenase deficiency in a patient with congenital lysine intolerance. Nature (London) 211: 854–855.

Busk R T, Dukes P C 1975 Progeny, pregnancy and phenylketonuria. New Zealand Medical Journal 82: 226–229.

Campbell A G M, Rosenberg L E, Snodgrass P J, Nuzum C T 1973 Ornithine transcarbamylase deficiency: a cause of lethal neonatal hyperammonemia in males. New England Journal of Medicine 288: 1–6.

Carson N A J, Scally B G, Neill D W, Carre I J 1968 Saccharopinuria: a new inborn error of lysine metabolism. Nature (London) 218: 679.

Carton D, DeSchrijver K, Kint J, VanDurme J, Hooft C 1969 Argininosuccinicaciduria. Neonatal variant with rapid fatal course. Acta Paediatrica Scandinavica 58: 528–534.

Cathelineau L, Saudubray J-M, Polonovski C 1974 Heterogeneous mutations of the structural gene of human ornithine carbamyltransferase as observed in five personal cases. Enzyme 18: 103–113.

Cederbaum S D, Shaw K N F, Valente M 1977 Hyperargininemia. Journal of Pediatrics 90: 569.

Childs B, Nyhan W L, Borden M, Bard L, Cooke R E 1961 Idiopathic hyperglycinemia and hyperglycinuria: new disorder of amino acid metabolism I. Pediatrics 27: 522–538.

Clow C L, Laberge C, Scriver C R 1975 Neonatal hypertyrosinemia and evidence for deficiency of ascorbic acid in Arctic and subarctic peoples. Canadian Medical Association Journal 113: 624–626.

Colombo J P, Bachmann C, Terheggen H G, Lavinha F, Lowenthal A (ed) 1976 Argininemia. In: The ureau cycle, S Grisolia, R Baguena, and F Mayor, New York, Wiley-Interscience, p 415–424.

Colombo J P, Richterich R, Donath A, Spahr A, Rossi E 1964 Congenital lysine intolerance with periodic ammonia intoxication. Lancet 1: 1014–1015.

Committee for Improvement of Hereditary Disease Management 1976 Management of maple syrup urine disease in Canada. Canadian Medical Association Journal 115: 1005–1013.

Connelly J L, Danner D J, Bowden J A 1968 Branched-chain α-keto acid metabolism I. Isolation, purification and partial characterization of bovine liver α-keto-isocaproic acid and α-keto-β-methylvaleric acid dehydrogenase. Journal of Biological Chemistry 243: 1198–1203.

Dancis J, Hutzler J, Cox R P, Woody N L 1969 Familial hyperlysinemia with lysine-ketoglutarate reductase deficiency. Journal of Clinical Investigation 48: 1447–1452.

Dancis J, Hutzler J, Rokkones T 1967 Intermittent branched-chain ketonuria: variant of maple syrup urine disease. New England Journal of Medicine 276: 84–89.

Dancis J, Hutzler J, Tada K, Wada Y, Morikawa T, Arakawa T 1967 Hypervalinemia. A defect in valine transamination. Pediatrics 39: 813–817.

Dancis J, Levitz M 1978 Abnormalities of branched chain amino acid metabolism. In: The metabolic basis of inherited diseases, J Stanbury, J Wyngaarden and D Frederickson (eds), New York, McGraw-Hill Inc.

Danks D 1978 Malignant hyperphenylalaninemia: current status. Journal of Inherited Metabolic Disease 2: 49.

DeGroot C J, Troelstra J A, Hommes F A 1970 The enzymatic defect of the nonketotic form of hyperglycinemia. Pediatric Research 4: 238–243.

DeMars R, LeVan S L, Trend B L, Russell L B 1976 Abnormal ornithine carbamyltransferase in mice having the sparse-fur mutation. Proceedings of the National Academy of Sciences of the United States of America (Washington) 73: 1693–1697.

Dobson J C, Kushida E, Williamson M, Friedman E G (PKU collaborative study) 1976 Intellectual performance of 36 phenylketonuria patients and their nonaffected sibships. Pediatrics 58: 53–58.

Efron M L 1965 Familial hyperprolinemia: report of a second case, associated with congenital renal malformations, hereditary hematuria and mild mental retardation, with demonstration of an enzyme defect. New England Journal of Medicine 272: 1243–1254.

Efron M L, Bixby E M, Pryles C V 1965 Hydroxyprolinemia II. A rare metabolic disease due to a deficiency of the enzyme 'hydroxyproline oxidase.' New England Journal of Medicine 272: 1229–1309.

Erbe R W (ed) 1977 Prenatal diagnosis of inherited disease, entry 74. In: Biological handbooks II, human health and disease, P L Altman and D D Katz, Bethesda, Md, FASEB, p 91–P.

Fellman J H, Buist N R M, Kennaway N G, Swanson R E 1972 The source of aromatic ketoacids in tyrosinemia and phenylketonuria. Clinica Chimica Acta 39: 243–246

Firgaira F, Cotton R G H, Danks D M 1979 Human dehydropteridine reductase: a method for the measurement of activity in cultured cells and its application to malignant hyperphenylalaninemia. Clinica Chimica Acta 95: 47

Fleisher L D, Longhi R C, Tallan H H, Beratis N G, Hirschhorn K, Gaull G E 1974 Homocystinuria: investigations of cystathionine synthase in cultured fetal cells in the prenatal determination of genetic status. Journal of Pediatrics 85: 667.

Følling A 1934 Uber ausscheidung von phenylbrenztraubensaure in den harn als stoffwechselanomalie in verbindung mit imbezillitat. Zeitschrift Physiol Chem 277: 169–176.

Fowler B, Kraus J, Packman S, Rosenberg L E 1978 Homocystinuria. Evidence for three distinct classes of cystathionine β-synthase mutants in cultured fibroblasts. Journal of Clinical Investigation 61: 645–653.

Freeman J M, Finklestein J D, Mudd S H 1975 Folate-responsive homocystinuria and 'schizophrenia': a defect in methylation due to deficient 5,10-methylenetetrahydrofolate reductase activity. New England Journal of Medicine 292: 491–496.

Friedman P A, Fisher D B, Kang E S, Kaufman S 1973 Detection of hepatic phenylalanine 4-hydroxylase in classical phenylketonuria. Proceedings of the National Academy of Sciences of the United States of America 70: 552–556.

Frimpter G W, Haymovitz A, Horwith M 1963 Cystathioninuria. New England Journal of Medicine 268: 333–339.

García-Castro J, Isales-Forsythe C M, Levy H L, Shih V E, Laó-Vélez C R, González-Rios M C, Reyes de Torres L C 1982 Prenatal diagnosis of non-ketotic hyperglycinemia. The New England Journal of Medicine 306(2): 79–81

Gaull G E, Rassin D K, Solomon G E, Harris R C, Sturman J A 1970 Biochemical observations on so-called hereditary tyrosinemia. Pediatric Research 4: 337–344.

Gelehrter T D, Snodgrass P J 1974 Lethal neonatal deficiency of carbamyl phosphate synthetase. New England Journal of Medicine 290: 430–433.

Gentz J, Jagenburg R, Zetterstrom R 1965 Tyrosinemia, an inborn error of tyrosine metabolism with cirrhosis of the liver and multiple renal tubular defects (de Toni-Debre-Fanconi syndrome). Journal of Pediatrics 66: 670–696.

Gerritsen T, Waisman H A 1966 Hypersarcosinemia: an inborn error of metabolism. New England Journal of Medicine 275: 66.

Ghadimi H, Binnington V I, Pecora P 1965 Hyperlysinemia associated with retardation. New England Journal of Medicine 273: 723–729.

Ghadimi H, Partington M W 1967 Salient features of histidinemia. American Journal of Diseases of Children 113: 83–87.

Giorgio A J, Luhby A L 1969 A rapid screening test for the detection of congenital methylmalonic aciduria in infancy. American Journal of Clinical Pathology 52: 374–379.

Glick N R, Snodgrass P J, Schafer I A 1976 Neonatal argininosuccinicaciduria with normal brain and kidney but absent liver argininosuccinate lyase activity. American Journal of Human Genetics 28: 22–30.

Goldsmith L A, Kang E, Bienfang D C, Jimbow K, Gerald P, Baden H P 1973 Tyrosinemia with plantar and palmar keratosis and keratitis. Journal of Pediatrics 83: 798–805.

Gompertz D, Goodey P A, Saudubray J M, Charpentier C, Chignolle A 1974 Prenatal diagnosis and methylmalonic aciduria. Pediatrics 54: 511–513.

Goodman S 1980 An introduction to gas chromatography – mass spectrometry and the inherited organic acidemias. American Journal of Human Genetics 32: 781–792.

Goodman S L, Browder J A, Hiles R A, Miles B S 1972 Hydroxylysinemia-a disorder due to a defect in the metabolism of free hydroxylysine. Biochemical Medicine 6: 344–354.

Goodman S L, Mace J W, Turner B, Garrett W J 1973 Antenatal diagnosis of argininosuccinicaciduria. Clinical Genetics 4: 236–240.

Gravel R A, Lam F K, Scully K J, Hsia Y E 1977 Genetic complementation of propionyl CoA carboxylase deficiency in cultured fibroblasts. American Journal of Human Genetics 24: 378–388.

Gravel R A, Mahoney M J, Ruddle F H, Rosenberg L E 1975 Genetic complementation in heterokaryons of human fibroblasts defective in cobalamin metabolism. Proceeding of the National Academy of Sciences of the United States of America (Washington) 72: 3181–3185.

Hanley W B, Linsao L S, Netley C 1971 The efficacy of dietary therapy for phenylketonuria. Canadian Medical Association Journal 104: 1089–1092.

Harker L A, Ross R, Slichter S J, Scott C R 1976 Homocystine-induced arteriosclerosis: the role of endothelial cell injury and platelet response in its genesis. Journal of Clinical Investigation 58: 731–741.

Hill A, Nordin P M, Zaleski W A 1970 Dietary treatment of tyrosinosis. Journal of the American Dietetic Association 56: 308–312.

Hillman R E, Otto E F 1974 Inhibition of glycine-serine interconversion in cultured human fibroblasts by products of isoleucine catabolism. Pediatric Research 8: 941–945.

Hollowell J G Jr, Hall W K, Coryell M E, McPherson J Jr, Hahn D A 1969 Homocystinuria and organic aciduria in a patient with vitamin B_{12} deficiency. Lancet 2: 1428.

Holtzman N A, Meek A G, Mellits E D, Kallman C H 1974 Neonatal screening for phenylketonuria III. Altered sex ratio: extent and possible causes. Journal of Pediatrics 85: 175–181.

Holtzman N A, Mellits E D, Kallman C 1974 Neonatal screening for phenylketonuria II. Age dependence of initial phenylalanine in infants with PKU. Pediatrics 53: 353–357.

Howell R R, Stevenson R E 1971 The offspring of phenylketonuric women. Social Biology 18: 519–529.

Hsia D Y –Y 1970 Phenylketonuria and its variants. Progress in Medical Genetics 7: 29–68.

Hsia Y E, Scully K, Lilljeqvist A-Ch, Rosenberg L E 1970 Vitamin B_{12} dependent methylmalonicaciduria. Pediatrics 46: 497.

Hudson F P, Morduant V L, Leaky I 1970 Evaluation of treatment begun in first three months of life in 184 cases of phenylketonuria. Archives of Disease in Childhood 45: 5–12

Huntley C C, Stevenson R E 1969 Maternal phenylketonuria. Course of two pregnancies. Obstetrics and Gynecology 34: 694–700.

Jacoby L B, Shih V E, Niermeijer M F, Boue J 1980 Prenatal diagnosis of citrullinemia. American Journal of Human Genetics 31: 42A (abstract).

Jervis G A 1953 Phenylpyruvic oligophrenia: deficiency of phenylalanine oxidizing system. Proceedings of the Society for Experimental Biology and Medicine 82: 514–515.

Jeune M, Collombel C, Michel M, David M, Guibault P, Guerrier G, Albert J 1970 Hyperleucinisoleucinemie par defaut partiel de transamination associee a une hyperprolinemie de Type 2. Observation familiale d une double aminoacidopathie. Semaine des hôpitaux de Paris (Annales de pédiatrie) 17: 85–99.

Justice P, O'Flynn M E, Hsia D Y 1967 Phenylalanine-hydroxylase activity in hyperphenylalaninemia. Lancet 1: 928–930.

Kaiser-Kupfer M I, De Monasterio F M, Valle D, Walser M, Brusilow S 1980 Gyrate atrophy of the choroid and retina: improved visual function following reduction of plasma ornithine by diet. Science 210: 1128–1131.

Kang E S, Kaufman S, Gerald P S 1970 Clinical and biochemical observations of patients with atypical phenylketonuria. Pediatrics 45: 83–92.

Kang E S, Snodgrass P J, Gerald P S 1978 Methylmalonyl CoA racemase defect: another cause of methylmalonic aciduria. Pediatric Research 6: 875–879.

Kaufman S 1958 Phenylalanine hydroxylation cofactor in phenylketonuria. Science 128: 1506–1508.

Kaufman S 1976 The phenylalanine hydroxylating system in phenylketonuria and its variants. Biochemical Medicine 15: 42–54.

Kaufman S, Holtzman N A, Milstien S, Butler I J, Krumkolz A 1975 Phenylketonuria due to a deficiency of dihydropteridine reductase. New England Journal of Medicine 293: 785–790.

Kennaway N G, Harwood P J, Ramberg D A, Koler R D, Buist N R M 1975 Citrullinemia: enzymatic evidence for genetic heterogeneity. Pediatric Research 9: 554.

Kim Y J, Rosenberg L E 1974 Studies of the mechanism of pyridoxine responsive homocystinuria II. Properties of normal and mutant cystathionine synthase from cultured fibroblasts. Proceedings of the National Academy of Sciences of the United States of America (Washington) 71: 4821–4825.

Knox W E 1972 Phenylketonuria. In the metabolic basis of inherited disease. J B Stanbury, J B Wyngaarden, and D S Fredrickson (eds) New York, McGraw-Hill Book Co.. Inc., p 266–295.

Koch J, Stokstad E L R, Williams H E, Smith L H 1967 Deficiency of 2-oxo-glutarate glyoxylate carboligase activity in primary hyperoxaluria. Proceedings of the National Academy of Sciences of the United States of America (Washington) 57: 1123–1129.

Komrower G M, Sardharwalla I B (ed) 1971 The dietary

treatment of homocystinuria. In: Inherited disorders of sulphur metabolism, N A Carson and D N Raine, London, Livingstone, p 254–263.

Kretchmer N, Levine S Z, McNamara H, Barnett H L 1956 Certain aspects of tyrosine metabolism in the young I. The development of the tyrosine oxidizing system in human liver. Journal of Clinical Investigation 35: 236–244.

La Du B N (ed) 1967 The enzymatic deficiency in tyrosinemia. In: Symposium on treatment of amino acid disorders. D Y Y Hsia. American Journal of Diseases of Children 113: 54–57.

La Du B N, Gjessing L R 1978 Tyrosinosis and tyrosinemia. In the metabolic basis of inherited disease, 4th ed. J B Stanbury, J B Wyngaarden and D S Fredrickson, New York, McGraw-Hill Book Co., Inc., p 256–267.

La Du B N, Howell R R, Jacoby G A, Seegmiller J E, Sober E K, Zannoni V G, Canby J P, Ziegler L K 1963 Clinical and biochemical studies on two cases of histidinemia. Pediatrics 32: 216–227.

Langenbeck U, Grimm T, Rudiger H W, Passarge E 1975 Heterozygote tests and genetic counseling in maple syrup urine disease. An application of Baye's theorem. Humangenetik 27: 315–322.

Lenke R R, Levy H L 1980 Maternal phenylketonuria and hyperphenylalaninemia. New England Journal of Medicine 303: 1202–1208.

Levy H L, Karolkewicz V, Houghton S A, MacCready R A 1970 Screening the 'normal' population in Massachusetts for phenylketonuria. New England Journal of Medicine 282: 1455–1458.

Levy H L, Mudd S H, Schulman J D, Dreyfus P M, Abeles R H 1970 A derangement in B_{12} metabolism associated with homocystinemia, cystathioninemia, hypomethioninemia and methylmalonic aciduria. American Journal of Medicine 48: 390–397.

Levy H L, Shih V E, MacCready R A (ed) 1972 Massachusetts metabolic disorders screening program. In: Early diagnosis of human genetic defects, M Harris, Washington, D C, U S Government Printing Office, p 47–66.

Levy H L, Shih V E, Madigan P M 1974 Routine newborn screening for histidinemia. Clinical and biochemical results. New England Journal of Medicine 291: 1214–1219.

Mahoney M J, Hart A C, Steen V D, Rosenberg L E 1975 Methylmalonic acidemia: biochemical heterogeneity in defects of 5'-deoxyadenosyl cobalamin synthesis. Proceedings of the National Academy of Sciences of the United States of America (Washington) 72: 2799–2803.

Medes G 1932 A new error of tyrosine metabolism: tyrosinosis. The intermediary metabolism of tyrosine and phenylalanine. Biochemical Journal 26: 917–940.

Menkes J H, Welcher D W, Levi H S, Dallas J, Gretsky N E 1972 Relationship of elevated blood tyrosine to the ultimate intellectual performance of premature infants. Pediatrics 49: 218–224.

Mitoma C, Auld R M, Udenfriend S 1957 On the nature of enzymic defect in phenylpyruvic oligophrenia. Proceedings of the Society for Experimental Biology and Medicine 94: 634–635.

Mohyuddin F, Rathbun J C, McMurray W C 1967 Studies on amino acid metabolism in citrullinuria. American Journal of Diseases of Children 113: 152–156.

Morris M D, Fisher D A, Fiser R 1966 Late-onset branched-chain keto aciduria (maple syrup urine disease). Lancet 86: 149–152.

Morrow G III, Barness L A, Cardinale G J, Abeles R H, Flanks J G 1969 Congenital methylmalonic acidemia: enzymatic evidence for two forms of the disease. Proceedings of the National Academy of Sciences of the United States of America (Washington) 63: 191–197.

Morrow G III, Schwarz R H, Hallock J A, Barness L A 1970 Prenatal detection of methylmalonic acidemia. Journal of Pediatrics 77: 120–123.

Mudd S H, Edwards W A, Loeb P M, Brown M S, Laster L 1970 Homocystinuria due to cystathionine synthase deficiency: the effect of pyridoxine. Journal of Clinical Investigation 49: 1762–1773.

Mudd S H, Finkelstein J D, Irreverre F, Laster L 1964 Homocystinuria: an enzymatic defect. Science 143: 1443–1445.

Mudd S H, Irreverre F, Laster L 1967 Sulfite oxidase deficiency in man: demonstration of the enzymatic defect. Science 156: 1599–1601.

Mudd S H, Levy H L 1978 Disorders of transsulfuration. In: The metabolic basis of inherited disease, 4th edn. J B Wyngaarden and D S Fredrickson, New York, McGraw-Hill Books Company, Inc., p 458–503.

Narisawa K, Wada Y, Saito T, Suzuki H, Kudo M, Arakawa T, Katushima N, Tsuboi R 1977 Infantile type of homocystinuria with $N^{5,10}$-methylenetetrahydrofolate reductase defect. Tohoku Journal of Experimental Medicine 121: 185–194.

Nyhan W L, Fawcett N, Ando T, Rennert O M, Julius R L 1973 Response to dietary therapy in B_{12} unresponsive methylmalonic acidemia. Pediatrics 81: 539.

O'Donnell J J, Sandman R P, Martin S R 1977 Deficient L-ornithine: 2-oxoacid aminotransferase in cultured fibroblasts from a patient with gyrate atrophy of the retina. Biochemical and Biophysical Research Communications 79: 396–399.

Pelkonen R, Kivirikko K I 1970 Hydroxyprolinemia. New England Journal of Medicine 283: 451–456.

Perry T L (ed) 1971 Treatment of homocystinuria with a low methionine diet and supplemental L-cystine. In: Inherited disorders of sulphur metabolism. N A Carson and D N Raine, London, Livingstone, p 245–253.

Perry T L, Hansen S, Tischler B, Bunting R 1967 Determination of heterozygosity for phenylketonuria on the amino acid analyzer. Clinica Chimica Acta 18: 51–56.

Partington M W, Delahaye D J, Masotti R E, Read J H, Roberts B 1968 Neonatal tyrosinemia. A follow-up study. Archives of Diseases in Childhood 43: 195–199.

Partington M W, Scriver C R, Sass-Kortsak E 1967 Conference on hereditary tyrosinemia. Canadian Medical Association Journal 97: 1045–1101.

Rama Rao B S, Subhash M N, Marayanan H S 1974 Hydroxyprolinemia: case report. Indian Pediatrics 11: 829–830.

Reed L J, Cox D J 1966 Macromolecular organization of enzyme systems. Annual Review of Biochemistry 35: 57–84.

Ricciuti F C, Gelehrter T D, Rosenberg L E 1976 X chromosome inactivation in human: confirmation of X–linkage of ornithine transcarbamylase. American Journal of Human Genetics 28: 332–338.

Rosenberg L E 1980 Disorders of amino acid metabolism. In: Metabolic control and disease, P E Bondy and L E Rosenberg (ed), Philadelphia, W B Saunders Company.

Rosenberg L E 1978 Disorders of propionate, methylmalonate and cobalmin metabolism. In: The metabolic basis of inherited diseases, J Stanbury, J Wyngaarden and D Frederickson (ed), New York, McGraw-Hill Inc.

Rosenberg L E, Patel L, Lilljeqvist A 1975 Absence of an intracellular cobalmin – binding protein in cultured fibroblasts from patients with defective synthesis of 5'-deoxyadenosylcobalmin and methylcobalmin. Proceedings of the National Academy of Sciences of the United States of America 72: 4617.

Rosenberg L E, Tanaka K 1977 Metabolism of amino acids and organic acids. In: The year in metabolism, Freinkel (ed), Plenum Med Pub.

Rosenblatt D, Mohyuddin F, Scriver C R 1970 Histidinemia discovered by urinary screening after renal transplantation. Pediatrics 46: 47–53.

Rosenblatt D, Scriver C R 1968 Heterogeneity in genetic control of phenylalanine metabolism in man. Nature 218: 677–678.

Sarharwalla I B, Fowler B, Robins A J, Komrower G M 1974 Detection of heterozygotes for homocystinuria: study of sulfur containing amino acids in plasma and urine after L-methionine loading. Archives of Diseases in Childhood 49: 553.

Schafer I A, Scriver C R, Efron M L 1962 Familial hyperprolinemia, cerebral dysfunction and renal anomalies occuring in a family with hereditary nephropathy and deafness. New England Journal of Medicine 267: 51–60.

Schulman J D, Lustberg T J, Kennedy J L, Museles M, Seegmiller J E 1970 A new variant of maple syrup urine disease (branched-chain ketoaciduria). American Journal of Medicine 49: 118–124.

Scott C R, Clark S H, Teng C C, Swedberg K R 1970 Clinical and cellular studies of sarcosinemia. Journal of Pediatrics 77: 805–811.

Scott CR, Dassell S W, Clark S H, Teng C C, Swedberg K R 1970 Cystathioninemia: a benign genetic condition. Journal of Pediatrics 76: 571–577.

Scott C R, Teng C C, Goodman S I, Greensher A, Mace J W 1972 X–linked transmission of ornithine transcarbamylase deficiency. Lancet II: 1148.

Scriver C R (ed) 1977 Hereditary and acquired amino acidopathies: entry 75. In: Biological handbooks II, human health and disease, P L Altman and D D Katz, Bethesda, Md, FASEB, p 97–105.

Scriver C R, Davies E 1967 Investigation in vivo of the biochemical defect in hereditary tyrosinemia and tyrosyluria. In conference on hereditary tyrosinemia. M Partington, C R Scriver and A Sass-Kortsak (ed) Canadian Medical Association Journal 97: 1076–1078.

Scriver C R, Efron M L 1978 Disorders of proline and hydroxyproline metabolism. In: The metabolic basis of inherited disease, 4th edn. J B Stanbury, J B Wyngaarden and D S Fredrickson, New York, McGraw-Hill Book Company, Inc., p 336–361.

Scriver C R, Larochelle J, Silverberg M 1967 Hereditary tyrosinemia and tyrosyluria in a French Canadian geographic isolate. American Journal of Diseases of Children 113: 41–46.

Scriver C R, Mackenzie S, Clow C L, Delvin E 1971 Thiamine-responsive maple syrup urine disease. Lancet 1: 310–312.

Shepard T H, Lee L W, Krebs E G 1960 Primary hyperoxaluria II. Genetic studies in a family. Pediatrics 25: 869–871.

Shih V E 1978 Urea cycle disorders and other congenital hyperammonemic syndromes. In: The metabolic basis of inherited disease, 4th edn. J B Wyngaarden and D S Fredrickson, New York, McGraw-Hill Book Company, Inc, p 362–386.

Shih V E, Abrams J F, Johnson J L, Carney M, Mandell R, Robb R M, Cloherty J P, Rajagopalan K V 1977 Sulfite oxidase deficiency: biochemical and clinical investigations of

a hereditary metabolic disorder in sulfur metabolism. New England Journal of Medicine 297: 1022–1028.

Short E M, Conn H O, Snodgrass P J, Campbell A G M, Rosenberg L E 1973 Evidence for X--linked dominant inheritance of ornithine transcarbamylase deficiency. New England Journal of Medicine 288: 7–12.

Simell O, Takki K 1973 Raised plasma-ornithine and gyrate atrophy of the choroid and retina. Lancet 1: 1031–1033.

Smith I, Wolff O H 1974 Natural history of phenylketonuria and influence of early treatment. Lancet ii: 540–544.

Snyderman S E, Norton P M, Roitman E, Holt E L Jr 1964 Maple syrup urine, with particular reference to dietotherapy. Pediatrics 34: 454–472.

Snyderman S E, Sansariag C, Chen W J, North P M, Phansalker S V 1977 Argininemia. Journal of Pediatrics 90: 563–568.

Sweetman L, Packman S, Yoshino M, Cowan M, Wara D, Ammann, A, Nyhan W 1979 Biotin responsive multiple carboxylase deficiency. Pediatric Research 13: 426 (abstract).

Tada K, Narisawa K, Yoshida T, Konno T, Mochizuki K, Arakawa T, Yoshida T, Kikuchi G 1969 Hyperglycinemia: a defect in glycine cleavage reaction. Tohoku Journal of Experimental Medicine 98: 289–296.

Takki K, Simell O 1974 Genetic aspects in gyrate atrophy of the choroid and retina with hyperornithinemia. British Journal of Ophthalmology 58: 907–916.

Tedesco T A, Mellman W J 1967 Argininosuccinate synthetase activity and citrulline metabolism in cells and cultured from a citrullinemic subject. Proceedings of the National Academy of Sciences of the United States of America (Washington) 57: 829–834.

Terheggen H G, Schwenk A, Lowenthal A, VanSande M, Colombo J P 1969 Argininemia with arginase deficiency. Lancet 2: 748–749.

Thoene J, Beach B, Kulovich S, Batshaw M, Walser M, Brusilow S, Nyhan W 1975 Keto acid treatment of neonatal citrullinemia. American Journal of Human Genetics 27: 88A (abstract).

Tomlinson S, Westall R G 1964 Argininosuccinicaciduria, argininosuccinase and arginase in human blood cells. Clinical Science 26: 261–269.

Toniguichi K, Gjessing L R 1965 Studies on tyrosinosis 2. Activity of transaminase, parahydroxyphenylpyruvate oxidase and homogentisic acid oxidase. British Medical Journal 1: 968–969.

Trijbels J M F, Sengers R C A, Bakkeren J A J M, DeKort A F M, Deutman A F 1977 L-ornithine-ketoacid-transaminase deficiency in cultured fibroblasts of a patient with hyperornithinemia and gyrate atrophy of the choroid and retina. Clinica Chimica Acta 79: 371–377.

Valle D, Kaiser-Kupfer M I, Del Valle L A 1977 Gyrate atrophy of the choroid and retina: deficiency of ornithine aminotransferase in transformed lymphocytes. Proceedings of the National Academy of Sciences of the United States of America (Washington) 74: 5159–5161.

Valle D L, Phang J M, Goodman S I 1974 Type II hyperprolinemia: absence of Δ'-pyrroline-5-carboxylic acid dehydrogenase activity. Science 185: 1053–1054.

Van Der Zee S P M, Trijbels J M F, Monnens L A H, Hommes F A, Schretlen E D A M 1971 Citrullinemia with rapidly fatal neonatal course. Archives of Diseases in Childhood 46: 847–851.

Wada Y, Tada K, Minagawa A, Yoshida T, Morikawa T, Okamura T 1963 Idiopathic valinemia: probably a new entity of inborn error of valine metabolism. Tohoku Journal of Experimental Medicine 81: 46–55.

Wadman S K, Van Der Heiden C, Ketting D, Van Sprang F J 1971 Abnormal tyrosine and phenylalanine metabolism in patients with tyrosyluria and phenylketonuria: gas-liquid chromatographic analysis of urinary metabolites. Clinica Chimica Acta 34: 277–287.

Wallace H W, Moldave K, Meister A 1957 Studies on conversion of phenylalanine to tyrosine in phenylpyruvic oligophrenia. Proceedings of the Society for Experimental Biology and Medicine 94: 632–633.

Walser M, Batshaw M, Sherwood G, Robinson B, Brusilow S 1977 Nitrogen metabolism in neonatal citrullinemia. Clinical Science and Molecular Medicine 53: 173–181.

Wick H, Bachmann C, Baumgartner R, Brechbuhler T, Colombo J P, Wiesmann U, Mihatsch M J, Ohnacker H 1973 Variants of citrullinemia. Archives of Diseases in Childhood 48: 636–641.

Williams H E, Smith L H Jr, 1968 L-glyceric aciduria. A new genetic variant of primary hyperoxaluria. New England Journal of Medicine 278: 233–239.

Wolf B, Rosenberg L E 1978 Heterozygote expression in propionyl CoA carboxylase deficiency differences between major complementation groups. Journal of Clinical Investigation 62: 931–936.

Woody N C, Hutzler J, Dancis J 1966 Further studies of hyperlysinemia. American Journal of Diseases of Children 112: 577–580.

Woody N C, Snyder C H, Harris J A 1965 Histidinemia. American Journal of Diseases of Children 110: 606–613.

Zannoni V G, La Du B N 1963 Determination of histidine-deaminase in human stratum corneum and its absence in histidinemia. Biochemical Journal 88: 160–162.

89

Disorders of carbohydrate metabolism

W. G. Ng, T. F. Roe and G. N. Donnell

INTRODUCTION

Inborn errors of carbohydrate metabolism discussed in this chapter include disaccharidase deficiencies, disorders of monosaccharide metabolism, glycogen storage diseases and gluconeogenic disorders. Additional detailed information may be sought in *Inherited Disorders of Carbohydrate Metabolism* (Burman et al, 1980) and *The Metabolic Basis of Inherited Disease* (Stanbury et al, 1978).

DISACCHARIDASE DEFICIENCIES

The major sources of dietary carbohydrate in man are starch and the disaccharides lactose and sucrose. In adults starch constitutes 60% of the carbohydrate ingested; however, in newborns and young infants the primary carbohydrate is lactose (milk sugar). Sucrose consumption varies widely with the choice of infant formulae and other eating habits. The normal digestive process involves splitting of disaccharides by intestinal hydrolytic enzymes (lactase, sucrase, isomaltase and maltase) into monosaccharides prior to absorption (Fig. 89.1).

Defective intestinal absorption of dietary sugars leads to clinical manifestations, such as flatulence, abdominal cramps, diarrhea, and perianal irritation. Levels of enzymes involved in the hydrolysis of disaccharides may be depressed either on a genetic or acquired basis. The latter situation results from damage to the brush border cells of the small intestine consequent to infection or other injuries. When enzymatic hydrolysis is impaired, ingested disaccharide accumulates and provides a growth medium for intestinal bacteria which produce carbon dioxide, hydrogen, and organic acids. The stools tend to be sour, foamy, loose and watery with an acidic pH. A diagnosis of disaccharidase deficiency may be suspected from the history of symptoms developing in association with the ingestion of a particular sugar and a laboratory finding of disaccharides in the urine. Direct confirmation may be obtained by measuring enzyme activity in intestinal mucosal cells removed on peroral small bowel biopsy. Indirect confirmation of the diagnosis can be made by a disaccharide tolerance test. Disaccharidase deficiency is suggested if the blood glucose curve is flat upon ingestion of the suspect disaccharide.

Lactase deficiency

Lactase deficiency is a rare disorder in infants and young children. The disorder is thought to be of genetic origin and inherited as an autosomal recessive trait (Townley, 1966); however, the number of documented cases reported are insufficient to support this hypothesis clearly.

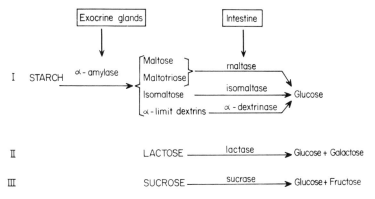

Fig. 89.1 Digestion of carbohydrates

Another disorder, distinct from inherited lactase deficiency, has been described which begins in early infancy with vomiting and diarrhea. Lactose, sucrose and amino acids are excreted in the urine in increased amounts (Durand, 1958). Death may result unless lactose is removed from the diet. Autopsy findings include atrophic enteritis and degenerative change in the renal tubule. The basic cause is unknown.

Late-onset (adult type) lactase deficiency differs from that encountered in infants. Symptoms usually do not occur until adult life, but occasionally may start at an earlier age. This form of lactase deficiency is common in Jews, Blacks, American Indians, Eskimos and Japanese. Some surveys indicate that more than 60% of adults in these racial groups may have a deficiency of the enzyme lactase. It is not known whether genetic predisposition leads to loss of lactase activity with increasing age or whether a post weaning decrease in intestinal lactase occurs because of dietary change. Thus, the term, hypolactasia' has also been used to describe this condition (Schmidt & Schmidt, 1979).

Sucrase-isomaltase deficiency

The mode of inheritance of this condition appears to be autosomal recessive. An incidence of 0.2% has been reported for North American (Petersen & Herber, 1967) and 10% for Greenland Eskimos (McNair et al, 1972). Clinical manifestations described above tend to be more severe in the younger child and depend upon the amount of ingested sugar. Absence of sucrase activity is generally associated with absence of isomaltase activity in intestinal cells. Whereas sucrase-isomaltase occurs as an enzyme complex of two distinct subunits, each acting independently on its specific substrate (Conklin et al, 1975), genetic deficiency usually results in the absence of cross-reacting material detected by radioimmunoassay, suggesting either a major structural alteration or lack of production of the enzyme molecule (Gray et al, 1976).

GLUCOSE-GALACTOSE MALABSORPTION

This is a rare disorder in which an acute, profuse, watery diarrhea develops in newborn infants following initial feeding (Abraham et al, 1967). Intestinal disaccharidase activities are normal. Fructose is absorbed normally, but glucose and galactose are not. There is no significant rise in blood glucose levels following an oral glucose-galactose tolerance test. The stool usually contains large amounts of reducing sugars (>2 g %). Diarrhea may be decreased by feeding of a diet composed of casein, butterfat and fructose. All patients have mild defects in renal tubular reabsorption of glucose. The basic defect is probably at the carrier-mediated transport process. Four cases have been presented in detail (Burke & Danks, 1966), and additional cases have been described later. Pedigree analysis of a consanguinous Swedish family going back to ten generations suggested the defect has an autosomal recessive mode of inheritance (Melin & Meeuwisse, 1969).

DISORDERS OF GALACTOSE METABOLISM

Galactose metabolism

Galactose, a component of lactose, is an important nutrient for newborn infants and young children. In human breast milk the lactose content is about 7 gm/dl, and in cow's milk the concentration is approximately 5 gm/dl. In the newborn infant lactose may provide as much as 40% of the caloric intake, but only 3–4% in the adult because of lower milk intake. Galactose also is a constituent of many glycoproteins, glycolipids and mucopolysaccharides. The principal pathway for metabolism of galactose has been designated as the 'Leloir Pathway' (Fig. 89.2). Galactose is phosphorylated to galactose-1-phosphate by the enzyme galactokinase. Galactose-1-phosphate is exchanged for the glucose-1-phosphate moiety of uridine diphosphate glucose

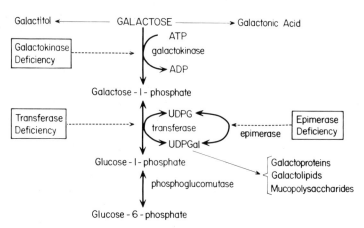

Fig. 89.2 Pathways of galactose metabolism

(UDPG) to form uridine diphosphate galactose (UDPGal) by galactose-1-phosphate uridyltransferase (transferase). The glucose-1-phosphate released leads into the glucose pathway. UDPGal formed is converted to UDPG by the enzyme UDPGal-4-epimerase (epimerase). The sum of these three enzymatic reactions involving galactokinase, transferase, and epimerase is

Galactose + ATP = Glucose-1-phosphate + ADP

UDPGal also is utilized for synthesis of complex galactose-containing carbohydrates. A small amount of galactose is converted to galactitol by aldose reductase and to galactonic acid by galactose dehydrogenase.

All of the three galactose enzymes in the major pathway are widely distributed in tissues, including erythrocytes, leucocytes, skin fibroblasts, liver, kidney, brain and cultured amniotic fluid cells. The gene loci in man for galactokinase, transferase, and epimerase are on chromosomes #17, #9, and #1, respectively (Orkwiszewski et al, 1974; Mohandas et al, 1977; Lin et al, 1979).

Galactokinase deficiency

Clinical aspects

Galactokinase deficiency was first reported by Gitzelmann in 1965. The patient was a 42 year-old man originally described as having galactose diabetes at 9 years of age. Additional patients were reported subsequently. The major clinical manifestations are cataracts and pseudotumour cerebri, both appearing early in infancy. In contrast to the transferase defect, hepatomegaly, jaundice, mental retardation are not usually features of this disorder; yet, isolated reports of one or more of these findings have been made in patients with galactokinase deficiency. Hyperbilirubinaemia was observed in one child (Cook et al, 1971); in another, hepatosplenomegaly (Thalhammer et al, 1968). Generalized seizures and mental deterioration in a 17 year-old patient (Pickering & Hall, 1972) and severe mental retardation in two sibs have also been described (Segal et al, 1979). How these manifestations relate to the basic enzymatic defect is still unclear.

Biochemical aspects

Ingestion of lactose will raise blood galactose concentrations to values as high as 100 mg/dl. As a consequence, galactose appears in the urine. Galactitol and galactonic acid are produced in increased amounts due to diversion of galactose into these secondary pathways and they also appear in the urine. It is thought that the accumulation of galactitol is the cause of cataract formation and cerebral oedema. In contrast to classical galactosaemia (transferase deficiency), amino aciduria and proteinuria are absent. The diagnosis of galactokinase deficiency can be confirmed by measurement of activity of the enzyme in erythrocytes. One should be aware that the activity is

high in the blood of newborns and decreases with age (Ng et al, 1965).

Treatment

Early detection is important because the cataracts can be averted by removing lactose from the diet. Treatment is simple and consists of exclusion of lactose and other sources of galactose from the diet.

Genetic aspects

Galactokinase deficiency is transmitted as an autosomal recessive trait. Parents of affected children exhibit intermediate values of erythrocyte galactokinase activity. Based upon results of newborn screening programs, the frequency of occurrence has been estimated at about 1:250 000. This is in contrast to the findings of a carrier frequency in the general population of approximately 1 in 100 giving an estimated incidence of 1:40 000 (Mayes & Guthrie, 1968). A low activity galactokinase variant (Philadelphia) has been described among Blacks (Tedesco et al, 1977). The presence of this variant in the population renders carrier identification difficult. Galactokinase activity is present in cultured amniotic fluid cells; this provides a means for prenatal diagnosis. Families at risk should receive counselling with the pregnant mother advised to restrict intake of lactose to protect the affected fetus. It is of interest that cataracts were found in offspring of a mother who was heterozygous for galactokinase deficiency (Winder, 1981).

Galactose-1-phosphate uridyltransferase deficiency (galactosaemia)

Clinical aspects

Galactosaemia probably was first described in 1908 by von Reuss, but it was not until 1956 that Kalckar and his associates established the defect in activity of the enzyme galactose-1-phosphate uridyltransferase. Untreated patients show distinctive manifestations early in life. The infant appears normal at birth, and symptoms usually do not develop until milk feedings are given. Food may be refused; vomiting is common, and diarrhea occurs occasionally. Other manifestations include lethargy, hypotonia, jaundice, hepatomegaly and susceptibility to infection. Later, in untreated patients, cataracts become evident, and physical and mental retardation occur. The clinical course of many infants is fulminant, and death occurs early from inanition, infection and hepatic failure. In some individuals the course is much milder and may even escape early detection.

Biochemical aspects

Galactosaemia may be suspected on clinical grounds, but laboratory confirmation is essential. Many of the tests formerly used for diagnosis depended upon ingestion of galactose. This approach should not be employed because it is hazardous to the patient. Direct enzyme assay in erythrocytes can be carried out readily to confirm the diagnosis. On a galactose-containing diet, affected individuals excrete large amounts of galactose, galactitol and galactonic acid in the urine. Gross generalized amino aciduria and proteinuria are also evident. The erythrocyte galactose-1-phosphate level is elevated. It is believed that this compound produces hepatic damage, whereas galactitol accounts for the formation of cataracts.

There are many reliable methods for measurement of erythrocyte transferase activity; affected individuals exhibit either little or no activity in their red blood cells. Earlier blood transfusions in patients will interfere with or invalidate the interpretation of the assay because transferase is present in the donor cells. Under this circumstance, studies on both parents to determine heterozygosity can be helpful in reaching a presumptive diagnosis. Neonatal screening has been initiated effectively in many countries. Methods depend upon the measurement of galactose and/or galactose-1-phosphate by microbiological assays (Guthrie, 1968) or measurement of transferase activity by a fluorometric technique (Beutler & Baluda, 1966). The microbiological assays will detect both galactokinase and transferase defects, whereas the enzyme assay is limited to recognition of the transferase defect. Due to the high frequency of Duarte variants (described later), the Duarte-galactosaemia compound heterozygotes (D/G) are not infrequently picked up in neonatal screening programmes utilizing the fluorescent spot test. Infants who are D/G compound heterozygotes have 20–25% of normal activity and often show significant elevations of erythrocyte galactose-1-phosphate. Some of the values approximate those found for affected galactosaemia patients. The children are asymptomatic, and the necessity for dietary treatment is not established.

Treatment
Treatment is directed toward minimizing the accumulation of galactose and its metabolites in body tissues by excluding milk and milk-containing products from the diet. Various milk substitutes are available (casein hydrolysates, soybean formulas). While a galactose-free diet is the basis of treatment, supplementary measures often are required in the neonate to correct secondary manifestations, such as hypoglycaemia, hyperbilirubinaemia, hypoprothrombinaemia, Gram-negative sepsis and anaemia. The infections respond poorly to antibiotic therapy unless dietary therapy also is initiated. The immediate effects of dietary treatment are dramatic with reversal of the acute manifestations. Galactose restriction is compatible with good general health and normal patterns of physical development. Treated patients as a group can achieve normal intelligence scores. On the other hand, poor dietary control may lead to mental and physical retardation. Although galactosaemic men and women have had normal offspring, a large number of female patients have ovarian hypofunction (Kaufman et al, 1979) while gonadal function in adult males appears to be normal.

Genetic aspects
Galactosaemia has been found in all races. The frequency of occurrence of galactosaemia based upon newborn screening results is approximately 1:60 000. The disorder is transmitted as an autosomal recessive condition. Carriers can be identified and exhibit about one-half of normal erythrocyte transferase activity. However, transferase polymorphism renders identification of carriers difficult unless electrophoretic analysis is carried out simultaneously with activity measurements.

Several biochemical variants of transferase have been described. Some are asymptomatic; others associated with disease. The two most common variants are the Duarte (Beutler et al, 1965) and the Los Angeles (Ng et al, 1973). These are not associated with any clinical symptoms of disease. Both variant enzymes can be distinguished from the normal by their banding pattern on electrophoresis. The Duarte variant is a low-activity variant; erythrocyte transferase activity in the homozygote is similar to that for the galactosaemia heterozygote, about one-half normal. The Los Angeles variant has a slightly higher than normal activity. The frequencies of the occurence of Duarte variant/normal heterozygotes and the Los Angeles/normal heterozygotes are 10–12% and 5%, respectively. A third asymptomatic transferase variant designated as the 'Berne variant' exhibits decreased activity and slower electrophoretic mobility than normal (Scherz et al, 1976). Several transferase variants have been described which are associated with clinical manifestations similar to classical galactosaemia. These include the Negro (Segal, 1969), Indiana (Chacko et al, 1971), Rennes (Schapira & Kaplan, 1969), Chicago (Chacko et al, 1977), and atypical galactosaemia (Matz et al, 1975; Lang et al, 1980). Different physicochemical properties have been described for each variant enzyme, but no attempt has been made to compare one to another in the same study. Symptoms of the 'Rennes' and the 'Indiana' variants are said to be more severe than the 'Negro'. All of these very low activity variants can be identified upon neonatal screening (Ng et al, 1978) but require special biochemical approaches to be differentiated from classical galactosaemia. Recently, the authors have studied a 6 month-old patient with bilateral lenticular cataracts suspected of galactokinase deficiency. The defect turned out to be a variant form of transferase deficiency (less than 5% of normal activity).

Prenatal diagnosis of galactosaemia is feasible and has successfully been performed in a number of instances

(Ng et al, 1977). Galactitol concentration in amniotic fluid of an affected fetus was shown to be elevated (Allen et al, 1980). Prenatal diagnosis in this disorder may have the value in determining the need for dietary restriction of lactose during pregnancy.

Uridine diphosphate galactose-4-epimerase deficiency
Deficiency of uridine diphosphate galactose-4-epimerase is not usually associated with any known clinical problem. The decrease in epimerase activity is confined to the red cells and is not manifest in nucleated cells, such as liver, cultured skin fibroblasts and lymphocytes (Gitzelmann et al, 1976). The deficiency is attributed to the presence of an unstable variant enzyme requiring higher NAD concentration for maximum activity. The mode of inheritance is autosomal recessive in which the heterozygote exhibits about one-half normal erythrocyte epimerase activity. The erythrocyte galactose-1-phosphate concentration in early infancy may reach levels as high as 50 mg/dl, and affected individuals may be suspected of having galactosaemia on screening with the use of the microbiological assay. No treatment is required. Recently a case of epimerase deficiency with symptoms similar to classical galactosaemia was reported (Holton et al, 1981). The patient improved after restriction of galactose feeding.

DISORDERS OF FRUCTOSE METABOLISM

Fructose metabolism
Fructose is a monosaccharide found in honey, fruits and other plant tissues. In combination with glucose it forms the disaccharide sucrose. It also exists in a number of oligosaccharides, such as raffinose (a trisaccharide) and stachyose (a tetrasaccharide). The latter is found abundantly in legumes. Ingested sucrose is hydrolyzed by intestinal sucrase to glucose and fructose. The oligosaccharides raffinose and stachyose, which also contain galactose and glucose, are not digested in man.

The liver plays a dominant role in the metabolism of fructose; other organs metabolize fructose, but to a lesser extent (Fig. 89.3). The overall process results in conversion of the sugar to glycolytic intermediates leading either to the formation of glucose or to lactic acid. In the liver, fructose is phosphorylated to fructose-1-phosphate (F-1-P) in the presence of fructokinase. This enzyme is also present in kidney and in intestinal mucosa. Fructokinase is not present in muscle, adipose tissue and blood cells, and in these tissues fructose is phosphorylated to fructose-6-phosphate by hexokinase (Herman & Zakim, 1968). In the liver, F-1-P is further metabolized to D-glyceraldehyde and dihydroxyacetone phosphate by F-1-P aldolase or 'aldolase B'. Aldolase B differs from aldolases A and C in that the latter isozymes act principally on fructose-1,6-diphosphate. In the seminal vesicles, the lens of the eye and peripheral nerves, fructose can be metabolized to sorbitol. In normal subjects, in vivo radioisotopic studies (Landau et al, 1971) have shown that fructose is converted to glucose solely by way of F-1-P. Sorbitol does not appear to be an intermediate. In two patients with hereditary fructose intolerance due to F-1-P aldolase deficiency, it was estimated that 12–20% of fructose was metabolized by way of fructose-6-phosphate.

In man, deficiencies in hepatic fructokinase and F-1-P aldolase have been described. Inactivity of fructokinase is responsible for essential fructosuria (fructosaemia), whereas deficiency of F-1-P aldolase results in hereditary fructose intolerance. Fructose-1,6-diphosphatase deficiency is sometimes included among the disorders of fructose metabolism, but it seems more appropriate to

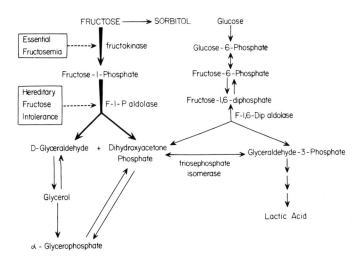

Fig. 89.3 Pathways of fructose metabolism

list it as one of the gluconeogenic disorders described later in this chapter.

Essential fructosuria (fructosaemia)

The incidence of this benign condition is estimated as 1:130 000 in the general population (Froesch, 1978). However, essential fructosuria usually causes no symptoms and the incidence may be somewhat higher. Transmission follows an autosomal recessive pattern. The genetic defect is a deficiency of hepatic fructokinase (Schapira et al, 1961/62). Ingested fructose is not well metabolized by the liver and reaches high level in the blood with overflow into the urine. The presence of the sugar in the urine can readily be demonstrated. No treatment is necessary.

Hereditary fructose intolerance (HFI)

Clinical aspects

The clinical manifestations in individuals with HFI may vary with the age at which fructose is introduced into the diet and with quantity of sugar ingested. In infants, ingestion of fructose may produce findings similar to those found in galactosaemia, e.g. failure to thrive, vomiting, hepatomegaly, oedema, hyperbilirubinaemia and seizures. Because many formulae contain sucrose, the opportunities of an affected infant for exposure to fructose are increased accordingly. In older children and in adults with HFI, ingestion of fructose lowers the blood glucose level precipitously. Pallor, vomiting, sweating, and even coma may be manifest. It is typical for these individuals to develop a strong aversion for all sweets as a protective mechanism.

Biochemical aspects

The biochemical defect in HFI is a deficiency of liver fructose-1-phosphate aldolase. Enzyme activity is usually less than 10% of normal when F-1-P is utilized as the assay substrate, and between 10 and 50% of normal when fructose-1,6-diphosphate is the substrate. The enzyme deficiency also can be demonstrated in intestinal mucosa. Blood cells cannot be utilized for diagnosis since the enzyme is not present in leukocytes or erythrocytes.

Whereas the diagnosis of HFI can be suspected on clinical grounds, laboratory confirmation is essential. Untreated patients ingesting fructose in their diet excrete large amounts of this sugar in their urine and also show a gross generalized amino aciduria. A fructose tolerance test is a useful first step in facilitating diagnosis before assay of the enzyme, which requires either a biopsy sample of liver or intestinal mucosa. Administration of fructose, either orally or parenterally, is followed by a fall in the blood glucose level and serum inorganic phosphate presumably due to its utilization in the formation of fructose-1-phosphate; the rise in uric acid is thought to result from rapid degradation of purine nucleotides to uric acid. The hypoglycaemia is related to inhibition of glycogenolysis by F-1-P (van den Berghe et al, 1973).

HFI may be confused biochemically with tyrosinosis in early infancy insofar as elevation of blood tyrosine and methionine levels have been observed in some cases, presumably because of liver damage (Grant et al, 1970). The gross generalized amino aciduria is akin to that seen in galactosaemia patients and may result from toxic action of F-1-P on the proximal renal tubules. Observation of frustosuria, however, serves to distinguish HFI from galactosaemia or tyrosinosis.

Treatment

The clinical manifestions in young infants with HFI may be severe, and prompt elimination of fructose from the diet is important. Major sources of fructose include cane sugar, honey, fruits and formulae utilizing sucrose as the source of carbohydrate. The prognosis for treated patients is good. Liver and kidney damage is reversed, and neurological residuals are uncommon. The use of fructose infusion as a source of calories in hospitalized patients must be approached with caution until it is known that the patient does not have HFI.

Genetic aspects

The frequency of occurrence of HFI in the general population is not known because many patients with HFI may go unrecognized. An incidence of 1:20 000 has been reported for Switzerland (Gitzelmann et al, 1973). The defect is inherited as an autosomal recessive trait. Heterozygote detection has been complicated by relative inaccessibility of tissue for enzyme assay and the inability to differentiate normals from heterozygotes by parenteral loading with fructose (Beyreiss et al, 1968). Biochemical studies of F-1-P aldolase from liver biopsies of 5 patients with HFI using antibody techniques suggest that genetic heterogeneity probably is common (Gitzelmann et al, 1974).

ESSENTIAL PENTOSURIA

Essential pentosuria is a benign disorder encountered principally in Jews and is inherited as an autosomal recessive trait. The urine contains L-xylulose which is excreted in increased amounts because of a block in the conversion of xylulose to xylitol. The condition is usually discovered accidentally and no treatment is required.

GLYCOGEN STORAGE DISEASES

Glycogen metabolism

Glycogen is the principal storage form of carbohydrate in animal cells; it is present in virtually every type of tissue. Glycogen is a polymer composed of highly branched chains of glucose molecules. The glucose units are linked in the 1–4 positions, whereas the branch points are attached in 1–6 linkages. Glycogen molecules are relatively large, spherical structures, and their aggregations are easily recognizable by electron microscopy in cell cytoplasm. Liver has the highest glycogen content of all tissues, usually 3–5 g/100g. Skeletal muscle normally contains 1–1.5 g/100g. The glycogen content of liver increases following carbohydrate-rich meals and decreases during periods of fasting. During a fast, liver glycogen is degraded to glucose which is released into the circulation to maintain glucose homoeostasis.

The regulation of glycogenolysis in the liver is complex (Fig. 89.4). The most clearly defined mechanism involves activation of the enzyme adenyl cyclase (AC) by the hormones glucagon or epinephrine. This increases the cyclic adenosine monophosphate (cAMP) level in the cytosol which in turn activates protein kinase, phosphorylase kinase and phosphorylase in rapid sequence by phosphorylation of these enzymes (Hers, 1976). Phosphorylase acts upon the terminal units of the glycogen chains liberating glucose-1-phosphate (Glu-1-P). Debrancher enzyme removes branch points and liberates free glucose. Approximately 7% of the glycosyl units are released as free glucose.

Several other factors have been shown to affect the activity of phosphorylase. Vasopressin (Keppens & de Wulf, 1975) and angiotensin II (Keppens & de Wulf, 1976) both activate phosphorylase without increasing cAMP. Ionic calcium enhances, and potassium ion inhibits phosphorylase activation. Insulin acts at several levels to inhibit phosphorylase activity (van de Werve et al, 1977). An amylase is present in hepatocytes which removes oligosaccharide chains, 3–5 units long, from

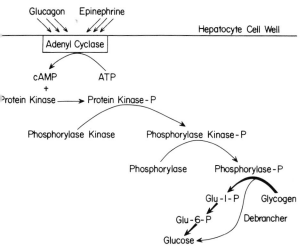

Fig. 89.4 Sequential activation of the enzymes in glycogenolysis

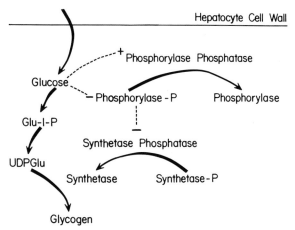

Fig. 89.5 Regulation of glycogen synthesis

glycogen. Lysosomal acid maltase breaks down these oligosaccharides and provides an alternate pathway for glycogen catabolism.

The rate of glycogen synthesis increases when the concentrations of glucose and insulin rise in the blood, and the glucagon level falls. When the concentration of glucose in the hepatocyte increases, binding of glucose to phosphorylase (Fig. 89.5) causes partial inactivation of that enzyme (Stalmans et al, 1974). At the same time, binding of glucose to phosphorylase phosphatase enhances the conversion of phosphorylase to the inactive form. The decrease in active phosphorylase diminishes inhibition of glycogen synthetase phosphatase (Stalmans et al, 1971), thereby promoting the conversion of glycogen synthetase to the active (dephosphorylated) form. Insulin sitmulates the activation of glycogen synthetase, apparently through inactivation of phosphorylase (Wittens & Avruch, 1978). A fall in glucagon concentration in blood also leads to deactivation of phosphorylase and inhibition of glycogenolysis.

Glycogen synthesis involves the following steps:

1. Glu-1-P + UTP ———— UDPG + PP
   (UDPG pyrophosphorylase)
2. UDPG + glycogen$_{(n)}$———— glycogen$_{(n+1)}$+ UDP
   (glycogen synthetase)

Glycogen synthetase adds glucosyl units to the ends of the chains. Brancher enzyme adds new branch points and initiates the formation of additional branch chains.

The disorders of glycogen metabolism, generally named glycogen storage diseases (GSD), result from deficiencies of various enzymes in the catabolic pathways of glycogen metabolism. They can be divided into those disorders in which hepatomegaly is the dominant feature, and those in which muscle involvement is paramount. Glycogen storage diseases originally were named numerically: GSD type I (glucose-6-phosphatase deficiency) through GSD type VI (hepatic phosphorylase deficiency). The authors prefer to designate the disorders according to the enzyme deficiency.

GSD with marked hepatomegaly

Glucose-6-phosphatase deficiency (GSD type Ia, von Gierke's disease).

Clinical aspects. This disorder, described in 1929 by von Gierke, was the first abnormality of glycogen metabolism to be recognized. Clinical manifestations usually appear in the first six months of life. The infants are mildly obese and have abdominal distension and hepatomegaly, but no splenomegaly. Brief periods of fasting (3–4 hours) result in severe hypoglycaemia and acidosis. Perspiration is excessive, and older children complain of heat intolerance. Epistaxis and easy bruising are common. Bowel movements tend to be loose. Renomegaly is characteristic, but renal function is normal in childhood. Affected infants and children are prone to severe lactic acidosis during minor infections and until recently, the mortality rate was high. In older untreated children, growth is slow, and sexual development is incomplete.

Uric acid production is increased, and its renal clearance is decreased. As a consequence, gout and urinary tract stones are seen in many affected children. Hyperlipidaemia is invariably present and may cause cutaneous xanthoma. Hepatic adenomata often develop by adolescence (Howell et al, 1976; Miller et al, 1978), and several patients have died of hepatocellular carcinoma (Zangenek et al, 1969), suggesting that the adenomata are premalignant lesions. Uric acid nephropathy and/or diffuse interstitial nephritis (Hollings, 1963), nephrotic syndrome and renal failure (Sonobe et al, 1976), may occur during the second or third decade of life. Other complications are bony fractures, neurologic deficits and seizures, acute pancreatitis (Michels & Beaudet, 1980) and pulmonary hypertension (Pizzo, 1980). There is variability in the severity of manifestations in GSD type I. A few patients are mildly affected and may be discovered as adults with hepatomegaly and gout (Stamm & Webb, 1975).

Biochemical aspects. The production of glucose by glycogenolysis and gluconeogenesis is markedly reduced because of glucose-6-phosphatase deficiency in liver and kidney (Fig. 89.6). Normal plasma glucose concentration cannot be maintained in the postprandial state; this results in inhibition of insulin, and enhancement of glucagon release from the pancreas. This stimulates glycogen breakdown in the liver but, in the absence of Glu-6-phosphatase, lactic and pyruvic acids are produced in excess instead of glucose (Sadeghi-Nejad et al, 1974). The laboratory findings are characteristic. Blood obtained after a brief fasting period reveals hypoglycaemia (10–30 mg/dl) and elevated lactic acid levels (50–100 mg/dl). Hyperlipidaemia and hyperuricemia are

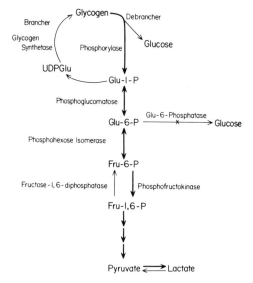

Fig. 89.6 Glycogen metabolism and enzyme deficiency (Glu-6-phosphatase) in GSD type I

almost always present. Glucagon administration causes little, if any, rise in blood glucose but a marked rise in blood lactate. Other types of GSD which are clinically similar to GSD type I (Debrancher and phosphorylase deficiencies) have normal fasting blood lactate levels (Fernandes et al, 1969). Fructose-1,6-diphosphatase deficiency is also similar to GSD type I, and measurement of hepatic enzyme activities is necessary for differential diagnosis. In GSD type I, the histologic abnormalities in liver include steatosis, glycogenosis and mild periportal fibrosis. Glu-6-phosphatase activity is absent in both liver and kidney. More than one enzyme deficiency in the same patient has been reported (Service et al, 1978); however, it is not clear whether a double enzyme defect or adaptive inactivation of one of the enzymes is involved (Moses et al, 1966).

Treatment. Frequent feedings of carbohydrate during the daytime and the infusion of a concentrated glucose solution at night via nasogastric tube or by gastrostomy (Greene et al, 1976) are used to maintain euglycaemia. This regimen reduces the elevated blood levels of lactate, uric acid and lipids. There also is marked improvement in growth and strength (Greene et al, 1979). The long term effects of this therapy on hepatoma formation and other complications remain to be determined (Roe et al, 1979). Allopurinol may be needed for controlling hyperuricaemia.

Genetic aspects. Glu-6-phosphatase is inherited as an autosomal recessive disease. The incidence is estimated to be 1:200 000 births but may be higher in some population groups. A method for prenatal diagnosis has not been established. Glu-6-Phosphatase activity is reported to be present in placenta (Matalon et al, 1977) and in amniotic fluid epithelial cells (Negishi et al, 1977), but not in fibroblasts cultured from amniotic fluid.

Glycogen storage disease type Ib
Some individuals with all of the clinical and biochemical manifestations of Glu-6-phosphatase deficiency have normal activity of this enzyme when their liver tissue is assayed after freezing. However, when the assay is performed on fresh tissue, and efforts are made to avoid disruption of the endoplasmic reticulum, Glu-6-phosphatase activity cannot be demonstrated (Narisawa et al, 1978). It is thought that GSD type Ib is the result of a transport defect in the system which carries Glu-6-P into the lumen of the tubules of the endoplasmic reticulum (Lange et al, 1980). Glu-6-phosphatase is believed to be located on the luminal surface of these tubules. Neutropenia and recurrent mouth lesions are characteristic of GSD type Ib, but are not seen in type Ia (Beaudet et al, 1980; McCabe et al, 1980). The inheritance pattern appears to be autosomal recessive.

Amylo-1,6-glucosidase (debrancher) deficiency (GSD type III, limit dextrinosis, Cori's disease)

Clinical aspects. The clinical manifestations can be recognised during infancy. Abdominal distension due to hepatomegaly is moderate or marked; splenomegaly is minimal or absent. Hypoglycaemia is usually mild and often accompanied by ketonuria after overnight fasting. Muscular hypotonia is common and may be the primary complaint. There is no bleeding tendency, heat intolerance, loose stools, rapid breathing or enlargement of the kidneys. Most of these children survive childhood without difficulty. Slow growth and abdominal enlargement improve as they mature but muscular weakness may increase (Brunberg et al, 1971). Hepatic failure and hepatoma have not been reported in adult patients.

Biochemical aspects. Absence of debrancher enzyme results in glycogen accumulation in the liver and in many other tissues, including leucocytes and erythrocytes. The tendency for hypoglycaemia is minimized by gluconeogenesis and the availability of the outer tiers of the glycogen molecules for degradation to glucose.

Marked elevation of serum transaminase activity is common, but there is no other evidence of hepatic dysfucntion. Hyperlipidaemia may be present but hyperuricaemia is usually absent. Blood lactate levels are normal in the fasting state and there is no rise in blood glucose or lactate values following glucagon administration. A characteristic increase in blood lactate following the oral administration of glucose, fructose or galactose (2 g/kg) has been described (Fernandes et al, 1969).

Histological examination of the liver shows increased fat and glycogen in the hepatocytes and mild periportal fibrosis. Debrancher deficiency can be confirmed by demonstrating absence of enzyme activity in liver and in muscle. Cultured fibroblasts may be used to confirm debrancher deficiency. Erythrocytes and leucocytes also have been used for diagnosis, but the results have been equivocal (Deckelbaum et al, 1972).

Treatment. Therapy is directed toward preventing hypoglycaemia by frequent feedings and avoidance of prolonged periods of fasting. Limitation of fat intake for those individuals with hyperlipidaemia seems prudent. In most intances, growth is only moderately decreased. In those patients who have marked growth retardation, nightly intragastric glucose infusion therapy can be used to promote growth.

Genetic aspects. The genetics of GSD type III may be more complex than is presently known. Amylo-1,6-glucosidase (debrancher) and another enzyme, oligo-1,4 1,4-glucan transferase are both associated with the same cellular protein (Brown & Illingworth, 1964). Deficiency of either or both activities would be expected to result in the same clinical picture. These two enzyme activities are presumably under separate genetic control. Absence of debrancher activity in liver is usually associated with the same deficiency in muscle; however, deficiency of this enzyme limited to the liver also has been described. The overall incidence of this disease is estimated to be approximately 1:200 000 (Huijing, 1973), but it is much more common in Israel (Levin et al, 1967). Debrancher enzyme determination in amniotic fluid fibroblasts should provide a means of prenatal diagnosis.

Hepatic phosphorylase (GSD type VI), phosphorylase kinase (GSD type IX), and phosphorylase activating system deficiencies (including protein kinase deficiency, GSD type X)

Clinical aspects. These disorders are less well defined than GSD types I and III; however, their clinical appearance is similar to those disorders (de Barsy & Lederer, 1980) and usually recognizable in the first 2 years of life. Affected children exhibit abdominal enlargement because of hepatomegaly, mild adiposity, hypotonia and growth failure. Hypoglycaemia is either mild or absent. Lactic acidosis, bleeding tendency and loose bowel movements are not seen. Although growth is retarded in childhood, normal height and complete sexual development are eventually achieved. Abdominal distension and hepatomegaly may decrease or disappear by adolescence.

Biochemical aspects. Deficiency of phosphorylase (or one of the enzymes that leads to its activation) obstructs glycogen degradation in the liver, and absence of fasting hypoglycaemia is related to the fact that phosphorylase activity usually is only partially deficient and hepatic gluconeogenesis is intact.

Laboratory studies reveal a moderate elevation of serum transaminase values and hyperlipidaemia. Fasting blood glucose, lactic and uric acid levels are normal. Blood lactate values rise following meals and after glucose, galactose or fructose ingestion. Glucagon administration is reported to cause a minimal glycaemic response in patients with phosphorylase deficiency but a normal glycemic response in phosphorylase kinase deficiency (Koster et al, 1973). In the authors' experience with these disorders, response to glucagon has been variable. Liver tissue obtained by biopsy shows steatosis, glycogenosis, and minimal periportal fibrosis. Enzyme assay reveals 75–90% reduction in phosphorylase activity in both phosphorylase or phosphorylase activating system deficiency. The phosphorylase activating system is considered to be defective if liver tissue does not activate purified phosphorylase. If liver phosphorylase cannot be activated by purified phosphorylase kinase, phosphorylase itself is considered abnormal. Phosphorylase and phosphorylase kinase activities in muscle are usually normal in these disorders, and the cause of the hypotonia is not clear. Protein kinase (cyclic 3'5'-AMP dependent kinase) deficiency is reported to involve both liver and muscle (Hug et al, 1970).

Treatment. Hypoglycaemia is not a problem, therefore no special feeding programme is necessary. Because of liver enlargement, activities which might lead to abdominal trauma, such as contact sports, should be limited.

Genetic aspects. All of the enzyme deficiencies of the phosphorylase system are inherited as autosomal recessive defects, with the exception of phosphorylase kinase deficiency. Both autosomal recessive (Hug, et al, 1969; Lederer et al, 1975) and X–linked recessive inheritance (Huijing and Fernandez, 1969) of phosphorylase kinase deficiency have been reported. The incidence of these disorders considered as a group is of the same order as GSD type I (1:200 000).

The authors are not aware of reports of prenatal diagnosis for these disorders. Detection of the carrier state (mothers of the patients) of X–linked phosphorylase kinase deficiency has been reported (Huijing, 1970).

Brancher deficiency (GSD type IV amylopectinosis, Andersen's disease)

Clinical aspects. Brancher deficiency is one of the rarest and least studied of the glycogen storage diseases. Affected infants begin to show evidence of disease within the first year of life, and death by 2–4 years appears to be the usual outcome. Features of hepatic failure and portal hypertension appear including growth failure, jaundice, splenomegaly and a prominent abdominal venous pattern. Hypotonia is common, and hypoglycaemia is absent (Andersen, 1952).

Biochemical aspects. An abnormal form of glycogen, with long chains and infrequent branch points accumulates in many cell types, including hepatocytes, skeletal

and myocardial muscle cells, fibroblasts, leucocytes and nerve cells. Hepatic cirrhosis is presumed to result from the abnormal glycogen. Carbohydrate and glucagon tolerance tests usually are normal, provided that liver failure is not severe at the time of testing.

Deficiency of brancher enzyme can be demonstrated in liver, in leucocytes (Brown & Brown, 1966) and in cultured skin fibroblasts (Howell, et al, 1971). In histologic sections of liver, staining of the abnormal glycogen with iodine produces a distinctive blue color. This disease must be differentiated from other forms of liver failure in infancy, such as neonatal hepatitis, biliary atresia, polycystic disease of liver and kidney, and alpha-1-antitrypsin deficiency.

Treatment. No form of therapy has been successful.

Genetic aspects. This disorder is inherited as an autosomal recessive defect. Heterozygotes appear to be identifiable by enzyme assay of cultured skin fibroblasts. The enzyme is normally present in cultured amniotic fluid cells, and these cells may be useful for prenatal diagnosis.

GSD primarily involving muscle

Acid alpha-glucosidase (AAG) deficiency (GSD type II, Pompe's disease, acid maltase deficiency, alpha-1,4-glucosidase deficiency)

Clinical aspects. AAG deficiency was first recognized in severely affected infants. Subsequently 2 and possibly 3 clinical syndromes of muscle involvment associated with AAG deficiency have been identified (Tanaka et al, 1979). In these disorders, glycogen accumulates in a variety of tissues. Involvement of cardiac muscle is most significant for the affected infant (Kahana et al, 1964).

In the infantile form of GSD type II, manifestations appear between birth and 6 months of age. The clinical features are hypotonia, macroglossia, moderate hepatosplenomegaly, cardiomegaly and congestive heart failure. The condition is progressive, leading to death by 1–3 years of age. Characteristic electrocardiographic abnormalities include rapid pulse conduction (short PR interval), wide amplitude QRS complex and changes of left ventricular hypertrophy. Histologic examination reveals glycogen accumulation in virtually every cell type. The excess glycogen is characteristically found within membrane-bound structures (lysosomes) as well as free in the cytoplasm.

The late-onset forms of GSD type II (Engle et al, 1973) may be manifest in childhood or in the second or third decades of life. Skeletal muscle weakness, decreased exercise tolerance and decreased respiratory reserve are the usual clinical features. Hepatomegaly and cardiomegaly usually are absent. Death may result from complications of respiratory insufficiency.

The infantile form of GSD type II is distinct clinically, but severe skeletal muscle weakness may dominate the clinical picture, and it may be confused with neuromuscular disorders of infancy, such as Werdnig-Hoffman disease. The late-onset form(s) may be confused with other causes of muscular weakness in children and adults. Tests of carbohydrate tolerance and metabolism are normal in all of the forms.

Biochemical aspects. Alpha-1,4- and alpha-1,6-glucosidase activities are normally associated with a single lysosomal protein (Brown et al, 1970). These activities promote hydrolysis of glycogen to glucose, and absence of these enzymes results in glycogen accumulation within lysosomes.

AAG deficiency is demonstrable in liver, muscle, and cultured skin fibroblasts. The results of enzyme assay in mixed leucocyte preparations must be interpreted with caution. Only isolated lymphocytes or cultured lymphocytes, but not granulocytes (i.e. polymorphonuclear cells), are suitable for diagnosis and carrier detection (Taniguchi et al, 1978). Granulocytes contain 'renal' maltase which is active in patient's cells (Dreyfus & Poenaru, 1980). Thus, some patients may have normal acid maltase activity in mixed leucocyte preparations if these preparations contain predominantly granulocytes (Potter et al, 1980).

The difference between the infantile and late-onset forms may be due to a more complete deficiency of enzyme activity in the infantile form (Beratis et al, 1978a). A cross-reacting material (CRM) negative and a CRM positive form of infantile GSD type II have been reported (Beratis et al, 1978b).

Treatment. There is no specific therapy for this enzyme deficiency. The administration of purified α-glucosidase was not effective (Hug, 1974; Tyrrell, 1976).

Genetic aspects. The infantile and late-onset forms are inherited as autosomal recessive disorders. The carrier state can be identified by assay of cultured fibroblasts. Prenatal diagnosis is possible (Salafsky & Nadler, 1971).

Myophosphorylase (MP) deficiency (GSD type V, McArdle disease)

Clinical aspects. Glycogen MP deficiency usually becomes manifest in late adolescence or in the second decade of life (McArdle, 1951). The principal symptoms are pain and stiffness of muscles during exercise (Fattah et al, 1970). Strenuous activity can result in myoglobinuria. Several instances of acute renal failure due to rhabdomyolysis have been reported (Grunfeld et al, 1972). Muscle groups which are stressed may become swollen and tender. In later life, chronic muscle weakness may develop (Engle et al, 1963).

Biochemical aspects. The manifestations result from deficient energy production in muscle. During muscle activity, glycogen normally is broken down, and the energy for muscle contraction is derived from glycolysis.

Glycogen degradation is blocked in MP deficiency, and the defect in glycolysis is reflected in the absence of lactate production by muscle during ischaemic exercise.

Other disorders of muscle metabolism have similar clinical features, and therefore muscle biopsy for enzyme analysis may be necessary for diagnosis. Muscle histology shows damaged fibres, increased glycogen content and absence of MP activity. MP activity may be present in regenerating fibres due to the presence of a fetal-type isozyme. This isozyme has been demonstrated in cultured muscle cells from affected individuals (Meienhofer et al, 1977). Phosphorylase activity in liver is normal in this disease.

Treatment. The treatment for McArdle disease is to avoid strenuous activity. Because the muscle symptoms result from lack of substrate (particularly fatty acids), the symptoms can be minimized by warming-up exercises which mobilize fatty acids from fat stores (Porte et al, 1966).

Genetic aspects. This is a rare disorder, inherited as an autosomal recessive trait (Schmid & Hammaker, 1961). Two varieties of enzyme deficiency have been found, one lacking the enzyme protein and the other with an apparently inactive enzyme protein (Feit & Brooke, 1976). Prenatal diagnosis is not practical because muscle tissue is needed for the assay. Furthermore, prenatal diagnosis may be complicated by the presence of the fetal isozyme which is under separate genetic control.

Muscle phosphofructokinase (PFK) deficiency (GSD type VII)

Clinical aspects. The clinical features of PFK deficiency are very similar to those of McArdle disease (Tarui, 1965). Exercise tolerance is limited by muscle cramps and pain. Symptoms usually begin during childhood and may be very mild or very severe. Strenuous exercise may be followed by muscle pain, malaise, nausea and myoglobinuria (Tobin et al, 1973).

Biochemical aspects. Laboratory studies show elevation of muscle enzyme values (muscle aldolase, creatine phosphokinase, lactate dehydrogenase and oxaloacetate transaminase) in the serum. The reticulocyte count is mildly increased, but there is no anaemia. Muscle fibres show increased glycogen content and vacuolar and degenerative changes. The activity of PFK is absent in muscle and reduced in erythrocytes. The PFK molecule appears to be a tetramer. The muscle isozyme is composed of 4 identical (M) subunits, whereas erythrocyte PFK is made up of two different subunits (M and R). In PFK deficiency disease, the M subunit is absent and the residual PFK activity in erythrocytes reflects presence of the R subunit (Layzer & Rasmussen, 1974).

Treatment. Treatment of PFK deficiency is the same as that of MP deficiency: avoidance of strenuous exercise.

Genetic aspects. PFK deficiency is rare. It appears to be inherited as an autosomal recessive disorder.

Other glycogenoses

Hepatic glycogenosis with Fanconi's renal tubular defect and vitamin D-resistant rickets. This infrequently reported syndrome is recognized in infants on the basis of rickets, hepatomegaly and growth failure associated with increased renal clearance of glucose, amino acids, protein, phosphate and uric acid (Garty et al, 1974). Affected patients have either low or normal fasting plasma glucose levels and normal fasting blood lactate values. After oral administration of galactose, there is an excessive rise in blood lactate. The glycaemic response to glucagon is variable. Histologic findings show increased glycogen content in liver and muscle and steatosis of liver. Rickets is severe but improves with oral phosphate and vitamin D therapy in pharmacologic doses. Pathogenesis of this disorder is unknown; no enzyme deficiency has been identified.

Hepatic glycogenosis with renal glycosuria. The only patient reported thus far was a mentally retarded girl with marked hepatomegaly and renal glycosuria without other renal tubular dysfunctions. Fasting plasma glucose levels were normal. The glycogen content was increased in liver, muscle, erythrocytes and leucocytes. No enzyme defect was identified (Gutman et al, 1965).

Glucose phosphate isomerase (GPI) deficiency. The features of this disorder include severe haemolytic anaemia, hepatomegaly and muscle weakness. Liver and erythrocytes contain excessive amounts of glycogen. GPI activity is decreased in many tissues including erythrocytes and leucocytes (Van Biervliet & Staal, 1977).

Glycogenosis of liver and brain with progressive neurologic deterioration (GSD type VIII). In 1967, Hug et al described a child with hepatomegaly and progressive neurologic deterioration. The glycogen content of liver and brain was increased, and hepatic phosphorylase was in the inactive form. The phosphorylase activating system was normal. No other enzyme abnormality was identified.

GLUCONEOGENIC DISORDERS ASSOCIATED WITH LACTIC ACIDOSIS

Metabolism

The maintenance of carbohydrate homeostasis in the human body is a complex process and involves the interaction of many factors. In fasting conditions blood glucose is derived mainly from glycogen breakdown (glycogenolysis) and from the conversion of lactic acid and certain amino acids to glucose (gluconeogenesis).

Gluconeogenesis takes place primarily in the liver and kidneys. The metabolic process is in part under endocrine control. During a prolonged fast, the levels of glu-

cocorticoids may be increased. These hormones increase the synthesis of pyruvate carboxylase, glucose-6-phosphatase, and aminotransferase, participants in the gluconeogenic pathway. Gluconeogenic amino acids, such as alanine, aspartic acid and glutamic acid are converted to pyruvate, oxaloacetate and α-ketoglutarate, respectively and subsequently feed into the pathway culminating in the formation of glucose (Fig. 89.7). During fasting, epinephrine and glucagon increase, accelerating the glycogenolytic process through the activation of adenyl cyclase (as described in the section on glycogen metabolism). At the other end of the glycolytic pathway, pyruvate kinase is inactivated by a cyclic AMP protein kinase diminishing the coversion of triose phosphate to pyruvate and lactate.

In addition to pyruvate kinase, gluconeogenesis is also tightly regulated by other key enzymes which are sensitive to allosteric control. Pyruvate carboxylase, which plays a primary role in conversion of pyruvate to oxaloacetate, is activated by acetyl CoA. When excess acetyl CoA builds up in cells, glucose synthesis is enhanced. Phosphoenolpyruvate carboxykinase also is necessary for phosphoenolpyruvate formation from oxaloacetate. Other key enzymes in regulating the gluconeogenic pathway are fructose-1,6-diphosphatase and glucose-6-phosphatase. The former is stimulated by citrate and inhibited by AMP. Glucose-6-phosphatase and fructose-1,6-diphosphatase are known to be present only in liver, kidney, and intestinal tissues, whereas the pyruvate carboxylase and phosphoenolpyruvate carboxykinase have been shown to be present in other tissues, including cultured skin fibroblasts. Genetic defects have been encountered in each of these enzymes in man. Hypoglycaemia and lactic acidosis are the most common clinical manifestations. Lactic acidosis frequently may be found in sick infants and children secondary to hypoxia, shock or other disorders. For example, mitochondrial damage observed in Reye's syndrome leads to lactic acidosis (Robinson et al, 1977). Whatever the cause, persistent lactic acidosis usually needs prompt medical attention.

Fructose-1,6-diphosphatase deficiency

Clinical aspects

Symptoms usually begin in early infancy with the clinical manifestation of hypoglycaemia, hyperlactic acidaemia and ketoacidosis (Baker & Winegrad, 1970). The onset often follows an infection. In some patients the onset is delayed and the clinical picture is similar to that of ketotic hypoglycaemia. The most common physical finding is hepatomegaly, resulting from fatty metamorphosis. Despite the metabolic defect, growth and intellectual development may proceed normally. Fructose-1,6-diphosphatase deficiency may be confused with glycogen storage disease type I, because of similarity of

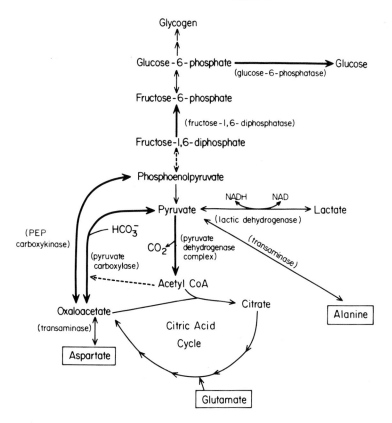

Fig. 89.7 The gluconeogenic pathway

clinical features and of laboratory findings. Confirmation of diagnosis is based upon measurement of fructose-1,6-diphosphatase activity in liver tissue.

Biochemical aspects
Prolonged fasting in the affected patient induces severe hypoglycaemia, lactic acidosis and hyperalaninaemia. The ingestion of glycerol, fructose and alanine produces hypoglycaemia, an increase in lactate and a fall in serum inorganic phosphate. Serum uric acid also may increase. The glycaemic responses to glucagon and galactose administration have been variable.

The biochemical defect is a deficiency in fructose-1,6-diphosphatase activity. This enzyme normally is present in liver, kidney and intestinal tissue. However, it also has been reported to be present in muscle (Krebs & Woodford, 1965), platelets (Karpatkin et al, 1970) and lymphocytes (Fong et al, 1979). It has not yet been established whether study of these tissues ·will truly reflect the patient's overall biochemical and genetic status.

Treatment
Treatment consists of frequent small feedings, in order to prevent hypoglycaemia, and limiting fructose and sor-

bitol intake. It has been suggested that folic acid may increase synthesis of fructose-1,6-diphosphatase (Greene et al, 1972), and its use in affected children should be tested clinically.

Genetic aspects
Fructose-1,6-diphosphatase deficiency is a rare condition inherited as an autosomal recessive trait. In three parents of affected children, intermediate values of enzyme activity were found in the liver (Gitzelmann et al, 1973; Saudubray et al, 1973). If these findings can be extended to platelets or cultured lymphocytes, the identification of carriers would be facilitated greatly.

A family in which both the mother and a 19 month-old daughter were affected has been reported (Tauton et al, 1978). Fructose-1,6-diphosphatase activity in liver and intestinal mucosa was about 25% of normal. Both patients had symptomatic hypoglycaemia. The mother was unable to do her housework without having to stop several times to rest. She had unexplained episodes of crying, chilly sensations and dizziness occurring some two to five hours after meals. Biochemical studies of the liver enzyme from the mother did not reveal any difference in migration upon polyacrylamide gel electrophoresis or in K_m for fructose-1,6-diphosphate.

Pyruvate carboxylase deficiency

Clinical aspects

Clinical manifestations usually appear soon after birth. Metabolic acidosis, failure to thrive, hypotonia, anorexia, and hyporeflexia have been observed. Death within one to two months of age is the rule, in spite of intensive care (Saudubray et al, 1976). Patients surviving the initial problems exhibit retarded growth, seizures, hypotonia, and continuing metabolic acidosis. Laboratory findings include severe lactic acidosis, ketonaemia, hyperammonaemia and in some cases hypoglycaemia. It has been suggested that pyruvate carboxylase deficiency also is associated with Leigh's disease (Hommes et al, 1968). Though the two disorders may involve the same enzyme deficiency, they are now clinically considered to be separate entities.

Biochemical aspects

The enzyme deficiency has been demonstrated in liver tissue. The assay is complicated by its dependency upon the presence of the allosteric activator, acetyl CoA. Furthermore, the enzyme is also labile. Low activities of the enzyme found in liver obtained at autopsy may reflect lability rather than a primary genetic defect. Human leucocytes and cultured skin fibroblasts also exhibit pyruvate carboxylase activity. The enzyme activity in these cells is deficient in affected patients and is intermediate in known carriers (Atkin et al, 1979; Atkin, 1979). The enzyme also is present in cultured amniotic cells, thus offering the potential for prenatal diagnosis.

Treatment

Drastic supportive measures are usually needed. Metabolic acidosis (lactic acidosis) should be corrected promptly. Peritoneal dialysis may be helpful in reversing the clinical consequences of the metabolic defect. Biotin, thiamine and lipoic acid have been used in some patients with questionable benefit. Inclusion of glutamate and aspartic acid in the diet as sources of oxaloacetate has been helpful.

Genetic aspects

Pyruvate carboxylase deficiency is inherited as an autosomal recessive disorder. Only a few cases have been reported, and no data is available regarding the frequency of occurrence.

Phosphoenolpyruvate carboxykinase deficiency

Phosphoenolpyruvate carboxykinase deficiency is rare. One patient had persistent neonatal hypoglycaemia, severe cerebral atrophy, optic nerve atrophy and fatty liver and kidneys. The enzyme defect was demonstrated in liver (Vidnes & Sovik, 1976). Another patient presented at four months of age with failure to thrive, hepatomegaly, hypotonia, developmental delay, lactic acidaemia and fasting hypoglycaemia. Cultured skin fibroblasts showed 19% of normal activity of phosphoenolpyruvate carboxykinase (Robinson et al, 1979).

Deficiencies of pyruvate dehydrogenase complex (PDHC)

Clinical aspects

The extremely variable clinical expression in this grouping suggests both clinical and biochemical heterogeneity. Patients have been described with one or more of the following findings: microcephaly, slow mental and physical development, seizures, optic atrophy of variable degree, cerebellar ataxia along with severe lactic acidosis. Partial deficiency of the enzyme complex also has been observed in patients with spinocerebellar degeneration and in Friedreich's ataxia (Kark & Rodriguez-Budelli, 1979). Patients do not usually have hypoglycaemia, and PDHC has not been considered as a group of key enzymes in gluconeogenesis.

Biochemical aspects

PDHC comprises three principal enzymes (E_1 = pyruvate dehydrogenase or pyruvate decarboxylase, E_2 = dihydrolipoyl transacetylase and E_3 = dihydrolipoyl dehydrogenase) and five different coenzymes (thiamine pyrophosphate, lipoic acid, coenzyme A, flavine adenine dinucleotide and nicotinamide adenine dinucleotide). In addition, a specific kinase for inactivation and a phosphatase for activation of the pyruvate dehydrogenase have been demonstrated. The sequence of the PDHC reactions is as follows (Lehninger, 1975):

(1) $E_1TPP + CH_3COCOOH \rightarrow CO_2 + E_1TPP\text{-}CHOHCH_3$
(2) $E_1TPP\text{-}CHOHCH_3 + E_2lipoic \ (ox) \rightarrow E_1TPP + CH_3COE_2lipoic$
(3) $CH_3COE_2lipoic + CoASH \rightarrow CH_3COSCoA + E_2lipoic \ (red)$
(4) $E_2lipoic \ (red) + E_3FAD \rightarrow E_2lipoic \ (ox) + E_3FADH_2$
(5) $E_3FADH_2 + NAD^+ \rightarrow E_3FAD + NADH + H^+$

Because of the complexity of this enzyme system, it is important to have available reliable methods for each enzyme assay to pinpoint the basic defect. PDHC activity is present in cultured skin fibroblasts, and therefore, this tissue should be a good source for investigation. Caution is needed to avoid mycoplasma contamination because an unusually large amount of pyruvate dehydrogenase activity has been demonstrated in infected cultures (Clark et al, 1978). A single case with dihydrolipoyl dehydrogenase defect (Robinson et al, 1977) and several cases with pyruvate dehydrogenase deficiency have been reported (Stromme et al, 1976; Cedarbaum et al, 1976). In affected patients, the levels of pyruvate, lactate and alanine are increased in blood and urine. In milder cases, random samples of blood or urine may show normal amounts of lactate. Oral glucose loads or high carbohydrate intake may induce elevations in blood lactic acid and aggravate the symptoms.

Treatment

Administration of thiamine and/or lipoic acid has not been helpful. Intravenous glucose administration should be done with caution because it can cause severe lactic acidosis. It is recommended that diet should be high in fats and low in carbohydrates (Cedarbaum et al, 1976). While this diet may be helpful in saving the patient's life, it has not prevented the mental deterioration in severe cases.

Genetic aspects

Available data suggest that deficiencies of PDHC are inherited as autosomal recessive disorders. Because of the several enzymes and cofactors involved, the specific biochemical cause should be demonstrated so as to ascertain the particular mode of inheritance.

The frequency of occurrence of PDHC deficiencies may be greater than now realized. Any patient who has died as a result of lactic acidosis can be suspected of having disorder in the PDHC system. Prenatal diagnosis should be possible because the enzyme system is present in cultured amniotic cells.

REFERENCES

Abraham J M, Levin B, Oberholzer V G, Russell A 1967 Glucose-galactose malabsorption. Archives of Diseases in Childhood 42: 592–597

Allen J T, Gillett M, Holton J B, King G S, Pettit B R 1980 Evidence of galactosemia in utero. Lancet 1: 603

Anderson D H 1952 Studies on glycogen disease with report of a case in which the glycogen was abnormal. In: Najjar V A (ed) Carbohydrate metabolism: a symposium on the clinical biochemical aspects of carbohydrate utilization in health and disease, Johns Hopkins Press, Baltimore, ch 1, p 28

Atkin B M 1979 Carrier detection of pyruvate carboxylase deficiency in fibroblasts and lymphocytes. Pediatric Research 13: 1101–1104

Atkin B M, Utter M F, Weinberg M B 1979 Pyruvate carboxylase and phosphoenolpyruvate carboxykinase activity in leukocytes and fibroblasts from a patient with pyruvate carboxylase deficiency. Pediatric Research 13: 38–43

Baker L, Winegard A I 1970 Fasting hypoglycemia and metabolic acidosis associated with deficiency of hepatic fructose-1,6-diphosphatase activity. Lancet 2: 13–16

Beaudet A L, Anderson D C, Michels V V, Arion W J, Lange A J 1980 Neutropenia and impaired neutrophil migration in type IB glycogen storage disease. Journal of Pediatrics 97: 906–910

Beratis N G, Labadie G U, Hirschhorn K 1978a Characterization of the molecular defect in infantile and adult alpha-glucosidase deficiency fibroblasts. Journal of Clinical Investigation 62: 1264–1274

Beratis N G, Labadie G U, Hirschhorn K 1978b Genetic heterogeneity in acid alpha-glucosidase deficiency. American Journal of Human Genetics 30: 23 A

Beutler E, Baluda M C 1966 A simple spot screening test for galactosemia. Journal of Laboratory and Clinical Medicine 68: 137–141

Beutler E, Baluda M C, Sturgeon P, Day R 1965 A new genetic abnormality resulting in galactose-1-phosphate uridyltransferase deficiency. Lancet 1: 353–354

Beyreiss K, Willgerodt H, Theile H 1968 Untersuchungen bei heterozygoten merkmalsträgern für fructoseintoleranz. Klinische Wochenschrift 46: 465–468

Brown B I, Brown D H 1966 Lack of an alpha-1,4-glucan:alpha-1,4- glucan 6-glucosyl transferase in a case of type IV glycogenosis. Proceedings of the National Academy of Sciences (USA) 56: 725–729

Brown B I, Brown D H, Jeffrey P L 1970 Simultaneous absence of alpha-1,4-glucosidase and alpha-1,6-glucosidase

activities (pH 4) in tissue of children with type II glycogen storage disease. Biochemistry 9: 1423–1428

Brown D H, Illingworth B 1964 The role of olio-1,4→1,4-glucantransferase and amylo-1,6-glucosidase in the debranching of glycogen. In: Whelan W J (ed) Control of glycogen metabolism, Little Brown, Boston, p 139–150

Brunberg A J, McCormick W F, Schochet S S 1971 Type III glycogenosis, an adult with diffuse muscle weakness and muscle wasting. Archives of Neurology 25: 171–178

Burke V, Danks D M 1966 Monosaccharide malabsorption in young infants Lancet 1: 1177–1180

Burman D, Holton J B, Pennock C A (eds) 1980 Inherited disorders of carbohydrate metabolism, MTP Press limited, Falcon House, Lancaster, England

Cederbaum S D, Blass J P, Minkoff N, Brown W J, Cotton M E, Harris S H 1976 Sensitivity to carbohydrate in a patient with familial intermittent lactic acidosis and pyruvate dehydrogenase deficiency. Pediatric Research 10: 713–720

Chacko C M, Christian J C, Nadler H L 1971 Unstable galactose-1-phosphate uridyltransferase: a new variant of galactosemia. Journal of Pediatrics 78: 454–460

Chacko C M, Wappner R S, Brandt I K, Nadler H L 1977 The Chicago variant of clinical galactosemia. Human Genetics 37: 261–270

Clark A F, Farrell D F, Burke W, Scott C R 1978 The effect of mycoplasma contamination on the in vitro assay of pyruvate dehydrogenase activity in cultured fibroblasts. Clinica Chimica Acta 87: 119–124

Conklin K A, Yamashiro K M, Gray G M 1975 Human intestinal sucrase-isomaltase: identification of free sucrase and isomaltase and cleavage of hybrid into active distinct subunits. Journal of Biological Chemistry 250: 5735–5741

Cook J G H, Don N A, Mann T P 1971 Hereditary galactokinase deficiency. Archives of Disease in Childhood 46: 465–469

de Barsy Th, Lederer B 1980 Type VI glycogenosis: identification of subgroups. In: Burman D, Holton J B, Pennock C A (eds) Inherited disorders of carbohydrate metabolism, MTP Press Limited, Falcon House, Lancaster, England, ch 19, p 369–380

Deckelbaum R J, Russell A, Shapira E, Cohen T, Agam G, Gutman A 1972 Type III glycogenosis: atypical enzyme activities in blood cells in two siblings. Journal of Pediatrics 81: 955–961

Dreyfus J C, Poenaru L 1980 White blood cells and the

diagnosis of α-glucosidase deficiency. Pediatric Research
14: 342–344

Durand P 1958 Lacttosuria idiopatica in una paziente con
diarrea cronica ed acidosi. Minerva Pediatrica 10: 706

Engle A G, Gomez M R, Seybold M D, Lambert E H 1973
The spectrum and diagnosis of acid maltase deficiency.
Neurology 23: 95–106

Engle W K, Eyerman E L, Williams H E 1963 Late onset
type of skeletal muscle phosphorylase deficiency. New
England Journal of Medicine 268: 135–141

Fattah S, Rubulis A, Faloon W 1970 McArdle's disease:
metabolic studies in a patient and review of the syndrome.
American Journal of Medicine 48: 693–699

Feit H, Brooke M H 1976 Myophosphorylase deficiency: two
different molecular etiologies. Neurology 26: 963–967

Fernandes J, Huijing F, van de Kamer J H 1969 A screening
method for liver glycogen diseases. Archives of Disease in
Childhood 44: 311–317

Fong W F, Hynic I, Lee L, McKendry J B R 1979 Increase
of fructose-1,6-diphosphatase activity in cultured human
peripheral lymphoctyes and its suppression by
phytohemagglutinin. Biochemical and Biophysical Research
Communications 88: 222–228

Froesch E R 1978 Essential fructosemia and hereditary
fructose intolerance. In: Stanbury J B, Wyngaarden J B,
Fredrickson D S (eds) The metabolic basis of inherited
diseases, 4th edn. McGraw-Hill, New York, ch 6,
p 121–136

Garty R, Cooper M, Tabachnik E 1974 The Fanconi
syndrome associated with hepatic glycogenosis and
abnormal metabolism of galactose. Journal of Pediatrics
85: 821–823

Gitzelmann R 1965 Deficiency of erythrocyte galactokinase in
a patient with galactose diabetes. Lancet 2: 670–671

Gitzelmann R, Baerlock K, Prader A 1973 Hereditäre
Störungen in fructoseund galaktose-stoffwechsel.
Monatsschrift für Kinderheilkunde 121: 174–180

Gitzelmann R, Steinmann B, Bally C, Lebherz H G 1974
Antibody activation of mutant human fructose diphosphate
aldolase B in liver extracts of patients with hereditary
fructose intolerance. Biochemical and Biophysical Research
Communications 59: 1270–1277

Gitzelmann R, Steinmann B, Mitchell B, Haigis E 1976
Uridine diphosphate galactose 4-epimerase deficiency. IV.
Report of eight cases in three families. Helvetica Paediatrica
Acta 31: 441–452

Grant D B, Alexander F W, Seakins J W T 1970 Abnormal
tyrosine metabolism in hereditary fructose intolerance. Acta
Paediatrica Scandinavica 59: 432–434

Gray G M 1978 Intestinal disaccharidase deficiencies and
glucose malabsorption. In: Stanbury J B, Wyngaarden J B,
Fredrickson D S (eds) The metabolic basis of inherited
disease, 4th edn. McGraw-Hill, New York, ch 64,
p 1526–1536

Gray G M, Conklin K A, Townley R R W 1976 Sucrase-
isomaltase deficiency. New England Journal of Medicine
294: 750–753

Greene H L, Slonim A E, O'Neil J A Jr, Burr I M 1976
Continuous nocturnal intragastric feeding for management
of type I glycogen-storage disease. New England Journal of
Medicine 294: 423–425

Greene H L, Slonim A E, O'Neil J A Jr, Burr I M 1979
Type I glycogen storage disease: a metabolic basis for
advances in treatment. In: Barness L A (ed) Advances in
Pediatrics Vol 26 Year Book Medical Publishers, Chicago,
ch 3, p 64–92

Greene H L, Stifel F B, Herman R H 1972 Ketotic
hypoglycemia due to hepatic fructose-1,6-diphosphatase
deficiency: treatment with folic acid. American Journal of
Diseases of Children 124: 415–418

Grunfeld J, Ganeval D, Chanard J, Fardeau M, Dreyfus J
1972 actue renal failure in McArdle's syndrome. New
England Journal of Medicine 286: 1237–1242

Guthrie R 1968 Screening for inborn errors of metabolism in
the newborn infant – a multiple test program. Birth Defects
Original Article Series 6: 92

Gutman A, Rachmilewitz E, Stein O, Eliakim M, Stein Y
1965 Glycogen storage disease, report of a case with
generalized glycogenosis without demonstrable enzyme
defect. Israel Journal of Medical Science 1: 14–25

Hansen T L, Christensen E 1979 Studies on pyruvate
carboxylase from cultured human fibroblasts and amniotic
fluid cells. Journal of Inherited Metabolic Disease
2: 23–28

Herman R H, Zakim D 1968 Fructose metabolism IV.
Enzyme deficiencies: essential fructosuria, fructose
intolerance, and glycogen-storage disease. American Journal
of Clinical Nutrition 21: 693–698

Hers H G 1976 The control of glycogen metabolism in the
liver. In: Snell E E, Boyer P D, Meister A, Richardson C C
(eds) Annual Review of Biochemistry Vol 45, Annual
Reviews Inc., Palo Alto, U.S.A., P 167–189

Hollings E H 1963 Gout and glycogen storage disease. Annals
of Internal Medicine 58: 654–663

Holton J B, Gillett M G, MacFaul R, Young R 1981
Galactosemia: a new severe variant due to uridine
diphosphate galactose-4-epimerase deficiency. Archives of
Disease in Childhood 56: 885–887

Hommes F A, Polman H A, Reerink J D 1968 Leigh's
encephalomyelopathy: an inborn error of gluconeogenesis.
Archives of Disease in Childhood 43: 423–426

Howell R R, Kaback M M, Brown B I 1971 Type IV
glycogen storage disease: branching enzyme deficiency in
skin fibroblasts and possible heterozygote detection. Journal
of Pediatrics 78: 638–642

Howell R R, Stevenson R E, Ben-Menachem Y, Phyliky R L,
Berxy D H 1976 Hepatic adenomata with type I glycogen
storage disease. Journal of the American Medical
Association 236: 1481–1484

Hug G 1974 Enzyme therapy and prenatal diagnosis in
glycogenosis type II. American Journal of Diseases of
Children 128: 607–609

Hug G, Schubert W K, Chuck G 1969 Deficient activity of
dephosphophosphorylase kinase and accumulation of
glycogen in the liver. Journal of Clinical Investigation
48: 704–714

Hug G, Schubert W K, Chuck G 1970 Loss of cyclic 3'5'-
AMP dependent kinase and reduction of phosphorylase
kinase in skeletal muscle of a girl with deactivated
phosphorylase and glycogenosis of liver and muscle.
Biochemical and Biophysical Research Communications
40: 982–988

Hug G, Schubert W K, Chuck G, Garancis J C 1967 Liver
phosphorylase; deactivation in a child with progressive
brain disease, elevated hepatic glycogen and increased
urinary catecholamines. American Journal of Medicine
42: 139–145

Huijing F 1970 Glycogen storage disease type VIa: low
phosphorylase kinase activity caused by a low enzyme-
substrate affinity. Biochimica et Biophysica Acta
206: 199–201

Huijing F 1973 Genetic defects of glycogen metabolism and

its control. Annals of the New York Academy of Science 210: 290–302

Huijing F, Fernandez J 1969 X–chromosome inheritance of liver glycogenosis with phosphorylase kinase deficiency. American Journal of Human Genetics 21: 275–284

Kahana D, Telem C, Steinitz K, Solomon M 1964 Generalized glycogenosis: report of a case with deficiency of alpha glucosidase. Journal of Pediatrics 65: 243–251

Kalckar H M, Anderson E P, Isselbacher K J 1956 Galactosemia, a congenital defect in a nucleotide transferase: a preliminary report. Proceedings of the National Academy of Sciences U S A 42: 49–51

Kark R A P, Rodriguez-Budell M 1979 Pyruvate dehydrogenase deficiency in spinocerebellar degenerations. Neurology 29: 126–131

Karpatkin S, Charmatz A, Langer R M 1970 Glycogenesis and glyconeogenesis in human platelets. Incorporation of glucose, pyruvate and citrate into platelet glycogen; glycogen synthetase and fuctose-1,6-diphosphatase activity. Journal of Clinical Investigation 49: 140–149

Kaufman F, Kogut M D, Donnell G N, Koch R 1979 Ovarian failure in galactosemia. Lancet 2: 737–738

Keppens S, de Wulf H 1975 The activation of liver glycogen phosphorylase by vasopressin. FEBS Letters 51: 29–32

Keppens S, de Wulf H 1976 The activation of liver glycogen phosphorylase by angiotensin II. FEBS Letters 68: 279–282

Koster J F, Fernandez J, Slee R G, van Berkel Th J C, Hulsmann W C 1973 Hepatic phosphorylase deficiency: a biochemical study. Biochemical and Biophysical Research Communications 53: 282–290

Krebs H A, Woodford M 1965 Fructose-1,6-diphosphatase in striated muscle. Biochemical Journal 94: 436–445

Landau B R, Marshall J S, Craig J W, Hostetler K Y, Genuth S M 1971 Quantitation of the pathways of fructose metabolism in normal and fructose intolerant subjects. Journal of Laboratory and Clinical Medicine 78: 608–618

Lang A, Groeb H, Bellkuhl B, Von Figura K 1980 A new variant of galactosemia: galactose-1-phosphate uridyltransferase sensitive to produce inhibition by glucose-1-phosphate. Pediatric Research 14: 729–734

Lange A J, Arion W J, Beaudet A L 1980 Type Ib glycogen storage disease is caused by a defect in the glucose-6-phosphate translocase of the microsomal glucose-6-phosphatase system. Journal of Biological Chemistry 255: 8381–8384

Layzer R B, Rasmussen J 1974 The molecular basis of muscle phosphofructokinase deficiency. Archives of Neurology 31: 411–417

Lederer B, van Hoof F, van den Berghe G, Hers H 1975 Glycogen phosphorylase and its converter enzymes in hemolysates of normal human subjects and of patients with type VI glycogen-storage disease. Biochemical Journal 147: 23–35

Lehninger A L 1975 Biochemistry, 2nd edn. Worth Publishers, Inc., New York, p 451

Levin S, Moses S W, Chayoth R, Jagoda N, Steinitz K 1967 Glycogen storage disease in Israel: a clinical, biochemical and genetic study. Israel Journal of Medical Sciences 3: 397–410

Lin M S, Oizumi J, Ng W G, Alfi O S, Donnell G N 1979 Assignment of the gene for uridine diphosphate galactose-4-epimerase to human chromosome 1 by human-mouse somatic cell hybridization. Somatic Cell Genetics 5: 363–371

Matalon R, Michals K, Justice P, Deanching M N 1977 Glucose-6-phosphatase activity in human placenta: a possible detection of heterozygote for glycogen storage disease type I. Lancet 1: 1360–1361

Matz D, Enzenauer J, Meune F 1975 Uber einen fall von atypischer galaktosamie. Humangenetik 27: 309–313

Mayes J S, Guthrie R 1968 Detection of heterozygotes for galactokinase deficiency in a human population. Biochemical Genetics 2: 219–230

McArdle B 1951 Myopathy due to a defect in muscle glycogen breakdown. Clinical Science 10: 13–33

McCabe E R, Melvin T R, O'Brien D, Montgomery R R, Robinson W A, Bhasker C, Brown B I 1980 Neutropenia in a patient with type IB glycogen storage disease: in vitro response to lithium chloride. Journal of Pediatrics 79: 944–946

McNair A, Gudmand-Hayer E, Jarnum S, Orrild L 1972 Sucrose malabsorption in Greenland. British Medical Journal 2: 19–21

Meienhofer M C, Askanas V, Proux-Daegelen D, Dreyfus J, Engel K 1977 Muscle-type phosphorylase activity present in muscle cells cultured from three patients with myophosphorylase deficiency. Archives of Neurology 34: 779–780

Melin K, Meeuwisse G W 1969 Glucose-galactose malabsorption: a genetic study. Acta Paediatrica Scandinavica, Supplement 188: 19–24

Michels V V, Beaudet A L 1980 Hemorrhagic pancreatitis in a patient with glycogen storage disease type I. Clinical Genetics 17: 220–222

Miller J H, Gates G F, Landing B H, Kogut M D, Roe T F 1978 Scintigraphic abnormalities in glycogen storage disease. Journal of Nuclear Medicine 19: 354–358

Mohandas T, Sparkes R S, Sparkes M S, Shulkin J D 1977 Assignment of the human gene for galactose-1-phosphate uridyltransferase to chromosome 9: studies with Chinese hamster-human somatic cell hybrids. Proceedings of the National Academy of Sciences U S A 74: 5628–5631

Moses S W, Levin S, Chayoth R, Steinitz K 1966 Enzyme induction in a case of glycogen storage disease. Pediatrics 38: 111–121

Narisawa K, Igarashi Y, Otomo H, Tada K 1978 A new variant of glycogen storage disease type I probably due to a defect in glucose-6-phosphatase transport system. Biochemical and Biophysical Research Communications 83: 1360–1364

Negishi H, Benke P J 1977 Epithelial cells and von Gierke's disease. Pediatric Research 11: 936–939

Ng W G, Bergren W R, Donnell G N 1973 A new variant of galactose-1-phosphate uridyltransferase in man: the Los Angeles variant. Annals of Human Genetics 37: 1–8

Ng W G, Donnell G N, Bergren W R 1965 Galactokinase activity in human erythrocytes of individuals at different ages. Journal of Laboratory and Clinical Medicine 66: 115–121

Ng W G, Donnell G N, Bergren W R, Alfi O, Golbus M S 1977 Prenatal diagnosis of galactosemia. Clinica Chimica Acta 74: 227–235

Ng W G, Kline F, Lin J, Koch R, Donnell G N 1978 Biochemical studies of a human low-activity galactose-1-phosphate uridyl transferase variant. Journal of Inherited Metabolic Disease 1: 145–151

Orkwiszewski K G, Tedesco T A, Croce C M 1974 Assignment of the human gene for galactokinase to chromosome 17. Nature 252: 60–62

Peterson M L, Herber R 1967 Intestinal sucrase deficiency. Transactions of the Association of American Physicians 80: 275–283

Pickering W R, Howell R R 1972 Galactokinase deficiency: clinical and biochemical findings in a new kindred. Journal of Pediatrics 81: 50–55

Pizzo C J 1980 Type I glycogen storage disease with focal nodular hyperplasia of the liver and vasoconstrictive pulmonary hypertension. Pediatrics 65: 341–343

Porte D, Crawford D, Jennings D B, Aber C, McIlroy M 1966 Cardiovascular and metabolic responses to exercise in McArdle's syndrome. New England Journal of Medicine 275: 406–412

Potter J L, Robinson H B Jr, Kramer J D, Schafer I A 1980 Apparent normal leukocyte acid maltase activity in glycogen storage disease type II (Pompe's disease). Clinical Chemistry 26: 1914–1915

Robinson B H, Gall D G, Cutz E 1977a Deficient activity of hepatic pyruvate dehydrogenase and pyruvate carboxylase in Reye's syndrome. Pediatric Research 11: 279–281

Robinson B H, Taylor J, Kahler S 1979 Mitochondrial phosphoenolpyruvate carboxykinase deficiency in a child with lactic acidemia, hypotonia and failure to thrive. American Journal of Human Genetics 31: 60A

Robinson B H, Taylor J, Sherwood W G 1977b Deficiency of dihydrolipoyl dehydrogenase (a component of the pyruvate dan α-ketoglutarate dehydrogenase complexes), a cause of congenital chronic lactic acidosis in infancy. Pediatric Research 11: 1198–1202

Roe T F, Kogut M D, Buckingham B A, Miller J, Gates G, Landing B 1979 Hepatic tumors in glycogen storage disease type I. Pediatric Research 13: 481

Sadeghi-Nejad A, Presente E, Binkiewicz A, Senior B 1974 Studies in type I glycogenosis of the liver. Journal of Pediatrics 85: 49–54

Salafsky I S, Nadler H L 1971 Alpha-1,4-glucosidase activity in Pompe's disease. Journal of Pediatrics 79: 794–798

Saudubray J M, Drefus J C, Cepanec C, Lelo'ch H, Trung P H, Mozziconadi P 1973 Acidose lactique, hypoglycemie et hepatomegalie par deficit hereditaire en fructose-1,6-diphosphatase hepatique. Archives Francaises de Pediatrie 30: 609–632

Saudubray J M, Marsac C, Charpentier C, Cathelineau L, Besson Leaud M, Leroux J P 1976 Neonatal congenital lactic acidosis with pyruvate carboxylase deficiency in two siblings. Acta Paediatrica Scandinavica 65: 717–724

Schapira F, Kaplan J 1969 Electrophoretic abnormality of galactose-1-phosphate uridyltransferase in galactosemia. Biochemical and Biophysical Research Communications 33: 451–455

Schapira F, Schapira G, Dreyfus J C 1961/62 La lesion enzymatique de la fructosurie benigne. Enzymologia Biologica et Clinica 1: 170–175

Scherz R, Pflugshaupt R, Butler R 1976 A new genetic variant of galactose-1-phosphate uridyl transferase. Human Genetics 35: 51–55

Schmid R, Hammaker L 1961 Hereditary absence of muscle phosphorylase (McArdle's syndrome). New England Journal of Medicine 264: 223–225

Schmidt E, Schmidt F W 1979 Clinical aspects of gut enzymology. Journal of Clinical Chemistry and Clinical Biochemistry 17: 693–704

Segal S 1969 The Negro variant of congenital galactosemia. In: David Hsia (ed) Galactosemia, Charles C. Thomas, Springfield, Illinois, ch 23, p 176–185

Segal S, Rutman J Y, Frimpter G W 1979 Galactokinase deficiency and mental retardation. Journal of Pediatrics 95: 750–752

Service F J, Veneziale C M, Nelson R A, Ellefson R D, Go V L W 1978 Combined deficiency of glucose-6-phosphatase and fructose-1,6-diphosphatase. American Journal of Medicine 64: 696–706

Sonobe H, Ogawa K, Takahashi I 1976 Familial nephropathy associated with hepatic type of glycogen storage disease. Acta Pathologica Japan 26: 727–738

Stalmans W, de Wulf H, Hers H 1971 The control fo liver glycogen synthetase phosphatase by phosphorylase. European Journal of Biochemistry 18: 582–587

Stalmans W, Laloux M, Hers H 1974 The interaction of liver phosphorylase a with glucose and AMP. European Journal of Biochemistry 49: 415–427

Stamm W E, Webb D I 1975 Partial deficiency of hepatic glucose-6-phosphatase in an adult patient. Archives of Internal Medicine 135: 1107–1109

Stanbury J B, Wyngaarden J B, Fredrickson D S (eds) 1978 The metabolic basis of inherited disease, 4th edn. McGraw-Hill, New York

Stromme J H, Borud O, Moc P J 1976 Fetal lactic acidosis in a newborn attributable to a congenital defect of pyruvate dehydrogenase. Pediatric Research 10: 60–66

Tanaka K, Shimazu S, Oya N, Tomisawa M, Kusunoki T, Soyama K, Ono E 1979 Muscular form of glycogenosis type II (Pompe's disease).Pediatrics 63: 124–129

Taniguchi N, Kato E, Yoshida H, Iwaki S, Ohki T, Koizumi S 1978 Alpha-glucosidase activity in human leucocytes: choice of lymphocytes for the diagnosis of Pompe's disease and the carrier state. Clinica Chimica Acta 89: 293–299

Tarui S 1965 Phosphofructokinase deficiency in skeletal muscle: a new type of glycogenosis. Biochemical and Biophysical Research Communications 19: 517–523

Taunton O D, Greene H L, Stifel F B, Hofeldt F D, Lufkin E G, Hagler L, Herman Y, Herman R H 1978 Fructose-1,6-diphosphatase deficiency, hypoglycemia, and response to folate therapy in a mother and her daughter. Biochemical Medicine 19: 260–276

Tedesco T A, Miller K L, Rawnsley B E, Adams M C, Markus H B, Orkwiszewski K G, Mellman W J 1977 The Philadelphia variant of galactokinase. American Journal of Human Genetics 29: 240–247

Thalhammer O, Gitzelmann R, Pantlitschko M 1968 Hypergalactosemia and galactosuria due to galactokinase deficiency in a newborn. Pediatrics 42: 441–445

Tobin W E, Huijing F, Porro R S, Salzman R T 1973 Muscle phosphofructokinase deficiency. Archives of Neurology 28: 128–130

Townley R R W 1966 Disaccharidase deficiency in infancy and childhood. Pediatrics 38: 127–141

Tyrrell D A, Ryman B E 1976 Use of liposomes in treating type II glycogenosis. British Medical Journal 811: 88–89

van Bierolet J-P, Staal G E 1977 Excessive hepatic glycogen storage in glucosephosphate isomerase deficiency. Acta Paediatrica Scandinavica 66: 311–315

van de Werve G, Hue L, Hers H 1977 Hormonal and ionic control of the glycogenolytic cascade in rat liver. Biochemical Journal 162: 135–142

van den Berghe G, Hue L, Hers H G 1973 Effect of the administration of fructose on the glycolytic action of glucagon, an investigation of the pathogency of hereditary fructose intolerance. Biochemical Journal 134: 637–645

Vidnes J, Sovik O 1976 Gluconeogenesis in infancy and childhood. III Deficiency of the extra mitochondrial form of hepatic phosphoenol pyruvate carboxykinase in a case of

persistent neonatal hypoglycemia. Acta Paediatrica
Scandinavica 65: 307–312
von Reuss A 1980 Zuckerausscheidung in Singlingsalter.
Wiener Medizinische Wochenschrift 58: 799–803
Winder A F 1981 Laboratory screening in the assessment of
human cataract. Transactions of the Ophthalmological
Societies of the United Kingdom 101: 127–130

Wittens L A, Avruch J 1978 Insulin regulation of hepatic
glycogen synthase and phosphorylase. Biochemistry
17: 406–410
Zangeneth F, Limbeck G A, Brown B I 1969 Hepatorenal
glycogenosis and carcinoma of the liver. Journal of
Pediatrics 74: 73–83

90

Disorders of purine and pyrimidine metabolism

J. E. Seegmiller

INTRODUCTION

Concretions of the urinary tract have long claimed the interest of chemists and physicians and first brought human aberrations of purine metabolism to medical attention (Scheele, 1776; Marcet, 1817). The isolation of uric acid in a kidney stone led to the identification of monosodium urate in a gouty tophus and increased concentrations of urate in the serum of gouty patients by A. B. Garrod in 1848. Although gout was classed as an inborn error of metabolism by A. E. Garrod in 1923, no single enzyme defect is responsible for this disease. Instead evidence of heterogeneity has been found with both genetic and environmental factors contributing to the hyperuricaemia responsible for gout. Our knowledge of specific hereditary abnormalities in purine metabolism began less than two decades ago with the identification of the enzyme defect responsible for xanthinuria (Engelman et al, 1964; Ayvazion, 1964) and subsequent identification of the enzyme responsible for Lesch-Nyhan disease and its variants (Seegmiller et al, 1967) which led to identification of enzyme defects responsible for gouty arthritis. The past decade has seen a burgeoning of additional disorders of purine metabolism responsible for such widely different clinical conditions as immunodeficiency disease, a new type of kidney stones, haemolytic anaemia and an exercise intolerance (Fig. 90.1).

Our knowledge of human disorders of pyrimidine metabolism began in a similar manner with identification of a patient whose urine formed a crystalline deposit on cooling which was identified as orotic acid. This led to identification of the specific enzyme defects associated with this disorder (Huguley et al, 1959). More recently, a deficiency of pyrimidine 5'-nucleotidase associated with a congenital primary haemolytic anaemia has been found. A number of reviews have been published (Thompson & Seegmiller, 1979; Seegmiller et al, 1979; Seegmiller, 1979a; Seegmiller, 1979b; Seegmiller, 1980a; Seegmiller et al, 1980; Wyngaarden & Kelley, 1976; Seegmiller, 1980b; Seegmiller, 1980c; Newcomb, 1975; Mitchell & Kelley, 1980; Boss & Seegmiller, 1979; Muller et al, 1977a; Muller et al, 1977b).

PURINE METABOLISM

Gout

Gout is a form of arthritis caused by the deposition, in and about the joints, of needle-shaped crystals of monosodium urate monohydrate from hyperuricaemic supersaturated body fluids. The deposits of monosodium urate and the surrounding inflammatory and granulomatous response provides the characteristic pathology that differentiates gout from other forms of arthritis and from its prodromal state of hyperuricaemia.

Hyperuricaemia

The hyperuricaemia, responsible for gout, results from a heterogeneous group of environmental, physiological and genetic abnormalities and their interaction. In some patients, the hyperuricaemia results primarily from a genetically-determined excessive synthesis of the purine precursors of uric acid. In others, the purine synthesis is normal and a diminished renal excretion of uric acid is responsible. In still others, both mechanisms contribute. The hyperuricaemia itself is entirely asymptomatic, although it may be a risk factor for development of such disorders as cardiovascular disease and diabetes mellitus (Fessel, 1980; Fessel et al, 1973). Patients with only a modest degree of hyperuricaemia may remain asymptomatic throughout life.

Acute gout

The degree and duration of hyperuricaemia may well be the determinants of the chance formation of the first seed crystal and thereby the age at which sufficient crystals accumulate for the first acute attack to develop. Over the years the attacks become more frequent and eventually can progress to chronic articular symptoms with permanent damage and deformity of the joint, resulting from the progressive erosion of joint surfaces by enlarging deposits of monosodium urate crystals, known as tophi. Many gouty patients also develop some evidence of renal dysfunction which, if progressive, can lead to life-threatening uraemia as the most serious complication of the disease. A portion of the renal damage can be

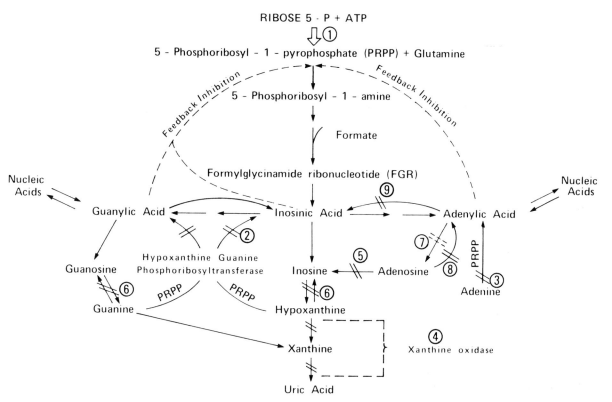

Fig. 90.1 Known enzyme defects in human purine metabolism. (1) Increased phosphoribosylpyrophosphate synthetase activity in patients with overproduction of uric acid and gout. (2) Gross deficiency of hypoxanthine guanine phosphoribosyltransferase in children with Lesch-Nyhan disease and partial deficiency of the same enzyme in patients with overproduction of uric acid and gout. (3) Adenine phosphoribosyltransferase deficiency in patients with kidney stones composed of 2-8 dioxyadenine that are often confused with uric acid stones. (4) Xanthine oxidase deficiency in patients with xanthinuria who are at increased risk for xanthine calculi of the urinary tract and, in occasional patients, myalgia from xanthine crystals in the muscle. (5) Adenosine deaminase deficiency associated with severe combined immunodeficiency disease. (6) Purine nucleoside phosphorylase deficiency associated with isolated defect in T cells. (7) Purine 5′-nucleotidase activity is low in lymphocytes of patients with agammaglobulinaemia that may be secondary to loss of B cells. (8) Adenosine kinase deficiency has so far been developed only in the human lymphoblast cell lines. Its counterpart in patients is yet to be identified. (9) Myoadenylate deaminase deficiency is associated in some patients with development of weakness and muscle cramps after vigorous exercise and failure to show a rise in venous blood ammonia in response to muscle exercise.

attributed to uric acid renal lithiasis, or less commonly calcium oxalate stones. In addition, vascular changes in the kidney, hypertension and cardiovascular disease can also contribute to the overall pathology. Recent studies suggest sub-clinical lead poisoning as a major cause of renal dysfunction in patients with gout (Batuman et al, 1981; Reif et al, 1981).

Hyperuricaemia and gout are found in association with an ever-increasing number of other clinical disorders. Included are endocrine disorders of hypothyroidism, both hypo- and hyperparathyroidism, hypoadrenal states, myeloproliferative disorders, idiopathic hypercalciuria and psoriasis. The possibility of their being the first manifestations of one of these underlying disorders should always be considered and should lead to a complete medical evaluation to rule out these other disorders. In the present section, we will limit our discussion to the genetically-determined enzyme defects, in both carbohydrate and purine metabolism, that lead to purine overproduction as a cause of hyperuricaemia and gouty arthritis. The insight detailed studies of these disorders has given as to the normal regulatory process of purine metabolism will also be discussed.

Accompanying the increased understanding of the precise mechanisms leading to gouty arthritis has been the development of rational approaches to therapeutic intervention. The result has been a dramatic improvement in the control of this disease, so that essentially all gouty patients can anticipate a life relatively unhampered by gouty arthritis, provided they follow medical advice and maintain continuous medical supervision. A number of reviews of gouty arthritis and hyperuricaemia have recently been published (Seegmiller, 1980a; Seegmiller et al, 1980; Boss & Seegmiller, 1979; Wyngaarden & Kelly, 1976; Becker & Seegmiller, 1974; Kelley & Weiner, 1978; McCarty, 1974).

Clinical features. The presenting symptoms of acute gouty arthritis are usually sufficiently distinctive to allow its presumptive diagnosis and its differentiation from other forms of arthritis. The typical presentation consists of a monoarticular arthritis involving a peripheral joint, which shows evidence of intense inflammation consisting of redness, warmth, swelling and acute tenderness, which is far greater than is seen in most other forms of arthritis. The common presenting site is in the first metatarsophalangeal joint, which is the site of the greatest degree of physiological trauma with walking. Precipitating events may be unusual exercise, emotional upset or surgical trauma. Quite often a site of old injury determines the location for the most troublesome attacks of gout. Simkin (1977) has proposed an ingenious mechanism for concentration of urate in the first metatarsophalangeal joint based on the slower diffusion of urate from a traumatic effusion in this joint from excessive exercise. If untreated, the acute attack will gradually recede spontaneously over a period of one to two weeks with complete restoration of function, but attacks will inevitably recur in the same or different joints at increasing frequency, which can eventually lead to a chronic smouldering inflammation which is usually associated with aggressive erosion of the joints, leading to permanent joint damage.

Diagnosis. The most important differential diagnosis is the distinction of gouty from septic arthritis. The latter disease can lead to substantial degrees of joint destruction within a relatively short time. A most direct method of distinguishing these two disorders is by the introduction of a needle into the joint space and removal of joint fluid after sterile preparation. It should be cultured, the remaining portion centrifuged and the sediment examined, with a portion stained for bacteria and the remaining portion examined under a microscope in a haemocytometer chamber. The use of cross-polarizing filters attached to an ordinary microscope will allow the ready identification of the needle-shaped crystals of monosodium urate due to their rotation of polarized light. The introduction of a red retardation filter allows the ready distinction to be made between the negatively birefringent needle-shaped crystals of monosodium urate characteristic of gouty arthritis and the positively birefringent trapezoidal or irregularly shaped crystals of calcium pyrophosphate which are diagnostic of chondrocalcinosis or 'pseudo gout' (McCarty, 1974).

A search should also be made for gouty tophi in other parts of the body, particularly over the helix of the ears and over the points of insertion of tendons of elbows, knees or feet. If such a tophus is identified, a diagnosis

of gout can quickly be made by introducing a needle and examining the contents of the needle in a drop of saline under a microscope to reveal the same needle-shaped crystals typical of gouty arthritis. The subsequent demonstration of hyperuricaemia provides additional confirmation of the clinical impression. Demonstration of crystals in fluid from the asymptomatic first metatarsophalangeal joint has proven helpful in arriving at a diagnosis (Weinberger et al, 1979). Occasionally patients will be found with serum urate concentrations in the upper range of normal during the acute attack of gout. These usually return to the hyperuricaemic range when the stress of the acute attack is relieved.

Treatment. General measures for treatment include rest, elevation of the affected joint and administration of analgesics including narcotics, which is justified since this is a self-limited disease, to control the severe pain while more specific measures are being instituted. The patient should be encouraged to develop the habit of drinking at least three litres of water per day to decrease the tendency for formation of kidney stones which are commonly found in gouty patients. The acute attack responds readily to colchicine given at a dose of 0.5 mg every hour to the point of nausea, vomiting, or diarrhoea. It also responds readily to phenylbutazone, indomethacin and a wide variety of newer anti-inflammatory drugs (Boss et al, 1979; Seegmiller, 1980a).

Treatment aimed at lowering the serum urate concentration should be deferred until the acute attack of gout has been brought under control. Otherwise, experience has shown that it can lead to further exacerbation and delay in recovery from the acute attack.

Classification of gout

The period of recovery, while the patient's gout is being brought under control with prophylactic daily colchicine 0.5 mg two to three times daily as tolerated to prevent recurrences, is a convenient time to evaluate the patient's 24-hour excretion of uric acid and creatinine. Drugs such as aspirin, allopurinol or uricosuric drugs and alcoholic drinks, which are known to alter uric acid production or excretion, are stopped and the patient started on a diet virtually free of purines for a six-day period. During the last three days of the diet, the 24-hour urine is collected in a container containing 3 ml of toluene or 1/4 gram of thymol crystals, as preservative, to allow assessment of the degree of uric acid production. The urine should be stored at room temperature and analyzed for both uric acid and creatinine, after care has been taken to completely dissolve, by warming and agitation, any sediment of uric acid that may be present in the bottle.

The upper range of normal excretion for an adult male is 600 mg/24 hours. Patients excreting quantities in excess of this amount are producing excessive amounts of uric acid and should be started on allopurinol after recovery from the acute attack. Allopurinol not only blocks uric acid production by inhibiting the enzyme xanthine oxidase but also diminishes excessive purine synthesis in most patients, except those with Lesch-Nyhan disease or its variants. Other indications for using allopurinol are intolerance of a uricosuric drug, recurrent calculi of the urinary tract composed of uric acid or evidence of impaired renal function. Daily colchicine will suppress the tendency for gout patients to have an exacerbation of their disease during the first weeks to months of initiation of therapy with a drug designed to lower the serum urate concentration to the normal range. Patients should be warned of this possibility and instructed to increase the dose of colchicine at the first sign of an impending attack. Patients excreting less than 600 mg per day should be started on probenicid at a dose of 1/2 tablet (0.25 grams) daily with a gradual increase over the course of a week to a maintenance dose of 0.5 grams twice daily with additional increases in dosage as needed to maintain the serum urate concentration in the normal range. Subsequent follow-up should be done at intervals of 6 months for routine checks on renal function, haematology and serum urate to prevent recurrence of the disease. This approach to treatment is to maintain the serum urate in the normal range and is most gratifying to the patient who can thereby live an essentially normal life without incapacitation from gouty arthritis.

Enzyme defects associated with gout

The primary genetically-determined enzyme defects leading to gouty arthritis so far identified have all been associated with a marked overproduction of uric acid. Since an excessive production of uric acid is found in only 10 to 15% of gouty patients (Watts, 1977), known enzyme defects probably account for less than 5% of gouty patients. The assessment of 24-hour excretion of uric acid as a routine part of the evaluation of gouty patients has the added advantage of identifying those in whom a more detailed examination for enzyme abnormalities may be appropriate.

Purine over-production and gout in glycogen storage disease type 1

A marked hyperuricaemia and modest over-production of uric acid can lead to the development of gouty arthritis in early adult life, which has been found in over 40 patients with hepatic glucose-6-phosphatase deficiency (glycogen storage disease type 1) (Seegmiller, 1980a; Alepa et al, 1967; Kelley et al, 1968; Lockwood et al, 1969). Clinical features include hepatomegaly, retarded rate of growth and sexual development, bleeding tendencies with frequent epistaxis, early development of severe cardiovascular disease and an eating pattern in adult life of frequent small starchy meals rather than full meals. Blood shows a marked lactic acidaemia, hyperur-

icaemia, marked hyperlipidaemia and fasting hypoglycaemia. A number of theories have been proposed to account for the hyperuricaemia. The lactic acidaemia interferes with renal excretion of uric acid but, in addition, patients show evidence of an increased rate of purine synthesis (Alepa et al, 1967; Kelley et al, 1968; Jakovcic &Sorenson, 1967; Roe & Kogut, 1977). Greene et al (1978) provided evidence of ATP depletion and an accelerated purine nucleotide breakdown. Correction of hyperuricaemia by continuous nocturnal drip suggests a role for carbohydrate deprivation in its genesis (Benke & Gold, 1977; Greene et al, 1977).

Lesch-Nyhan disease

In its most severe presentation this disease is a most incapacitating neurological disorder, limited to males who present with the choreoathetosis, spasticity, mild mental retardation, 'cerebral palsy' and compulsive self-mutilation manifested by biting away of lips and tongue and ends of the fingers (Lesch & Nyhan, 1964). Affected children also produce markedly excessive quantities of uric acid which forms the basis for a relatively simple screening test, in which the ratio of uric acid to creatinine in the morning urine sample is measured (Kaufman et al, 1968; McInnes et al, 1972). Although most patients also show an elevation of serum urate, particularly in later stages of the disease, this test cannot be used to rule out this disorder as around five to ten percent show a normal serum urate.

The primary abnormality resides in a structural gene on the X–chromosome coding for the synthesis of the enzyme hypoxanthine-guanine phosphoribosyltransferase, which is grossly deficient in this disorder (Seegmiller et al, 1967; Seegmiller, 1976). Less severe deficiencies of the same enzyme show a clinical expression with attenuation or even absence of the neurological dysfunction, but an excessive purine synthesis remains giving rise to severe gouty arthritis with onset in early adult life and, in most cases, with the production of kidney stones composed of uric acid (Kelley et al, 1967; Kelley et al, 1969; Seegmiller, 1976; Seegmiller, 1980c). Recurrence of the severe forms of the disease in families carrying the gene can now be prevented through monitoring of pregnancies and prenatal diagnosis (Fujimoto et al, 1968; Boyle et al, 1970; Van Heeswijk et al, 1972; Seegmiller, 1974). Several reviews have been published (Kelley et al, 1969; Seegmiller, 1976; Seegmiller, 1980a; Seegmiller, 1980b; Nyhan, 1977; Wyngaarden & Kelley, 1976).

Clinical features

Although the biochemical abnormality is present prenatally, as shown by demonstration of the HRT deficiency in amniotic cells (Fujimoto et al, 1968), at birth children with this disease appear entirely normal. The first indication of the disease to many mothers is the passage of brownish to red-orange sand in the nappies, particularly noticeable when the infant becomes dehydrated. Some of the infants are very irritable with episodes of screaming, suggesting the possibility of renal colic. Most infants show normal development during the first few months of life. The first indication of impaired motor development is inability to support the head at 4 to 6 months of age with hypotonicity during the next year of life. Voluntary movements of both athetoid and choreoform types are present by the latter part of the first year of life, with an increase in muscle tone as the first extrapyramidal sign. Pyramidal symptoms consisting of increased deep tendon reflexes, a sustained ankle clonus, scissoring of the lower extremities and extensor plantar responses are usually present by one year of age. An increased incidence of dislocation of the hips and club feet may in some way be related to the early hypotonicity.

Motor and physical development of affected children are grossly impaired with subnormal height and weight. Some of them show dysphagia and vomiting as prominent symptoms. An occasional patient is able to sit in a normal manner during the first year of life, which is subsequently lost with the onset of the neurological symptoms. They have a characteristic dysarthric speech, although they can usually make themselves understood to those who are caring for them. Severely affected children are never able to walk (Nyhan, 1977).

Behaviour abnormalities
A compulsive aggressiveness and a self mutilation are the most variable features of the disease and are expressed in these children by biting away their lips, tongue and ends of their fingers, if given the opportunity. Biting can, in some cases, begin with the eruption of incisors. In other patients it may be delayed until early adolescence. In any given patient it can be highly variable in expression, with the patient going through periods when he shows extensive self-mutilation and other periods when this no longer is a problem. Self-mutilation tends to be correlated, at least in some cases, with emotional stress. In addition, some older children develop opisthotonic spasms which appear to be at least semivoluntary. An accompanying laryngeal spasm and stridor sometimes produces a temporary cyanosis. If the patient's head is in range of a hard object at the time of a spasm he may injure it. Children also sometimes throw themselves from the bed if left unattended or injure themselves on sharp edges of wheelchairs that are left unpadded.

Aggressive acts against others are also included in the bizarre behaviour of these children. This can take the form of biting, hitting, spitting or kicking. Physician's eye glasses are common targets for their aggression, so it is best for the examining physician to transfer them to his pocket before examining such a child. They often pinch or strike attendants in areas of sexual significance and become verbally aggressive, often with a remarkable shocking vocabulary of profanity and words that are socially unacceptable. Frequent projectile vomiting is also used by older children as one of their weapons, especially when the child becomes upset emotionally.

Even though this bizarre behaviour would be expected to alienate individuals about them, invariably these children are favourite patients of ward personnel and are charming and very responsive individuals. The children are fully aware and sensitive to their environment. They show a remarkably good sense of humour. They smile and laugh easily and appear to have far greater intelligence than their scores on intelligence tests would indicate.

Some, but not all, of the patients with less severe deficiencies of the HPRT enzyme with resulting minimal neurological dysfunction also show a compulsive behaviour. The unusual behaviour of one such patient included a compelling urge to put his hand in the cog wheels of machines which he had done on at least one occasion and lost the tip of a middle finger. He also recounted having an uncontrollable impulse to jump from a motorcycle or automobile while travelling at high speed, which had resulted in severe injuries to himself and his vehicles (Geerdink et al, 1973).

Lesch-Nyhan disease and its variants are the first well-documented example of a compulsive stereotyped form of behaviour that is associated with a biochemical aberration. Since a harmless biting of lips and fingernails is a relatively common response to stress in members of the normal population, the genetic and biochemical changes could be merely producing an exaggerated response to this environmental stress.

Pathology
Autopsies reported on at least 11 patients have shown no characteristic anatomical finding in histological preparations that could be of value in characterizing the disease. Kidneys are a target for damage, leading to cardiovascular disease and death in uraemia. The most far-advanced gouty nephropathy seen at the National Institutes of Health was observed in one of Dr Nyhan's original patients who died at age 12, despite his having experienced only one acute attack of gout in the knee (Seegmiller, 1968).

Biochemical features
The most extreme degree of excessive purine synthesis yet encountered in the human is found in children with Lesch-Nyhan disease. The 24-hour uric acid excretion is four to eight times that of normal individuals (Lesch & Nyhan, 1964; Seegmiller et al, 1967; Seegmiller, 1976). The urine also contains increased amounts of the uric acid precursors 4-amino-5-imidazole carboxamide (Newcombe, 1970) and hypoxanthine (Balis et al, 1967).

Hyperuricaemia is the eventual outcome of this overproduction but may take a number of years to develop in some patients.

Primary enzyme defect. A gross deficiency of the enzyme hypoxanthine-guanine phosphoribosyltransferase (HPRT) is found in all patients with Lesch-Nyhan disease (Seegmiller et al, 1967; Seegmiller, 1976). In patients with the most severe enzyme defect, activity is virtually absent from all cells of the body. In patients with less severe deficiencies, the HPRT activity in dialyzed erythrocyte lysates may range from less than .01 to 10 or 20% of the normal, using hypoxanthine as a substrate (Kelley et al, 1967a; Kelley et al, 1969; Seegmiller, 1980c).

A concurrent increase in the activity of the analogous enzyme concerned with conversion of adenine to its nucleotide, adenine phosphoribosyltransferase (APRT), is a consistent finding in erythrocytes of all patients who show a severe HPRT deficiency (Seegmiller et al, 1976; Seegmiller, 1976), but is not found in their fibroblasts. This increase is not found in erythrocytes of patients with a partial HPRT deficiency (Emmerson et al, 1977).

HPRT activity in fibroblasts of affected children is invariably substantially higher than is found in their erythrocytes with values of around 1 to 3% of the activity found in normal fibroblasts (Fujimoto & Seegmiller, 1970; Kelley & Mead 1971). In no patient has a complete deficiency of the enzyme been observed in the patient's cultured fibroblasts.

Heterozygote detection

All pedigrees have shown a pattern of inheritance consistent with X–linkage. Definitive proof came with the demonstration by radioautography of both normal and mutant phenotypes in fibroblasts grown from skin biopsies of the mothers and remains a very reliable method for heterozygote detection (Rosenbloom et al, 1967). Such a finding is entirely consistent with the single X–inactivation hypothesis proposed independently by Lyon (1961) and Beutler (1962). Demonstration of the presence of both normal and mutant cells can also be done by cloning or by selection for the mutant phenotype in the mother's fibroblasts with thioguanine or 6-azaguanine (Salzmann et al, 1968; Migeon et al, 1968; Felix & DeMars, 1971; Fujimoto et al, 1971). Heterozygotes can also be detected by assaying hair roots (Gartler et al, 1971; Bakay et al, 1980).

Instead of the one-third new mutations expected, examination of 47 kindred revealed only four probands with new mutations (Francke et al, 1976).

Erythrocytes of mothers of severely HPRT-deficient children invariably show an activity of HPRT in the normal range. A selective advantage of the normal stem cell over the mutant phenotype at some stage of fetal or cellular development seems to be the most satisfactory explanation. Only in heterozygotes of partial HPRT deficiency have normal and mutant erythrocytes been demonstrated (Emmerson et al, 1977).

Properties of normal and mutant enzymes

HPRT has been purified up to 13 000-fold from human erythrocytes (Milman et al, 1977; Krenitsky, 1969). Magnesium and sulphhydryl groups are required for its activity and its substrates are magnesium phosphoribosylpyrophosphate (PRPP) and either hypoxanthine or guanine. It reacts with xanthine at a rate only 0.3% of that of hypoxanthine (Kelley et al, 1967b). It also reacts with 6-mercaptopurine, 8-azaguanine, allopurinol and 6-thioguanine to form the respective ribonucleotides, but fails to react with adenine, uric acid, uracil, azathioprine, or oxypurinol (Krenitsky et al, 1969).

The purified native enzyme is composed of two or three subunits of molecular weight 25 000. The reported molecular weights of the native enzyme range from 68 000 (Kelley & Arnold, 1973) to 81 000 (Ghangas & Milman, 1977). In one HPRT-deficient clone from a HeLa cell line with a missense mutation, a new protein spot was detected at the same molecular weight as the subunit, but a different position on isoelectric focusing (Milman et al, 1976). Post-transcriptional alterations in the enzyme undoubtedly give rise to the three to four peaks observed on isoelectric focusing (Kelley et al, 1969; Bakay & Nyhan, 1971).

Considerable heterogeneity in mutations has been described. The majority of patients with the complete syndrome show no cross-reactive material (Bakay et al, 1976). In some patients the mutation had produced decreased activity by reason of a decreased affinity for one of the substrates, resulting in essentially normal activity at concentrations of PRPP and guanine ten-fold greater than those generally used in the assay (Henderson et al, 1976). A variety of other types of mutations in this enzyme have also been described and are referred to in reviews (Seegmiller, 1980a).

Mechanism of purine overproduction

The excessive rates of purine synthesis observed in patients are also found in their fibroblasts (Seegmiller et al, 1967; Rosenbloom et al, 1968) and lymphoblasts (Lever et al, 1974), providing hypoxanthine is present in the medium. If hypoxanthine is omitted from the medium, then normal cells increase their rate of purine synthesis to values quite comparable to that seen in HPRT-deficient lymphoblasts (Hershfield & Seegmiller, 1977). The most reasonable explanation for the excessive rate of purine synthesis is the increased amounts of phosphoribosylpyrophosphate (PRPP) accumulating as a result of the HPRT mutation. Fibroblasts cultured from affected patients show a two- to three-fold accumulation of PRPP and their erythrocytes a ten-fold accumulation over normal values (Rosenbloom et al, 1968; Kelley et al, 1970). PRPP is a rate-limiting substrate for the presumed rate-determining reaction of purine biosynthesis catalyzed by the enzyme phosphoribosylpyrophosphate glutamine amidotransferase (Wood & Seegmiller, 1973; Wood et al, 1973). Further support for this concept comes from the correlation of increased intracellular PRPP in fibroblasts and excessive rates of purine synthesis as a result of a different mutation found in other families with gouty arthritis consisting of increased activity of the enzyme PRPP synthetase (see below). Both types of mutation produce an increase in intracellular PRPP in cultured fibroblasts that are associated with an excessive rate of uric acid synthesis (Rosenbloom et al, 1968; Becker, 1976).

Treatment

General measures for treatment include avoidance of dehydration, assurance of high fluid intake and making certain that nutrition is adequate. Many of these children take a very long time to eat and in an understaffed institution may actually be malnourished. Sites of chronic irritation in the mouth from sharp edges of teeth can be eliminated by a dentist, hands can be kept away from the mouth and yet be left free for use by constructing loose fitting wrap-around fabric splints for the elbows containing wooden or plastic ribs in a fabric pocket and secured in place with the tightness desired by Velcro fasteners. These children seem to be incapable of learning from punishment, but they do respond to positive experiences and some success in behaviour modification has been achieved by simply turning away from the child when their aberrant behaviour is in evidence (Jochmus et al, 1977; Nyhan, 1977).

Drugs now available are very effective in preventing the damage to kidneys produced by the excessive amounts of uric acid excreted in the urine. Allopurinol, at doses up to 10 mg/kg body weight per day, produces a striking decrease in uric acid content of both urine and serum, but fails to decrease the total purine synthesis as is seen in other types of purine over-production. Hypoxanthine and xanthine replace the deficit in uric acid in urine. Established renal calculi composed of uric acid can thereby be substantially reduced in size. A high fluid intake of at least 50 ml/kg per day will diminish the chance of forming urinary concretions composed of xanthine that have been noted occasionally in children treated with allopurinol.

Unfortunately, no rational therapy has yet been found satisfactory for treating the neurological dysfunction. Children treated with diazepam (Valium) are more tractable and less spastic. Hydroxytryptophan has been reported to reduce self-mutilation in children in Japan (Mizumo & Yugari, 1974; Mizumo & Yugari, 1975) but was not effective in reducing the self-mutilating behav-

iour in numerous other studies (Frith et al, 1976; Ciaranello et al, 1976; Anderson et al, 1976; Nyhan, 1977). A transient beneficial effect has been found with administration of combinations of the peripheral decarboxylase inhibitor carbidopa, immipramine and hydroxytryptophan (Nyhan, 1977).

Prenatal diagnosis

Until a more effective therapy for the neurological aspects of this disease is developed, prevention of the disease by monitoring pregnancies is indicated. This is best done by identifying heterozygous females among the relatives of an index case (Seegmiller, 1974). Index cases are readily detected by demonstrating a high ratio of uric acid to creatinine in morning urine samples (Kaufman et al, 1968). Our centre has monitored 25 pregnancies at risk for carrying an affected fetus and has identified 7 affected fetuses, each sufficiently early that the parents' desire to terminate the pregnancy could be met.

Increased phosphoribosyl pyrophosphate (PRPP) synthetase

The excessive production of uric acid found in six families with gouty arthritis has now been traced to an increased activity of phosphoribosyl-pyrophosphate (PRPP) synthetase. The increased intracellular concentration of PRPP found in fibroblasts or lymphoblasts cultured from patients with this disorder provides another example, with a different mutation, of the relation of concentration of this substance with rate of purine biosynthesis de novo (Rosenbloom et al, 1968; Becker, 1976). This correlation provides additional evidence in support of the concept outlined above of the central role of PRPP concentrations in governing the rate of purine synthesis de novo in vivo.

Clinical presentation

In all families an excessive rate of purine synthesis was in evidence, ranging from 1.0 to 2.4 grams/24 hours while maintained on a diet virtually free of purines. In addition, a high incidence of renal calculi composed of uric acid was also present in these families (Seegmiller, 1980a). Other clinical features in one family include deafness (see below) (Becker et al, 1980a; Becker et al, 1980b).

Heterogeneity in mutations

As with patients of Lesch-Nyhan disease, considerable heterogeneity has already been detected in mutations at the PRPP synthetase locus. The patient (described by Sperling et al, 1972a; Zoref et al, 1975; Sperling et al, 1972b) showed an enhanced rate of PRPP synthetase activity only at very low levels of inorganic phosphate added to red cell lysates. At higher phosphate concentrations the enzyme showed a normal activity. It also showed a diminished response to the feedback inhibitor, adenosine diphosphate (Zoref et al, 1975). The same defect was found in two additional family members over two generations.

A different mutation in the PRPP synthetase locus was responsible for the overproduction of uric acid and gouty arthritis of two brothers described by Becker et al (1972; Becker et al, 1973a; Becker et al, 1973b; Becker et al, 1973c; Becker & Seegmiller, 1975; Becker, 1976). The mutant enzyme showed a three-fold increase in enzyme activity at all concentrations of phosphate in the lysate with normal kinetics except for a three-fold increase in V_{max}. The mutant enzyme showed an increased specific activity as shown by the presence of normal amounts of cross-reacting materials on testing with antibodies to purified enzyme (Becker et al, 1973c), thus delineating a most unusual type of mutation. Mutant enzyme showed a difference in electrophoretic migration from that of normal, providing evidence that it results from a mutation in a structural gene coding for the enzyme. The brothers showed an incorporation of ^{14}C-glycine into urinary uric acid that was $2\frac{1}{2}$ to 3 times normal.

Genetics
Both the HPRT enzyme and PRPP synthetase enzyme are located in close proximity on the X–chromosome. X–linkage, first suspected from pedigree studies, was later confirmed by demonstrations of normal and mutant cell populations in fibroblasts cultured from heterozygous females (Zoref et al, 1977a; Zoref et al, 1977b; Yen et al, 1978). More definitive studies mapping the adjacent locations on the X–chromosome utilized the techniques of somatic cell genetics (Goss & Harris, 1975; Becker et al, 1979). PRPP synthetase was mapped on the long arm of the human X–chromosome between the alpha galactosidase locus and the HPRT locus. This demonstration provides the first example of a gene coding for two enzymes in a metabolic sequence being found on the same chromosome of the mammalian cell.

Properties of mutant enzyme
PRPP synthetase isolated from human erythrocytes is composed of subunits of 33 200 MW which undergo reversible association (Becker et al, 1975; Myer & Becker, 1977; Becker et al, 1977). The monomer or aggregates of up to eight units show only minimal if any activity. The full activity is found only in aggregates of 16 and 32 subunits and for their formation magnesium ion, inorganic orthophosphate, magnesium ATP, reaction products or nucleotide inhibitors are required.

Other defects in phosphoribosylpyrophosphate synthetase
Two different reports of a deficiency in PRPP synthetase have appeared. A severe deficiency of PRPP synthetase was first reported in a child with hypouricaemia and

mental retardation who showed a remarkable and unexplained recovery of enzyme activity after treatment with adrenocorticotrophic hormone (Wada et al, 1974; Iinuma et al, 1975). A decrease to 30% of normal (Valentine et al, 1972) was later found to be a secondary response to a three- to four-fold increase in intracellular concentration of pyrimidine-5'-nucleotides from a gross deficiency of pyrimidine-5'-nucleotidase (Valentine et al, 1974) (see section below).

Hereditary xanthinuria
A gross hereditary deficiency of the enzyme xanthine oxidase results in the substitution of the precursors xanthine and hypoxanthine for uric acid as the end products of purine metabolism (Ayvazian, 1964). The formation of xanthine stones of the urinary tract is the principle clinical problem of patients with xanthinuria and occurred in 40% of a series of 42 patients (Seegmiller, 1980a). It was associated with a sulphite oxidase deficiency in one patient, who presented with mental retardation, seizures, nystagmus, dislocated lens, enophthalmus and developmental asymmetry of the skull (Duran et al, 1978; van der Heiden et al, 1979; Johnson et al, 1980). Additional clinical problems observed in four patients were muscle symptoms, myalgia or arthralgia, particularly after exercise; with crystals composed of xanthine or hypoxanthine demonstrated in the muscles of three. Since the first report of xanthine urinary calculi (Marcet, 1817) well over 60 additional reports of calculi have appeared.

Diagnosis
The majority of patients are discovered from routine use of blood chemistry panels which reveal a serum urate that is usually less than 1.0 mg/dl in an individual who is otherwise healthy and taking none of the drugs known to lower serum urate concentrations. The diagnosis is confirmed by demonstrating the excretion of less than 100 mg of uric acid per day in the 24-hour urine, along with several hundred milligrams of hypoxanthine and xanthine, as compared to around 0.2 mg per 24 hours for the normal individual. Of these oxypurines, 50 to 90% is xanthine.

Heterogeneity in xanthinuria is suggested in the mutations leading to the clinical presentation of xanthinuria and is shown by the markedly variable ratios of uric acid to oxypurines that have been described indicating different degrees of severity. This procedure should also distinguish xanthinuria from other causes of hypouricaemia. In patients with a renal tubular defect, uric acid rather than oxypurines will be the major component of urine. In those with hypouricaemia from purine nucleoside phosphorylase deficiency (see below), the purine nucleosides will be present in the urine, rather than oxypurines or uric acid.

A wide variety of methods are available for the demonstration of xanthine in the urine, including paper chromatography (Dent & Philpot, 1954; Thompson, 1960), column chromatography (Bradford et al, 1968), paper electrophoresis (Englemann et al, 1964) or by enzyme assay using xanthine oxidase and uricase (Chalmers & Watts, 1969; Klinenberg et al, 1967). Demonstration of the enzyme defect has been done using biopsy of intestinal epithelium or liver (Ayvazian, 1964; Seegmiller, 1980a), but is not routinely required for the diagnosis.

Treatment

A high fluid intake and avoidance of dehydration provides the simplest and most rational approach to management. In patients with recurrent xanthine stones a restriction of the purine content of the diet should be of benefit and alkalinization of the urine may help prevent recurrence. Attempts have been made to substitute the more soluble hypoxanthine for xanthine by administration of allopurinol (Englemann et al, 1964; Holmes et al, 1974). Subsequent studies, however, have failed to confirm a beneficial effect (Salti et al, 1976; Simmons et al, 1974; Simmons et al, 1975).

Deficiency of adenine phosphoribosyltransferase (APRT)

Of the first six known cases of homozygous deficiency of adenine phosphoribosyltransferase (APRT), four presented with calculi of the urinary tract composed of 2-8-dihydroxyadenine, a substance not previously reported in human calculi. The clinical presentation in each case has been in childhood and the stone has initially been identified on the basis of qualitative tests as uric acid. A clinical observation that could be of help to the urologist in identifying this condition is that uric acid stones are hard and tend to be yellow, whereas 2-8-dihydroxyadenine stones are friable and grey-blue on crushing. The simplest test for detection of 2-8-dihydroxyadenine is to determine the ultraviolet absorption spectrum at pH 2 and compare it with that of uric acid and a known standard of 2-8-dihydroxyadenine. The later can be produced by the prolonged action of xanthine oxidase on adenine. Confirmation of the diagnosis is found by demonstrating increased amounts of adenine in the urine and the virtual absence of APRT in dialyzed lysates of erythrocytes of the affected patient (Cartier & Hemet, 1974; Debray et al, 1976; Simmonds et al, 1976; VanAcker et al, 1977a; VanAcker et al, 1977b; Simmonds et al, 1977; Simonds et al, 1978; Cartier et al, 1980; VanAcker et al, 1980). No impairment of immune function has been found (Stevens et al, 1980) and both homozygotes and heterozygotes show values for uric acid in the serum and urine in the normal range. This is an example of a disease in which the heterozygous state was detected before the homozygous state was identified (Kelley et al, 1968). The reported frequency of heterozygotes is one in 233 individuals (Johnson et al, 1977). Rational treatment is with allopurinol.

Immunodeficiency diseases associated with defects in purine metabolism

The discovery, within the past decade, of specific defects in each of three sequential enzymes of purine metabolism in association with three specific types of immunodeficiency disease has added a new dimension to studies of biochemical factors regulating this complex system (Fig. 90.2). Two of these deficiencies definitely represent abnormal gene products, adenosine deaminase deficiency and purine nucleoside phosphorylase deficiency. The purine-5′-nucleotidase deficiency in patients with agammaglobulinaemia may well be a secondary result of immaturity or loss of B cells.

Adenosine deaminase deficiency

A gross deficiency of the enzyme adenosine deaminase was reported by Giblett et al (1972) in two unrelated children with severe combined immunodeficiency disease. Since that time over three dozen families with adenosine deaminase deficiency have been identified. All patients show a virtually complete impairment of T-cell function with varying degrees of B-cell dysfunction depending on the family or the stage of the disease (Seegmiller, 1980a; Meuwissen & Pollara, 1974). As a consequence, these children are vulnerable to infections of viral, bacterial and fungal origin and if untreated can succumb to overwhelming infections within the first year or so of life. About one-half of the patients with an autosomal recessive type of severe combined immunodeficiency disease are estimated to have a deficiency of adenosine deaminase (Hirschhorn, 1977).

Diagnosis. Adenosine deaminase deficiency should be suspected in all patients who show recurrent infections during the first year of life. Absence of the thymus shadow on X–ray and absence of tonsils or palpable lymph nodes further supports this presumption. Many patients also show a bony abnormality of the thorax with flaring of the costochondral junction, but this has not proven to be a consistent or specific finding. Confirmation of the defect is shown by demonstrating the virtual absence of adenosine deaminase in red cells, fibroblasts or lymphocytes cultured from affected children. In one patient with an ADA deficiency a gross deficiency of ecto-5′-nucleotidase has also been described, which presumably was secondary to the B-cell immaturity and dysfunction (Boss et al, 1981). Occasional patients have been found in whom the ADA deficiency is limited to erythrocytes and reflects an unstable enzyme. Such individuals do not have impairment of the immune system (Hirschhorn et al, 1979).

Mechanism of pathology. The proposed mechanism of

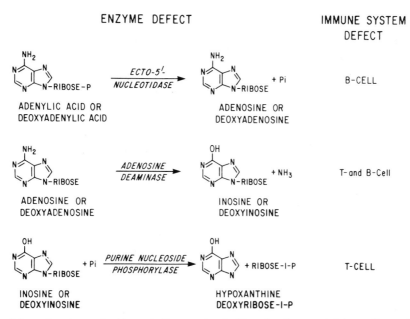

ENZYME DEFECT

IMMUNE SYSTEM
DEFECT

ADENYLIC ACID OR
DEOXYADENYLIC ACID   →[ECTO-5′-NUCLEOTIDASE]→   ADENOSINE OR
DEOXYADENOSINE   + Pi   B-CELL

ADENOSINE OR
DEOXYADENOSINE   →[ADENOSINE DEAMINASE]→   INOSINE OR
DEOXYINOSINE   + NH_3 T-and B-Cell

INOSINE OR
DEOXYINOSINE   + Pi   →[PURINE NUCLEOSIDE PHOSPHORYLASE]→   HYPOXANTHINE
DEOXYRIBOSE-1-P   + RIBOSE-1-P   T-CELL

Fig. 90.2 Enzyme defects of purine nucleotide catabolism associated with various immunodeficiency diseases. Low purine-5′-nucleotidase may well be a secondary effect and reflect the paucity and immaturity of B cells rather than being the direct product of the mutant gene.

suppression of the immune system is shown in Figure 90.3. Both adenosine and deoxyadenosine are substrates for adenosine deaminase. However, adenosine kinase has a higher affinity for adenosine, thereby providing an alternative pathway for its utilization (Schnebli et al, 1967). The kinase for deoxyadenosine shows a much lower affinity. Consequently, ADA-deficient children excrete, in the urine, substantial amounts of deoxyadenosine, some 6000 times that found in normal urine (Simmonds et al, 1978; Kuttesch et al, 1978; Goldblum et al, 1978). Erythrocytes and lymphocytes of affected children show a 10- to 20- fold increase in intracellular concentration of deoxyATP (Coleman et al, 1978; Donofrio et al, 1978; Cohen et al, 1978). In model systems, T-cell lines of human lymphoblasts show a greater susceptibility than B-cell lines to deoxyATP accumulation and its accompanying growth inhibition (Carson et al, 1977; Carson et al, 1978). Impairment of growth was traced to a decreased rate of destruction of deoxyATP. This, in turn, was related to the lower activities of purine ecto-5′-nucleotidase in T cells than in B cells (Carson et al, 1977; 1978; Thompson et al, 1980).

The deoxyATP, in both the bacterial and mammalian system, is a potent allosteric inhibitor of all activities of the enzyme ribonucleoside diphosphate reductase which is responsible for synthesis of deoxyribonucleotide in all cells (Reichard, 1972; Reichard, 1978). In support of this concept is the ability of other deoxynucleosides to overcome the inhibition of mitogen-stimulated lymphocytes

produced by a potent ADA inhibitor, deoxycoformycin and small amounts of deoxyadenosine (Bluestein et al, 1978; Bluestein et al, 1980).

Another theory for the mechanism of immunosuppression includes a permanent inhibition of the enzyme S-adenosyl-homocysteine hydrolase by deoxyadenosine that could lead to accumulation of S-adenosyl-homocysteine with a resulting inhibition of methylation reactions by S-adenosylmethionine (Hershfield, 1979; Hershfield et al, 1979). A modest accumulation of cyclic AMP has been observed in lymphocytes of ADA-deficient patients (Schmalsteig et al, 1977). The susceptibility to growth inhibition by adenosine and an ADA inhibitor of a lymphoid cell line deficient in enzymes involved in cAMP toxicity argues against this mechanism (Ullman et al, 1976). The possible role of the latter two mechanisms in affected children remains to be assessed.

Treatment. Bone marrow transplantation from a histocompatible donor remains the treatment of choice (Goode & Hanson, 1978). However, a transient restoration of immune function has been achieved in about half the patients by infusion at 4- to 6-week intervals of irradiated erythrocytes (Polmar et al, 1975).

Purine nucleoside phosphorylase deficiency
A report of a severe deficiency of the enzyme purine nucleoside phosphorylase (PNP) in a child with an isolated defect of T-cell function by Giblett et al (1975) was followed by identification of additional patients, all of

whom showed evidence of gross impairment of T-cell function (Hamet et al, 1977; Griscelli et al, 1976; Wadman et al, 1976; Siegenbeck et al, 1976; Stoop et al, 1977). Two patients have been reported who died of vaccinia infection and one with a varicella infection, pointing out the great susceptibility of these children to common viral infections. Two patients with PNP deficiencies have presented with neurological problems consisting of a tetraparesis in one case (Stoop et al, 1977) and a tremor and ataxia in the other (Rich et al, 1979).

Instead of excreting uric acid in the urine, these patients excrete phenomenally large amounts of the expected ribonucleoside substrates for the missing enzymes, inosine and guanosine. Totally unexpected was the presence of remarkable quantities of the corresponding deoxynucleosides, deoxyinosine and deoxyguanosine which constituted around one-third of the total nucleosides excreted (Cohen et al, 1976). On a molar basis, the amount of purines excreted was comparable to the amount produced by children with Lesch-Nyhan disease (above). Since this enzyme deficit prevents these children from making hypoxanthine, a possible explanation for the excessive purine synthesis is found in the phenomenal increase in purine synthesis produced in normal cells deprived of hypoxanthine (Hershfield & Seegmiller, 1977).

One family has been described with a less severe deficiency of purine nucleoside phosphorylase associated with a clinical presentation of familial autoimmune haemolytic anaemia (Rich et al, 1979; Rich et al, 1980; Fox et al, 1977; Gelfand et al, 1978; Edwards et al, 1978).

Treatment. As with patients with ADA deficiency, transfusion of irradiated erythrocytes has produced a transient return of immunological function in two patients with PNP deficiency (Ammann et al, 1978; Zegers et al, 1979; Staal et al, 1980; Rich et al, 1980).

Mechanism of immunosuppression. The rationale for immunosuppression in this disease is very similar to that for ADA deficiency (Fig. 90.3), with the exception that deoxyguanosine leads to the deoxyGTP accumulation within the cells of the immune system. This nucleotide triphosphate then becomes the active inhibitor of the ribonucleoside diphosphate reductase leading to inhibition of production of deoxynucleosides of guanine, uracil and cytosine, thus preventing DNA synthesis (Cohen et al, 1978). Further evidence for this concept has been found in the resistance to deoxyguanosine toxicity of mouse T-lymphoma cells traced to ribonucleoside diphosphate resistant to allosteric inhibition by deoxyGTP (Gudas et al, 1978; Seegmiller, 1980a).

Significance for tumour therapy. The mechanism deduced for the immunosuppression of either ADA or PNP deficiency points the way for possible use of inhibitors of these same enzymes possibly with their deoxynucleosides as specific therapy for conditions resulting from over-active T cells. The most potent inhibitor known for ADA is deoxycoformycin with a Ki of 2.5 × 10^{-12} M (Johns & Adamson, 1976; Adamson et al, 1977; Agarwal et al, 1979). Inhibition of ADA by the potent ADA inhibitor deoxycoformycin has been used for treatment of T-cell leukemia with some promising results (Yu et al, 1979; Smyth et al, 1979; Koller et al, 1980; Mitchell et al, 1979; Yu et al, 1980; Yu et al, 1981). Although a more potent inhibitor of purine nucleoside phosphorylase has been described than was previously available (Willis et al, 1980) even more potent and specific inhibitors would undoubtedly be useful.

Decreased ecto-purine-5'-nucleotidase
A decrease in activity of the membrane-bound enzyme ecto-purine-5'-nucleotidase has been reported in lymphocytes from peripheral blood of patients with both acquired and hereditary forms of agammaglobulinaemia and as an accompaniment of malignant lymphomas (Johnson et al, 1977; Quagliata et al, 1974; Edwards et al, 1978). The evidence now available favours the view of the low activity reflecting immaturity and scarcity of B cells rather than a primary product of an abnormal gene. A complete absence of the enzyme activity was not found in any of the patients, and in normal controls a wide range of values was found. A possible explanation for the wide range of values in controls has been suggested by the report of Boss et al (1980) showing a decrease in the activity of this enzyme in both T and B lymphocytes with advancing age after mid-life. In normal individuals, T-cells show about one-third the activity of this enzyme found in B-cells. Some evidence has been presented that the enzyme activity may reflect a degree of B-cell immaturity (Boss et al, 1979). Concurrence of low ecto-5'-nucleotidase activity in a patient with adenosine deaminase deficiency has also been found (Boss et al, 1981).

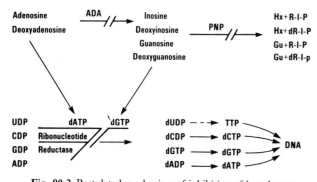

Fig. 90.3 Postulated mechanism of inhibition of lymphocyte proliferation in genetic deficiency of adenosine deaminase (ADA) or nucleoside phosphorylase (PNP).

X–linked agammaglobulinaemia

Affected males show a paucity of B cells and low activities of ecto-5'-nucleotidase in peripheral blood lymphocytes. All attempts at producing long-term cultures from their peripheral blood lymphocytes have been unsuccessful. However, some of the lymphoblast lines established from peripheral blood lymphocytes of female relatives showed a low ecto-5'-nucleotidase activity during the initial phase of the cultures. However, the activity rapidly increased with prolonged culture. This observation suggested the possible identification in this manner of carriers for the gene (Thompson et al, 1980). The low activity of this enzyme in T cells may be the basis for their greater susceptibility to deoxyadenosine toxicity (see ADA deficiency above).

Myoadenylate deaminase deficiency

A gross deficiency of the enzyme adenylic acid deaminase has been found in muscle cells, but not erythrocytes or leucocytes, of five patients with exercise intolerance leading to weakness and muscle cramps as their major symptoms. They also showed decreased muscle mass, hypotonia and non-specific abnormal electromyograms. In some patients an increase in serum creatine phosphokinase was found and venous ammonia failed to rise after muscle exercise. The defects seem to be limited only to AMP deaminase generated within muscle and is not found in erythrocytes or in cultured fibroblasts or lymphoblasts (Fishbein et al, 1978). The same defect was found in 6 of 256 biopsies examined, but only two of the six patients had exercise related symptoms (Shumate et al, 1979). AMP deaminase was also found to be low in muscle tissue of patients with an early onset form of Duchenne muscular dystrophy (Kar & Pearson, 1973). One patient with myoadenylate deficiency also had gouty arthritis (Dimauro et al, 1980). His cultured fibroblasts showed a normal activity. An overactivity of the corresponding enzyme of liver has been proposed on theoretical grounds as a possible basis for excessive purine synthesis and gouty arthritis by Hers & Van den Berghe (1979).

Deficiency of adenylate kinase

Two sibs from consanguinous parents of an Arabian family showed a severe non-spherocytic haemolytic anaemia associated with a severe deficiency of the enzyme adenylate kinase (Szeinberg et al, 1969; Szeinberg, 1969). This enzyme is normally involved in the synthesis of ADP from AMP so that its deficiency could well interfere with generation of ATP. However, the possible role in their anaemia of the glucose-6-phosphate dehydrogenase deficiency, also found in their erythrocytes, must be considered.

Other abnormalities

An increase in adenosine deaminase activity was found in erythrocytes of 12 members affected with haemolytic anaemia in a family of 23, spanning three generations. They showed splenomegaly, a reticulocytosis averaging 6%, a negative Coomb's test for autoimmune haemolytic anaemia and no evidence of haemoglobinopathy (Valentine et al, 1977). It was inherited in a dominant pattern and affected 5 of 10 males and 8 of 13 females. A low ATP content of the erythrocytes, as a result of this enhanced enzyme activity, seems to be the basis for the chronic haemolysis. The possibility of treatment with the very potent inhibitor of adenosine deaminase, deoxycoformycin, should be considered (Mitchell & Keller, 1980).

Other unidentified disorders of purine metabolism

Several families have been described with increased rates of purine synthesis associated with neurological dysfunction. These include a child originally thought to have autistic behaviour (Nyhan et al, 1969; Becker et al, 1978) but who, on repeated examinations several years later, had an increased activity of phosphoribosylpyrophosphate synthetase and deafness (Becker et al, 1980a; Becker et al, 1980b). An association of uric acid synthesis with ataxia, weakness, deafness and renal insufficiency with varying degrees of disability have been reported in a large family (Rosenberg, 1970). A girl with an encephalopathy, self-mutilation and excessive uric acid production, but no hyperuricaemia, has also been reported by Hooft et al (1968).

DISORDERS OF PYRIMIDINE METABOLISM

Hereditary orotic aciduria

A severe inherited deficiency of two enzymes of pyrimidine metabolism, orotate phosphoribosyltransferase and orotidine 5'-phosphate decarboxylase, characterizes the metabolic abnormality of hereditary orotic aciduria. The resulting interruption of the biosynthesis of pyrimidine nucleotides in affected patients results in the excretion in their urine of large amounts of orotic acid, the substrate for the first of the missing enzymes. On cooling the urine, crystalline deposits of orotic acid form along the wall of the container.

Clinical symptoms

Twelve patients have now been described, 11 of which are summarized in a recent review (Seegmiller, 1980a). Affected patients appear normal at birth but in the first year of life develop a severe megaloblastic anaemia resistant to usual forms of treatment, with an accompanying retardation of physical and mental development (Huguley, 1959). The original patient died from an overwhelming varicella infection at the age of two years, suggesting the possibility of T-cell dysfunction (see PNP deficiency above). In one recently-diagnosed patient evidence of immune dysfunction was found (Perignon, personal communication).

Treatment

Since these children are incapable of making pyrimidines, they are the counterpart of auxotrophic bacteria and have a new dietary requirement of pyrimidines. The administration of uridine, at a dose of 1.5 g per day, produced a dramatic decline in orotic acid excretion as a result of feed-back inhibition and produced a prompt reticulocyte response and development of a normal appearance of bone marrow within 20 days. The children resumed growth. This dietary supplement, adjusted at intervals for increases in body requirements, seems to be a fully adequate form of treatment (Becroft & Phillips, 1965; Becroft & Phillips, 1969; Hagard & Lockhart, 1967).

Orotic aciduria associated with defects in urea synthesis

Genetically-determined human deficiencies in each of the five enzymes involved in urea synthesis have been found (Levine & Hoogenraad, 1974). In each case hyperammonaemia was a prominent feature of the clinical disorder which also included vomiting, lethargy and coma. In the few cases that have been examined so far an orotic aciduria has been found (Beaudry et al, 1975; McLeod et al, 1972). Presumably, the orotic aciduria arises from excessive carbamyl phosphate formed in the mitochondria in response to the hyperammonaemia which then leaks into the cytoplasm where it becomes a precursor for pyrimidine nucleotide synthesis.

Deficiency of pyrimidine 5'-nucleotidase in patients with non-spherocytic haemolytic anaemia

A selective autosomal recessively inherited deficiency of the enzyme pyrimidine 5'-nucleotidase limited to erythrocytes results in a non-spherocytic haemolytic anaemia. Increased concentrations of pyrimidine nucleotides are present in all erythrocytes (Valentine et al, 1974; Vives-Corrons et al, 1976; Ben-Bassat, 1976; Rochant, 1975; Torrance, 1977; Miewa, 1977). A decrease of activity of this same enzyme is seen as a very sensitive index of lead poisoning (Valentine et al, 1976).

Xeroderma pigmentosum

A defect in some stage in excision and repair of thymidine dimers of DNA induced by ultraviolet light is the fundamental defect found in patients with xeroderma pigmentosum. Their clinical presentation includes abnormalities of pigmentation on exposed areas of the skin, produced by sunlight, and numerous malignancies in the same area of the skin (Cleaver, 1968; Robbins et al, 1974; Robbins et al, 1976; Cleaver et al, 1978). It is inherited in an autosomal recessive manner and heterogeneity of the genetic lesion involved is shown by correction of the defect by cell fusion of fibroblasts cultured from patients from different families. Five complementation groups have been so identified (Kramer et al, 1975). No fully effective treatment has been devised, other than prevention of exposure to sunlight and the removal of superficial dermis with an electric dermatome to retard development of malignant tumours (Epstein et al, 1972).

REFERENCES

Adamson R H, Zaharevitz D W, Johns D G 1977 Enhancement of the biological activity of adenosine analogs by the adenosine deaminase inhibitor 2'-deoxycoformycin. Pharmacology 15: 84–89

Agarwal R P, Spector T, Parks P E 1979 Tight-binding inhibitors: IV. Inhibition of adenosine deaminase by various inhibitors. Biochemical Pharmacology 26: 259–267

Alepa F P, Howell R R, Klinenberg,J R, Seegmiller J E 1967 Relationships between glycogen storage disease and tophaceous gout. American Journal of Medicine 42: 58–66

Ammann A J, Wara D W, Allen T 1978 Immunotherapy and immunopathologic studies in a patient with nucleoside phosphorylase deficiency. Clinical Immunology and Immunopathology 10: 262–269

Anderson L T, Herrmann L, Dancis J 1976 The effect of 1-5-hydroxytryptophan on self-mutilation in Lesch-Nyhan disease: A negative report. Neuropaediatrie 7: 439–442

Ayvazian J H 1964 Xanthinuria and hemochromatosis. New England Journal of Medicine 270: 18–22

Bakay B, Becker M A, Nyhan W L 1976 Reaction of antibody to normal human hypoxanthine phosphoribosyltransferase with products of mutant genes. Archives of Biochemistry and Biophysics 177: 415–426

Bakay B, Nyhan W L 1971 The separation of adenine and hypoxanthineguanine phosphoribosyltransferase isoenzymes by disc gel electrophoresis. Biochemical Genetics 5: 81–90

Bakay B, Tucker-Pian C, Seegmiller, J E 1980 Detection of Lesch-Nyhan Syndrome carriers: Analysis of hair roots for HPRT by agarose gel electrophoresis and autoradiography. Clinical Genetics 17: 1–6

Balis M E, Krakoff I H, Berman P H, Dancis J 1967 Urinary metabolities in congenital hyperuricosuria. Science 156: 1122–1123

Batuman V, Maesaka J K, Haddad B, Tepper E, Landy E, Wedeen R P 1981 The role of lead in gout nephropathy. New England Journal of Medicine 304: 520–523

Beaudry M A, Letarte J, Collu R, Leboeuf G, Ducharme J R, Melancon S B, Dallairf L 1975 Chronic hyperammonemia with orotic aciduria: Evidence of pyrimidine pathway stimulation. Diabetic Metabolism 1: 29–37

Becker M A 1976 Patterns of phosphoribosylpyrophosphate and ribose-5-phosphate concentration and generation in fibroblasts from patients with gout and purine overproduction. Journal of Clinical Investigation 57: 308–318

Becker M A, Kostel P J, Meyer L J 1975 Human phosphoribosylpyrophosphate synthetase: Comparison of purified normal and mutant enzymes. Journal of Biological Chemistry 250: 6822–6830

Becker M A, Meyer L J, Wood A W, Seegmiller J E 1972 Gout associated with increased PRPP synthetase activity. Arthritis and Rheumatism 15: 430A

Becker M A, Meyer L J, Wood A W, Seegmiller J E 1973a Purine over-production in man associated with increased phosphoribosylpyrophosphate synthetase activity. Science 179: 1123–1126

Becker M A, Kostel P J, Meyer L J, Seegmiller J E 1973b Human phosphoribosylpyrophosphate synthetase: Increased enzyme specific activity in a family with gout and excessive purine synthesis. Proceedings of the National Academy of Sciences USA 70: 2749–2752

Becker M A, Meyer L J, Huisman W H, Lazar C S, Adams W B 1977 Human phosphoribosylpyrophosphate synthetase: Relation of activity and quaternary structure. In: Muller M M, Kaiser E, Seegmiller J E (eds) Advances in Experimental Medicine and Biology, 76a, Plenum Press, New York, 71–79

Becker M A, Meyer L J, Wood A W, Seegmiller J E 1973c Gout with purine overproduction due to increased phosphoribosylpyrophosphate synthetase activity. American Journal of Medicine 55: 232–242

Becker M A, Raivio K O, Bakay B, Adams W B, Nyhan W L 1978 Superactive phosphoribosylpyrophosphate (PRPP) synthetase with altered regulatory and catalytic functions. Abstracts of 29th Annual Meeting of the American Society of Human Genetics, p 22a

Becker M A, Raivio K O, Bakay B, Adams W B, Nyhan W L 1980a Superactive phosphoribosylpyrophosphate synthetase with altered regulatory and catalytic properties. In: Rapado A, Watts R W E, DeBruyn C H M M (eds) Advances in Experimental Medicine and Biology 122A: Plenum Press, New York, p 387–392

Becker M A, Raivio K O, Bakay B, Adams W B, Nyhan W L 1980b Variant human phosphoribosylpyrophosphate synthetase altered in regulatory and catalytic functions. Journal of Clinical Investigation 65: 109–120

Becker M A, Seegmiller J E 1974 Genetic aspects of gout. In: Annual Review of Medicine, Annual Reviews, Inc. 25: 15–28

Becker M A, Seegmiller J E 1975 Recent advances in the identification of enzyme abnormalities underlying excessive purine synthesis in man. Arthritis and Rheumatism 18: 687–694

Becker M A, Yen R C K, Itkin P, Goss S J, Seegmiller J E, Bakay B 1979 Regional localization of the gene for human phosphoribosylpyrophosphate synthetase on the X–chromosome. Science 203: 1016–1019

Becroft D M O, Phillips L I 1965 Hereditary orotic aciduria and megaloblastic anaemia: a second case, with response to uridine. British Medical Journal 1: 547–552

Becroft D M O, Phillips L I, Simmonds A 1969 Hereditary orotic aciduria: long-term therapy with uridine and a trial of uracil. Pediatric Pharmacology Therapy 75: 885–891

Ben-Bassat I, Brok-Simoni F, Kende G, Holtzmann F, Ramot

B 1976 A family with red cell pyrimidine 5′nucleotidase deficiency. Blood 47: 919–922

Benke P J, Gold S 1977 Purine metabolism in therapy of Von Gierke's disease. Pediatric Research 1: 837a

Beutler E 1962 Biochemical abnormalities associated with hemolytic states. In: Weinstein I M, Beutler E (eds) Mechanisms of Anemia, McGraw-Hill Book Co., New York p 195–236

Bluestein H G, Thompson L F, Albert D A, Seegmiller J E 1980 Altered deoxynucleoside triphosphate levels paralleling deoxynucleoside toxicity in adenosine deaminase inhibited human lymphocytes. In: Rapado A, Watts R W E, DeBruyn C H M M, (eds) Advances in Experimental Medicine and Biology, Plenum Press, New York, 122A: 427–432

Bluestein H G, Willis R C, Thompson L F, Matsumoto S, Seegmiller J E 1978 Accumulation of deoxyribonucleotides as a possible mediator of immunosuppression in hereditary deficiency of adenosine deaminase. Transactions of the Association of American Physicians SCI: 394–402

Boss G R, Seegmiller J E 1979 Hyperuricemia and gout: Recent developments in classification, complications and management. New England Journal of Medicine 300: 1459–1468

Boss G R, Thompson L F, O'Connor R D, Ziering R W, Seegmiller J E 1981 Ecto-5′-nucleotidase deficiency: Association with adenosine deaminase deficiency and non-association with deoxyadenosine toxicity. Clinical Immunology & Immunopathology 19: 1–7

Boss G R, Thompson L F, Spiegelberg H L, Pichler W J, Seegmiller J E 1980 Age dependency of lymphocyte ecto-5′-nucleotidase activity. Journal of Immunology 125: 679–682

Boss G R, Thompson L F, Spiegelberg H L, Waldman T A, O'Connor R D, Hamburger R N, Seegmiller J E 1979 Lymphocyte ecto-5′-nucleotidase activity as a marker of B-cell maturation. Transactions of the Association of American Physicians XCII: 309–315

Boyle J A, Raivio K O, Astrin K H, Schulman J D, Graf M L, Seegmiller J E, Jacobsen C B 1970 Lesch-Nyhan syndrome: Prevention control by prenatal diagnosis. Science 169: 688–689

Bradford M J, Krakoff I H, Leeper R, Balis M E 1968 Study of purine metabolism in a xanthinuric female. Journal of Clinical Investigation 47: 1325–1332

Carson D A, Kaye J, Matsumoto S, Seegmiller J E, Thompson L 1979 Biochemical basis for the enhanced toxicity of deoxyribonucleosides toward malignant human T cell lines. Proceedings of the National Academy of Sciences USA 76: 2430–2433

Carson D A, Kaye J, Seegmiller J E 1978 Differential sensitivity of human leukemic T cell lines and B cell lines to growth inhibition by deoxyadenosine. Journal of Immunology 121: 1726–1731

Cartier M P, Hamet M 1974 A new metabolic disease: The complete deficit of adenine phosphoribosyltransferase and lithiasis of 2,8-dihydroxyadenine. C R Academy of Science, Paris 279: 883–886

Cartier P, Hamet M, Vincens A, Perignon J L, 1980 Complete adenine phosphoribosyltransferase (APRT) deficiency in two siblings: Report of a new case. In: Rapado A, Watts R W E, DeBruyn C H M M (eds). Advances in Experimental Medicine and Biology, Plenum Press, New York, 122A: 343–348

Chambers R A, Watts R W E 1969 The separate determination of xanthine and hypoxanthine in urine and blood plasma by an enzymatic differential spectrophotometric method. Analyst 94: 226–233

Ciaranello R D, Anders T F, Barchas J D, Berger P A, Cann H M 1976 The use of 5-hydroxytryptophan in a child with Lesch-Nyhan syndrome. Child Psychiatry in Human Development 7: 127–133

Cleaver J E 1968 Defective repair replication of DNA in xeroderma pigmentosum. Nature 218: 652–656

Cleaver J E 1978 Xeroderma Pigmentosum. In: Stanbury J B, Wyngaarden J B, Frederickson D S (eds) The Metabolic Basis of Inherited Disease, McGraw-Hill, San Francisco, p 1072–1095

Cohen A, Doyle D, Martin D W, Ammann A J 1976 Abnormal purine metabolism and purine overproduction in a patient deficient in purine nucleoside phosphorylase. New England Journal of Medicine 295: 1449–1454

Cohen A, Gudas L J, Ammann A J, Staal G E J, Martin D W 1978 Deoxyguanosine triphosphate as a possible toxic metabolite in immunodeficiency associated with purine nucleoside phosphorylase deficiency. Journal of Clinical Investigation 61: 1405–1409

Cohen A, Hirschhorn R, Horowitz S D, Rubinstein A, Polmar S H, Hong R, Martin D W 1978 Deoxyadenosine triphosphate as a potentially toxic metabolite in adenosine deaminase deficiency. Proceedings of the National Academy of Sciences USA 75: 472–476

Coleman M S, Donofrio J, Hutton J J, Hahn L, Daoud A, Lampkin B, Dyminski J 1978 Identification and quantitation of adenine deoxynucleotides in erythrocytes of a patient with adenosine deaminase deficiency and severe combined immunodeficiency. Journal of Biological Chemistry 253: 1619–1626

Debray H, Cartier P, Temstet A, Cendron J 1976 Child's urinary lithiasis revealing a complete deficit in adenine phosphoribosyltransferase. Pediatric Research 10: 762–766

Dent C E, Philpot G R 1954 Xanthinuria, an inborn error (or deviation) of metabolism. Lancet 1: 182–185

Dimauro S, Miranda A F, Hays A P, Franck W A, Hoffman G S, Schoenfeldt R S, Singh N 1980 Myoadenylate deaminase deficiency. Journal of Neurological Science 47: 191–202

Donofrio J, Coleman J S, Hutton J J, Daoud A, Lampkin B, Dyminsky J 1978 Overproduction of adenine deoxynucleosides and deoxynucleotides in adenosine deaminase deficiency with severe combined immunodeficiency disease. Journal of Clinical Investigation 62: 884–887

Duran M, Korteland J, Beemer F A, van der Heiden C, de Bree P K, Brink M, Wadman S K, Lombeck I 1979 Variability of sulfituria: Combined deficiency of sulfite oxidase and xanthine oxidase. In: Homes F A (eds) Models for the Study of Inborn Errors of Metabolism, Amsterdam, Elsevier/North Holland

Edwards N L, Magilavy D B, Cassidy J T, Fox I H 1978 Lymphocyte ecto-5′-nucleotidase deficiency in congenital agammaglobulinemia. Clinical Research 26: 513A

Emmerson B T, Johnson L A, Gordon R B 1977 HGPRT-positive and HGPRT-negative erythrocytes in heterozygotes for HGPRT deficiency. In: Muller M M, Kaiser E, Seegmiller J E (eds) Advances in Experimental Medicine and Biology, Plenum Press, New York, p 359–360

Engelman K, Watts R W E, Klinenberg J R, Sjoerdsma A, Seegmiller J E 1964 Clinical, physiological and biochemical studies of a patient with xanthinuria and pheochromocytoma. American Journal of Medicine 37: 839–861

Epstein E H, Burk P G, Cohen I K, Decker P 1972 Dermatome shaving in the treatment of xeroderma pigmentosum. Archives of Dermatology 105: 589–590

Fessel W J 1980 High uric acid as an indicator of cardiovascular disease. The American Journal of Medicine 68: 401–404

Fessel W J, Siegelaub A B, Johnson E S 1973 Correlates and consequences of asymptomatic hyperuricemia. Archives of Internal Medicine 132: 44–54

Felix J S, DeMars R 1971 Detection of females heterozygous for the Lesch-Nyhan syndrome by 8-azaguanine-resistant growth of cultured human fibroblasts. Journal of Laboratory and Clinical Medicine 77: 596–604

Fishbein W N, Armbrustmacher V W, Griffin J L 1978 Myoadenylate deaminase deficiency: A new disease of muscle. Science 200: 545–548

Fox I H, Andres, C M, Gelfand E W, Biggar D 1977 Purine nucleoside phosphorylase deficiency: Altered kinetic properties of a mutant enzyme. Science 197: 1084–1086

Franke U, Felsenstein J, Gartler S M, Migeon B R, Dancis J, Seegmiller J E, Bakay B F, Nyhan W L 1976 The occurrence of new mutants in the X–linked recessive Lesch-Nyhan disease. American Journal of Human Genetics 28: 123–137

Frith C D, Johnstone E C, Joseph M H, Powell R J, Watts R W E 1976 Double-blind clinical trial of 5-hydroxytryptophan in a case of Lesch-Nyhan syndrome. Journal of Neurology, Neurosurgery and Psychiatry 39: 656–662

Fujimoto W Y, Seegmiller J E 1970 Hypoxanthine-guanine phosphoribosyltransferase deficiency: Activity in normal, mutant, and heterozygote cultured human skin fibroblasts. Proceedings of the National Academy of Sciences USA 65: 577–584

Fujimoto W Y, Seegmiller J E, Uhlendorf B W, Jacobson C B 1968 Biochemical diagnosis of an X–linked disease in utero. Lancet 2: 511–512

Garrod A B 1848 Observations on certain pathological conditions of the blood and urine in gout, rheumatism and Bright's disease. Transactions of the Medical Society of London 31: 83–98

Garrod A E 1923 Inborn errors of metabolism. Oxford, London

Gartler S M, Scott R C, Goldstein J L, Campbell B, Sparkes R 1971 Lesch-Nyhan syndrome: Rapid detection of heterozygotes by use of hair follicles. Science 172: 572–574

Geerdink R A, DeVries W H M, Willemse J, Oei T L, DeBruyn C H M M 1973 An atypical case of hypoxanthine-guanine phosphoribosyltransferase deficiency (Lesch-Nyhan syndrome). Clinical Genetics 4: 348–352

Gelfand E W, Dosch H M, Biggar W D, Fox I H 1978 Partial purine nucleoside phosphorylase deficiency: Studies of lymphocyte function. Journal of Clinical Investigation 61: 1071–1081

Ghangas G S, Milman G 1977 Hypoxanthine phosphoribosyltransferase: Two dimensional gels from normal and Lesch-Nyhan hemolysates. Science 196: 1119–1120

Giblett E R, Anderson J E, Cohen F, Pollara B, Meuwissen H J 1972 Adenosine-deaminase deficiency in two patients with severely impaired cellular immunity. Lancet 2: 1067–1069

Giblett E R, Ammann A J, Wara D W, Sandman R, Diamond L K 1975 Nucleoside-phosphorylase deficiency in a child with severely defective T-cell immunity and normal B-cell immunity. Lancet 1: 1010–1013

Goldblum R M, Schmalstieg F C, Nelson J A, Mills G C 1978 Adenosine deaminase (ADA) and other enzyme abnormalities in immune deficiency states. In: Summit R L, Bergsma D (eds) Cell Surface Factors, Immune

Deficiencies. Twin Studies, National Foundation of March of Dimes Birth Defects, Original Article Series, New York, XIV: 73–84

Good R A, Hansen M A 1976 Primary immunodeficiency disease. Advances in Experimental Medicine and Biology 73B: 155–178

Goss J, Harris H 1975 New method for mapping genes in human chromosomes. Nature, London 255: 680–684

Greene H L, Slonim A E, O'Neill J A, Burr I M 1977 Continuous noctural intragastric feeding for management of Type 1 glycogen-storage disease. New England Journal of Medicine 294: 423–425

Greene H L, Wilson F A, Hefferan P, Terry A B, Moran J R, Slonim, A E, Claus T H, Burr I M 1978 ATP depletion, a possible role in hyperuricemia in glycogen storage disease Type 1. Journal of Clinical Investigation 62: 321–328

Griscelli C, Hamet M, Ballet J J 1976 Third Workshop Internal Cooperative Group for Bone Marrow Transplantation in Manhattan, New York

Gudas L J, Ullman B, Cohen A, Martin D W 1978 Deoxyguanosine toxicity in a mouse T lymphoma: Relationship to purine nucleoside phosphorylase-associated immune dysfunction. Cell 14: 531–538

Haggard M E, Lockhart L H 1967 Megaloblastic anemia and orotic aciduria. A hereditary disorder of pyrimidine metabolism responsive to uridine. American Journal of Disabled Children 113: 733–740

Hamet M, Griscelli C, Cartier P, Ballet J, DeBruyn C, Hosli P 1977 A second case of inosine phosphorylase deficiency with severe T-cell abnormalities. In: Muller M M, Kaiser E, Seegmiller J E (eds) Advances in Experimental Medicine and Biology 76A, Plenum Press, New York, p 477–480

Henderson J F, Dossetor J B, Dasgupta M K, Russel A S 1976 Uric acid lithiasis associated with altered kinetics of hypoxanthine-guanine phosphoribosyltransferase. Clinical Biochemistry 9: 4–8

Hers H G, Van den Berghe 1979 Enzyme defect in primary gout. Lancet 1: 585–586

Hershfield M S 1979 Apparent suicide inactivation of human lymphoblast S-adenosylhomocysteine hydrolase by 2′-deoxyadenosine and adenine arabinoside. Journal of Biological Chemistry 254: 22–25

Hershfield M S, Kredich N M 1979 In vivo inactivation of erythrocyte S-adenosylhomocysteine hydrolase by 2′-deoxyadenosine in adenosine deaminase-deficient patients. Journal of Clinical Investigation 63: 807–811

Hershfield M S, Seegmiller J E 1977 Regulation of de novo purine synthesis in human lymphoblasts: Similar rates of de novo synthesis during growth by normal cells and mutants deficient in hypoxanthine-guanine phosphoribosyltransferase activity. Journal of Biological Chemistry 252: 6002–6010

Hirschhorn R, 1977 Defects of purine metabolism in immunodeficiency disease. In: Schwartz R S (ed) Progress in Clinical Immunology, Grune & Stratton, San Francisco, p 67–83

Hirschhorn R H, Roegner V, Jenkins T, Seaman C, Piomelli S, Borkowsky W 1979 Erythrocyte adenosine deaminase deficiency without immunodeficiency: Evidence for an unstable mutant enzyme. Journal of Clinical Investigation 64: 1130–1139

Holmes E W, Mason D H, Goldstein L I, Blount R E, Kelley W N 1974 Xanthine oxidase deficiency: Studies of a previously unreported case. Clinical Chemistry 20: 1076–1079

Hooft C, Van Nevel C, DeSchaepdryver A F 1968

Hyperuricosuric encephalopathy without hyperuricemia. Archives of Disabled Children 43: 734–737

Huguley C M, Bain J A, Rivers S L, Scoggins R B 1959 Refractory megablastic anemia associated with excretion of orotic acid. Blood 14: 615–634

Iinuma K, Wada Y, Onuma A, Tanabu M 1975 Electroencephalographic study of an infant with phosphoribosylpyrophosphate synthetase deficiency. Tohoku Journal of Experimental Medicine 116: 53–55

Jakovcic S, Sorensen L B 1967 Studies of uric acid metabolism in glycogen storage disease associated with gouty arthritis. Arthritis and Rheumatism 10: 129–134

Jochmus I, Koch A, Wilhelmstroop-Meyer A 1977 Verhaltenstherapie der autoagressionen beim Lesch-Nyhan-Syndrom. Mschr Kinderheilk 125: 839–841

Johns D G, Adamson R H 1976 Enhancement of the biological activity of cordycepin (3′-deoxyadenosine)by the adenosine deaminase inhibitor 2′-deoxycoformycin. Biochemical Pharmacology 25: 1441–1444

Johnson J L, Waud W R, Rajagopalan K V, Duran M, Beemer F A, Wadman S K 1980 Inborn errors of molybdenum metabolism: Combined deficiencies of sulfite oxidase and xanthine dehydrogenase in a patient lacking the molybdenum cofactor. Proceedings of the National Academy of Sciences USA 77: 3715–3719

Johnson L A, Gordon R B, Emmerson B T 1977 Adenine phosphoribosyltransferase: A simple spectrophotometric assay and the incidence of mutation in the normal population. Biochemical Genetics 15: 265–272

Johnson S M, Asherson G L, Watts R W E, North M E, Allsop J, Webster A B D 1977 Lymphocyte-purine 5′-nucleotidase deficiency in primary hypogammaglobulinaemia. Lancet 1: 168–170

Kar N C, Pearson C M 1973 Muscle adenylic acid deaminase activity. Neurology 23: 478–482

Kaufman J M, Greene M L, Seegmiller J E 1968 Urine uric acid to creatinine ratio. A screening test for inherited disorders of purine metabolism. Journal of Pediatrics 73: 583–592

Kelley W N, Arnold W J 1973 Human hypoxanthine-guanine phosphoribosyltransferase: Studies on the normal and mutant forms of the enzyme. Federation Proceedings 32: 1656–1659

Kelley W N, Greene M L, Fox I H, Rosenbloom F M, Levy R I, Seegmiller J E 1970 Effects of orotic acid on purine and lipoprotein metabolism in man. Metabolism 19: 1025–1035

Kelley W N, Greene M L, Rosenbloom F M, Henderson J F, Seegmiller J E 1969 Hypoxanthine-guanine phosphoribosyltransferase deficiency in gout. A review. Annals of Internal Medicine 70: 155–206

Kelley W N, Levy R I, Rosenbloom F M, Henderson J F, Seegmiller J E 1968 Adenine phosphoribosyltransferase deficiency: A previously undescribed genetic defect in man. Journal of Clinical Investigation 47: 2281–2289

Kelley W N, Meade J C 1971 Studies on hypoxanthine-guanine phosphoribosyltransferase in fibroblasts from patients with the Lesch-Nyhan syndrome: Evidence for genetic heterogeneity. Journal of Biological Chemistry 246: 2953–2958

Kelley W N, Rosenbloom F M, Henderson J F Seegmiller J E, 1967a A specific enzyme defect in gout associated with overproduction of uric acid. Proceedings of the National Academy of Sciences USA 57: 1735–1739

Kelley W N, Rosenbloom F M, Henderson J F, Seegmiller J E, 1967b Xanthine phosphoribosyltransferase in man: Relationship to hypoxanthine-guanine phosphoribosyltransferase. Biochemical and Biophysical Research Communications 28: 340–345

Kelley W N, Rosenbloom F M, Seegmiller J E, Howell R R 1968 Excessive production of uric acid in Type 1 glycogen storage disease. Journal of Pediatrics 72: 488–496

Kelley W N, Weiner I M (eds) 1978 Uric Acid. Springer-Verlag, New York, p 639

Klinenberg J R, Goldfinger S, Bradley K H, Seegmiller J E 1967 An enzymatic spectrophotometric method for the determination of xanthine and hypoxanthine. Clinical Chemistry 13: 834–841

Koller C A, Mitchell B S, Grever M R, Mejias E, Malspeis L, Metz E N 1980 Treatment of acute lymphoblastic leukemia with 2'-deoxycoformycin: Clinical and biochemical consequences of adenosine deaminase inhibition. Cancer Treatment 64: 1949–1952

Kraemer K H, De Weerd-Kastelein E A, Robbins J H, Keijzer W, Barrett S F, Petinga R A, Bootsma D 1975 Five complementation groups in xeroderma pigmentosum. Mutation Research 33: 327–340

Krenitsky T A, Papainnou R, Elion G B 1969 Human hypoxanthine phosphoribosyltransferase. I. Purification, properties, and specificity. Journal of Biological Chemistry 244: 1263–1270

Kuttesch J F, Schmalstieg F C, Nelson J A 1978 Analysis of adenosine and other adenine compounds in patients with immunodeficiency diseases. Journal of Liquid Chromatography 1: 97–109

Lesch M, Nyhan W L 1964 A familial disorder of uric acid metabolism and central nervous system function. American Journal of Medicine 36: 561–570

Lever J E, Nuki G, Seegmiller J E 1974 Expression of purine overproduction in a series of 8-azaguanine-resistant diploid human lymphoblast lines. Proceedings of the National Academy of Sciences USA 71: 2679–2683

Levine R L, Hoogenraad N J, Kretchmer N 1974 A review: Biological and clinical aspects of pyrimidine metabolism. Pediatric Research 8: 724–734

Lockwood D H, Merimee T J, Edgar P J, Greene M L, Fujimoto W Y, Seegmiller J E, Howell R R 1969 Insulin secretion in type 1 glycogen storage disease. Journal of American Diabetes Association 18: 755–758

Lyon M F 1961 Gene action in the X-chromosome of the mouse. Nature 190: 372–373

Macleod P, Mackenzie S, Scriver C R 1972 Partial ornithine carbamyl transferase deficiency: An inborn error of the urea cycle presenting as orotic aciduria in a male infant. Canadian Medical Association Journal 107: 405–408

Marcet A 1818 An essay on the chemical history and medical treatment of calculous disorders. London

McCarty D J 1974 Crystal deposition joint disease. Annual Review of Medicine 25: 279–288

McInnes R, Lamm P, Clow C L, Scriver C R 1972 A filter paper sampling method for the uric acid: Creatinine ratio in urine. Normal values in the newborn. Pediatrics 49: 80–84

Meuwissen H J Pollara B 1978 Combined immunodeficiency and inborn errors of purine metabolism. Blut 37: 173–181

Meyer L J, Becker M A 1977 Human erythrocyte phosphoribosylpyrophosphate synthetase. Dependence of activity on state of subunit association. Journal of Biological Chemistry 252: 3919–3925

Miewa S, Nakashima K, Fujii H, Matsumoto M, Nomura K 1977 Three cases of hereditary hemolytic anemia with pyrimidine 5'-nucleotidase deficiency in a Japanese family. Human Genetics 37: 361–364

Migeon B R, DerKaloustian V M, Nyhan W L, Young W J, Childs B 1968 X-linked hypoxanthine-guanine phosphoribosyltransferase deficiency: heterozygote has two clonal populations. Science 160: 425–427

Milman G, Krauss S W, Olsen A S 1977 Tryptic peptide analysis of normal and mutant form of hypoxanthine phosphoribosyltransferase from HeLa cells. Proceedings of the National Academy of Sciences USA 74: 926–930

Milman G, Lee E, Ghangas G S, McLaughlin J R, George M 1976 Analysis of HeLa cell hypoxanthine phosphoribosyltransferase mutants and revertants by two-dimensional polyacrylamide gel electrophoresis: Evidence for silent gene activation. Proceedings of the National Academy of Sciences USA 73: 4589–4593

Mitchell B S, Kelley W N 1980 Purinogenic immunodeficiency diseases: Clinical features and molecular mechanisms. Annals of Internal Medicine 92: 826–831

Mitchell B S, Koller C A, Heyn R 1979 Disappearance of acute T cell lymphoblastic leukemia following therapy with 2'-deoxycoformycin. Blood 54: 253

Mizuno T I, Yugari Y 1974 Self-mutilation in the Lesch-Nyhan syndrome. Lancet 1: 761

Mizuno T, Yugari Y 1975 Prophylactic effect of 1-5-hydroxytryptophan on self-mutilation in the Lesch-Nyhan syndrome. Neuropaediatrie 6: 13–23

Muller M M, Kaiser E, Seegmiller J E (eds) 1977a In: Advances in Experimental Medicine and Biology, Vol. 76A, Plenum Press, New York, p 641

Muller M M, Kaiser E, Seegmiller J E (eds) 1977b In: Advances in Experimental Medicine and Biology, Vol. 76B, Plenum Press, New York, p 373

Newcombe D S, 1975 Inherited biochemical disorders and uric acid metabolism. University Park Press, Baltimore, p 282

Newcombe, D S 1970 The urinary excretion of aminoimidazolecarboxamide in the Lesch-Nyhan syndrome. Pediatrics 46: 508–512

Nyhan W 1977 Behavior in the Lesch-Nyhan syndrome. In: Chess S, Thomas A (eds) Annual Progress in Child Psychiatry and Child Development, 10th Annual Edition, p 175–194

Nyhan W L, James J A, Teberg A J, Sweetman L, Nelson L G 1969 A new disorder of purine metabolism with behavioral manifestations. Journal of Pediatrics 74: 20–27

Nyhan W L, Johnson H G, Kaufman I A, Jones K L 1980 Serotonergic approaches to the modification of behavior in the Lesch-Nyhan syndrome. Applied Research in Mental Retardation 1: 25–40

Polmar S H, Wetzler E M, Stern R C, Hirschhorn R 1975 Restoration of in vitro lymphocyte responses with exogenous adenosine deaminase in a patient with severe combined immunodeficiency. Lancet 2: 743–746

Quagliata F, Faig D, Conklyn M, Silber R 1974 Studies on the lymphocyte 5'-nucleotidase in chronic lymphocytic leukemia, infectious mononucleosis, normal subpopulations, and phytohemagglutinin-stimulated cells. Cancer Research 34: 3197–3202

Reichard P 1972 Control of deoxyribonucleotide synthesis in vitro and in vivo. Advances in Enzyme Regulation 10: 3–16

Reichard P 1978 From deoxynucleotides to DNA synthesis. Federation Proceedings 37: 9–14

Reif M C, Constantiner A, Levitt M F 1981 Chronic gouty nephropathy: A vanishing syndrome? New England Journal of Medicine 304: 535–536

Rich K C, Arnold W J, Palella T, Fox I H 1979 Cellular immune deficiency with autoimmune hemolytic anemia in purine nucleoside phosphorylase deficiency. American Journal of Medicine 67: 172–176

Rich K C, Mejias E, Fox I H 1980 Purine nucleoside

phosphorylase deficiency: Improved metabolic and immunologic function with erythrocyte transfusions. New England Journal of Medicine 303: 937–977

Robbins J H, Kraemer K H, Andrews A D 1976 Inherited DNA repair defects in H. sapiens: Their relation to UV-associated processes in xeroderma pigmentosum. In: Yuhas J M, Tennant R W, Regan J D (eds) Biology of Radiation Carcinogenesis, Raven Press, New York

Robbins J H, Kraemer K H, Lutzner M A, Festoff B W, Coon H G 1974 Xeroderma pigmentosum: An inherited disease with sun sensitivity, multiple cutaneous neoplasms, and abormal DNA repair. Annals of Internal Medicine 80: 221–248

Rochant H, Dreyfus B, Rosa R, Boiron M, 1975 First case of pyrimidine 5'-nucleotidase deficiency in a male. International Society of Hematology, European & African Third Meeting, London, August 24–28, Abstract 19

Roe T E, Kogut M D 1977 The pathogenesis of hyperuricemia in glycogen storage disease Type 1. Pediatric Research 11: 664–669

Rosa R, Rochant H, Dreyfus B, Valentin E, Rosa J 1977 Electrophoretic and kinetic studies of human erythrocytes deficient in pyrimidine 5'-nucleotidase. Human Genetics 38: 209–215

Rosenberg A L, Bergstrom L, Troost B T, Bartholomew B A 1970 Hyperuricemia and neurologic deficits, a family study. New England Journal of Medicine 282: 992–997

Rosenbloom F M, Henderson J F, Caldwell I C, Kelley W N, Seegmiller J E 1968 Biochemical bases of accelerated purine biosynthesis de novo in human fibroblasts lacking hypoxanthine-guanine phosphoribosyltransferase. Journal of Biological Chemistry 243: 1116–1173

Rosenbloom F M, Kelley W N, Henderson J F, Seegmiller J E 1967 Lyon hypothesis and X–linked disease. Lancet 2: 305–306

Rosenbloom F M, Kelley W N, Miller J, Henderson J F, Seegmiller J E 1967 Inherited disorder of purine metabolism: Correlation between central nervous system dysfunction and biochemical defects. Journal of American Medical Association 202: 175–177

Salti I S, Kattuah N, Alam S, Wehby V, Frayha R 1976 The effect of allopurinol on oxypurine excretion in xanthinuria. Journal of Rheumatology 3: 201–204

Salzmann J, DeMars R, Benke P 1968 Single-allele expression at an X–linked hyperuricemia locus in heterozygous human cells. Proceedings of the National Academy of Sciences USA 60: 545–552

Scheele K W 1931 Examen Chemicum Calculi Urinarn, Opuscula II, p 73, 1776. Cited from Levene P A, Bass L W 1931 Nucleic Acids, New York, Chemical Catalog Company

Schmalstieg F C, Nelson J A, Mills G C, Monahan T M, Goldman A S, Goldblum R M 1977 Increased purine nucleotides in adenosine deaminase-deficient lymphocytes. Journal of Pediatrics 91: 48–51

Schnebli H P, Hill D L, Bennett L L 1967 Purification and properties of adenosine kinase from human tumor cells of type H. Ep. No 2. Journal of Biological Chemistry 242: 1997–2004

Seegmiller J E 1974 Amniotic fluid and cells in the diagnosis of genetic disorders. In: Natelson S, Scommegna A, Epstein M B (eds) Amniotic Fluid: Physiology, Biochemistry, and Clinical Chemistry John Wiley and Sons, New York 1: 291–316

Seegmiller J E 1976 Inherited deficiency of hypoxanthine-guanine phosphoribosyltransferase in X–linked uric aciduria (the Lesch-Nyhan syndrome and its variants). In: Harris H,

Hirschhorn K (eds) Advances in Human Genetics, Plenum Press, New York, p 75–163

Seegmiller J E 1979a Abnormalities of purine metabolism in human immunodeficiency diseases. In: Baier H P, Drummond G I (eds) Physiological and Regulatory Functions of Adenosine and Adenine Nucleotides, Raven Press, New York, p 395–408

Seegmiller J E 1979b Disorders of purine and pyrimidine metabolism. In: Freinkel N (ed) Contemporary Metabolism, Plenum Medical Book Company, New York, 1: 1–85

Seegmiller J E 1980a Diseases of purine and pyrimidine metabolism. In: Bondy P K, Rosenberg L E (eds)Metabolic Control and Disease, Eighth Edition, W B Saunders Company, Philadelphia, p 777–937

Seegmiller J E 1980b Possible mechanisms of immunodeficiency disease associated with hereditary defects in enzymes of purine degradation. In: Seligman M, Hitzig W H (eds) Primary Immunodeficiencies INSERM Symposium, Elsevier/North-Holland Biomedical Press, p 269–277

Seegmiller J E 1980c Human aberrations of purine metabolism and their significance for rheumatology. Annals of Rheumatic Diseases 39: 103–117

Seegmiller J E, Bluestein H, Thompson L, Willis R, Matsumoto S, Carson D 1979 Primary aberrations of purine metabolism associated with impairment of the immune response. In: Hommes F A (ed) Models for the Study of Inborn Errors of Metabolism, Elsevier/North-Holland Biomedical Press, p 153–168

Seegmiller J E, Rosenbloom F M, Kelley W N 1967 Enzyme defect associated with a sex-linked human neurological disorder and excessive purine synthesis. Science 155: 1682–1684

Seegmiller J E, Thompson L, Bluestein H, Willis R, Matsumoto S, Carson D 1980 Nucleotide and nucleoside metabolism and lymphocyte function. In: Gelfand E W, Dosch H M (eds) Biological Basis of Immunodeficiency, Raven Press, New York, p 251–268

Shumate J B, Katnik R, Ruiz M, Kaiser K, Frieden C, Brooke M H, Carroll J E 1979 Myoadenylate deaminase deficiency. Muscle and Nerve 213–216

Siegenbeek van Heukelom L H, Staal G E J, Stoop J W, Zegers B J M 1976 An abnormal form of purine nucleoside phosphorylase in a family with a child with severe defective T-cell and normal B-cell immunity. Clinica Chimica Acta 72: 117–124

Simkin P A 1977 The pathogenesis of podagra. Annals of Internal Medicine 86: 230–233

Simmonds H A, Levin B, Cameron J S 1974 Variations in allopurinol metabolism by xanthinuric subjects. Clinical Sciences and Molecular Medicine 47: 173–178

Simmonds H A, Levin B, Cameron J S 1975 Variations in allopurinol metabolism by xanthinuric subjects. Clinical Sciences and Molecular Medicine 49: 81–82

Simmonds H A, Panayi G S, Corrigall V 1978 A role for purine metabolism in the immune response: Adenosine-deaminase activity and deoxyadenosine catabolism. Lancet 1: 60–63

Simmonds H A, Rose G A, Potter C F, Sahota A, Barratt T M, Williams D I, Arkell D G, Van Acker K J, Cameron J S 1978 Adenine phosphoribosyltransferase deficiency presenting with supposed 'uric acid' stones: pitfalls of diagnosis. Proceedings of the Royal Society of Medicine 71: 791–795

Simmonds H A, Van Acker K J, Cameron J S, McBurney A 1977 Purine excretion in complete adenine phosphoribosyltransferase deficiency: Effect of diet and allopurinol therapy. In: Muller M M, Kaiser E, Seegmiller J E (eds) Advances of Experimental Medicine and Biology 76B, Series: Purine Metabolism in Man II: Physiological, Pharmacological, and Clinical Aspects, Plenum Press, New York, p 304–311

Simmonds H A, Van Acker K J, Cameron J S, Snedden W 1976 The identification of 2,8-dihydroxyadenine, a new component of urinary stones. Biochemical Journal 157: 485–487

Smyth J F, Chassin M M, Harrap K R, Adamson R H, Johns D G 1979 2-deoxycoformycin (DCF) : Phase 1 trial and clinical pharmacology. Proceedings of the American Society of Clinical Oncology 20: 187

Sperling O, Boer P, Persky-Brosh S, Kanarek E, DeVries A 1972 Altered kinetic property of erythrocyte phosphoribosylpyrophosphate synthetase in excessive purine production. European Journal of Clinical Biological Research 17: 703

Sperling O, Eilam G, Persky-Brosh S, DeVries A 1972 Accelerated erythrocyte 5-phosphoribosyl-1-pyrophosphate synthesis. A familial abnormality associated with excessive uric acid production and gout. Biochemical Medicine 6: 310–316

Staal G E J, Stoop J W, Zegers B J M, Siegenbeek van Heukelom L H, Van der Vlist M J M, Wadman S K, Martin D W 1980 Erythrocyte metabolism in purine nucleoside phosphorylase deficiency after enzyme replacement therapy by infusion of erythrocytes. Journal of Clinical Investigation 65: 103–108

Stevens W J, Peetermans M E, Van Acker K J 1980 Immunological evaluation of a family deficient in adenine phosphoribosyltransferase (APRT). In: Rapado A, Watts R W E, DeBruyn C H M M (eds) Purine Metabolism in Man-III. Advances in Experimental Medicine and Biology, Plenum Press, New York, 122a: 355–359

Stoop J W, Zegers B J M, Hendricks G F M, Siegenbeek van Heukelom L H, Staal G E J, de Bree P K, Wadman S K, Ballieux R E 1977 Purine nucleoside phosphorylase deficiency associated with selective cellular immunodeficiency. New England Journal of Medicine 296: 651–655

Szeinberg A, Gavendo S, Cahane D 1969 Erythrocyte adenylate-kinase deficiency. Lancet 1: 315–316

Szeinberg A, Kahana D, Gavendo S, Zaidman J, Ben-Ezzer J 1969 Hereditary deficiency of adenylate kinase in red blood cells. Acta Haematologica 42: 111–126

Thompson L F, Boss G R, Spiegelberg H L, Bianchino A, Seegmiller J E 1980 Ecto-5'-nucleotidase activity in lymphoblastoid cell lines derived from heterozygotes for congenital X–linked agammaglobulinemia. Journal of Immunology 125: 190–193

Thompson L F, Seegmiller J E 1979 Adenosine deaminase deficiency and severe combined immunodeficiency disease. In: Meister A (ed) Advances in Enzymology, John Wiley & Sons, Inc. p 167–210

Thompson R V 1960 Purines and pyrimidines and their derivatives. In: Chromatographic and Electrophoretic Techniques, Interscience Publishers, Inc., New York, 1: 231–235

Torrance J D, Karabus C D, Shinier M, Meltzer M, Katz J, Jenkins T 1977a Haemolytic anaemia due to erythrocyte pyrimidine 5'-nucleotidase deficiency. South African Medical Journal 52: 671–677

Ullman B, Cohen A, Martin D W 1976 Characterization of a cell culture model for the study of adenosine deaminase-

and purine nucleoside phosphorylase-deficient immunologic disease. Cell 9: 205–211

Valentine W N, Anderson H M, Paglia D E, Jaffe E R, Konrad P N, Harris S R 1972 Studies on human erythrocyte nucleotide metabolism. II Nonspherocytic hemolytic anemia, high red cell ATP, and ribosephosphate pyrophosphokinase (RPK, E.C.2.7.6.1) deficiency. Blood 39: 674–684

Valentine W N, Fink K, Paglia D E, Harris S R, Adams W S 1974 Hereditary hemolytic anemia with human erythrocyte pyrimidine 5'-nucleotidase deficiency. Journal of Clinical Investigation 54: 866–879

Valentine W N, Paglia D E, Fink K, Madokoro G 1976 Lead poisoning: Associated with haemolytic anemia, basophilic stippling, erythrocyte pyrimidine 5'-nucleotidase deficiency, and intraerythrocytic accumulation of pyrimidine. Journal of Clinical Investigation 58: 926–932

Valentine W N, Paglia D E, Tartaglia A P, Gilsanz F 1977 Hereditary hemolytic anemia with increased red cell adenosine deaminase (45- to 70-fold) and decreased adenosine triphosphate. Science 195: 783–785

Van Acker K J, Simmonds H A, Cameron J S 1977a Complete deficiency of adenine phosphoribosyltransferase: Report of a family. In: Muller M M, Kaiser E, Seegmiller J E (eds) Advances in Experimental Medicine and Biology, 76A, Plenum Press, New York, p 295–302

Van Acker K J, Simmonds H A, Potter C, Cameron J S 1977b Complete deficiency of adenine phosphoribosyltransferase. Report of a family. New England Journal of Medicine 297: 127–132

Van Acker K J, Simmonds H A, Potter C F, Sahota A 1980 Inheritance of adenine phosphoribosyltransferase (APRT) deficiency. In: Rapado A, Watts R W E, DeBruyn C H M M (eds) Purine Metabolism in Man-III. Advances in Experimental Medicine and Biology, Plenum Press, New York, 122A: 349–353

van der Heiden C, Beemer F A, Brink W, Wadman S K, Duran M 1979 Simultaneous occurrence of xanthine oxidase and sulfite oxidase deficiency. A molybdenum dependent inborn error of metabolism? Clinical Biochemistry 12: 206–208

Van Heeswijk P J, Blank C H, Seegmiller J E, Jacobson C B 1972 Preventive control of the Lesch-Nyhan syndrome. Obstetrics and Gynecology 40: 109–113

Vives-Corrons J L, Montserrat-Costa E, Rozman C 1976 Hereditary hemolytic anemia with erythrocyte pyrimidine 5'-nucleotidase deficiency in Spain. Clinical, biological and family studies. Human Genetics 34: 285–292

Wada Y, Nishimura Y, Tanabu M, Yoshimura Y, Iinuma K, Yoshida T, Arakawa T 1974 Hypouricemic mentally retarded infant with a defect of 5-phosphoribosyl-1-pyrophosphate synthetase of erythrocytes. Tohoku Journal of Experimental Medicine 113: 149–157

Wadman S K, De Bree P K, Van Gennip A H, Stoop J W, Zwegers B J M, Staal G E J, Siegenbeek van Heukelom L H 1976 Urinary purines in a patient with a severely defective T-cell immunity and a purine nucleoside phosphorylase deficiency. Clinical Chemistry and Clinical Biochemistry 14: 326–331

Watts R W E 1977 Chairman panel discussion: Hyperuricemia as a risk factor. In: Muller M M, Kaiser E, Seegmiller J E (eds) Advances in Experimental Medicine and Biology 76A, Plenum Press, New York, p 342–364

Weinberger A, Schumacher H R, Agudelo C A 1979 Urate crystals in asymptomatic metatarsophalangeal joints. Annals of Internal Medicine 91: 56–57

Willis R C, Robbins R K, Seegmiller J E 1980 An in vivo and in vitro evaluation of 1-B-D-ribofuranosyl-1,2,4-triazole-3-carboxamidine: An inhibitor of human lymphoblast purine nucleoside phosphorylase. Molecular Pharmacology 18: 287–295

Wood A W, Becker M A, Seegmiller J E 1973 Purine nucleotide synthesis in lymphoblasts cultured from normal subjects and a patient with Lesch-Nyhan syndrome. Biochemical Genetics 9: 261–274

Wood A W, Seegmiller J E 1973 Properties of 5-phosphoribosyl-1-pyrophosphate amidotransferase from human lymphoblasts. Journal of Biological Chemistry 248: 138–143

Wyngaarden J B, Kelley W N 1976 Gout and hyperuricemia. Grune & Strutton, New York, p 55

Yen, R C K, Adams B, Lazar C, Becker M A 1978 Evidence for X–linkage of human phosphoribosylpyrophosphate synthetase. Proceedings of the National Academy of Sciences USA 75: 482–485

Yu A L, Bakay B, Kung F H, Nyhan W L 1981 The effect of 2'-deoxycoformycin on the metabolism of purines and the survival of malignant cells in a patient with T-cell leukemia. Cancer Research 41: 2677–2682

Yu A, Kung F, Bakay B, Nyhan W L 1979 Preliminary clinical trial of deoxycoformycin in human T-cell leukemia. Journal of Clinical Chemistry and Clinical Biochemistry 17: 451–452

Yu A L, Kung F H, Bakay B, Nyhan W L 1980 In vitro and in vivo effect of deoxycoformycin in human T-cell leukemia. In: Rapado A, Watts R W E, DeBruyn C H M M (eds) Purine Metabolism in Man-III, Plenum Press, New York, p 373–379

Zegers B J M, Stoop J W, Staal G E J, Wadman S K 1979 An approach to the restoration of T-cell function in a purine nucleoside phosphorylase deficient patient. Ciba Foundation Symposium 68: 231–247

Zoref E, DeVries A, Sperling O 1975 Mutant feedback-resistant phosphoribosylpyrophosphate synthetase associated with purine overproduction and gout. Phosphoribosylpyrophosphate and purine metabolism in cultured fibroblasts. Journal of Clinical Investigation 56: 1093–1099

Zoref E, DeVries A, Sperling O 1977a Evidence for X–linkage of phosphoribosylpyrophosphate synthetase in man. Studies with cultured fibroblasts from a gouty family with mutant feedback-resistant enzyme. Human Heredity 1: 73–80

Zoref E, DeVries A, Sperling O 1977b X–linked pattern of inheritance of gout due to mutant feedback-resistant phosphoribosylpyrophosphate synthetase. In: Muller M M, Kaiser E, Seegmiller J E (eds) Advances in Experimental Medicine and Biology, 76A, Plenum Press, New York, p 287–292

91

Disorders of organic acid metabolism

S. I. Goodman

INTRODUCTION

Organic acidaemias are a group of inborn errors of (usually) amino acid metabolism in which the diagnostic accumulated compounds are acids that, because they do not contain an amino group, do not react with ninhydrin. They were first reported in 1961, albeit unknowingly, when idiopathic hyperglycinaemia was described as a syndrome of mental retardation, hyperglycinaemia, and episodic ketoacidosis, neutropenia and thrombocytopenia induced by protein intake or infection (Childs et al, 1961). It became realized some years later that the clinical and biochemical features of this disease, which had become known as ketotic hyperglycinaemia, were usually caused by organic acidaemias, and in particular by methylmalonic acidaemia (Rosenberg et al, 1968), propionic acidaemia (Hsia et al, 1971), and 2-methyl-3-hydroxybutyric acidaemia (Hillman & Keating, 1974).

Isovaleric acidaemia was the first organic acidaemia to be recognized, in large part because industrial chemists recognized the odour surrounding a particular patient as being due to a short-chain fatty acid (Budd et al, 1967). The description of this condition led to a search for others, usually by combined gas chromatography-mass spectrometry (GC-MS), and to the rapid delineation of the remaining disorders described in this section.

The ability of GC-MS to simultaneously separate and identify the components of complex mixtures has made it the method most widely used to indentify and investigate organic acidaemias. GC alone will exclude disease in most (80–90%) patients, and can be performed in any well equipped clinical laboratory. Large peaks in other samples, while usually due to drugs and food additives and not to the abnormal acids of disease, will necessitate referral to a laboratory with enough experience in organic acid analysis by GC-MS to ensure rapid and accurate diagnosis.

Clinical features vary but, in general, organic acidaemia should be suspected, and urine organic acids examined (the compounds are not effectively reabsorbed from the glomerular filtrate by the renal tubule) in the following situations:

1. Clinical features of ketotic hyperglycinaemia (see above)
2. Presence of an unusual odour
3. Acute disease in infancy, especially when associated with metabolic acidosis, hypoglycaemia, or hyperammonaemia
4. Chronic or recurrent metabolic acidosis, with or without an anion gap
5. Progressive extrapyramidal disease in childhood
6. Reye syndrome when recurrent, familial, or in infancy.

Pedigree date and/or enzyme measurements in obligate heterozygotes have shown that most organic acidaemias are inherited as autosomal recessive traits, but in a few instances, as in methylmalonic acidaemia due to the *cbl* D defect, pedigree data is too scanty and knowledge of the primary defect too uncertain to exclude X–linked inheritance. Prenatal diagnosis is relatively simple because the enzyme defects are usually expressed in cultured amniotic cells, and because the affected fetus often excretes large and easily detected amounts of abnormal organic acids into the amniotic fluid.

ISOVALERIC ACIDAEMIA

Clinical course

The clinical course of isovaleric acidaemia, first recognized in 1966 because of the distinctive 'cheesey', 'sour,' or 'sweaty feet' odour of isovaleric acid (Budd et al 1967; Tanaka et al 1966), varies considerably. Some patients develop poor feeding, acidosis, seizures, and the characteristic odour during the first few days of life, with coma and death following quite soon if the diagnosis is not made and appropriate treatment begun (Newman et al 1967; Budd et al 1967). Others show only episodes of vomiting, lethargy, encephalopathy, pancytopenia, and odour precipitated by infections or protein ingestion (Ando et al, 1971). Developmental retardation is common. Fatty changes in the liver and kidneys are often found at autopsy. The disorder is due to deficiency of isovaleryl-CoA dehydrogenase (Rhead & Tanaka, 1980),

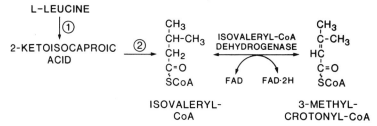

Fig. 91.1 Early steps in oxidation of L-leucine. (1) Leucine: 2-ketoglutarate transaminase. (2) Branched-chain ketoacid decarboxylase. Electrons pass from the FAD of isovaleryl-CoA dehydrogenase into the electron transport chain via an electron transfer flavoprotein (ETF).

an enzyme in L-leucine metabolism which oxidizes iso-valeryl-CoA to 3-methylcrotonyl-CoA (Fig. 91.1).

Pathogenesis

The primary metabolites of isovaleryl-CoA which are accumulated are isovalerylglycine (Tanaka & Isselbacher, 1967), 3-hydroxyisovaleric acid (Tanaka et al, 1968), and isovaleric acid. The first, produced by glycine-N-acylase catalyzed conjugation in the liver, is excreted at all times, while the latter two, which are produced by ω-oxidation and de-esterification, appear only when isovaleryl-CoA accumulation exceeds the glycine conjugating capacity of the liver, as after a protein load or during infection. The relationship of the compounds to the clinical and post-mortem findings is not well understood.

Diagnosis and differential diagnosis

Diagnosis is suggested by the clinical course and odour, and confirmed by demonstrating isovalerylglycine in urine and deficiency of isovaleryl-CoA dehydrogenase in tissues. Several of the same clinical and organic acid findings may occur in glutaric acidaemia type II, but other organic acids are usually present, and the tissue activity of isovaleryl-CoA dehydrogenase is normal.

Treatment

Diets low in protein or leucine reduce the accumulation of isovaleryl-CoA and appear to decrease the number and severity of acute episodes while permitting normal intellectual development (Levy et al, 1973). Oral glycine probably increases the liver's capacity to form isovaleryl-glycine, which is probably less toxic than isovaleric acid itself, and several catastrophically sick infants have been treated with it with remarkable effect (Cohn et al, 1978).

Genetics

Family studies, in which males and females are affected with approximately equal frequency, suggest inheritance as an autosomal recessive trait. Neither carrier detection nor prenatal diagnosis have been reported but, since almost complete deficiency of isovaleryl-CoA dehydrogenase can be demonstrated in mutant fibroblasts, both should be possible.

3-METHYLCROTONYLGLYCINAEMIA

Clinical course and heterogeneity

3-Methylcrotonylglycinaemia was first described in 1970 in a 4½-month-old girl with feeding problems, developmental delay, severe hypotonia, and an odour like that of cat's urine (Eldjarn et al, 1970; Stokke et al, 1972). It has since been described in a few patients with similar courses (Gompertz et al, 1973; Keeton & Moosa, 1976) as well as in several others with additional findings of acidosis and/or alopecia and a candida-like rash (Gompertz et al, 1971; Roth et al, 1976; Cowan et al, 1979).

The organic acids characteristic of the disease are 3-methylcrotonylglycine and 3-hydroxyisovaleric acid, which derive from glycine conjugation and hydration of 3-methylcrotonyl-CoA, suggesting a block in 3-methylcrotonyl-CoA carboxylase (Fig. 91.2). Substantial differences in clinical manifestations, organic acid excretion, and tissue enzyme activity of different patients suggest that the disorder has several different causes. Isolated

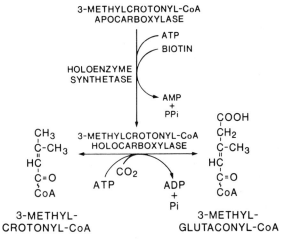

Fig. 91.2 Carboxylation of 3-methylcrotonyl-CoA and its relation to the activity of holocarboxylase synthetase. Holocarboxylase (holoenzyme) synthetase attaches biotin to this and several other apocarboxylases.

deficiency of 3-methylcrotonyl-CoA carboxylase has been described only once, in a three-month-old girl whose diagnosis remains in doubt because enzyme activity was not examined in cultured fibroblasts and because she excreted 2-oxoglutaric acid instead of 3-methylcrotonyl-glycine (Finnie et al, 1976). Fibroblasts from some patients with alopecia, rash, and acidosis are deficient in propionyl-CoA carboxylase and pyruvate carboxylase as well as in 3-methylcrotonyl-CoA carboxylase when grown in biotin-poor medium (Saunders et al, 1979; Bartlett & Gompertz, 1976), and the defect in these cells, which belong to the *bio* complementation group of propionic acidaemia, may be in holocarboxylase synthetase (Fig. 91.2). Fibroblasts from other patients, usually those with somewhat later onset of alopecia and mucocutaneous candidiasis, low carboxylase activities in peripheral leukocytes and low serum and/or urine concentrations of biotin, contain normal carboxylase activities (Cowan et al, 1979), and the defect in these patients may be in intestinal absorption of biotin.

Pathogenesis
The alopecia and candida-like skin rash observed in combined carboxylase deficiency states, i.e. forms of 3-methylcrotonylglycinaemia that are presumed due to holocarboxylase synthetase deficiency and to deficient biotin uptake from the gut, also occur in severe biotin deficiency (Scott, 1958), but their pathogenesis even in the deficiency state is not clear.

Diagnosis
Diagnosis is suggested by 3-methylcrotonylglycine and/or 3-hydroxyisovaleric acid in the urine of a child with appropriate clinical features, and evaluation should then include a careful search for organic acids derived from propionyl-CoA and pyruvate (3-hydroxypropionic, methylcitric, and lactic), examination of carboxylase activities in cultured fibroblasts, and biotin determinations in serum and urine. As similar clinical and laboratory features may occur in severe biotin deficiency, a careful evaluation should be made of the adequacy of biotin intake and the possibility that biotin loss in the stool is excessive.

Treatment
Biotin in large doses, e.g. 10 mg/day, produces rapid clinical improvement and almost complete disappearance of abnormal organic acids from the urine (Cowan et al, 1979; Keeton & Moosa, 1976; Gompertz et al, 1973; Gompertz et al, 1971).

Genetics
Family studies suggest that all forms of 3-methylcrotonylglycinaemia are transmitted as autosomal recessive traits, but the lack of information on the primary defects precludes heterozygote detection. Prenatal diagnosis, while perhaps possible by demonstrating abnormal organic acids in amniotic fluid and (in some forms) defective 3-methylcrotonyl-CoA carboxylase activity in cultured amniotic cells, has not been reported.

3-HYDROXY-3-METHYLGLUTARIC ACIDAEMIA

Clinical course
Hydroxymethylglutaric acidaemia was first described in a seven-month-old boy who developed apnea and cyanosis, hepatomegaly, acidosis, and severe hypoglycaemia without ketonuria shortly after an attack of diarrhea and vomiting (Faull et al, 1976), and additional patients have presented in infancy, with hypoglycaemia and acidosis (Schutgens et al, 1979), and at the age of two years, with what appeared to be Reye syndrome (Robinson et al, 1980). It is due to deficiency of hydroxymethylglutaryl-CoA lyase (Wysocki & Hähnel, 1976a), an enzyme of leucine oxidation which is also involved in the synthesis of ketone bodies (Fig. 91.3).

Pathogenesis
The most prominent organic acids in this condition are 3-hydroxy-3-methylglutaric, 3-methylglutaconic and 3-

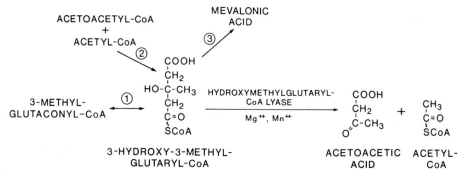

Fig. 91.3 The reaction catalyzed by hydroxymethylglutaryl-CoA lyase. (1) Methylglutaconyl-CoA hydratase. (2) Hydroxymethylglutaryl-CoA synthetase. (3) Hydroxymethylglutaryl-CoA reductase. (Reproduced with permission of Alan R. Liss, Inc.)

hydroxyisovaleric (Wysocki et al, 1976; Faull et al, 1976; Duran et al, 1978; Robinson et al, 1980), and especially after protein ingestion and in situations that normally favour ketone body formation. Moreover, because ketone bodies cannot be made, metabolic adjustments based on their oxidation by tissues are compromised.

Diagnosis and differential diagnosis
The diagnosis should be entertained in all patients with hypoglycaemia without ketosis in infancy and childhood, and confirmed by the organic aciduria and hydroxymethylglutaryl-CoA lyase deficiency in tissues. The observation that the same organic aciduria can occur without lyase deficiency in fibroblasts (Truscott et al, 1979) makes enzyme diagnosis mandatory.

Treatment
Biochemical control might be expected from a low protein (or leucine) diet together with measures to prevent catabolism and ketosis. One patient with the disorder had no attacks of acidosis for fourteen months after diagnosis (Wysocki & Hähnel, 1978) suggesting that the approach is indeed effective.

Genetics
Hydroxymethylglutaric acidaemia is inherited as an autosomal recessive trait, and heterozygote detection is possible by demonstrating intermediate lyase activity in leucocytes (Wysocki & Hähnel, 1976b). 3-Methylglutaconic acid excretion in maternal urine increased during a pregnancy with an affected fetus (Duran et al, 1979), and prenatal diagnosis can likely also be made by analyzing organic acids in amniotic fluid and/or by assaying hydroxymethylglutaryl-CoA lyase in cultured amniotic cells.

2-METHYL-3-HYDROXYBUTYRIC ACIDAEMIA

Clinical course
2-Methyl-3-hydroxybutyric acidaemia was first described in a six-year-old boy with episodes of acidosis and encephalopathy appearing after upper respiratory tract infections (Daum et al, 1973), and several additional patients have now been described (e.g. Gompertz et al, 1974). The disease usually presents beyond the first year of life and, without treatment, mental retardation or death during an episode of ketoacidosis is common. One patient developed hyperammonaemia and features of ketotic hyperglycinaemia in infancy (Hillman & Keating, 1974), however, and another was apparently well, suffering only from intermittent headaches, at the age of 15 years (Halvorsen et al, 1979).

This condition is apparently due to deficiency of the potassium-dependent acetoacetyl-CoA thiolase which catalyzes the cleavage of both 2-methylacetoacetyl-CoA and acetoacetyl-CoA (Robinson et al, 1979) (Fig. 91.4).

Pathogenesis
The acids which accumulate include normal ketone bodies, e.g. 3-hydroxybutyric and acetoacetic, and 2-methyl-3-hydroxybutyric and 2-methylacetoacetic, which derive in part from metabolite backup and in part from the entry of 2-methylacetoacetyl-CoA into the hydroxymethylglutaryl-CoA cycle. Tiglyl-CoA, which is excreted as the glycine conjugate in this condition as well as in propionic acidaemia and methylmalonic acidaemia, may cause hyperglycinaemia by inhibiting the conversion of glycine to serine (Hillman & Otto, 1974).

Diagnosis and differential diagnosis
Diagnosis is suggested by the clinical course and a consistent pattern of urine organic acids, and should be

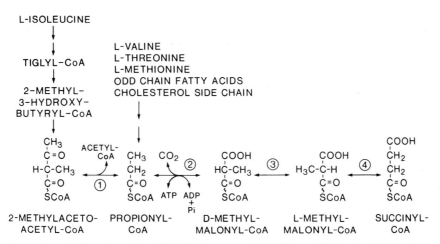

Fig. 91.4 Formation and metabolism of propionyl-CoA. (1) Acetoacetyl-CoA thiolase. (2) Propionyl-CoA carboxylase. (3) Methylmalonyl-CoA racemase. (4) Methylmalonyl-CoA mutase. Adenosylcobalamin is the specific coenzyme for methylmalonyl-CoA mutase.

confirmed whenever possible by demonstrating tissue deficiency of acetoacetyl-CoA thiolase. Because 2-methyl-3-hydroxybutyric acid is often excreted in normal ketosis (Landaas, 1975), diagnosis during acute episodes may be difficult unless tiglylglycine is present and the disorder should not be ruled out unless oral L-isoleucine loading fails to produce 2-methyl-3-hydroxybutyric aciduria.

Treatment

A low protein diet decreases the frequency and severity of episodes of acidosis and permits normal growth and development (Daum et al, 1973; Hillman & Keating, 1974; Gompertz et al, 1974).

Genetics

Family studies, which show approximately equal numbers of males and females to be affected, unaffected parents to excrete 2-methyl-3-hydroxybutyric acid after isoleucine loads (Daum et al, 1973; Gompertz et al, 1974), and parental consanguinity (Daum et al, 1973), suggest inheritance as an autosomal recessive trait. Heterozygote detection and prenatal diagnosis are probably possible but have not been reported.

PROPIONIC ACIDAEMIA

Clinical course and heterogeneity

Propionic acidaemia was first described in 1968 in an infant who died with severe metabolic acidosis and a serum propionic acid concentration of $5.4 \times 10^{-3}M$ (Hommes et al, 1968), and many additional patients have been reported since that time. The disorder may present in the first week of life with feeding difficulties, lethargy, vomiting and life-threatening acidosis, hypoglycaemia, and hyperammonaemia, or the course may be chronic, with poor feeding, failure to thrive, and episodes of vomiting, ketoacidosis, hyperglycinaemia and neutropenia triggered by infection or protein ingestion (Wadlington et al, 1975; Shafai et al, 1978). Seizures and developmental retardation are common. Postmortem examination often shows fatty infiltration of the liver.

Propionic acidaemia fibroblasts are deficient in propionyl-CoA carboxylase (Fig. 91.4) (Hsia et al, 1971), and can be divided into three main complementation groups, one of which, designated bio, is discussed in the section on 3-methylcrotonylglycinaemia. Two groups of cells, termed pcc A and pcc C, are deficient in propionyl-CoA carboxylase alone (Gravel et al, 1977; Wolf et al, 1978). Heterozygous carriers of pcc A mutations, but not pcc C mutations, show intermediate activity of propionyl-CoA carboxylase in leucocytes and fibroblasts, results which can be explained if the enzyme is composed of

non-identical subunits, one of which is produced in considerable excess but both of which are needed for activity (Wolf & Rosenberg, 1978).

Pathogenesis

The metabolites of propionyl-CoA most characteristic of propionic acidaemia are 3-hydroxypropionic, methylcitric , and propionic acid (Ando et al, 1972a; Ando et al, 1972b). The first is apparently formed by β-oxidation, the second by citrate synthetase catalyzed condensation with oxaloacetic, and the latter by simple de-esterification. The pathogenesis of the clinical phenotype is not clear. Marked hyperammonaemia probably contributes appreciably to the severe encephalopathy of patients presenting as newborns, possibly because propionyl-CoA inhibits the synthesis of N-acetylglutamate, the major allostearic activator of carbamyl phosphate synthetase (Coude et al, 1979). The cause of vomiting, encephalopathy, hypoglycaemia, and the post-mortem findings in patients without hyperammonaemia is more obscure. The contention that mitochondrial toxicity plays a role in pathogenesis is supported by observations that methylcitrate inhibits the citrate-malate shuttle as well as several enzymes of citrate and isocitrate metabolism (Cheema-Dhadli et al, 1975), and that propionate inhibits mitochondrial oxidation of pyruvate and 2-ketoglutarate (Gregersen, 1979).

Diagnosis

Diagnosis will be suggested by the clinical presentation and a consistent pattern of urine organic acids, but should be confirmed whenever possible by examining activities of propionyl-CoA, 3-methylcrotonyl-CoA, and pyruvate carboxylase in peripheral leucocytes and cultured fibroblasts.

Treatment

Acute therapy is directed to treating shock, acidosis, hypoglycaemia and hyperammonaemia with fluids, bicarbonate, glucose and even exchange transfusion and/or dialysis. Biotin should be tried in large doses, i.e. 10 mg/day, but it only rarely reduces organic acidaemia in patients who do not have combined carboxylase deficiency. In biotin non-responders, i.e. the vast majority of patients, treatment involves dietary restriction of propiogenic amino acids or protein. Some patients do well on such a regimen, achieving normal growth and development albeit with ketoacidosis complicating acute infections (Brandt et al, 1974), but most do not.

Genetics

All forms of propionic acidaemia are inherited as autosomal recessive traits, but only carriers of the pcc A mutation can be identified by intermediate tissue activity of propionyl-CoA carboxylase. Prenatal diagnosis of pcc

A and *pcc C* disease is possible by showing propionyl-CoA carboxylase deficiency in cultured amniotic cells (Gompertz et al, 1975) and/or accumulation of methyl-citrate in amniotic fluid (Sweetman et al, 1979).

METHYLMALONIC ACIDAEMIA

Clinical course and heterogeneity

Since almost simultaneous initial descriptions of methylmalonic acidaemia in 1967 by groups in Norway (Stokke et al, 1967) and Great Britain (Oberholzer et al, 1967), it has been one of the most frequently reported and extensively investigated human inborn error of metabolism. The clinical presentation, course, and postmortem findings are virtually identical to those of propionic acidaemia (Rosenberg et al, 1968). Hyperammonaemia has been observed with increasing frequency, particularly in acutely ill infants (Packman et al, 1978). The course may be quite different in patients with the *cbl C* and *cbl D* defects, most of whom present during infancy with seizures, hypotonia, microcephaly or profound developmental retardation, and eventually develop megaloblastic anaemia (Levy et al, 1970; Dillon et al, 1974; Carmel et al, 1980). Some, however, present with only mild developmental delay (Anthony & McLeay, 1976; Goodman et al, 1970). Thrombophlebitis and pulmonary embolism have complicated the course of one patient with the *cbl D* mutation (Goodman, unpublished).

The metabolic block in methylmalonic acidaemia is at methylmalonyl-CoA mutase, and Fig. 91.5 shows that this can be caused by defects in the mutase itself as well as by those of adenosylcobalamin biosynthesis. Five genetic complementation groups have now been defined in methylmalonic acidaemia fibroblasts. One, *mut*, contains cells with mutations in the apomutase, two, *cbl C* and *cbl D*, contain cells deficient in biosynthesis of methylcobalamin and adenosylcobalamin, and two, *cbl A* and *cbl B*, are deficient only in the synthesis of adenosylcobalamin (Gravel et al, 1975; Willard et al, 1979). Some *mut* lines contain no detectable mutase activity while activity can be restored to others by the addition of adenosylcobalamin (Willard & Rosenberg, 1977). The only patient reported with methylmalonyl-CoA racemase deficiency (Kang et al, 1972) in fact belongs to the *mut* group (Willard & Rosenberg, 1979). *Cbl B* lines are deficient in ATP:cob(I)alamin adenosyl transferase and, since only some of these cell lines recover mutase activity when grown in the presence of hydroxycobalamin, there is heterogeneity even within this group (Fenton & Rosenberg, 1978; Willard & Rosenberg, 1979). The specific defects in the remaining groups are not known, but the *cbl A* defect probably involves the reduction of cob(III)alamin to cob(I)alamin (Fenton & Rosenberg, 1978).

Pathogenesis

Methylmalonic acid, the compound most characteristic of the methylmalonic acidaemias, derives from de-ester-

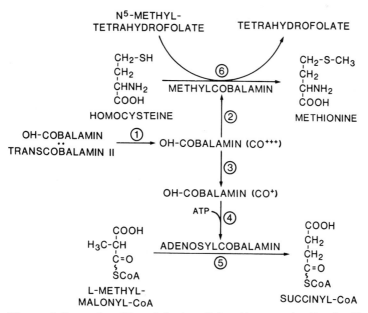

Fig. 91.5 Relationship of B_{12} metabolism to that of L-methylmalony-CoA and homocysteine. Details of Steps (1) and (2) are not known. Step (3) involves transport into the mitochondrion and reduction of Co^{+++} to Co^+. (4) ATP: cob(I)alamin adensoyl transferase. (5) L-methylmalonyl-CoA mutase. (6) N^5-methyltetrahydrofolate: homocysteine methyltransferase. (Reproduced with permission of Alan R. Liss, Inc.)

ification of the mutase substrate. Derivatives of propionyl-CoA, i.e. 3-hydroxypropionate and methylcitrate, are also accumulated, as are abnormal ketone bodies derived from the entry of propionyl-CoA into the hydroxymethylglutaryl-CoA cycle. Defective synthesis of methylcobalamin in *cbl C* and *cbl D* patients causes N^5-methyltetrahydrofolate: homocysteine methyltransferase deficiency, and thus homocystinaemia and homocystinuria.

Because propionyl-CoA accumulates in this disorder, many of the points made in the discussion of propionic acidaemia also pertain to methylmalonic acidaemia. Hypoglycaemia has been attributed to inhibition of pyruvate carboxylase by methylmalonyl-CoA (Utter et al, 1974) and to inhibition of mitochondrial transport of malate, 2-ketoglutarate, and isocitrate by methylmalonic acid (Halperin et al, 1971). The megaloblastosis which is often observed in patients with the *cbl C* and *cbl D* defects is probably due to the trapping of folic acid as N^5-methyltetrahydrofolate (Carmel et al, 1980).

Diagnosis

Diagnosis is suggested by the clinical course and the presence of large quantities of methylmalonic acid in urine. A careful search for homocystinaemia and/or homocystinuria should always be made; when present, it is accompanied by low methionine and high cystathionine in serum and not, as in cystathionine synthetase deficisicy, by high methionine and low cystathionine. Whenever possible, tissue enzymes should be assayed and the defect assigned to a complementation group.

Excretion of methylmalonic acid in B_{12} deficiency is usually not as pronounced as in the inherited disorders. The only reported patient in whom this was not so was the breast-fed, 6-month-old son of a woman who had eaten no animal protein for 8 years; in addition to methylmalonic acidaemia, the child had homocystinuria, a very low serum B_{12}, megaloblastic anaemia, and marked central nervous system disturbances (Higginbottom et al, 1978).

Treatment

As in propionic acidaemia, treatment is directed first to treating shock, acidosis, hypoglycaemia and hyperammonaemia. Therapy with B_{12} should be tried but its effects are so apt to be confused with those of vomiting and failure to feed that responsiveness to B_{12} should also be assessed later, during a period of relatively constant protein intake.

B_{12}-responsiveness has been examined rigorously in few patients, but the impression is that those with *cbl* defects usually respond and that those with *mut* defects do not. In some B_{12} responders, hydroxocobalamin (1 mg/day × 2–5 days) has a greater and more sustained effect than the same dose of cyanocobalamin (Goodman

et al, 1972) but, since both may eventually cause toxic symptoms, it may be best to combine cobalamin therapy with moderate protein restriction. Homocystinuria in *cbl C* and *cbl D* patients does not respond to B_{12} as well as methylmalonic aciduria, and betaine hydrochloride, which promotes transmethylation of homocysteine by betaine: homocysteine methyltransferase, may be useful in such cases (Goodman, unpublished).

Treatment of B_{12}-nonresponders is by restriction of protein or propiogenic amino acids to amounts which just permit normal growth and development. Although striking successes with dietary treatment have been reported (Nyhan et al, 1973), most patients do not do well and often die during episodes of ketoacidosis (Kaye et al, 1974; Duran et al, 1978).

One woman with an affected B_{12}-responsive fetus was given large doses of cyanocobalamin during the last nine weeks of pregnancy and her methylmalonic acid excretion, which had been increasing, began to decrease. The infant was treated with B_{12} and a low-protein diet immediately after birth, apparently with a favourable outcome (Ampola et al, 1975). The relevance of these observations is in question, however, as it has not yet been shown that the fetus suffers irreversible damage in utero.

Genetics

All forms of congenital methylmalonic acidaemia appear to be transmitted as autosomal recessive traits, although X–linked inheritance of the *cbl D* defect has not been excluded. Intermediate activity of methylmalonyl-CoA mutase and ATP:cob(I)alamin adenosyltransferase in fibroblasts can be used to characterize heterozygous carriers of *mut* and *cbl B* disease (Fenton & Rosenberg, 1978; Willard & Rosenberg, 1978), but carriers of the other mutations cannot yet be distinguished. All forms can probably be diagnosed in utero by demonstrating defective conversion of methylmalonyl- to succinyl-CoA in cultured amniotic cells (Willard & Rosenberg, 1976), but prenatal diagnosis of the *cbl C* and *cbl D* forms has not been reported to date. The amniotic fluid methylmalonic acid concentration has been elevated in several affected fetuses (Morrow et al, 1970; Mahoney et al, 1975; Ampola et al, 1975).

GLUTARIC ACIDAEMIA

Course and heterogeneity

Glutaric acidaemia may be one of the more common organic acidaemias but its course is so different from most of these disorders that the diagnosis can easily be missed. The disorder presents after a 3-month to 2-year period of normal development either with hypotonia and loss of head control or with an acute episode of vomiting

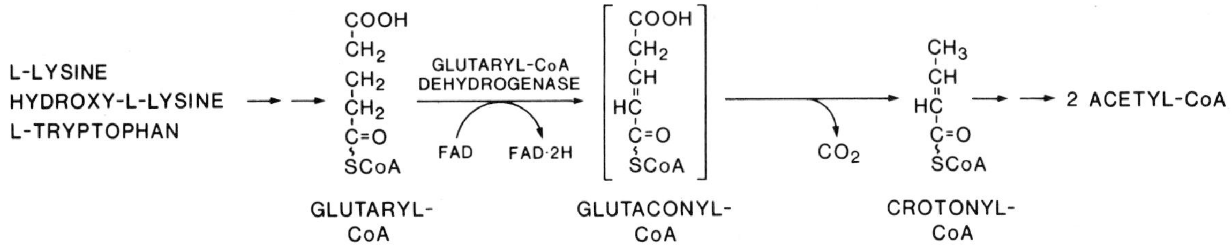

Fig. 91.6 The reaction catalyzed by glutaryl-CoA dehydrogenase, which probably dehydrogenates and decarboxylates the substrate. If glutaconyl-CoA is an intermediate, it is probably not readily dissociated from the enzyme. Electrons pass from the FAD of glutaryl-CoA dehydrogenase into the electron transport chain at coenzyme Q, probably through the electron transfer flavoprotein (ETF). (Reproduced with permission of Alan R. Liss, Inc.)

and encephalopathy following a relatively minor infection. Seizures, abnormal movements, hypoglycaemia, hepatomegaly and acidosis may be noted during the episode. Whatever the presentation, extrapyramidal symptoms e.g. dystonia, athetosis, and chorea, develop and progress (Goodman et al, 1975; Kyllerman & Steen, 1977; Whelan et al, 1979). Death may occur during an episode of acidosis and hypoglycaemia. The course is more attenuated when the mutant enzymes have more residual activity (Gregersen et al, 1977; Brandt et al, 1978; Christensen & Brandt, 1978). Fatty changes in the viscera and neuronal loss in the putamen and lateral aspects of the caudate have been described at autopsy (Goodman et al, 1977).

This disorder is due to deficiency of glutaryl-CoA dehydrogenase (Fig. 91.6), the enzyme which oxidizes glutaryl-CoA, an intermediate of lysine, hydroxylysine and tryptophan metabolism, to crotonyl-CoA (Goodman et al, 1975).

Pathogenesis

The organic acids characteristic of glutaric aciduria are glutaric, 3-hydroxyglutaric and glutaconic. The first and second are usually present (Stokke et al, 1975; Goodman et al, 1977; Gregersen & Brandt, 1978), but the third is present only occasionally, especially during ketoacidosis. Perhaps relevant to the pathogenesis of striatal degeneration is the observation that all three acids are powerful inhibitors of neuronal glutamate decarboxylase (Stokke et al, 1976), the enzyme responsible for the synthesis of GABA.

Diagnosis

Diagnosis should be suspected in any child with progressive dyskinesis and will be confirmed by the presence of glutaric aciduria and deficient tissue activity of glutaryl-CoA dehydrogenase. The main disorder from which the organic acid findings must be distinguished is glutaric acidaemia type II (see below), in which additional organic acids are excreted and tissue activity of glutaryl-CoA dehydrogenase is normal.

Treatment

Treatment is seldom successful, perhaps because irreversible striatal changes are already present at diagnosis. Restriction of dietary protein or glutarigenic amino acids reduce glutaric acid excretion but have little clinical effect. Riboflavin produced clinical improvement and a modest decrease in glutaric aciduria in two Danish patients (Brandt et al, 1979), but had no effect in one patient observed by the author. Lioresal$_R$, the *p*-chlorophenyl analogue of GABA, has improved some patients (Brandt et al, 1979), and had no effect on others.

Genetics

Glutaric acidaemia is inherited as an autosomal recessive trait, and leucocytes of heterozygotes contain intermediate activities of glutaryl-CoA dehydrogenase (Goodman & Kohlhoff, 1975). Prenatal diagnosis is possible by demonstrating enzyme deficiency in amniotic cells in culture and/or large amounts of glutaric acid in amniotic fluid (Goodman et al, 1980b).

GLUTARIC ACIDAEMIA TYPE II

Clinical course and heterogeneity

Glutaric acidaemia type II was first described in 1976 in a baby who died at 3 days of age with profound hypoglycaemia, metabolic acidosis, the 'smell of sweaty feet,' and a complex organic aciduria which, while dominated by glutaric acid, also contained many compounds not seen in glutaric acidaemia (Przyrembel et al, 1976). Several additional patients have been described since that time; one with symptoms like the first, one a 4½-year-old girl with episodes of hypoglycaemia, encephalopathy and hyperammonaemia associated with infections, and one a nineteen-year-old woman with episodic vomiting and severe hypoglycaemia (Tanaka et al, 1977; Dusheiko et al, 1978; Goodman et al, 1980a).

Pathogenesis

The organic acids accumulated in glutaric acidaemia type II include various combinations of glutaric, 2-hydroxyglutaric, isovalerylglycine, 3-hydroxyisovaleric, ethylmalonic and hexanoylglycine, most of which appear to derive from acyl-CoA esters normally oxidized by FAD-containing dehydrogenases. Accumulation of sarcosine has also been noted (Goodman et al, 1980a).

Substrate oxidation is impaired in whole cells (Przyrembel et al, 1976; Mantagos et al, 1979) but the activities of the acyl-CoA dehydrogenases are normal (Rhead & Tanaka, 1979; Goodman et al, 1980a). The primary defect is not known, but is generally believed to lie either in electron transfer from dehydrogenases into or through the electron transport chain or in the transfer of acyl-CoA moieties between various cell compartments. There is no subunit common to all these dehydrogenases, and tissue conversion of riboflavin to FAD, the common coenzyme, is apparently normal (Goodman et al, 1980a).

Diagnosis and differential

Diagnosis is suggested by the clinical phenotype and confirmed by the organic aciduria (which has been observed only in this disease and in Jamaican vomiting sickness) and by normal tissue activities of the acyl-CoA dehydrogenases.

Treatment

To date, treating affected infants with bicarbonate and a low carbohydrate and protein diet has not prevented an early fatal outcome. If the condition is due to a defect in electron transport, and if the accumulated substrates are toxic, treatment with methylene blue may be justified.

Genetics

Patients have been of both sexes and all families have had more than one affected child, suggesting inheritance as an autosomal recessive trait. Neither carrier detection nor prenatal diagnosis have been reported; the latter may be possible, however, by demonstrating the abnormal organic acids in amniotic fluid.

PYROGLUTAMIC ACIDAEMIA (5-OXOPROLINAEMIA)

Clinical course and heterogeneity

Pyroglutamic acidaemia was first described in an 18-year-old man with chronic metabolic acidosis, mental retardation ataxia, and spastic quadriplegia (Jellum et al, 1970; Kluge et al, 1972). Four additional patients have been described, all of whom developed severe metabolic acidosis and evidence of haemolysis, i.e. indirect hyperbilirubinaemia, anaemia, and reticulocytosis, in infancy. The haemolytic anaemia tends to become compensated, but metabolic acidosis is persistent and requires treatment (Hagenfeldt et al, 1974; Larson et al, 1974; Spielberg et al, 1977). The condition is due to deficiency of glutathione synthetase (Wellner et al, 1974).

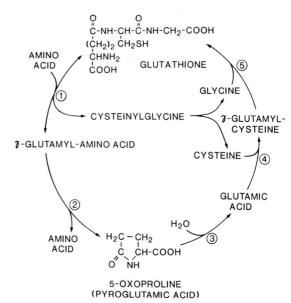

Fig. 91.7 The gamma-glutamyl cycle. (1) γ-Glutamyltranspeptidase. (2) γ-Glutamyl-cyclotransferase. (3) 5-Oxoprolinase. (4) β-Glutamylcysteine synthetase. (5) Glutathione synthetase. (Reproduced with permission of Alan R. Liss, Inc.)

Pathogenesis

The γ-glutamyl cycle, a series of reactions concerned with the synthesis and breakdown of glutathione, is shown in Fig. 91.7. It is not clear why pyroglutamic acid is excreted in glutathione synthetase deficiency instead of γ-glutamylcysteine, but it is thought that decreased levels of glutathione may release γ-glutamylcysteine synthetase from feedback inhibition, and that γ-glutamylcysteine is then formed and converted to pyroglutamic acid faster than it can be hydrolyzed by 5-oxoprolinase (Wellner et al, 1974).

One of the postulated functions of glutathione in the cell is to maintain membrane integrity, and haemolytic anaemia in pyroglutamic acidaemia may be due to glutathione deficiency. Indeed, in a form of glutathione synthetase deficiency in which the mutant enzyme is active but unstable, deficiency of glutathione is more marked in erythrocytes than in nucleated cells, and haemolytic anaemia occurs without pyroglutamic acidaemia (Mlohler et al, 1970; Spielberg et al, 1978). The observation that amino acid transport is normal in pyroglutamic acidaemia (Larsson et al, 1974; Spielberg et al, 1977) does not support a major role for the γ-glutamyl cycle in carrier mediated transport of amino acids.

Diagnosis and differential diagnosis

The serum and urine concentrations of pyroglutamic are so high in this condition that diagnosis is fairly simple, provided that the patient is not receiving Nutramigen, a formula which can contain as much as 6 mg pyroglutamic acid/g powder (Oberholzer et al, 1975). As 5-oxoprolinase deficiency could also conceivably cause pyroglutamic acidaemia, diagnosis should be confirmed by enzyme assay whenever possible.

Treatment
Treatment of acidosis with bicarbonate is simple and appears to permit normal growth and development.

Genetics
Pyroglutamic acidaemia is inherited as an autosomal recessive trait, with glutathione synthetase activity in tissues of heterozygous carriers being intermediate between those of patients and controls (Wellner et al, 1974; Spielberg et al, 1977). Prenatal diagnosis has not been reported but may be possible by demonstrating glutathione synthetase deficiency in cultured amniotic cells or increased pyroglutamic acid in amniotic fluid; amniotic fluid of one affected fetus contained about 15 times the normal concentration of pyroglutamic acid at term (Larsson et al, 1974).

REFERENCE

Ampola M G, Mahoney M J, Nakamura E, Tanaka K 1975 Prenatal therapy of a patient with vitamin-B_{12}-responsive methylmalonic acidaemia. New England Journal of Medicine 293: 313–317

Ando T, Klingberg W G, Ward A N, Rasmussen K, Nyhan W L 1971 Isovaleric acidaemia presenting with altered metabolism of glycine. Pediatric Research 5: 478–486

Ando T, Rasmussen K, Nyhan W, Hull D 1972a 3-Hydroxypropionate: Significance of β-oxidation of propionate in patients with propionic acidaemia and methylmalmonic acidaemia. Proceedings of the National Academy of Science USA 69: 2807–2811

Ando T, Rasmussen K, Wright J M, Nyhan W L 1972b Isolation and identification of methylcitrate, a major metabolic product of propionate in patients with propionic acidaemia. Journal of Biological Chemistry 247: 2200–2204

Anthony M, McLeay A C 1976 A unique case of derangement of vitamin B_{12} metabolism. Proceedings of the Australian Association of Neurologists 13: 61–65

Bartlett K, Gompertz D 1976 Combined carboxylase defect: Biotin-responsiveness in cultured fibroblasts. Lancet 2: 804

Brandt N J, Brandt S, Christensen E, Gregersen N, Rasmussen K 1978 Glutaric aciduria in progressive choreoathetosis. Clinical Genetics 13: 77–80

Brandt N J, Gregersen N, Christensen E, Grøn I H, Rasmussen K 1979 Treatment of glutaryl-CoA dehydrogenase deficiency (glutaric aciduria): Experience with diet, riboflavin and GABA analogue. Journal of Pediatrics 94: 669–673

Brandt I K, Hsia Y E, Clement D H, Provence S A 1974 Propionic-acidaemia (ketotic hyperglycinaemia): Dietary treatment resulting in normal growth and development. Pediatrics 53: 391–395

Budd M A, Tanaka K, Holmes L B, Efron M L, Crawford J D, Isselbacher K J 1967 Isovaleric acidaemia: Clinical features of a new genetic defect of leucine metabolism. New England Journal of Medicine 277: 321–327

Carmel R, Bedros A A, Mace J W, Goodman S I 1980 Congenital methylmalonic aciduria-homocystinuria with megaloblastic anaemia: Obeservations on response to hydroxyocobalamin and on the effect of homocysteine and methionine on the deoxyuridine suppression test. Blood 55: 570–579

Cheema-Dhadli S, Leznoff C C, Halperin M L 1975 Effect of 2-methylcitrate on citrate metabolism: Implications for the management of patients with propionic acidaemia and methylmalonic aciduria. Pediatric Research 9: 905–908

Childs B, Nyhan W L, Borden M A, Bard L, Cooke R E 1961 Idiopathic hyperglycinaemia and hyperglycinuria, a new disorder of amino acid metabolism. I. Pediatrics 27: 522–538

Christensen E, Brandt N J 1978 Studies on glutaryl-CoA dehydrogenase in leukocytes, fibroblasts and amniotic fluid cells. The normal enzyme and the mutant form in patients with glutaric aciduria. Clinica Chimica Acta 88: 267–276

Cohn R M, Yudkoff M, Rothman R, Segal S 1978 Isovaleric acidaemia: Use of glycine therapy in neonates. New England Journal of Medicine 299: 996–999

Coude F X, Sweetman L, Nyhan W L 1979 Inhibition by propionyl-coenzyme A of N-acetylglutamate synthetase in rat liver mitochondria. Journal of Clinical Investigation 64: 1544–1551

Cowan M J, Packman S, Wara D W, Ammann A J, Yoshino M, Sweetman L, Nyhan W 1979 Multiple biotin-dependent carboxylase deficiencies associated with defects in T-cell and B-cell immunity. Lancet 2: 115–118

Daum R S, Scriver C R, Mamer O A, Delvin E, Lamm P, Goldman H 1973 An inherited disorder of isoleucine catabolism causing accumulation of α-methylacetoacetate and α-methyl-β-hydroxybutyrate, and intermittent metabolic acidosis. Pediatric Research 7 149–160

Dillon M J, England J M, Gompertz D, Goodey P A, Grant D B, Hussein H A-A, Linnell J C, Matthews D M, Mudd S H, Newns G H, Seakins J W T, Uhlendorf B W, Wise I J 1974 Mental retardation, megaloblastic anaemia, methylmalonic aciduria, and abnormal homocysteine metabolism due to an error in B_{12} metabolism. Clinical Science and Molecular Medicine 47: 43–61

Duran M, Ketting D, Wadman S K, Jakobs C, Schutgens R B H, Veder H A 1978a Organic acid excretion in a patient with 3-hydroxy-3-methylglutaryl-CoA lyase deficiency: facts and artefacts. Clinica Chimica Acta 90: 187–193

Duran M, Bruinvis L, Ketting D, Wadman S K 1978b Deranged isoleucine metabolism during ketotic attacks in patients with methylmalonic acidaemia. Journal of Inherited Metabolic Disease 1: 105–107

Duran M, Schutgens R B H, Ketel A, Heymans H, Berntssen M W J, Ketting D, Wadman S K 1979 3-Hydroxy-3-methylglutaryl coenzyme A lyase deficiency: Postnatal management following prenatal diagnosis by analysis of maternal urine. Journal of Pediatrics 95: 1004–1007

Dusheiko G, Kew M C, Joffe B I, Lewin J R, Mantagos S, Tanaka K 1979 Recurrent hypoglycaemia associated with glutaric aciduria type II in an adult. New England Journal of Medicine 301: 1405–1409

Eldjarn L, Jellum E, Stokke O, Pande H, Waaler P E 1970 β-Hydroxyisovaleric aciduria and β-methylcrotonylglycinuria: A new inborn error of metabolism. Lancet 2: 521–522

Faull K, Bolton P, Halpern B, Hammond J, Danks D M, Hähnel R, Wilkinson S P, Wysocki S J, Masters P L 1976 Patient with defect in leucine metabolism. New England Journal of Medicine 294: 1013

Fenton W A, Rosenberg L E 1978 Genetic and biochemical analysis of human cobalamin mutants in cell culture. Annual Review of Genetics 12: 223–248

Finnie M D A, Cottrall K, Seakins J W T, Snedden W 1976 Massive excretion of 2-oxoglutaric acid and 3-hydroxyisovaleric acid in a patient with a deficiency of 3-methylcrotonyl-CoA carboxylase. Clinica Chimica Acta 73: 513–519

Gompertz D, Draffan G H, Watts J L, Hull D 1971 Biotin-responsive β-methylcrotonylglycinuria. Lancet 2: 22–24

Gompertz D, Bartlett K, Blair D, Stern C M M 1973 Child with a defect in leucine metabolism associated with β-hydroxyisovaleric aciduria and β-methylcrotonylglycinuria. Archives of Disease in Childhood 48: 975–977

Gompertz D, Saudubray J M, Charpentier C, Bartlett K, Goodey P A, Draffan D H 1974 A defect in L-isoleucine metabolism associated with α-methyl-β-hydroxybutyric and α-methylacetoacetic aciduria: Quantitative in vivo and in vitro studies. Clinica Chimica Acta 57: 269–281

Gompertz D, Goodey P A, Thom H, Russell G, Johnston A W, Mellor D H, MacLean M W, Ferguson-Smith M E, Ferguson-Smith M A 1975 Prenatal diagnosis and family studies in a case of propionic-acidaemia. Clinical Genetics 8: 244–250

Goodman S I, Moe P G, Hammond K B, Mudd S H, Uhlendorf B W 1970 Homocystinuria with methylmalonic aciduria: Two cases in a sibship. Biochemical Medicine 4: 500–515

Goodman S I, Keyser A J, Mudd S H, Schulman J D, Turse H, Lewy J 1972 Responsiveness of congenital methylmalonic-aciduria to derivatives of vitamin B$_{12}$. Pediatric Research 6: 138

Goodman S I, Kohlhoff J G 1975 Glutaric Aciduria: Inherited deficiency of glutaryl-CoA dehydrogenase activity. Biochemical Medicine 13: 138–140

Goodman S I, Markey S P, Moe P G, Miles B S, Teng C C 1975 Glutaric aciduria: A 'new' disorder of amino acid metabolism. Biochemical Medicine 12: 12–21

Goodman S I, Norenberg M D, Shikes R H, Breslich D J, Moe P G 1977 Glutaric aciduria: Biochemical and morphologic considerations. Journal of Pediatrics 90: 746–750

Goodman S I, McCabe E R B, Fennessey P V, Mace J W 1980a Multiple acyl-CoA dehydrogenase deficiency (Glutaric aciduria type II) with transient hypersarcosinaemia and sarcosinuria; possible inherited deficiency of an electron transfer flavoprotein. Pediatric Research 14: 12–17

Goodman S I, Gallegos D A, Pullin C J, Halpern B, Truscott R J W, Wise G, Wilcken B, Ryan E D, Whelan D T 1980b Antenatal diagnosis of glutaric acidaemia. American Journal of Human Genetics 32: 695–699

Gravel R A, Mahoney M J, Ruddle F H, Rosenberg L E 1975 Genetic complementation in heterokaryons of human fibroblasts defective in cobalamin metabolism. Proceedings of the National Academy of Science USA 72: 3181–3185

Gravel R A, Lam K F, Scully K J, Hsia Y E 1977 Genetic complementation of propionyl-CoA carboxylase deficiency in cultured human fibroblasts. American Journal of Human Genetics 29: 378–388

Gregersen N 1979 Studies on the effects of saturated and unsaturated shortchain monocarboxylic acids on the energy metabolism of rat liver mitochondria. Pediatric Research 13: 1227–1230

Gregersen N, Brandt N J, Christensen E, Grøn I, Rasmussen K, Brandt S 1977 Glutaric aciduria: Clinical and laboratory findings in two brothers. Journal of Pediatrics 90: 740–745

Gregersen N, Brandt N J 1979 Ketotic episodes in glutaryl-CoA dehydrogenase deficiency (glutaric aciduria). Pediatric Research 13: 977–981

Hagenfeldt L, Larsson A, Zetterström R 1974 Pyroglutamic aciduria: Studies in an infant with chronic metabolic acidosis. Acta Paediatrica Scandinavica 63: 1–8

Halperin M L, Schiller C M, Fritz I B 1971 The inhibition by methylmalonic acid of malate transport by the dicarboxylate carrier in rat liver mitochondria. Journal of Clinical Investigation 50: 2276–2282

Halvorsen S, Stokke O, Jellum E 1979 A variant form of 2-methyl-3-hydroxybutyric and 2-methylacetoacetic aciduria. Acta Paediatrica Scandinavica 68: 123–128

Higgenbottom M C, Sweetman L, Nyhan W L 1978 A syndrome of methylmalonic aciduria, homocystinuria, megaloblastic anaemia and neurologic abnormalities in a vitamin B$_{12}$-deficient breast-fed infant of a strict vegetarian. New England Journal of Medicine 299: 317–323

Hillman R E, Otto E F 1974 Inhibition of glycine-serine interconversion in cultured human fibroblasts by products of isoleucine catabolism. Pediatric Research 8: 941–945

Hillman R E, Keating J P 1974 Beta-ketothiolase deficiency as a cause of the 'ketotic hyperglycinaemia syndrome.' Pediatrics 53: 221–225

Hommes F A, Kuipers J R G, Elema J D, Jansen J F, Jonxis J H P 1968 Propionicacidaemia, a new inborn error of metabolism. Pediatric Research 2: 519–524

Hsia Y E, Scully K J, Rosenberg L E 1971 Inherited propionyl-CoA carboxylase deficiency in 'ketotic hyperglycinaemia.' Journal of Clinical Investigation 50: 127–130

Jellum E, Kluge T, Börreson H C, Stokke O, Eldjarn L 1970 Pyroglutamic aciduria – A new inborn error of metabolism. Scandinavian Journal of Clinical and Laboratory Investigation 26: 327–335

Kang E S, Snodgrass P J, Gerald P S 1972 Methylmalonyl Coenzyme A racemase defect: Another cause of methylmalonic aciduria. Pediatric Research 6: 875–879

Kaye C I, Morrow G, Nadler H L 1974 In vitro 'responsive' methylmalonic acidaemia: A new variant. Journal of Pediatrics 85: 55–59

Keeton B R, Moosa A 1967 Organic aciduria: Treatable cause of floppy infant syndrome. Archives of Disease in Childhood 51: 636–638

Kluge T, Børreson H C, Jellum E, Stokke O, Eldjarn L, Fretheim B 1972 Esophageal hiatus hernia and mental retardation: Life-threatening postoperative metabolic acidosis and potassium deficiency linked with a new inborn error of nitrogen metabolism. Surgery 71: 104–109

Kyllerman M, Steen G 1977 Intermittently progressive dyskinetic syndrome in glutaric aciduria. Neuropädiatrie 8: 397–404

Landaas S 1975 Accumulation of 3-hydroxyisobutyric acid, 2-methyl-3-hydroxybutyric acid and 3-hydroxyisovaleric acid in ketoacidosis. Clinica Chimica Acta 64: 143–154

Larsson A, Zetterström R, Hagenfeldt L, Andersson R, Dreborg S, Hörnell H 1974 Pyroglutamic aciduria (5-oxoprolinuria), an inborn error in glutathione metabolism. Pediatric Research 8: 852–856

Levy H L, Mudd S H, Schulman J D, Dreyfus P M, Abeles R H 1970 A derangement in B$_{12}$ metabolism associated with homocystinemia, cystathioninemia, hypomethioninemia and methylmalonic aciduria. American Journal of Medicine 48: 390–397

Levy H L, Erickson A M, Lott I T, Kurtz D J 1973 Isovaleric acidaemia: Results of family study and dietary treatment. Pediatrics 52: 83–94

Mantagos S, Genel M, Tanaka K 1979 Ethylmalonic-adipic aciduria: In vivo and in vitro studies indicating deficiency of activities of multiple acyl-CoA dehydrogenases. Journal of Clinical Investigation 64: 1580–1589

Mohler D N, Majerus P W, Minnich V, Hess C E, Garrick M D 1970 Glutathione synthetase deficiency as a cause of hereditary hemolytic disease. New England Journal of Medicine 283: 1253–1257

Morrow G, Schwarz R H, Hallock J A, Barness L A 1970 Prenatal detection of methylmalonic acidaemia. Journal of Pediatrics 77: 120–123

Newman C G H, Wilson B D R, Callaghan P, Young L 1967 Neonatal death associated with isovalericacidaemia. Lancet 2 439–442

Nyhan W L, Fawcett N, Ando T, Rennert O M, Julius R L 1973 Response to dietary therapy in B$_{12}$ unresponsive methylmalonic acidaemia. Pediatrics 51: 539–548

Oberholzer V G, Levin B, Burgess E A, Young W F 1967 Methylmalonic aciduria: An inborn error of metabolism leading to chronic metabolic acidosis. Archives of Disease in Childhood 42: 492–504

Oberholzer V G, Wood C B S, Palmer T, Harrison B M 1975 Increased pyroglutamic acid levels in patients on artificial diets. Clinica Chimica Acta 62: 299–304

Packman S, Mahoney M J, Tanaka K, Hsia Y E 1978 Severe hyperammonaemia in a newborn infant with methylmalonyl-CoA mutase deficiency. Journal of Pediatrics 92: 769–771

Przyrembel H, Wendel U, Becker K, Bremer H J, Bruinvis L, Ketting D, Wadman S K 1976 Glutaric aciduria type II: Report on a previously undescribed metabolic disorder. Clinica Chimica Acta 66: 227–239

Rhead W, Tanaka K 1979 Evidence for normal isovaleryl and butyryl-CoA dehydrogenase activity in fibroblast mitochondria from patients with glutaric aciduria type II. American Journal of Human Genetics 31: 59A Abstr.

Rhead W J, Tanaka K 1980 Demonstration of a specific mitochondrial isovaleryl-CoA dehydrogenase deficiency in fibroblasts from patients with isovaleric acidaemia. Proceedings of the National Academy of Science USA 77: 580–583

Robinson B H, Sherwood W G, Taylor J, Balfe J W, Mamer O A 1979 Acetoacetyl-CoA thiolase deficiency: A cause of severe ketoacidosis in infancy simulating salicylism. Journal of Pediatrics 95: 228–233

Robinson B H, Oei J, Sherwood G, Slyper A H, Heininger J, Mamer O A 1980 Hydroxymethylglutaryl-CoA lyase deficiency: Features resembling Reye syndrome. Neurology 30: 714–718

Rosenberg L E, Lilljeqvist A, Hsia Y E 1968 Methylmalonic aciduria: An inborn error leading to metabolic acidosis, long-chain ketonuria and intermittent hyperglycinaemia. New England Journal of Medicine 278: 1319–1322

Roth K, Cohn R, Yandrasitz J, Preti G, Dodd P, Segal S 1976 Beta-methylcrotonic aciduria associated with lactic acidosis. Journal of Pediatrics 88: 229–235

Saunders M, Sweetman L, Robinson B, Roth K, Cohn R, Gravel R A 1979 Biotin-responsive organicaciduria: Multiple carboxylase defects and complementation studies with propionicacidaemia in cultured fibroblasts. Journal of Clinical Investigation 64: 695–1702

Scott D 1958 Clinical biotin deficiency (egg white injury). Acta Medica Scandinavica 162: 69–70

Schutgens R B H, Heymans H, Ketel A, Veder H A, Duran M, Ketting D, Wadman S K 1979 Lethal hypoglycaemia in a child with a deficiency of 3-hydroxy-3-methylglutarylcoenzyme A lyase. Journal of Pediatrics 94: 89–91

Shafai T, Sweetman L, Weyler W, Goodman S I, Fennessey P V, Nyhan W L 1978 Propionic acidaemia with severe hyperammonaemia and defective glycine metabolism. Journal of Pediatrics 92: 84–86

Spielberg S P, Kramer L I, Goodman S I, Butler J, Tietze F, Quinn P, Schulman J D 1977 5-Oxoprolinuria: Biochemical observations and case report. Journal of Pediatrics 91: 237–241

Spielberg S P, Garrick M D, Corash L M, Butler J D, Tietze F, Rogers L, Schulman J D 1978 Biochemical heterogeneity in glutathione synthetase deficiency. Journal of Clinical Investigation 61: 1417–1420

Stokke O, Eldjarn L, Norum K R, Steen-Johnsen J, Halvorsen S 1967 Methylmalonic acidaemia: A new inborn error of metabolism which may cause fatal acidosis in the neonatal period. Scandinavian Journal of Clinical and Laboratory Investigation 20: 313–328

Stokke O, Eldjarn L, Jellum E, Pande H, Waaler P E 1972 Beta-methylcrotonyl-CoA carboxylase deficiency: A new metabolic error in leucine degradation. Pediatrics 49: 726–735

Stokke O, Goodman S I, Thompson J A, Miles B S 1975 Glutaric aciduria: Presence of glutaconic and β-hydroxyglutaric acids in urine. Biochemical Medicine 12: 386–391

Stokke O, Goodman S I, Moe P G 1976 Inhibition of brain glutamate decarboxylase by glutarate, glutaconate, and β-hydroxyglutarate: Explanation of the symptoms in glutaric aciduria? Clinica Chimica Acta 66: 411–415

Tanaka K, Budd M A, Efron M L, Isselbacher K J 1966 Isovaleric acidaemia: A new genetic defect of leucine metabolism. Proceedings of the National Academy of Science USA 56: 236–242

Tanaka K, Isselbacher K J 1967 The isolation and identification of N-isovalerylglycine from urine of patients with isovaleric acidaemia. Journal of Biological Chemistry 242: 2966–2972

Tanaka K, Orr J C, Isselbacher K J 1968 Identification of β-hydroxyisovaleric acid in the urine of a patient with isovaleric acidaemia. Biochimica et Biophysica Acta 152: 638–641

Tanaka K, Mantagos S, Genel M, Seashore M R, Billings B A, Baretz B H 1977 New defect in fatty-acid metabolism with hypoglycaemia and organic aciduria. Lancet 2: 986–987

Truscott R J W, Halpern B, Wysocki S J, Hähnel R, Wilcken B 1979 Studies on a child suspected of having a deficiency in 3-hydroxy-3-methylglutaryl-CoA lyase. Clinica Chimica Acta 95: 11–16

Utter M F, Keech D B, Scrutton M G A 1964 A possible role for acetyl CoA in the control of glyconeogenesis. In: Weber G (ed) Advances in Enzyme Regulation, vol 2, Pergamon, New York p 49–68

Wadlington W B, Kilroy A, Ando T, Sweetman L, Nyhan W L 1975 Hyperglycinaemia and propionyl CoA carboxylase deficiency and episodic severe illness without consistent ketosis. Journal of Pediatrics 86: 707–712

Wellner V P, Sekura R, Meister A, Larsson A 1974 Glutathione synthetase deficiency, an inborn error of metabolism involving the γ-glutamyl cycle in patients with

5-oxoprolinuria (pyroglutamic aciduria). Proceedings of the National Academy of Science USA 71: 2505–2509

Whelan D T, Hill R, Ryan E D, Spate M 1979 L-Glutaric acidaemia: Investigation of a patient and his family. Pediatrics 63: 88–93

Willard H F, Ambani L M, Hart C, Mahoney M J, Rosenberg L E 1976 Rapid prenatal and postnatal detection in inborn errors of propionate, methylmalonate, and cobalamin metabolism: A sensitive assay using cultured cells. Human Genetics 32: 277–283

Willard H F, Rosenberg L E 1977 Inherited deficiencies of human methylmalonyl CoA mutase activity: Reduced affinity of mutant apoenzyme for adenosylcobalamin. Biochemical and Biophysical Research Communications 78: 927–934

Willard H F, Mellman I S, Rosenberg L E 1978 Genetic complementation among inherited deficiencies of methylmalonyl-CoA mutase activity: Evidence for a new class of human cobalamin mutant. American Journal of Human Genetics 30: 1–13

Willard H F, Rosenberg L E 1979a Inherited deficiencies of methylmalonyl CoA mutase activity: Biochemical and genetic studies in cultured skin fibroblasts. In: Hommes F A (ed) Models for the Study of Inborn Errors of Metabolism, Elsevier, New York p 297–310

Willard H F, Rosenberg L E 1979b Inborn errors of cobalamin metabolism: Effect of cobalamin supplementation in culture on methylmalonyl CoA mutase activity in normal and mutant human fibroblasts. Biochemical Genetics 17: 57–75

Wolf B, Hsia Y E, Rosenberg L E 1978 Biochemical differences between mutant propionyl-CoA carboxylases from two coplementation groups. American Journal of Human Genetics 30: 455–464

Wolf B, Rosenberg L E 1978 Heterozygote expression in propionylcoenzyme A carboxylase deficiency. Journal of Clinical Investigation 62: 931–936

Wysocki S J, Wilkinson S P, Hähnel R, Wong C Y B, Panegyres P K 1976 3-Hydroxy-3-methylglutaric aciduria, combined with 3-methylglutaconic aciduria. Clinica Chimica Acta 70: 399–406

Wysocki S J, Hähnel R 1976a 3-Hydroxy-3-methylglutaric aciduria: Deficiency of 3-hydroxy-3-methylglutaryl coenzyme A lyase. Clinica Chimica Acta 71: 349–351

Wysocki S J, Hähnel R 1976b 3 Hydroxy-3-methylglutaric aciduria: 3-hydroxy-3-methylglutaryl-coenzyme A lyase levels in leukocytes. Clinica Chimica Acta 73: 373–375

Wysocki S J, Hähnel R 1978 3-Methylcrotonylglycine excretion in 3-hydroxy-3-methylglutaric aciduria. Clinica Chimica Acta 86: 101–108

92

Disorders of copper metabolism

D. M. Danks

GENERAL BACKGROUND

Copper is an essential micronutrient for man and animals, being a component of a number of important enzymes (Evans, 1973; Underwood, 1977; Mason, 1980; Danks, 1981). Table 92.1 lists those enzymes or cellular functions for which copper has been proved essential.

Table 92.1 Copper enzymes in man.

Common name	Functional role	Known or expected consequence of deficiency
Cytochrome oxidase	Electron transport chain	Uncertain
Superoxide dismutase	Free radical detoxification	Uncertain
Tyrosinase	Melanin production	Failure of pigmentation
Dopamine β hydroxylase	Catecholamine production	Neurological effects, type uncertain
Lysyl oxidase	Cross-linking of collagen and elastin	Vascular rupture
Caeruloplasmin	Ferroxidase ?other roles	Anaemia
Enzyme not known	Cross-linking of keratin (disulphide bonds)	Pili torti

This list is probably not yet complete as other enzymes appear to contain copper. The consequences of nutritional copper deficiency observed in man and animals correspond quite well to those which would be expected in the light of these functions (Table 92.2) (Danks, 1980). The precise effects differ between species as does the order in which these effects develop on a deficient diet.

The adult human body contains 70 to 100 mg of copper and the daily requirement is of the order of 1 to 5 mg. Absorption occurs in the upper small intestine by active processes which have not been fully defined. An equivalent amount is excreted in the bile and very little of this biliary copper is reabsorbed. Renal losses are very small, filtered copper being reabsorbed efficiently. A moderate amount of copper is present in sweat and in very hot climates this may become significant to the copper balance.

Copper absorbed from the intestine is transported by serum albumin bound to the amino-terminal tripeptide and is largely taken up by the liver. Some of this copper reappears in the plasma over the next 48 hours in caeruloplasmin, a ferroxidase which may or may not also serve a copper transport role (Frieden, 1980).

Copper must be delivered to the intracellular sites of synthesis of the various copper-enzymes. Copper ions are very reactive and highly toxic and could not be tolerated free in body tissues. A very efficient system of specific transport processes must exist ensuring that copper ions

Table 92.2 Effects seen in nutritional copper deficiency in man, sheep, rats, pigs, and in Menkes syndrome.

Effect	Man	Sheep	Rai	Pig	Menkes syndrome
Anaemia	++	++	++	++	−
Neutropenia	+	+	+	+	−
Abnormal hair structure	±	++	+	+	++
Depigmentation	±	+	+	+	+
Arterial rupture	?	−	+	++	++
Myocardial fibrosis	?	−	+	+	−
Osteoporosis	+	±	+	++	+
Emphysema	?	−	+	−	+
Cerebellar ataxia	−	+*	+*	+*	+
Other brain damage	−	+*	+*	+	++

* Seen only after fetal copper deficiency

are always held complexed to larger molecules which deliver the copper to the sites where it is required. Genes must code for each of these transport molecules and one can therefore anticipate a considerable number of genetic defects affecting copper homeostasis and availability.

To date just two genetic defects are known in man. Wilson disease was discovered in 1912 and was shown to be related to copper homeostasis in 1948 (Cuming, 1948). Menkes syndrome was described in 1962 (Menkes et al, 1962) and first shown to be related to copper metabolism in 1972 (Danks et al, 1972b).

Availability of mice affected by mutations apparently homologous to those causing Menkes syndrome and the use of tissue culture studies have advanced the understanding of Menkes syndrome. Neither of these advantages has been available to those studying Wilson disease, but recent discoveries offer exciting possibilities, mentioned below.

References throughout this chapter are to recent articles which review a particular topic. No attempt is made to cite first observations of particular findings.

WILSON DISEASE

Clinical features

Clinical presentation is generally with liver disease or with neurological disturbance (Strickland et al, 1973; Dobyns et al, 1979). Hepatic symptoms may occur at any age, but are most frequently seen in childhood between the ages of 8 and 16 years (Odievre et al, 1974; Sass-Kortsak, 1975). Presentation with neurological symptoms before the age of 14 years is very unusual and is most frequent between the ages of 20 and 40 years.

Almost any symptom of liver disease may be seen, but acute presentation is surprisingly frequent for a basic process which is undoubtedly very slow and gradual in its effects. Some children are diagnosed only in the second or third episode of acute jaundice, earlier episodes being ascribed to hepatitis – a tragic situation if the final episode is fulminant and fatal. Haemolysis is often a prominent feature of the more severe acute hepatic episodes and some patients present with haemolysis unaccompanied by other features of liver failure (Iser et al, 1974). However, liver disease is always found on investigation of such patients.

Dysarthria and deterioration of coordination and voluntary movement are the most frequent neurological symptoms. These are often accompanied by involuntary movements and by disorders of posture and tone. A concomitant loss of intellectual function and/or disturbances of behaviour may or may not be seen at the onset, but always develops later. Untreated these symptoms progress to bulbar palsy and death.

Osteoarthropathy (Canelas et al, 1978; Golding & Walshe, 1977), renal tubular acidosis and renal calculi

(Wiebers et al, 1979) are seen quite frequently and may occasionally be the presenting feature. Kayser-Fleischer rings provide the most valuable diagnostic sign of Wilson disease, but do not cause any symptoms. They comprise golden-brown granular pigmentation of the outer crescent of the iris at the limbus. Sometimes they can be observed with the naked eye, but slit lamp examination is required in many patients to detect this sign. Anaemia (Hoagland & Goldstein, 1978) and cataracts (Wiebers et al, 1977) are occasionally symptoms.

Regardless of the mode of presentation, some degree of liver disease is always present if evidence is sought.

Laboratory and cell culture findings

Typically serum caeruloplasmin is greatly reduced and the non-caeruloplasmin copper concentration is increased. The nett effect is a moderate reduction in the total serum copper level. Urinary copper excretion is increased and the excretion is very greatly augmented after administration of penicillamine. Liver copper concentration is greatly increased. Typical figures are quoted in Table 92.3.

The ultimate test for Wilson disease at the present time is the demonstration of a gross reduction of incorporation of copper isotope into caeruloplasmin (Sternlieb & Scheinberg, 1979). Total plasma radioactivity continues to fall over 48 hours after intravenous injection of copper 64 in patients with Wilson disease. A secondary rise in radioactivity is seen in normal subjects from four hours through to 48 hours due to appearance of labelled caeruloplasmin. Intermediate results (i.e. smaller secondary rise) are seen in some heterozygotes for Wilson disease and in patients with copper retention secondary to other forms of liver disease (Vierling et al, 1978).

Many other tests reveal the damaging effects of the disease on the various organs affected and are useful in diagnosis. Some results are relatively specific and others quite nonspecific. Any or all liver functions may be deranged; no particular pattern of derangement is characteristic. Generalised aminoaciduria, glucosuria and defective urinary acidification are frequent and similar

Table 92.3 Typical copper measurements in Wilson disease.

	Wilson disease	Normal (adults)
Serum caeruloplasmin		
OD units per ml	0–0.25	0.25–0.49
mg/l	0–200	200–400
Serum copper		
μmol/l	3–10	11–24
Urinary copper		
(μg per 24 hours)		
Untreated	100–1 000	<40
On penicillamine –	1 500–3 000	100–600
250 mg 6 hourly		

to those found in many other diseases damaging renal tubules. Anaemia (normochromic), neutropenia and thrombocytopenia are occasionally seen (Hoagland & Goldstein, 1978). Some microscopic findings in liver biopsies were proposed to be rather specific (e.g. marked glycogen accumulation in hepatocyte nuclei) but most authors now agree that the changes are variable and non-specific (Sternlieb, 1978; Sternlieb, 1980).

Investigation of patients with neurological symptoms generally includes e.e.g. which only rarely gives a specific result (Westmoreland et al, 1974) and CT scan in which increased radiolucency of the basal ganglia has been described as an important finding in support of the diagnosis (Nelson et al, 1979).

Fibroblastic cells grown from skin biopsies from patients have recently been found to accumulate abnormally high concentrations of copper (Goka et al, 1976; Chan et al, 1980; Camakaris et al, 1980a). Some variability of this phenomenon in different flasks of the same culture have been observed and more work is required to standardise test conditions (Camakaris et al, 1980a). These findings give promise of a new diagnostic test and of a means of understanding the basic defect in copper transport.

Diagnosis

Wilson disease is an important condition because it is one of the very few treatable causes of chronic liver disease and of chronic brain degeneration. Clinicians must therefore keep it in mind (BMJ Editorial, 1978; Sternlieb, 1978; Cartwright, 1978). It is numerically significant in both these clinical complexes. Indeed, it is the most frequent single cause of cirrhosis in later childhood, causing approximately 20% of all cases of cirrhosis which develop between the ages of 4 and 16 years (Sass-Kortsak, 1975).

Paediatricians should, therefore, take the attitude that chronic liver disease presenting after 4 or 5 years of age is due to Wilson disease until proved otherwise. A similar attitude to adult patients is probably justified, but is harder to promote because the high frequency of alcoholic liver disease tends to obscure the situation. Wilson disease can cause effects indistinguishable from chronic active hepatitis (Scott et al, 1978), and presentation with cirrhosis is possible even in late middle age (Fitzgerald et al, 1975).

The classical diagnostic tests (examination for Kayser-Fleischer rings, measurement of serum copper, of caeruloplasmin and 24 hour urinary excretion of copper) will identify 95% of adult cases, but fail in approximately 15–20% of childhood cases (Sternlieb, 1978; Werlin et al, 1978). The copper content of a needle liver biopsy should therefore be measured in every child with chronic liver disease. A sample of about 5 mg should be analysed to avoid erroneous interpretation due to uneven distribution of copper in the liver. Copper levels above 500 μg/g dry weight are usually diagnostic, but such levels may occur in some other forms of liver disease and copper 64 studies may be needed to finalise the diagnosis. Only by taking this aggressive attitude will the tragic failure to diagnose Wilson disease be eliminated.

Treatment

Penicillamine is a very effective drug for the treatment of Wilson disease, using 1 to 3 g daily in adult patients or in older children. Dosage is monitored by 24 hour urinary excretion of copper which should be kept in the range of 1 to 3 mg daily. Serious complications were frequent when DL-penicillamine was used, but are not very frequent with pure D-penicillamine. A nephrotic syndrome was very frequent and is still encountered occasionally. Thrombocytopenia and skin rashes are the most common complication. A short course of prednisolone may control these effects, but they may persist and necessitate withdrawing the drug. Bone marrow aplasia can occur.

When serious complications of penicillamine therapy develop and persist, other chelating drugs have to be considered (e.g. triethylene tetramine). Dietary restriction of copper intake is not necessary, although foods with very high copper content (shellfish and crustaceans) should be avoided.

Two other methods of treatment have been proposed. Zinc competes with copper for intestinal absorption and good control has been claimed with long term zinc therapy (Hoogenraad et al, 1978). Sauna baths have been suggested as a means of promoting copper excretion in the sweat (Sunderman et al, 1974).

Penicillamine has an effect on clinical features only after several weeks (neurological features) or several months (liver disease). Consequently it is very difficult to save patients who present in a fulminant episode of liver failure (Sternlieb, 1980). A method of removing copper rapidly during acute fulminant liver failure is needed. Peritoneal dialysis is moderately effective as is exchange transfusion (Hamlyn et al, 1977). Albumin infusion may increase the binding of the large amount of non-caeruloplasmin copper present in these episodes. All too often these measures prove insufficient.

In neurological cases which are diagnosed only after considerable damage has occurred, and while awaiting a response to penicillamine, L-dopa may be useful as a symptomatic measure.

Genetics and genetic heterogeneity

Inheritance is autosomal recessive and is indicated by the occurrence of the disease in sibs with the expected segregation ratio and by parental consanguinity (Bearn, 1960; Strickland et al, 1973). The incidence is not known accurately. Experience in Melbourne suggests a figure in the range 1 in 50 000 to 1 in 100 000 live births.

The range of disease effects and severity is wide and allelic heterogeneity is almost certain. However, the most striking difference – that between hepatic and neurological presentation – does not seem to be explained by allelic variation. Many families have been described in which one sib has presented with liver manifestations and another with neurological onset. Females more often present with liver disease and males with neurological features (Strickland et al, 1973). A particularly mild neurological form has been described in New York among Jewish immigrants from Eastern Europe (Bearn, 1960).

Heterozygotes do not have any clinical manifestations. Approximately 10% show lowered levels of serum copper and caeruloplasmin. An intermediate secondary rise in plasma radioactivity after copper 64 is seen in heterozygotes as a group but cannot be used to identify individual heterozygotes.

Genetic counselling

Sibs of a patient with Wilson disease have a 1 in 4 risk of developing the disease. These sibs should be examined for liver or neurological disease and for Kayser-Fleischer rings and by measuring serum copper, serum caeruloplasmin and urinary copper. Patients older than the index case may be assumed to be unaffected if no abnormalities are detected. Younger sibs should be investigated more fully using liver biopsy or copper 64 studies if initial tests are normal.

Investigation of potential heterozygotes has little value, because available tests are not reliable and cannot be interpreted when applied to individuals with low a priori risks of being heterozygotes (e.g. spouses of aunts or uncles who may be heterozygotes).

The risk to offspring of affected individuals is low. Over 50 pregnancies have been reported in patients in good clinical health on penicillamine treatment, without serious symptoms during pregnancy and with normal babies (Scheinberg & Sternlieb, 1975; Walshe, 1977). Two reports have described babies with unusual connective tissue changes born to women on penicillamine therapy for cystinuria and rheumatoid arthritis respectively (Mjolnerod et al, 1971; Linares et al, 1979). Interference with collagen cross-linking by penicillamine was blamed. Other reports suggest that such occurrences are rare (Scheinberg & Sternlieb, 1975; Walshe, 1977; Lyle, 1979). For the present it seems reasonable to continue penicillamine during pregnancy if the maternal disease has been treated for a relatively short time. In long treated patients no clinical effects are seen during rests from therapy for 6 or 9 months and cessation during pregnancy might be preferable.

Prenatal diagnosis/presymptomatic diagnosis

Prenatal diagnosis has not been possible, but the recent findings in cultured cells raise this possibility. However, many would doubt the place of prenatal diagnosis in a disease of late onset for which effective treatment is available.

Mass screening of newborn babies has been suggested and simple methods of measuring serum caeruloplasmin do exist. However, the very low levels seen in normal newborn babies make recognition at this age very difficult. Early symptomatic diagnosis of first cases in families through constant awareness should be sufficient.

Pathogenesis

The basic biochemical defect is unknown. It is not a defect in the structure of caeruloplasmin, and genetically determined deficiency of caeruloplasmin does not cause liver or brain disease (Edwards et al, 1979). The two most fundamental defects are slow production of caeruloplasmin and severe interference with biliary excretion of copper. Presumably the defect lies in some step common to both these processes. The difficulty of studying these processes in the liver and the lack of a satisfactory animal model have hindered research. Work with cell cultures (see above) and Bedlington terriers (see below) may change this situation.

Copper accumulates progressively in Wilson disease and the sub-cellular distribution changes during the course of the disease. Suggestions that this distribution allows distinction between toxic and non-toxic copper accumulation are less firmly expressed now than a decade ago (Goldfischer et al, 1968; Sternlieb, 1980).

The rate of accumulation, and other unknown factors, influence the degree of liver damage. Intercurrent virus infections may play a part in precipitating symptomatic liver disease. If liver damage is not too severe the patient lives on and copper 'overflows' from the liver to the brain, eyes, kidney, myocardium and many other tissues. This overflow can also occur in copper accumulation secondary to other forms of liver disease (Sternlieb, 1980). This fact and the improvement seen after liver transplantation support the idea that the extrahepatic effects are secondary to overflow from the liver.

Haemolytic crises are associated with very high levels of non-caeruloplasmin plasma copper. It is likely that some acute hepatic insult (e.g. an intercurrent virus infection) releases more copper than can be complexed in the plasma and induces acute copper poisoning with haemolysis, and further liver damage.

Animal models

Attempts to mimic Wilson disease by chronic copper poisoning of laboratory animals are very artifical and unsatisfactory as models for the disease. Recent findings in Bedlington terriers with a recessively inherited disease involving hepatic copper accumulation (Twedt et al, 1979) and progressive liver disease are encouraging, and may allow more rapid progress of our knowledge of Wilson disease.

MENKES SYNDROME

Clinical features

The full clinical syndrome comprises abnormal hair, progressive cerebral degeneration, hypopigmentation, bone changes, arterial rupture and thrombosis, and hypothermia (Danks et al, 1972a).

Premature delivery is very frequent, as is neonatal hyperbilirubinaemia. Hypothermia is common in the neonatal period and even in older babies. At this stage the child's appearance is usually normal with fine normal hair. However, some patients have trichorrhexis nodosa and monilethrix at this age. Neonatal symptoms may resolve and the baby may seem normal during the next two or three months, although growth may be slow. By about three months of age the more flagrant symptoms of developmental delay, loss of early developmental skills and convulsions appear. Cerebral degeneration then dominates the clinical picture with various vascular complications, particularly intracranial, and death occurs between the age of 6 months and 3 years in most cases.

The hair becomes tangled, lustreless and greyish with a stubble of broken hairs palpable over the occiput and temporal regions where the hair rubs on sheets. Pili torti is found microscopically (Figs. 92.1 and 92.2). The facies is quite characteristic with pudgy cheeks and abnormal eyebrows, and is recognisable even in babies who have no hair. Skeletal X–rays show osteoporosis and widening of the flared metaphyses with spiky protrusions at the edges, which may fracture (Kozlowski & McCrossin, 1979). Rib fractures are common. Wormian bones are usually seen in the skull. The combination of these bony changes with a subdural haematoma may lead to the erroneous diagnosis of child abuse. Studies to demonstrate the brain substance (CT scan or air studies) may show macroscopic patches of brain destruction. Arteriograms show elongation, tortuosity and variable calibre of major arteries throughout the brain, viscera and limbs, with areas of localised dilatation and other areas of marked narrowing (Danks et al, 1972a). Emphysema, bladder diverticulae and retinal tears have been described.

One very mildly affected patient has been described who presented at the age of 2 years with mild mental retardation and marked cerebellar ataxia (Procopis et al, 1980). Pili torti was present, bone changes were very mild and arteriography showed generalised elongation and uniform dilatation of arteries. CT scan was normal.

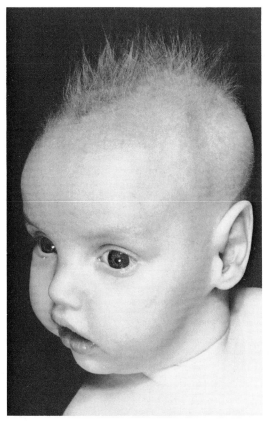

Fig. 92.1 Typical appearance of baby with Menkes syndrome aged 5 months.

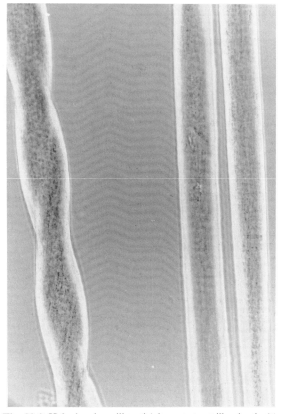

Fig. 92.2 Hair showing pili torti (phase contrast illumination).

Laboratory and cell culture findings

Serum copper and caeruloplasmin levels are very low. Interpretation is complicated by the changing values for these measurements during the first year in normal babies who are born with very little caeruloplasmin (and therefore very low serum copper levels) and achieve adult levels by about 2 years. The rise is rapid in the first weeks and after 2 to 4 weeks the low levels in affected babies are obvious. Real difficulty exists when testing a newborn boy in an affected family. Diagnosis cannot be made with confidence until two weeks (Grover et al, 1979).

Liver content of copper is grossly reduced and duodenal or jejunal biopsy shows greatly increased copper content (Danks et al, 1972b). Oral copper 64 is poorly absorbed; copper 64 given intravenously is cleared from plasma and incorporated into caeruloplasmin quite normally (Lucky & Hsia, 1979). Typical copper measurements are shown in Table 92.4.

Table 92.4 Typical copper measurements in Menkes syndrome at usual age of diagnosis.

	Menkes disease (3–12 months)	Normal (3–12 months)
Serum caeruloplasmin		
OD units per ml	<0.08	>0.25
mg/l	<50	>200
Serum copper μmol/l	<6	>12
Liver copper		
μg/g dry weight	10–20	140–70
Duodenal copper		
μg/g dry weight	50–80	7–29

Disturbances of copper handling in cultured cells comprise the most definitive test for the disease (Camakaris et al, 1980b; Chan et al, 1978; Prins & van den Hamer, 1980). Cells (fibroblastic, amniotic or lymphoid) show increased copper content, increased sensitivity to killing by copper added to culture medium, increased retention of copper 64 added to culture medium for 24 hours, and markedly decreased release of this copper 64 if cells are then grown for a further 24 hours in medium free of isotope. Typical results are shown in Table 92.5. These finding are influenced by the phase of fibroblastic cell growth at the time of testing. Use of confluent cultures which have been held in a non-dividing state by reducing the fetal calf serum in the medium gives most reproducible results in our experience. Special care is needed in prenatal diagnosis using amniotic cells.

Reduced levels of various copper enzyme activities have been demonstrated. Light and electron microscopy show changes in elastin in the aortic wall which are consistent with defective cross-linking (Oakes et al, 1974). Hair keratin analyses show defective disulphide bonding (Danks et al, 1972b).

Diagnosis

Diagnosis can be made with great confidence by the clinical features. Microscopic examination of the hair is very helpful, even in a mild case. Low levels of serum copper and caeruloplasmin will clinch the diagnosis. Assay of copper in gut mucosal or liver biopsies may be used. Studies of cell cultures comprise the ultimate test, showing marked abnormality even in the mild case (Procopis et al, 1980).

Treatment

No form of treatment has yet been shown to be truly effective. Copper has been administered parenterally in a number of different forms – copper sulphate, copper chloride, copper EDTA, copper glycinate, copper histidinate, and copper albumin complex. Copper nitriloacetate is the only form of copper which has proved to be absorbed from the intestine (Grover et al, 1979). All these forms of treatment have corrected the hepatic copper deficiency and restored normal levels of serum copper. Some improvement in physical condition has resulted, but has not prevented fatal outcome or prevented the continuing cerebral degeneration. Restoration of normal brain copper levels has not been achieved (Grover et al, 1979).

It is likely that many of the effects of the disease are

Table 92.5 Findings of Menkes syndrome in cultured cells (fibroblastic or amniotic) used diagnostically in our laboratory (Camakaris et al 1980).

	Normal cells	Menkes cells
Copper content (μg per 10^6 cells)		
in normal medium	0.023 ± 0.013★	0.282 ± 0.091★
with added copper (6 μg per ml)	0.113 ± 0.074★	0.770 ± 0.156★
^{64}Cu content after 24 hours (μg ^{64}Cu per 10^6 cells)	0.004 ± 0.001★	0.060 ± 0.019★
^{64}Cu efflux over subsequent 24 hours in culture (percentage of content at 24 hours)	70–90%	0–5%

★ Standard deviation

already established in utero and that postnatal treatment cannot be fully effective. However, the search should be continued for some chemical form of copper which can bypass the disturbance in copper transport and deliver the copper to the copper enzymes which require it, even in the brain.

Since some of the more serious effects of the disease may be the result of defective catecholamine synthesis, trials of monoamine oxidase inhibitors may be warranted.

Genetics and genetic heterogeneity

Numerous pedigrees show X–linked recessive inheritance, further supported by the mosaic skin depigmentation seen in a Negro heterozygous female (Volpintesta, 1974), and the pili torti seen in some heterozygotes. Mental retardation has been described in one Japanese girl, the sister of a severely affected male (Iwakawa et al, 1979).

Experience in Melbourne in 1966–71 suggested an incidence of 1 in 35 000 (Danks et al, 1972a). Extension to 1980 would modify this figure to 1 in 100 000.

The mildly affected boy described recently (see above) presumably represented an allelic variant.

Heterozygotes may show abnormalities in cultured cells similar to those seen in affected males, but X–chromosome inactivation confounds the situation quite seriously. In fact, only about half of obligate heterozygotes are identified by studies on a single skin biopsy (Camakaris et al, 1980b; Horn, 1980). Use of 2 or 3 biopsies from separate sites improves the diagnostic ability considerably, as does cloning of the fibroblastic cells grown from a biopsy (Horn et al, 1980). Development of a test using hair roots seems desirable. At present one can say that presence of pili torti, of mosaic skin pigmentation or of abnormal cell culture results demonstrate heterozygosity in a female relative, but one cannot exclude heterozygosity with confidence.

Prenatal diagnosis

Any or all of the disturbances of copper metabolism in cultured cells which are described above can be used for prenatal diagnosis. Experience in Melbourne supports the idea of using all four characteristics and taking great care to standardise the cell culture conditions. Copper 64 retention after 24 hours has been used alone by other groups (Horn, 1976), but is particularly susceptible to alteration according to the phase of cell culture and to the copper content of the medium in our experience. Release of copper 64 during a subsequent 24 hours in media without isotope is least affected by culture variables and is the most reliable single test in our laboratory.

Prenatal diagnosis should probably be concentrated in a few laboratories heavily involved with research on cellular copper metabolism until more experience has accumulated.

Pathogenesis

The primary defect causes accumulation of copper in cells in a form unavailable to the sites of copper enzyme synthesis (Danks, 1977; Horn et al, 1978; Prins & van den Hamer, 1980). The precise fault in copper transport within the cells is not yet identified.

Because copper transport is defective in the intestinal mucosa, profound copper deficiency develops. This is aggravated by defective reabsorption of copper from the urinary filtrate. Even that copper which is absorbed is bound up in unavailable sites in many tissues. The effective copper deficiency is much greater than the levels measured in various tissues would suggest.

Before birth copper deficiency is probably less severe (Danks, 1977) but is presumably still present since symptoms are apparent at birth.

The actual clinical features can be explained by failure of the various copper enzymes listed in Table 92.1 and they match up rather closely with the effects of copper deficiency listed in Table 92.2. The absence of anaemia and neutropenia is remarkable and unexplained.

Animal models

The *mottled* mutants in the mouse exhibit disturbances of copper metabolism which are so similar to those of Menkes syndrome that homology of the loci is proposed, especially because both loci are X–chromosomal (Hunt, 1974; Danks, 1977). Of the mottled variants, presumed to be allelic, *brindled* is nearest to typical Menkes syndrome in severity; *blotchy* is less severe. Research on these animals has advanced understanding of the human disease very greatly (Danks, 1977; Prins & van den Hamer, 1980; Hunt & Port, 1979).

Other possible genetic defects of copper metabolism

Since the distribution of copper throughout the body, including absorption and excretion, must involve many separate gene-controlled functions, there must be many genetic diseases of copper transport yet to be discovered. These should be sought among diseases with abnormal hair, with depigmentation, with arterial degeneration and with each of the individual symptoms that are known to occur in copper deficiency (Table 92.2). Other diseases of copper accumulation may also exist.

Liver diseases associated with hepatic copper retention

Since the majority of copper excreted from the body is put out in the bile one might expect that copper retention would be seen secondary to a number of forms of liver disease. This is the case, but the occurrence of copper retention is not as predictable as one might expect. In particular it should be a constant feature of diseases with complete obstruction to bile flow, like extrahepatic biliary atresia. While some patients show gross copper retention others have normal levels of liver copper. The levels of liver copper are very variable in most forms of liver disease with occasional patients showing high levels (Smallwood et al, 1968; Reed et al, 1972). The reason for these differences must be sought in future work which will also need to evaluate the role of copper chelation in the treatment of these patients.

A few forms of liver disease are proving to show a more consistent occurrence of hepatic copper retention, and deserve very careful scrutiny for the possibility that a disturbance of copper transport is basic to the cause of the disease.

Primary biliary cirrhosis has been known to show massive copper accumulation in liver cells for a number of years, but only recently have trials of penicillamine therapy been published (Deering et al, 1977). These have shown quite encouraging results. A rather specific secondary interference with copper excretion is most probable (Sternlieb, 1980) but the possibility of a primary defect in copper transport must not be dismissed. Genetic factors are not established as important in primary biliary cirrhosis.

Indian childhood cirrhosis has recently been shown to be consistently associated with hepatic copper retention (Tanner et al, 1978; Sternlieb, 1980) and as yet no trials of penicillamine therapy or studies of copper transport in cultured cells have been reported. Genetic factors are considered important in the cause of this particular form of childhood liver disease and a primary defect in copper transport is somewhat more likely.

Several patients with different forms of *neonatal cholestatic liver disease* have been shown to accumulate large amounts of copper in the liver (Evans et al, 1978; Smith & Danks, 1978; Kaplinsky et al, 1980). The cases reported are rather heterogeneous in their basic features and more studies will be needed to see whether any particular forms of neonatal liver disease are involved. At present the two particular forms that warrant closest attention are the recessively inherited condition of neonatal cholestatic jaundice and lymphoedema described by Aagenes (1974) and the arterio-ductular hypoplasia syndrome (Alagille et al, 1975). One child with the former syndrome developed extreme hepatic copper accumulation before dying of cirrhosis at the age of five years and had also deposited enough copper in the basal ganglia to produce signs of lenticular degeneration very similar to those in Wilson disease (Smith & Danks, 1978). More patients with this condition should be studied. In arterio-ductular hypoplasia copper retention is frequent, but is perhaps more likely to be secondary. This condition shows autosomal dominant inheritance.

NOTES ADDED IN PROOF

Further studies on our own patients have shown that plasmaphoresis is much more effective than peritoneal dialysis in removing copper during acute haemolytic/liver failure crises in Wilson disease; that monoamine oxidase inhibitors have produced no clinical improvement in two patients with Menkes syndrome even in doses which raised the blood pressure; and that fibroblastic cell cultures from patients with Indian childhood cirrhosis take up and release copper normally.

Walshe (1982) has published extensive experience indicating that triethylene tetramine is as effective as penicillamine in treating Wilson disease and may cause toxic effects less often. Horn (1981) has published data regarding 42 amniotic cell studies in fetuses at risk of Menkes syndrome. Cutis laxa of the X–linked type appears to involve lysyl oxidase deficiency disturbed copper transport in vivo (low serum copper and caeruloplasmin) (Byers et al, 1980) and in vitro (high copper levels in cultured cells) (Kuivaniemi et al, 1982; observations in our own laboratory).

REFERENCES

Åagenaes O 1974 Hereditary recurrent cholestasis with lymphoedema – Two new families. Acta Paediatrica Scandinavica 63: 465–471

Alagille D, Odievre M, Gautier M, Dommergues J P 1975 Hepatic ductular hypoplasia associated with characteristic facies, vertebral malformations, retarded physical, mental and sexual development, and cardiac murmur. Journal of Pediatrics 86: 63–71

Bearn A G 1960 Genetic analysis of Wilson's disease. Annals of Human Genetics 24: 33

Byers P H, Siegel R C, Holbrook K A, Narayanan A S, Bornstein P, Hall J G 1980 X–linked cutis laxa: defective cross-link formation in collagen due to decreased lysyl oxidase activity. New England Journal of Medicine 303: 61–65

Camakaris J, Ackland L, Danks D M 1980a Abnormal copper metabolism in cultured cells from patients with Wilson's disease. Journal of Inherited Metabolic Diseases 3: 155–158

Camakaris J, Danks D M, Ackland L, Cartwright E, Borger P, Cotton R G H, 1980b Altered copper metabolism in cultured cells from human Menkes' syndrome and mottled mouse mutants. Biochemical Genetics 18: 117–131

Canelas H M, Carvalho N, Scaff M, Vitule A, Barbosa E R, Azevedo E M 1978 Osteoarthropathy of hepatolenticular degeneration. Acta Neurologica Scandinavica 57: 481–487

Cartwright G E 1978 Diagnosis of treatable Wilson's disease. New England Journal of Medicine 298: 1347–1350

Chan W Y, Cushing W, Cofeman M A, Rennert O M 1980 Genetic expression of Wilson's disease in cell culture: a diagnostic marker. Science 208: 299–300

Chan W Y, Garnica A D, Rennert O M 1978 Cell culture

studies of Menkes' kinky hair disease. Clinica Chimica Acta 88L 495–507

Cumings J N 1948 The copper and iron content of brain and liver in the normal and in hepato-lenticular degeneration. Brain 71: 410–415

Danks D M 1977 Copper transport and utilisation in Menkes' syndrome and in mottled mice. Inorganic Perspectives in Biology and Medicine 1: 73–100

Danks D M 1980 Copper deficiency in humans. Excerpta Medica Amsterdam (Ciba Symposium 79) 209–220

Danks D M, Campbell P E, Stevens B J, Mayne V, Cartwright E 1972a Menkes' kinky hair syndrome: an inherited defect in copper absorption with widespread effects. Pediatrics 50: 188–201

Danks D M, Stevens B J, Campbell P E, Gillespie J M, Walker-Smith J, Blomfield J, Turner B 1972b Menkes' kinky-hair syndrome. Lancet i: 1100–1103

Deering T B, Dickson E R, Fleming C R, Geall M G, McCall J T, Baggenstoss A H 1977 Effects of D-penicillamine on copper retention in patients with primary biliary cirrhosis. Gastroenterology 72: 1208–1212

Dobyns W B, Goldstein N P, Gordon H 1979 Clinical spectrum of Wilson's disease (Hepatolenticular degeneration). Mayo Clinic Proceedings 54: 35–42

Editorial 1978 British Medical Journal 1384–1385

Edwards C Q, Williams D M, Cartwright G E 1979 Hereditary hypoceruloplasminemia. Clinical Genetics 15: 311–316

Evans G W 1973 Copper homeostasis in the mammalian system. Physiological Reviews 53: 535–570

Evans J, Newman S, Sherlock S 1978 Liver copper levels in intrahepatic cholestasis of childhood. Gastroenterology 75: 875–878

Fitzgerald M A, Gross J B, Goldstein N P, Wahner H W, McCall J T 1975 Wilson's disease (hepato-lenticular degeneration) of late adult onset. Mayo Clinic Proceedings 50: 438–442

Frieden E 1980 Caeruloplasmin: a multi-functional metallo protein of vertebrate plasma. Excerpta Medica Amsterdam (Ciba Symposium 79)

Goka T J, Stevenson R E, Hefferan P M, Howell R R 1976 Menkes' disease: a biochemical abnormality in cultured human fibroblasts. Proceedings of the National Academy of Sciences USA 73: 604–606

Goldfischer S, Sternlieb I 1968 Changes in the distribution of hepatic copper in relation to the progression of Wilson's disease (hepatolenticular degeneration). American Journal of Pathology 53: 883–894

Golding D N, Walshe J M 1977 Arthropathy of Wilson's disease: study of clinical and radiological features in 32 cases. Annals of Rheumatic Disease 36: 99–111

Grover W D, Johnson W C, Henkin R I 1979 Clinical and biochemical aspects of trichopoliodystrophy. Annals of Neurology 5: 65–71

Hamlyn A N, Gollan J L, Douglas A P, Sherlock S 1977 Fulminant Wilson's disease with haemolysis and renal failure: copper studies and assessment of dialysis regimens. British Medical Journal 2: 660–663

Hoagland H C, Goldstein N P 1978 Hematologic (cytopenic) manifestations of Wilson's disease (Hepatolenticular degeneration). Mayo Clinic Proceedings 53: 498–500

Hoogenraad T U, Van den Hamer C J A, Koevoet R, de Ruyter Korver E G W M 1978 Oral zinc in Wilson's disease. Lancet ii: 1262

Horn N 1976 Copper incorporation studies on cultured cells for prenatal diagnosis of Menkes' disease. Lancet i: 1156–1158

Horn N 1980 Menkes X–linked disease: heterozygous phenotypic uncloned fibroblast cultures. Journal of Medical Genetics 17: 257–761

Horn N 1981 Menkes X–linked disease: prenatal diagnosis of hemizygous males and heterozygous females. Prenatal Diagnosis 1: 107–120

Horn N, Mooy P, McGuire V M 1980 Menkes' X–linked disease: two clonal cell populations in heterozygotes. Journal of Medical Genetics 17: 262–266

Hunt D M 1974 Primary defect in copper transport underlies mottled mutants in the mouse. Nature 249: 852–854

Hunt D M, Port A E 1979 Trace element binding in the copper deficient mottled mutants of the mouse. Life Sciences 24: 1453–61

Iser J H, Stevens B J, Stening G F, Hurley T H, Smallwood R A 1974 Hemolytic anemia of Wilson's disease. Gastroenterology 67: 290–293

Iwakawa Y, Niwa T, Tomita M et al. 1979 Menkes' kinky hair syndrome: report on an autopsy case and his female sibling with similar clinical manifestations. Brain Development (Tokyo) 11: 260–266

Kaplinsky C, Sternlieb I, Javitt N, Rotem Y 1980 Familial cholestatic cirrhosis associated with Kayser-Fleischer rings. Pediatrics 65: 782–788

Kozlowski K, McCrossin R 1979 Early osseous abnormalities in Menkes' kinky-hair syndrome. Pediatric Radiology 8: 191–194

Kuivaniemi H, Peltonen L, Palotie A, Kaitila I, Kivirikko K I 1982 Abnormal copper metabolism and deficient lysyl oxidase activity in a heritable connective tissue disorder. Journal of Clinical Investigation 69: 730–733

Linares A, Zarranz J J, Rodriguez-Alarcon J, Diaz-Perez J L 1979 Reversible cutis laxa due to maternal D-penicillamine treatment. Lancet ii: 43

Lucky A W, Hsia Y E 1980 Distribution of ingested and injected radiocopper in two patients with Menkes' kinky-hair disease. Pediatric Research 13: 1280–1284

Lyle W H 1978 Penicillamine in pregnancy. Lancet i: 606–607

Mason K E 1979 A conspectus of research on copper metabolism and requirements in man. Journal of Nutrition 109: 1979–2066

Menkes J H, Alter M, Steigleder G K, Weakley D R, Sung J H 1962 A sex-linked recessive disorder with retardation of growth, peculiar hair and focal cerebral and cerebellar degeneration. Pediatrics 29: 764–779

Mjølnerød O K, Rasmussen K, Dommerud S A, Gjeruldsen S T 1971 Congenital connective-tissue defect probably due to D-penicillamine treatment in pregnancy. Lancet i: 673–675

Nelson R F, Guzman D A, Grahovac Z, Howse D C N 1979 Computerized cranial tomography in Wilson's disease. Neurology 29: 866–868

Oakes B W, Danks D M, Campbell P E 1976 Human copper deficiency: ultrastructural studies of the aorta and skin in a child with Menkes' syndrome. Experimental and Molecular Pathology 25: 82–98

Odievre M, Vedrenne J, Landrieu P, Alagille D 1974 Les formes hepatiques 'pures' de la maladie de Wilson chez l'enfant: à propos de dix observations. Archives Francais de Pediatrie 31: 215–222

Prins H W, Van den Hamer C J A 1980 Abnormal copper-thionein synthesis and impaired copper utilisation in mutated brindled mice: model for Menkes' disease. The Journal of Nutrition 110: 151–157

Reed G B, Butt E M, Landing B H 1972 Copper in childhood

liver disease: A histologic, histochemical and chemical survey. Archives of Pathology 93: 249–255

Sass-Kortsak A 1975 Wilson's disease: a treatable cause of liver disease in children. Pediatric Clinics of North America 22: 963–984

Scott J, Gollan J L, Samourian S, Sherlock S 1978 Wilson's disease, presenting as chronic active hepatitis. Gastroenterology 74: 645–651

Smallwood R A, Williams H A, Rosenoer V M, Sherlock S 1968 Liver copper levels in liver disease: studies using neutron activation analysis. Lancet ii: 1310–1313

Smith A L, Danks D M 1978 Secondary copper accumulation with neurological damage in child with chronic liver disease. British Medical Journal 2: 1400–1401

Sternlieb I 1978 Diagnosis of Wilson's disease. Gastroenterology 74: 787–789

Sternlieb I, Scheinberg I H 1979 The role of radiocopper in the diagnosis of Wilson's disease. Gastroenterology 77: 138–142

Sternlieb I 1980 Copper and the liver. Gastroenterology 78: 1615–1628

Strickland G T, Frommer D, Leu M-L, Pollard R, Sherlock S, Cumings J N 1973 Wilson's disease in the United Kingdom and Taiwan. Quarterly Journal of Medicine XLII: 619–38

Sunderman P W, Hohnadel P C, Evenson M A, Wannamaker B B, Dahl B S 1974 Excretion of copper in sweat of patients with Wilson's disease during sauna bathing. Annals of Clinical Laboratory Science 74: 407–412

Tanner M S, Portmann B, Mowat A P, Williams R, Pandit A N, Mills C F et al. 1979 Increased hepatic copper concentration in Indian childhood cirrhosis. Lancet ii: 4524–4526

Twedt D C, Sternlieb I, Gilbertson D U M 1979 Clinical morphologic and chemical studies on copper toxicosis of Bedlington terriers. Journal of American Veterinary Association 175: 269–275

Underwood E J 1977 Trace Elements in Human and Animal Nutrition 4th edn. Academic Press, New York

Vierling J M, Shrager M A, Rumble W F, Aamodt R, Berman M D, Jones E A 1978 Incorporation of radiocopper into ceruloplasmin in normal subjects and in patients with primary biliary cirrhosis and Wilson's disease. Gastroenterology 74: 652–660

Volpintesta E J 1974 Menkes' kinky hair syndrome in a black infant. American Journal of Diseases of Children 128: 244–246

Walshe J M 1977 Pregnancy in Wilson's disease. Quarterly Journal of Medicine XLVI: 73–83

Walshe J M 1982 Treatment of Wilson's disease with trientine (triethylene tetramine). Lancet i: 643–648

Werlin S L, Grand R J, Perman J A, Watkins J B 1978 Diagnostic dilemmas of Wilson's disease: diagnosis and treatment. Pediatrics 62: 47–51

Westmoreland B F, Goldstein N P, Klass D W 1974 Wilson's disease: electroencephalographic and evoked potential studies. Mayo Clinic Proceedings 49: 401–404

Wiebers D O, Hollenhorst R W, Goldstein N P 1977 The ophthalmologic manifestation of Wilson's disease. Mayo Clinic Proceedings 52: 409–416

Wiebers D O, Wilson D M, McLeod R A, Goldstein N P 1979 Renal stones in Wilson's disease. American Journal of Medicine 67: 249–254

93

Disorders of iron metabolism: idiopathic haemochromatosis and atransferrinaemia

M. Simon

There are many inherited disorders of iron metabolism. Most of them – notably those associated with the haemoglobinopathies, with certain anaemias and with the porphyrias – are dealt with in other chapters of this book. In this chapter we shall be concerned with a relatively common disease, idiopathic haemochromatosis, and a very rare disease, congenital atransferrinaemia. Possible relations between idiopathic haemochromatosis and refractory idiopathic sideroblastic anaemia will also be touched on.

IDIOPATHIC HAEMOCHROMATOSIS

Definition

Idiopathic haemochromatosis, a condition involving and probably arising from an iron overload state affecting several organs, is a hereditary disease transmitted as an autosomal recessive trait and is controlled by a gene situated on the sixth chromosome near to the A-locus of the HLA system. Fibrosis of certain organs, particularly the liver, should no longer be included in the definition of the disease, since ideally the diagnosis should be established before the onset of fibrosis. Haemochromatosis was first described by Trousseau in 1865 and given its present name following the studies of Von Recklinghausen in 1889.

Classification of the different forms of haemochromatosis

Idiopathic haemochromatosis is the 'prototype' of iron overload diseases. A number of variants exist, so much so that for a time it was questioned (MacDonald, 1964) whether in fact the original disease was an entity distinct from these variants. The following classification is proposed (Simon et al, 1980a):

A. Familial idiopathic haemochromatosis
B. Secondary forms of haemochromatosis
1. Associated with anaemia
   a. aplastic anaemia in which the iron overload is due to excessive oral intake of iron and especially multiple transfusions performed to correct the anaemia;

   b. haemolytic anaemia, such as congenital spherocytosis, with generally minimal iron overload;
   c. anaemia with increased but ineffective erythropoiesis involving increased iron absorption and requiring transfusions, such as sideroblastic anaemia, pyridoxine-responsive or not, and especially thalassaemia, which is in all probability the major cause of severe iron overload and in which the elevated iron stores are the chief cause of mortality;
2. Associated with cirrhosis.
   a. uncomplicated cirrhosis, particularly that which is secondary to alcohol abuse
   b. cirrhosis treated by portacaval shunt surgery
3. Due to dietary factors, notably the consumption of iron-rich beverages (Bantu siderosis)
4. Due to oral or parenteral iron therapy in haemodialysed patients
5. Due to other causes, notably
   a. porphyria cutanea tarda, in which iron overloading is a mild and not constant feature
   b. congenital atransferrinaemia.

Transfusional iron overload states are not considered by certain investigators (Powell et al, 1980) under the heading of haemochromatosis, since they involve mainly the reticuloendothelial system rather than parenchymal tissue and do not cause marked tissue damage.

Many of the secondary iron overload states listed above are associated with inherited conditions dealt with elsewhere in this book.

Clinical features of idiopathic haemochromatosis

Organic and metabolic manifestations
Skin pigmentation is pronounced, often grey but sometimes brown, is diffuse but affects mainly exposed areas of skin. Mucosal pigmentation may be seen, with slate-grey patches in the mouth. About half the patients show cutaneous atrophy, ichthyosiform changes and flattening of the nails or true spoon nail (Chevrant-Breton et al, 1977). Loss of body hair is common.

In advanced forms of the disease pronounced hepatomegaly is a constant finding. The liver is firm, portal hypertension is rare and liver tests may be normal or show a slight elevation in serum transaminases and a fall in sulphobromophthalein excretion.

Glucose tolerance is commonly decreased and diabetes mellitus, mainly of the insulin-dependent type, used to be seen in about 60% of cases (Dymock et al, 1972; Simon et al, 1973a). This diabetes is partly a consequence of the pancreatic and hepatic lesions. Some investigators maintain that it arises through the same genetic mechanism underlying common diabetes (Balcerzack et al, 1966; Saddi & Feingold, 1974), but others consider that such a mechanism may play only a minor role in the diabetes of haemochromatosis patients (Stocks & Powell; Simon et al, 1978; Simon & Bourel, 1979a).

Hypogonadism is the main endocrine abnormality and can be attributed, on the basis of a reduced response to luteinizing hormone releasing hormone (LHRH) or the Clomiphene stimulation test, to gonadotrophin deficiency (Tourniaire et al, 1974; Guillon et al, 1975; Walsh et al, 1976). Abnormalities of other pituitary functions or of adrenal or thyroid glands are rare and generally mild. A few cases of hypoparathyroidism have been described. Plasma parathyroid hormone concentration is often slightly increased (Pawlotsky et al, 1975).

Heart disease is most commonly revealed by electrocardiographic abnormalities consisting of a decrease in QRS amplitude and T-wave flattening or inversion. Myocardial disease is seen clinically in 15 to 20% of cases and produces congestive heart failure and/or arrhythmias such as atrial fibrillation or even ventricular tachycardia or fibrillation (Mattheyses et al, 1978).

Bone demineralization is common (Delbarre, 1960) and one half to two thirds of patients suffer from joint disease (Schumacher, 1964). This takes the form either of attacks of pseudogout, or more often a moderate chronic rheumatic disease affecting mainly the metacarpophalangeal joints of the second and third fingers and the hips. Radiography shows chondrocalcinosis, especially to the knees, and/or appearances of subchondral joint disease, particularly of the metacarpophalangeal joints. Many joints may be affected.

Other manifestations of the disease include: easy fatigability, abdominal pain, increased pancreatic and or biliary secretion in response to secretin stimulation, vitamin A and C deficiency.

Biochemical and histological tests of iron overload

Tests of iron overload were recently reviewed by Brissot et al (1981). Serum iron is elevated, usually above 36 μmol/l (200 μg/100 ml). Concentrations above 28.5 μmol/l (160 μg/100 ml) are suggestive of haemochromatosis. Transferrin saturation is at or near 100%.

The intravenous or intramuscular injection of one gramme or more of desferrioxamine provokes a marked increase in urinary iron excretion, exceeding 27 μmol (1500 μg) per 24 hours in females and 36 μmol (2000 μg) per 24 hours in males, but in actual practice often exceeding 180 μmol (10000 μg) per 24 hours. Serum ferritin measured by immunoradiometric assay (Addison et al, 1972) exceeds 200 μg/l in females and 300 μg/l in males (Worwood, 1979), and levels above 2000 μg/l are not uncommon.

These tests can give false-positive results in the presence of hepatic cytolysis or of haemolysis. The desferrioxamine test can give false-negative results in cases of vitamin C deficiency. Inflammation lowers serum iron and raises serum ferritin.

Histological examination of a liver biopsy specimen reveals marked iron deposition in hepatocytes and Kupffer cells. Evidence of fibrosis and, in advanced cases, of cirrhosis is also seen. Hepatic iron concentration measured biochemically (Barry & Sherlock, 1971) is proportional to total body iron: normally it does not exceed 3.6 μmol (200 μg)/100 mg dry weight but it may reach 90 μmol (5000 μg)/100 mg in patients with haemochromatosis.

HLA associations

The finding of an association with certain HLA antigens, notably HLA-A3, B7 and B14, is indicative of a genetic component in idiopathic haemochromatosis (Simon et al, 1975; Simon et al, 1976a). However, these antigens are clearly not specific and are absent in a quarter of haemochromatosis patients.

Overall picture, natural history and treatment

Major manifestations of the disease are found in 8 or 9 cases out of 10 in men, who also exhibit earlier onset of the disease – usually around the forties – than women. Mortality may ensue through heart failure or carcinoma of the liver, which may develop, once cirrhosis has set in, even after correction of iron overload. Hence the need for early detection of mild cases with only skin hyperpigmentation and hepatic involvement without cirrhosis, or of still latent or subclinical cases detected by family studies. In clinically mild cases complete cure is possible; in latent cases, the disease can be prevented altogether.

Treatment consists essentially of weekly phlebotomies removing 400 to 500 ml of blood at each session until excess iron is removed. Further phlebotomy sessions are done at less frequent intervals to prevent subsequent iron build-up. A response to phlebotomy is seen in the patient's general state of health, skin changes, liver abnormalities and sometimes also the heart condition. Other aspects of the disease show little or no response. Survival is greatly increased (Bomford & Williams, 1976).

Pathogenesis of idiopathic haemochromatosis

The extremes of the idiopathic haemochromatosis spectrum are now well documented: at one end, the allele responsible for the disease, and at the other, its expression as clinical and biochemical features. Between these two extremes there is much variation which has been the subject of considerable speculation.

Does iron deposition play a part in the pathogenesis of idiopathic haemochromatosis ?

The degree of iron overload in an organ does not always correspond exactly to the severity of tissue damage. Nevertheless, there are sound arguments in favour of the pathogenic role of iron: 1) Parenchymal iron overload states in man, whatever the cause, are associated with similar clinical features; 2) Phlebotomy therapy improves the clinical picture and prolongs survival in advanced cases (Powell, 1970; Bomford & Williams, 1976) and, as far as can be judged at present, cures or prevents the disease in mild or latent cases respectively; 3) Removal of excess iron by phlebotomy totally restores to normal certain biochemically measurable factors, such as excess biliary or pancreatic secretion following secretin stimulation (Simon et al, 1973) or ascorbic acid deficiency (Brissot et al, 1978); 4) In a recent study (Awai et al, 1979), the administration of nitrilotriacetate iron to rabbits and rats produced iron overloading of the liver and pancreas, and diabetes, which resolved after phlebotomy therapy.

As for the mechanism of tissue damage, recent hypotheses invoke the rupture of overloaded lysosomes (Peters et al, 1977) and the action of free radicals (Aisen et al, 1977). So far, though, little is known about this.

Hypotheses to explain the basic disorder of iron metabolism

An abnormality of iron absorption and/or storage can be assumed to be present. This occurs in at least two sites: the intestinal mucosa and the liver. Biopsy specimens of intestinal mucosa removed from haemochromatosis patients have been found to take up more iron than specimens from normal individuals (Cox & Peters, 1978). Iron administered to haemochromatosis patients was found to be deposited in the liver – even after removal of excess iron and in iron deficiency states – before being used for erythropoiesis (Pollycove et al, 1971; Batey et al, 1978).

Defective production of ferritin by intestinal cells has been postulated by Crosby (1963). It is true that in patients with idiopathic haemochromatosis the concentration of ferritin in the intestinal mucosa is comparatively low. However, it is also low in patients with secondary haemochromatosis and it increases with iron administration (Halliday et al, 1978). Liver ferritin synthesis is not altered in the early stages of idiopathic haemochromatosis (Beaumont et al, 1980).

The possibility of a reticuloendothelial disorder being involved has its proponents. Astaldi et al (1966) and Cat-

tan et al (1967) have noted an abnormally low concentration and abnormal distribution of iron in villous macrophages. The findings of certain iron kinetic studies have been taken to indicate an iron storage deficiency of the reticuloendothelial system in haemochromatosis patients (Fillet, 1977), but these findings have not been confirmed by other investigators (Stefanelli et al, 1980).

Essentially, what is required is to find the abnormal gene product and therefore the basic cause of the disorder.

Genetics

The genetics of haemochromatosis has been the subject of several recent reviews (Simon et al, 1980a; Simon et al, 1981).

Historical background

Sheldon's inborn error of metabolism theory, postulated in 1935, was widely disputed right up to the sixties (MacDonald, 1964). A number of successive observations, however, gradually lent weight to the view of the disease being an inherited trait: iron absorption was found to be increased among certain relatives of idiopathic haemochromatosis patients; instances of familial occurrence of haemochromatosis were reported, and major disturbances in biochemical body iron parameters were seen among relatives of patients with idiopathic haemochromatosis but not among those of patients with haemochromatosis secondary to alcoholic liver disease; the eating habits of haemochromatosis patients were found to differ little or not at all from those of control subjects.

Every conceivable mode of inheritance has been advanced. While the arguments in favour of an autosomal recessive trait have gradually gained strength, up till quite recently they were far from achieving universal acceptance. What clinched the matter and finally proved the hereditary nature of the disease and its recessive mode of transmission was the discovery of an association with certain HLA antigens (Simon et al, 1975; Simon et al, 1977a).

Proof of recessive inheritance

Phenotype studies

Williams et al (1962) observed that the most pronounced forms of iron overload, measured in liver biopsy specimens, occurred in the proband generation. Walsh et al (1964) reported abnormal iron overload tests in 25% of sibs but much more rarely among parents and offspring. Saddi and Feingold (1974) noted identical unsaturated transferrin levels among parents and offspring of haemochromatosis patients, these levels being midway between those found in probands, at one extreme, and in control subjects, at the other. Moreover, abnormally high urinary iron excretion after desferrioxamine was seen in certain sibs but not in members of other generations. In this study, segregation analysis was consistent with a recessive mode of transmission.

Recessive inheritance was established statistically by Simon et al (1977b) in a study of 97 families. They separated out minor cases (i.e. those with little or no clinical evidence of disease, increased serum iron and transferrin saturation, and iron excretion following desferrioxamine increased but remaining below 4000 μg (72 μmol)/24 hr) from major cases. They then compared the distribution of each of these two categories among sibs and offspring using the same age groups in each generation for comparison (Table 93.1). The major cases, assumed to correspond to the homozygous state, were significantly more common among sibs – a finding consistent with a recessive mode of transmission. When, on the other hand, the major and minor cases were taken together, assuming they corresponded to different degrees of expression of an allele in the heterozygous state, these were also significantly more common among the sibs, a finding which is incompatible with a dominant mode of transmission, which would have given an equal frequency in the two generations.

Genotype studies

1. Association of haemochromatosis with HLA antigens. An association of idiopathic haemochromatosis with certain HLA-A and B locus antigens was first suggested in 1975 in a study of 20 cases (Simon et al, 1975) and then demonstrated in the series extended to 51 cases (Simon et al, 1976a). Since then, this association has been the subject of numerous reports (summarized in Table 93.2). An excess of HLA-A3 is found consistently, this antigen being present in around 70 to 75% of patients compared with around 25% of normal controls. B7 is also increased in frequency, but less so and with greater variability from one series to another. B14 was found to be very significantly increased in some series but not in others.

Up to now, no C-locus antigen defined to date has shown an excess in haemochromatosis patients (Fauchet

et al, 1977; Lloyd et al, 1978). An excess, although not reaching significance, has been found for an as yet poorly defined antigen, DRw6, and for Dw6 (Fauchet et al, 1979), as well as for the properdin BfF allele (Fauchet et al, 1980b).

2. Family studies. Figure 93.1 illustrates that if a haemochromatosis locus exists and is closely linked to the HLA complex, the disease producing allele will be in haplotype association with particular HLA alleles. In accordance with recessive inheritance, affected sibs should have the same two HLA haplotypes as the proband, that is, they should be HLA-identical to the proband. This was in fact the case in the first family studies reported by Simon et al in 1976(b) and was confirmed statistically very soon afterwards (Simon et al, 1977a). Subsequent reports have all corroborated these early studies (Lipinski et al, 1978; Lloyd et al, 1978; Basset et al, 1979). The frequency of diseased sibs HLA-identical to their probands is very significantly higher than would be expected both by chance in the absence of linkage, and in the case of dominant inheritance with linkage (Simon et al, 1981). This proves that the haemochromatosis locus is linked to the HLA complex and points conclusively to a recessive mode of transmission for the disease.

3. Studies of unrelated subjects. These studies were based on the supposition that an HLA allele, HLA-A3 as it turns out, in frequent haplotype association with the haemochromatosis allele would be distributed differently among haemochromatosis patients, depending on whether the haemochromatosis allele itself had to be present in the homozygous or heterozygous state to produce the disease. These studies very soon provided evidence of a recessive mode of inheritance (Simon et al, 1977a; Simon et al, 1977b), confirmed by applying the formulae proposed by Thomson and Bodmer (1977) to currently available data (Table 93.3).

4. Exceptions to the general rule are seen, such as diseased sibs who are only half-HLA-identical to the proband or, exceptionally, HLA-nonidentical. Pseudodominant inheritance from one generation to the

Table 93.1 Frequencies of iron overload: comparison between generations II and III by similar age groups. (From Simon et al, Clinical Genetics, 1977 11: 327–341 and published with permission)

| Age group | Generation | Iron overload | | | Comparison between generations for frequencies of | |
		major	minor	absent	major overloads: recessive hypothesis	major + minor overloads: dominant hypothesis
25–45 years	II	13	9	61	$P = 0.0007$	$P = 0.032$
	III	0	7	50		
30–40 years	II	6	4	30	$P = 0.035$	$P = 0.017$
	III	0	1	27		

P = exact Fisher's probability (one-tailed).

Table 93.2 HLA antigens in unrelated patients with idiopathic haemochromatosis.

Authors	Country	Number of unrelated patients	A3 Patients n	A3 Patients %	A3 Controls %	A3 pc <	B14 Patients n	B14 Patients %	B14 Controls %	B14 pc <	B7 Patients n	B7 Patients %	B7 Controls %	B7 pc <
Walters et al (1975)	Ireland	7	7	100			1				6	86	21	
Shewan et al (1976)	Scotland	6	5	83			1				5	83		
Bomford et al (1977)	England	35	24	69	31	15×10^{-3}	7	20	6	NS	12	34	20	NS
Morris et al (1977)	Australia	10	6	60	20		2	20	7		5	50	21	
Henke et al (1978)	Germany	11	6	55			0	0			5	45		
Laukens et al (1978)	Belgium	12	10	83	25	10^{-2}	0	0	7.5		8	75	15	10^{-3}
Lipinski et al (1978)	France	48	36	75	26	10^{-8}	11	23	9	5×10^{-2}	18	38	19	5×10^{-2}
Dirska et al (1978)	Germany	22	16	73	30	5×10^{-3}	0	0	5	NS	10	45	19	NS
Kuhnl et al (1978)	Germany	35	26	74	21	10^{-4}	1	3	6	NS	21	60	22	10^{-4}
McCarthy et al (1979)	Ireland	20	12	60	24	3×10^{-2}	4	20	12.6	NS	12	60	27	10^{-5}
Powell et al (1979)	Australia	78	56	72	22	10^{-8}	7	9	9	NS	46	59	24	10^{-5}
Valberg (1980)	Canada	23	13	57	25	10^{-3}	5	22	8	7×10^{-2}	14	61	22	10^{-4}
Ritter et al (1980)	Sweden	40	27	68	32	10^{-4}	10	25	2.4	10^{-3}	14	35	28	NS
Simon et al (1980)	Brittany	258	188	73	28	10^{-10}	76	29	10	10^{-10}	109	42	26	10^{-4}
Total		605	432	71.4			125	20.7			285	47.1		

n: number of patients   pc: p value multiplied by the number of antigens tested

From Simon et al, In: HLA in Endocrine and Metabolic Disorders. Farid N (ed) Academic Press, New York, 1981 and published with permission

Table 93.3 258 unrelated haemochromatosis patients broken down into A3 homozygous, A3 heterozygous, or lacking A3. From Simon et al, In: HLA in Endocrine and Metabolic Disorders. Farid N (ed) Academic Press, New York, 1981 and published with permission

	A3 homozygotes	A3 heterozygotes	non-A3 patients
Expected numbers for dominant inheritance:	26.8	161.2	70
for recessive inheritance:	59.2	128.8	70
Observed numbers:	63	125	70

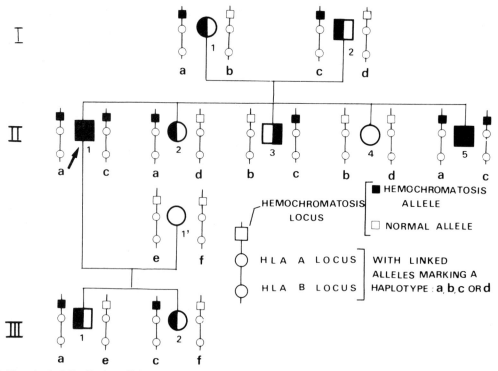

Fig. 93.1 Hypothetical distribution of haemochromatosis alleles, each in combination with a particular HLA haplotype, among relatives of a patient with idiopathic haemochromatosis (person II-I). The topographic relations between the presumed haemochromatosis locus and the HLA loci are diagrammatic approximations.
■ homozygous male; ◐ heterozygous female; ○ 'gene free' female.
Reprinted by permission of the New England Journal of Medicine 301: 169–174 (1979).

next has also been observed. Such exceptions can be explained by genetic recombination between the haemochromatosis allele and the marker HLA haplotype – a rare event because of their close linkage– and, more commonly, by homozygous-heterozygous matings (Simon et al, 1979; Simon et al, 1980b). Figure 93.2 illustrates such a mating: the proband (II 1) is the daughter of a patient who died from haemochromatosis (I 2). She inherited a second allele, linked to the HLA-A3, B14 haplotype, from her mother, who in fact showed signs of mild iron overload. These exceptions, once elucidated, are entirely consistent with recessive inheritance.

Relationship between idiopathic haemochromatosis and other conditions in the light of HLA data

Haemochromatosis and insulin-dependent diabetes. As mentioned above, the possibility has been raised that the genetic mechanism postulated for common diabetes might be involved in the pathogenesis of the diabetes associated with haemochromatosis. In a study of 155 haemochromatosis patients the frequency of the HLA antigens alleged to be 'markers' of a genetic background unfavourable (in the case of B7) or favourable (in the case

of B8, B15, B18, Cw3, Dw3, Dw4, DR3 and DR4) to the onset of common insulin-dependent diabetes differed little according to whether the patients had overt diabetes, reduced glucose tolerance, or normal glucose tolerance (Simon et al, 1978). This seems to weaken the case for common insulin-dependent diabetes being related to the diabetes of haemochromatosis.

Idiopathic haemochromatosis and haemochromatosis secondary to alcoholism. HLA markers related to idiopathic haemochromatosis are not increased in cases of haemochromatosis classed, according to the findings of dietary surveys and clinical and biochemical studies, under the heading of haemochromatosis due to alcoholic liver disease (Simon et al, 1977c). In this form of haemochromatosis, which involves only mild iron overload, the frequency of related HLA markers is well below that found with homozygosity for idiopathic haemochromatosis and does not even attain the level associated with heterozygosity for idiopathic haemochromatosis. However, this does not rule out the possibility of alcoholism contributing to expression of the heterozygous state.

Idiopathic haemochromatosis and idiopathic refractory sideroblastic anaemia. Cartwright et al (1980) have reported that five out of seven individuals they examined

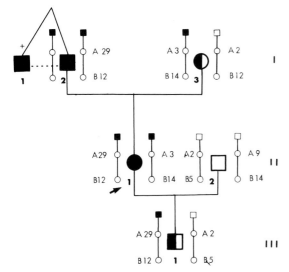

Fig. 93.2 A family with pseudo-dominant transmission. (From Simon et al, Nouv Presse Méd, 1979, 8: 421–424 and published with permission)

who had this type of anaemia were carriers of the HLA-A3 antigen and that in two families sideroblastic anaemia was found to coexist with idiopathic haemochromatosis, at least in the putative heterozygous state. They postulated heterozygosity for haemochromatosis not only as a cause of the iron overload state in these anaemias but also of the anaemia itself. As the proponents of this interesting hypothesis admit, it remains to be proved.

HLA antigens and iron overload in haemodialysed patients. Bregman et al (1980) have reported a high prevalence of the 'haemochromatosis alleles' A3, B7 and B14, taken together, in patients on maintenance haemodialysis. This finding needs confirmation.

Other considerations concerning the haemochromatosis allele

How many linked genes code for haemochromatosis: one or two? A two gene hypothesis has been advanced (Bomford et al, 1977; Eddleston &Williams, 1978). According to this hypothesis one gene, in haplotype association with HLA-A3, is responsible for increased plasma to storage iron exchange and is not expressed biochemically. The other is responsible for increased iron absorption and is expressed by elevated serum iron levels. A study of HLA markers and biochemical expression in 247 heterozygotes (Simon et al, 1980c) produced no evidence to support this hypothesis but pointed fairly convincingly to the existence of a single gene.

Where is the haemochromatosis gene located? Several linkage studies (Simon et al, 1977a; Lipinski et al, 1978; Cartwright et al, 1979; Kidd, 1979; Fauchet et al, 1980a) suggest with a very high probability that the haemochromatosis locus is situated on the sixth chromosome

less than one centimorgan from the A-locus of the HLA complex. Whether the haemochromatosis locus is on the same side of the A-locus as the B-locus or on the opposite side, which is more likely, has not been determined (Simon et al, 1980a).

Present knowledge of HLA markers and the haemochromatosis allele. There are two HLA haplotypes that occur preferentially in combination with the haemochromatosis allele. These are A3, B7 and A3, B14. From the data in Table 93.2 these two haplotypes are seen to be unevenly distributed throughout the world. Certain haplotypes may be preferentially found in certain areas, such as A11, B35, which is common in a particular areas of Brittany. Current data on the association between HLA markers and the haemochromatosis allele in the populations studied so far are consistent with origin of the disease through a single mutational event, the differentiation of associated HLA haplotypes having occurred through recombination between the haemochromatosis locus and the HLA complex, and within the HLA complex itself. This is only one of many possible hypotheses (Simon et al, 1980a; Simon et al, 1981).

Phenotypic expression of the haemochromatosis allele. In homozygotes, phenotypic expression is almost constant and most often pronounced in males, it is less frequent and usually moderate in females. At the present time there is no known test specific for the heterozygous state. Biochemical tests for iron overload are abnormal in 20% (Beaumont et al, 1979; Simon et al, 1980c) to 30% (Cartwright et al, 1979) of heterozygotes. The greatest deviations from normal are found (with varying frequency depending probably on local environmental circumstances) for serum ferritin (Beaumont et al, 1979) or serum iron and percent transferrin saturation (Cartwright et al, 1979).

Detection and prevention

In certain parts of the world where the disease is common, mass screening, by including serum iron determination in routine health check-ups, would be justified. Elsewhere, cases could only be traced through family studies. A comparison has been made between serum ferritin measurement and HLA typing to determine which would be the better for this purpose (Basset et al, 1979). In fact, genotype studies – which have proved extremely important – and phenotype studies are not mutually exclusive but rather complementary and together would offer maximum efficacy without increasing the overall cost: HLA typing determines the risk, whereas phenotypic tests detect the physical realization of that risk, and need not be repeated in low risk relatives. Conversely, if phenotypic tests reveal frank haemochromatosis in a theoretically low-risk individual, they are valuable in pointing to the presence of a possible 'new' haemochromatosis allele marker which could then be used to determine the risk to other members of the same family.

In a typical family (Fig. 93.1), an HLA-identical sib is homozygous, a half-HLA-identical sib heterozygous, and a non-HLA-identical sib would carry no disease allele. In the rare case – especially rare where the disease itself is uncommon – of a third disease allele in a family (through a homozygous-heterozygous mating), a half-HLA-identical sib may be homozygous and a non-HLA-identical sib heterozygous. In order to establish the status of the offspring of a patient with haemochromatosis, all of whom must be at least heterozygous, both HLA genotyping and phenotypic tests must be performed on the patient's mate (Fig. 93.2) in order to find out if he or she is carrying a haemochromatosis allele that would determine the homozygous state in 50% of their children.

Repeated phlebotomy is the treatment of choice in a homozygote with phenotypic expression of the disease. A heterozygous individual needs dietary counselling (avoidance of alcoholic drinks, for example) with very occasional phenotypic surveillance (say every five or ten years). An allele-free individual requires no surveillance and can be reassured that he or she is not at risk either of developing haemochromatosis or of transmitting susceptibility to it. In many cases this approach should prevent a disease which is at best disabling and at worst leads to death from heart failure or cancer of the liver.

CONGENITAL ATRANSFERRINAEMIA

Acquired transferrin deficiency, such as that due to protein-poor nutrition (Lahey et al, 1958) and in which outcome is related to the degree of the deficiency, is fairly common. A number of transferrin variants, without associated disease, are known (Kirk, 1968). Only a very small number of cases, however, of congenital atransferrinaemia have been reported (Heilmeyer et al, 1961; Cap et al, 1968; Sakata, 1969; Goya et al, 1972; Loperena et al, 1974).

The original case report by Heilmreyer et al (1961) outlined the clinical, biochemical and genetic features of the disease. The patient was a 7 year-old girl with a history of anaemia from the age of three months for which numerous transfusions had been performed. The anaemia was associated with a tendency to infection, poor growth, skin hyperpigmentation, hepatomegaly and heart disease. Serum iron and serum transferrin were extremely low. Iron absorption was fairly elevated and plasma iron turnover greatly increased. Death was sudden. At autopsy, lesions were found similar to those associated with haemochromatosis, with iron deposition and fibrosis of the heart, pancreas and liver. Both parents had low serum transferrin levels and could be considered heterozygous in accordance with a recessive mode of transmission. Similar findings have been described in the few other reported cases.

In the patient described by Goya et al (1972) it could be established that the congenital disorder involved the synthesis and not the breakdown of transferrin. Monthly administration of transferrin-rich plasma fractions has proved effective in correcting the anaemia.

ACKNOWLEDGEMENT

The author would like to express his thanks to those whose contribution was essential in personal works about genetics of haemochromatosis, especially to M. Bourel, R. Fauchet, B. Genetet and J. L. Alexandre, C. Beaulont, P. Bot, P. Brissot, G. Edan, J. P. Hespel, M. Jollant, L. Le Mignon, M. Le Reun, C. Scordia.

REFERENCES

Addison G M, Beamish M R, Hales C N, Hodgkins M, Jacobs A, Llewellin P 1972 An immunoradiometric assay for ferritin in the serum of normal subjects and patients with iron deficiency and iron overload. Journal of Clinical Pathology 75: 326–329

Aisen P 1977 Some physiochemical aspects of iron metabolism. In: Iron Metabolism, Ciba Foundation Symposium 51 (New Series), Elsevier North Holland, Amsterdam. p 1–18

Astaldi G, Meardi G, Lisinot T 1966 The iron content of jejunal mucosa obtained by Crosby's biopsy in hemochromatosis and hemosiderosis. Blood 28: 70–82

Awai M, Narasaki M, Yamanoi Y, Seno S 1979 Induction of diabetes in animals by parenteral administration of ferric nitrilotriacetate. American Journal of Pathology 95: 663–673

Balcerzak S P, Westerman M P, Lee R E, Doyle A P 1966 Idiopathic hemochromatosis. A study of three families. American Journal of Medicine 40: 857–873

Barry M, Sherlock S 1971 Measurement of liver iron concentration in needle-biopsy specimens. Lancet 1: 100–103

Basset M L, Halliday J W, Powell L W, Doran T, Bashir H 1979 Early detection of idiopathic haemochromatosis: relative value of serum-ferritin and HLA typing. Lancet 2: 4–7

Batey R, Pettit J E, Nicholas A W, Sherlock S, Hoffbrand D M 1978 Hepatic iron clearance from serum in treated hemochromatosis. Gastroenterology 75: 856–859

Beaumont C, Simon M, Smith P, Worwood M 1980 Hepatic and serum ferritin concentrations in patients with idiopathic hemochromatosis. Gastroenterology 79: 877–883

Bomford A, Williams R 1976 Long term results of venesection therapy in idiopathic haemochromatosis. Quarterly Journal of Medicine 45: 611–627

Bomford A, Eddleston A L W F, Kennedy L A, Batchelor L H, Williams R 1977 Histocompatibility antigens as markers of abnormal iron metabolism in patients with idiopathic haemochromatosis and their relatives. Lancet 1: 327–329

Bregma H, Gelfan M C, Winchester J F, Manz H J, Knepshield J H, Schreiner G E 1980 Iron overload associated myopathy in patients on maintenance haemodialysis: a histocompatibility linked disorder. Lancet 2: 882–885

Brissot P, Deugnier Y, Le Treut A, Renouard F, Simon M, Bourel M 1978 Ascorbic acid status in idiopathic hemochromatosis. Digestion 17: 479–487

Brissot P, Herry D, Verger J P, Messner M, Renouard F, Ferrand B, Simon M, Bourel M 1981 Assessment of liver iron content in 271 patients: reevaluation of direct and indirect methods. Gastroenterology 80: 557–565

Cartwright G E, Edwards C Q, Skolnick M H, Amos D B 1980 Association of HLA-linked hemochromatosis with idiopathic refractory sideroblastic anemia. Journal of Clinical Investigation 65: 989–992

Cartwright G E, Edwards C Q, Kravitz K, Skolnick M, Amos D B, Johnson A, Buskjaer L 1979 Hereditary hemochromatosis: phenotypic expression of the disease. New England Journal of Medicine 301: 175–179

Cattan D, Marche C, Jori G P, Debray C 1967 Le stock martial des villosites duodéno-jéjunales. L'absorption martiale vue par l'histologie. Nouvelle revue française d'hématologie 7: 259–270

Chevrant-Breton J, Simon M, Bourel M, Ferrand B 1977 Cutaneous manifestations of idiopathic hemochromatosis. Archives of Dermatology 113: 161–165

Cox T M, Peters T J 1978 Uptake of iron by duodenal biopsy specimens from patients with iron-deficiency anemia and primary haemochromatosis. Lancet 1: 123–124

Crosby W H 1963 The control of iron balance by the intestinal mucosa. Blood 22: 441–449

Delbarre F 1960 Ostéoporose des hémochromatoses. Semaine de Hôpitaux de Paris 36: 3279–3284

Dymock I W, Cassar J, Pyke D A, Oakley W G, Williams R 1972 Observations on the pathogenesis, complications and treatment of diabetes in 115 cases of haemochromatosis. American Journal of Medicine 52: 203–210

Eddleston A L W F, Williams R 1978 HLA and liver disease. British Medical Bulletin 34: 295–300

Fauchet R, Simon M, Genetet B, Bourel M 1980a Idiopathic hemochromatosis. In: Terasaki P (ed) Histocompatibility testing. Eighth International Histocompatibility Workshop, UCLA Tissue Typing Laboratory, Los Angeles. p 707–710

Fauchet R, Genetet N, Genetet B, Simon M, Bourel M 1979 HLA determinants in idiopathic hemochromatosis. Tissue Antigens 14: 10–14

Fauchet R, Hauptmann G, Simon M, Bourel M, Mayer S, Genetet B 1980b Markers of factor B (Bf) and C4 in idiopathic hemochromatosis. Eighth International Histocompatibility worshop, Los Angeles

Fauchet R, Simon M, Genetet B, Kerbaol M, Bansard J Y, Genetet N, Bourel M 1977 HLA-A, B, C, D and lymphocyte B antigen typing in idiopathic haemochromatosis with the study of five families. Tissue Antigens 10: 206

Fillet G 1977 Le fer dans l'organisme. Masson, Paris

Guillon J, Charbonnel B, Le Mort J P, Brizard A 1975 Testostérone dihydritestosterone, LH, FSH plasmatiques, test LH-RH dans l'hémochromatose idiopathique. Revue française d'endocrinologie clinique, nutrition et métabolisme 16: 299–305

Halliday J W, Mack U, Powell L W 1978 Duodenal ferritin content and structure. Relation with body iron stores in man. Archives of Internal Medicine 138: 1109–1113

Kidd K K 1979 Genetic linkage and hemochromatosis. New England Journal of Medicine 301: 209–210

Lipinski M, Hors J, Saleun J P, Saddi R, Passa P, Lafaurie S, Feingold N, Dausset J 1978 Idiopathic hemochromatosis: linkage with HLA. Tissue Antigens 11: 471–474

Lloyd D A, Adams P, Sinclair N R, Stiller L R, Valberg L S 1978 Histocompatibility antigens as markers of abnormal iron metabolism in idiopathic hemochromatosis. Canadian Medical Association Journal 119: 1051–1056.

MacDonald R A 1964 Hemochromatosis and hemosiderosis. Thomas Books, Springfield

Mattheyses M, Hespel J P, Brissot P, Daubert J C, Hita de Nercy Y, Lancien G, Le Treut A, Pony J C, Simon M, Ferrand B, Gouffault J, Bourel M 1978 Myocardiopathie de l'hémochromatose. Archives des maladies du coeur et des vaisseaux 71: 371–379

Pawlotsly Y, Simon M, Hany Y, Brissot P, Bourel M 1975 High plasma parathyroid hormone levels and osteoarticular changes in primary haemochromatosis. Scandinavian Journal of Rheumatology 4, suppl 8

Peters T J, Selden C, Seymour C A 1976 Lysosomal disruption in the pathogenesis of hepatic damage in primary and secondary haemochromatosis. Ciba Foundation Symposium 51: 317–329

Pollycove M, Fawwaz R A, Winchell H S 1971 Transient hepatic deposition of iron in primary hemochromatosis with iron deficiency following venesection. Journal of Nuclear Medicine 12: 28–30

Powell L W, Basset M L, Halliday J W 1980 Hemochromatosis. Gastroenterology 78: 374–381

Powell L W, Campbell C B, Wilson E 1970 Intestinal mucosal uptake of iron and iron retention in idiopathic haemochromatosis as evidence for a mucosal abnormality. Gut 11: 727–731

Saddi R, Feingold J 1974a Idiopathic haemochromatosis. An autosomal recessive disease. Clinical Genetics 5: 234–241

Saddi R, Feingold J 1974b Idiopathic haemochromatosis and diabetes mellitus. Clinical Genetics 5: 242–247

Schumacher H R 1964 Hemochromatosis and arthritis. Archives of Rheumatology 7: 41–50

Simon M, Bourel M 1979a L'hémochromatose idiopathique: I-Aspects cliniques, biologiques et thérapeutique. Nouvelle Presse Médicale 8: 855–859

Simon M, Bourel M 1979b L'hémochromatose idiopathique: II-Aspects pathogéniques et génétiques, dépistage et prévention. Nouvelle Presse Médicale 8: 1083–1087

Simon M, Bourel M, Fauchet R, Genetet B 1976a Association of HLA-A3 and HLA-B14 antigens with idiopathic haemochromatosis. Gut 17: 332–334

Simon M, Bourel M, Genetet B, Fauchet R 1977a Idiopathic hemochromatosis. Demonstration of recessive inheritance and early detection by family typing. New England Journal of Medicine 297: 1017–1021

Simon M, Alexandre J L, Bourel M, Le Marec B, Scordia C 1977b Heredity of idiopathic haemochromatosis: a study of 106 families. Clinical Genetics 11: 327–341

Simon M, Alexandre J L, Fauchet R, Genetet B, Bourel M 1980a The genetics of hemochromatosis. In: Steinberg A G, Bearn A G, Motulsky A G, Childs B (eds) Progress in Medical Genetics IV, Saunders, Philadelphia. p 135–168

Simon M, Pawlotsky Y, Bourel M, Fauchet R, Genetet B 1975 Hemochromatose idiopathique. Maladie associée à l'antigène tissulaire HL-A3? Nouvelle Presse Médicale 4: 1432

Simon M, Vongsavanthong S, Hespel J P, Lecornu M, Bourel M 1973a Diabète et hémochromatose. I – Le diaète dans l'hémochromatose. A propos de 130 cas personnels d'hémochromatose. Semaine de Hôpitaux de Paris 49: 2125–2132

Simon M, Bourel M, Genetet B, Fauchet R, Edan G, Brissot P 1977c Idiopathic hemochromatosis and iron overload in alcoholic liver disease: differentiation by HLA phenotype. Gastroenterology 73: 655–658

Simon M, Fauchet R, Le Mignon L, Hespel J P, Beaumont C, Bourel M 1980b Recessive inheritance of idiopathic haemochromatosis: exceptions that confirm the rule. Iron Club Meeting. Sheffield, abstracts

Simon M, Fauchet R, Hespel J P, Brissot P, Genetet B, Bourel M 1981 Idiopathic hemochromatosis and HLA. In: Farid N (ed) HLA in Endocrine and Metabolic Disorders, Academic Press, New York. p 291–323

Simon M, Gosselin M, Kerbaol M, Delanoe G, Trebaul L, Bourel M 1973b Functional study of exocrine pancreas in idiopathic haemochromatosis, untreated and treated by venesections (32 cases). Digestion 8: 485–496

Simon M, Alexandre J L, Fauchet R, Genetet N, Scordia C, Jollant M, Hespel J P, Bourel M 1978 Le diabète de l'hémochromatose idiopathique n'est pas favorisé (sauf à titre fortuit) par l'hérédité diabétique. In: Journées ann Diabetol Hôtel-Dieu, Flammarion, Paris, p 33–43

Simon M, Hespel J P, Fauchet R, Brissot P, Hita de Nercy Y, Edan G, Genetet B, Bourel M 1979 Hérédité récessive de l'hémochromatose idiopathique; deux observations de transmission pseudo-dominante reconnue comme récessive par étude de la surcharge en fer et des génotypes HLA dans les familles. Nouvelle Presse Médicale 8: 421–424

Simon M, Bourel M, Alexandre J L, Brissot P, Hita de Nercy Y, Scordia C, Fauchet R, Genetet N, Genetet B 1976b Hérédité de l'hémochromatose: sa liaison avec le système HLA. Nouvelle Presse Médicale 5: 1762

Simon M, Fauchet R, Hespel J P, Beaumont C, Brissot B, Hery B, Hita de Nercy Y, Genetet B, Bourel M 1980c Idiopathic hemochromatosis. A study of biochemical expression in 247 heterozygous members of 63 families. Evidence for a single major HLA-linked gene. Gastroenterology 78: 703–708

Stefanelli M, Bentley D P, Cavill I 1980 Quantification of iron release from RES in man. Iron Club Meeting. Sheffield, abstracts

Stocks A E, Powell L W 1973 Carbohydrate intolerance in idiopathic haemochromatosis and cirrhosis of the liver. Quarterly Journal of Medicine 42: 733–749

Thomson G, Bodmer W 1977 The genetic analysis of HLA and disease associations. In: Dausset G, Svejgaard M (ed) HLA and Disease, Munksgaard, Williams and Wilkins, Copenhagen, Baltimore. p 84–93

Tourniaire J, Fevre M, Mazenod B, Ponsin G 1974 Effects of clomiphene citrate and synthetic LHRH on serum luteinizing hormone (LH) in men with idiopathic hemochromatosis. Journal of Clinical Endocrinology and Metabolism 38: 1122–1124

Trousseau A 1865 Clinique Médicale de l'Hôtel-Dieu de Paris. Baillère, Paris

Von Recklinghausen F D 1889 Uber Haëmochromatose. Berliner Klinische Wochenschrift 26: 925

Walsh R J, Perkins K W, Blackurn C R B 1964 Xth Congress of Internal Society of Haematology Abstract F 16, Munksgaard, Copenhagen

Walsh C H, Wright A D, Williams J, Holder G 1976 A study of pituitary function in patients with idiopathic hemochromatosis. Journal of Clinical Endocrinology and Metabolism 43: 866–872

Williams R, Scheuer P J, Sherlock S 1962 The inheritance of idiopathic haemochromatosis. A clinical and liver biopsy study of 16 families. Quarterly Journal of Medicine 31: 249–265

Worwood M 1979 Serum ferritin. CRC Critical Reviews in Clinical Laboratory Sciences 10: 171–204

ATRANSFERRINAEMIA

Cap J L, Mayerava V Y 1968 Kongenitalna atransferinemia u ll mesacneho dietata. Ceskoslovenska Pediatrie 23: 1020–1075

Goya N, Miyazake S, Kodate S Y, Uskio B 1972 A family of congenital atransferrinemia. Blood 40: 239–245

Heilmeyer L, Keller W, O Vivell, Keiderling W, Betke K, Wohler F, Schultze H E 1961 Congenital transferrin deficiency in a seven year old girl. German Medical Monthly 6: 385

Kirk R L 1968 The world distribution of transferrin variants and some unsolved problems. Acta Geneticae Medicae et Gemellologiae 17: 613

Lahey M E, Behar M, Viteri F, Scrimshaw N S 1958 Values for copper, iron and iron-binding capacity in the serum in kwashiorkor. Pediatrics 22: 72–79

Loperena L, Dorantes S, Medrano E, Berron R, Vega L, Cuaron A, Rodriguez C, Marquez J L 1974 Atransferrinemia hereditaria. Boletin médico del Hospital Infantil Vol XXXI, no 3

Sakata T 1969 A case of congenital atransferrinemia. Shonika Shinnryo 32: 1523–1529

94

The mucopolysaccharidoses

J. Spranger

The genetic mucopolysaccharidoses are hereditary, progressive disorders caused by the excessive intralysosomal accumulation of glycosaminoglycans (acid mucopolysaccharides) in various tissues. Glycosaminoglycans are long-chain complex carbohydrates consisting of a variety of uronic acids, amino sugars and neutral sugars. They are usually linked to proteins to form proteoglycans. Proteoglycans are major constituents of the ground substance of connective tissue. They are also present in mitochondria, nuclear and cell membranes (Kraemer & Smith, 1974; Dietrich et al, 1976).

The major glycosaminoglycans are chondroitin-4-sulphate, chondroitin-6-sulphate, heparan sulphate, dermatan sulphate, keratan sulphate and hyaluronic acid. In the organism these substances are degraded by the sequential action of lysosomal enzymes leading to a stepwise shortening of the glycosaminoglycan chain (Fig. 94.1). Absent activity of a lysosomal enzyme results in the gradual accumulation of partially degraded glycosaminoglycan molecules in lysosomes. Distended lysosomes accumulate in the cell (Fig. 94.2) and interfere with normal cell function.

Some clinical manifestations of the mucopolysaccharidoses such as coarse facial features, thick skin, corneal clouding and organomegaly can be regarded as the direct expression of glycosaminoglycan accumulation in tissue. Others, such as mental retardation, growth deficiency, skeletal dysplasia are the result of defective cell function. Joint contractures and herniae point to an interference of accumulated glycosaminoglycans with other metabolic substances such as collagen or fibronectin.

Different mucopolysaccharidoses are caused by different enzyme deficiencies leading to the accumulation of biochemically different glycosaminoglycan degradation products. As a general rule, the impaired degradation of heparan sulphate is more closely associated with mental deficiency and the impaired degradation of dermatan sulphate, chondroitin sulphates and keratan sulphate with mesenchymal abnormalities. Some of the salient features of the mucopolysaccharidoses are summarized in Table 94.1.

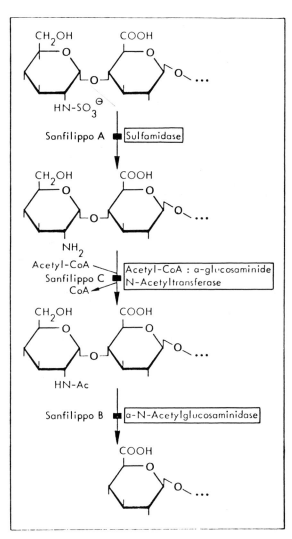

Fig. 94.1 Enzymatic degradation of N-sulphoglucosaminyl residues in heparan sulphate by the sequential action of three lysosomal enzymes. The deficiency of any of these three enzymes leads to clinically indistinguishible forms of mucopolysaccharidosis III: Sanfilippo disease A, B or C

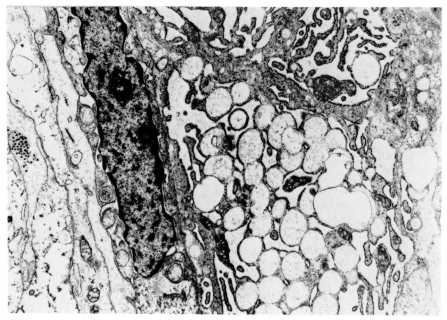

Fig. 94.2 The cytoplasm of an osteoblasts from a patient with mucopolysaccharidosis II is filled with numerous membrane bound vacuoles containing a fine granular material (buffered glutaraldehyde × 6000)

MUCOPOLYSACCHARIDOSIS I-H (HURLER DISEASE)

Hurler disease is characterized by the combination of progressive mental degeneration with a peculiar clinical phenotype. The characteristic 'Hurler phenotype' consists of gross facial features, enlarged and deformed skull, small stature, corneal opacities, hepatosplenomegaly, valvular heart defects, thick skin, joint contractures and herniae (Fig. 94.3).

The clinical features become more apparent with age. In infancy nonspecific signs are found such as a slightly enlarged head, chronic rhinitis and herniae. A diagnosis may be suspected on the basis of broad ribs and coarse bone structure in a routine chest film. It can be confirmed by demonstrating an elevated urinary excretion of glycosaminoglycans and appropriate enzyme studies. By the end of the first year of life the Hurler phenotype becomes evident. Growth is still normal at that age but slows down thereafter. The disorder is progressive and usually leads to death before the age of 14 years. Death commonly occurs from cardiac failure due to valvular incompetence and chronic respiratory infections. The patients are severely demented but usually retain a certain degree of emotional contact.

Complications include chronic upper respiratory infections, large herniae, cardiac insufficiency and increased cranial pressure due to impaired spinal fluid circulation caused by thickened leptomeninges and subarachnoidal cysts. Torsion of the enlarged spleen has been observed.

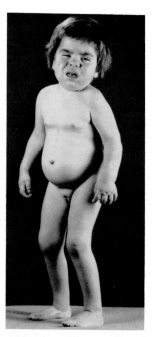

Fig. 94.3 3 year old patient with mucopolysaccharidosis I-H. Note coarse facial features, dense hair, disproportionately short trunk, protuberant abdomen and multiple flexion contractures of the joints.

Table 94.1 The genetic mucopolysaccharidoses

Number	Eponym	Main clinical features	Defective enzyme	Assay in	Genetics
MPS I-H	Pfaundler-Hurler	Severe Hurler phenotype, mental retardation, corneal clouding, death usually before age 14 years	α-L-iduronidase	L,F,Ac	AR
MPS I-S	Scheie	Stiff joints, corneal clouding, aortic valve disease, normal intelligence, survive to adulthood	α-L-iduronidase	L,F,Ac	AR
MPS I.H/S	Hurler-Scheie	Phenotype intermediate between I-H and I-S; genetic heterogeneity possible in this group, but at least some patients Hurler-Scheie double heterozygotes	α-L-iduronidase	L,F,Ac	AR
MPS II-XR	Hunter	Severe course: similar to MPS I-H but usually clear cornea. Mild course: milder clinical phenotype, later manifestation and survival to adulthood without or with mild mental retardation. Deafness.	Iduronate sulphate sulphatase	S,L,Ac? Af?	XR
MPS II-AR	Hunter	Same as MPS II-XR	Iduronate sulphate sulphatase	S,L,Ac? Af?	AR
MPS III-A	Sanfilippo A	Behavioural problems, aggression,	Heparan-S-sulphaminidase	L,F,Ac	AR
MPS III-B	Sanfilippo B	progressive dementia, seizures,	N-ac-α-D-glucosaminidase	S,F,Ac	AR
MPS III-C	Sanfilippo C	survival to second or third decade of life possible, considerable	Ac-CoA-glucosaminide N-acetyltransferase	F,Ac?	AR
MPS III-D	Sanfilippo D	intrafamilial variability, mild dysmorphism, coarse hair, clear corneae, usually normal height.	N-ac-glucosamine-6-sulphate sulphatase	L,F	AR
MPS IV-A	Morquio A	Short-trunk type of dwarfism, fine corneal opacities, characteristic bone dysplasia, final height below 125 cm	Galactosamine-6-sulphate sulphatase	F,Ac?	AR
MPS IV-B	Morquio B	Same as IV-A but milder, adult height over 120 cm.	β-galactosidase	L,F,Ac	AR
MPS V	No longer used	formerly Scheie disease			
MPS VI	Maroteaux-Lamy	Hurler phenotytpe with marked corneal clouding and normal intelligence. Mild, moderate and severe expression in different families (?allelic mutations)	N-acetyl-galactosamine α-4-sulphate sulphatase (Arylsulphatase B)	S,L,F, Ac	AR
MPS VII	Sly	Highly variable. Dense inclusions in granulocytes	β-glucuronidase	S,L,F, Ac	AR

L = Leucocytes   S = Serum   F = Cultured fibroblasts   Ac = Cultured amniotic cells   Af = Amniotic fluid
AR = autosomal recessive   XR = X-chromosomal recessive

X–rays show a pattern of skeletal abnormalities called 'dysostosis multiplex'. Its major features are a large skull with a deep, elongated, J-shaped sella, oar-like ribs, deformed, hook-shaped lower thoracic and upper lumbar vertebrae, pelvic dysplasia, shortened tubular bones with expanded diaphyses and dysplastic epiphyses (Fig. 94.4). The bone structure is coarse and irregular. The abnormalities become more distinct with age.

Blood smears show abnormal cytoplasmic inclusions in lymphocytes. The urinary excretion of dermatan sulphate and heparan sulphate is increased. The diagnosis is confirmed by assay in leucocytes and cultured fibroblasts of the enzyme alpha-L-iduronidase.

Mucopolysaccharidosis I-H is inherited as an autosomal recessive trait. Prenatal diagnosis is possible by measuring the iduronidase activity and the incorporation

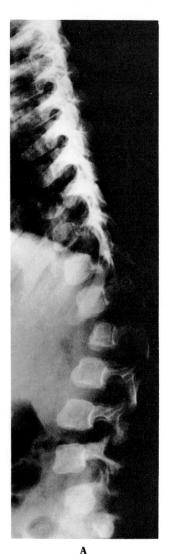

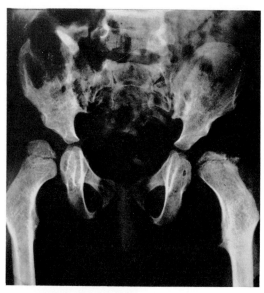

B

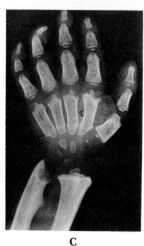

Fig. 94.4 Dysostosis multiplex. (A) 4 years. The vertebral bodies have an ovoid shape which is abnormal for this age. There is an ossification defect in the anterosuperior aspect of the bodies of L-2 to L-4. L-2 is hypoplastic and dorsally displaced. (B) 4 years. The basilar portions of the iliac bones are hypoplastic, the acetabular fossae are shallow and the iliac wings are flared. The capital femoral epiphyses are small, and the femoral necks are broad and in valgus position. (C) 8 years. The tubular bones are abnormally short, wide and deformed. The proximal and middle phalanges are bullet-shaped. The second to fifth metacarpals are narrow at their bases. The epiphyses are irregular. The carpal bones are small. The distal articular surfaces of the ulna and radius are slanted towards each other. The bone trabeculation is coarse and the cortices are thin.

A   **C**

of labelled sulphate in glycosaminoglycans of cultured amniotic cells.

No causal therapy is available. Attempts at enzyme replacement using plasma transfusions have failed. The effect of fibroblast transplantation is presently being evaluated (Gibbs et al, 1980). Reversal of clinical features and biochemical improvement has been reported in a one-year-old boy with Hurler disease after bone marrow transplantation (Hobbs et al, 1981).

MUCOPOLYSACCHARIDOSIS I-S (SCHEIE DISEASE)

Scheie disease is a milder manifestation of iduronidase deficiency than Hurler disease. It is rarely diagnosed before the age of six years. Its major clinical features are coarse but not Hurler-like facial features, corneal clouding and joint contractures, notably of the fingers. Heart murmurs are caused by stenosis and/or regurgitation at the heart valves, mostly of the aorta. Some patients are deaf. They are of normal or almost normal height and their intelligence is unimpaired. Their life expectancy is generally good, depending on the rate of progression of cardiac disease. Complications include retinopathy, glaucoma, the carpal tunnel syndrome, pes cavus and herniae.

X–rays show minimal changes of dysostosis multiplex with broad ribs, small carpal bones with proximal convergence of the finger rays and mild hypoplasia of the lower portions of the iliac bones of the pelvis. The urinary excretion of dermatan sulphate and heparan sulphate is increased.

Mucopolysaccharidoses I-H and I-S are probably

allelic mutations involving the alpha-L-iduronidase locus. Cell fusion studies show no complementation of Hurler and Scheie cells (Galjaard, 1979). The different severity of Hurler and Scheie disease may be caused by a higher residual activity of alpha-L-iduronidase towards its natural substrates in the latter.

Therapeutic measures include operative procedures for correction of the carpal tunnel syndrome, glaucoma and aortic disease. Corneal transplants may become necessary.

MUCOPOLYSACCHARIDOSIS I-H/S (HURLER-SCHEIE COMPOUND)

Given a gene frequency of 1 in 330 for Mucopolysaccharidosis I-H and 1 in 700 for Mucopolysaccharidosis I-S there must be patients carrying both the Hurler and the Scheie gene (McKusick et al, 1972). The frequency of these double heterozygotes in the population is estimated as $2 \times (1:330) \times (1:700) = 1:115\,000$ (versus $1:100\,000$ for Hurler disease and $1:500\,000$ for Scheie disease).

The phenotype of these patients would be expected to be less severe than that for MPS I-H and more severe than that for MPS I-S. A number of such patients has been observed (e.g. Spranger et al, 1974; Leisti et al, 1976; Stevenson et al, 1976). They are short, have corneal opacities, joint contractures, hepatomegaly, abnormal heart valves and other features of Mucopolysaccharidosis I-H. In contrast to the latter they are less severely retarded, have puckish rather than Hurler-like facial features and may survive into adulthood. Their skeletal abnormalities are less severe than in Hurler disease. Destruction of the sellar region, probably caused by arachnoid cysts, seems to be relatively common (Winters et al, 1976; McKusick et al, 1978).

The genetic concept of Mucopolysaccharidosis I-H/S requires that the incidence of parental consanguinity is not increased. However, in at least four families with alpha-L-iduronidase deficiency and an intermediate Hurler-Scheie phenotype parental consanguinity has been recorded (Jensen et al, 1978; Kohn et al, 1978; Kaibara et al, 1979). Some patients look different from the so-called I-H/S compound cases (Babarik et al, 1974; Danes, 1974). Thus there may be other (allelic?) forms of alpha-L-iduronidase deficiency in addition to the I-H/S compound, Hurler and Scheie disease.

MUCOPOLYSACCHARIDOSIS II (HUNTER DISEASE)

The clinical features of mucopolysaccharidosis II are similar to those of mucopolysaccharidosis I-H with the notable exception of the cornea which is generally clear.

Only rarely are corneal opacities found in a child with Hunter disease. Conversely, clear corneae are the exception in Hurler disease (Gardner & Hay, 1974; Spranger et al, 1978). Nodular skin lesions giving the skin a pebbled appearance are seen in some patients and are probably unique to mucopolysaccharidosis II.

The disease may take a rapid, an intermediate or a slow course. Patients with a *rapid course* are almost as severely affected as patients with Hurler disease, with first manifestations in late infancy, rapid physical and mental deterioration and death in early puberty.

In its *mild form* the disease is detected later and the patients survive to adulthood. They are slightly short, heavy built with moderately coarse facial features, hoarse voice, joint contractures notably of the fingers, median nerve entrapment, enlarged liver and spleen, and herniae. Hearing defects are almost invariably present. Atypical retinitis pigmentosa and chronic papilloedema with impairment of vision are commonly found. Heart disease due to valvular thickening, myocardial and ischaemic factors is a problem. Patients with the mild form are mentally normal. In the adult patients reported by Karpati et al (1974) multiple nerve entrapment and moderate shortness of stature were the only clinical symptoms.

X-ray studies show dysostosis multiplex in a milder and more slowly progressive form than in mucopolysaccharidosis I-H. In adult patients the only pathologic findings may be small carpal bones and mild dysplasia of the pelvis and femoral heads with premature arthrosis (Grossman & Dorst, 1973). The urine contains large amounts of heparan sulphate and dermatan sulphate.

Mucopolysaccharidosis II is an X–linked recessive condition caused by a deficiency of the enzyme iduronate sulphate sulphatase. The enzyme activity can be determined in serum, lymphocytes and cultured fibroblasts. Prenatal diagnosis is possible by measurement of iduronate sulphate sulphatase in amniotic fluid and by S^{35} incorporation studies in cultured amniotic cells (Liebaers & Neufeld, 1975; Liebaers et al, 1977).

Severe and mild forms have been described in the same family (Yatziv et al, 1977) and the different severity of the manifestations is probably the expression of variability. In most families, however, the affected males are affected to a similar degree. Carrier detection is difficult but can be attempted by iduronate sulphate sulphatase determination in hair roots (Nwokoro & Neufeld, 1979).

Autosomal recessive inheritance of mucopolysaccharidosis II has been observed (Neufeld et al, 1977). The affected females had the typical Hunter phenotype.

Therapeutically, fibroblast transplantation has been claimed to result in mild corrective changes of excreted urinary glycosaminoglycans and some clinical improvement (Dean et al, 1980).Symptomatic measures are indicated as in other mucopolysaccharidoses.

MUCOPOLYSACCHARIDOSIS III (SANFILIPPO DISEASE)

Mucopolysaccharidosis III is clinically characterized by comparatively mild dysmorphism and progressive dementia. First clinical symptoms usually appear after the second year of life. They relate to behavioural problems and include sleep disturbances, lack of concentration, short attention span, impulsiveness. Later, hyperactivity and aggressiveness occur. Psychomotor skills are gradually lost. The patients stop speaking. Convulsions occur. The most prominent clinical feature is abundant and coarse, often blond hair (Fig. 94.5). The patients are of normal height and their corneae are clear. Liver and spleen are not or only mildly enlarged.

The course of the disease is relentless and leads to a vegetative state. Most patients die before the age of 20 years from aspiration pneumonia. Intrafamilial variability may be considerable. Some patients are retarded from infancy, others may attend the first grades of school. Some patients die before the age of 10, others survive into middle adulthood (Kamp, 1979).

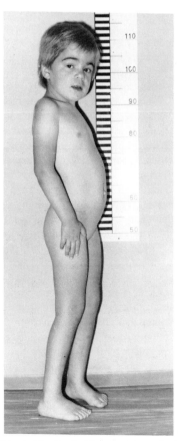

Fig. 94.5 5 year old patient with mucopolysaccharidosis III. The hair is abundant. The facial features are slightly coarse. The patient is of normal height.

There are mild skeletal changes of dysostosis multiplex with thickened calvaria, ovoid vertebral bodies and hypoplasia of the lower portions of the pelvic ilia. Peripheral lymphocytes contain conspicuous inclusions. The urinary excretion of heparan sulphate and chondroitin sulphates is elevated.

The disorder is caused by the deficiency of any of multiple lysosomal enzymes involved in the degradation of heparan sulphate (Fig. 94.1): sulphamidase (mucopolysaccharidosis III-A), alpha-N-acetyl-glucosaminidase (mucopolysaccharidosis III-B) and acetyl-CoA-alpha-glucosaminide-N-acetyl-transferase (mucopolysaccharidosis III-C). Clinically, the three enzyme deficiencies cannot be differentiated. They are inherited as autosomal recessive disorders. Mucopolysaccharidosis III-A seems to be more common than mucopolysaccharidoses III-B and III-C. Prenatal diagnosis is possible. A fourth type of Sanfilippo disease, MPS III-D, has recently been described (Gatti et al, 1982). It is caused by a deficiency of N-ac-glucosamine-6-sulphate sulphatase, an enzyme that acts specifically to remove sulphate from position 6 of N-ac-glucosamine in heparan sulphate (not shown in Fig. 94.1).

Therapy is symptomatic. Control of hyperactivity is difficult and may require a combination of sedatives and psychorelaxants including haloperidol. Barbiturates are frequently without effect.

MUCOPOLYSACCHARIDOSIS IV (MORQUIO DISEASE)

The main clinical features of Morquio disease are a short-trunk type of dwarfism with normal intelligence and without Hurler-like facial characteristics. Historically, the disorder has been confused with numerous spondyloepiphyseal dysplasias. It was clearly defined by Maroteaux et al (1963).

The first signs appear in the second or third year of life. Thoracic deformity, kyphosis and/or genu valgum and growth retardation are noted. Other features gradually develop until finally a characteristic pattern of clinical findings has emerged with a prominent lower face, enamel hypoplasia of the teeth, short neck, protruding upper sternum, accentuated spinal curves, genu valgum, prominent and loose joints and short fingers (Fig. 94.6A). Slit-lamp examination shows fine corneal opacities and audiometry reveals hearing loss. Adult height is below 120 cm in mucopolysaccharidosis IV-A and between 120 cm and 140 cm in mucopolysaccharidosis IV-B.

The most important complication is spinal cord compression at the upper cervical level due to atlanto-axial instability. This is caused by a combination of odontoid hypoplasia and ligamentous hyperlaxity. The first symptoms of a cervical myelopathy are easy fatigu-ability. Later subtle neurologic signs develop. If unde-tected, the condition may lead to quadriplegia. Spinal cord compression may also occur at the level of D-12 to L-2 where anterior hypoplasia of the vertebral bodies leads to an acute kyphosis with encroachment upon the spinal canal. Other complications are multiple arthroses and aortic regurgitation which develops in some patients.

X–ray studies show a characteristic spondyloepiphy-seal bone dysplasia with platyspondyly, anterior hypo-plasia of the vertebral bodies at the thoracolumbar junction, odontoid hypoplasia, hypoplastic basilar por-tions of the ilia of the pelvis, genua valga, marked epi-physeal dysplasia and shortening of the tubular bones (Fig. 94.6B). Children excrete excessive amounts of ker-atan sulphate in the urine. This is not the case in adults with Morquio disease. Failure to detect keratan sulphate in the urine is either caused by the older age of the patient or by improper biochemical technique: keratan sulphate is notoriously difficult to detect in the urine.

Morquio disease is heterogeneous. The more severe type IV-A is caused by the deficiency of N-acetyl-gal-

actosamine-6-sulphate-sulphatase (Singh et al, 1976). The milder type IV-B is caused by the deficiency of a β-galactosidase with specificity for keratan sulphate and chondroitin sulphates (Arbisser et al, 1977).

Both disorders are inherited as autosomal recessive traits. Prenatal diagnosis should be possible by appro-priate enzyme assay in cultured amniotic cells.

The most important therapeutic measure is the pre-vention of cervical myelopathy. Preventive fusion of the cervical spine is recommended (Kopits et al, 1972; Lip-son, 1977). Genua valga are corrected by osteotomy. Dental care and hearing aids are important.

MUCOPOLYSACCHARIDOSIS VI (MAROTEAUX-LAMY DISEASE)

Patients with mucopolysaccharidosis VI have a Hurler-like phenotype with normal intelligence. There is a mild and a severe form.

The *severe form* manifests itself in early childhood with thoracic deformities, lumbodorsal kyphosis, herniae and genua valga. Coarse facial features develop. Growth is retarded and ceases at about 10 years. Macrocephaly and hydrocephaly are found in some patients and are caused by thickened meninges, possibly arachnoidal cysts lead-ing to impaired flow and reabsorption of spinal fluid. Other complications are optic atrophy, buphthalmos, cardiac insufficiency and the carpal tunnel syndrome. The patients may survive into their third decade of life. They are severely handicapped by visual loss, joint con-tractures and by social problems stemming from their unusual appearance. Their mental performance remains relatively normal.

The *mild form* is recognized later and the patients may live into late adulthood. In its mildest expression, stiff-ness of the hands, corneal opacities, herniae and body height below 160 cm with only slightly coarse facial fea-tures are the only symptoms. More commonly, adoles-cents and adults with the mild form have distinctly Hurler-like facial features, dense corneal clouding, short stature, joint contractures, organomegaly and cardiac involvement.

Radiographs show dysostosis multiplex, the severity of which corresponds to the degree of clinical involve-ment. Dense granulations are found in neutrophils of peripheral blood smears. The urine contains excessive amounts of dermatan sulphate.

The disease is caused by a deficiency of the enzyme N-acetyl-galactosamine-4-sulphate sulphatase (arylsulpha-tase B). It is inherited as an autosomal recessive trait. The mild and severe forms have been claimed to be caused by allelic mutations. Some patients exhibit signs of intermediate severity, and the different forms may also be caused by variability of expression of the same

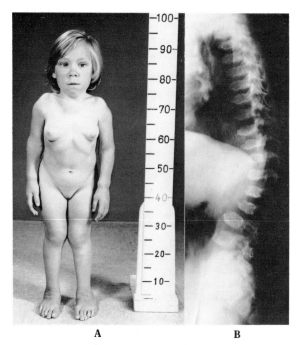

Fig. 94.6 (A) 12 year old girl with mucopolysaccharidosis IV, Morquio disease. The spine is disproportionately short. The lower half of the face is slightly accentuated. The joints are prominent and there are genua valga. (B) The vertebral bodies are flattened, more markedly in their dorsal than in their anterior portions. There is anterior pointing. At the lumbodorsal junction the anterior portions of the vertebral bodies are slightly hypoplastic. In some patients the hypoplasia is more marked with a resultant kyphosis and narrowing of the spinal canal at this level.

gene mutation. Prenatal diagnosis has been performed (Kleijer et al, 1976).

Therapeutic measures include shunting procedures to relieve increased intracranial pressure, corneal grafting, operative treatment of the carpal tunnel syndrome and hip replacement in adults with severe coxarthrosis. Replacement of defective heart valves may be considered in patients with the mild form of the disease.

MUCOPOLYSACCHARIDOSIS VII

Mucopolysaccharidosis VII is caused by a deficiency of the enzyme β-glucuronidase. The clinical symptoms of the few published cases vary and a definite clinical description is not possible at present. Titration patterns resulting from an enzyme immunoassay support the assumption of genetic heterogeneity (Bell et al, 1977). Variability of intrafamilial expression has also been observed (Guibaud et al, 1979).

In its mildest form, thoracic kyphosis and mild scoliosis are the only clinical findings (Danes & Degnan, 1974; Gitzelmann et al, 1978). One patient with this mild form had, in addition, fibromuscular dysplasia of the aorta and minimal coarsening of the face (Beaudet et al, 1975).

Other patients have more severe manifestations. They attract medical attention in later infancy or early childhood because of slightly coarse facial features, hepatosplenomegaly, herniae, thoracic deformities and thoracolumbar kyphosis (Beaudet et al, 1975; Gehler et al, 1974; Guibaud et al, 1979; Pfeiffer et al, 1977). The patients are mentally moderately retarded. Recurrent respiratory infections are a major problem.

One patient seems to be an example of a severe form of the disease (Beaudet et al, 1975). He presented with neonatal jaundice and hepatosplenomegaly. He had multiple herniae, gross corneal clouding, severely delayed psychomotor development, recurrent infections and died at 2.9 years of age.

Radiographs show minimal flattening of the vertebral bodies in mild cases and more pronounced changes of dysostosis multiplex in more severely affected patients. Dense Alder-type inclusions are found in peripheral granulocytes, and the original description of the so-called Alder anomaly may very well have been made in siblings with β-glucuronidase deficiency (Alder, 1944). Increased amounts of glycosaminoglycans are found in the urine. The diagnosis is established by determination of β-glucuronidase activity in serum, leucocytes or fibroblasts.

The β-glucuronidase deficiencies are probably inherited as autosomal recessive conditions. The structural locus for β-glucuronidase has been assigned to chromosome 7 (Grzeschik, 1975; Lalley et al, 1975). Prenatal diagnosis has been performed (Maire et al, 1979).

REFERENCES (* denotes General Reference)

Alder A 1944 Über konstitutionell bedingte Granulationsveränderungen der Leukozyten. Helvetica Paediatrica Acta 11: 161–165

Arbisser A I, Donelly K A, Scott C I, DiFerrante N, Singh J, Stevenson R E, Aylesworth A S, Howell R R 1977 Morquio-like syndrome with beta galactosidase deficiency and normal hexosamine sulphatase activity: mucopolysaccharidosis IVB. American Journal of Medical Genetics 1: 195–205

Babarik A, Benson P F, Dean M F, Muir H 1974 Chondroitin-sulphaturia with alpha-L-iduronidase deficiency. Lancet 1: 464–465

Beaudet A L, DiFerrante N A, Ferry G D, Nichols B L, Mullins C E 1975 Variation in the phenotypic expression of B-glucuronidase deficiency. Journal of Pediatrics 86: 388–394

Bell C E, Sly W S, Brot F E 1977 Human β-glucuronidase deficiency mucopolysaccharidosis. Journal of Clinical Investigation 59: 97—n105

*Cantz M, Gehler J 1976 The mucopolysaccharidoses: inborn errors of glycosaminoglycan catabolism. Human Genetics 32: 233–255

Danes B S 1977 Variant of iduronidase deficient mucopolysaccharidoses. Further evidence for genetic heterogeneity. Journal of Medical Genetics 14: 346–351

Danes B S, Degnan M 1974 Different clinical and biochemical phenotypes associated with β-glucuronidase deficiency. Birth Defects: Original Article Series 10: No 12, 251–257

Dean M F, Muir H, Benson P, Button L 1980 Enzyme replacement therapy in the mucopolysaccharidoses by fibroblast transplantation. Birth Defects: Original Article Series 16: No 1, 445–456

Dietrich C P, Sampaio L O, Toledo O M S 1976 Characteristic distribution of sulphated mucopolysaccharides in different tissues and in their respective mitochondria. Biochemical and Biophysical Research Communications 71: 1–10

*Galjaard H 1980 Genetic metabolic diseases, 1st Edn, Elsevier North Holland, Amsterdam. Ch 3, p 114

Gardner R J M, Hay H R 1974 Hurler's syndrome with clear corneas. Lancet II: 845

Gatti R, Borrone C, Durand P et al 1982 Sanfilippo type D disease: clinical findings in two patients with a new variant of mucopolysaccharidosis III. European Journal of Pediatrics 138: 168–171

Gehler J, Cantz M, Tolksdorf M, Spranger J, Gilbert E, Drube H 1974 Mucopolysaccharidosis VII: β-glucuronidase deficiency. Humangenetik 23: 149–158

Gibbs D A, Spellacy E, Roberts A E, Watts R W E 1980 The treatment of lysosomal storage diseases by fibroblast transplantation: some preliminary observations. Birth Defects: Original Article Series 16: No 1, 457–474

Gitzelmann R, Wiesmann U N, Spycher M A, Herschkowitz

N, Giedion A 1978 Unusually mild course of β-glucuronidase deficiency in two brothers (mucopolysaccharidosis VII). Helvetica Paediatrica Acta 33: 413–428

Grossman H, Dorst J P 1973 The mucopolysaccharidoses and mucolipidoses. Progress in Pediatric Radiology. Karger, Basel 4: 495–544

Grzeschik K H 1975 Assignment of human genes: β-glucuronidase to chromosome 7, adenylate kinase 1 to 9, a second enzyme with enolase activity to 12, and mitochondrial IDH to 15. Gene Mapping Conference Baltimore 3: 142–148

Guibaud P, Maire I, Goddon R, Teyssier G, Zabot M T, Mandon G 1979 Mucopolysaccharidose type VII par déficit en β-glucuronidase. Etude d'une famille. Journal de Génétique Humaine 27: 29–43

Hobbs J R, Barret A J, Chambers D et al 1981 Reversal of clinical features of Hurler's disease and biochemical improvement after treatment by bone-marrow transplantation. Lancet II: 709–712

Jensen O A, Pedersen C, Schwartz M, Vestermark S, Warburg M 1978 Hurler/Scheie phenotype. Report of an inbred sibship with tapetoretinal degeneration and electron-microscopic examination of the conjunctiva. Ophthalmologica, Basel 176: 194–204

Kaibara N, Eguchi M, Shibata K, Takagishi K 1979 Hurler-Scheie phenotype: a report of two pairs of inbred sibs. Human Genetics 53: 37–41

Karpati G, Carpenter S, Eisan A A, Wolfe L S, Feindel W 1974 Multiple peripheral nerve entrapments. An unusual phenotypic variant of the Hunter syndrome (mucopolysaccharidosis II) in a family. Archives of Neurology 31: 418–422

Kleijer W J, Wolffers G M, Hoogeveen A, Niermeijer M F 1976 Prenatal diagnosis of Maroteaux-Lamy syndrome. Lancet II: 50

Kohn G, Bach G, Lasch E, ElMassri M, Legum C, Cohen M M 1978 A new phenotypic variant of alpha-L-iduronidase deficiency. Monographs of Human Genetics 10: 7–10

Kopits S E, Perovic M N, McKusick V A, Robinson R A, Bailey J A 1972 Congenital atlantoaxial dislocations in various forms of dwarfism. Journal of Bone and Joint Surgery 54-A: 1349–1350

Kraemer P M, Smith D A 1974 High molecular-weight heparan sulphate from the cell surface. Biochemical and Biophysical Research Communications 56: 423–429

Lalley P A, Brown J A, Eddy R L, Haley L L, Shows T B 1975 Assignment of the gene for β-glucuronidase (β-GUS) to chromosome 7 in man. Gene Mapping Conference Baltimore 3: 184–187

Leisti J, Rimoin D L, Kaback M, Shapiro L J, Matalon R 1976 Allelic mutations in the mucopolysaccharidoses. Birth Defects: Original Article Series 12: 6, 81–91

Liebaers I, Neufeld E F 1975 Iduronate sulphatase deficiency in serum and lymphocytes of Hunter patients. Abstract, Annual Meeting, American Society of Human Genetics, Baltimore, October 8–11

Liebaers I, DiNatale P, Neufeld E F 1977 Iduronate sulphatase in amniotic fluid: an aid in the prenatal diagnosis of the Hunter syndrome. Journal of Pediatrics 90: 423–425

Lipson S J 1977 Dysplasia of the odontoid process in Morquio's syndrome causing quadriparesis. The Journal of Bone and Joint Surgery 59-A: 340–344

Maire I, Mandon G, Zabot M T, Mathieu M 1979 β-Glucuronidase deficiency: enzyme studies in an affected family and prenatal diagnosis. Journal of Inherited Metabolic Diseases 2: 29–34

Maroteaux P, Lamy M 1963 La maladie de Morquio. Etude clinique, radiologique et biologique. Presse Médicale 71: 2091–2094

*McKusick V A 1972 Heritable disorders of connective tissue, 4th edn Mosby Saint Louis. Ch 11, p 521–686

McKusick V A, Howell R R, Hussels, I E, Neufeld E F, Stevenson R E 1972 Allelism, non-allelism and genetic compounds among the mucopolysaccharidoses. Lancet I: 993–996

*McKusick V A, Neufeld E F, Kelly T E 1978 The mucopolysaccharide storage diseases. In: Stanbury J B, Wyngaarden J B, Fredrickson D S (ed) The metabolic basis of inherited disease, 4th edn McGraw-Hill, New York. Ch 53, p 1290

*Neufeld E F 1974 The biochemical basis for mucopolysaccharidoses and mucolipidoses. Progress in Medical Genetics 10: 81–101

Neufeld E F, Liebaers I, Epstein C J, Yatziv S, Milunsky A, Migeon B R 1977 The Hunter syndrome in females: is there an autosomal recessive form of iduronate sulphatase deficiency? American Journal of Human Genetics 2: 455–461

Nwokoro N, Neufeld E F 1979 Detection of Hunter heterozygotes by enzymatic analysis of hair roots. American Journal of Human Genetics 31: 42–49

Pfeiffer R A, Kresse H, Bäumer N, Sattinger E 1977 Beta-glucuronidase deficiency in a girl with unusual clinical features. European Journal of Pediatrics 126: 155–161

*Rampini S U 1976 Klinik der Mukopolysaccharidosen. Enke, Stuttgart

Singh J, DiFerrante N, Niebes P, Tavella P 1976 N-acetylgalactosamine-6-sulphate sulphatase in man. Absence of the enzyme in Morquio disease. Journal of Clinical Investigation 57: 1036–1040

*Spranger J 1972 The systemic mucopolysaccharidoses. Ergebnisse der Inneren Medizin und Kinderheilkunde, Springer, Berlin, Heidelberg, New York 32: 165–265

Spranger J, Gehler J, O'Brien J F, Cantz M 1974 Chondroitin-sulphaturia with alpha-L-iduronidase deficiency. Lancet II: 1082

Spranger J, Cantz M, Gehler J, Liebaers I, Theiss W 1978 Mucopolysaccharidosis II (Hunter disease) with corneal opacities. European Journal of Pediatrics 129: 11–16

Stevenson R E, Howell R R, McKusick V A, Suskind R, Hanson J W, Elliott D E, Neufeld E F 1976 The iduronidase-deficient mucopolysaccharidoses: clinical and roentgenographic features. Pediatrics 57: 111–122

Van de Kamp J J P 1979 The Sanfilippo syndrome. Pasmans, 'S-Gravenhage

Winters P R, Harrod M J, Molenich-Heetred S A, Kirkpatrick J, Rosenberg R N 1976 Alpha-L-iduronidase deficiency and possible Hurler-Scheie genetic compound. Neurology 26: 1003–1007

Yatziv S, Erickson R P, Epstein C J 1977 Mild and severe Hunter syndrome (MPS II) within the same sibships. Clinical Genetics 11: 319–326

95

The oligosaccharidoses (formerly mucolipidoses)

J. G. Leroy

INTRODUCTION

The term mucolipidoses was introduced into the literature in the first comprehensive paper (Spranger & Wiedemann, 1970) on a number of hereditary disorders clinically related to both the mucopolysaccharidoses and the sphingolipidoses. Excessive urinary excretion of acid mucopolysaccharides (AMPS) is not observed in the mucolipidoses but dysostosis multiplex in varying degrees is reminiscent of the mucopolysaccharidoses, while macular cherry-red spot and demyelination in peripheral nerves in some of the entities provide links with the sphingolipidoses. Although useful as a concept, 'mucolipidosis' is a misnomer in the chemical sense because in most of the entities originally included there is no true storage of either mucopolysaccharides or lipids. There is ample evidence now that either directly or indirectly the metabolism of the carbohydrate in glycoproteins and glycolipids is adversely affected in the mucolipidoses, resulting in excess presence and excretion of oligosaccharides. Therefore the term oligosaccharidosis is proposed as a substitute for the common name mucolipidosis.

In Table 95.1 are listed the disorders which fit the definition of oligosaccharidosis. Most of the entities were already in the original list of mucolipidoses. Examples of recent entries are: sialidosis type 2, the Goldberg-Wenger syndrome and the Berman syndrome.

GENERAL CONSIDERATIONS ON GENETICS AND MANAGEMENT

Each one of the nosological entities among the oligosaccharidoses is inherited as an autosomal recessive trait with a recurrence risk of 1 in 4 for sibs of probands. All known primary metabolic defects involve lysosomal acid hydrolases (Table 95.1). Effective treatment is not available. Results of recent research on the oligosaccharidoses have explained why enzyme substitution therapy, as attempted in the past in some mucopolysaccharidoses and in some lipidoses, has been clinically ineffective (Sly,

1980). Although understanding of intracellular routing of endogenous lysosomal hydrolases and their receptor mediated endocytosis has considerably improved, the multiple and complex requisites for effective enzyme substitution therapy are unlikely to be met in the near future. Management of the oligosaccharidoses thus becomes an object for preventive medicine. Such prevention paradoxically finds its retrospective foundation in early diagnosis in the proband and its practical strategies in genetic counselling and prenatal diagnosis. Fetal monitoring by assay of the relevant lysosomal hydrolase in cultured amniotic fluid cells is available, even in both I-cell disease and pseudo-Hurler polydystrophy where advantage can be taken of the fact that many acid hydrolases are secondarily affected by the primary defect. Elective abortion is of ever increasing importance within the scheme of prevention.

Prospective preventive measures like mass screening programmes remain unrealistic. Detection of heterozygosity, though usually possible in the patients' parents, is not reliable in other relatives, because the ranges of specific enzyme activities in heterozygotes and homozygous normals overlap. Supportive management of the patients cannot be effective without simultaneous guidance to their parents and healthy sibs. It must include all modern clinical measures to deal with complications, and constant attention to their basic right to human happiness.

DISORDERS DUE TO DEFECTIVE RECOGNITION MARKER(S) ON LYSOSOMAL HYDROLASES

I-cell disease (mucolipidosis II)

Clinical manifestations

I-cell disease (ICD) is a slowly progressive disorder with clinical onset at birth and fatal outcome in childhood. The neonate with ICD has a low birth weight. His facies is plump and swollen, his skin thick and particularly stiff about the ears. Congenital herniae are consistently present in males. One or more orthopaedic abnormalities are common: clubfoot, dislocation of the hip(s), thoracic de-

Table 95.1 The oligosaccharidoses (mucolipidoses).

Synonymous designations of entities		Intracellular enzyme deficiency	
Current	Proposed	Primary	Secondary
(Mucolipidosis I)			
Infantile dysmorphic sialidosis (Sialidosis type 2)	Dysmorphic sialidosis Sialidosis type Spranger syndrome	glycoprotein sialidase	—
Normosomatic sialidosis Cherry-red spot–myoclonus syndrome (Sialidosis type 1)	Sialidosis type 2	glycoprotein sialidase	—
I-cell disease (Mucolipidosis II)		glucNac-1-phospho-* transferase	multiple acid hydrolases
Pseudo-Hurler polydystrophy (Mucolipidosis III)		glucNac-1-phospho-* transferase (possibly partial)	multiple acid hydrolases
Sialidase with β-galactosidase deficiency (juvenile dysmorphic sialidosis)	Goldberg-Wenger syndrome	stabilizing glycoprotein	glycoprotein sialidase β-D-galactosidase
Pseudo-G_{M1}-gangliosidosis	Infantile pseudo-gangliosidosis	stabilizing glycoprotein?	glycoprotein sialidase β-D-galactosidase
(Mucolipidosis IV)	Berman syndrome	ganglioside sialidase (?)	—
Mannosidosis	—	α-D-mannosidase	—
Fucosidosis	—	α-L-fucosidase	—
Mucosulphatidosis Multiple sulphatase deficiency	—	multiple sulphatases?	multiple sulphatases?

* Complete name of enzyme: UDP-N-acetylglucosamine: glycoprotein N-acetylglucosamine-1-phosphotransferase.
( ): designation no longer recommended.
The β-galactosidase deficiency states in infants and adolescents, also true oligosaccharidoses, are traditionally discussed with the sphingolipidoses.

formity or kyphosis. Despite generalized hypotonia the range of movement in the shoulders is already limited.

Unlike Hurler syndrome (MPS-IH) there is no temporary acceleration of skeletal growth around one year of age. Instead, growth decelerates within six months from birth and often ceases before fifteen months. Growth failure is always severe and a final height of 80 cm is rarely exceeded. Head size is proportional to stature. Stiffening of all joints occurs from the first year of life. Psychomotor retardation is extreme in some patients but rather mild in others. Upper respiratory infection and otitis recur frequently. Breathing is noisy. The facies resembles that of patients with MPS-IH but shows consistent differences: small orbits and hypoplastic supra-orbital ridges, prominence of the eyes, tortuous pattern of prominent periorbital veins, telangiectatic capillaries over midface and cheeks, impressive gingival swelling and prominent mouth. Hepatosplenomegaly is moderate or absent. The corneae are clear but haziness is found on slit lamp examination (Leroy et al, 1971). In the longer surviving patients, coarsening of facial features, broadening of hands and wrists and cardiac murmurs are common. The abdomen is protuberant with an umbilical hernia often present (Fig. 95.1A).

Bronchopneumonia and congestive heart failure are the usual causes of death.

Patients with ICD must be distinguished from those with either G_{M1}-gangliosidosis type 1, or infantile pseudogangliosidosis (see below). Confusion is less likely with MPS-IH patients or with children with either infantile dysmorphic sialidosis or nephrosialidosis (see below).

Within the clinical phenotype of ICD there exists more variation than is usually encountered in biochemically well defined autosomal recessive disorders. However affected sibs have very similar clinical features possibly indicating genetic heterogeneity between families.

Radiographic features

The radiological abnormalities in MPS-IH and in G_{M1}-gangliosidosis type 1 are qualitatively indistinguishable

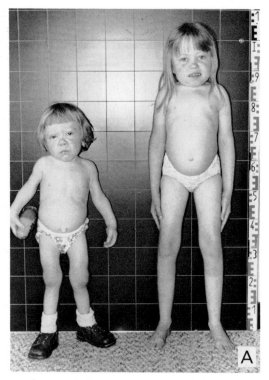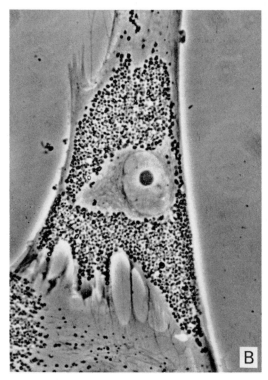

Fig. 95.1 (A) 3½ year-old patient with I-cell disease (left of figure) and next to her a 10 year-old girl with pseudo-Hurler polydystrophy. (B) Living inclusion cell (I-cell) as observed in the phase contrast microscope. A juxtanuclear zone, probably including the Golgi apparatus, is free of granular inclusions.

from those in ICD. Excessive periosteal new bone formation along the long tubular bones before one year of age is a feature shared with the patient having infantile G_{M1}-gangliosidosis. In ICD 'dysostosis multiplex', a term introduced to summarize the general radiographic findings in these and related disorders, is quantitatively most severe at any given time in the clinical course. Excellent radiographic descriptions are available (Spranger et al, 1974; Maroteaux, 1974). Radiographs most informative in making a diagnosis include lateral skull, lateral spine, anteroposterior thorax and pelvis, humerus and hands with wrists.

Laboratory findings: 'The I-cell phenomenon'; diagnosis
The name 'I-cell' disease originated from the observation in the phase contrast microscope of a large number of cytoplasmic granular inclusions in the patients' skin fibroblasts cultured in vitro (Fig. 95.1B). These cells were called 'Inclusion cells' or 'I-cells' and the corresponding disorder I-cell disease (Leroy & DeMars, 1967). The cytoplasmic inclusions are swollen lysosomes with pleomorphic contents as shown by electron microscopy (DeMars & Leroy, 1967; Tondeur et al, 1971; Hanai et al, 1971). The original definition of the 'I-cell' phenomenon was a morphological one. It was soon extended by

several biochemical findings, some of which are also apparent in vivo. In 'I-cells' the activity of a large number of lysosomal acid hydrolases is considerably decreased or absent (Leroy & Spranger, 1970; Leroy et al, 1972). These include the glycoprotein and ganglioside sialidases (Cantz & Messer, 1979; Pallman et al, 1980). The activity of the same acid hydrolases is greatly increased in the culture media of I-cells and also in the patients' extracellular fluids (Wiesmann et al, 1971a & b). In postmortem tissues the specific activity of β-D-galactosidase and of various sialidases is reduced, but that of other acid hydrolases is within normal limits (Leroy et al, 1972; Eto et al, 1979; Cantz & Messer, 1979; Pallman et al, 1980). Findings in leucocytes are inconsistent but probably similar.

Except for its presence also in pseudo-Hurler polydystrophy (see below) and although clearly a secondary effect of the genetic defect in each disorder, the I-cell phenomenon is of great diagnostic significance in ICD. The diagnosis made or suspected clinically is confirmed by the ten- to one hundred fold increase in serum hydrolase activity and also by the demonstration of the I-cell phenomenon in cultured skin fibroblasts.

The secondarily impaired degradation of glycoproteins is sufficiently extensive in vivo to result in excessive urinary excretion of several sialyloligosaccharides in ICD (Humbel, 1975). Although of considerable scientific interest (Strecker et al, 1977) this is only of limited value in diagnosis because a qualitatively similar abnormality is observed in the sialidoses.

Histopathology and chemical pathology

In an 8 month-old patient with severe psychomotor deficit, the single most characteristic pathological feature was the presence of a large number of cytoplasmic, unit membrane-bound vacuoles in connective tissue cells, irrespective of the organ in which they were located. Such abnormal cells were particularly abundant in skin, gums, heart valves and the zones of endochondral and membranous bone formation. Pericytes of capillaries, adventitial cells and Schwann and perineurial cells were affected. In the renal glomeruli there was foamy transformation only in the visceral and not in the parietal cells of Bowman's capsule. Changes in neurons and glial cells were minimal, inconsistent and possibly of a secondary nature. The heterogeneous osmiophilic bodies in hepatocytes were considered of questionable significance. Küpffer cells did not contain such dense bodies and appeared normal (Martin et al, 1975).

Although there is a need for more well controlled anatomical studies, these data indicate that in ICD connective tissue cells are primarily affected. Whereas in cultured fibroblasts the cytoplasmic granules are filled with pleomorphic material, the corresponding in vivo inclusions in mesenchymal cells are either empty or contain only sparse granulo-fibrillar material.

On the one hand there is neither histochemical nor biochemical evidence of significant storage of lipids, mucopolysaccharides or lipid- and protein-bound sialic acid in brain and visceral organs in ICD (Leroy et al, 1972; Dacremont et al, 1974; Martin et al, 1975; Berra et al, 1979; Eto et al, 1979). On the other hand I-cells accumulate $^{35}SO_4$-containing compounds including mucopolysaccharides (Schmickel et al, 1975) and lipids (Leroy et al, 1972) in addition to free and bound sialic acid (Thomas et al, 1976). Apparently the multiple enzyme deficiencies in I-cells, isolated in vitro from other tissues, result in storage of metabolites.

The I-cell phenomenon is not overt in postmortem organs, although the primary enzyme deficiency (see below) is expressed in these parenchymatous tissues (Waheed et al, 1982).

The primary metabolic defect

In cell strains derived from the patients' parents a small number of I-cells is consistently observed (DeMars & Leroy, 1967). In the serum of these obligate heterozygotes there is a slight but definite increase of several acid hydrolases (Van Elsen & Leroy, 1973; Van Elsen et al, 1976). This indicates that the I-cell phenomenon must be a direct consequence of the primary metabolic defect. Important progress on the nature of this defect stems from the in vitro observation of mutual complementation of faulty ^{35}S-AMPS degradation in cocultivated mutant cell strains from donors with genetically different mucopolysaccharidoses. This complementation was explained by intercellular exchange of distinct corrective factors subsequently identified as lysosomal hydrolases involved in AMPS breakdown, with the implication that these enzymes can be secreted by one cell in culture and taken up again by another (for a review see Neufeld, 1974). Uptake of extracellular enzymes is achieved through receptor-mediated pinocytosis. Also by this mechanism I-cells can take up extracellular bovine β-D-glucuronidase and human α-L-iduronidase (Hickman & Neufeld 1972). Once captured, the exogenous enzymes are maintained in I-cells and display a normal turnover rate, thus disproving the earlier hypothesis of excessive leakage from I-cells because of some membrane defect (Wiesmann et al, 1971a & b). However, α-L-iduronidase and β-D-glucuronidase obtained from I-cell culture medium are not taken up by indicator MPS-IH or MPS VII fibroblasts respectively, nor is ICD N-acetyl-β-D-hexosaminidase (hex) pinocytosed by a G_{M2}-gangliosidosis Sandhoff type cell strain. From this observation it has been surmised that the ICD primary metabolic defect is responsible for the lack in lysosomal hydrolases of a common recognition marker essential for their adsorption to specific receptors and subsequent internalization. Moreover, this observation led to Neufeld's secretion-recapture hypothesis about physiologic routing of lysosomal enzymes and their final targeting to lysosomes. Intercellular transfer of acid hydrolases is probably of only minor importance in human fibroblasts (Reuser et al, 1976; von Figura & Weber, 1978; Vladutiu & Ratazzi, 1979). However, studies of adsorptive uptake of lysosomal enzymes have identified the carbohydrate nature of their common recognition marker. Treatment with sodium iodonate does not alter the catalytic activity of normal hex but completely prevents pinocytosis (Hickman et al, 1974). Among preparations of lysosomal enzymes from non-ICD sources a 'high uptake' form, a more acidic glycoprotein equipped with the recognition marker, but also a 'low uptake' form without this marker can be distinguished. The latter form cannot be pinocytosed by normal fibroblasts (Glaser et al, 1975). Mannose-6-phosphate and phosphorylated mannans were found to be the most effective inhibitors of adsorptive pinocytosis of hydrolases, indicating that phosphorylated mannose is a likely part of the recognition site. Pretreatment with alkaline phosphatase converts the 'high uptake' form into the 'low uptake' form, abolishes receptor-mediated pinocytosis and underscores the role of the phosphate group(s) (Kaplan et al, 1977; Sando & Neufeld, 1977; Ullrich et al, 1978). Direct chemical analysis has also demonstrated the presence of mannose-6-phosphate in high mannose type oligosaccharides specifically released from urinary α-N-acetyl-glucosaminidase (von Figura & Klein, 1979), bovine testicular β-D-galactosidase (Distler et al, 1979) and human splenic β-glucuronidase (Natowicz et al, 1979) following treatment of the purified enzymes with endo β-N-acetylglucosaminidase H. According to Sly and Stahl (1978) the recognition marker is of crucial importance in intracellular segregation of precursor lysosomal enzymes and secretory proteins. Von Figura and Weber (1978) interpret their data as meaning that lysosomal enzymes in normal fibroblasts are cycled via the cell surface in a receptor-bound form before reaching the lysosomal apparatus, thus minimizing their release into the culture medium. Irrespective of the stage in their intracellular transport and processing at which the recognition role of mannose-6-phosphate is physiologically important, receptor-associated lysosomal enzymes are found at the normal cell surface and not at the surface of I-cells (von Figura & Voss, 1979). The failure of I-cells to retain their lysosomal hydrolases thus relates to a failure of these enzymes to bind to the plasma membrane. Hex in I-cells and I-cell medium is very deficient in phosphoester linked phosphate (Bach et al, 1979a). In I-cells phosphorylation and processing of the newly synthesized precursor proteins which are of larger molecular size than the mature intracellular hydrolases, does not occur. Large amounts of unphosphorylated enzymes are encountered in the culture medium. In control fibroblasts only small amounts of phosphorylated precursor are found extracellularly. Intralysosomal enzymes are fully processed and loose their phosphate recognition marker (Hasilik & Neufeld, 1980 a & b), which is needed to gain access to lysosomes but not to be retained (Sly & Stahl, 1978). A major portion of the $^{32}P_i$ groups in newly phosphorylated high mannose-type oligosaccharides in biosynthetic intermediates of lysosomal enzymes appear to be blocked by N-acetylglucosamine which renders the mannose-6-phosphate containing carbohydrate chains insensitive to alkaline phosphatase (Tabas & Kornfeld, 1980; Hasilik et al, 1980). During maturation of the acid hydrolase precursors a microsomal α-N-acetyl-glucosaminyl phosphodiesterase in rat liver and human fibroblasts can remove these blocking N-acetyl-glucosamine residues and thereby expose the mannose-6-phosphate recognition marker (Waheed et al, 1981; Varki & Kornfeld, 1980). This 'deblocking' enzyme is normal in I-cells.

The mere finding of the phosphodiesters suggested their formation by enzymatic transfer of N-acetylglucosamine-1-phosphate onto C_6 of mannose. It has recently been shown that glycopeptide of thyroglobulin and β-hexosaminidase dephosphorylated by acid hydrolysis and acting as acceptors can be phosphorylated by an enzyme in microsomes from rat liver, human

placenta, postmortem organs and normal human fibroblasts, in the presence of UDP-N-acetylglucosamine acting as the donor molecule. This reaction is highly deficient in fibroblasts and parenchymatous organs from patients with I-cell disease or pseudo-Hurler polydystrophy. Thus the primary defect in these disorders is a deficiency in UDP-N-acetylglucosamine: lysosomal hydrolase N-acetylglucosamine-1-phosphotransferase (Hasilik et al, 1981; Reitman et al, 1981; Waheed et al, 1982).

Pseudo-Hurler polydystrophy (mucolipidosis III)
This disorder has been delineated by Maroteaux (1966) and was called mucolipidosis III (Spranger & Wiedemann, 1970) before its biochemical alignment with ICD was known.

Clinical manifestations
Complaints of physical slowness, joint stiffness and slow mental development about the age of three years mark the clinical onset. The patient's facies is plump, and the range of movement in shoulders and hips already reduced. Growth rate is slower than normal and the head circumference remains proportional to stature, which is below normal in adults. The corneae are clear by inspection but show opacities on slit lamp examination. Liver and spleen are usually not enlarged (Kelly et al, 1975; Leroy & Van Elsen, 1975). Mental deficiency in ML III patients is mild and non-progressive (Fig. 95.1A). The course of the disease is very slow with increasing joint stiffness. ML III patients of advanced age have been reported (Langer quoted in Kelly et al, 1975) but insufficient data on life expectancy are available.

There is generalized osteoporosis. Bone age is considerably delayed. Dysostosis multiplex though variable between patients is generally mild, except for the severe and progressive lesions in the hips (Kelly et al, 1975; Spranger et al, 1974), where secondary arthritic changes are a considerable problem. Stiffness in the shoulders is of soft tissue origin. Urinary excretion of AMPS is normal. That of sialyl-oligosaccharides is excessive, complex and indistinguishable from that found in ICD urine (Humbel, 1975; Strecker et al, 1977; Sewell, 1980). This finding is nevertheless of orienting value for diagnosis.

Diagnosis; the relationship between ML III and ICD (ML II)
The I-cell phenomenon is apparent in ML III fibroblasts as in ICD cultures. Thus ML III derived cells are also I-cells. The activity of many acid hydrolases is considerably reduced in the cells and elevated in the conditioned culture media (Thomas et al, 1973; Berman et al, 1974a). The residual activity of β-D-galactosidase (Leroy & O'Brien, 1976) and of sialidase (Den Tandt & Leroy, 1980) is higher in 'I-cells' from ML III patients than in those from ICD donors. Contrary to findings in

ICD, in oligosaccharides isolated from ML III acid hydrolases a small amount of phosphorylation is encountered (Hasilik & Neufeld, 1980). It is tempting to correlate these findings with the milder clinical phenotype in ML III. Of direct diagnostic importance is the fact that in serum of ML III patients there is also a greatly increased activity of many acid hydrolases.

The dividing line between ML III patients and 'ICD' patients with mild mental handicap and protracted course may not be clear, but differences in growth rate, final height and degree of dysostosis multiplex form the strongest grounds for distinguishing between the two disorders.

The presence of the I-cell phenomenon in both disorders points towards a closely related pathogenesis, as has been proved by the finding of the same enzyme defect (Reitman et al, 1981). Complementation between ICD and ML III cell strains on the one hand, and between strains from different donors for either ICD or ML III on the other, has not been observed (Gravel et al, 1981). These results, based on a limited number of cell strains, favour the hypothesis that ICD and ML III are produced by homozygosity for different mutant alleles (tentatively symbolized by ml^2 and ml^3 in Table 95.2) at the single gene locus $|ML|$. Accordingly, genetic heterogeneity within either nosological entity would appear unlikely. However, earlier results by Champion and Shows (1977) were interpreted as favouring the existence of such heterogeneity. Using more extensive experimental data, Shows claims to be able to distinguish up to three complementation groups within ICD. The majority of patients would represent one group, only two patients a second, and only one a possible third group. Within ML III this author categorizes six patients in one, and two in a second complementation group (Shows, personal communication). If true, at least more than one $|ML|$ locus would have to be postulated.

Results of in vitro hybridization of pairs of I-cell strains will be more conclusive once the primary enzyme defect(s) themselves can be studied in this manner.

THE SIALIDOSES

Dysmorphic sialidosis Synonyms: Mucolipidosis I (ML I); Sialidosis type 1 (formerly sialidosis type 2); Spranger syndrome

Initially named lipomucopolysaccharidosis when first delineated in 1968 by Spranger, and renamed mucolipidosis I (ML I) upon introduction of the concept of the mucolipidoses (Spranger & Wiedemann, 1970), this disorder is the prototype among the sialidoses. Dysmorphic sialidosis, late infantile dysmorphic sialidosis, and less ideally sialidosis type 1, are acceptable alternative names for ML I, and together with the eponym Spran-

Table 95.2 Proposed gene loci and mutant alleles (minimal number) in the oligosaccharidoses with deficiency of glycoprotein sialidase and β-galactosidase.

Locus (tentative)	Clinical entity	Genotype (homozygous mutant)	Deficiency	
			sialidase (type)	β-galactosidase (type)
$|ML|$‡	I-cell disease (ML I)	ml^2/ml^2	yes★	yes★
	Pseudo-Hurler polydystrophy (ML III)	ml^3/ml^3	(secondary)	(secondary)
$|SIAL|$	Dysmorphic sialidosis; sialidosis type I; ML I	$sial^1/sial^1$		
	Normosomatic sialidosis; CRSM-syndrome; sialidosis type 2	$sial^2/sial^2$	yes (primary)	no
$|SG|$	Goldberg-Wenger syndrome (childhood type) (adolescence type)	sg^-/sg^- (multiple) alleles?)	yes (primary?) (secondary)	yes (secondary)
	Pseudo-gangliosidosis (infantile)			
$|GAL|$†	GM_1-gangliosidosis 1	gal^1/gal^1	no	yes (primary)
	GM_1-gangliosidosis 2	gal^2/gal^2		
	Gal⁻ chronic type	gal^3/gal^3		
	Gal⁻ Morquio type (MPS IVB)	gal^4/gal^4		

★ : among many other secondary enzyme deficiencies.
† : not discussed *in extenso* with the oligosaccharidoses.
‡ : more than one locus, with several alleles each, equally possible.

ger syndrome are preferable to the designation sialidosis type 2 (Lowden & O'Brien, 1979).

Clinical manifestations

Complaints of slow psychomotor development usually come in late infancy, when coarse facial features and thoracolumbar kyphosis are also noted. At first puffy face, depressed nasal bridge and broad maxilla are reminiscent of MPS-IH or hypothyroidism. Developmental landmarks are reached with delay. Intellectual development and physical growth are slower than normal, with height being below the third percentile between the ages of 3 and 5 yrs, when similarity of the facies with that in the Hurler syndrome becomes more striking. The lower median part of the nose has a bulbous shape with anteverted nostrils. Gingival hypertrophy is mild to moderate. The teeth are widely spaced, the tongue is enlarged and the maxillary part of the face prominent. The thoracic cage is barrel shaped, with pectus excavatum and thoracolumbar kyphosis. Hepatomegaly, although an early feature in some patients, is inconsistent or absent in others. Splenomegaly is rare. Herniae can be present. Sensorineural deafness is already present in early childhood. Ophthalmologic examination reveals a cherry-red macular spot, often strabismus and inconsistently cataract and corneal opacity. The clinical picture is only fully developed in late childhood, with the appearance of progressive ataxia and nystagmus, and by muscle wasting and loss of strength. Subsequently a coarse tremor and myoclonic jerks complete the neurologic syndrome. Mental deterioration is not a feature and seizures have not been observed, but sensory deficits, irregular deep tendon reflexes and decreased nerve conduction velocity are consistent indications of peripheral nerve involvement. Of interest is that limitation of large joint movements is only minimal and that the small joints of the hands are not affected. Progression of dysmorphic sialidosis is very slow. The patients become chair-bound from adolescence. Adverse effects of the neurologic deficits and pneumonia have been considered the causes of death in adolescence or early adulthood (Spranger et al, 1977; Kelly & Graetz, 1977; Winter et al, 1980).

Radiographic findings

The radiological manifestations of ML I can also be summarized by the term dysostosis multiplex. They progress slowly to a moderate degree of abnormality. The skull is mildly dolichocephalic and shows progressive thickening of the calvaria and sclerosis at the base. The vertebral bodies, initially of biconvex configuration, have irregular end plates. Ossification defects in the lower thoracic and upper lumbar region result in antero-inferior beaking of a few vertebrae. Kyphosis is prominent. Moderate scoliosis is often observed in addition to flaring of the iliac wings and mildly dysplastic acetabula. Short tubular bones show osteopenia and irregularly distributed coarse trabeculation (Spranger et al, 1974; Winter et al, 1980).

Histopathology and chemical pathology; diagnosis

Peripheral lymphocytes contain abnormal vacuoles. In bone marrow smears histiocytic cells have a foamy cytoplasm. Histopathologic changes are noticed in neurons as well as in mesenchymal and visceral cells. Hepatocytes as well as Küpffer cells are filled with cytoplasmic vacuoles and granules. Electron micrographs show enlarged membrane bound lysosome-like organelles filled with reticulo-granular material. These vesicular structures fill major portions of the cytoplasm (Freitag et al quoted in Spranger et al, 1977). At present the data on kidney pathology in ML I are still insufficient.

The discovery of an increased urinary excretion of several oligosaccharides (Humbel, 1975) led to the structural elucidation of these compounds as glycoprotein derived sialyloligosaccharides in which sialic acid residues occupy the terminal non-reducing position (Strecker et al, 1977 and Strecker's earlier work quoted therein). The urinary oligosaccharide pattern is typical in sialidosis patients and valuable in orienting further diagnostic study (Sewell, 1980). Similar oligosaccharides are less excessively excreted in ICD and in ML III urine. The latter observation among others leads to the now rejected hypothesis that sialidase deficiency would be the primary defect in ICD. More importantly, the pursuit of that hypothesis has led to the discovery that a profound deficiency of glycoprotein sialidase is the primary enzyme defect in sialidosis type 1 and in the other sialidoses (Cantz et al, 1977). As a consequence, the degradation of $\alpha 2 \rightarrow 3$ and $\alpha 2 \rightarrow 6$ neuraminosyl linkages in the sialoglycan parts of glycoprotein is impaired. The normal activity in ML I brain is explained by interference by the sialidase active towards gangliosides, which in brain and in cultured fibroblasts is unaffected (Pallman et al, 1980). On the contrary, in ICD both types of sialidase are secondarily impaired by the primary defect (Cantz & Messer, 1979).

The demonstration in fibroblasts of a deficiency of sialidase active towards water-soluble substrates establishes the diagnosis in the sialidoses. Here this deficiency is not associated with deficient intracellular activity of several other lysosomal hydrolases. Parents of patients with dysmorphic sialidosis, have intermediate sialidase activity (Cantz et al, 1977). The enzyme defect in patients can also be demonstrated in leucocytes.

Storage products have not been amply studied in sialidosis I. In brain there is an increase of lipid-bound and protein-bound sialic acid and of all gangliosides (Berra et al, 1979). The accumulation of free and bound sialic acid in sialidosis fibroblasts matches that in I-cells (Cantz & Messer, 1979).

Recently defined sialidoses

Almost simultaneously with the discovery of the primary metabolic defect in sialidosis type 1 (ML I) a deficiency of acid sialidase was found to be the enzyme defect in the cherry-red spot – myoclonus syndrome (CRSM syndrome) (O'Brien, 1977) and subsequently also in a condition called nephrosialidosis (Maroteaux et al, 1978). Because of the enzyme defect which these entities appear to share, and because of the accumulation and excessive urinary excretion of sialylated glycoproteins and oligosaccharides in each one of them, the common name sialidosis has been proposed (Durand et al, 1977). It should be reserved exclusively for the clinical conditions due to the isolated primary deficiency of glycoprotein sialidase (Lowden & O'Brien, 1979). The term sialidosis therefore does not include either ICD and ML III, or the syndromes associated with a combined deficiency of sialidase and β-galactosidase, although in all of these, excessive oligosacchariduria is observed.

Normosomatic sialidosis

Synonyms : Cherry-red spot–myoclonus (CRSM) syndrome; Sialidosis type 2 (formerly sialidosis type 1).

Sialidosis type 2 is here proposed as a synonym for the CRSM syndrome or normosomatic sialidosis instead of sialidosis type 1. The latter label has been introduced only recently in order to align the CRSM syndrome with ML I (Lowden & O'Brien, 1979) but in comparing them, such terminology is neither in line with the chronology of clinical delineation, nor with the age of onset or overall severity of the two disorders.

The designation CRSM syndrome correctly refers to the main clinical features: slowly progressive reduction of visual acuity with onset in some patients before ten years of age, and a crippling often generalized action myoclonus appearing in the second decade of life. A macular cherry-red spot is almost consistently found, but the time of its first appearance cannot be determined without prospective observations in younger sibs of probands. Seizures in these patients are not associated with loss of consciousness and probably represent repetitive bursts of generalized severe myoclonus. CRSM syndrome patients consistently have nystagmus. Initially some of them complain of burning pains in the limbs. Cerebellar ataxia is also reported but is hard to evaluate in the presence of much abnormal extrapyramidal activity. Important negatives in this syndrome are: absence of dysostosis multiplex even in patients with mild scoliosis; absence of psychomotor retardation and mental deficiency except for terminal deterioration; absence of corneal clouding even on slit-lamp examination and absence of facial coarsening. For a review to the original literature see Lowden and O'Brien (1979). Patients with the CRSM syndrome were recently reported by Rapin et al (1978), Thomas et al (1978) and Thomas et al

(1979). Patients with visual disturbance and cherry-red spot only and thus without any extrapyramidal sign (Durand et al, 1977) probably do not represent a separate entity, because in some patients a long time-lag between the onset of reduced vision and that of myoclonus is observed. Recently, peripheral neuropathy has been documented in the CRSM syndrome, thus linking also pathologically this entity to ML I (Steinman et al, 1980). The residual activity of sialidase is higher in fibroblasts from CRSM syndrome than in those from ML I patients (O'Brien & Warner, 1980). The parents of patients, have intermediate levels of sialidase activity (Thomas et al, 1978). Sialidosis type 1 (ML I) and sialidosis type 2 (CRSM syndrome) must be due to the homozygous state for either mutant allele $sial^1$ or $sial^2$ at a single locus symbolized here by $|SIAL|$ and assumed to determine the structure and function of acid lysosomal sialidase active towards water-soluble substrates (Table 95.2). This hypothesis finds its strongest basis in the lack of mutual enzymatic complementation in somatic cell hybrids between ML I and CRSM-strains (Hoogeveen et al, 1980).

Nephrosialidosis

The name nephrosialidosis has been given to the disorder initially described in two sibs with early appearing and severe clinical features of ML I associated with glomerular nephropathy, the latter being the cause of death in the older sib. Sialidase was deficient in both, and β-D-galactosidase was normal (Maroteaux et al, 1978, Den Tandt & Leroy, 1980). A somewhat similar patient has been reported recently (Aylsworth et al, 1980). The deficiency of sialidase was nearly complete against both the $2 \rightarrow 3$ and $2 \rightarrow 6$ isomers of ^{3}H-sialyllactitol and therefore not different from the deficiency in ML I. Because of the current lack of information on kidney pathology in ML I patients, it may be premature to consider nephrosialidosis as a separate clinical entity and to accept the existence of still another mutant allele ($sial^{ne}$) and a third homozygous mutant genotype at the $|SIAL|$ locus. It is equally possible that in nephrosialidosis the more severe part of the spectrum of clinical expression due to homozygosity of the $sial^1$ allele, is represented.

SYNDROMES ASSOCIATED WITH A COMBINED DEFICIENCY OF SIALIDASE AND β-D-GALACTOSIDASE

Within the oligosaccharidoses there are patients who have symptoms of both sialidosis and primary β-D-galactosidase deficiency. A rather severe deficiency of β-D-galactosidase in skin and conjunctival tissues was found by Goldberg et al (1971) who first described such a patient. Wenger et al (1978) have recently demonstrated that glycoprotein sialidase is also markedly reduced in similar patients. Two clinically different phenotypes can at present be distinguished. Firstly, a disorder with onset in childhood or adolescence which is named here the Goldberg-Wenger syndrome. Secondly, a severe disorder in neonates or infants with a rapidly fatal course, clinically indistinguishable from G_{M2}-generalized gangliosidosis type 1 (Gravel et al, 1979; Lowden et al, 1981). This disease, referred to here as infantile pseudo-gangliosidosis, is also associated with a combined deficiency of sialidase and β-galactosidase.

Evidence from somatic cell genetics strongly indicates that all patients with the combined enzyme deficiency, whatever the age of onset of their disease, belong to a single complementation group (Hoogeveen et al, 1980), governed by mutant alleles at a distinct gene locus, symbolized by |SG| (abbreviation of sialidase and galactosidase). The deficiency of β-D-galactosidase is found neither in all tissues, nor in plasma. The deficiency, where encountered, is less complete than in patients with isolated primary β-galactosidase deficiency. In obligate heterozygotes, β-D-galactosidase is normal, but sialidase activity is intermediate.

Recent experimental work suggests that the |SG| gene locus directs the synthesis of a nonenzymic phosphoglycoprotein of 32 000 daltons, which is secreted in the culture medium of normal cells and other mutants but not in that of fibroblasts derived from patients with the Goldberg-Wenger syndrome. This 'corrective factor' apparently is needed for protection of β-galactosidase against excessive proteolytic degradation and for stabilization as well as catalytic activation of sialidase (Hoogeveen et al, 1981; d'Azzo, 1982).

At present it is impossible to speculate on the number of different mutant alleles responsible for the conditions in the reported patients with the Goldberg-Wenger syndrome who differ mainly in age of onset ranging from less than 2 years (Andria et al, 1978) up to 18 years (Miyatake et al, 1979). Intrafamily variation between patients is smaller than interfamily differences, which favours the hypothesis of at least a small number of different homozygous mutant genotypes and of allelic heterogeneity.

The Goldberg-Wenger syndrome

The first proband presented as a patient with 'a new syndrome which combines clinical features of several storage diseases, but which is nonetheless unique'.

From several observations reported in the literature the following composite clinical picture can be drawn of patients with the Goldberg-Wenger syndrome. Clinical onset is most often early in the second decade of life but can occur even in childhood (Goldberg et al, 1971; Andria et al, 1978). The main signs and symptoms are

in four areas: (1) slowly progressive action myoclonus, related extrapyramidal movements and sometimes seizures; (2) decreasing visual acuity and cherry-red spot in the macula; (3) mild dysostosis multiplex, mild coarsening of facial features and moderately short stature; (4) moderate impairment of intellectual functioning, a constant feature though unusual in the initial stages of the disease. Hearing loss is occasionally present and angiokeratoma more consistently reported. There is no hepatomegaly in juvenile and adult patients. Nystagmus has not been observed. On slit-lamp examination most patients show corneal opacities. In addition to the patients already referred to, others have been reported by Koster et al (1976), Suzuki et al (1977) (four out of six cases) and Okada et al (1979).

In the past the Goldberg-Wenger syndrome has been confused with either or both ML I and the CRSM syndrome. See Table 95.3 for distinctive features. The differential diagnosis between the Goldberg-Wenger syndrome and the chronic disease type of primary β-D-galactosidase deficiency with onset in late childhood or adolescence is equally relevant (Wenger et al, 1980; Stevenson et al, 1977). Still another clinical variant of primary β-galactosidase deficiency is mentioned in Tables 95.2 and 95.3 by the designation gal⁻ Morquio-type. Mental retardation is absent in the latter type of patient with radiographic features reminiscent of the Morquio syndrome. Therefore this disorder, which has been described either as spondyloepiphyseal dysplasia (O'Brien et al, 1976) or grouped among the mucopolysaccharidoses as MPS IV B (Arbisser et al, 1977, Graebe et al, 1980) is easily distinguished from the Goldberg-Wenger syndrome.

Infantile pseudo-gangliosidosis

Three unrelated neonates presenting with a condition clinically almost indistinguishable from G_{M1}-gangliosidosis type 1 but with extensive oedema and ascites, have recently been diagnosed as having a combined deficiency of glycoprotein sialidase and β-galactosidase. One patient died as a newborn, the two others at six and eight months of age. They had a plump facies, depressed nasal bridge, cloudy corneae, macular cherry-red spot and conjunctival telangiectasia with similar lesions over the lower abdomen. In the longer surviving patients respiratory infection recurred frequently and both congestive heart failure and renal failure were the compounding causes of death in addition to anaemia and thrombocytopenia. Radiographically the skeletal changes were identical to those in G_{M1}-gangliosidosis and ICD. Large numbers of vacuolated leucocytes were present in peripheral blood smears. Urinary excretion of AMPS was normal, that of sialylated oligosaccharides excessive and typical. In the fibroblasts cultured from each patient the I-cell phenomenon was absent but glycoprotein sialidase was nearly

Table 95.3 Features of differential diagnostic significance in the late onset oligosaccharidoses.

Feature	Deficiency:	Pseudo-Hurler polydystrophy (ML III)	Normosomatic sialidosis (CRSM syndrome)	Goldberg-Wenger syndrome	Gal⁻ Chronic type	Gal⁻ Morquio type (MPS IV B)
		multiple acid hydrolases	sialidase	sialidase β-D-galactosidase	β-D-galactosidase	
Macular cherry-red spot		−	+	+	−	−
Corneal clouding (clinical inspection)		−	−	±	−	+
Myoclonus		−	++	+	−	−
Other neurologic symptoms		−	−	−	+(1)	+
Dysostosis multiplex		+(2)	−	+(2)	+(3)	+(3)
Facial coarsening		+	−	+	−	−
Mental Deficiency		±	−	+	++	−

(1) Rigidity; mild pyramidal signs; speech difficulty
(2) Mild
(3) Type spondyloepiphyseal dysostosis: mild to moderate

inactive. The level of β-galactosidase was much reduced, but less so than in G_{M1}-gangliosidosis cells. Sialic acid was found in large excess in the mutant fibroblasts. In cultured cells the activity of sialidase was intermediate between that in controls and in the patients, but β-galactosidase was normally active. Pairwise co-culture of, and somatic cell hybrid formation between, the cells from each of these probands and I-cells or G_{M1}-gangliosidosis fibroblasts showed complementation in all instances (Gravel et al, 1979; London et al, 1981). Complementation studies with cells from patients with the Goldberg-Wenger syndrome have not yet been performed.

THE BERMAN SYNDROME (MUCOLIPIDOSIS IV; ML IV)

From the time of its delineation by Berman et al (1974) this disorder has been aligned with the mucolipidoses, because of features shared with the mucopolysaccharidoses and the lipidoses. Until now it has been encountered in a few patients only in the Ashkenazi Jewish population. Following an uneventful neonatal period, signs of slowing psychomotor development are evident before the patients' first birthday. In some of them corneal clouding, a consistent and prominent feature of the disorder, is present from infancy. Loss of acquired motor skills occurs during the second year. A stable level of low grade environmental contact and severe mental deficiency is reached soon thereafter. Subsequently the disorder manifests little progression. Neurologic examination

reveals moderate hypotonia with hyperactive tendon reflexes and normal sensivity. Retinal degeneration has been observed. Lack of sufficient patient reports largely precludes any representative clinical description. The following negatives are noteworthy; there is neither facial coarsening, nor macrocephaly; skin, joint or bony abnormalities are not found; skeletal growth is unaffected; there is no true organomegaly, no excessive urinary excretion of acid mucopolysaccharides and no radiologic abnormalities of the skeleton (Berman et al, 1974; Merin et al, 1975; Tellez-Nagel et al, 1976).

The electron microscopic findings can be summarized as follows. Hepatocytes contain grossly abnormal lysosomal organelles filled with membranous cytoplasmic bodies of irregular structure and content, in addition to abnormally large amounts of glycogen and smooth endoplasmic reticulum. In contrast, the inclusions in Küpffer cells have a vacuolar appearance. Membranous lamellar inclusions and irregular vacuoles are present also in epithelial cells and fibroblasts in the conjunctiva (Berman et al, 1974). In neurons, oligodendrocytes, endothelial and perithelial cells, numerous dense bodies are found. Tellez-Nagel et al (1976) distinguish two types of typical inclusion in addition to bodies also encountered in gangliosidosis and lipofuscinosis.

In both grey and white matter the total ganglioside content is increased.

In fibroblasts a large number of lamellated multivesicular membranous bodies similar to those in hepatocytes are seen with the electron microscope. Vacuoles sometimes with loose granular content are equally abundant.

Under the phase contrast microscope the cultured skin fibroblasts are different from 'I-cells'. Because in amniotic cells cultured from at risk pregnancies inclusions similar to those in fibroblasts from patients have been found, prenatal diagnosis has been successful even before the elucidation of the primary genetic defect (Kohn et al, 1977). All lysosomal acid hydrolases routinely tested are normally active. In cultured ML IV fibroblasts increased levels of monosialo-G_{M3} and disialo-G_{D3} gangliosides and of sulphated mucopolysaccharides and hyaluronic acid are found (see references in Bach et al, 1979b) generating the hypothesis that a deficiency of a ganglioside sialidase is responsible for this syndrome. Bach et al (1979b) have already presented data in support of a reduced activity of solubilized ganglioside sialidase, probably of lysosomal origin, in ML IV fibroblasts. The activity of neuraminlactose sialidase appears unaffected in this disorder. Similar results were found in mutant amniotic cells (Bach et al, 1980). The final answer to the nature of the primary defect in ML IV may have to await the complete characterization and proper intracellular localization of the various cellular sialidases.

MANNOSIDOSIS

The nosological delineation of mannosidosis has almost coincided with the discovery of the responsible metabolic defect by Öckerman (1967a & b).

Clinical and radiographic features

The neonatal period is uneventful in mannosidosis, but even during the patients' first year of life recurrent respiratory infections and otitis require hospital admissions. Sitting up unaided and crawling usually occur at the normal time. Psychomotor progress slows in the second year and walking is achieved with delay or, in some instances, not at all as in the first recorded patient. Belated onset of speech and psychomotor retardation are the usual reasons for clinical evaluation. In childhood, signs and symptoms are: normal stature, macrocephaly, prominent forehead, plump facies, clear corneae, persistent epicanthic folds, low nasal bridge, noisy breathing, thick lips and prominent jaw and mouth. Joint mobility is minimally impaired. The abdomen is protuberant with an umbilical hernia as a rule. In boys inguinal herniae or hydroceles are common. Hepatosplenomegaly is mild to moderate in young patients, but disappears in adolescence. Thoracolumbar kyphosis, hearing loss of both the conductive and the sensorineural type, clumsy broad-based gait and deficiency of motor skills are almost always present. Although hypotonia is common, deep tendon reflexes are usually increased in the lower limbs. Occasionally hypertonia is found. Speech and language remain at an elementary level. This is probably related to both hearing difficulties and mental deficiency. The

patients' disposition is usually agreeable, but sudden episodes of anger or aggressiveness and periods of sleep disturbance are regularly reported. Ophthalmologic examination does not reveal any retinal changes but regularly detects cataract.

In most instances the clinical course is rather mild and barely progressive, with slowly coarsening facial and general body features. Data on life expectancy are scarce. Apparently most patients survive well into adulthood and are found among the mentally retarded with normal stature and hearing defects (Loeb et al, 1969; Autio et al, 1973; Farriaux et al, 1975; Booth et al, 1976; Kristler et al, 1977). Some patients are more severely affected (Aylsworth et al, 1976) and have a fatal course in childhood due to complications like attacks of vomiting, restlessness, dehydration and ketoacidosis (Kjellman et al, 1969) or refractory viral infection with respiratory failure, as in one patient with associated cellular immunodeficiency (Desnick et al, 1976). In sibs reported from Israel (Bach et al, 1978) corneal clouding was apparent. These patients, possibly examples of a variant mannosidosis, also showed marked limitation of joint mobility. In general the number of case reports is still too limited to assess fully the possibility of clinical heterogeneity.

Radiographic findings can be summarized as mild and slowly progressive dysostosis multiplex. Thickening and sclerosis of the calvaria and macrocephaly are the most consistent findings. Long tubular bones including clavicles and ribs, are undermodeled. The lumbar gibbus is associated with antero-inferior beaking of some lumbar vertebrae. The metacarpals and phalanges show slightly widened diaphyses, proximal pointing and coarse trabeculation. There is mild iliac flaring and coxa valga.

Deficiency of acid α-D-mannosidase; formal diagnosis

The diagnosis of mannosidosis is based on the demonstration in tissue or body fluids of a severe deficiency of lysosomal α-D-mannosidase with optimal activity near pH 4.5. In postmortem tissues of the original patient the large residual activity (Kjellman et al, 1969) was mainly due to isozymes active at more neutral pH (Carroll et al, 1972; Poenaru & Dreyfus, 1973). Precautions against other α-mannosidases which may interfere with the enzyme assay are particularly relevant when the artificial p-nitrophenyl- or 4-methylumbelliferyl-mannoside substrates are used.

The activity of α-D-mannosidase can be determined most easily in total homogenates of leucocytes and/or cultured fibroblasts, where at pH 4.2 interference of neutral isozymes is negligible and the specific activity of lysosomal α-D-mannosidase in mannosidosis is but a few per cent of that in controls. Similar results in cultured amniotic fluid cells and postmortem organs respectively establish prenatal diagnosis or confirmation of mannosidosis. By DEAE-cellulose chromatography normal tissue acid α-D-mannosidase is resolved into two components called A and B (Phillips et al, 1974a). Both are activated by Zn^{2+} and inhibited by Co^{2+} and EDTA. Both are deficient in mannosidosis, where the corresponding mutant enzyme is activated by Co^{2+} (Desnick et al, 1976; Halley et al, 1980). The neutral enzyme peak C is eluted at slightly higher salt concentration. This cytosolic enzyme is unaffected in mannosidosis and activated by Co^{2+}. There is no immunological cross-reaction between the C form and antibodies raised against the acidic forms of α-D-mannosidase (Phillips et al, 1975).

In human plasma or serum, the 'intermediate' form of α-D-mannosidase is predominant and the lysosomal enzyme much less abundant. The former is thermolabile at 56° C and most active at pH 5.5–6.0 (Hirani et al, 1977), but the latter is thermostable. Serum or plasma lysosomal mannosidase can be measured at its pH optimum of 4.6 most reliably only after thermoinactivation (56° C) of the samples dialysed against phosphate buffered saline (Hirani & Winchester, 1980; Van Elsen & Leroy, 1981). In some instances, an apparent increase in the K_m value of the mutant α-D-mannosidase has been found (Beaudet & Nichols, 1976; Desnick et al, 1976; Halley et al, 1980). Too few patients have been studied in this way to correlate differences in enzyme substrate affinity with clinical heterogeneity.

A neurodegenerative disorder with autosomal recessive inheritance, also known as mannosidosis, exists in Angus cattle (Phillips et al, 1974b) and has been detected in cats (Burditt et al, 1980). Deficiency of the lysosomal α-D-mannosidase is the responsible metabolic defect in both animal models.

Histopathology and chemical pathology

Vacuolization in peripheral lymphocytes is very prominent in all patients reported. In liver tissue numerous clear vacuoles of varying sizes are seen in hepatocytes and even more so in Küpffer cells. In the former the contents of the cellular inclusions exist in histiocytes of bone marrow, in endothelial cells of sinusoid vessels and in lymphocytes of spleen and lymph nodes (Kjellman et al, 1969; Loeb et al, 1968; Autio et al, 1973; Desnick et al, 1976; Kistler et al, 1977). Throughout the central nervous system the cytoplasm of neurons is distended, being packed with an abundance of single membrane-bound vacuoles with remarkably clear, sparsely dispersed reticulogranular material (Kjellman et al, 1969; Desnick et al, 1976). The severe morphologic changes in hepatocytes and neurons are not due to storage of large macromolecules but to accumulation of abnormal amounts of mannose-containing oligosaccharides derived from improperly degraded carbohydrate chains in glycoproteins (Öckerman, 1969). That mannosidosis must be considered an oligosaccharidosis is shown by the dem-

onstration of excessive urinary excretion of mannose containing-oligosaccharides (Fig. 95.2) by simple screening tests of silicagel thin layer chromatography (Humbel, 1975; Sewell, 1980). With more refined methods of analytical chemistry the structure of the oligosaccharides excreted has been worked out in detail (Strecker, 1977) thus relating the mannose-rich metabolites to the lysosomal enzyme defect.

FUCOSIDOSIS

This disorder was originally recognized as an atypical mucopolysaccharidosis (Durand et al, 1966; Durand et al, 1968) with normal urinary excretion of AMPS. With the demonstration that the vacuoles in peripheral lymphocytes and liver are abnormally swollen lysosomes, a search among the lysosomal hydrolases for the responsible metabolic defect led to the finding of a profound deficiency in tissues and body fluids of α-L-fucosidase (Van Hoof & Hers, 1968).

Clinical and radiographic findings

An initial symptom free interval of six to twelve months is followed by frequent upper respiratory infections at the time when delay in psychomotor development becomes overt. Physical examination at this stage reveals a slightly coarse facies, thickened lips and tongue, thick skin and generalized hypotonia with depressed deep tendon reflexes. Some patients never learn to walk alone. Abundant sweating with increased salinity of the sweat has been noticed in young patients. Subcutaneous and epidermal changes are discussed later. Slowing of linear growth occurs from about the age of two years (Loeb et al, 1969b; Durand et al, 1969; Patel et al, 1972). Mild hepatosplenomegaly, inconsistently observed in early childhood, is absent in older patients. Mild thoracolumbar kyphosis and cardiomegaly are more often radiographic than clinical findings. The corneae are clear and the opthalmologic findings normal except for some tortuosity and irregularity of calibre in the retinal vessels (Libert et al, 1977). Before three years of age, and earlier in some patients, the clinical course is characterized by progressive loss of motor skills, apathy, hypertonia and spasticity with hyperreflexia, sometimes seizures, increasing mental deterioration and finally dementia and decerebrate rigidity. Patients with this natural course extending over only a few years (Durand et al, 1969) or a slightly longer period (Loeb et al, 1969) succumb to complications of their neurodegenerative disease. Patients manifesting these various features have been considered examples of fucosidosis type 1 (Tondeur, 1977).

The observation of several patients with severe mental deficiency, an almost non-progressive disease, mild

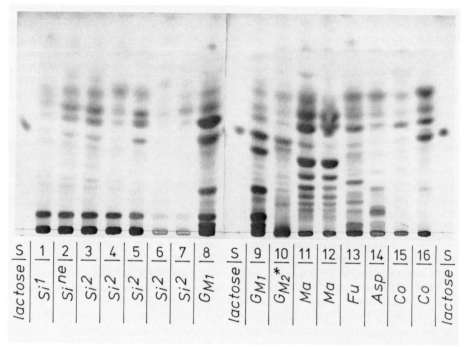

Fig. 95.2 Thin-layer chromatograms of urinary oligosaccharides. (Courtesy of Dr G. Strecker, Lille, France). Silica gel 60 (Merck) plates; development in n-butanol/acetic acid/water (2 : 1: 1; v/v); compounds visualized with orcinol (Humbel, 1975).

S	: Standard
1, 5	: Dysmorphic sialidosis
2	: Nephrosialidosis
3, 4 6, 7 }	: Normosomatic sialidosis
8, 9	: G_{M1} gangliosidosis type 1
10	: G_{M2} gangliosidosis (*type Sandhoff)
11, 12	: Mannosidosis
13	: Fucosidosis
14	: Aspartylglucosaminuria (not discussed in text.)
15, 16	: Control urine

radiographic abnormalities, angiokeratoma and telangiectasia, reported when in their teens or twenties (Patel et al, 1972; Gatti et al, 1973; Kousseff et al, 1973; Borrone et al, 1974; MacPhee et al, 1975), prompted the suggestion of a second phenotype, fucosidosis type 2. These patients, surviving beyond adolescence and into early adulthood, probably represent the majority of cases. Late in their disease they have recurrent attacks of dehydration due to inability to control body temperature (Patel et al, 1972).

As more information becomes available on the overall course of fucosidosis, the extent of the clinical spectrum and the frequency of signs and symptoms, the hypothesis of two distinct clinical phenotypes can hardly be maintained. Vascular markings and skin lesions are not exclusively seen in older patients with slow evolution. Even in early childhood extensive subcutaneous telangiectasia may be found especially on the thenar and hypothenar eminences, on the lateral aspect of the sole and also over

the thorax. Pinhead-sized skin lesions similar to angiokeratoma in Fabry disease may also develop on many regions of the body even during childhood (Patel et al, 1972; Kousseff et al, 1973; Gatti et al, 1973). Patients with either type of disease have been observed in one large pedigree (Durand et al, 1976). In somatic cell hybridization experiments with fibroblast cultures derived from either type of patient, no mutual complementation is observed (Beratis et al, 1976), indicating that allelic mutations at a single gene locus would be the most likely explanation if indeed two clinically different types of fucosidosis exist.

Radiographic changes are either absent or mild in young patients. Skeletal age lags behind the patients' chronologic age. Lumbar vertebrae are either slightly hypoplastic or normal in the presence of dorsolumbar kyphosis. Thus true dysostosis multiplex is not encountered in fucosidosis. Instead, mild spondyloepiphyseal dysplasia is often found in longer surviving subjects.

α-L-Fucosidase deficiency; formal diagnosis

Assay of α-L-fucosidase in leucocytes using the fluorescent 4-methyl-umbelliferyl-α-L-fucopyranoside as a substrate is at present the method of choice for establishing or excluding the diagnosis of fucosidosis (Robinson & Thorpe, 1974). The profound deficiency of α-L-fucosidase found in tissues (Patel et al, 1972; Matsuda et al, 1973; MacPhee et al, 1975; Borrone et al, 1974) is similar in both patients with rapidly advancing disease and those with the more protracted course, although critical comparison of results obtained in different laboratories with different methods of enzyme assay is impossible.

α-L-Fucosidase deficiency has been shown in liver, brain, kidney and other visceral organs (Van Hoof & Hers, 1968; Loeb et al, 1968; Robinson & Thorpe, 1974) and in cultured fibroblasts (Zielke et al, 1972; Matsuda et al, 1973). No material cross-reacting against anti-'wild-type' fucosidase antibodies has been detected in liver (Alhadeff et al, 1975) and fibroblasts (Thorpe & Robinson, 1978) of patients. The normal intracellular enzyme has a broad pH optimum about 5.5. A multiplicity of molecular forms can be revealed by various resolution techniques which partly explains the peculiar pH optimum. In fucosidosis all isozymes of α-L-fucosidase, identified by isoelectric focusing and known to differ slightly in sialic acid content, are deficient (Alhadeff et al, 1974).

Determination of α-L-fucosidase activity in serum is of no value in the diagnosis of fucosidosis because in about 12% of normal individuals the average serum enzyme activity is only about 5% of that in the rest of the population (Ng et al, 1976). In these normal individuals with variant α-L-fucosidase in serum, the enzyme in leucocytes has normal activity.

Pathological findings

Weakly PAS positive vacuoles are found in peripheral lymphocytes. In hepatocytes studied with the electron microscope two types of unit-membrane bound cytoplasmic vacuoles are seen: one type has very light, loosely structured contents; the other type is filled with rounded osmiophilic lamellar structures. The Küpffer cells contain similar vacuole-like structures. Also histiocytes, glomerular endothelium, epithelial and other cell types in conjunctiva and skin (irrespective of the presence of angiokeratoma) as well as bronchial and rectal mucosa endothelial cells are swollen by similar lysosome-like structures (Libert et al, 1977). In brain, neuronal and myelin loss is considerable. In the small proportion of neurons left, large unit-membrane bound vacuoles are consistently observed.

Fucose-containing oligosaccharides are excreted excessively in the urine (Strecker, 1977). Simple screening by thin layer chromatography can distinguish the pattern of oligosaccharide excretion in fucosidosis from that in other oligosaccharidoses, provided the appropriate known samples are included in the study (Humbel, 1975) (Fig. 95.2). In brain and liver, fucose containing glycosylceramide is considerably increased (Dawson, 1972). In fucosidosis, increased antigenicity of the fucose containing blood group substances would be expected and has actually been observed (Staal et al, 1977).

The complexity of the products stored is part of the reason why enzyme study is the most important means of establishing the diagnosis, although urinary screening for oligosaccharides and electron microscopic study of skin or conjunctiva biopsy specimens are important in directing the efforts of the biochemistry laboratory.

MUCOSULPHATIDOSIS; MULTIPLE SULPHATASE DEFICIENCY

The first patients with this apparently rare disorder were described by Austin who subsequently found a deficiency of several sulphatases (Austin et al, 1965). The clinical phenotype is a composite of features encountered in some of the mucopolysaccharidoses and components also seen in metachromatic leucodystrophy.

Clinically, the disorder manifests itself late in the first year of life with psychomotor retardation, moderate hepatosplenomegaly, recurrent respiratory infections, inguinal herniae in males, radiographic features of dysostosis multiplex, and increased urinary excretion of AMPS. Information on urinary oligosaccharide excretion is not yet available. The skin can show scaling. Neurodegenerative symptoms are apparent before two years of age with loss of acquired skills, progressive quadriplegia, ataxia, nystagmus, convulsions, decrease and loss of vision and hearing. The corneae are clear. Ophthalmologic examination shows loss of retinal pigment, grey maculae and atrophy of the optic nerve disks. The disorder ends fatally before adolescence and sometimes in early childhood.

A few patients have been described with multiple sulphatase deficiencies. The diagnosis can be made formally by demonstrating deficiencies of lysosomal arylsulphatases A and B and of microsomal arylsulphatase C. Several other sulphatases have also been found deficient. For the data on chemical pathology, histopathology and molecular aspects of the sulphatases involved, the reader is referred to well documented reviews (Austin, 1973; Dulaney & Moser, 1978).

REFERENCES

Alhadeff J A, Miller A L, Wenger D A, O'Brien J S 1974 Electrophoretic forms of human liver α-L-fucosidase and their relationship to fucosidosis (mucopolysaccharidosis F). Clinica Chimica Acta 57: 307–313

Alhadeff J A, Miller A L, Wenaas H, Vedvick T, O'Brien J S 1975 Human liver α-L-fucosidase. Purification, characterisation and immunochemical studies. Journal of Biological Chemistry 250: 7106–7113

Andria G, Del Giudice E, Reuser A J J 1978 Atypical expression of β-galactosidase deficiency in a child with Hurler-like features but without neurological abnormalities. Clinical Genetics 14: 16–23

Arbisser A I, Donnelli K A, Scott C I, Di Ferrante N, Singh J, Stevenson R E, Aylsworth A S, Howell R R 1977 Morquio-like syndrome with β-galactosidase deficiency and normal hexosamine sulfatase activity: Mucopolysaccharidosis IV B. American Journal of Medical Genetics 1: 195–205

Austin J H 1973 Studies in metachromatic leukodystrophy. XII. Multiple sulfatase deficiency. Archives of Neurology 28: 258–264

Austin J, Armstrong D, Shearer L 1965 Metachromatic form of diffuse cerebral sclerosis. V The nature and significance of low sulfatase activity : a controlled study of brain, liver and kidney in four patients with MLD. Archives of Neurology 13: 593–614

Autio S, Norden N E, Öckerman P A, Riekkinen P, Rapola J, Louhimo T 1973 Mannosidosis : clinical, fine-structural and biochemical findings in three cases. Acta Paediatrica Scandinavica 62: 555–565

Aylsworth A S, Taylor H A, Stuart C M, Thomas G H 1976 Mannosidosis : phenotype of a severely affected child and characterization of α-mannosidase activity in cultured fibroblasts from the patient and his parents. Journal of Pediatrics 88: 814–818

Aylsworth A S, Thomas G H, Hood J L, Libert J 1980 A severe infantile sialidosis: clinical biochemical and microscopic features. Journal of Pediatrics 96: 662–668

Bach G, Kohn G, Lasch E E, Massri M E, Ornoy A, Sekeles E, Legum C, Cohen M M 1978 A new variant of mannosidosis with increased enzymatic activity and mild clinical manifestation. Pediatric Research 12: 1010–1015

Bach G, Bargal R, Cantz M 1979a I-cell disease : deficiency of extracellular hydrolase phosphorylation. Biochemical and Biophysical Research Communications 91: 976–981

Bach G, Zeigler M, Schaap T, Kohn G 1979b Mucolipidosis type IV: ganglioside sialidase deficiency. Biochemical and Biophysical Research Communications 90: 1341–1347

Bach G, Zeigler M, Kohn G 1980 Biochemical investigations of cultured amniotic fluid cells in Mucolipidosis type IV. Clinica Chimica Acta 106: 121–128

Beaudet A L, Nichols B L 1976 Residual altered α-mannosidase in human mannosidosis. Biochemical and Biophysical Research Communications 68: 292–297

Beratis N G, Turner B M, Hirschhorn K 1976 Reply: on genetic variants in fucosidosis. Journal of Pediatrics 89: 690

Berman E R, Kohn G, Yatziv S, Stein H 1974a Acid hydrolase deficiencies and abnormal glycoproteins in Mucolipidosis III. Clinica Chimica Acta 52: 115–124

Berman E R, Livni H, Shapira E, Merin S, Levij S I 1974b Congenital corneal clouding with abnormal systemic storage bodies: a new variant of mucolipidosis. Journal of Pediatrics 84: 519–526

Berra B, Di Palma S, Lindi C, Sandhoff K 1979 Content of gangliosides and protein-bound sialic acid in post-mortem brain of patients with mucolipidosis I and II (ML I and ML II). Cell and Molecular Biology 25: 281–284

Booth C W, Chen K K, Nadler H L 1976 Mannosidosis : clinical and biochemical studies in a family of affected adolescents and adults. Journal of Pediatrics 88: 821–824

Borrone G, Gatti R, Trias X, Durand P 1974 Fucosidosis : clinical, biochemical, immunologic and genetic studies in two new cases. Journal of Pediatrics 84: 727–730

Burditt L J, Chotai K, Hirani S, Nugent P G, Winchester B G 1980 Biochemical studies on a case of feline mannosidosis. Biochemical Journal 189: 467–473

Cantz M, Gehler J, Spranger J 1977 Mucolipidosis I : increased sialic acid content and deficiency of an α-N-acetyl-neuraminidase in cultured fibroblasts. Biochemical and Biophysical Research Communications 74: 732–738

Cantz M, Messer H 1979 Oligosaccharide and ganglioside neuraminidase activities of mucolipidosis I (sialidosis) and mucolipidosis II (I-cell disease) fibroblasts. European Journal of Biochemistry 79: 113–118

Carroll N, Dance N, Masson P K, Robinson D, Winchester B G 1972 Human mannosidosis. The enzymic defect. Biochemical and Biophysical Research Communications 49: 579–583

Champion M J, Shows T B 1977 Correction of human mucolipidosis II enzyme abnormalities in somatic cell hybrids. Nature 270: 64–66

Dacremont G, Kint J A, Cocquyt G 1974 Brain sphingolipids in I-cell disease (mucolipidosis II). Journal of Neurochemistry 22: 599–602

Dawson G 1972 Glycosphingolipid abnormalities in liver from patients with glycosphingolipid and mucopolysaccharide storage diseases. In: Volk B W, Aronson S M (eds) Sphingolipids, Sphingolipidoses and Allied Disorders, Plenum Press, New York. p 395–413

d'Azzo A 1982 Multiple lysosomal enzyme deficiency in man. Doctorial Thesis. Rotterdam, The Netherlands

DeMars R I, Leroy J G 1967 The remarkable cells cultured from a human with Hurler's syndrome : An approach to visual selection for in vitro genetic studies. In vitro 2: 107–118

Den Tandt W R, Leroy J G 1980 Deficiency of neuraminidase in the sialidoses and the mucolipidoses. Human Genetics 53: 383–388

Desnick R J, Sharp H L, Grabowski G A, Brunning R D, Quie P G, Sung J H, Gorlin R J, Ikonne J U 1976 Mannosidosis: clinical, morphologic, immunologic and biochemical studies. Pediatric Research 10: 985–996

Distler J, Hieber V, Sahagian G, Schmickel R, Jourdian G W 1979 Identification of mannose-6-phosphate in glycoproteins that inhibit the assimilation of β-galactosidase by fibroblasts. Proceedings of the National Academy of Sciences USA 76: 4235–4239

Dulaney J T, Moser H W 1978 Sulfatide lipidosis : metachromatic leucodystrophy. In: Stanbury J B, Wyngaarden J B, Fredrickson D S (eds) The Metabolic Basis of Inherited Disease, 4th edn McGraw-Hill, New York. p 770–809

Durand P, Borrone C, Della Cella G 1966 A new mucopolysaccharide lipid storage disease. Lancet ii: 1313

Durand P, Borrone C, Della Cella G, Philippart M 1968 Fucosidosis. Lancet i: 1198

Durand P, Borrone C, Della Cella 1969 Fucosidosis.

Journal of Pediatrics 75: 665–674

Durand P, Borrone C, Gatti R 1976 On genetic variants in fucosidosis. Journal of Pediatrics 89: 688–690

Durand P, Gatti R, Cavalieri S, Borrone C, Tondeur M, Michalski J C, Strecker G 1977 Sialidosis (Mucolipidosis I). Helvetica Paediatrica Acta 32: 391–400

Eto Y, Owada M, Katagawa T, Kokubun Y, Rennert O W 1979 Neurochemical abnormality in I-cell disease : chemical analysis and a possible importance of β-galactosidase deficiency. Journal of Neurochemistry 32: 397–405

Farriaux J P, Legouis I, Humbel R, Dhondt J L, Richard P, Strecker G, Fourmaintraux A, Ringel J, Fontaine G 1975 La Mannosidose. A propos de 5 observations. La Nouvelle Presse Médicale 4: 1867–1870

Gatti R, Borrone C, Trias X, Durand P 1973 Genetic heterogeneity in fucosidosis. Lancet ii: 1024

Glaser J H, Roozen K J, Brot F E, Sly W S 1975 Multiple isoelectric and recognition forms of human β-glucuronidase activity. Archives of Biochemistry and Biophysics 166: 536–542

Goldberg M, Cotlier E, Fichenscher L G, Kenyon K, Enat R, Borowsky S A 1971 Macular cherry-red spot, corneal clouding and β-galactosidase deficiency. Archives of Internal Medicine. 128: 387–398

Gravel R A, Lowden J A, Callahan J W, Wolfe L S, Ng Yin Kin N M K 1979 Infantile sialidosis: a phenocopy of type 1 G_{M1} gangliosidosis distinguished by genetic complementation and urinary oligosaccharides. American Journal of Human Genetics 31: 669–679

Gravel R A, Gravel Y L, Miller A L, Lowden J A 1981 Genetic complementation analysis of I-cell disease and pseudo-Hurler polydystrophy. In: Callahan J W, Lowden J A (eds) Lysosomes and lysosomal storage diseases, Raven Press, New York

Groebe H, Krins M, Schmidberger H, von Figura K, Harzer K, Kresse H, Paschke E, Sewell A, Ullrich K 1980 Morquio syndrome (mucopolysaccharidosis IV B) associated with β-galactosidase deficiency. Report of two cases. American Journal of Human Genetics 32: 258–272

Halley D J J, Winchester B G, Burditt L J, d'Azzo A, Robinson D, Galjaard H 1980 Comparison of the α-mannosidases in fibroblast cultures from patients with mannosidosis and mucolipidosis II and from controls. Biochemical Journal 187: 541–543

Hanai J, Leroy J G, O'Brien J S 1971 Ultrastructure of cultured fibroblasts in I-cell disease. American Journal of Diseases of Children 122: 34–38

Hasilik A, Neufeld E F 1980a Biosynthesis of lysosomal enzymes in fibroblasts. Synthesis as precursors of higher molecular weight. Journal of Biological Chemistry 255: 4937–4945

Hasilik A, Neufeld E F 1980b Biosynthesis of lysosomal enzymes in fibroblasts. Phosphorylation of mannose residues. Journal of Biological Chemistry 255: 4946–4950

Hasilik A, Klein U, Waheed A, Strecker G, von Figura K 1980 Phosphorylated oligosaccharides in lysosomal enzymes: identification of p-N-acetylglucosamine (1)-phospho (6) mannose diester groups. Proceedings of the National Academy of Sciences USA 77: 7074–7078

Hasilik A, Waheed A, von Figura K 1981 Enzymatic phosphorylation of lysosomal enzymes in the presence of UDP-N-acetylglucosamine. Absence of the activity in I-cell fibroblasts. Biochemical Biophysical Research Communications 98: 761–767

Hickman S, Neufeld E F 1972 A hypothesis for I-cell disease: defective hydrolases that do not enter lysosomes.

Biochemical Biophysical Research Communications 49: 992–999

Hickman S, Shapiro L J, Neufeld E F 1974 A recognition marker required for uptake of a lysosomal enzyme by cultured fibroblasts. Biochemical Biophysical Research Communications 57: 55–61

Hirani S, Winchester B G, Patrick A D 1977 Measurement of the α-mannosidase activities in human plasma by a differential assay. Clinica Chimica Acta 81: 135–144

Hirani S, Winchester B G 1980 Plasma α-D-mannosidase in mucolipidosis II and mucolipidosis III. Clinica Chimica Acta 101: 251–256

Hoogeveen A T, Verheyen F W, d'Azzo A, Galjaard H 1980 Genetic heterogeneity in human neuraminidase deficiency Nature 285: 500–502

Hoogeveen A, d'Azzo A, Brossmer R, Galjaard H 1981 Correction of combined β-galactosidase/neuraminidase deficiency in human fibroblasts. Biochemical Biophysical Research Communications 103: 292–300

Humbel R 1975 Biochemical screening for mucopolysaccharidosis, mucolipidosis and oligosaccharidosis. Helvetica Paediatrica Acta 30: 191–200

Kaplan A, Fischer D, Achard D, Sly W 1977 Phosphohexosyl recognition is a general characteristic of pinocytosis of lysosomal glycosidases by human fibroblasts. Journal of Clinical Investigation 60: 1088–1093

Kelly T E, Thomas G H, Taylor H A, McKusick V A, Sly W S, Glaser J H, Robinow M, Luzzati L, Espiritu C, Feingold M, Bull M J, Ashenhurst E M, Ives E J 1975 Mucolipidosis III (pseudo-Hurler polydystrophy): clinical and laboratory studies in a series of 12 patients. Johns Hopkins Medical Journal 137: 156–175

Kelly T E, Graetz G 1977 Isolated acid neuraminidase deficiency : a distinct lysosomal storage disease. American Journal of Medical Genetics 1: 3–46

Kistler J P, Lott I T, Kolodny E H, Friedman R B, Nersasian R, Schnur J, Mihm M C, Dvorak A, Dickersin R 1977 Mannosidosis : new clinical presentation, enzyme studies and carbohydrate analysis. Archives of Neurology 34: 45–51

Kjellman B, Gamstorp I, Brun A, Öckerman P A, Palmgren B 1969 Mannosidosis : a clinical and histopathologic study. Journal of Pediatrics 75: 366–373

Kohn G, Livni N, Ornoy A, Sekeles E, Beyth Y, Legum C, Bach G, Cohen M M 1977 Prenatal diagnosis of mucolipidosis IV by electron microscopy. Journal of Pediatrics 90: 62–66

Koster J F, Niermeyer M F, Loonen M C B, Galjaard H 1976 β-galactosidase deficiency in an adult : a biochemical and somatic cell genetic study on a variant of G_{M1}-gangliosidosis. Clinical Genetics 9: 427–432

Kousseff B G, Beratis N G, Danesino C, Hirschhorn K 1973 Lancet ii: 1387–1388

Leroy J G, DeMars R I 1967 Mutant enzymatic and cytological phenotypes in cultured human fibroblasts. Science 157: 804–806

Leroy J G, Spranger J W 1970 I-cell disease (cont.) New England Journal of Medicine 283: 598–599

Leroy J G, Spranger J W, Feingold M, Opitz J M, Crocker A C 1971 I-cell disease: a clinical picture. Journal of Pediatrics 79: 360–365

Leroy J G, Ho M-W, MacBrinn M C , Zielke K, Jacob J, O'Brien J S 1972 I-cell disease : biochemical studies. Pediatric Research 6: 752–759

Leroy J G, Van Elsen A F 1975 Natural history of a mucolipidosis. Twin girls discordant for ML III. Birth Defects : Original Article Series XI(6): 325–334

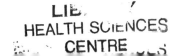

Leroy J G, O'Brien J S 1976 Mucolipidosis II and III : different residual activity of beta-galactosidase in cultured fibroblasts. Clinical Genetics 9: 533–539

Libert J, Tondeur M, Martin J J 1977 La fucosidose : aspects anatomopathologiques et microscopie électronique. In: Farriaux J P (ed) Les oligosaccharidoses, Crouan & Roques, Lille. p 51–58

Loeb H, Tondeur M, Toppet M, Cremer N 1969a Clinical, biochemical and ultrastructural studies of an atypical form of mucopolysaccharidosis. Acta Paediatrica Scandinavica 58: 220–228

Loeb H, Tondeur M, Jonniaux G, Mockel-Pohl S, Vamos-Hurwitz 1969b Biochemical and ultrastructural studies in a case of mucopolysaccharidosis 'F' (Fucosidosis). Helvetica Paediatrica Acta 24: 519–537

Lowden J A, O'Brien J S 1979 Sialidosis : a review of human neuraminidase deficiency. American Journal of Human Genetics 31: 1–18

Lowden J A, Cutz E, Skomorowski M A 1981 Infantile type 2 sialidosis with β-galactosidase deficiency. In: Tettamanti G, Durand P, Di Donato S (eds) Sialidases and Sialidoses, Edi. Ermes, Milan, p 261–280

MacPhee G B, Logan R W, Primrose D A A 1975 Fucosidosis: how many cases undetected? Lancet ii: 462–463

Maroteaux P 1982 Maladies osseuses de l'enfant. 2nd Edition. Flammarion, Paris.

Maroteaux P, Humbel R, Strecker G, Michalski J C, Maude R 1978 Un nouveau type de sialidose avec atteinte rénale : la néphrosialidose. Archives Françaises de Pédiatrie 35: 819–829

Martin J J, Leroy J G, Farriaux J-P, Fontaine G, Desnick R J, Cabello A 1975 I-cell disease (mucolipidosis II). A report on its pathology. Acta Neuropathologica (Berlin) 33: 285–305

Matsuda I, Arashima S, Anakura M, Ege A, Hayata I 1973 Fucosidosis. Tohuku Journal of Experimental Medicine 109: 41–48

Merin S, Livni N, Berman E R, Yatziv S 1975 Mucolipidosis IV. Ocular, systemic and ultrastructural findings. Investigative Ophthalmology 14: 437–448

Miyatake T, Atsumi Y, Obayaski T, Mizuno Y, Ando S, Ariga T, Matsui-Nakamura K, Yamada T 1979 Adult type neuronal storage disease with neuraminidase deficiency. Annals of Neurology 6: 232–244

Natowicz M R, Chi M M-Y, Lowry O H, Sly W S 1979 Enzymatic identification of mannose-6-phosphate on the recognition marker for receptor-mediated pinocytosis of β-glucuronidase by human fibroblasts. Proceedings of the National Academy of Sciences USA 76: 4322–4326

Neufeld E F 1974 The biochemical basis for mucopolysaccharidoses and mucolipidoses. Progress in Medical Genetics 10: 81–101

Ng W G, Donnell G N, Koch R, Bergren W R 1976 Biochemical and genetic studies of plasma and leucocyte α-L-fucosidase. American Journal of Human Genetics 28: 42–50

O'Brien J S 1977 Neuraminidase deficiency in the cherry red spot-myoclonus syndrome. Biochemical Biophysical Research Communications 79: 1136–1141

O'Brien J S, Gugler E, Giedeon A, Wiesmann U, Herschkowitz N, Meier C, Leroy J 1976 Spondyloepiphyseal dysplasia, corneal clouding, normal intelligence and acid β-galactosidase deficiency. Clinical Genetics 9: 495–504

O'Brien J S, Warner T G 1980 Sialidosis: delineation of subtypes by neuraminidase assay. Clinical Genetics 17: 35–38

Öckerman P A 1967a A generalized storage disorder resembling Hurler's syndrome. Lancet ii: 239–241

Öckerman P A 1967b Deficiency of beta-galactosidase and alpha-mannosidase: primary enzyme defects in gargoylism and a new generalized disease. Acta Paediatrica Scandinavica 177: 35–36

Öckerman P A 1969 Mannosidosis: isolation of oligosaccharide storage material from brain. Journal of Pediatrics 75: 360–365

Okada S, Yutaka T, Kato T, Ikehara C, Yabuuchi H, Okawa M, Inui M, Chiyo H 1979 A case of neuraminidase deficiency associated with a partial β-galactosidase defect. European Journal of Pediatrics 130: 239–249

Pallman B, Sandhoff K, Berra B, Miyatake T 1980 Sialidase in brain and fibroblasts in three patients with different types of sialidosis. In: Svennerholm L, Mandel P, Dreyfus H, Urban P F (eds) Structure and function of gangliosides, Plenum Press, New York. p 401–414

Patel V, Watanabe I, Zeman W 1972 Deficiency of α-L-fucosidase. Science 176: 426–427

Phillips N C, Robinson D, Winchester B G 1974a Human liver α-D-mannosidase activity. Clinica Chimica Acta 55: 11–19

Phillips N C, Robinson D, Winchester B G, Jolly R D 1974b Mannosidosis in Angus Cattle. Biochemical Journal 137: 363–371

Phillips N, Robinson D, Winchester B 1975 Immunological characterization of human liver α-D-mannosidase. Biochemical Journal 151: 469–475

Poenaru L, Dreyfus J C 1973 Electrophoretic heterogeneity of human α-mannosidase. Biochimica et Biophysica Acta 303: 171–174

Rapin I, Goldfischer S, Katzman R, Engel J, O'Brien J S 1978 The cherry-red spot-myoclonus syndrome. Annals of Neurology 3: 234–242

Reitman M L, Vaski A, Kornfeld S 1981 Fibroblasts from patients with I-Cell disease and pseudo-Hurler polydystrophy are deficient in uridine 5'-diphosphate N-acetylglucosamine: glycoprotein N-acetylglucosaminylphospho-transferase activity. Journal of Clinical Investigation 67: 1574–1579

Reuser A, Halley D, de Wit E, Hoogeveen A, van der Kamp M, Mulder M, Galjaard H 1976 Intercellular exchange of lysosomal enzymes : enzyme assays in single human fibroblasts after cocultivation. Biochemical Biophysical Research Communications 69: 311–318

Robinson D, Thorpe R 1974 Fluorescent assay of α-L-fucosidase. Clinica Chimica Acta 55: 65–69

Sando G N, Neufeld E F 1977 Recognition and receptor-mediated uptake of a lysosomal enzyme, α-L-iduronidase, by cultured human fibroblasts. Cell 12: 619–627

Schmickel R D, Distler J, Jourdian G W 1975 Accumulation of sulfate-containing acid mucopolysaccharides in I-cell fibroblasts. Journal of Laboratory and Clinical Medicine 86: 672–682

Sewell A C 1980 Urinary oligosaccharide excretion in disorders of glycolipid, glycoprotein and glycogen metabolism. European Journal of Pediatrics 134: 183–194

Sly W S 1980 Multiple recognition forms of human β-glucuronidase and their pinocytosis receptors: implications for enzyme therapy. Birth Defects: Original Article Series 16(1): 115–128

Sly W, Stahl P 1978 Receptor-mediated uptake of lysosomal enzymes. In: Silverstein S C (ed) Transport of Macromolecules in Cellular Systems, Dahlem Konferenzen, Abakon Berlin. p 229–244

Spranger J W, Wiedemann H-R 1970 The genetic mucolipidoses. Humangenetik 9: 113–139

Spranger J, Langer L O, Wiedemann H-R 1974 Bone dysplasias, Fisher, Stuttgart

Spranger J, Gehler J, Cantz M 1977 Mucolipidosis I-a sialidosis. American Journal of Medical Genetics 1: 21–29

Staal G E J, Van Der Heyden McM, Troost J, Moes M, Borst-Eilers E 1977 Fucosidosis and Lewis substances. Clinica Chimica Acta 76: 155–157

Steinman L, Tharp B R, Dorfman L J, Forno L S, Sogg R L, Kelts K A, O'Brien J S 1979 Peripheral neuropathy in the cherry-red spot-myoclonus syndrome (sialidosis type I). Annals of Neurology 7: 450–456

Stevenson R E, Taylor H A, Parks S E 1978 β-galactosidase deficiency: prolonged survival in three patients following early central nervous system deterioration. Clinical Genetics 13: 305–313

Strecker G 1977 Glycoproteines et glycoprotéinoses. In: Farriaux J P (ed) Les Oligosaccharidoses. Crouan & Roques, Lille. p 13–30

Strecker G, Peers M-C, Michalski J-C, Hondi-Assah T, Fournet B, Spik G, Montreuil J, Farriaux J-P, Maroteaux P, Durand P 1977 Structure of nine sialyloligosaccharides accumulated in urine of eleven patients with three different types of sialidosis. European Journal of Biochemistry 75: 391–403

Suzuki Y, Nakamura N, Fukuoka K, Shimada Y, Uono M 1977 β-galactosidase deficiency in juvenile and adult patients. Human Genetics 36: 219–229

Tabas I, Kornfeld S 1980 Biosynthetic intermediates of β-glucuronidase contain high mannose oligosaccharides with blocked phosphate residues. Journal of Biological Chemistry 255: 6633–6639

Tellez-Nagel I, Rapin I, Iwamoto T, Johnson A B, Norton W T, Nitowsky H 1976 Mucolipidosis IV. Clinical, ultrastructural, histochemical and chemical studies of a case including a brain biopsy. Archives of Neurology 33: 828–835

Thomas G H, Taylor H A, Reynolds L W, Miller C S 1973 Mucolipidosis III (pseudo-Hurler polydystrophy) Multiple lysosomal enzyme abnormalities in serum and cultured fibroblast cells. Pediatric Research 7: 751–756

Thomas G H, Tiller G E, Reynolds L W, Miller C S, Bace J W 1976 Increased levels of sialic acid associated with a sialidase deficiency in I-cell disease (Mucolipidosis II) fibroblasts. Biochemical Biophysical Research Communications 71: 188–195

Thomas G H, Tipton R E, Ch'ien L T, Reynolds L W, Miller C S 1978 Sialidase (α-N-acetyl-neuraminidase) deficiency: the enzyme defect in an adult with macular cherry-red spots and myoclonus without dementia 13: 369–379

Thomas P K, Abrams J D, Swallow D, Stewart G 1979 Sialidosis type 1: cherry red spot-myoclonus syndrome with sialidase deficiency and altered electrophoretic mobilities of some enzymes known to be glycoproteins. Journal of Neurology, Neurosurgery and Psychiatry 42: 873–880

Thorpe R, Robinson D 1978 Purification and serological studies of human α-L-fucosidase in the normal and fucosidosis states. Clinica Chimica Acta 86: 21–30

Tondeur M, Vamos-Hurwitz E, Mockel-Pohl S, Dereume J P, Cremer N, Loeb H 1971 Clinical, biochemical and ultrastructural studies in a case of chondrodystrophy presenting the I-cell phenotype in tissue culture. Journal of Pediatrics 79: 366–378

Tondeur M 1977 La fucosidose. In Farriaux J P (ed) Les Oligosaccharidoses, Crouan & Roques, Lille, p 43–49

Ullrich K, Mersmann G, Weber E, von Figura K 1978 Evidence for lysosomal enzyme recognition by human fibroblasts via a phosphorylated carbohydrate moiety. Biochemical Journal 170: 643–650

Van Elsen A F, Leroy J G 1973 I-cell disease (mucolipidosis II). Serum hydrolases in obligate heterozygotes. Humangenetik 20: 119–123

Van Elsen A F, Leroy J G, Vanneuville F J, Vercruyssen A L 1976 Isoenzymes of serum N-acetyl-beta-D-glucosaminidase in the I-cell disease heterozygote. Human Genetics 31: 75–81

Van Elsen A F, Leroy J G 1981 α-D-Mannosidases in serum of patients with I-cell disease (ICD). Clinica Chimica Acta 112: 159–165

Van Hoof F, Hers H-G, 1968 Mucopolysaccharidosis by absence of α-fucosidase. Lancet i: 1198

Varki A, Kornfeld S 1980 Identification of a rat liver α-N-acetylglucosaminyl phosphodiesterase capable of removing 'Blocking' α-N-acetylglucosamine residues from phosphorylated high mannose oligosaccharides of lysosomal enzymes. Journal of Biological Chemistry 255: 8398–8401

Vladutiu G D, Ratazzi M C 1979 Excretion reuptake route of β-hexosaminidase in normal and I-cell disease cultured fibroblasts. Journal of Clinical Investigation 63: 595–601

von Figura K, Weber E 1978 An alternative hypothesis of cellular transport of lysosomal enzymes in fibroblasts. Biochemical Journal 176: 943–950

von Figura K, Klein U 1979 Isolation and characterization of phosphorylated oligosaccharides from α-N-acetylglucos-aminidase that are recognized by cell-surface receptors. European Journal of Biochemistry 94: 347–354

von Figura K, Voss B 1979 Cell-surface-associated lysosomal enzymes in cultured human skin fibroblasts. Experimental Cell Research 121: 267–276

Waheed A, Pohlman R, Hasilik A, von Figura K 1981 Subcellular location of two enzymes involved in the synthesis of phosphorylated recognition markers in lysosomal enzymes. Journal of Biological Chemistry 256: 4150–4152

Waheed A, Pohlman R, Hasilik A, von Figura K, van Elsen A, Leroy J 1982 Deficiency of UDP-N-acetylglucosamine: lysosomal enzyme N-acetylglucosamine-1-phosphotransferase in organs of I-cell patients. Biochemical Biophysical Research Communications 105: 1052–1058

Wenger D A, Tarby T J, Wharton C 1978 Macular cherry-red spot and myoclonus with dementia: coexistent neuraminidase and β-galactosidase deficiencies. Biochemical Biophysical Research Communications 82: 589–595

Wenger D A, Sattler M, Mueller O T, Myers G G, Schneiman R S, Nixon G W 1980 Adult G_{M1} gangliosidosis: clinical and biochemical studies on two patients and comparison to other patients called variant or adult G_{M1} gangliosidosis. Clinical Genetics 17: 323–334

Wiesmann U N, Lightbody J, Vassella F, Herschkowitz N N 1971a Multiple lysosomal enzyme deficiency due to enzyme leakage? New England Journal of Medicine 284: 109–110

Wiesmann U N, Vassella D, Herschkowitz N N 1971b I-cell disease: leakage of lysosomal enzymes into extracellular fluids. New England Journal of Medicine 285: 1090–1091

Winter R M, Swallow D M, Baraitser M, Purkiss P 1980 Sialidosis type 2 (acid neuraminidase deficiency): clinical and biochemical features of a further case. Clinical Genetics 18: 203–210

Zielke K, Veath M L, O'Brien J S 1972 Fucosidosis: deficiency of α-L-fucosidase in cultured skin fibroblasts. Journal of Experimental Medicine 136: 197–199

96

The gangliosidoses and related lipid storage diseases

A.K. Percy

INTRODUCTION

Recent clinical and biochemical advances have dramatically expanded our understanding of the gangliosidoses and related disorders. As a group, these disorders share the following features in common: (1) they are genetic; (2) they are characterized, with notable exceptions, by degenerative processes affecting the central and/or peripheral nervous system; (3) they involve the tissue storage in abnormal concentration of a normal lipid or glycolipid and in some cases a glycoprotein or mucopolysaccharide as well; and (4) the molecular defect in many of them is the deficiency of a lysosomal acid hydrolase. The gangliosides and related sphingolipids have been implicated in a group of lipid storage diseases called the sphingolipidoses. The spingolipidoses will be described in the context of the accumulated sphingolipid and the relevant biochemical defect (Brady, 1978; Pilz et al, 1979; Sandhoff & Christomanou, 1979; Svennerholm, 1969). A separate group of CNS storage diseases, the neuronal ceroid lipofuscinoses, is less well understood in terms of a specific biochemical abnormality (Zeman & Siakotos, 1973). Four clinically distinct entities will be discussed. Finally, five other disorders of lipid metabolism involving tissue storage will be outlined (Lowden & O'Brien, 1979; Percy et al, 1979).

HISTORICAL ASPECTS

The gangliosidoses and related sphingolipidoses represent the culmination of clinical and laboratory observations extending back 100 years. Clinical and pathological descriptions for each of these disorders have been available for many years. Our understanding of the molecular basis of these disorders however, has only occurred in the last quarter century. One of these disorders, Tay-Sachs disease, provides a perspective. With his description, in 1881, of a child with generalized weakness and cherry-red macular degeneration, Waren Tay signaled a century of àctivity involving many biomedical disciplines

and culminating in our present understanding of the sphingolipidoses.

Following the identification and characterization of the stored lipid utilizing improved techniques in lipid chemistry (Svennerholm, 1962), the biochemical lesion could then be defined (Okada & O'Brien, 1969). This biochemical definition however, did not represent the end of this story. Rather the need for interdisciplinary collaboration has expanded with the awareness of heterogeneity within many of these disorders and with the clinical implications relative to accurate clinical diagnosis, genetic counselling and prenatal detection.

CLINICAL CONSIDERATIONS

Pathogenetic correlations

The disorders of lipid storage share a common biochemical pathogenesis. The storage or accumulation of a specific compound might represent excess synthesis and/or deficient degradation of the accumulated material. In each disorder with a defined biochemical lesion, lipid storage is the result of deficient activity of a specific degradative enzyme with one exception, G_{M3}-gangliosidosis. In particular, the sphingolipidoses represent the deficiency of a specific lysosomal (degradative) enzyme with the resultant intracellular (lysosomal and cytoplasmic) accumulation of sphingolipid or other lipid material.

Lipids are important constituents of all biological membranes participating critically in cell structure and function. Individual lipid constituents exhibit considerable variability from tissue to tissue, particularly, among the specialized membranes of the nervous system. As might be anticipated, the lipid storage diseases, especially, the sphingolipidoses, reflect the tissue distribution of the disease-related lipid.

In general, the sphingolipidoses involving the central nervous system may be divided into two groups, one group predominantly affecting the white matter or myelin-containing portion of the nervous system and thus called *leukodystrophies*, the second impinging on neuronal or gray matter processes. Storage of sphingolipids which predominate in the white matter, namely galactosyl-cer-amide and sulphatide, is representative of diseases in the former group. Since the leukodystrophies generally have their onset during infancy and early childhood, the prin-cipal initial manifestations of these white matter disor-ders are delay or decline in motor development and abnormalities of gait along with upper motor neuron or long tract findings. Disorders of the second group are represented by the gangliosidoses and are accompanied by early symptoms including seizures, intellectual diffi-culties, and visual abnormalities. This clinical formula-tion of entities involving gray or white matter pertains only during first stages of the disease. As the process advances, dysfunction of the nervous system dissemi-nates and specificity of white or gray matter involvement is lost. The concept, however, may focus the diagnostic process during the initial clinical assessment (Freeman & McKhann, 1969).

Biochemical basis

The stored materials in most of the disorders considered in this chapter belong to a class of compounds known as sphingolipids. A preliminary understanding of the struc-ture of these compounds is necessary for an appreciation of the clinical-biochemical correlations.

Definition and tissue localization

The sphingolipids are a group of compounds sharing a common basic component called ceramide (Fig. 96.1). Ceramide is a long chain amino alcohol to which is attached a fatty acid covalently linked to the amino group. The individual sphingolipids are formed by the addition of specific groups to the terminal alcohol posi-tion of ceramide. The unique physicochemical charac-teristics of each sphingolipid derives from this particular side chain. With the single exception of sphingomyelin, one or more of the hexose units, glucose, galactose or N-acetylgalactosamine , is added to the alcohol group. Sev-eral of the sphingolipids are uncharged at physiological pH, but three types, the sulphatides, the sphingomye-lins, and the gangliosides have a charged group(s) under physiological conditions. The fatty acid chain length may vary from 14 to 26 carbon units particularly in neural tissue where longer chain fatty acids are found predom-inantly.

The gangliosides, a sub-group of the sphingolipids are characterized by N-acetyl-neuraminic acid (NANA, sialic acid) linked covalently to the hexose units. Gan-gliosides vary in two respects: (1) length of sugar side chain may vary from two to four hexose groups, and (2) the number of NANA groups per molecule may vary

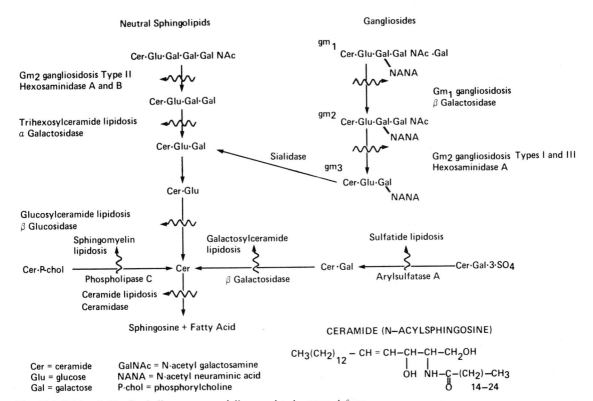

Fig. 96.1 Sphingolipids. Catabolic sequence and disease-related enzyme defects.

from one to four. At least ten chemically-distinct gangliosides have been identified.

The sphingolipids are ubiquitous in human tissues (Mårtensson, 1969), principally as components of cellular membranes. The concentration of the individual sphingolipids varies greatly from tissue to tissue. For example, the neutral sphingolipid, glucosylceramide is a common constituent of liver and spleen yet is not present in significant quantity in neural tissue (Svennerholm et al, 1963). Hence, the principal clinical manifestations of glucosylceramidosis (Gaucher disease) involve the liver and spleen. Conversely, galactosylceramide and sulphatides are prominent constituents of the nervous system, particularly of myelin, and to a lesser extent, of kidney. Disorders involving these lipids affect the nervous system predominantly. Globoside is the major glycosphingolipid in kidney and erythrocytes. Sphingomyelin is prominent in all human membranes.

Gangliosides with four hexose units attached to the ceramide and one or more NANA derivatives are major components of neurons and neuronal membranes and may be integrally involved in synaptic transmission. The smallest ganglioside, G_{M3}, predominates in non-neutral tissues, where it may comprise more than 70% of the total ganglioside fraction (Svennerholm, 1970).

Metabolic interrelations
As one might suspect from the common chemical backbone , the sphingolipids are closely linked in terms of their metabolism. Biosynthesis reflects enzyme-mediated addition of the various relevant substituents to ceramide in sequential fashion utilizing appropriate uridyl or cytidyl nucleotides. Sphingolipid degradation is also stepwise involving specific hydrolases acting at the free terminal, non-reducing end of the sugar chain. Should any one hydrolase be missing, or be present in rate-limiting amounts, degradation cannot proceed. Total degradation of a glycosphingolipid, thus, requires the action, sequentially and in concert, of a series of enzymes each having a very high degree of specificity for the terminal sugar and for the anomeric configuration of the glycosidic bond (Fig. 96.1).

Beginning in 1964, a deficiency in the activity of each of these degradative enzymes has been linked with a human genetic disorder. A specific catabolic enzyme deficiency interrupts the metabolic sequence and the sphingolipid preceding the defective enzyme accumulates. In general, this accumulation occurs in the tissue(s) where the relevant sphingolipid or one of its precursors is a prominent constituent. That is, storage of neural sphingolipids invariably results in neural dysfunction whereas deposition of predominantly extra-neural sphingolipids manifests visceral involvement and may even spare the central nervous system. Regardless, the sphingolipid accumulation within the cell occurs, at least in part, within the *lysosomes*, the subcellular site of the degradative (hydrolytic) enzymes.

Lysosomes are important subcellular organelles containing enzymes which perform vital housekeeping chores within the cell by degrading or hydrolyzing complex compounds to small molecules which can then be recycled or eliminated. Lysosomes, identified by de Duve and coworkers (1955), are intracellular organelles which are membrane-bound and which contain a repertoire of hydrolytic enzymes optimally-active at acid pH. These enzymes are primarily involved in the degradation of intralysosomal macromolecules which represent either the turnover of normal cellular constituents or are molecules imbibed by pinocytosis. Having postulated that some human diseases might be due to the deficient activity of a lysosomal hydrolase resulting in intralysosomal accumulation of various molecules, Hers (1963) demonstrated the deficiency of an acid glucosidase in Type II glycogen storage disease. Similar deficiencies were soon described for the sphingolipid storage diseases. Austin et al (1965) reported deficiency of arylsulphatase A in metachromatic leukodystrophy, and Brady and coworkers (1965) found a reduced level of glucocerebrosidase activity in Gaucher's disease. Since that time, hydrolase deficiencies in most of the other 'lipid storage' diseases have been established.

THE SPHINGOLIPIDOSES

The storage of each major sphingolipid (Fig. 96.1) has now been associated with a clinical disorder (Table 96.1). Dysfunction of the central nervous system is a prominent feature in each disorder with the exception of Fabry disease , and variant forms of Gaucher and Niemann-Pick disease.

Presently, there are nine distinct diseases representing accumulation of a specific sphingolipid. One or more variant forms (Table 96.1) differing in age at onset, in clinical presentation as reflected in the tissues involved, and in clinical course have been identified for several of these disorders. Differences in enzyme substrate specificity, tissue distribution, or residual activity may account for the observed variability in these disorders.

Present nomenclature is based on the disease-related lipid and the known metabolic interrelationship of the sphingolipids. While the familiar eponyms are included, the biochemical classification better describes this family of disorders.

Gangliosidoses

G_{M1} gangliosidoses
G_{M1} gangliosidoses are characterized by the accumulation of the ganglioside, G_{M1} (Fig. 96.1). Presently, two forms

Table 96.1 Sphingolipidoses: clinical and biological features

Disease	Clinical features	Stored material	Enzyme defect
I. G_{M1}-gangliosidosis *Type I*: Onset – infancy Death by age 2	psychomotor deterioration Hurler-like appearance hepatomegaly	G_{M1}-ganglioside asialo G_{M1}-ganglioside, keratansulfate	β-galactosidase isoenzymes A, B, C
Type II Onset – 6–12 mos. Death by age 3–10	psychomotor deterioration	Same	β-galactosidase isoenzymes B, C
II. G_{M2}-gangliosidosis *Type I* – Tay-Sachs Onset – 6–12 mos. Death by age 5	psychomotor deterioration cherry-red maculae seizures	G_{M2} ganglioside asialo G_{M2}–analogue	Hexosaminidase A
Type II – Sandhoff Onset – 6–12 mos. Death by 5 yrs.	psychomotor deterioration cherry-red maculae visceromegaly	G_{M2}–ganglioside asialo G_{M2}-analogue globoside in viscera	Hexosaminidase A & B
Type III – Juvenile Onset – 2–5 yrs Death by age 15	psychomotor deterioration gait disturbance	G_{M2}–ganglioside asialo-G_{M2}-analogue	Hexosaminidase A
III. G_{M3}-gangliosidosis Onset at birth Death in infancy	psychomotor deterioration seizures macroglossia	G_{M3}–ganglioside	galactosamine transferase
IV. Sphingomyelin lipidosis *Type I* – infantile (85%) Onset in infancy Death by age 4	psychomotor deterioration hepatosplenomegaly	sphingomyelin	sphingomyelinase (phospholipase C)
Type II – adult Onset in childhood Prolonged survival	hepatomegaly pulmonary infections	sphingomyelin (brain spared)	sphingomyelinase (phospholipase C)
Type III – late infantile Onset – 1–6 yr Death by adolescence	hepatosplenomegaly initially psychomotor deterioration gait difficulties	sphingomyelin	unknown
Type IV – Nova Scotia Onset – 1–6 yr Death by adolescence	same as Type III	sphingomyelin	unknown
V. Sulphatide lipidosis *Type I* – late infantile Onset – 12–24 mos. Death by age 5–6	psychomotor deterioration gait difficulty hypotonia	sulphatide (cerebroside sulphate)	sulphatide sulphatase (arylsulphatase A)
Type II – juvenile Onset – 4–8 yrs Death in teens	cerebellar ataxia psychomotor deterioration	same	same
Type III – adult Onset – 15 yrs or older Prolonged survival	dementia, depression long tract signs	same	same
Type IV Onset – 12–18 mos. Death by age 10–12	psychomotor deterioration hepatosplenomegaly skeletal deformities	sulphatide cholesterol sulphate mucopolysaccharide sulphate	multiple sulphatase deficiencies
VI. Galactosylceramide lipidosis Onset in infancy	psychomotor deterioration	galactosylsphingosine	galactosylceramide

Table 96.1 (cont'd)

Disease	Clinical features	Stored material	Enzyme defect
Death by age 2	cortical blindness optic atrophy	(psychosine) globoid cells contain galactosylceramide	β-galactosidase
VII. **Trihexosylceramide lipidosis** Onset – adolescence to adulthood Prolonged survival	peripheral neuropathy cutaneous angiectases renal and cardiac disease X-linked	trihexosylceramide	α-galactosidase
VIII. **Glucosylceramide lipidosis** *Type I* – adult (80%) Onset – by adolescence	hepatosplenomegaly	glucosylceramide brain spared	glucosylceramide β-glucosidase
Type II – infantile (15%) Onset – infancy Death by age 2	psychomotor deterioration extensor spasms hepatosplenomegaly	glucosylceramide	same
Type III – juvenile (Sweden) Onset – 4–8 yr. Death by age 10–15	hepatosplenomegaly initially dementia	glucosylceramide	same
IX. **Ceramide lipidosis** Onset – early infancy Death by age 2	subcutaneous granulomas pulmonary infiltrates psychomotor deterioration	ceramide G_{M3}–ganglioside in viscera	ceramidase

of G_{M1}-gangliosidosis have been recognized (Landing et al, 1964; O'Brien et al, 1972).

Type I G_{M1}-gangliosidosis (generalized gangliosidosis) is a devastating disease which appears in infancy with death usually resulting before the second birthday. The disease is marked by severe bony abnormalities resembling the appearance of the child with Hurler syndrome, hepatosplenomegaly and profound motor and mental retardation. Initial complaints consist of feeding difficulties or failure to thrive. The infants are hypoactive or hypotonic, appear to have both facial and peripheral edema, frontal bossing, and a depressed nasal bridge with hypertelorism. The gums are commonly hypertrophied and the tongue enlarged. Pigmentary changes of the macula resembling the cherry-red spot of Tay-Sachs disease occur in about half the cases described. There is an exaggerated startle response to noise. Mental and motor development is severely retarded from birth, the infants showing little interest in their environment. Initially, bony changes are mainly observed in the long bones of the extremities as periosteal new bone formation, but with progression of the disease, involvement of the vertebral bodies becomes prominent. There is also widening of the long bones reflecting enlargement of the marrow space secondary to cellular lipid storage. In addition, as the disease progresses, flexion contractures

of the joints appear, especially involving the fingers, knees, and elbows. Characteristically, the hands appear very broad with short stubby fingers. Macrocephaly may develop later on although not nearly as severe or impressive as seen in Tay-Sachs disease. The pathology of Type I, G_{M1}-gangliosidosis includes vacuolation of the peripheral lymphocytes, the accumulation of histiocytes in the visceral organs, mainly the liver and spleen, and the accumulation of intracytoplasmic material in cells of bone marrow. The most devastating lipid accumulation occurs in neurons throughout the nervous system and may, indeed, be seen in the ganglion cells of the rectum. Viewed by electron microscopy this stored material is noted within the lysosomes resembling the membranous cytoplasmic bodies first described in Tay-Sachs disease.

Type II G_{M1}-gangliosidosis differs from Type I in that the symptoms and signs do not appear until late infancy and death may not result until the end of the first decade. Bony involvement is mild and in the usual case, mental and motor development may appear normal through the first year of life. Initially, gait disturbance or ataxia occurs followed by the loss of attempts at speech. No organomegaly or evidence of macular degeneration is noted. Progressive weakness and hypotonia follow with the eventual development of seizures. By the end of the second year interest in the environment is usually lost and deterioration to a vegetative state after this point is fairly rapid. Pathological findings in Type II G_{M1}-gangliosidosis are very similar to those described for Type I, although usually less extensive. Despite the absence of organomegaly, there is evidence of histiocyte accumulation in the liver.

Biochemical defect. The chemical abnormalities described for G_{M1}-gangliosidosis are similar for each type; namely, G_{M1}-ganglioside is stored in the central nervous system (Fig. 96.1). In addition, mucopolysaccharide (a keratan sulfate-like compound) can be found in the visceral organs in both Type I and Type II patients (Suzuki, 1968). The G_{M1}-ganglioside has been isolated from the visceral organs of Type I patients, but similar isolations have not been made for Type II. The biochemical defect is the failure to cleave the terminal galactose from the G_{M1}-ganglioside molecule (Fig. 96.1). In both disorders there is a profound deficiency in the activity of the enzyme, β-galactosidase, which is responsible for removing this terminal galactose (Okada & O'Brien, 1968; O'Brien et al, 1972). Observations from liver and cultured fibroblasts suggest that the deficiency is less profound in Type II disease, although the level of deficiency is similar in brain for the two types. The β-galactosidase activity represents a family of enzymes (isoenzymes) and separation of these isoenzymes reveals at least three distinct zones of activity. There is general agreement that two of these isoenzymes are absent in G_{M1}-gangliosidosis whereas the third, isoenzyme A, may or may not be present. While isoenzyme A is detectable in Type I disease, in Type II disease it is, in fact, increased. The existing isoenzyme A activity may be sufficient to confine the major pathophysiologic changes to the nervous system in Type II disease. At the present time, this remains the only explanation for these two different types of G_{M1}-gangliosidosis (Singer & Shafer, 1972; O'Brien, 1975).

In addition to these two types of β-galactosidase deficiency diseases, several patients with variant forms of β-galactosidase deficiency and variable clinical manifestations have been described (Wenger et al, 1980). Precise molecular explanations for these findings are presently unavailable.

G_{M2} gangliosidoses

Type I G_{M2}-gangliosidosis (Tay-Sachs disease) is, perhaps, the most familiar sphingolipidosis affecting the nervous system. This disorder occurs commonly in Jewish families, particularly those from eastern Europe (Ashkenazi). The carrier frequency for this autosomal recessive gene is approximately 3.0% of Jewish individuals descended from European regions. About 1/3600 infants of Ashkenazi (Eastern European) Jewish ancestry has Tay-Sachs disease and about 1/30 individuals in this group is a carrier of the mutant gene. Tay-Sachs disease is not restricted to the Jewish population, however, having been reported in virtually every ethnic and racial group. It is a particularly devastating disease which presents in the period of infancy, often around the fifth or sixth month of life, and is usually fatal within 5 years. These infants may appear normal initially, but within six months are characterized by apathy, hypotonia ,and delayed psychomotor development. As in G_{M1}-gangliosidosis these infants exhibit an exaggerated startle response to noise. This feature is commonly the indication for seeking medical attention. Physical examination includes cherry-red spots in the macular areas of the retinae (Fig. 96.2). This represents lipid storage in the ganglion cells of the retina obscuring the choroidal vessels lying behind (Fig. 96.3). In the foveal region of the retina where the ganglion cells are sparse the vascularity of the underlying choroid then projects as the cherry-red spot. This disease progresses fairly rapidly with early psychomotor retardation, blindness usually by 12 to 18 months, and the appearance of seizures. There is no hepatosplenomegaly. Macrocephaly, a common feature of this disease, particularly in children who survive past the first year of life, is a reflection of glial proliferation and is not a representation of lipid storage *per se*. Pathological features of this disorder are principally those of swollen, stuffed neurons (Fig. 96.4) and secondary gliosis. Despite a lack of clinical evidence of extraneural involvement, there are lipid-laden cells identifiable in liver, spleen, and lung. Electron microscopy reveals membranous cytoplasmic bodies composed of concentric layers of dense membranes located throughout the cytoplasm of the involved neurons representing lipid-laden lysosomes.

A juvenile form of G_{M2}-gangliosidosis, sometimes called the juvenile form of Tay-Sachs disease, is more aptly denoted as G_{M2}-gangliosidosis, Type III (Brett et al, 1973). This form appears between the ages of two and five as a progressive deterioration of psychomotor behavior and an insidious disturbance of gait. Death usually

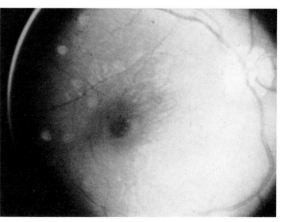

Fig. 96.2 Cherry-red macula.

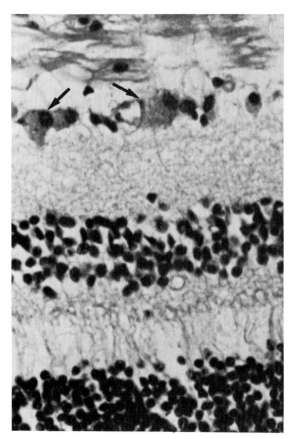

Fig. 96.3 Lipid-laden retinal ganglion cells. Hematoxylin and eosin.

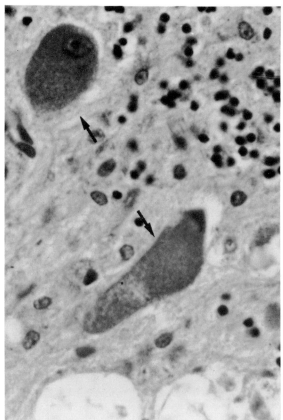

Fig. 96.4 Lipid-laden neurons from brain of patient with Gm_2–gangliosidosis. Luxol fast blue-hematoxylin and eosin.

occurs within fifteen years. No predilection for Jewish individuals is evident. Physical examination is similar to that in Type I G_{M2}gangliosidosis with the notable absence of macrocephaly and cherry-red maculae. Optic atrophy or retinitis pigmentosa may be seen instead. Pathological examination reveals similar, although generally less extensive, neuronal storage of lipid than in Type I.

Biochemical defect. Types I and III G_{M2}-gangliosidosis are characterized by storage of the G_{M2}-ganglioside (Fig. 96.1). Normally a very minor ganglioside component, in this disease the G_{M2}-ganglioside is increased enormously representing greater than 90% of the ganglioside fraction in neural tissue. G_{M2}-ganglioside is also increased in liver and spleen when compared to normal tissue. In addition, the *asialo* form of the G_{M2}-ganglioside, that is G_{M2}-ganglioside minus the NANA group (Fig. 96.1), is also present in excess and may represent up to 5% of the total glycolipid fraction in brain.

The enzymatic defect in G_{M2}-gangliosidosis is characterized by failure to hydrolyze the terminal amino sugar from the G_{M2}-ganglioside (Fig. 96.1). This enzyme is known as a hexosaminidase and occurs as two major

forms, or isoenzymes, designated A and B. Total hexosaminidase activity, representing the hydrolytic action of both hexosaminidase A and B may be elevated in tissues from children with Types I and III G_{M2}-gangliosidosis. Hexosaminidase A is virtually absent, however, with a compensatory increase in hexosaminidase B accounting for the normal or elevated levels of total hexosaminidase activity (Okada & O'Brien, 1969). In the juvenile form or Type III, there is partial deficiency of the hexosaminidase A isoenzyme perhaps accounting for the delayed onset and longer course of this form.

Type II G_{M2}-gangliosidosis (Sandhoff disease) is considered separately from Type I and III because the clinical and biochemical findings differ (Sandhoff et al, 1968). Age at onset and progression of disease resemble Type I. This disease is not seen predominantly in Jewish individuals, but is accompanied by psychomotor retardation, blindness with cherry-red maculae, and exaggerated startle response to noise. Enlargement of the liver and spleen is prominent and represents the principal clinical difference from Type I.

Biochemical defect. Type II manifests the striking accumulation, particularly in neural tissue, of G_{M2}-ganglioside and the asialo-form of G_{M2} (Fig. 96.1). This asialo-form may represent as much as one-third of the total glycolipid fraction of the brain. In addition to G_{M2} storage, globoside, the common neutral glycolipid of red blood cells and kidney (Fig. 96.1), accumulates in the abdominal organs, namely the liver, kidney, and spleen. Globoside, you will note, has the same terminal amino sugar as G_{M2}-ganglioside. The biochemical abnormality of Type II G_{M2}-gangliosidosis is total deficiency of hexosaminidase activity. Both isoenzyme A and B activities are absent in tissues of individuals with the disorder whereas hexosaminidase S, a minor isoenzyme, is increased (Sandhoff et al, 1971).

G_{M2}-variants

Additional types of G_{M2}-gangliosidosis have been described. One, termed the AB variant, is characterized by the onset of dementia, gait difficulties, and seizures in a six year old child without macular or visual abnormalities. Neuronal membranous cytoplasmic bodies typical of Tay-Sachs disease were seen at postmortem examination. The enzymatic lesion is particularly interesting. Total hexosaminidase activity using an artificial substrate was normal or increased and, activity of the A isoenzyme with the same substrate was about 50% of control values but hexosaminidase activity was absent with the natural substrate, G_{M2}-ganglioside. The exact nature of the enzymatic defect is not resolved at present, but may involve the absence of an *activating* substance essential for the binding of G_{M2} to the hexosaminidase molecule (Conzelmann & Sandhoff, 1978). O'Neill et al (1978) described an adult AB variant presenting with seizures, dementia, and normal pressure hydrocephalus. Hexosominidase A and B were normal using artificial substrate. Another reported variant featuring cherry red maculae and cerebellar ataxia, without seizures or dementia appears to be an adult form of Type II (Oonk et al, 1979). Hexosaminidase B activity is absent and hexosaminidase A is severely deficient. A third variant (chronic form) with slow progression of cerebellar ataxia and distal muscle wasting and without seizures, dementia, or macular changes revealed normal total hexosaminidase activity and profoundly reduced hexosaminidase A activity in serum (Johnson et al, 1977). In leucocytes, hexosaminidase activity was about 50% of control values.

Yet another variant (adult) was identified in the course of a Tay-Sachs screening programme. A young adult, in good health, was noted to have a profound deficiency in serum and fibroblast hexosaminidase A activity. Subsequently, he has developed typical features of amyotrophic lateral sclerosis including muscle weakness, wasting and fasciculations. Rectal biopsy revealed neuronal inclusions similar to those noted in classical Tay-Sachs disease (Yaffe et al ,1979).

Table 96.2 G_{M2}-Gangliosidoses heterogeneity of hexosaminidase deficiency diseases

Type	Clinical features	Biochemical abnormality	Subunit notation*
I. Late infantile (Tay-Sachs)	Blindness, seizures, psychomotor deterioration	Hex A deficiency, B increased	$\alpha_0\,\beta_2$ $\beta_2\,\beta_2$
II. Sandhoff	Similar to Type I, visceromegaly	Hex A and B deficiency	$\alpha_2\,\beta_0$ $\beta_0\,\beta_0$
III. Juvenile	Ataxia, spasticity, seizures, psychomotor deterioration, anterior horn cell disease	Hex A deficiency	$\alpha_0\,\beta_2$ $\beta_2\,\beta_2$
IV. Juvenile Sandhoff	Cerebellar ataxia, cherry red maculae, intact mentation	Hex A and B deficiency	$\alpha_2\,\beta_0$ $\beta_0\,\beta_0$
V. AB variant	Similar to Type I	Hex A and B increased with artificial substrate	$\alpha_2\,\beta_2$ $\beta_2\,\beta_2$
VI. Adult	ALS – like syndrome	Hex A deficiency	$\alpha_0\,\beta_2$ $\beta_2\,\beta_2$
VII. Chronic	Spinocerebellar degeneration, distal muscle wasting, dystonia, intact mentation	Hex A deficiency	$\alpha_0\,\beta_2$ $\beta_2\,\beta_2$

* Hexosaminidase subunit representation

Isoenzyme	Subunit Structure
Hexosaminidase A	$\alpha_2\,\beta_2$
Hexosaminidase B	$\beta_2\,\beta_2$
Hexosaminidase S	$\alpha_2\,\alpha_2$

At least, seven forms of G_{M2}-gangliosidosis (Table 96.2) have been described. Types I, II, VI, and VII may be linked to mutations at the α-subunit locus, Types III and IV at the β-subunit locus. Type V appears to represent a mutation at a separate locus distinct from the α and β loci. This formulation results from the assignment of genes for hexosaminidase (Hex) A and B to separate chromosomes (Gilbert et al, 1975) and subunit structure representation (Beutler & Kuhl, 1975) in which the Hex A is denoted by $\alpha_2 \beta_2$, Hex B by $\beta_2\beta_2$, and Hex S by $\alpha_2\alpha_2$.

G_{M3}-gangliosidosis

G_{M3}-gangliosidosis is a disorder recently described in two males within a single family (Max et al, 1974). Respiratory difficulty and seizures began within the first days of life. Lethargy, poor feeding, macroglossia, and gingival hyperplasia were noted. The infant was hypotonic, developed little and had frequent generalized seizures. Death occurred at three months of age. The brain from one child contained large amounts of G_{M3}-ganglioside and virtually no G_{M2} or G_{M1} ganglioside. A novel biosynthetic defect in ganglioside production was noted. Activity of UDP-GalNAc: G_{M3} N-acetylgalactosaminyltransferase which converts G_{M3} to G_{M2} ganglioside was severely diminished in his brain and liver. The genetics of this disorder are unclear, but X–linked recessive transmission is possible.

Other sphingolipidoses

Sphingomyelin lipidoses (Niemann-Pick disease)

This group of disorders is characterized by an abnormal accumulation of sphingomyelin (Fig. 96.1). Four clinical forms have been described, but deficient enzyme activity has been noted in only two (Brady et al, 1966).

The infantile or acute form (Type I), representing about 80% of sphingomyelin lipidosis cases, appears in early infancy with failure to thrive and hepatomegaly. Psychomotor deterioration is prominent leaving the child devastated by 12 months of age. Death results by age 4. As with Tay-Sachs disease, this form is especially common in eastern European Jews (Ashkenazi). A characteristic, although not diagnostic finding, is the appearance of foam cells in the bone marrow. Approximately one-half the patients have cherry-red maculae. Pathological findings are generalized with foam cells appearing throughout the reticuloendothelial system. Neuropathological findings include marked neuronal storage, numerous foam cells representing lipid storage in glial cells, and glial proliferation. Electron microscopy of the foam cells reveals multi-laminated concentric cytoplasmic inclusions.

Type II has been called the chronic form because of the absence of neurological involvement and because of an apparently prolonged survival. Enlargement of liver and spleen is evident in early childhood. The earliest diagnosed patients are now in their 30's without neurological impairment.

Type III and IV are clinically similar and there is no compelling pathological or biochemical reason to separate them. Type IV signifies a cluster of cases in Nova Scotia all traced to a single mutation in ancestors of French Acadians (Winsor & Welch, 1978). Both types appear in early childhood (age 1 to 6) with death by adolescence. Hepatosplenomegaly is the prominent finding initially, but evidence of neurological involvement soon appears, manifested as gait disturbance and gradual intellectual deterioration.

Biochemical defect. Each type of sphingomyelin lipidosis is marked by the abnormal accumulation of sphingomyelin in most tissues. In Type I, the accumulation is so extensive that sphingomyelin may represent 2–5% of the body weight (Kamoshita et al, 1969). Because of its clinical course, Type II has not yet been examined thoroughly. Nonetheless, sphingomyelin content of liver and spleen is several-fold greater than in controls. Sphingomyelin accumulation in Types III and IV is less significant (Philippart et al, 1969). There is a 3–4 fold increase in spleen; in the liver, sphingomyelin content may be normal. Activity of the enzyme, sphingomyelinase, is deficient in Types I and II. The different clinical course of these two types is not explained by any quantitative difference in sphingomyelinase deficiencies, each form having similar residual activities (Gal et al, 1980). Sphingomyelinase activity in Types III and IV is normal, thus no clear explanation for sphingomyelin accumulation exists. One could question whether these two forms, in fact, represent a sphingomyelin lipidosis. Two recent reports, however, do suggest abnormal sphingomyelin degradation in the Type III disorder.

Prenatal diagnosis of Type III was aided by the reduction of sphingomyelinase activity in fetal tissues to 33–50% of control levels whereas postnatal tissues yielded control level activities (Harzer et al, 1978). These authors experienced difficulty in solubilizing sphingomyelinase from Type III tissues suggesting, that in the intact cell, the enzyme may be relatively inaccessible to its substrate. Christomanou (1980) provided evidence for a deficient sphingomyelinase and glucocerebrosidase activating factor (heat-stable and non-enzymic) in Type III tissues and concluded that previous in vitro analyses utilizing exogenous detergents had masked this deficiency.

Sulphatide lipidoses (metachromatic leukodystrophy – MLD)

This disorder is represented by four clinical forms, three of which differ in age at onset, rate of progression and clinical findings, but share a quantitatively similar deficiency of the lysosomal hydrolase, arylsulphatase A. The fourth is a separate entity, clinically and biochemically. The late infantile form (Type I), most common of the four, usually presents from 12–24 months. Progressive loss of motor milestones and gait difficulty with hypotonia are first noted and, subsequently, a decline in speech and mentation. Cherry-red maculae have been described. Death usually occurs by age 6. Diagnosis may be aided by finding an increase in CSF protein and a decrease in nerve conduction velocity (Hagberg et al, 1960).

A juvenile form (Type II) occurs between 4–8 years with cerebellar ataxia and gait dysfunction progressing to death in the second decade (Haberland et al, 1973; Haltia et al, 1980). An adult form (Type III) appears in the late teens or later with a psychosis or dementia and evidence of long tract involvement. Survival may be prolonged well into adult life (Percy et al, 1977).

Pathological studies are abundant for the late infantile form but are less extensive for the two delayed forms. The late infantile and juvenile forms manifest involvement predominantly of white matter, nerve tracts, and peripheral nerves. Loss of myelin, glial proliferation, and the appearance of metachromatically-staining material is characteristic (Fig. 96.5). In addition, metachromatic material may be identified in peripheral nerve, liver, gall bladder, spleen, kidney, pancreas, lung, and lymph nodes. While the cerebral cortex is relatively spared in the late infantile and juvenile forms, significant neuronal storage of metachromatic material is seen in adult cases. Segmental demyelination is invariably present in peripheral nerve. Electron microscopy of brain and nerve reveals granular cytoplasmic inclusions which are multilaminated (Fig. 96.6).

Biochemical defect. The metachromatic material stored in this disorder is the sulphated derivative of galactosylceramide called sulphatide (Fig. 96.1). Sulphatide accumulates in both neural and non-neural tissues in this disorder due to a deficiency in the activity of the lysosomal enzyme, sulphatide sulphatase (Mehl & Jatzkewitz, 1963). This enzyme appears identical with one of the arylsulphatase isoenzymes, arylsulphatase A (Austin et al, 1963). The reduction of arylsulphatase A activity in each form is profound and quantitatively similar whether employing the natural or artificial substrate (Percy & Kaback, 1971). While the clinical-biochemical discrepancy is not resolved by in vitro enzyme analyses, tissue culture studies reveal differences which could explain the clinical variations noted. When cultured skin fibroblasts are incubated in the presence of sulphatide, cells from patients with sulphatidosis Type I have little ability to remove the sulphatide; cells from patients with Type II disease are somewhat better, and those from Type III patients are better still (Porter et al, 1971).

The fourth form of metachromatic leukodystrophy is termed multiple sulphatase deficiency disease. This condition is genetically and biochemically perplexing. These patients have significant defects in the activity of a variety of sulphatases. Arylsulphatase A, arylsulphatase B, iduronate sulphatase and heparan-N-sulphatase, all lysosomal enzymes involved in glycolipid or mucopolysaccharide catabolism, are reduced in these patients as is the microsomal enzyme, steroid sulphatase (Murphy et al, 1971). Since distinct autosomal and X–chromosomal genes are

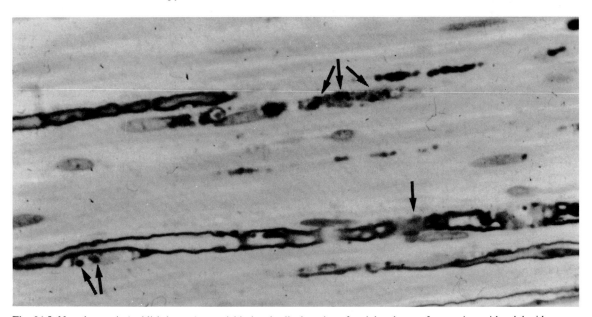

Fig. 96.5 Metachromatic (reddish-brown) material in longitudinal section of peripheral nerve from patient with sulphatide lipidosis. Methylene blue.

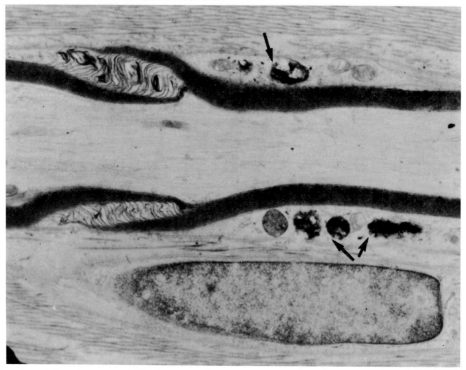

Fig. 96.6 Densely-staining storage material in Schwann cell cytoplasm adjacent to myelin sheath. Electron micrograph of peripheral nerve from patient with sulphatide lipidosis.

involved in the coding for these enzyme proteins, the precise location of the genetic lesion is unclear. Clinically, these children are similar to juvenile or late infantile MLD patients but in addition have hepatosplenomegaly and increased urinary mucopolysaccharide excretion. Many of these patients then show features both of a lipidosis and a mucopolysaccharidosis. Under suitable conditions, cultured skin fibroblasts from such patients reveal significant activities of arylsulphatase A suggesting that in the intact cell the enzyme is synthesized but for as yet unknown reasons may not be accessible to its substrate (Fluharty et al, 1978).

A further variant was recently described in which arylsulphatase A activity was about 50% of control levels (or in the heterozygote range) using both natural and artificial substrates (Shapiro et al, 1979). The patient developed symptoms at age 4 with seizures, mental deterioration, and initial hypotonia and hyporeflexia progressing to spasticity. Cultured skin fibroblasts were unable to hydrolyze exogenous sulphatide whereas cells from the mother behaved as control preparations. Deficiency of 'activating factor' for sulphatide degradation could explain these findings.

Galactosylceramide lipidosis (Krabbe disease)
The appearance of multinucleate or globoid cells in brain characterizes this disorder. Hence, the term globoid cell leukodystrophy has been synonymous with Krabbe dis-

ease. Onset is in the first six months and progression is relentless leading to death by age 2. Feeding difficulty, irritability and failure of psychomotor development are noted clinically resulting in spasticity, cortical blindness, optic atrophy, and deafness. The peripheral nerves are also involved as indicated by decreased nerve conduction velocity. Cerebrospinal fluid protein is almost always elevated. Pathological findings are confined to the nervous system. The brain is small and of rubbery consistency. Gray matter is relatively spared; white matter is almost devoid of myelin (Fig. 96.7). Glial cell proliferation (gliosis) is profound and numerous macrophages and multinucleate globoid cells are noted (Fig. 96.8).

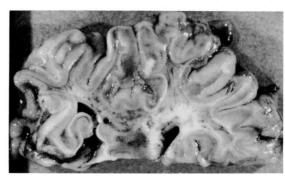

Fig. 96.7 Virtual absence of white matter in brain from patient with galactosylceramide lipidosis.

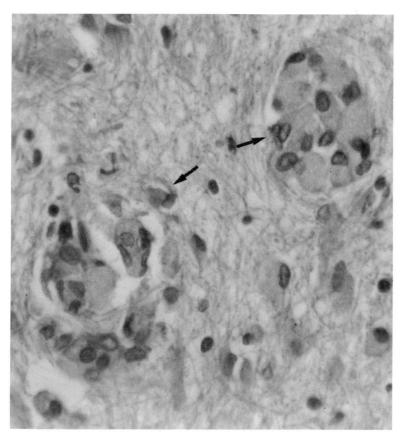

Fig. 96.8 Typical multinucleate 'globoid' cells in brain from patient with galactosylceramide lipidosis. Hematoxylin and eosin.

Peripheral nerves are marked by segmental demyelination without evidence of globoid cells.

Electron microscopy of the globoid cells reveals cytoplasmic inclusions which have a hollow tubular appearance similar to, but distinct from those seen in glucosylceramide lipidosis. Typical globoid cells have been produced experimentally by intracerebral injection of galactosylceramide or by culturing retinal cells in the presence of galactosyl- or glucosylceramide (Austin, 1963; Sourander et al, 1966).

Biochemical defect. Galactosylceramide lipidosis is a unique disorder of sphingolipid catabolism. Instead of lipid storage there is an absolute deficiency of galactosylceramide as well as the other sphingolipids. However, when the globoid cells are isolated, chemical analysis reveals a relative accumulation of galactosylceramide. This observation and the previously described experiments inducing globoid cells prompted the analyses which revealed deficient galactosylceramide β-galactosidase activity (Fig. 96.1). This β-galactosidase enzyme is distinct from the enzyme involved in G_{M1}-gangliosidosis (Suzuki & Suzuki, 1970). Recently, Svennerholm et al (1980) reported a 100-fold accumulation of galactosyl-sphingosine (psychosine), the deacylated galactosylceramide, in white matter from affected infants. The cytopathic effect of galactosylsphingosine on oligodendroglia could explain the absolute deficiency of galactosylceramide.

A variant form of galactosylceramide lipidosis has been described with onset in childhood from age 4 to 8. The principal findings are gait disturbance and progressive psychomotor deterioration. Pathological findings are similar to the infantile form and the deficiency of galactosylceramide β-galactosidase activity is quantitatively similar. The clinical course is somewhat longer, however, with death in the second decade. In contrast to the infantile form, peripheral nerve function as measured by nerve conduction velocity was normal in this juvenile variant (Young et al, 1972).

A further variant was described by Dunn et al (1976). This child had the early onset of signs and symptoms , a prolonged course, and typical enzymatic abnormalities but lacked globoid cells on histologic examination.

Trihexosylceramide lipidosis (Fabry disease).
This disorder is the only sphingolipid disorder which

generally spares the central nervous system and the only sphingolipidosis inherited as an X–linked recessive. This disease has its onset in childhood or adolescence and may run a variable course. Death usually occurs in middle adulthood, or at least by the end of the fifth decade. Pathological manifestations of this disease are predominantly noted in the skin, kidneys, and cornea. The disease may appear as episodes of burning pain, particularly in the distal extremities, often associated with fever and elevation of the erythrocyte sedimentation rate. Cutaneous vascular lesions called *angiokeratoma corporis diffusum* may also represent the initial manifestations. These lesions are usually symmetrical especially occurring over the abdomen, lower back, the buttocks, hips, and thighs, as well as the genitalia. Lesions have also been noted in the mouth and conjunctivae. The skin lesions are actually dilated vessels or angiectases with diffuse lipid infiltration of vascular endothelium. Exceptional patients may have central nervous system involvement presenting with manifestations of cerebrovascular insufficiency (Lou & Reske-Nielsen, 1971). Peripheral oedema is often present without tangible explanation. Recently, reduced motor nerve conduction velocities were noted in 8 of 12 affected males and one-third of obligate carriers (Sheth & Swick, 1979). Signs of renal dysfunction usually do not appear until adulthood, but ultimately, the complications of chronic renal failure ensue. Death usually results either from renal failure itself or from the cardiac and/or cerebral complications of hypertension or vascular disease. Many female carriers, by Lyonization, show some involvement although in an attentuated form, most commonly manifested as hazy clouding of the cornea (Bird & Lagunoff, 1978). Survival of female carriers may be normal, although they often succumb to the same complications as the hemizygous males (Burda & Winder, 1967).

Pathological examinations reveal a generalized involvement of the endothelial lining of the blood vessels and reticuloendothelial system, epithelial tissues of cornea, kidney, and skin and in the ganglion cells of the autonomic nervous system and the Schwann cells of the peripheral nervous system (Sima & Robertson, 1978). Motor neurons themselves are ordinarily spared. Electron microscopy (EM) reveals cytoplasmic inclusions in lysosomes with a laminated structure and regular periodicity distinct from the inclusions seen in the other sphingolipidoses. CNS neuronal inclusions have been noted in the amygdala by EM (Grunnet & Spilsbury, 1973).

Biochemical defect. Fabry disease is marked by the accumulation of trihexosylceramide (Fig. 96.1) and digalactosylceramide in most tissues of the body. Both compounds accumulated have as the terminal disaccharide , two galactose units linked in an alpha configuration.

This is pertinent in that the enzymatic defect consists of markedly reduced α-galactosidase activity (Brady et al, 1967). Digalactosylceramide is present in human tissues in very small amounts under normal circumstances and only in this disorder does it increase abnormally. Renal transplantation has been employed as a rational mode of intervention (Clarke et al, 1972). Results are promising, but it is not clear whether the transplant provides a source of the deficient enzyme or whether the improvement is merely a reflection of normalization of renal function.

Glucosylceramide lipidoses (Gaucher disease)

Glucosylceramide lipidosis occurs in three clinically-distinct forms, each involving the accumulation of glucosylceramide: Type I-Adult or chronic form (CNS spared), Type II-Infantile form (early CNS involvement) and Type III-Juvenile form (late CNS involvement).

The adult or chronic form (Type I) represents about 80% of the total cases. This form is, like Tay-Sachs and Niemann-Pick disease, associated with eastern European Jews (Ashkenazi). Symptoms often occur in childhood, and usually by adolescence, with progressive splenomegaly and evidence of hypersplenism (pancytopenia). Affected individuals usually reach adulthood, and those with later onset may have normal life expectancy. The chronicity of the disease is denoted by massive hepatosplenomegaly and by bony lesions. These bony lesions consist of expansion of the bone marrow space and pathological fractures. CNS pathology consists of perivascular storage with intense glio-mesodermal fibrillary reaction and typical Gaucher cells but with no neuronal storage (Soffer et al, 1980). The infantile form, Type II (about 15% of reported cases), is a fulminant disease, appearing in infancy, usually with failure to thrive, recurrent pulmonary infections and hepatosplenomegaly. Neurological signs occur early in infancy and progress rapidly resulting in spasticity, strabismus, and persistent extension of head and neck (extensor rigidity). Seizures may appear as well while cherry-red maculae are generally absent. Death occurs usually by age 2. The characteristic pathological finding is the appearance of Gaucher cells throughout the reticuloendothelial system especially in bone marrow and visceral organs. These are reticuloendothelial cells containing cytoplasmic fibrillary tangles simulating wrinkled tissue paper. Perivascular Gaucher cells are visible in brain along with evidence of neuronal storage and degeneration. Electron microscopy of Gaucher cells reveals numerous inclusions which resemble hollow tubules.

The juvenile form (Type III) is represented mainly by a cluster of cases from Sweden. Splenomegaly may be noted during the first year of life, but development may be normal until intellectual deterioration becomes manifest from age 4 to 8. Death comes usually by age 15. Pathological findings generally resemble those of Type II.

Biochemical defect. Glucosylceramide lipidosis is marked by the accumulation of glucosylceramide. Glucosylceramide is stored in extra-neural organs in each form of Gaucher disease, but only in Type II (infantile form) does the sphingolipid accumulate in brain.

Glucosylceramide (Fig. 96.1) occupies a strategic position in the degradation pathway of globoside and gangliosides. Brady and coworkers (1965) found glucosylceramide β-glucosidase activity to be deficient in glucosylceramide lipidosis. This observation was particularly significant. It clearly defined for the first time a sphingolipid hydrolase deficiency and prompted the intense investigative interest which has resolved the primary enzymatic deficiency in each sphingolipid storage disease.

Type I and II have residual enzyme activity (glucosylceramide β-glucosidase) which is inversely proportional to the rate of progression of the disorder. The infantile form has little detectable activity while the adult or chronic form has from 5–15% of control levels (Brady, 1966). Reduced enzyme activity has been described in Type III patients representing about 15–20% of control levels (Hultberg et al, 1973; Hultberg, 1978; Nishimura & Barranger, 1980).

Ceramide lipidosis – lipogranulomatosis (Farber Disease)
Lipogranulomatosis is a very unusual and devastating disorder of early infancy recently added to the sphingolipidosis category (Crocker et al, 1967). Irritability, a weak, hoarse cry, lymphadenopathy, joint swelling, multiple subcutaneous nodules, and severe psychomotor retardation characterize this disorder. Cherry-red maculae have been noted. The clinical course is relentlessly progressive with recurrent fever and pulmonary infiltrates. Death usually occurs by age 2. Pathological changes are generalized. Diffuse extraneural granulomas involve skin, lung, liver, spleen, and joint capsules. The granulomas typically contain lipid-laden cells (histiocytes). Neuropathological findings include neuronal storage, glial proliferation, and foci of myelin loss. Retinal ganglion cells accumulate lipid material as well.

Biochemical defect. Two types of sphingolipid accumulate in lipogranulomatosis. There is a mild elevation of ganglioside, mainly G_{M3}, or haematoside (Fig. 96.1) in *visceral* organs. Brain ganglioside levels appear normal. The major sphingolipid stored is ceramide (Fig. 96.1) which is increased 10-fold in kidney and 60-fold in liver. Ceramide levels in gray matter appear normal while a 5-fold increase is noted in white matter. The postulated defect in ceramide catabolism (Fig. 96.1) has been confirmed by delineation of ceramidase deficiency in kidney, liver, and cultured fibroblasts (Sugita et al, 1972; Dulaney et al, 1976).

NEURONAL CEROID LIPOFUSCINOSES

The ceroid lipofuscinoses, a clinically well-described but pathophysiologically poorly-understood group of neurodegenerative diseases, are similar to the sphingolipidoses in many respects. Yet, the chemical nature of the 'stored' material is not known nor is the specific enzyme deficiency. There are four recognizable clinical disorders with an autosomal recessive inheritance pattern (Table 96.3 and Fig. 96.9).

Type I is an infantile form of neuronal ceroid lipofuscinosis described extensively in the Finnish population.

Table 96.3 Neuronal ceroid lipofuscinoses: clinical and biological features

Variant	Age at onset	Prognosis	Clinical features	Pathology
Infantile (Finnish)	1–2 years	rapid progression death by age 10	psychomotor deterioration, microcephaly, ataxia, myoclonus, retinal atrophy and blindness	lack of cerebral cortical neurons; inclusions in lymphocytes, neutrophils, and in brain macrophages and astrocytes (autofluorescent)
Late Infantile (Jansky-Bielchowsky)	2–4 years	rapid progression death by age 10	seizures, dementia, ataxia, retinitis pigmentosa, macular degeneration	autofluorescent lipopigment and curvilinear bodies in brain and liver
Juvenile (Batten-Spielmeyer-Sjögren-Vogt)	5–10 years	slow progression death by age 20	visual loss, dementia, retinitis pigmentosa, seizures and ataxia	autofluorescent lipopigment and curvilinear bodies in brain
Adult (Kufs)	teens to adulthood	very slow progression	slowly progressive dementia, seizures (occasionally)	autofluorescent lipopigment inclusions in brain

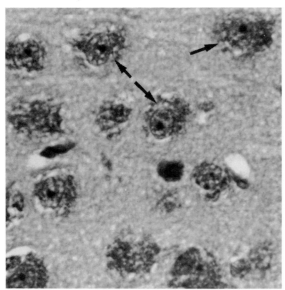

Fig. 96.9 Neuronal cytoplasmic accumulation of lipofuscin in neuronal ceroid lipofuscinosis. Luxol fast blue-hematoxylin and eoslin.

Profound mental and motor deterioration and blindness appear at age 1–2 years. Progression is relentless with death in the first decade. Pathologically, severe microcephaly with brain atrophy and an absence of cerebral cortical neurons are noted (Hagberg et al, 1974). Brain lipids are dramatically reduced (Svennerholm et al, 1975; Bourre et al, 1979).

Type II, Jansky-Bielschowsky disease, usually begins at age two to four with seizures. Death occurs by age eight. Dementia, blindness with optic atrophy, retinitis pigmentosa and macular degeneration are commonly seen. Diffuse cortical atrophy was noted by computed tomography (Valvanis et al, 1980). Type III, Batten-Spielmeyer-Sjögren-Vogt disease, usually appears later in childhood and has a somewhat more indolent course. Visual symptoms are particularly common in this disease, blindness being a relatively early finding. Macular degeneration with 'salt and pepper' pigmentary retinal changes are characteristic. Peripheral blood lymphocytes frequently show vacuolization, a finding occasionally observed in Jansky-Bielschowsky patients. Progressive dementia over ten years or more precedes death in the second decade. The fourth type of neuronal ceroid lipofuscinosis, Kufs disease, starts as a slowly progressive dementia at age 15–20. Seizures are occasionally seen, but visual or retinal changes are rare. Interestingly, instances of Kufs disease have been found in families in which Jansky-Bielschowsky or Spielmeyer-Sjögren-Vogt disease has occurred. The precise genetic mechanism accounting for these three clinical syndromes (Types II-IV) is therefore uncertain, and clarification awaits further

biochemical advances. Pathologically, the last three disorders are characterized by autofluorescent lipopigments in a number of viscera and in the brain (Fig. 96.10). By electron microscopy this pigment is found within granules appearing in a characteristic curvilinear 'fingerprint' pattern (Aguas et al, 1980).

The molecular defect in these disorders remains elusive. The origin of the autofluorescent lipofuscin is thought to represent peroxidation of tissue lipids with polymerization of the resulting products. A deficiency of leukocyte peroxidase activity was described six years ago in patients with the Batten variant (Armstrong et al, 1974). Subsequent studies from different centers contradicted these initial findings. Since a reduction in cellular peroxidase activity might explain the lipopigment accumulation, interest in this area has been rekindled with recent reports of glutathione peroxidase deficiencies in erythrocytes from patients with the Type I (Finnish) and Type III (Batten) forms (Westermarck & Sandholm, 1977; Jensen et al, 1978). Alternatively, the autofluorescent material was shown to contain retinoyl complexes and not peroxidized polyunsaturated fatty acids (Wolfe et al, 1977).

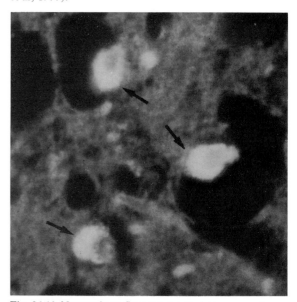

Fig. 96.10 Neuronal autofluorescent material in neuronal ceroid lipofuscinosis.

OTHER LIPIDOSES

Five disorders of lipid metabolism involving tissue storage will be described briefly (Table 96.4). These are phytanic acid lipidosis (Refsum disease); Wolman disease and cholesterol ester lipidosis, which appear to share a common enzymatic deficiency; cholestanol lipidosis (cerebrotendinous xanthomatosis), and cherry-red spot-myoclonus syndrome.

Table 96.4 Other inherited lipidoses: clinical and biological features

Clinical syndrome	Onset	Prognosis	Clinical features	Stored material	Enzyme defect
Phytanic acid lipidosis (Refsum disease)	Adolescence	Prolonged survival treatable with diet, plasmapheresis	ataxia, deafness polyneuropathy, retinitis pigmentosa	phytanic acid	fatty acid α-oxidation, probably initial α-hydroxylase
Triglyceride and cholesterol ester lipidosis (Wolman Disease)	Infancy	Death by 3 mos.	adrenal calcification, marasmus, hepatosplenomegaly	cholesterol esters and triglycerides	acid lipase
Cholesterol ester lipidosis	Childhood	Normal life expectancy	hepatomegaly, foam cells in bone marrow	cholesterol esters and triglycerides	acid lipase
Cholestanol lipidosis (Cerebrotendinous Xanthomastosis)	Late childhood to early adolescence	Prolonged survival (age 30–50)	xanthomas, cataracts, dementia, ataxia	cholestanol and cholesterol	cholesterol 26-hydroxylase
Cherry-red spot-myoclonus syndrome	5–10 years	Prolonged survival	cherry-red maculae, gait difficulties, intention myclonus, intellect normal	oligosaccharides glycoproteins	α-sialidase

Phytanic acid lipidosis (Refsum disease)

Phytanic acid lipidosis, a clinically-complex, potentially-treatable disorder transmitted as an autosomal recessive, often appears in childhood and usually by age 20. It was originally called heredopathia atactica polyneuritiformis because of the prominent cerebellar ataxia and peripheral neuropathy (Refsum, 1960). The mode of onset is variable and may involve extremity weakness, unsteadiness of gait, failing vision particularly at night, or anosmia. The complete clinical syndrome includes cerebellar ataxia, retinitis pigmentosa, symmetrical motor and sensory peripheral neuropathy, epiphysial dysplasia as manifested in a shortened fourth metatarsal bone, syndactyly, hammer toes, cartilage degeneration, and pes cavus. Clinical investigations reveal elevated CSF protein, decreased nerve conduction velocity, and conduction defects in the EKG. Remissions and exacerbations, the latter often as a result of intercurrent febrile illness, surgical procedures or pregnancy, are typical with an overall pattern of progressive disability. Pathological findings include hypertrophic interstitial peripheral neuropathy with demyelination, retinal degeneration, and glial proliferation in brain.

Biochemical defect. Plasma phytanic acid (normally present only in trace amounts) may represent 5 to 30% of the total fatty acid fraction and tissue phytanic acid may account for 50% of total fatty acids. Phytanic acid levels in peripheral nerves usually exceed those in the central nervous system (MacBrinn & O'Brien, 1968).

Phytanic acid is a natural product, the major source being chlorophyll-containing foods and foods derived from ruminant animals, namely, cows. Hence, phytanic acid lipidosis is unique among the lipid storage disorders in that the accumulating material is derived from exogenous sources and does not represent accretion of a normal membrane constituent. Metabolism of phytanic acid by the usual fatty acid β-oxidation pathway is precluded by the methyl side-group, thus, an initial α-oxidation step is required. A defect in this α-oxidation step was noted in patients with phytanic acid lipidosis and intermediate levels were found in obligate heterozygotes (Stokke et al, 1961; Steinberg & Hutton, 1972).

Since phytanic acid is obtained from dietary sources, a diet low in phytanic acid offers a potential mode of therapy. Improvement of affected patients has been noted in terms of reduced plasma phytanic acid levels and amelioration of the peripheral neuropathy. No improvement was noted in cerebellar or cranial nerve function. Early institution of dietary restriction might delay or even prevent disease onset. Plasma phytanic acid levels may be lowered acutely by plasmaphoeresis (Lundberg et al, 1972; Gibberd et al, 1979).

Triglyceride and cholesterol ester lipidosis

Two clinical entities, one with limited survival, the other with normal life expectancy, are associated with the accumulation of cholesterol esters and triglycerides.

The first disorder, Wolman disease (Abramov et al, 1956; Crocker et al, 1965) is a devastating autosomal recessive disorder of early infancy with death by twelve to eighteen months. Failure to thrive with poor feeding and malabsorption, hepatosplenomegaly, and adrenal enlargement with calcifications are noted at onset. Primary central nervous system involvement is unusual. Lipid-laden histiocytes are seen in the bone marrow and in most organs including occasional histiocytic collections in brain. The second disorder, cholesterol ester lipidosis, has been described in only a half dozen families. Moderate hepatomegaly (liver function normal) occurs in childhood and foam cells are found in the bone marrow, liver and intestine. Disability is minimal and life expectancy appears normal. In addition, three affected siblings have been described with a clinical picture intermediate between Wolman disease and cholesterol ester lipidosis (Beaudet et al, 1977).

Biochemical defect. These disorders are characterized by tissue accumulation of cholesterol esters and triglycerides. In liver, the magnitude of increase is similar in each disorder. Brain lipid analyses from patients with Wolman disease reveal no consistent abnormality. Plasma cholesterol and triglyceride levels have usually been normal in Wolman disease and increased along with low density lipoproteins in cholesterol ester lipidosis. In each disorder, the proportion of esterified cholesterol in the plasma appears normal.

Acid phosphatase (a lysosomal hydrolase) activity in the limiting membrane of stored lipid material suggested defective lysosomal function in Wolman disease. Deficient activity of an acid lipase or esterase has been noted histochemically in liver and peripheral blood smears (Lake, 1971), and biochemically in liver, spleen, leukocytes, and fibroblasts (Patrick and Lake, 1969). Wolman patients exhibited no evidence of acid lipase activity. In contrast, the patients designated as cholesterol ester lipidosis had about 15–20% control activity (Beaudet et al, 1974). Heterozygote detection has been established in leucocytes and fibroblasts.

In summary, these observations suggest that Wolman disease and cholesterol ester lipidosis represent phenotypic variants of a similar, although quantitatively, different biochemical defect in acid lipase activity as reflected in cholesterol ester and triglyceride storage.

Cholestanol lipidosis (cerebrotendinous xanthomatosis)

Cholestanol lipidosis is an extremely unusual disorder (10–15 cases) involving the clinical constellation of dementia, xanthomas, cataracts, and progressive neurological dysfunction (Menkes et al, 1968). Onset is usually in childhood in the form of a dementia followed by the appearance of cataracts and xanthomas. Progressive neurological dysfunction leads to death by age 30–35. Xanthomas are most commonly found on the Achilles tendon but may also be found on triceps tendons, tibial tuberosity, or extensor tendons of the fingers. With advanced disease, pain and vibratory sensation may be lost and distal muscular atrophy is evident.

Pathological changes in the brain include glial proliferation, myelin loss and foam cells in perivascular spaces. Cerebral grey matter is spared while the white matter is devastated. Granulomas virtually replace cerebellar white matter. Xanthomas consist of birefringent crystals with multinucleate giant cells and mononuclear cells.

Biochemical defect. Cholestanol levels are markedly increased in all tissues. While the usual plasma lipids are normal, plasma cholestanol may be increased severalfold. Interestingly, the tendon xanthomas reveal cholesterol storage predominantly with mild elevation of cholestanol. Cholesterol levels in brain are increased only slightly. Cholestanol (dihydrocholesterol) is itself derived from a minor pathway of cholesterol catabolism. No direct enzymatic evidence of defective cholestanol catabolism is available. However, recent reports indicate that one of the final steps in the conversion of cholesterol to bile acids is impaired in this disorder resulting in diminished cellular capacity to catabolize cholesterol. Increased levels of cholestanol would arise in response to shunting cholesterol from its usual bile acid pathway to the cholestanol pathway. Oftebro et al (1980) reported an absence of cholesterol 26-hydroxylase activity in liver mitochondria while Salen et al (1979) had previously noted a reduction of liver microsomal 24-hydroxylase activity to 25% of control levels. Definitive confirmation will resolve this discrepancy.

Cherry-red spot-myoclonus syndrome (sialidosis type I)

The cherry-red spot-myoclonus syndrome is a slowly progressive disorder with onset in childhood and survival into adulthood (Rapin et al, 1975). The principal clinical features are cherry-red maculae and intention myclonus (myoclonic movements occurring during voluntary movement) without significant intellectual problems. Recent information provides clinical, electrophysiological and morphological evidence of a sensorimotor peripheral neuropathy (Steinman et al, 1980). Deficiency of the lysosomal enzyme, sialidase (neuraminidase), in cultured fibroblasts has been described with intermediate sialidase activity in cells from obligate heterozygotes (Thomas et al, 1978). However, the exact nature of the lysosomal inclusions may be mucopolysaccharides and glycoproteins and, thus, this syndrome may *not* represent a lipid storage disorder (Rapin et al, 1978).

GENETICS

Each of the sphingolipidoses with the exception of trihexosylceramide lipidosis (Fabry disease) is transmitted as an autosomal recessive trait which requires that each parent must be a carrier or obligate heterozygote for the disease-related recessive gene. Fabry disease, on the other hand, is inherited as an X–linked recessive, and as a result the female heterozygote may, by Lyonization (Lyon, 1962), manifest signs and symptoms as in the affected male.

With the advent of appropriate enzymological assays for each of these disorders, it is now possible to screen high-risk individuals for heterozygosity. That is, determination of the disease-related enzyme activity in potential carriers for a given disorder should yield values which are intermediate between the affected level and the normal control range. In general, activity of the disease-related enzyme in the heterozygote is 30 to 60 per cent of normal control values while affected individuals manifest less than ten percent of the disease-related enzyme activity. By this method, it has possible to provide some measure of genetic counselling for each of these disorders. The ramifications of this genetic counselling will be discussed below.

PATIENT EVALUATION

A thorough history and physical assessment are essential in evaluating the patient with an inherited lipid storage disorder. Significant historical data may be derived from a detailed family history such as evidence of consanquinity or previous children with similar difficulties. One should specifically ask about untimely childhood deaths from unknown or ill-defined causes in this or previous generations. Occasionally, the parents will describe a previous child who was given the diagnosis of 'progressive cerebral palsy' or 'progressing encephalitis'. Since cerebral palsy is non-progressive, such a description should alert the clinician.

In many instances, the lipid storage disorders profoundly affect psychomotor development. When acquired skills are lost or expected milestones are never achieved, little doubt exists about the progressive nature of the disease process. However, it is often difficult to decide whether a plateau in development represents normal variation or evidence of psychomotor delay. As a rule, the pattern of development in the child with a non-progressive central nervous system disorder resulting, for example, from the impact of neonatal hypoxia or asphyxia will be continuous but at a slower rate than normal. The child with a lipid storage disorder affecting the central nervous system may appear to exhibit a similar pattern at first glance, but as the disease process progresses, serial assessments will show that the actual rate of development is slowing.

The physical examination may also provide important clues. The presence of organomegaly suggests a storage disease. Bony abnormalities or dysmorphic facial features are encountered in patients with the mucolipidoses and with the sphingolipidosis, G_{M1}-gangliosidosis. Ophthalmologic findings include corneal changes (trihexosylceramide lipidosis), cherry-red maculae (G_{M1}-gangliosidosis, G_{M1}-gangliosidosis-Tay-Sachs disease, sphingomyelin lipidosis-type I, sialidosis Type I, and, rarely, sulphatide

lipidosis), optic atrophy (sphingolipidoses), and retinal pigmentary changes (neuronal ceroid lipofuscinoses, phytanic acid lipidosis-Refsum disease). Since the peripheral nerves may also be involved, one may see the interesting if not confusing combination of hypotonia and hyporeflexia and Babinski signs. Cerebellar ataxia and nystagmus may be prominent features of sulphatide lipidosis or the infantile forms of neuronal ceroid lipofuscinosis.

Definitive diagnosis of those diseases for which the biochemical lesion is known can be accomplished by demonstrating deficient activity of the disease-related enzyme in appropriate tissues such as leucocytes or cultured skin fibroblasts. Enzymatic assays are now available for the rapid and accurate diagnosis of the sphingolipidoses, phytanic acid lipidosis (Refsum disease) the cholesterol ester lipidoses, and sialidosis Type I. When a definitive diagnosis is established , it is crucial that other family members (parents and sibs) be tested.

Prior to the development of definitive biochemical methodologies, diagnosis depended on tissue biopsy and appropriate histological examination. Using peripheral nerve, rectal myenteric plexus, or brain, characteristic inclusions were identified along with other neuropathologic findings. For those diseases which can be established in leucocytes or cultured skin fibroblasts by relevant enzyme testing, nerve or brain biopsy is no longer acceptable. Skin biopsies should be employed when a diagnosis cannot be established clinically or biochemically and then only under carefully controlled conditions where professional expertise will guarantee proper handling of the tissue (Martin & Jacobs, 1973; O'Brien et al, 1975; Farrell and Sumi, 1977).

Brain biopsy demands even more stringent controls requiring the multidisciplinary approach which will insure skilled histology, electron microscopy, neurochemistry, and neurobiochemistry. Brain biopsy should not be conducted in hospitals lacking such a multidisciplinary capability. The goal of brain biopsy in otherwise ill-defined neurodegenerative diseases must be to provide a diagnosis, if possible ,and to guide the physician in counselling the family relative to prognosis and to possible genetic implications. The family needs to understand that the procedure is unlikely to benefit the child directly, but may provide important information regarding the disease process itself and, thereby, enhance our future approaches to patients with these problems.

PREVENTION

Where an identifiable at-risk population can be defined, as in Tay-Sachs disease, and carriers identified with easily available tissue, population screening is a rational undertaking. Programs currently in force have screened in excess of 200 000 individuals and monitored more than 600 at-risk pregnancies for Tay-Sachs disease (Kaback et al, 1977). For the other disorders of sphingolipid metabolism, we are presently dependent on the detection of index cases. Unless there is previous evidence of one of these disorders, an affected individual must be identified and the diagnosis established before the other members of that family could receive the benefits of genetic counselling.

PRENATAL DIAGNOSIS

In the last few years, each of the sphingolipidoses has been detected in a mid-trimester fetus and the diagnosis has been confirmed in aborted tissues. Since the probability of the fetus being affected for these disorders is one in four and since the abortion procedure utilizing hypertonic saline or prostaglandins is without major difficulty, the monitoring of pregnancies of at-risk couples has become an integral part of genetic counselling. In instances where the family desires additional, phenotypically-normal children, the physician can now provide and insure the realization of this possibility.

THERAPY

Effective treatment is currently unavailable for the sphingolipidoses. This can be stated unequivocally in relation to those disorders which affect the nervous system. Individuals with trihexosylceramide lipidosis (Fabry disease) have been treated effectively with renal transplantation (Clarke et al, 1972). Since the life-threatening aspects of this disorder involve chronic renal insufficiency, renal transplantation is a potentially favourable mode of therapy. The observed lowering of blood sphingolipid levels may be due to graft-produced enzyme, but also may be in part due to improved glomerular filtration and effects of immunosuppressive therapy. Similar, although less extensive , studies have been performed with splenic transplantation in Gaucher patients (Groth et al, 1972) and hepatic transplantation in Niemann-Pick disease (Delvin et al, 1974).

Specific enzyme replacement therapy has not yet been achieved for any of the lysosomal storage diseases. Enthusiasm for this modality arose following the demonstration that defective mucopolysaccharide metabolism could be normalized in cell culture systems by exposure to appropriate 'corrective factors' or enzymes. Numerous theoretical and practical difficulties exist including large scale isolation of the relevant lysosomal enzymes, potential immunological complications after repeated injection and in the case of those disorders with

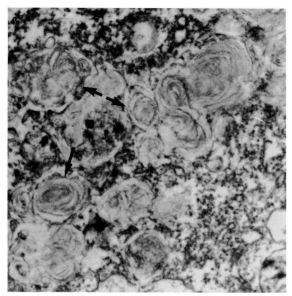

Fig. 96.11 Membranous inclusions in anterior horn cell from fetus (20 wk. gestation) with Gm_2–gangliosidosis. Reproduced from Percy et al (1973).

prominent central nervous system involvement, the physical-chemical blood brain barrier. In an attempt to circumvent these problems laboratory models have been developed to explore chemical alteration of the blood brain barrier enabling brain uptake of the lysosomal hydrolases (Barranger et al, 1977) and a variety of alternative delivery systems involving entrapment of the enzymes in liposomes (Reynolds et al, 1978) or autologous erythrocyte membranes (Hiler et al, 1973). The latter maneuvers are directed at reducing antigenicity and, for patients with lysosomal storage diseases sparing the CNS, may represent an effective alternative.

Pathological alterations in central nervous system both by light and electron microscopy (Fig. 96.11) have been noted in affected fetuses aborted at 20 weeks gestation (Percy et al, 1973). Unless these changes are found to be reversible, appropriate therapy may have to commence during intrauterine life. The availability of a number of animal models of lysosomal storage diseases provides the opportunity to evaluate these critical questions and it seems likely that progress will be made in this area in the future (Baker et al, 1979; Pritchard et al, 1980; and Wenger et al, 1980).

ACKNOWLEDGEMENT

Dawna Armstrong, M D, Department of Pathology, Baylor College of Medicine, Houston, Texas kindly assisted with the illustrative reproductions.

REFERENCES

Detailed information regarding the disorders discussed above may be found in following review articles: Stanbury J B, Wyngaarden J B, Fredrickson D S (eds) 1978 The metabolic basis of inherited disease, 4th edition McGraw Hill, New York. ch 31–40

Abramov A, Schorr S, Wolman M 1956 Generalized xanthomatosis with calcified adrenals. American Journal of Diseases of Children 91: 282–286

Aquas A P, Moura Nunes J F, Hasse Ferreira A D, Vital J P 1980 Neuronal ceroidlipofuscinosis: ultrastructural study of lymphocytic dense bodies. Neurology 30: 976–980

Armstrong D, Dimmitt S, Van Vormer D E 1974 Studies in Batten's disease I: Peroxidase deficiency in granulocytes. Archives of Neurology 30: 144–152

Austin J 1963 Studies in globoid (Krabbe) leukodystrophy. Archives of Neurology 9: 207–231

Austin J, Armstrong D, Shearer L 1965 Metachromatic form of diffuse cerebral sclerosis V. The nature and significance of low sulfatase activity. Archives of Neurology 13: 593–614

Baker H J, Reynolds G D, Walkley S U, Cox N R, Baker G H 1979 The gangliosidoses: comparative features and research applications. Veterinary Pathology 16: 635–649

Barranger J A, Pentchev P G, Rapoport S I, Brady R O 1977 Augmentation of brain lysosomal enzyme activity following enzyme infusion with concomitant alteration of the blood-brain barrier. Annals of Neurology 1: 496

Beaudet A L, Ferry G D, Nichols Jr B L, Rosenberg H S 1977 Cholesterol ester storage disease: Clinical, biochemical, and pathological studies. Journal of Pediatrics 90: 910–914

Beaudet A L, Lipson M H, Ferry G D, Nichols Jr B L 1974 Acid lipase in cultured fibroblasts: cholesterol ester storage disease. Journal of Laboratory and Clinical Medicine 84: 54–61

Beutler E, Kuhl W 1975 Subunit structure of human hexosaminidase verified: interconvertibility of hexosaminidase isozymes. Nature 258: 262–263

Bird T D, Lagunoff D 1978 Neurologic manifestations of Fabry disease in female carriers. Annals of Neurology 4: 537–540

Brady R O 1978 Sphingolipidoses. Annual Review of Biochemistry 46: 687–713

Brady R O, Kanfer J N, Shapiro D 1965 Metabolism of glucocerebrosides. II evidence of an enzymatic deficiency in Gaucher's disease. Biochemical and Biophysical Research Communications 18: 221–225

Brady R O, Kanfer J N, Mock M, Fredrickson D S 1966 The metabolism of sphingomyelin. II evidence of an enzymatic deficiency in Niemann-Pick disease. Proceedings of the National Academy of Sciences USA 55: 366–369

Brady R O, Gal A E, Bradley R M, Mårtenson E, Warshaw A L, Laster L 1967 Enzymatic defect in Fabry's disease, ceramidetrihexosidase deficiency. New England Journal of Medicine 276: 1163–1167

Brett E M, Ellis R B, Haas L, Ikonne J U, Lake B D, Patrick A D, Stephens R 1973 Late onset G_{M2}-gangliosidosis. Archives of Diseases in Childhood 48: 775–785

Burda C D, Winder P R, 1967 Angiokeratoma corporis diffusum universale (Fabry's disease) in female subjects. American Journal of Medicine 42: 293–301

Christomanou, H 1980 Niemann-Pick disease, Type C: Evidence for the deficiency of an activating factor stimulating sphingomyelin and glucocerebroside degradation. Hoppe-Seyler's Zeitschrift Für Physiologische Chemie 361: 1489–1502

Clarke J T R, Guttman R D, Wolfe L S, Beaudoin J G, Morehouse D D 1972 Enzyme replacement therapy by renal allotransplantation in Fabry's diease. New England Journal of Medicine 287: 1215–1218

Conzelmann E, Sandhoff K 1978 A B variant of infantile G_{M2}-gangliosidoeis: deficiency of a factor necessary for stimulation of hexosaminidase A-catalyzed degradation of ganglioside G_{M2} and glycolipid G_{A2}. Proceedings of the National Academy of Sciences USA 75: 3979–3983

Crocker A C, Vawter G F, Neuhauser E B D, Rosowsky A 1965 Wolman's disease: three patients with a recently described lipidosis. Pediatrics 35: 627–640

Crocker A C, Cohen J, Farber S 1967 The 'Lipogranulomatosis' syndrome; review with report of patient showing milder involvement, in: Aronson S M, Volk B W (ed) Inborn Disorders of Sphingolipid Metabolism, Pergammon Press, Oxford. pp 485–503

DeDuve C, Pressman B C, Gianetto R, Wattiaux R, Appelmans F 1955 Tissue fractionation studies. intracellular distribution patterns of enzymes in rat-liver tissue. Biochemical Journal 60: 604–617

Delvin E, Glorieux F, Daloze P, Gorman J, Block P 1974 Niemann-Pick type A: enzyme replacement by liver transplantation. American Journal of Human Genetics 26: 25A

Dulaney J T, Milunsky A, Sidbury J R, Hobolth N, Moser H W 1976 Diagnosis of lipogranulomatosis (Farber's disease) by use of cultured fibroblasts. Journal of Pediatrics 89: 59–61

Dunn H G, Dolman C L, Farrell D F, Tischler B, Hasinoff C, Woolf L I 1976 Krabbe's leukodystrophy without globoid cells. Neurology 26: 1035–1041

Farrell D F, Sumi S M 1977 Skin punch biopsy in the diagnosis of juvenile neuronal ceroid-lipofuscinosis. Archives of Neurology 34: 39–44

Fluharty A L, Stevens R L, Davis L L, Shapiro L J, Kihara H 1978 Presence of arylsulfatase A (ARS A) in multiple sulfatase deficiency disorder fibroblasts. American Journal of Human Genetics 30: 249–255

Freeman J M, McKhann G M 1969 Degenerative diseases of the central nervous system. Advances in Pediatrics 16: 121–175

Gal A E, Brady R O, Barranger J A, Pentchev P G 1980 The diagnosis of type A and type B Niemann-Pick disease and detection of carriers using leucocytes and a chromogenic analogue of sphingomyelin. Clinica Chimica Acta 104: 129–132

Gibberd F B, Page N G R, Billimoria J D, Retsas S 1979 Heredopathia atactica polyneuritiformis (Refsum's disease) treated by diet and plasma exchange. Lancet 1: 575–578

Gilbert F, Kucherlapati R, Creagan R P, Murnane M J, Darlington G J, Ruddle F H 1975 Tay-Sachs' and Sandhoff's diseases: the assignment of genes for hexosaminidase A and B to individual human chromosomes. Proceedings of the National Academy of Sciences USA 72: 263–267

Groth C G, Blomstrand R, Hagenfeldt L, Ockerman P A, Samuelsson K, Svennerholm L 1972 Metabolic changes following splenic transplantation in a case of Gaucher's Disease in: Volk B W and Aronson S M (ed) Sphingolipids, Sphingolipidoses, and Allied Disorders Plenum Press, New York pp 633–639

Grunnet M L, Spilsbury P R 1973 The central nervous system in Fabry's disease. Archives of Neurology 28: 231–234

Haberland C, Brunngraber E, Witting L,Daniels A 1973 Juvenile metachromatic leucodystrophy. Acta Neuropathologica 26: 93–106

Hagberg B, Sourander P, Svennerholm L, Voss H 1960 Late infantile metachromatic leukodystrophy of the genetic type. Acta Paediatrica Scandinavica 49: 135–153

Hagberg B, Haltia M, Sourander P, Svennerholm L, Eeg-Olofsson O 1974 Polyunsaturated fatty acid lipidosis – infantile form of so-called neuronal ceroid lipofuscinosis 1: Clinical and morphological aspects. Acta Paediatrica Scandinavica 63: 752–763

Haltia T, Palo J, Haltia M, Icén A 1980 Juvenile metachromatic leukodystrophy. Archives of Neurology 37: 42–46

Harzer K, Schlote W, Peiffer J, Benz H U, Anzil A P 1978 Neuroviscidosis lipidosis compatible with Niemann-Pick disease type C. Acta Neuropathologica 43: 97–104

Hers H G 1963 α-Glucosidase deficiency in generalized glycogen storage disease (Pompe's disease). Biochemical Journal 86: 11–16

Hultberg B, Sjoblad S, Ockerman P A 1973 4-methylumbelliferyl-β-glucosidase in cultured human fibroblasts from controls and patients with Gaucher's disease. Clinica Chimica Acta 49: 93–97

Hultberg B 1978 β-glucosidase activities in the Norrbotten type of juvenile Gaucher's disease. Acta Neurologica Scandinavica 58: 89–94

Jensen G E, Shukla V K S, Gissel-Nielsen G, Clausen J 1978 Biochemical abnormalities in Batten's syndrome. Scandinavian Journal of Clinical and Laboratory Investigation 38: 309–318

Johnson W G, Chutorian A, Miranda A 1977 A new juvenile hexosaminidase deficiency disease presenting as cerebellar ataxia. Neurology 27: 1012–1018

Kaback M M, Nathan T J, Greenwald S 1977 Tay-Sachs disease: heterozygote screening and prenatal diagnosis – US experience and world perspective in: Kaback M (ed) Progress in Clinical and Biological Research in Tay-Sachs: Screening and Prevention, Alan R Liss Publishers, New York pp 13–36

Kamoshita S, Aron A, Suzuki K, Suzuki K 1969 Infantile Niemann-Pick disease ,a chemical study. American Journal of Diseases of Children 117: 379–394

Lake B D 1971 Histochemical detection of the enzyme deficiency in blood films in Wolman's disease. Journal of Clinical Pathology 24: 617–620

Landing B H, Silverman F N, Craig J M, Jacoby M D, Lahey M E, Chadwick D L 1964 Familial neurovisceral lipidosis. American Journal of Diseases of Children 108: 503–522

Lou H O C, Reske-Nielsen E 1971 The central nervous system in Fabry's disease. Archives of Neurology 25: 351–359

Lowden J A, O'Brien J S 1979 Sialidosis: a review of human neuraminidase deficiency. American Journal of Human Genetics 31: 1–18

Lu⟨…⟩ A, Lilja L G, Lundberg P O, Try K 1972 ⟨…⟩thia atactica polyneuritiformis (Refsum's disease). Neurology 8: 309–324

⟨…⟩2 Sex chromatin and gene action in the ⟨…⟩-chromosome. American Journal of Human ⟨…⟩–148

⟨…⟩rien J S 1968 Lipid composition of the

nervous system in Refsum's disease. Journal of Lipid Research 9: 552–561

Mårtensson E 1969 Glycosphingolipids of animal tissue. Progress in the Chemistry of Fats and Other Lipids 10: 367–407

Martin J J, Jacobs K 1973 Skin biopsy as a contribution to diagnosis in late infantile amaurotic idiocy with curvilinear bodies. European Neurology 10: 281–291

Max S R et al 1974 G_{M3} (hematoside) sphingolipodystrophy. New England Journal of Medicine 291: 929–931

Mehl E, Jatzkewitz H 1963 Uber ein Cerebrosid-schwefelsaureester spaltendes Enzym aus Schweineniere. Hoppe-Seylers Zeitschrift fur Physiologische Chemie 331: 292–294

Menkes J H, Schimschock J R, Swanson P D 1968 Cerebrotendinous xanthomatosis: The storage of cholestanol within the nervous system. Archives of Neurology 19: 47–53

Murphy J V, Wolfe H J, Balazs E A,Moser H W 1971 A patient with deficiency of arylsulfatases A, B, C and steroid sulfatase associated with storage of sulfatide, cholesterol sulfate and glycosaminoglycans in: Bernsohn J Grossman H (ed) Lipid Storage Diseases: Enzymatic Defects and Clinical Implications, Academic Press, New York pp 67–110

Nishimura R N, Barranger J A 1980 Neurologic complications of Gaucher's disease type 3. Archives of Neurology 37: 92–93

O'Brien J S 1975 Molecular genetics of G_{M1} β-galactosidase. Clinical Genetics 8: 303–313

O'Brien J S et al 1972 Juvenile G_{M1} gangliosidoses: clinical, pathological, chemical, and enzymatic studies. Clinical Genetics 3: 411–434

O'Brien J S, Bernett J, Veath M L, Paa D 1975 Lysosomal storage disorders: diagnosis by ultrastructural examination of skin biopsy specimens. Archives of Neurology 32: 592–599

Oftebro H, Björkhem I, Skrede S, Schreiner A, Pedersen J I 1980 Cerebrotendinous xanthomatosis: a defect in mitochondrial 26-hydroxylation required for normal biosynthesis of cholic acid. Journal of Clinical Investigation 65: 1418–1430

Okada S, O'Brien J S 1968 Generalized gangliosidosis: beta-galactosidase deficiency. Science 160: 1002–1004

Okada S, O'Brien J S 1969 Tay-Sachs disease: generalized absence of a beta-D-N-acetylhexosaminidase component. Science 165: 698–700

O'Neill B,Butler A B, Young E, Falk P M, Bass N H 1978 Adult-onset G_{M2}-gangliosidosis. Neurology 28: 1117–1123

Oonk J G W, Van der Helm H J, Martin J J 1979 Spinocerebellar degeneration: hexosaminidase A and B deficiency in two adult sisters. Neurology 29: 380–384

Patrick A D, Lake B O 1969 Deficiency of an acid lipase in Wolman's disease. Nature 222: 1067–1068

Percy A K, Kaback M M 1971 Infantile and adult-onset metachromatic leukodystrophy, biochemical comparisons and predictive diagnosis. New England Journal of Medicine 285: 785–787

Percy A K, McCormick U M, Kaback M M, Herndon R M 1973 Ultrastructure manifestations of G_{M1}- and G_{M2}-gangliosidosis in fetal tissues. Archives of Neurology 28: 417–419

Percy A K, Kaback M M, Herndon R M 1977 Metachromatic leukodystrophy: comparison of early- and late-onset forms. Neurology 27: 933–941

Percy A K, Shapiro L J, Kaback M M 1979 Inherited lipid storage diseases of the central nervous system. In: Gluck L (ed) Current Problems in Pediatrics, Vol 9(11) Yearbook Medical Publishers Inc, Chicago pp 1–51

Philippart M, Martin L, Martin J J, Menkes J H 1969 Niemann-Pick disease, morphological and biochemical studies in the visceral form with late central nervous system involvement (Crocker's group C). Archives of Neurology 20: 227–238

Pilz H, Heipertz R, Seidel D 1979 Basic findings and current developments in sphingolipidoses. Human Genetics 47: 113–134

Porter M T, Fluharty A L, Trammell G, Kihara H 1971 A correlation of intracellular cerebroside sulfatase activity in fibroblasts with latency in metachromatic leukodystrophy. Biochemical and Biophysical Research Communications 44: 660–666

Pritchard D H, Napthine D V, Sinclair A J 1980 Globoid cell leukodystrophy in polled Dorset sheep. Veterinary Pathology 17: 399–405

Rapin I, Katzman R, Engel Jr J 1975 Cherry red spots and progressive myoclonus without dementia: A distinct syndrome with neuronal storage. Transactions of the American Neurological Association 100: 39–42

Rapin I, Goldfischer S, Katzman R, Engel J, O'Brien J S 1978 The cherry-red spot-myoclonus syndrome. Annals of Neurology 3: 234–242

Refsum S 1960 Heredopathia atactica polyneuritiformis reconsideration. World Neurology 1: 334–337

Reynolds G D, Baker H J, Reynolds R H 1978 Enzyme replacement using liposome carriers in feline G_{M1}-gangliosidosis fibroblasts. Nature 275: 754–755

Sachs B 1887 On arrested cerebral development with special reference to its cortical pathology. Journal of Nervous and Mental Diseases 14: 541–553

Salen G, Shefer S, Cheng F W, Dayal B, Batta A K, Tint G S 1979 Cholic acid biosynthesis: the enzymatic defect in cerebrotendinous xanthomatosis. Journal of Clinical Investigation 63: 38–44

Sandhoff K, Andreae U, Jatzkewitz H 1968 Deficient hexosaminidase activity in an exceptional case of Tay-Sachs disease with additional storage of kidney globoside in visceral organs. Pathologia Europaea 3: 278–285

Sandhoff K, Harzer H, Wässle W, Jatzkewitz H 1971 Enzyme alterations and lipid storage in three variants of Tay-Sachs disease. Journal of Neurochemistry 18: 2469–2489

Sandhoff K, Christomanou H 1979 Biochemistry and genetics of gangliosidoses. Human Genetics 50: 107–143

Shapiro L J et al 1979 Metachromatic leukodystrophy without arylsulfatase A deficiency. Pediatric Research 13: 1179–1181

Sheth K J, Swick H M 1979 Peripheral nerve conduction in Fabry disease. Annals of Neurology 7: 319–323

Sima A A F, Robertson D M 1978 Involvement of peripheral nerve and muscle in Fabry's disease. Archives of Neurology 35: 291–301

Singer H S, Schafer I A 1972 Clinical and enzymatic variations in G_{M1}-generalized gangliosidosis. American Journal of Human Genetics 24: 454–463

Soffer D, Yamanaka T, Wenger D A, Suzuki K, Suzuki K 1980 Central nervous system involvement in adult-onset Gaucher's disease. Acta Neuropathologica 49: 1–6

Sourander P, Hansson H A, Olsson Y, Svennerholm L, 1966 Experimental studies on the pathogenesis of leukodystrophies, II the effect of sphingolipids on various cell types in cultures from the nervous system. Acta Neuropathologica 6: 231–242

Steinberg D, Hutton D 1972 Phytanic acid storage disease,

in: Volk B W, Aronson S M (ed) Sphingolipids Sphingolipidoses and Allied Disorders, Plenum Press, New York pp 515–532

Steinman L et al 1980 Peripheral neuropathy in the cherry-red spot-myoclonus syndrome (sialidosis type I). Annals of Neurology 7: 450–456

Stokke O, Try K, Eldjarn L 1961 α-Oxidation as an alternative pathway for the degradation of branched chain fatty acids in man, and its failure in patients with Refsum's disease. Biochimica et Biophysica Acta 144: 271–284

Sugita M, Dulaney J T, Moser H W 1972 Ceramidase deficiency in Farber's disease (lipogranulomatosis). Science 178: 1100–1102

Suzuki K 1968 Cerebral G_{M1}-gangliosidosis: chemical pathology of visceral organs. Science 159: 1471–1472

Suzuki K, Suzuki Y 1970 Globoid cell leukodystrophy (Krabbe's disease): deficiency of galactocerebroside β-galactosidase. Proceedings of the National Academy of Sciences USA 66: 302–309

Svennerholm E, Svennerholm L 1963 Neutral glycolipids of human blood serum, spleen, and liver. Nature 198: 688–689

Svennerholm L 1962 The chemical structure of normal human brain and Tay-Sachs ganglioside. Biochemical and Biophysical Research Communications 9: 436–446

Svennerholm L 1969 New principles for the classification of glycolipidoses. Metabolismo 5: 60–70

Svennerholm L 1970 Ganglioside Metabolism, in: Florkin M, Stotz E H (ed) Comprehensive Biochemistry; Vol 18 Elsevier, Amsterdam Chap IV

Svennerholm L, Zettergren L 1957 Infantile amaurotic idiocy. Acta Pathologica et Microbiologica Scandinavica 41: 127–134

Svennerholm L, Hagberg B, Haltia M, Sourander P, Vanier M T 1975 Polyunsaturated fatty acid lipidosis, II lipid biochemical studies. Acta Paediatrica Scandinavica 64: 489–496

Svennerholm L, Vanier M T, Månsson J E 1980 Krabbe Disease: a galactosylsphingosine (psychosine) lipidosis. Journal of Lipid Research 21: 53–64

Tay W 1881 Symmetrical changes in the region of the yellow spot in each eye of an infant. Transactions of the Ophthalmological Societies of the United Kingdom 1: 55–57

Thomas G H, Tipton R E, Ch'ien L T, Reynolds L W, Miller C S 1978 Sialidase deficiency: the enzyme defect in an adult with macular cherry-red spots and myoclonus without dementia. Clinical Genetics 13: 369–379

Valvanis A, Friede R L, Schubiger O, Hayek J 1980 Computed tomography in neuronal ceroid lipofuscinosis. Neuroradiology 19: 35–38

Wenger D A, Sattler M, Kudoh T, Snyder S P, Kingston R S 1980 Niemann-Pick disease: a genetic model in Siamese cats. Science 208: 1471–1473

Wenger D A, Sattler M, Mueller O T, Myers G G, Schneiman R S, Nixon G W 1980 Adult G_{M1}-gangliosidosis: clinical and biochemical studies on two patients and comparison to other patients called variant or adult G_{M1}-gangliosidosis. Clinical Genetics 17: 323–334

Westermarck T, Sandholm M 1977 Decreased erythrocyte glutathione peroxidase activity in neuronal ceroid lipofuscinosis (NCL) corrected with selenium supplementation. Acta Pharmacologica et Toxicologica 40: 70–74

Winsor E J T, Welch J P 1978 Genetic demographic aspects of Nova Scotia Niemann-Pick disease (type D). American

Journal of Human Genetics 30: 530–538
Wolfe L S, Ng Ying Kin N M K, Baker R R, Carpenter S,
    Anderman F 1977 Identification of retinoyl complexes as
    the autofluorescent component of the neuronal storage
    material in Batten disease. Science 195: 1360–1362
Yaffe M G et al 1979 An amyotrophic lateral sclerosis-like
    syndrome with hexosaminidase A deficiency: a new type of
    G_{M2}-gangliosidosis. Neurology 29: 611

Young E, Wilson J, Patrick A D, Crome L 1972
    Galactocerebrosidase deficiency in globoid cell
    leukodystrophy of late onset. Archives of Diseases in
    Childhood 47: 449–450
Zeman W, Siakotos A N 1973 The neuronal ceroid
    lipofuscinoses. In: Hers H G vanHoof F (ed) Lysosomes
    and storage diseases, Academic Press, New York
    pp 519–551

Pharmacogenetics

D.A. Price Evans

INTRODUCTION

Here we shall not deal primarily with metabolic disorders which give rise to spontaneous disease but rather with how the genetic constitution of patients determines to a considerable degree what happens when they receive drug medications.

Two main classes of polymorphism will be considered, those affecting drug metabolism and those influencing pharmacologic effect. In addition, HLA associated abnormal drug reactions, quantitative genetic studies and inter-ethnic variability in drug response will be considered.

SINGLE GENE PHENOMENA

Drug metabolism

All phenotypes common

Acetylation This polymorphism was found as a result of studying the fate of isoniazid in tuberculous patients. Some patients were found to have a relatively high plasma concentration at a standard time following a standard dose, whilst other patients had a relatively low plasma concentration under the same circumstances. An individual fell in the same class on repeated testing. Family studies disclosed the property to be controlled by two alleles at one autosomal locus.

It was suspected that these alleles might work by governing the acetylation of isoniazid. This suspicion was proved to be correct in two ways – (1) sulphadimidine (sulphamethazine) which only undergoes one biotransformation, viz. acetylation, was shown to have this enzymic conjugation controlled by the same alleles; (2) the degree of acetylation of isoniazid *in vitro* by liver tissue corresponded with the *in vivo* phenotype determined on the individual from whom the tissue was derived.

The enzyme governed by the alleles is N-acetyltransferase, present in liver and intestinal mucosa. It is not known whether the alleles control enzyme structure or rate of synthesis (see Evans, 1968).

Drug compounds which are polymorphically acetylated include:- isoniazid, sulphadimidine, sulphapyridine (especially as derived from salicylazo-sulphapyridine), hydralazine, dapsone, procaine amide and nitrazepam (following reduction of the nitro group to give an amine). Polymorphic acetylation of phenelzine has been put forward as an idea on the basis of its possessing a hydrazino-moiety the same as isoniazid and hydralazine. There is, however, no definite proof for this idea.

The importance of the acetylation polymorphism in practical therapeutics is shown in Table 97.1.

The ethnic distribution of the alleles controlling the acetylator polymorphism shows one interesting and unexplained fact. Along the Eastern littoral of Asia and associated islands is a 'cline'. The Eskimos are almost all rapid acetylators as are 90% of the Japanese. This percentage steadily falls towards the equator. No clear pattern has emerged with regard to allele frequencies in other geographic locations.

Since hydralazine-induced systemic lupus erythematosus (SLE) is a disorder of slow acetylators, surveys have been made of spontaneous SLE. It would appear however that patients with this disorder have a normal distribution of the alleles controlling the acetylation polymorphism.

Paroxonase The compound paroxon (0, 0-diethyl-0-p-nitrophenyl phosphate) is an organo-phosphorous anticholinesterase. It was formerly used in therapeutic practice for the treatment of glaucoma (Fagerlind et al, 1952).

In mammals the compound parathion is transformed in the liver by oxidative desulphuration into paroxon which is the active metabolite. Paroxon is then degraded into inactive moieties by the esterase paroxonase (EC 3.1.1.2) which is present in the plasma.

A genetic polymorphism for plasma paroxonase activity has been shown by Geldmacher-von-Mallinckrodt et al (1973) and by Playfer et al (1976) who used different assay techniques. Two phenotypes are recognisable, viz. persons with high and low enzymic activity. Low activity is an autosomal recessive character governed by an allele with a frequency of 0.7034 in the British white population (Fig. 97.1).

Table 97.1 Acetylator phenotypes in therapeutics.

Drug (i.e. enviromental factor)	Phenotype	Effect observed in the phenotype noted
Isoniazid	Slow	More prone to develop peripheral neuropathy on therapy with conventional doses
	Slow	More prone to phenytoin adverse effects when simultaneously being treated for tuberculosis with INH
	Slow	More prone to hepatotoxicity when being treated for tuberculosis with rifampicin and INH
	Rapid	Less favourable results of treating open pulmonary tuberculosis with a once-weekly isoniazid dosage regime
	Rapid	More prone to develop isoniazid-hepatitis
Hydralazine	Slow	Develop antinuclear antibodies and systemic lupus erythematosus-like syndrome
	Rapid	Require higher doses to control hypertension
Salicyl-azo-sulphapyridine	Slow	Increased incidence of various adverse reactions in healthy subjects and when drug used to treat ulcerative and Crohn's colitis
Dapsone	Rapid	Higher doses needed to control dermatitis herpetiformis (disputed)
	Slow	More adverse haematological effects

Genetic polymorphism of acetylation has been described for sulphadimidine, sulphapyridine, and the amine metabolite of nitrazepam produced in the body as a result of reduction, and for these drugs no firm association of a clinical event with either phenotype has been defined. Procaine amide has been shown to be polymorphically acetylated; and the correlation of clinical effects with plasma concentration makes it likely that the acetylator phenotype is relevant in clinical practice.

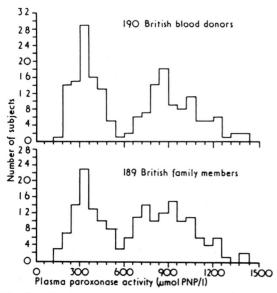

Fig. 97.1 The frequency distribution of plasma paroxonase activity in white British subjects (from Playfer et al, 1976).

Playfer et al (1976) also showed that there were large differences in the frequency distributions of plasma paroxonase activity in various ethnic groups. Agricultural and horticultural workers are occasionally exposed to parathion. It may be speculated (but is quite unproven) that persons genetically endowed with a high plasma paroxonase activity may be better able to withstand such exposure than individuals with the low activity phenotype.

As with most enzyme polymorphisms, the natural substrate and ecological significance are unknown.

Oxidation of debrisoquine Debrisoquine has been in clinical use for some years as a post-ganglionic sympathetic blocker type of antihypertensive. Studies of its metabolic fate revealed oxidation at a number of sites, by far the most important of which was on the carbon atom at the 4 position on the heterocyclic ring. The parent compound and the main metabolite can be simultaneously measured in urine in one gas chromatographic procedure.

Examination of the urine for debrisoquine and 4-hydroxydebrisoquine following a single small oral dose of the compound was performed in a population of healthy persons. Three out of 93 were shown to be in a category of their own, excreting only a very small amount of the metabolite (and much more of the unchanged drug) as compared to the other 90 persons. These 3 persons were termed 'poor metabolisers (PM)' and the remainder 'extensive metabolisers (EM)'. This polymorphism has been confirmed by studying large numbers of subjects (Fig. 97.2). An individual on re-testing falls in the same phenotypic class. The response is quantified as $\log_{10}$ metabolic ratio:-

$$\log_{10} \left[\frac{\text{conc. debrisoquine}}{\text{conc. 4-hydroxydebrisoquine}} \right]$$

Family studies have shown poor metabolisers to be homozygous for the allele controlling the recessive phenotype.

Hypotension has long been known to be an adverse effect of debrisoquine (the same as for many antihyper-

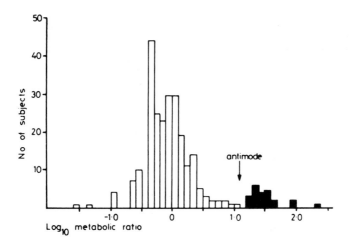

Fig. 97.2 The frequency distribution of $\log_{10}$ $\left[\dfrac{\text{concentration of urinary debrisoquine}}{\text{concentration of urinary 4-hydroxydebrisoquine}}\right]$ (from Evans et al, 1980).

tensives). An explanation for some of the cases of hypotension is afforded by the observation that PM subjects are more prone to hypotension than are EM subjects following a single therapeutic dose.

Preliminary results suggest that oxidation of the following compounds may be under the control of the 'debrisoquine' alleles:- guanoxan, phenacetin, phenytoin, metiamide and 4-methoxyamphetamine.

These suggestions will need to be confirmed by carrying out surveys on large numbers of subjects.

Sparteine Sparteine is an alkaloid formerly in clinical use as an anti-arrhythmic and oxytocic drug. In view of what follows, it is interesting to note that it was abandoned because of 'the unpredictability of its effects'. It has proved possible to measure sparteine and two of its metabolites (said to be dehydrated N-oxides) in the urine by a single gas chromatographic assay following a single small oral dose.

This procedure has been carried out in a standardised manner on a population of 360 subjects and it has been found that 5% lack the ability to produce the metabolites (Eichelbaum et al, 1979). It is suggested that these 'non-metabolisers' have a different genetically determined phenotype from the 'metabolisers', and that there is a genetic polymorphism in the metabolism of this compound. However, there are as yet no adequate family data to support this proposition.

It may be speculated (but there is no proof) that persons prone to adverse reactions following the therapeutic administration of sparteine in the past may well have been non-metabolisers.

A further point of interest is the relationship between the oxidation of debrisoquine and the metabolism of

sparteine. The apparent gene frequencies are similar and two preliminary reports suggest there may be some degree of common genetic control of the metabolism of the two compounds.

Ethanol It is a common observation that individuals differ markedly in their responses to ethanol. Recent studies have shed some light on the basis for this variability.

Of particular interest is the inter-ethnic difference in the pharmacologic effects of ethanol. Wolff (1972) showed 83% of 117 Oriental adults flushed after moderate amounts of beer, whereas flushing only occurred in 3% of occidentals tested the same way. Likewise, Ewing et al (1974) found 70% of 24 Orientals and only 13% of 24 occidentals flushed after ingesting ethanol.

Ewing et al (1974) suggested that the phenomenon might have a genetic basis, and tested the hypothesis that the flushing might be caused in Orientals by higher blood acetaldehyde levels. In the event this parameter showed a tendency to be higher in Orientals, but the difference between the two ethnic groups did not achieve statistical significance.

The rates at which individuals from different races metabolise ethanol have also been investigated. For example, Hanna (1978) found Chinese and Japanese subjects metabolised ethanol at a higher rate than Europeans. Reed (1978) surveyed data of this type and delineated certain problems of interpretation. However, the study of Reed et al (1976) compared both ethanol metabolism and acetaldehyde production in three different ethnic groups and showed both a higher ethanol metabolism and a higher acetaldehyde production in Chinese than in Caucasian subjects.

So there is a considerable body of evidence to suggest that Orientals show more pharmacologic effect than Europeans after alcohol ingestion and that they may metabolise ethanol to acetaldehyde at a higher rate.

Studies of liver enzymes *in vitro* must also be considered. The enzymes concerned are alcohol dehydrogenase (ADH) and acetaldehyde dehydrogenase.

A polymorphism for ADH was described on the basis of kinetic measurements by von Wartburg et al (1965). An 'atypical' enzyme was found in liver tissue in 2 out of 32 Europeans. This 'atypical' enzyme was shown to have a different molecular structure by possessing different pH optima, subtrate specificity and susceptibility to metal binding agents. It has a much greater capacity to metabolise ethanol than did the 'usual' form of the enzyme.

Later electrophoretic studies showed different liver alcohol dehydrogenases which were presumed by analogy with other enzymes to be under the control of three genetic loci. The 'atypical' form was shown to be due to a variant at ADH_2 (Smith et al, 1971).

'Atypical' liver ADH was found to occur in much higher frequency in the Japanese population than in the North European populations. For example, 85% of 40 Japanese livers possessed the atypical enzyme in the study of Harada et al (1980a).

Much less work has been done on acetaldehyde dehydrogenase. However, it has been shown that this enzyme, derived from human liver, also exhibits polymorphism *in vitro*. Harada et al (1980b) demonstrated the existence of four isozymes of liver acetaldehyde dehydrogenase. These isozymes have different Km values as well as showing differences on isoelectric focussing, evidence favouring the view that they have different molecular structures. Absence of the highly active band I isozyme was found in 52% of 40 Japanese – a phenomenon not observed in 68 Germans (Harada 1980a).

So we now have the problem of relating the *in vivo* pharmacologic and metabolic information with the *in vitro* enzymologic information on a population basis. As compared with Europeans, the Japanese for example, have more flushing after ethanol ingestion, with possibly a higher ethanol metabolism and acetaldehyde production, coupled with a higher incidence of 'atypical' ADH and absence of the highly active band I acetaldehyde dehydrogenase. So this naturally leads to the suggestion that the enzymic endowment leads to the *in vivo* observations.

When phenotyping can only be performed with liver tissue it is obviously difficult to correlate *in vivo* and *in vitro* observations in the same individuals. An early attempt was that of Edwards and Evans (1967) who estimated the ethanol metabolism of individuals scheduled for laparotomy and then 'typed' the ADH from small liver biopsies. Two individuals who possessed

'atypical' ADH did not have significantly shorter blood ethanol half-lives after a standard intravenous ethanol infusion.

However Harada et al (1980b) claim to have established a direct relationship in Japanese between lack of liver acetaldehyde dehydrogenase isozyme I and alcohol flushing.

The relationship of these genetic/enzymic observations to flushing produced by combinations of ethanol with chloropropamide and ethanol with metranidazole are at present obscure.

Some phenotypes rare

Pseudocholinesterase When succinyl choline (suxamethonium) was introduced into clinical practice as a short-term muscle relaxant, occasional patients were found who suffered from prolonged apnoea. Plasma pseudocholinesterase was known to hydrolyse the drug and so terminate its action. Therefore, the activity of this enzyme was investigated and the persons who suffered from the prolonged apnoea were found to have relatively low activities. In some individuals it became apparent that the low plasma activity was produced by a pathologic process, e.g. liver disease, poisoning by organophosphorous compounds, malnutrition, severe anaemia, hyperpyrexia, infectious diseases, cardiac failure, uraemia, catatonia and malignancy (Lehmann & Liddell, 1961). However, in many individuals such an explanation was not tenable and so the possibility arose that the low plasma enzyme activity was an inherited trait. Family studies of subjects with prolonged apnoea revealed healthy relatives who also had low plasma pseudocholinesterase activities (Lehmann & Simmons, 1958).

An important advance came about by studying the effects of enzyme inhibitors on plasma pseudocholinesterase. The action of dibucaine on the hydrolysis of benzoyl choline provided a standard test. The percentage inhibition of enzymic activity was termed the 'dibucaine number' (DN) (Kalow & Genest, 1957). In the families of subjects who had suffered prolonged apnoea following succinyl choline administration, the DN values were found to fall into three groups or modes. The probands had values around 20, their parents and some other relatives values around 50 to 60, whereas other family members and most of the population had values of about 80. Thus there were identified respectively 'abnormal' homozygotes, heterozygotes and 'normal' homozygotes. The nomenclature of the system was as follows. Enzymes were termed 'usual' U and 'atypical' A. The locus was termed the first esterase locus E_1. The alleles were termed E_1^u and E_1^a which were responsible for the structures of enzymes U and A respectively. It was noted that there was a tendency for a larger variance in the middle mode than in the others (Kalow & Staron, 1957).

Other inhibitors were then studied and fluoride ions were found to inhibit plasma pseudocholinesterase in a similar manner to dibucaine, that is to say considerable inhibition in most individuals, little inhibition of apnoeic subjects with heterozygotes intermediate. The percentage inhibition with fluoride was termed the fluoride number (FN). When a large number of relatives of apnoeic subjects were studied by both techniques it was found that separate small groups of individuals gave characteristic DN and FN values which indicated they were distinct phenotypes. This was the evidence for the existence of another allele E_1^f (Harris & Whittaker, 1961).

Further studies have revealed the existence of a fourth 'silent' allele which controls the structure of an enzyme with a very low activity. This allele is designated E_1^s (Liddell et al, 1962).

Genotypes which do not possess E_1^u have increased sensitivity to succinyl choline and are at risk of developing prolonged apnoea with customary doses. It is a fact however, that some individuals develop prolonged apnoea and do not have any pathological lesion which could be held responsible and who type $E_1^u E_1^u$ on the above tests. A recent study of such patients by Goedde et al (1979), using a new in vitro test which employs ^{14}C-labelled succinyl choline to assess plasma pseudocholinesterase, suggests the existence of further apnoea-prone genetic variants.

Individuals have been described with increased resistance to succinyl choline, due to their possessing a superactive variant of the enzyme and this is also a genetically determined character (Neitlich, 1966).

A second locus E_2 has been identified by electrophoretic studies of plasma pseudocholinesterase, but alleles at this locus do not influence the apnoea-proneness or other effects of the alleles at the E_1 locus (Harris et al, 1963).

Acatalasia Formerly catalase was considered to be essential to the functioning of mammalian cells. In 1946 however, a clinical observation by Professor Takahara showed that this presumption was not correct (see Takahara, 1952). A girl aged 11 years had been much afflicted by gangrene around the teeth of which she had lost several. Thereafter, caries involving the maxilla was followed by the development of an inflammatory mass in the maxillary sinus. After excising the inflammatory mass, Professor Takahara poured hydrogen peroxide on the raw surface as was his custom. Instead of frothing bright red, the wound became brownish-black. From this simple but startling observation, he deduced that the blood and tissues of this patient did not contain catalase. Subsequent biochemical investigations showed his deduction to have been correct. Subsequently further similar patients with oral gangrene were discovered in Japan and Korea.

An investigation of the genetics of the condition revealed that patients with the oral gangrene syndrome were homozygotes. Heterozygotes could be identified in Japanese pedigrees as a distinctly separate mode in a frequency distribution of blood catalase values.

For a while it was thought that acatalasia alleles were confined to the populations of Japan and surrounding countries. However, as a result of laborious searches, acatalasics were later discovered in Switzerland, Israel and Germany. There is some evidence for heterozygotes in Sweden and the U.S.A.

In the European families the clear-cut trimodal blood catalase distribution of the Japanese families was not found. Some heterozygotes were difficult to distinguish from normal homozygotes.

Generally speaking Caucasian acatalasics do not have the clinical picture shown by the original Japanese girl patient. However, one acatalasic child with oral gangrene and loss of teeth has been reported from East Germany.

Heterozygous individuals in acatalasic families could have an intermediate blood catalase activity either due to – (1) some cells having normal catalase activity and other cells having none, or (2) all cells having an intermediate enzyme activity. Two techniques have been applied to decide which is the true state of affairs. First, red cells were subjected to the action of hydrogen peroxide. In the absence of catalase the haemoglobin is more readily changed to methaemoglobin. The methaemoglobin was converted to cyanmethaemoglobin which was eluted out of the cells which contained it. If hypothesis (1) were correct this technique would show the blood to contain a mixture of two types of erythrocyte in heterozygotes. Secondly, antihuman catalase antibody was raised in rabbits and conjugated with fluorescein isothiocyanate. Smears of heterozygote blood were treated with this reagent. These techniques gave no evidence of mosaicism.

In all individuals, normal and acatalasics, the reticulocytes have more catalase activity than mature red cells. In acatalasics the catalase activity disappears very much more rapidly as the red cells age than is the case in normal individuals. This observation leads to the suggestion that acatalasics have an enzyme variant of greatly reduced stability.

Electrophoretic studies of catalase in normal homozygotes, heterozygotes and acatalasics have shown that the 'abnormal' catalase has a different electrophoretic activity from normal. Both forms are demonstrable in heterozygotes. The abnormal form has greater heat lability at 55°C in Swiss (but not in Japanese) acatalasics. On the other hand, in Japanese acatalasics the 'abnormal' catalase can be distinguished from the normal form by immunological techniques.

There thus appears to be definite evidence of the existence of different types of acatalasia. The natural role of the enzyme is thought to be to protect haemoglobin from being converted into methaemoglobin. There is at present no clue to the selective advantage to the heterozygote which Darwinian theory would predict as responsible for the existence and perpetuation of this seemingly stable genetic polymorphism (see Aebi & Suter, 1971).

Diphenylhydantoin (Phenytoin) This compound is metabolised by para-oxidation of one phenyl ring in the endoplasmic reticulum of the human liver cell. Three families have been described by Kutt et al (1971) in which the mother and one or more offspring seemed to have a relative inability to carry out this metabolic biotransformation. These individuals appear to be in quite a separate class from ordinary subjects, suggesting that they are expressing a distinct Mendelian character. The practical result is a high plasma steady state drug concentration and a long half-life. The high steady state concentration on conventional doses renders the subject unusually prone to the toxic effects of the drug, viz. ataxia, nystagmus, slurred speech, inattention etc.

Phenacetin A remarkable pedigree was described by Shahidi (1968) in which two individuals had a relative inability to de-ethylate phenacetin. Since this major pathway accepted less substrate, more of the drug was converted to minor metabolites such as phenetidine than is normally the case. These metabolites have a methaemoglobin-producing propensity, and it was in fact the clinical observation of methaemoglobinaemia which caused this family to be studied so intensively.

Bishydroxycoumarin (Dicoumarol) A single pedigree has been described (Vessell, 1975) in which individuals have a relatively inability to hydroxylate the compound. The consequence is a greater sensitivity than normal to the anticoagulant effect produced by ordinary dosages.

Pharmacological effects

All phenotypes common

Glucose-6-phosphate dehydrogenase deficiency This polymorphism first came to light as a result of studying persons who had developed haemolysis as an adverse reaction to treatment of their malaria with pamaquine and primaquine. Cross-transfusion experiments revealed that the cause was within susceptible individuals' erythrocytes; it was also found in these individuals that their haemoglobin concentration returned to normal after haemolysis even though they continued to ingest primaquine. The explanation for this lay in the fact that they produced a population of erythrocytes with a low mean age which was not as susceptible to haemolysis as older cells.

A genetic basis for this adverse reaction was suspected because it occurred more frequently in certain ethnic groups (e.g. Negroes) than others (e.g. those of Northern European extraction).

Within the susceptible erythrocyte there was a relative inability to maintain glutathione in a reduced state when the cell was confronted with an oxidant stress. This formed the basis of an *in vitro* test wherein an individual's red cells were incubated with acetyl phenylhydrazine and the glutathione was measured. This 'glutathione stability' test gave results which were bimodally distributed in males in the Negro population, suggesting that primaquine sensitivity was due to an allele on the X–chromosome.

Very soon it was realised that the deficiency was in the enzyme glucose-6-phosphate dehydrogenase (G6PD) and assays of the activity of this enzyme superseded the glutathione stability test as a phenotyping procedure.

A large number of other drugs in addition to primaquine are known to precipitate haemolysis in G6PD-deficient subjects. The ingestion of the bean *Vicia faba* can also produce the same effect and this is the basis of favism – an affliction described in antiquity.

Clinical observation revealed that Mediterranean G6PD-deficient individuals are more severely affected than Negro G6PD-deficient subjects after primaquine ingestion. When the purified enzyme was subjected to a number of biochemical procedures, e.g. electrophoresis, pH optimum, temperature stability, Michaelis constant with various substrates etc., it was found that there are in various populations a large number of different structural variants. The type responsible for G6PD-deficiency in Negroes (termed A-) is due to a single amino acid substitution as compared with the normal form, viz. asparagine is replaced by aspartic acid.

In the Negro form of deficiency, leucocyte G6PD activity is normal. In the Mediterranean and Chinese forms of the deficiency leucocyte G6PD activity is reduced.

The locus controlling G6PD is situated on the X–chromosome quite close to the locus for deuteranopia (estimated recombination fraction 5%).

The geographic distribution of G6PD-deficiency is similar to that of malaria – a fact which gave rise to the speculation that it might have a protective role. Support for this idea was derived from a finding in malarious heterozygotes. Due to Lyonisation, heterozygotes have some erythrocytes which are normal and some which are G6PD-deficient. It has been found that the latter type of cell is less frequently parasitized than the former (see Beutler 1978 for comprehensive review).

Negro and Mediterranean G6PD-deficient subjects are quite healthy provided their red cells are not subjected to chemical stresses. The situation is different in the rare Northern European kindred where a chronic non-spherocytic anaemia may have as its basis G6PD-deficiency (e.g. see McCann et al, 1980).

G6PD deficiency has been put to use in tumour research. For example, uterine myomas have been shown in heterozygotes to be either of one G6PD type or another, suggesting that such tumours arise from a single cell, whereas other tumours (e.g. colonic carcinoma) have shown both G6PD types suggesting a multicellular origin (see Fialkow, 1974).

PTC taste-testing The compound phenylthiocarbamide (PTC, phenylthiourea) was synthesized by Fox in 1932. He found that some persons experienced a distinctly bitter taste when crystals were placed on the tongue; whereas other persons detected only a very slight taste or none at all. Family studies revealed that non-tasters are homozygous for the allele controlling the recessive character and they form about 33% of the European population. In African and Chinese populations however, 'non-tasters' are less frequent. The polymorphism is detected by a number of compounds containing the S=C<configuration (Dawson et al, 1967), including methyl thiouracil, propyl thiouracil and thiopentone.

The following associations have been shown to exist between the PTC taste-testing polymorphism and various thyroid disorders:-

(1) a higher incidence of non-tasters among patients with adenomatous goitre (Kitchin et al, 1959; Harris et al, 1949),

(2) a higher incidence of tasters among patients with toxic diffuse goitre (Kitchin et al, 1959),

(3) a higher incidence of non-tasters among patients with athyrotic cretinism (Fraser, 1961).

In view of the embryologic relationship between tongue and thyroid, it is possible that cells in both tissues may have a similarity in their 'receptors' for the S=C<grouping.

Chlorpropamide-ethanol-flushing Some individuals flush when they consume ethanol with chlorpropamide. This response has been systematically investigated during the last few years. A simple phenotyping test is conducted using one 250 mg tablet of chlorpropamide followed by 40 ml of sherry. Scoring the responses can be (1) subjective, by history, (2) objective, by direct observation, and (3) objective, by measuring facial temperature. The phenotype of a given individual appears to remain constant on repeated testing. A few individuals who show chlorpropamide-alcohol flushing also experience nausea, giddiness, palpitations and breathlessness. About 5% have bronchial wheezing.

The genetics of chlorpropamide-alcohol flushing (CPAF) has been investigated and it has been deemed to be an autosomal dominant trait for two reasons. First, in every case in which the parents of affected subjects were tested, one has flushed. Second, persons who show CPAF have affected and normal offspring in about equal numbers. In other words there is direct transmission from parent to child.

CPAF occurs in about 10% of insulin-dependent dia-

betics and similarly in non-diabetic controls. However, about 50% of non-insulin dependent diabetics (NIDD) show CPAF (Leslie & Pyke, 1980). This statistical association between a genetically determined phenotype and NIDD appears particularly strong when there is a family history of NIDD.

There is also a relationship between CPAF and severe retinopathy in NIDD. This complication appears to arise particularly in CPAF-negative individuals. Similarly, large vessel disease (myocardial infarction, angina, intermittent claudication and absent foot pulses) is significantly more common in CPAF-negative individuals than in CPAF-positive NIDD patients (Barnett & Pyke, 1980). It would appear, therefore, that the CPAF phenotype has a prognostic value in NIDD.

A chance observation revealed that a known CPAF-positive individual had an intense facial flush after injection with an enkephalin analogue during an experiment. Following this it was found that the rise in skin temperature in CPAF-positive individuals was greater and longer than that produced in CPAF-negative individuals by an infusion of the prostaglandin DAMME (Sandoz, Fk 33824) (Leslie et al, 1979).

CPAF can be blocked by naloxone which is a point in favour of its being mediated by enkephalin action. However, there is also evidence that CPAF can be inhibited by aspirin and indomethacin. Since these agents inhibit prostaglandin synthesis the possibility is also raised that CPAF may be mediated by a prostaglandin. These speculations are of great importance because it is possible they may reveal the nature of the metabolic disturbances responsible for micro- and macrovascular complications in NIDD (Barnett et al, 1978).

Corticosteroid-induced ocular hypertension A disputed polymorphism of considerable clinical interest is that which some observers claim to have detected by instilling glucocorticoid eye drops into the conjunctival sac.

The impetus to this work arose from the facts that (1) it had long been known that glaucoma (due to raised intra-ocular tension) occurred in families, suggesting a genetic basis, and (2) soon after corticosteroid eye drops were introduced into clinical practice it was found that they could induce a steep rise in pressure within eyes which were previously normal.

The investigation of unrelated subjects by three groups of workers showed agreement as to the population distribution of the pressure changes produced by glucocorticoids (Becker, 1965; Armaly, 1965; Godel et al, 1972). These three groups of workers investigated families (208 offspring were investigated altogether) and found that the response of intra-ocular pressure to glucocorticoids exhibited three phenotypes corresponding to three genotypes produced by the segregation of two alleles at one autosomal locus (Becker & Kolker, 1966; Armaly, 1966; Feiler-Ofry, 1972). Of considerable clinical importance was the finding that possession of the allele determining the high pressure response to glucocorticoids appeared to confer a predisposition to develop glaucoma (Armaly, 1967; Francois et al, 1966; Becker & Kolker, 1966).

This rather attractive idea was shaken by the twin study of Schwartz et al (1972; 1973a; 1973b) who from their results concluded that (i) they could not regard the frequency distribution of intra-ocular pressure changes as deviating significantly from normal, (ii) concordance in monozygous twins was low (it should have been complete on a monogenic hypothesis), and (iii) heritability computations revealed that the genetic component of variance was small. Their view, therefore, was that intra-ocular pressure is under multifactorial control with a large environmental component.

It is a pity that such a promising line of research has ended in such confusion because of the enormous practical value such a simple predictive test for glaucoma might have had in families with this disease.

Some phenotypes rare

Malignant hyperthermia This is a fatal condition which supervenes unexpectedly in an otherwise fit subject during anaesthesia – usually with halothane and/or succinyl choline chloride (Britt & Kalow, 1968). Soon after induction of anaesthesia the muscles go into massive spasm and the body temperature quickly rises to a high level. The patient becomes acidotic and it is probably the cardiac effects of the acidosis which often cause sudden death.

Related individuals have suffered from this catastrophe and the disposition of these individuals within pedigrees suggests that it is inherited as a rare Mendelian dominant character.

In vitro studies performed with voluntary muscle strips obtained at biopsy from susceptible individuals have shown an abnormal contraction in response to halothane succinyl chlorine and caffeine (Moulds & Denborough, 1974a). The contraction was prevented by procaine. In a calcium-free bath muscle tissue from an affected person gave an initial sustained contraction when exposed to caffeine or halothane, but re-exposure to these agents when the muscle had relaxed following a change of bath liquid did not produce a second contracture. A second contracture could be produced however, if the bath liquid contained calcium. The suggestion has therefore been made that the calcium-storing sarcolemma and sarcoplasmic reticulum in malignant hyperthermia release abnormally large amounts of calcium in response to the action of the precipitating drug.

The investigation of muscle biopsies along the above lines has been proposed as a pre-operative screening test for relatives of subjects known to have suffered from malignant hyperthermia.

Some predictive value may also be obtained by a careful physical examination, since clinically evident myopathy of a minor degree may be present, and a serum creatine kinase, since this is raised in some susceptible subjects (Moulds & Denborough, 1974b).

Resistance to oral anticoagulants This rare Mendelian dominant character was discovered as a result of a clinical observation. A man who had sustained a myocardial infarction failed to show a lowering of his plasma prothrombin concentration following conventional doses of warfarin (O'Reilly et al, 1964). It transpired that the desired effect of the drug did occur when dosage was increased to a high level. His dose-response curve was in fact grossly displaced to the right as compared with ordinary patients. Otherwise he had no unusual features. In his pedigree other persons with the same phenotype were discovered. Later there was described a second independent much larger pedigree in which persons with the same phenotype occurred (O'Reilly, 1970). This 'warfarin resistance' is an autosomal dominant trait and is accompanied by resistance to other oral anticoagulants, e.g. dicoumarol (but not, of course, to heparin). The pharmacokinetics of warfarin is normal in resistant subjects.

It is clear that there is some mechanism in the liver producing 'anticoagulant resistant' individuals which is not affected to the same extent by a given concentration as in ordinary individuals. The precise nature of the biochemical mechanism controlled by this rare allele remains unknown.

Warfarin resistance in wild rats, which has been described from more than one focus in the U.K. and from the U.S.A. and Denmark, is also inherited as an autosomal dominant character. It would seem to be exactly analogous to the rare disorder in man.

Haemoglobin Zurich This unstable haemoglobin was originally discovered because a young girl and her father had suffered severe haemolysis following treatment with conventional doses of different sulphonamides (Frick et al, 1962).

The cause of the haemolysis was found to be within the red cells which showed inclusion bodies during the acute stage. Electrophoretic studies showed that the two patients possessed haemoglobin A and also an abnormal haemoglobin, named 'Zurich', which had a mobility intermediate between A and S. Structural studies showed that histidine, which usually occupies position 63 of the β chain, is replaced by arginine (Bachmann & Marti, 1962).

Subsequently ferrokinetic and Cr^{51}-tagged red cell survival studies showed that red blood cells from the original patients had a shorter life span than normal. Affected individuals also suffer from mild anaemia and episodic mild jaundice (when they have not been on drugs).

It appears, therefore, that haemoglobin Zurich is normally unstable, but when the patient has ingested sulphonamides the precipitation of the haemoglobin is greatly speeded up and a massive haemolysis results.

Some individuals with haemoglobin Zurich have not suffered from this low-grade haemolysis. On closer scrutiny these individuals turned out to be smokers. Haemoglobin Zurich has twice as much affinity for carbon monoxide as haemoglobin A, and it appears to be stabilised in smokers so protecting them from haemolysis (Zinkham, 1979).

Similar clinical manifestations would be expected with other unstable haemoglobins which have since been described. An example is haemoglobin H (formed of 4 β chains and no α chains) which has been described by Rigas and Koler (1961).

HLA AND ADVERSE REACTIONS

Many adverse reactions to drugs have an allergic or hypersensitivity basis. Their occurrence seems entirely unpredictable.

However, two examples have now been published which seem to form the basis of a new branch of pharmacogenetics in that they indicate a role for the HLA system (or some closely related genetic entity) in the predisposition to adverse reactions to drugs.

Firstly, 14 out of 15 individuals who developed proteinuria after auriothiomalate ('gold') therapy for rheumatoid arthritis were found to be of type DRw 3 which has a frequency of only about 8% in the Caucasian population (Wooley et al, 1980).

Secondly, patients with hydralazine-SLE, who have long been known to be slow acetylators, have now been found to be predominantly (75%) possessors of antigen DRw 4, which only occurs in about 25% of the general Caucasian population (Batchelor et al, 1980).

QUANTITATIVE GENETICS

The metabolism of many drugs is controlled by many genes (multifactorial inheritance). This conclusion is based on studies of drug metabolism in twins and other relatives.

Twin studies indicate a considerable degree of genetic control of the metabolism of various drugs – as revealed by their plasma half-lives or plasma steady state concentrations. These drugs include antipyrine, diphenylhydantoin, phenylbutazone, nortriptyline, amobarbital, dicoumarol, ethanol, lithium, tolbutamide and isoniazid.

An estimate of heritability (i.e. the contribution of additive genetic variance to the overall phenotypic variance) can be made by studying resemblance between relatives. Very few human pharmacogenetic studies of this kind have been published. Whittaker and Evans (1969) found that when plasma phenylbutazone half-lives were studied under particular circumstances the frequency distribution in the population was approximately normal (Fig. 97.3) and the regression of mean offspring values on mid-parent values indicated a heritability of about 0.66.

It seems clear that there are many feasible and informative experiments which can be performed by applying quantitative genetic techniques to human pharmacogenetic problems.

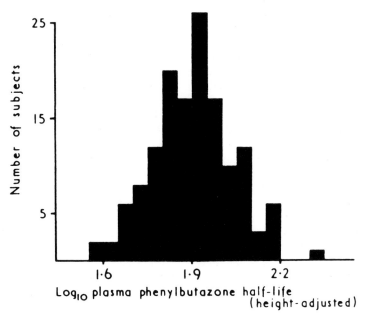

Fig. 97.3 The frequency distribution of $\log_{10}$ post-phenobarbitone plasma phenylbutazone half-lives adjusted to a standard height in 142 white British subjects including the members of 24 families (from Whittaker & Evans, 1970).

INTER-ETHNIC VARIABILITY

It is well known that alleles controlling blood groups, haemoglobins and enzyme polymorphisms differ widely in their distribution between ethnic groups. Practically every new genetic polymorphism that is discovered shows this phenomenon, a recent example being HLA. It is not surprising therefore, that the same is true of alleles controlling pharmacogenetic phenomena.

The alleles controlling the following aspects of drug metabolism show wide inter-ethnic variability in their frequency – acetylation, plasma pseudocholinesterase, ethanol dehydrogenation, methaemoglobin reductase and plasma paroxonase. Alleles controlling pharmacologic responses which differ greatly in their frequency in different ethnic groups include G6PD and PTC tasting.

Certain drugs whose biotransformations are known to be under a considerable measure of genetic control, have been found to show differences in their metabolism between ethnic groups. The interpretation of these observations where alleles cannot be recognised is fraught with danger. This is because environmental factors contribute to the variance, may differ considerably between ethnic groups, and are as yet unquantified. The study of Branch et al (1978) of antipyrine half-lives in (1) British white subjects in the U.K.,(2) Sudanese subjects in the Sudan and (3) Sudanese subjects in the U.K., showed that whilst there was a great difference between groups (1) and (2), groups (1) and (3) were very similar. On this basis an observation by Ziegler and Biggs (1977) that plasma tricyclic concentrations are higher in Black patients than in Caucasian patients will need critical examination before it can be ascribed with certainty to genetic differences between the two groups.

An interesting example is that of amobarbital which was advanced as 'a probe of drug oxidation' in man on the basis of its possession of the following properties:- pharmacologically inactive after a single test dose, fully absorbed without much 'first pass' effect, simple and repeatable pharmacokinetics, known metabolic fate, amenable to analysis with generally available methodology. The idea of using it as a probe was to see whether it could be used as a predictive tool for the way in which a particular person handled other drugs which were also known to be biotransformed by oxidation (Inaba et al, 1976). Further investigations using twins revealed that considerable genetic control was exercised on kinetic parameters which reflected the metabolic biotransformation of amobarbital (Endrenyi et al, 1976). It was later found that amobarbital is converted into two major metabolites, namely 3-hydroxyamobarbital (3-OHA) and an N-glucoside (ANG). In a comparison of medical students of Oriental and Caucasian origin at the University of Toronto, there was strong evidence to indicate that the Oriental group produced less 3-OHA and more ANG than did the Caucasians. It is possible that this ethnic difference has a genetic basis (even though amobarbital oxidation is inducible) since the distribution of this biotransformation was suggestively bimodal in the Orientals, amongst whom there were many 'poor oxidizers' (Kalow et al, 1979).

This topic of inter-ethnic differences is obviously an important one because it has practical implications in therapeutics.

CONCLUSIONS

Known pharmacogenetic alleles may well represent only a fraction of those which exist but are, as yet, undiscovered. Most of the cases examined using the techniques of quantitative genetics have shown genetic factors to be important in the metabolism of, and response to, various drugs. Therefore, it is clearly sensible to think of the possibility of a genetic explanation when an unusual adverse reaction is observed.

The family history may reveal the presence of a clinically important dominant character. In such a situation the patient may be at risk, e.g. from malignant hyperpyrexia or porphyria following anaesthesia. If such a suspicion is generated, then it is wise to carry out appropriate investigations not only on the patient but also on available relatives.

A novel adverse reaction may reveal a new allele. Knowledge of new alleles is in itself of value for a variety of subsequent genetic investigations. It must be emphasised that the key to making such advances lies in studying the relatives of the proband.

Clinical trials should be designed so that groups to be compared contain representative numbers of the different phenotypes in a polymorphism. A recent example raises the possibility of unlike groups having been compared in a large diabetic survey (Scott & Poffenbarger, 1979).

When a drug is released for use in a new population, then a new type of adverse reaction may be observed, or there may be a different incidence of known reactions.

The monitoring of plasma concentrations of drugs has been in existence for a long time (e.g. salicylates and sulphonamides), but is now feasible for a great variety of compounds. In the interpretation of such data there are a number of pharmacologic considerations of importance. One of the aims of the procedure, however, is to get an estimate of the inter-individual variability whose basis is to a considerable extent determined by heredity.

On a broader biologic basis the taking of a drug represents an environmental change. The phenotypes within a genetic polymorphism may respond to this environmental factor in different ways, e.g. some phenotypes may be more prone to adverse reactions whereas others may receive more benefit.

REFERENCES

Aebi H, Suter H 1971 In : Harris H, Hirschhorn K (eds) Advances in Human Genetics. Vol. 2. Plenum Press, New York. ch. 3, pp 143–199

Armaly M F 1965 Statistical attributes of steroid hypertensive response in the clinically normal eye. I. The demonstration of 3 levels of response. Investigative Ophthalmology 4: 187–197

Armaly M F 1966 The heritable nature of dexamethasone-induced ocular hypertension. Archives of Ophthalmology 75: 32–35

Armaly M F 1967 Inheritance of dexamethasone hypertension and glaucoma. Archives of Ophthalmology 77: 747–751

Bachman F, Marti H R 1962 Hemoglobin Zurich II. Physiochemical properties of the abnormal hemoglobins. Blood 20: 272–286

Barnett A H, Pyke D A 1980 Chlorpropamide-alcohol flushing and large vessel disease in non-insulin-dependent diabetes. British Medical Journal 281: 261–262

Barnett A H, Spiliopoulos A J, Pyke D A 1980 Blockade of chlorpropamide-alcohol flushing by indomethacin suggests an association between prostaglandins and diabetic vascular complications. Lancet 2: 164–166

Batchelor J R, Welsh K I, Tinoco R M, Dollery C T, Hughes C R V, Bernstein R, Ryan P, Naish P F, Aber G M, Bing R F, Russell G I 1980 Hydralazine-induced systemic lupus erythematosus: Influence of HLA-DR and sex on susceptibility. Lancet 1: 1107–1109

Becker B, Kolker A E 1966 Topical corticosteroid testing in conditions related to glaucoma. In: Schwartz B (ed) Corticosteroids and the Eye. Vol. 6 International Ophthalmology Clinics. Little Brown, Boston Mass. pp 1005–1015

Beutler E 1978 Glucose-6-phosphate dehydrogenase deficiency. In: Stanbury J B, Wyngaarden J B, Fredrickson D S (eds) Metabolic Basis of Inherited Disease 4th ed. McGraw-Hill, New York. Chapter 60, pp 1430–1451

Branch R A, Salih S Y, Homeida M 1978 Racial differences in drug-metabolising ability: a study with antipyrine in the Sudan. Clinical Pharmacology and Therapeutics 34: 283–286

Britt B A, Kalow W 1968 Hyper-rigidity and hyperthermia associated with anaesthesia. Annals of the New York Academy of Sciences 151: 947–958

Dawson W, West G B, Kalmus H 1967 Taste polymorphism to anetholtrithione and phenylthiocarbamate. Annals of Human Genetics, London 30: 273–276

Edwards J A, Evans D A P 1967 Ethanol metabolism in subjects possessing typical and atypical liver alcohol dehydrogenases. Clinical Pharmacology and Therapeutics 8: 824–829

Eichelbaum M, Spannbrucker N, Steincke B, Dengler H J 1979 Defective N-oxidation of sparteine in Man: A new pharmacogenetic defect. European Journal of Clinical Pharmacology 16: 183–187

Endrenyi L, Inaba T, Kalow W 1976 Genetic study of amobarbital elimination based on its kinetics in twins. Clinical Pharmacology and Therapeutics. 20: 701–714

Evans D A P 1968 Genetic variations in the acetylation of isoniazid and other drugs. Annals of New York Academy of Sciences 151: 723–733

Evans D A P, Mahgoub A, Sloan T P, Idle J R, Smith R L 1980 A family and population study of the genetic polymorphism of debrisoquine oxidation in a white British population. Journal of Medical Genetics 17: 102–105

Ewing J A, Rouse B A, Pellizzari E D 1974 Alcohol sensitivity and ethnic background. American Journal of Psychiatry 131: 206–210

Fagerlind L, Holmstedt B, Wallen O 1952 Preparation and determination of diethy-p-nitrophenyl phosphate (E 600) a drug used in the treatment of glaucoma. Svensk Farmaceutisk Tidskrift. 56: 303–309

Falconer D S 1960 Introduction to Quantitative Genetics. Reprinted (with amendments) 1964. Oliver and Boyd, Edinburgh

Feiler-Ofry V, Godel V, Stein R 1972 Systemic steroids and ocular fluid dynamics II The genetic nature of the ocular response and its different levels. Acta Ophthalmologica 50: 699–706

Fialkow P K 1974 The origin and development of human tumours studied with cell markers. New England Journal of Medicine 291: 26–35

Fox A L 1932 The relationship between chemical constitution and taste. Proceedings of the National Academy of Sciences (Washington) 18 : 115–120

Francois J, Heintz-de-Bree C, Tripathi R C 1966 The cortisone test and the heredity of primary open-angle glaucoma. American Journal of Ophthalmology 62: 844–852

Fraser G R 1961 Cretinism and taste sensitivity to phenylthiocarbamide. Lancet 1: 964–965

Frick P G, Hitzig W H, Betke K 1962 Hemoglobin Zurich I. A new hemoglobin anomaly associated with acute hemolytic episodes with inclusion bodies after sulphonamide therapy. Blood 20: 261–271

Geldmacher-von-Mallinckrodt M, Lindfort H H, Petenyi M, Flugel M, Fisher T, Hiller T 1973 Genetische determinierter Polymorphismus der menschlichen Serum-Paroxonase (EC 3.1.1.2) Humangenetik 17: 331–335

Godel V, Feiler-Ofry V, Stein R 1972 Systemic steroids and ocular fluid dynamics II. Systemic versus topical steroids Acta Ophthalmologica 50: 663–676

Goedde H W, Agarwal P, Benkmann H-G 1979 Pharmacogenetics of cholinesterase: New variants and suxamethonium sensitivity. Arztliche Laboratorium 25: 219–224

Hann J M 1978 Metabolic responses of Chinese, Japanese and Europeans to alcohol. Alcoholism: Clinical and Experimental Research 2: 89–92

Harada S, Misawa S, Agarwal D P, Goedde H W 1980a Liver alcohol dehydrogenase and aldehyde dehydrogenase in the Japanese: Isozyme variation and its possible role in alcohol intoxication. American Journal of Human Genetics 32: 8–15

Harada S, Agarwal D P, Goedde H W 1980b Electrophoretic and biochemical studies of human aldehyde dehydrogenase isozymes in various tissues. Life Sciences 26 : 1773–1780

Harris H , Kalmus H, Trotter W H 1949 Taste sensitivity to PTC in goitre and diabetes. Lancet 2: 1038–1039

Harris H, Hopkinson D A, Robson E B, Whittaker M 1963 Genetical studies on a new variant of serum cholinesterase detected by electrophoresis. Annals of Human Genetics (London) 26: 359–382

Harris H, Whittaker M 1961 Differential inhibition of human serum cholinesterase with fluoride. Recognition of two new phenotypes. Nature 191: 496–498

Inaba T, Tang B K, Endrenyi L, Kalow W 1976 Amobarbital – a probe of hepatic drug oxidation in Man. Clinical Pharmacology and Therapeutics 20: 439–444

Kalow W, Genest K 1957 A method for the detection of atypical forms of human serum cholinesterase. Determination of dibucaine numbers. Canadian Journal of Biochemistry and Physiology 35: 339–346

Kalow W, Staron N 1957 On distribution and inheritance of atypical forms of human serum cholinesterase as indicated by dibucaine numbers. Canadian Journal of Biochemistry and Physiology 35: 1305–1320

Kalow W, Tang B K, Kadar D, Endrenyi L, Chan F-Y 1979 A method for studying drug metabolism in populations: Racial differences in amobarbital metabolism. Clinical Pharmacology and Therapeutics 26: 766–776

Kitchin F D, Howel-Evans W, Clarke C A, McConnell R B, Sheppard P M 1959 PTC taste response and thyroid disease. British Journal of Medicine 1: 1069–1074

Kutt H 1971 Biochemical and genetic factors regulating dilantin metabolism in Man. Annals of the New York Academy of Sciences 179: 704–722

Lehmann H, Liddell J 1961 The cholinesterases. In: Evans F T, Gray T C (eds) Modern Trends in Anaesthesia 2 Butterworth, London. Chapter 8, pp. 164–205

Lehmann H, Simmons P H 1958 Sensitivity to suxamethonium. Lancet 2: 981–982

Leslie R D G, Barnett A H, Pyke D A 1979 Chlorpropamide-alcohol-flushing and diabetic retinopathy. Lancet 1: 997–999

Leslie R D G, Pyke D A 1980 Chlorpropamide-alcohol flushing as a drug-induced pseudo-allergic reaction. In: Dukor P, Kallos P, Schlumberger H D, West G B (eds) P A R Pseudo-allergic reactions. Involvement of Drugs and Chemicals, Vol. 1. Karger, Basel. pp. 294–301

Leslie R D G, Pyke D A, Stubbs W A 1979 Sensitivity to enkephalin as a cause of non-insulin dependent diabetes. Lancet 1: 341–343

Liddell J, Lehmann H, Silk E 1962 A 'silent' pseudocholinesterase gene. Nature 193 561–562

McCann S R, Smithwick A M, Temperley I J, Tipton K 1980 G6PD (Dublin): Chronic non-spherocytic haemolytic anaemia resulting from glucose-6-phosphate dehydrogenase deficiency in an Irish kindred. Journal of Medical Genetics 17: 191–193

Moulds R F W, Denborough M A 1974a Biochemical basis of malignant hyperpyrexia. British Medical Journal 2: 241–244

Moulds R F W, Denborough M A 1974b Identification of susceptibility to malignant hyperpyrexia. British Medical Journal 2: 245–247

Neitlich H W 1966 Increased plasma cholinesterase activity and succinyl choline resistance: A genetic variant. Journal of Clinical Investigation 45: 380–387

O'Reilly R A 1970 The second reported kindred with hereditary resistance to oral anticoagulant drugs. New England Journal of Medicine 282: 1448–1451

O'Reilly R A, Aggeler P M, Hoag M S, Leong L S, Kropatkin M L 1964 Hereditary transmission of exceptional resistance to coumarin anticoagulant drugs – the first reported kindred. New England Journal of Medicine 271 809–815

Playfer J R, Eze L C, Bullen M F, Evans D A P 1976 Genetic polymorphism and inter-ethnic variability of plasma paroxonase activity. Journal of Medical Genetics 13: 337–342

Reed T E 1978 Racial comparisons of alcohol metabolism. Background problems and results. Alcoholism: Clinical and Experimental Research 2: 83–87

Reed T E, Kalant H, Gibbins R J, Kapur B M, Rankin J G 1976 Alcohol and acetaldehyde metabolism in Caucasians, Chinese and Amerinds. Canadian Medical Association Journal 115: 851–852

Rigas D A, Koler R D 1961 Decreased erythrocyte survival in hemoglobin H disease as a result of the abnormal properties of hemoglobin H. The benefit of splenectomy. Journal of Hematology 18: 1–17

Schwartz J T, Reuling F H, Feinleib M, Garrison R J, Collie D J 1972 Twin heritability study of the effect of corticosteroids on intra-ocular pressure. Journal of Medical Genetics 9 : 137–143

Schwartz J T, Reuling F H, Feinleib M, Garrison R J, Collie D J 1973a Twin study on ocular pressure after topical dexamethasone I. Frequency distribution of pressure response. American Journal of Ophthalmology 76: 126–136

Schwartz J T, Rueling F H, Feinleib M, Garrison R J, Collie D J 1973b Twin study on ocular pressure following topically applied dexamethasone II. Inheritance of variation in pressure response. Archives of Ophthamology 90: 281–286

Scott J, Poffenbarger P L 1979 Tolbutamide pharmacogenetics and the UGDP controversy. Journal of the American Medical Association 242: 45–48

Shahidi N T 1968 Acetophenetidin-induced methaemoglobinaemia. Annals of the New York Academy of Sciences 151: 822–832

Smith M, Hopkins D A, Harris H 1971 Developmental changes and polymorphisms in human alcohol dehydrogenase. Annals of Human Genetics 34: 251–271

Takahara S 1952 Progressive oral gangrene probably due to lack of catalase in the blood (acatalasaemia). Lancet 2: 11011–1104

Vesell E S 1975 Pharmacogenetics – the individual factor in drug response. Triangle 14: 125–130

von Wartburg J P, Papenberg J, Aebi H 1965 An atypical human alcohol dehydrogenase. Canadian Journal of Biochemistry 43: 889–898

Whittaker J A, Evans D A P 1970 Genetic control of phenylbutazone metabolism in Man. British Medical Journal 4: 323–328

Wolff P H 1972 Ethnic differences in alcohol sensitivity. Science 175: 449–450

Wooley P H, Griffin J, Panayi G S, Batchelor J R, Welsh K I, Gibson T J 1980 HLA-DR antigens and toxicity to sodium auriothiomalate and D-penicillamine in rheumatoid arthritis. New England Journal of Medicine 303: 300–302

Zeiner A R 1978 Racial differences in circadian variation of ethanol metabolism. Alcoholism 2: 71–75

Ziegler V E, Biggs T J 1977 Tricyclic plasma levels. Effect of age, race, sex and smoking. Journal of the American Medical Association 238: 2167–2169

Zinkham W H 1979 Drug-induced hemolysis and smoking: Interaction between gene and environment. Item 48 in 24th Topics in Clinical Medicine. Johns Hopkins Hospital, Baltimore.

Cancer genetics

R.N. Schimke

INTRODUCTION

Cancer research has largely focused on the identification of environmental carcinogens. Indeed, scarcely a day passes without a pronouncement of some new agent (or some old agent newly studied) that has been causally implicated in human carcinogenesis, usually on the basis of studies in experimental animals. Until recently very little attention was paid to the possibility that man's genotype, or at least the genes in some men, might be the initiating factor and thereby provide fertile substrate for an environmental carcinogen. For obvious reasons, geneticists have concentrated on those unifactorial disorders in which malignancy is a regular enough occurrence to be noteworthy, having left consideration of common cancers to epidemiologists. It has been shown quite clearly that familial aggregation does exist even for common neoplasms and that this aggregation cannot be totally accounted for by the environment. Hence, there has been a recent quickening of interest in cancer genetics in man. The topic has been reviewed in some detail in a series of publications, and the interested reader should consult these for general background as well as more specific information on the diseases considered in this chapter. (Knudson et al, 1973; Lynch, 1976; Mulvihill et al, 1977a; Schimke 1978).

THE GENETIC AETIOLOGY OF CANCER

It is now quite clear that a variety of aneuploid states, single gene disorders and even polygenic conditions may predispose to malignancy, although the exact molecular mechanisms whereby these occur are rarely clear. In conditions such as xeroderma pigmentosum where the gene mutation is associated with defective DNA repair to ultraviolet light-induced damage, it is easy to visualize a cause and effect relationship. It is more difficult to account for heritable retinoblastoma or colon cancer since these are internal, presumably tissue specific neoplasms ,and in the case of retinoblastoma, even congenital. Even with the known heritable simple tumours such as familial retinoblastoma, it is necessary to account for decreased penetrance and variable expressivity.

Knudson and his colleagues (1973) have attempted to develop a comprehensive approach to cancer genetics in man. They have suggested that the development of any malignancy requires two mutational events which could be of a variety of types such as a single gene change or a chromosome rearrangement. With heritable tumours, the initial mutation would be germinal and the second somatic. The expected consequences of this reasoning would be that inherited tumours would tend to be multifocal (or bilateral when appropriate) and have an earlier age of onset. Decreased penetrance and less than complete monozygotic twin concordance could be explained by the absence of the somatic event even in a susceptible individual. Nonfamilial tumours would tend to be unifocal and have a later age of onset since two distinct somatic event would be required for tumour development. Implicit in this 'two-hit' hypothesis is the assumption that carcinogenesis is related to discrete ,random changes occurring at a constant average rate. The model has been criticized on mathematical grounds, and modifications of the basic premise have been offered as discussed elsewhere (Schimke, 1981). Whether ultimately correct or not, the model is heuristically useful.

Some malignancies are unicellular in origin,while others are not, as shown clearly by Fialkow (1977). It is not difficult to understand how a mutation in a single clone of cells could lead to malignancy. It is less easy to comprehend a tumour of multicellular origin, unless one involves cell-cell interaction, circulating oncogenic factors or unless the initial germinal mutation gave rise to multiple clones of defective cells, a possibility that has been suggested by Baylin et al (1978).

CANCER FAMILIES

Most of the tumours to be discussed in this chapter are site-specific; e.g., hereditary retinoblastoma, familial phaeochromocytoma and so forth. In addition to this, a number of families have been described in which there is a pattern of malignancies within the family, but not every individual necessarily has the same neoplasm. In general, the tumours in such families are the common malignancies seen in man but there are some unusual features. First of all, the tumour tends to occur at an earlier average age; e.g., colon carcinoma in the third or fourth decade versus the usual onset in the 60's or 70's. Secondly, it is not uncommon for an individual to have more than one primary tumour; e.g., both colon and endometrial carcinoma. Third, the tumours may be multicentric. Fourth, in these families usually more than 25% of the individuals in direct lineal descent from the proband are affected, the exact percentage obviously depending upon the age of these individuals. Fifth, for practical purposes, the cancer predisposition in these families behaves as an autosomal dominant trait with about 60% penetrance. Two cancer family syndromes have been tentatively identified, and it is quite likely that others exist (Table 98.1). The more common of the two is also appropriately called hereditary adenocarcinomatosis to indicate that the great bulk of affected individuals suffer from adenocarcinoma at various but rather predictable sites (Lynch et al, 1977). The other syndrome is less clearly delineated, since there is a broad array of tumours represented, the chief ones of which are breast carcinoma and sarcomas in adults and embryonal neoplasms in children (Lynch et al, 1978; Blattner et al, 1979).

This is not to say that other types of cancer families do not exist. For example, it appears that some members of families in which the proband has hereditary immunodeficiency have an increased incidence of malignancy particularly of the lymphoreticular system (Conley et al, 1980). Other families may have unique cancer-predisposing genes analogous to the so-called 'private' blood groups (Anderson, 1978). In still other instances, heterozygotes for certain rare recessive disorders, which in themselves predispose to cancer, may represent a population at increased risk for cancer. As will be seen, the majority of man's cancer predisposition seems to be inherited by an autosomal dominant mechanism. Yet there are a few diseases, all autosomal recessive, in which

Table 98.1 Cancer types seen in two probable varieties of cancer family syndrome

Type I	Type II
Endometrium	Breast
Ovary	Sarcoma
Breast	Embryonal
Prostate	Brain
Colon	Leukaemia
Stomach	Lymphoma
Pancreas	Adrenal
Skin	Thyroid
Melanoma	Bladder

Table 98.2 Neoplasms in some autosomal recessive disorders

Fanconi anaemia
Leukaemia
Oesophageal carcinoma
Skin carcinoma
Hepatoma
Ataxia-telangiectasia
Leukaemia
Lymphoma
Ovarian cancer
Gastric cancer
Brain tumours
Colon cancer
Bloom syndrome
Leukaemia
Carcinoma of tongue
Oesophageal carcinoma
Colon carcinoma
Xeroderma pigmentosum
Skin cancer
Melanoma
Leukaemia
Cancer of orophrynx
Werner syndrome
Sarcoma
Hepatoma
Breast carcinoma
Thyroid carcinoma
Leukaemia

the incidence of malignancy is quite high (Table 98.2). Virtually all of these have been found to have abnormalities in DNA repair after a variety of different insults (Arlet and Lehman, 1978), a topic discussed in more detail elsewhere in this volume. It is logical to assume that heterozygotes for these disorders might display partial defects in the same mechanisms to such an extent that they too would be at increased risk for the development of a tumour, although the number of families studied is small and the issue is controversial (Swift et al, 1980). Such partial defects have been uncovered in ataxia-telangiectasia (Chen et al, 1978) and Fanconi anaemia (Auerbach and Wolman, 1978). In the case of these latter two disorders, it has been estimated that, given the incidence of each in the population, about 1% of all cancer patients may be heterozygous for the Fanconi anaemia gene and another 2% heterozygous for ataxia-telangiectasia (Swift et al, 1974). Whether these predictions are accurate or not remains to be proved; nonetheless, it does appear that persons harbouring these genes certainly in homozygous and possibly in heterozygous forms are at increased risk for cancer and therefore constitute a special type of cancer family syndrome.

EMBRYONAL TUMOURS

There is increasing evidence that a substantial proportion of embryonal tumours in children develop because of a genetic predisposition (Schimke, in press). Moreover, the effect of the predisposing gene in some instances persists into later years, as manifested by an increased incidence of second malignancies.

Retinoblastoma

Retinoblastoma develops in roughly 1/20 000 infants. About 30% of all cases now appear to be hereditary, with transmission via an autosomal dominant mechanism with more than 90% penetrance (Knudson et al, 1973). About 2/3 of all gene carriers have bilateral disease, and the remaining 1/3 have only unilateral tumours. Ten to 12% of all sporadic unilateral cases actually might be heritable and this fact must be taken into consideration when counselling (Vogel, 1979). A small proportion of children with retinoblastoma have been found to have a chromosome abnormality which by high resolution banding has been shown to involve the long arm of chromosome 13, more specifically band 13q14 (Yunis & Ramsey, 1978). These children generally have retinoblastoma plus other congenital defects, generally the more complex the constellation of birth defects, the greater the size of the deletion. Most of these chromosomal errors are sporadic and the parents are normal. Exceptions have been reported, however, in which balanced parental translocations or inversions have resulted in multiple affected offspring (Riccardi et al, 1979; Sparkes et al ,1979). The deletion is permissive in the sense that not all individuals develop the tumour. In the familial settings, future pregnancies could be monitored by amniocentesis whereas in the standard heritable form of retinoblastoma, no such test is available at present. The locus for the enzyme esterase D is also in band 13q14, and studies of this enzyme polymorphism in affected families may be useful in defining small deletions beyond current powers of resolution (Sparkes et al, 1980).

Exactly what is lost in the 13q14 deletion is unknown. Riccardi et al (1979) have cautioned that one should be wary of considering genes lost through deletion in the same context as a point mutation; i.e., there may be no retinoblastoma gene *per se*, the tumour perhaps developing as a consequence of newly developed functional capacities generated by the cytogenetic alteration. For example, in one family in which multiple members had retinoblastoma associated with the 13q14 deletion the tumours were all unilateral, a finding in contrast to the usual heritable retinoblastoma where the majority of affected subjects have bilateral disease (Strong et al, 1980). Moreover, fluorescent banding studies in another family with retinoblastoma without 13q− showed discordant segregation of the affected parent's 13 chromosomes to each of two affected offspring, indicating that the 'pure' retinoblastoma gene (if such exists) is not on chromosome 13 or that meiotic recombination of the 13 chromosome is common, a seemingly unlikely event

since the relevant band is near the centromere (Knight et al, 1980).

Retinoblastoma has been described in few other chromosome syndromes but in view of the paucity of published reports, the findings are likely to be coincidental. This tumour has been noted, albeit uncommonly, in the cancer family syndrome; thus it is quite conceivable that the genetic mechanisms leading to the heritable form of retinoblastoma are heterogenous.

A proportion of surviving retinoblastoma patients have developed second malignancies, particularly in the head and neck area, usually attributable to the effects of local irradiation or intracarotid chemotherapy. Approximately 1/3 of the second malignancies arise outside the immediate treatment area, they are usually sarcomas, a favoured site being the femur, they tend to appear after a 7–15 year latent period, and are also more likely to develop in patients who have bilateral and/or familial disease (Matsunaga, 1980). Bladder carcinoma also seems to be unusually prevalent in older individuals in retinoblastoma families (Chan & Pratt, 1977) and some of these patients, on careful examination, have been found to have regressed retinal tumours (Howe & Manson, 1976). Pinealoma appears unusually frequent, again with bilateral retinoblastoma, an observation that, recognizing the vestigial photoreceptor function of the pineal, has given rise to the whimsical application of 'trilateral retinoblastoma' (Bader et al, 1980). The magnitude of the risk for second tumours may be as high as 10–15% (Abramson et al, 1979). It is conceivable that non-surgical therapy used for retinoblastoma might shorten the latent period for the development of the second malignancy or even hasten its development. On the basis or X–ray sensitivity studies of skin fibroblasts from retinoblastoma patients, Nove et al (1979) have suggested that there is a gene(s) in region 13q 14, distinct from but close to a postulated retinoblastoma locus that could render cells more radiosensitive. Consideration of both retinoblastomas and other tumours together as the total manifestations of a single mutant gene has tremendous long range consequences for patients and their families.

Wilms tumour

Wilms tumour comprises about 15% of all childhood neoplasms with half the tumours developing before age 3. About 1/3 of all cases may be hereditary, being transmitted as an autosomal dominant trait with roughly 60% penetrance (Knudson & Strong, 1972). Monozygotic twin concordance is about 50%, a figure compatible with the 'two-hit' hypothesis (Mauer et al, 1979). Most gene carriers probably have unilateral disease with as many as 1/3 of supposedly sporadic unilateral tumours being heritable. Bove and McAdams (1976) found coexistant anomalous metanephric differentiation in all bilateral and in 14 of 60 unilateral cases of Wilms tumour. Gallo (1978) reported similar findings in 12 of 61 cases, and of these 12, 4 subsequently developed tumours in the opposite kidney. If incomplete differentiation corresponds to a genetic defect in maturation, careful evaluation of the uninvolved renal parenchyma of all surgically removed kidneys would be of considerable importance since such foci might be equated with multifocal potentiality and, of course, multifocality is indicative of heritability.

Second tumours in survivors of Wilms tumour are not common, but it is only recently that mortality statistics have substantially improved. These tumours generally develop in the irradiated tumour bed or after treatment of metastases. Soft tissue sarcomas, hepatoblastomas, thyroid carcinoma, acute leukaemia and colon carcinoma have been reported (Meadows et al, 1977). Unfortunately in none of these reports of second tumours is information provided about other family history. It may well be the patient with the familial form of Wilms tumour is at greater risk for a second neoplasm. If this reasoning is correct, then patients with hereditary disease should be treated insofar as possible with surgery alone.

Patients with hemihypertrophy seem to have a greater incidence of embryonal malignancy (Müller et al, 1978). About 3% of patients with Wilms tumour have hemihypertrophy but data on the converse are not available. Hemihypertrophy is usually an isolated finding, but dominant pedigrees are known, and minor degrees probably go unnoticed. A family has been reported in which a woman with hemihypertrophy had three children with Wilms tumour (one bilateral, two unilateral) and another with a renal malformation (Meadows et al, 1974), the latter also being found with increased frequency with Wilms tumour (Bove & McAdams, 1976).

Another condition with associated Wilms tumour is congenital aniridia, an ocular defect reported in about 1% of Wilms tumour patients. Male patients may have pseudohermaphroditism, often severe enough that the sex of rearing is female. This complex appears to be due to an interstitial deletion of the short arm of chromosome 11, the deletion involving a part of the segment distal to the LDH-A locus, probably 11p13 (Riccardi et al, 1980). Wilms tumour is not invariable, even in similarly affected monozygotic twins, a finding also compatible with the idea that an additional environmental insult is necessary for tumour development. The 11p syndrome is generally sporadic, but an affected child has been described whose mother was found to have a chromosome shift on number 11 which led to meiotic misalignment and an 11p– deletion in her child (Hittner et al, 1979). In another family, two half-brothers and a maternal aunt were found to have the deleted segment secondary to anomalous segregation arising from a parental translocation between chromosomes 2 and 11 (Yunis & Ramsey, 1980). Isolated aniridia may occur as an autosomal dominant trait, but there is only a single case of associated Wilms tumour (Fraumeni & Glass, 1968) and nephroblastomas have not been reported with more complex dominant and recessive syndromes with aniridia. Similarly, Wilms tumours have been reported in a few patients with chromosome aneuploidy such as X0, a B/C translocation, and a survivor with trisomy 18 (Schimke, 1978). These are likely coincidental, although patients with Turner syndrome do have renal malformations which are independent predisposing causes, and nodular renal blastema has been described in autopsy protocols from individuals with trisomy 18 (Geiser & Schindler, 1969). A previously reported patient with a deletion of chromosome 8, aniridia and Wilms tumour has been found on restudy to be missing the 11p– segment as well (Francke et al, 1979).

Wilms tumour has been reported in Sotos syndrome, Klippel-Trenaunay syndrome, Beckwith-Widemann syndrome, and von Recklinghausen disease, conditions which feature growth disturbances of one form or another. The Beckwith-Wiedemann syndrome is probably an incompletely penetrant autosomal dominant trait with a high incidence of embryonal malignancy, particularly Wilms tumour, adrenal cortical carcinoma and hepatoblastoma (Sotelo-Avila, 1980). The association of Wilms tumour with neurofibromatosis may be related to the close proximity of the developing metanephric tissue to neuroectoderm.

Neuroblastoma

The neuroblastoma tumour cell is derived from the neural crest, a ubiquitous tissue that gives rise to a number of structures including the adrenal medulla and the autonomic ganglia (Schimke, 1977). While the adrenal is a favoured site, more than half the tumours are located outside these glands. Adequate genetic studies of neuroblastoma are lacking for two conflicting reasons. On the one hand, survival is poor, but paradoxically, some tumours, especially in females, mature to ganglioneuroma or ganglioneurofibromas and as such may never be detected except serendipitously (Wilson & Draper, 1974). In situ neuroblastomas are present in as many as 1/200 children at autopsy, an incidence far less than the 1/10 000 of frank tumours (Bolande, 1977). Comparatively few familial cases of neuroblastoma have been reported, although the tumour has been described in twins, in sibs and in two generations (Schimke, 1978). Autosomal dominant inheritance of the familial tumour would seem to be the most likely interpretation of the data. The gene defect could on occasion present as heterochromia iridis or as aganglionic megacolon (Knudson & Meadows, 1976).

The proportion of heritable cases of neuroblastoma is unknown but like the other embryonal neoplasms, the genetic form is more likely to be multifocal and become evident earlier. More than one tumour may be present at birth and the question arises as to whether the disease is already disseminated or represents multifocal, primary, and hence by definition, genetic disease. For example, a special group of children has been defined who present with small, commonly bilateral adrenal lesions, along with additional nodules in liver, skin and bone marrow, but who frequently show spontaneous regression of their tumours (Evans et al, 1980). Some feel that these patients actually have primary multifocal disease, not metastatic disease (Schimke, 1979). Others believe that the neuroblastoma nodules in this setting, termed stage IV-S, are not truly malignant but represent collections of neural crest tissue bearing only a germinal mutation (a single 'hit') that has interfered with their normal development (Knudson & Meadows, 1980).

Second tumours in neuroblastoma survivors include thyroid, renal and basal cell carcinoma, glioma and osteogenic sarcoma , virtually all of which arose in previously irradiated areas (Li, 1977; Meadows et al, 1977). One patient has been reported with congenital neuroblastoma, later multiple phaeochromocytomas and eventual multifocal renal cell carcinoma (Schimke, 1979).

Cytogenetic studies in neuroblastoma patients have not been rewarding as in the other embryonal neoplasms. Brodeur et al (1980a) found a deletion of the short arm of chromosome 1, among other abnormalities, in both neuroblastomas and in neuroblastoma cell lines. Excess numbers of small, paired chromatin bodies known as double minutes are also common. A single child with neuroblastoma and trisomy 13 has been reported (Feingold et al, 1971). Neuroblastoma has been seen in the fetal hydantoin syndrome (Seeler et al, 1979). It is conceivable that this substance is both teratogenic and oncogenic in certain susceptible individuals, since Wilms tumour has also been described in an infant exposed in utero (Taylor et al, 1980).

Hepatoblastoma and hepatoma

Hepatoblastoma is a rare tumour almost invariably developing before age two. There is very little evidence for a genetic aetiology, save for two reports of affected infant sibs (Fraumeni et al, 1969; Napoli and Campbell, 1977). The tumour has been reported with 'overgrowth'

Table 98.3 Genetic syndromes in which hepatoma may occur

Haemochromatosis
Fanconi anaemia
Ataxia-telangiectasia
Osler-Rendu-Weber syndrome
Tyrosinaemia
Alpha$_1$-antitrypsin deficiency
Familial cirrhosis
Byler disease
Werner syndrome

syndromes such as congenital hemihypertrophy (Miller et al, 1978), cerebral gigantism and the Beckwith-Wiedemann syndrome (Sotelo-Avila et al, 1980). In these situations, the genetics are those of the primary syndrome.

Hepatocellular carcinoma or hepatoma is also uncommonly familial, and when it occurs in relatives, it is almost invariably related to some prior hepatotoxic insult such as neonatal hepatitis, biliary atresia or cirrhosis of virtually any cause. Genetic syndromes in which hepatoma has been reported are listed in Table 98.3. It must be emphasized that hepatoma is an uncommon accompaniment of these conditions.

Teratomas

The majority of congenital teratomas develop in the sacrococcygeal area and few of them are malignant. In later childhood, they are generally gonadal in origin apparently arising by parthenogenesis from a single germ cell. The sacrococcygeal tumours may be discovered only incidentally, as in the kindreds described by Ashcraft et al (1975). Teratoma-free individuals who transmitted the autosomal dominant tendency had radiographically detectable sacral defects, anorectal abnormalities, or recurrent perianal abscesses, illustrating the extreme degree of variability of the gene defect. Hereditary teratomas may be more common than generally recognized, since many of them may be asymptomatic.

Individuals with the Klinefelter syndrome seem to be unusually prone to develop extragonadal teratomas (Sogge et al, 1979). The tumours may be functional, producing sufficient chorionic gonadotrophin to result in isosexual precocity in children.

Sarcomas

The relationship between sarcomas and other childhood neoplasms, particularly retinoblastoma, has been noted earlier. There is significant sib-sib correlation between osteogenic sarcoma, rhadbomyosarcoma, hamartomas and other unusual sarcomas (Miller, 1971). The earliest to appear is the rhabdomyosarcoma, but the tumour accounts for only about 2% of all deaths from cancer below age 15. It is rarely familial except as a facet of the cancer family syndrome.

The same is true in general with osteogenic sarcoma. For example, a man who had osteogenic sarcoma of the tibia at age 15 developed another such tumour of the mandible at age 40 (Epstein et al, 1970). He had two children with tumours, one an osteogenic sarcoma, the other an adreno-cortical carcinoma. In another family two sibs and their grandfather had sarcoma and a maternal aunt had leukaemia and breast cancer (Bottomley et al, 1971). The aunt had two children with acute leukaemia and another with an adrenal carcinoma. There are a few examples of familial osteogenic sarcoma occurring as isolated tumours, but not in sufficient quantity to construct a genetic hypothesis (Colyer, 1979). The tumours generally are not multiple and they develop during the adolescent growth spurt at the usual sites where rapid bone growth is taking place. The reports are mostly of sibs but two generation occurrence has been noted (Parry et al, 1979). In such families it is probably worthwhile to look for evidence of heritable conditions known to be associated with sarcomas, such as neurofibromatosis, multiple exostosis, osteogenesis imperfecta, fibrous dysplasia, and in older individuals, Paget disease. In one 3-year-old child with fibrous dysplasia and osteosarcoma, a 4q–/7pt chromosome rearrangement was found in peripheral lymphocytes (Brodeur et al, 1980b). Since the same finding was present in the child's mother, the cytogenetic alteration was probably coincidental. Mulvihill et al (1977b) described an American Indian family in which multiple sibs had varying combinations of limb anomalies, erythrocyte macrocytosis and childhood osteogenic sarcoma. The father had the limb deformities and macrocytosis. An abnormality in regulation of bone formation was postulated.

HAMARTOMA SYNDROMES

Neurofibromatosis

Neurofibromatosis is the prototype of the hamartoma syndromes, with an incidence of about 1/3000 births. The clinical features and the normal diagnostic criteria are well-described in standard medical texts and need not be recounted. A variety of tumours may complicate neurofibromatosis (Table 98.4) but the overall incidence of frank malignancy likely does not exceed a few percent (Schimke, 1979). Probably the most common tumours are those sarcomas that develop as a degenerative complication of the neurofibromas. Central nervous system tumours are next most frequent, the whole array of gliomas having been reported (Horton, 1976). In children, the CNS lesions may provide a clue to the diagnosis, since the characteristic skin changes are often not present in early life. In one reported series of meningiomas in children it was concluded that nearly a quarter were the direct result of neurofibromatosis (Merten et al, 1974).

Table 98.4 Some tumours described in patients with neurofibromatosis

Neurinoma	Phaeochromocytoma
Glioma	Paraganglioma
Ganglioneuroma	MEN syndromes
Schwannoma	Carcinoid
Meningioma	Leukaemia
Neuroblastoma	Nephroblastoma
Fibroma	Rhadbomyosarcoma
Sarcoma	Hepatoma

A separate central form of neurofibromatosis has been postulated, largely on the basis of patients with CNS tumours and few or no cutaneous findings, but the evidence is not conclusive. On the other hand, acoustic neuromas, which may complicate neurofibromatosis, appear also to exist as a separate autosomal dominant condition (Young et al, 1970).

Congenital fibromatosis is a disorder in children that may simulate neurofibromatosis (Baird & Worth, 1976). Affected individuals have fibrous, leiomyomatous tumour masses throughout the body that spontaneously regress, providing vital visceral function is not disturbed by their presence. It is inherited as an autosomal recessive trait.

Von Hippel-Lindau syndrome

The diagnostic hallmarks of this condition are hemangioblastomas of the retina and cerebellum, although these vascular tumours can develop anywhere in the brain or spinal cord. Cysts have been reported in a variety of organs, including the liver, kidney, pancreas and epididymis (Horton et al, 1976). Hypernephroma may develop in or adjacent to the renal cysts. In some families the renal cell carcinoma may be the only sign of the disease (Richard et al, 1973). Phaeochromocytomas also occur but much less commonly. Some patients with the syndrome have had nonfunctional pancreatic islet cell tumours, a topic discussed in detail later. Whether the patients with adrenal medullary and pancreatic tumours represent a distinct subgroup is not clear at present, although the parallel with the multiple endocrine neoplasia syndromes, particular types II and III, is obvious. Autosomal dominant inheritance is the accepted mode of genetic transmission for the von Hippel-Lindau syndrome.

Tuberous sclerosis

A wide variety of hamartomas characterize this disorder, notably in the brain, skin, retina, kidney and heart, although such tumours may be found in any organ. Malignant degeneration, usually sarcomatous in type, can occur, but probably in no more than a few percent of cases, and metastatic spread is rare. Even the characteristic brain tumours are histologically benign, although they often interfere with neurological function either by direct encroachment on vital structures or through obstructive hydrocephalus. More invasive brain tumours have been described, particularly in younger individuals, including glioblastomas and ependymomas (Horton, 1976). Optic gliomas may cause considerable visual disability. The kidney tumour is a mixed neoplasm, generally referred to an angiomyolipoma, that only rarely becomes truly malignant, although cystic degeneration and stone formation are common. The diagnostic skin lesions and the more rare cardiac rhabdomyomas are virtually never malignant. The trait is an autosomal dominant with considerable variation in expressivity.

Basal cell nevus syndrome

The chief feature of this disorder is the skin tumour, but other developmental abnormalities in the skeleton may be diagnostically useful since the basal cell nevi are not usually present in children (Gorlin and Sedano, 1972). Medulloblastomas are also seen. Interestingly, when children with the brain tumours are irradiated, basal cell carcinomas develop in an accelerated fashion in the irradiated scalp, neck and shoulder areas, whereas in non-irradiated affected adults, the nevi are more common in sun-exposed areas. Other tumours reported include meningioma, astrocytoma, rhabdomyosarcoma, fibrosarcoma, melanoma, ovarian fibroma and carcinoma, hamartomatous gastric polyps and mesenteric cysts (Southwick and Schwartz, 1979). It is inherited as a quite variable autosomal dominant.

Blue rubber bleb nevus syndrome

The name of this autosomal dominant syndrome is descriptive as affected patients have blister-like vascular nevi not only on the body surface but potentially in the viscera as well (Gorlin, 1976). The nevi may be painful, and tend to bleed, but are not malignant. Associated cancers have been described but neither with sufficient specificity or frequency for any firm conclusions to be made about the total neoplastic potential of the syndrome (Lichtig, 1971). A similar, but independent condition is familial angiolipomatosis, an autosomal recessive disorder, in which affected sibs have multiple subcutaneous tumours, particularly in the joint areas (Hapnes et al, 1980). There is no known malignant predisposition.

Cowden syndrome

Patients with this disorder are often quite striking in their physical appearance in that they have multiple papillomas of the oral cavity, hair follicle hamartomas, and angiomas, lipomas and cysts almost anywhere in the body (Gentry et al, 1975). Affected females have developed breast and uterine cancer, and both sexes reportedly have had colon and thyroid cancer (Mulvihill and McKeen, 1977). The disorder is a rare autosomal dominant. Patients without the typical facies may not be correctly diagnosed, so the overall incidence of malignancy is unknown.

Other Hamartoma syndromes

The Sturge-Weber syndrome is generally placed in this category, but it appears not to confer an increased risk of malignancy. Another neurocutaneous syndrome, the linear sebaceous nevus syndrome, has a high incidence of malignancy as attested by one study of 25 patients

(Andriola, 1976). The tumours have developed in diverse locations such as brain, skin, salivary glands, heart, oesophagus and jaw. Both these conditions are sporadic. Two other non-heritable hamartoma syndromes should be mentioned; the Klippel-Trenaunay-Weber (angio-osteohypertrophy) and the Maffucci syndromes. Bilateral Wilms tumours has been reported in the former (Ehrich et al, 1978) and while the association may have been coincidental, it has been mentioned that embryonal tumours tend to occur in syndromes involving aberrant growth patterns. Chondrosarcomas and angiosarcomas can develop in the Maffucci syndrome (enchondromas and hemangiomas) and, curiously, there seems to be an increased incidence of pituitary and perhaps other endocrine tumours as well (Schnall & Genuth, 1976; Lowell & Mathog, 1979). Other conditions that could easily be classified as hamartomatous conditions include the Gardner, Peutz-Jegher, and Turcot syndromes, but as all feature intestinal polyposis, they are discussed elsewhere in this book.

ENDOCRINE GLAND NEOPLASMS

Secretory tumours of any of the endocrine glands obviously have extensive physiologic implications, whether they are malignant or not. There is considerable controversy about the origin of endocrine tissue, many subscribing to the school of Pearse (1977) who considers that the entire endocrine system as well as other hormone secreting tissue such as the gastrointestinal tract (the paracrine system) is derived from neural crest, neuroectoderm or what has been termed neural-programmed ectoblast. Still others feel that whether cells, particularly neoplastic ones, have the capability to secrete hormones or not depends on other factors quite independent of their embryological source (Skrabenek, 1980; Odell and Wolfsen, 1980). The impetus for the initial uncritical acceptance of the common origin hypothesis largely emanated from study of the multiple endocrine neoplasia (MEN) syndromes, of which there are at least three, appropriately designed types I-III. Since types II and III have overlapping features, some prefer a IIa and IIb classification, although there are enough differences between the two that the former designation seems more appropriate. The entire topic of the MEN syndrome, their possible embryogenesis and their clinical presentation has been dealt with extensively (Rimoin & Schimke, in press).

MEN I (Wermer syndrome)

This condition consists of tumours or hyperplasia of, in order of decreasing frequency of involvement, parathyroids, pancreatic islet cells, pituitary, adrenal cortex and thyroid (Yamaguchi et al, 1980). The clinical presentation is variable depending upon the functional status of the various glands at the time of diagnosis. In some instances the affected individual is totally asymptomatic, the presence of the syndrome being detected only by systematic screening. More than 90% of the patients present with hypercalcaemia with or without complications, peptic ulcer, hypoglycaemia or symptoms referable to a pituitary tumour; e.g., headaches, visual disability or galactorrhoea-amenorrhoea. Less commonly they develop signs of acromegaly or Cushing syndrome or thyroid dysfunction. Tumours of the latter organ are unusual and are not medullary in type, this neoplasm being characteristic of MEN II and III. About 60% of affected family members have two glands involved, and 20% eventually have three or more. Generally speaking, the only consistent truly malignant part of the syndrome involves the islet cells, where the presentation may be that of insulinoma, the Zollinger-Ellison syndrome, the glucagonoma syndrome or pancreatic cholera (Schimke, 1976). Moreover, the islet cell tumours are prone to secrete a variety of ectopic hormones with a confusing array of symptoms. Other tumours described in MEN I include lipomas, schwanomas, thymomas and cutaneous leiomyomas.

Symptoms of the syndrome may develop at any age, but the condition is rare in childhood and uncommonly presents initially after age 60. As with the other MEN syndromes, MEN I is an autosomal dominant disorder with probably complete penetrance, but with considerable variability in expression. The basic genetic lesion is unknown and involvement of the various glands cannot be totally accounted for on the basis of present theories. Once the diagnosis is made, periodic screening studies must be undertaken in all first degree family members.

MEN II (Sipple syndrome)

Medullary thyroid carcinoma, phaeochromocytoma and parathyroid hyperplasia constitute the triad of findings characteristic of this syndrome. The thyroid tumour is actually derived from the parafollicular cells whose prime secretory product is calcitonin, the excessive secretion of which, while causing no symptoms, is extraordinarily useful in diagnosis. There is good evidence that parafollicular or C-cell hyperplasia probably always precedes frank malignancy by months or even years (Williams, 1979). The thyroid tumours once they develop are not surprisingly multifocal, and this is also true of the adrenal medullary neoplasms, although with the latter tumours, it is not uncommon for years to elapse between the detection of one tumour and the development of another (Schimke, 1976). The phaeochromocytomas may be extra-adrenal and are also preceded by premonitory adrenal medullary hyperplasia (Carney et al, 1975). The parathyroids are generally diffusely hyperplastic. As with islet cells, the medullary thyroid tumour may secrete a variety of substances besides calcitonin; e.g., ACTH,

serotonin, vasoactive intestinal polypeptide and so forth, again generating diagnostic confusion. Other tumours reported in MEN II include brain tumours, breast carcinoma, leukaemia and cancer of the pyriform sinus, but in no case is the association strong enough to be considered more than coincidental.

The thyroid tumour is ultimately malignant, although even with frank lymph node involvement, prolonged survival is not uncommon. The incidence of true malignancy of the adrenal medullary tumours is probably higher than with sporadic phaeochromocytomas. Peculiarly, they often do not respond to the usual provocative tests, and may actually be detected only incidentally, a factor that may account in part for the higher malignant potential.

Both the parafollicular cells and the adrenal medulla are derived from neural crest (Tischler et al, 1976) but there is no firm evidence that the parathyroids stem from the same source. Initially it was felt that parathyroid involvement was secondary to prolonged excessive calcitonin secretion but it now appears that hyperparathyroidism may precede at least the obvious presence of the thyroid tumour. Early stimulatory alterations in the chief cell micro-environment occasioned by C-cell hyperplasia cannot be totally excluded. MEN II is an autosomal dominant disorder with nearly complete penetrance by age 50.

Baylin et al (1978), using tissue from patients with MEN II who were also heterozygous for two electrophoretically distinguishable G6PD variants have established that the syndrome results from a clonal event in that each separate tumour focus has either the A or the B phenotype. This finding is in keeping with the 'two-hit' hypothesis in that a second somatic event would be necessary before a given cell would undergo malignant transformation and clonal growth. Further support for this hypothesis is derived from study of monozygotic twins who were concordant for thyroid carcinoma but discordant for phaeochromocytoma (Pohl et al, 1977).

Provocative testing with either or both calcium and pentagastrin is mandatory in individuals at risk for MEN II. These substances stimulate secretion of large amounts of calcitonin by the C-cells even during their preneoplastic stages, thereby allowing for curative thyroidectomy. Once basal serum calcitonin levels are elevated, the tumour is beyond the confines of the thyroid capsule.

MEN III (mucosal neuroma syndrome)

MEN III also includes medullary thyroid carcinoma and phaeochromocytoma, but in addition affected individuals have a rather striking habitus, including the virtually pathognomonic feature of mucosal neuromas, not only in the oropharynx but literally throughout the gastrointestinal tract (Schimke, 1972, 1973; Carney and Hayles, 1978). Other features that distinguish MEN III from

MEN II include the lack of consistent parathyroid involvement in the former disorder (Khairi et al, 1975) and the poorer prognosis, the mean survival being only to 27 years versus nearly 60 years in MEN II (Williams, 1977).

MEN III is also an autosomal dominant disorder, but calculations of penetrance are not possible as yet, since no systematic study of enough families has been undertaken to see whether mucosal neuromas could be present without the more malignant aspects of the syndrome. When these typical facies are present, it is important to remove the thyroid totally as soon as possible, since the tumour has been reported to be already malignant by age 2, and no therapy save for surgery has been shown to be consistently effective (Moyes and Alexander, 1977). The behaviour of the phaeochromocytoma in MEN III is similar to that in MEN II.

A better case for neural crest derivation of MEN III can be made than for either of the other well-recognized multiple endocrine adenoma syndromes. It would be of interest to see if the various neuromas as well as the component tumours in MEN III have a clonal origin.

Possible MEN syndromes

There are a host of reports of patients with two or more endocrine tumours, often of a type that suggests overlap of the recognized MEN syndromes. Virtually all of the cases are sporadic, and it is not clear that they are distinct syndromes.

One endocrine tumour association may be unique; i.e., that of phaeochromocytoma with pancreatic islet cell tumours, a combination of neoplasms that may be familial or occur sporadically. The phaeochromocytomas tend to be multiple and have an early age of onset. The islet cell tumours, which may be benign or malignant, have not been shown to be secretory, at least for any known hormones, a situation unlike that seen with MEN I where more than 75% of such lesions are functional (Carney et al, 1980). In the one affected family, the proband had multiple islet cell tumours and multicentric phaeochromocytomas, her daughter had a unilateral phaeochromocytoma, and her mother had bilateral phaeochromocytomas and a pituitary tumour (Janson et al, 1978). While it is tempting to consider this complex as MEN IV, it is interesting that about half the reported patients either had the von Hippel-Lindau syndrome, or had first degree relatives with this condition (Hull et al, 1979). In the family just noted, the proband had benign adenomas in both kidneys, findings reminiscent of the von Hippel-Lindau syndrome. Pancreatic adenomas, functional status unknown, have also been described in this condition (Horton et al, 1976). Conceivably, the von Hippel-Lindau syndrome may be more clinically variable than heretofore thought or, alternatively, it may be genetically heterogenous.

Other familial endocrine tumours

Familial examples of pituitary adenomas exclusive of MEN I are rare. Levin et al (1974) recorded brothers with acromegaly, and a mother-daughter pair have had the galactorrhoea-amenorrhoea syndrome (Linquette et al, 1967). The latter complex is commonplace in endocrine clinics and has been related by some clinicians to the extensive contemporary use of oral contraceptives; hence, no genetic interpretation of familial aggregation is possible.

There are numerous reports in the literature of familial hyperparathyroidism such that autosomal dominant inheritance seems assured (Marx et al, 1977). What is less clear is what proportion of these families actually have one of the MEN syndromes, the other facets not having become evident at the time the family is recorded. A reasonable estimate might be about one-third. Hyperparathyroidism has been reported in patients with papillary thyroid carcinoma on a nonfamilial basis. While external ionizing radiation has been implicated as a potential cause of both lesions, the evidence is far from convincing (LaVolsi & Feind, 1976).

Save for medullary thyroid cancer which is an integral feature of MEN II and III, there is very little support for an hereditary component in the aetiology of more common papillary or follicular tumours. Predisposing factors include goitre, particularly if it is long-standing, and external irradiation. Patients with the Gardner syndrome develop papillary thyroid cancer with unusual frequency and this tumour has been reported in the Cowden and the Werner syndrome. Both papillary and follicular neoplasms have been reported in the cancer family syndrome.

Pancreatic islet cell tumours, no matter what their secretory capacity, are only rarely familial except when part of MEN I or the aforementioned phaeochromocytoma-islet cell tumour complex. A father and daughter with insulinomas have been reported (Tragl & Mayr, 1977). In another family, one member had a glucagonoma and other individuals had elevated plasma levels of high molecular weight glucagon in a pattern consistent with autosomal dominant inheritance, but whether these family members actually had islet cell tumours is unknown (Boden & Owen, 1977). A familial form of nesidioblastosis has been recorded in sibs (Schwartz et al, 1979). Pathologically this abnormality is characterized by a diffuse and disorganized formation of new islet cells. Neonatal hypoglycaemia is the presenting feature and the clinical course may be relentless unless early subtotal pancreatectomy is performed, and even this may not be totally effective. Autosomal recessive inheritance of this peculiar entity is likely, but it is not strictly speaking a cancer syndrome.

Only about 10% of adult patients with adrenal cortical hyperfunction have primary adrenal disease. In children, however, adrenal carcinoma is much more likely, with the presenting features either of the Cushing syndrome or more commonly, of virilization (Gilbert & Cleveland, 1970). Earlier reports of familial occurrence of adrenal cortical tumours may well have represented untreated sibs with the mild, non-salt losing forms of the adrenogenital syndrome, conditions in which the pathologic anatomy of the adrenal glands is often quite bizarre due to the continued stimulation by ACTH. True malignancy in this setting is quite rare, as metastatic disease from such a source has not been successfuly documented. Other instances of familial adrenal cortical carcinoma seem to be part of the cancer family syndrome (Schimke, 1978). Familial Cushing syndrome due to bilateral nodular hyperplasia has been reported in four sibs from Cuba (Arce et al, 1978). Adrenal cortical tumours may complicate the Gardner and Beckwith-Wiedemann syndromes.

Embryonic tumours of the adrenal medulla have been discussed earlier. Phaeochromocytoma may be part of MEN II and III, of von Recklinghausen disease and the von Hippel-Lindau syndrome, all autosomal dominant disorders. In addition, the tumour has a separate hereditary basis in some instances, although also as an autosomal dominant trait. It has been estimated that nearly a quarter of all cases are hereditary with the hereditary form showing the expected features of frequent bilaterally and/or and extra-adrenal location (Knudson et al, 1973). This estimate includes all the entities mentioned earlier. The various paraganglia are embryologically related to the adrenal medulla, and it is not surprising to find tumours of structures such as the glomus jugulare or the carotid bodies in patients with familial phaeochromocytoma (Pollack, 1973). However, paragangliomas, or as some would prefer, chemodectomas, may occur on a familial basis in the absence of recognized phaeochromocytoma (Kahn, 1977).

Whether one considers the pineal gland as part of the endocrine system is questionable, although tumours of this gland in children on occasion adversely influence sexual maturation. Pineal hyperplasia associated with enlarged genitalia, unusual facies and insulin-resistant diabetes has been reported in sibs (West & Leonard, 1980). The occurrence of pinealoma patients with familial retinoblastoma has been mentioned earlier.

Carcinoid tumours are considered by some to be a form of endocrine neoplasia, predominantly because the tumours are secretory, but also because they occur as a component of MEN I and, in sporadic instances, with phaeochromocytoma. In these settings, the tumours are almost invariably foregut in location. Familial carcinoids independent of these other neoplasms are largely confined to the lower gastrointestinal tract and they are quite rare (Schimke, 1977).

REPRODUCTIVE SYSTEM

Testicular tumours

Testicular tumours are diagnosed in less than 1/50 000 males. Most are of the germ cell origin, except in children where teratomas and stromal tumours predominate. Gonadal teratomas usually develop parthenogenetically, especially in females. Nongonadal teratomas arise mitotically and thus have the same karotype as the host, although a tetraploid XXYY mediastinal lesion has been described (Kaplan et al, 1979). While familial examples of testicular teratomas are rare, bilateral lesions have been described in sibs, one pair of which had the Klinefelter syndrome (Gustavson et al, 1975; Shinohara et al, 1980). Interestingly enough, mediastinal teratomas (polyembryomas) also have been described in a few patients with the Klinefelter syndrome (Chaussain et al, 1979). Seminoma has also been noted in a patient with Klinefelter syndrome (Isurugi et al, 1979), but in this instance the gonad was cryptorchid, and it is well known that the incidence of malignancy in cryptorchid testes is increased at least 10–15 fold (Simpson & Photopoulos, 1976a). There are a number of genetic syndromes of which cryptorchidism is a feature; these are reviewed elsewhere (Rimoin & Schimke, in press).

Familial aggregation of testicular tumours independent of the above and of the intersex states have been reported, albeit infrequently. Probably less than 50 such families have been noted with the disease appearing in twins, sibs, and less commonly, two generations (Shinohara et al, 1980; Raghavan et al, 1980). There is a greater tendency for the tumours to be bilateral in these families and monozygotic twin concordance is high, bespeaking a simply inherited tendency for neoplasia in some families. Also supporting a prime genetic role is the documented ethnic difference between African Blacks and white Englishmen (30 fold higher in the latter), a difference that persists even after migration of the blacks from Africa. At the present time, however, no clearly defined mode of inheritance for testicular tumours has been established, although it is quite likely that bilateral tumours have a greater tendency to be heritable, perhaps as a sex-limited autosomal dominant trait.

Ovary

Ovarian cancer is about five times more common than testicular cancer. About 90% of the tumours are derived from germinal epithelium and they tend to occur in older women. No definitive environmental risk factors have been identified (Annegars et al, 1979). In contrast, a number of papers have documented multigeneration transmission of ovarian cancer (Simpson and Photopoulos, 1976a), but oddly enough, the tumours are uncommonly bilateral and the age of onset is usually similar to the non-familial cases.

In children, ovarian teratomas predominate and they do tend to be bilateral, frequently also undergoing torsion (Brown, 1979). A number of familial instances of teratomas have been described (Rimoin and Schimke, in press). Arrhenoblastomas and dysgerminomas have also been reported in females over two generations (Jensen et al, 1974). Ovarian fibromas have been recorded in four generations of a family (Dumont-Herskowitz et al, 1978). Perhaps 5–10% of ovarian tumours are due to simply inherited predisposing factors, behaving either as a sex-limited autosomal or an X–linked dominant trait. Table 98.5 summarizes some disorders in which gonadal tumours, either testicular or ovarian, may occur.

Gonadal tumours in intersex states

Gonadal tumours probably never occur in individuals with intersex states unless the gonad contains a Y–chromosome cell line (Simpson & Photopoulos, 1976b). The risk is variable, however, ranging from zero in XX males who are H-Y antigen positive to 20–30% in patients with XO/XY mosaicism or with H-Y positive, XY pure gonadal dysgenesis. Gonadal malignancy has been documented in true hermaphroditism, but it is rare. The risk for patients with the complete form of testicular feminization syndrome is probably about 10%, but those with the incomplete varieties, of which there are many, have not yet developed gonadal neoplasms. Inborn errors of steroid metabolism leading to sexual ambiguity do not seem to predispose to true malignancy in either sex. Testicular tumours in males with virilizing forms of the adrenogenital syndrome have been reported, but these disappear after cortisol therapy and are generally considered to be hypertrophied adrenal rest tissue.

Genital cancer

Cancer of the genitalia, exclusive of the uterus, is rare and genetic factors are of no aetiologic significance. There is no firm evidence that cancer of the cervix is at all genetic, except when it develops as a complication of the hereditary diseases dyskeratosis congenita and ectodermal dysplasia. Of greater interest to epidemiologists has been the association between maternal ingestion of

Table 98.5 Disorders in which gonadal tumours appear

XO/XY mosaicism
True hermaphroditism
XY pure gonadal dysgenesis
Testicular feminization
Cryptorchidism
Cancer family syndrome
Peutz-Jegher syndrome
Gardner syndrome
Basal cell nevus syndrome
Ataxia-telangiectasia
Stein-Leventhal syndrome

---

diethlstilboestrol and vaginal cancer in female offspring. A large cooperative study of such individuals revealed that 34% had vaginal changes, often referred to as vaginal adenosis, but the actual cancer incidence was low, being about 1/1000 women exposed (Robboy et al, 1979). The risk is age-related, in that the vast majority develop lesions prior to age 20.

Endometrial cancer has a more prominent genetic component, 16 of 154 patients in one series having an affected first degree relative (Lynch et al, 1967). Evaluation of the pedigrees revealed that about 10% of the multiply affected families contained members with other adenocarcinomas, a finding suggestive of the cancer family syndrome. Oestrogen use has been correlated with endometrial cancer, although the various studies are not in complete agreement (Hulka et al, 1980). It has been suggested that the use of both oestrogens and progesterone confers a protective effect. To what extent the use of unopposed oestrogen might interact with heritable factors is not known, but would be worthy of further study. Endometrial carcinoma has been reported in the Turner syndrome, and while most of the patients had received unopposed oestrogens, it is possible that the karotypic abnormality predisposes in some fashion to this malignancy (McCarty et al, 1978). Of note is a single case of vulvar carcinoma (Sanfilippo et al, 1979), and the absence of ovarian carcinoma in pure XO or patients with XO/XX mosaic karyotypes. Those with XO/XY and Turner phenotype are at substantial risk for gonadal neoplasms, but they should properly be considered as having mixed gonadal dysgenesis rather than the Turner syndrome. There is some evidence that individuals with the Turner syndrome may be unduly prone to tumours of neural crest derivatives (Wertelecki et al, 1970).

Uterine sarcomas have been reported in the Werner syndrome, and both endometrial and breast cancer have been seen in sclerotylosis. Uterine leiomyomas (fibroids) are so common that no good genetic studies have been performed.

Prostate

In situ prostate carcinoma may occur in 10–15% of males over the age of 50 (Lynch et al, 1966). Since cancer is, in general, a disease of older individuals, other tumours could easily develop in such men by chance alone; hence, no firm evidence for genetic factors has emerged. A statistical relationship between prostate cancer and breast, ovarian and endometrial cancer in female relatives was established in one study (Thiessen, 1974). All these tumours are part of the familial adenocarcinomatosis or cancer family syndrome, so that men with this kind of history may be at greater risk of having second tumours and of siring offspring with similar afflictions. It seems unlikely that such men constitute more than 1–2% of the entire prostate cancer population.

Breast cancer

In the United States, the average lifetime probability of a woman developing breast cancer is about 7%. The tumour accounts for more than 20% of all female neoplasms and is the leading cause of death in women (Anderson, 1977). The incidence rates have risen in Western countries since the turn of the century for unknown reasons. A host of adverse and protective circumstances have been associated with breast cancer, all of which are statistically interesting, but of little value in defining a high risk population much less an individual. Ethnic differences have been noted which appear to be related to environmental factors since they increase with migration from a low to a high incidence rate (MacMahon et al, 1975).

The first familial report of breast cancer was by Broca in 1886 who noted the disease in 10 of 24 female relatives. Other families with equally impressive numbers have been described, and it has been estimated that as many as 13% of all breast cancers are familial (Lynch et al, 1976). Even within this group, there is evidence of heterogeneity in that only about half of patients have had relatives with breast cancer alone, the remainder having a positive family history of breast carcinoma and/or other tumours; e.g., ovary, endometrium, colon and soft tissue sarcomas. Not surprisingly, the disease in families tends to appear earlier, even premenopausally and is often, if not initially, eventually bilateral (Anderson, 1977). The lifetime probability of developing breast cancer in the female progeny of a woman with premenopausal, bilateral disease is high enough to be consistent with autosomal dominant inheritance of a mammary tumour susceptibility gene (Petrakis, 1977; Lynch et al, 1978). In favour of this interpretation is a recent report suggesting linkage of such a gene with the glutamate-pyruvate transaminase locus (King et al, 1980). In other families notably those containing members with other tumours, no such linkage has been found.

Anderson (1974) noted that 8 of 234 (3.4%) pedigrees of breast cancer patients showed an associated adenocarcinoma at other sites, especially ovary, endometrium and colon, and an additional 14 (6%) showed aggregation of breast cancer with sarcomas, embryonal tumours and leukaemia. The data of Lynch et al (1976) suggest that about 30% of familial breast cancer occurs in families in which these other tumours appear as well. In general, these latter families conform to the two general types of cancer family syndrome mentioned earlier. It is also quite possible that other breast cancer syndromes exist, but these are not as yet well delineated (Jackson et al, 1979). Other estimates of the heritable fraction of breast cancer range from 8% (based on the incidence of bilaterality) to a theoretical prediction of 30% (Knudson et al, 1973).

Definition of that fraction of women with a genetic predisposition becomes exceedingly important, since environmental risk factors are so poorly defined. It is this group that should be screened more vigorously, although a case could be made for not using mammography (Land, 1980). As an example of possible radiation-facilitated breast carcinoma, Li et al (1981) described two affected sisters both of whom developed their tumours, four and eleven years respectively, after external radiation therapy for Hodgkin's disease. There was a strong family history of breast carcinoma. Fibrocystic disease is probably another reliable high-risk indicator (Hutchinson et al, 1980). There is also an increased likelihood for a woman with a unilateral breast cancer in a breast cancer kindred to develop disease on the opposite side (she indeed may already have *in situ* lesions) (Harris et al, 1978), such that the presence of both these factors, i.e., family history and fibrocystic disease, may well warrant prophylactic mastectomy. Interestingly, in breast cancer families the increased risk extends to and may be transmitted by males. Outside the confines of such families male breast cancer is uncommon and heritability is low in otherwise normal men (Marger et al, 1975). Males with the Klinefelter syndrome have a twenty-fold increased risk of mammary cancer, and the tumour has also been noted in true hermaphrodites, perhaps in both instances on the basis of abnormal estrogen levels and/or metabolism, although such has not been shown to be significant in women with breast carcinoma.

Breast carcinoma is a feature of the Cowden and Torre-Muir syndrome and it also has been reported in genetically determined immune deficiency states.

GASTROINTESTINAL CANCER

Gastrointestinal tumours, particularly of the colorectum, are among the most common neoplasms in man. In the past, much emphasis has been placed on those environmental factors that might predispose to malignancy. While such clearly exist, it is evident that heredity must also play a role, even in common cancers, although the genetic input varies with tumour site.

Oropharynx

While anatomic purists might quibble, the oropharnyx along with the rectum could be considered as the squamous cell extremes of the gastrointestinal tract. The heritable disorders that predispose to neoplasia in these structures are few and in general are associated with high cell turnover and/or abnormal DNA repair (Schimke, 1980). For example, in X–linked dyskeratosis congenita, leukoplakia of the oral and rectal mucosa may give rise to squamous cell carcinoma. The same tumour type has been reported in dominantly inherited ectodermal dysplasia, in both dominant and recessive epidermolysis bullosa, and in xeroderma pigmentosum and the Bloom syndrome. These latter two conditions are discussed in greater detail elsewhere in this volume.

Oesophagus

The bulk of oesophageal carcinoma is felt to develop because of nutritional deficiency and/or dietary peculiarities, largely because of the unusual geographic distribution of the disease, being more prevalent in central Africa and the Middle East. Hence, families with multiple affected individuals in these areas provide no insight into any potential genetic mechanisms. Ashley (1969), studying oesophageal cancer in Wales, concluded that the greater the Welsh ancestry the more likely the risk of developing the disease with an average two-fold risk over non-Welsh individuals living in Wales. The absolute risk is clearly low, given the population incidence of the disease.

Oesophageal cancer may complicate some rare genetic disorders, such as the previously mentioned dyskeratosis congenita and epidermolysis bullosa, and also the autosomal recessive Fanconi syndrome, another disorder in which DNA repair mechanisms are abnormal. Cancer of the oesophagus along with other GI cancers has been reported in common variable immunodeficiency for reasons not totally clear, although decreased immune surveillance is a plausible hypothesis (Spector et al, 1978). A similar rationale could be invoked for the increased incidence of oesophageal cancer in coeliac disease and in the more benign variant of scleroderma termed the CREST syndrome. In the latter condition recurrent acid reflux may be of greater aetiologic significance, and in the former nutritional deficiency may play a prominent role. Both coeliac disease and the CREST syndrome are reportedly autoimmune disorders, and like the other autoimmune diseases, the genetics are quite complex, with very little evidence for any major inherited component.

The most noteworthy genetic disease with oesophageal cancer is the late-onset form of tylosis. Virtually all patients with this rare, autosomal dominant disorder develop oesophageal malignancy by the seventh decade (Harper et al, 1970). Another autosomal dominant form of tylosis appears in infancy and does not predispose to any known malignancy. Sclerotylosis can be distinguished from either of the above conditions by additional atrophic skin changes beyond the palmer-plantar areas (Hunter et al, 1968). Oesophageal tumours have not been described in this condition but cancer of the tongue, tonsil, breast and uterus have been reported.

Stomach

There is some disagreement concerning the role of genetics in the development of gastric cancer (Lehtola, 1978; Anderson, 1978). While pedigrees purportedly showing autosomal dominant inheritance have been published, the data are equally compatible with a polygenic hypothesis. Specific environmental carcinogens have not been identified in man, although substances like ethanol

and certain nitroso compounds have been implicated. Histology may be significant, since heritability is greater with the diffuse rather than either the intestinal or undifferentiated cell types (Lehtola, 1978). Ethnic factors seem to be important, as does the simultaneous presence of blood group A and pernicious anaemia. The latter disorder is generally associated with anti-parietal cell antibodies, and patients not uncommonly have other evidence of autoimmune disease. Individuals with immune deficiency states, such as adult-onset common variable immunodeficiency and ataxia-telangiectasia seem to be predisposed to gastric cancer to such an extent as to perhaps constitute a subpopulation of individuals at increased risk for this neoplasm (Spector et al, 1978).

Gastric malignancy appears also to be more frequent in heterozygotes for the various autosomal recessive disorders with defective DNA repair. Gastric tumours may complicate some of the colon polyposis syndromes which are generally dominantly inherited. One apparently unique family has been described in which 10 members over 3 generations suffered only gastric polyposis with a high frequency of associated stomach cancers (Sandos & Magalhaes, 1980). There were no recognized intestinal polyps. Gastric cancer also has been reported in the cancer family syndrome. However, in the absence of any of these afore-mentioned risk factors, the absolute risk of a relative of a gastric cancer patient developing the same tumour is really quite low.

Benign stomach tumours have been noted in the basal cell nevus and Cowden syndromes (Schimke, 1980).

Small intestine

Tumours of the small bowel are rare, and when they occur are more likely to be one facet of more complex disorders such as the Gardner, Peutz-Jeghers or colon polyposis syndromes. In fact, the risk of small intestinal malignancy particularly in the periampullary structures is increased in the Gardner syndrome 100–200 fold (Pauli et al, 1980). Islet cell tumours and carcinoid tumours have been found in the duodenum in multiple endocrine neoplasia type I. Small bowel lymphomas have been described in multiple members of some families, but since most of these are male, the opinion has been advanced that those individuals have the Duncan syndrome, an X–linked selective immunodeficiency to Epstein-Barr virus.

Gallbladder

The most significant predisposing agent to gallbladder cancer is felt to be stones; yet the latter are so common and the former so rare that other factors must be of importance. Indians in the southwestern United States have a higher incidence of gallstones and a six-fold increase incidence of gallbladder cancer when compared to the non-Indian population. While shared environment; i.e., reservation living and a high fat, high car-bohydrate diet must be of significance, families have been reported in which detribalized individuals have developed the disease (Devon & Buechley, 1979). This might indicate that the Indian heritage adds to that risk conferred by the environment.

Liver

In nutritionally deprived areas of the world, both cir-rhosis and hepatocellular carcinoma are not uncommon. Elsewhere, if exposure to environmental hepatotoxins can be excluded familial aggregation of liver cancer is rare (Hagstrom & Baker, 1968). There are a number of heritable diseases involving the liver where carcinoma has developed (Table 98.3). Hepatitis B antigen may conceivably be transmitted from one generation to the next via the placenta giving rise to apparent dominant hepatoma (Ohbayashi et al, 1972). An unusual family has been described in which the affected individuals had var-ious combinations of liver cell adenomas or carcinomas and diabetes mellitus (Foster et al, 1973). Two younger female members also had sclerocystic ovaries along with hepatic adenomas and mild diabetes mellitus. Neither had been on oral contraceptives. Save for these few exceptions, the heritability of hepatic carcinoma should be considered quite low.

Pancreas

The incidence of adenocarcinoma of the pancreas appears to be increasing at about 15% per decade in the Western world. Suspected inciting agents are multiple but alco-hol, tobacco and certain industrial carcinogens have been most often incriminated. Calcific pancreatitis, either acquired or heritable seems to predispose. Pancreatic cancer has been reported in ataxia-telangiectasia and in the cancer family syndrome. Islet cell carcinomas are in integral feature of multiple endocrine neoplasia and may develop in the von Hippel-Lindau syndrome. Save for three families, two with affected sibs, the other with an involved father and son, familial aggregation of pan-creatic cancer is essentially nonexistent (Reimer et al, 1977).

Colorectum

Cancer of the colorectum is second only to lung cancer as a cause of morbidity and mortality in the Western world. Exclusive of the heritable polyposis syndromes, which account for less than 5% of all colon cancer, most cases are sporadic with a negative family history. How-ever, that genetic factors are operational to some extent is indicated by the results of one series where 26% of patients had a positive family history (Lovett, 1976) and surveys which suggest that the relatives of an index case have a 3-4 fold increased risk of developing colorectal cancer during their lifetime, i.e., if the lifetime proba-bility of large bowel cancer is 5%, an affected first degree

relative would increase the probability to at least 15% (Anderson, 1980a). However, these figures may be both an underestimate and an oversimplification. For exam-ple, pedigree studies of non-polyposis colorectal cancer patients have revealed some other markers that may indicate a greater liability to cancer in some families; e.g., earlier average age of onset in the index case, mul-tiple tumours, simultaneous or independent presence of endometrial carcinoma in a first degree female relative or gastric cancer in relatives of either sex, and a predom-inant right-sided location. It has been suggested that within the colorectal cancer patient category there are subgroups in whom the cancer liability behaves as auto-somal dominant trait with moderately high penetrance (Anderson, 1980a). These reputed entities are the cancer family syndrome or hereditary adenocarcinomatosis, hereditary gastrocolonic cancer, hereditary isolated colon cancer and the Torre-Muir syndrome, the latter clearly an autosomal dominant condition featuring sebaceous cysts, adenocarcinoma of the large and small bowel and uterus, squamous cell carcinoma of the mucous mem-branes and transitional cell carcinoma of the urinary sys-tem (Anderson, 1980b). Whether the former non-syndromic colorectal cancer families represent one or a series of entities is not clear, but there is evidence that in these families, the tumour develops in or prior to the fifth decade, the lesions are more likely to be right-sided (2/3 versus about 1/4 of sporadic cases) and they tend to be multiple about 20% of the time. Prolonged survival seems also to characterize this group of patients (Lynch et al, 1978). Whether one disease or many, it is possible that these families may well represent the bulk of patients at increased risk of colorectal cancer, the families of the remaining patients having essentially no greater risk than the general population. In other words, the population-based studies showing increased risk to relatives may represent a composite figure for a heterogeneous disease consisting of some patients with high risk and others with low risk. Clearly, detailed histories and prospective stud-ies are indicated to evaluate this possibility, since in the aggregate, these individuals could conceivably comprise 5–10% of the colon cancer patients. Marker studies, while perhaps not useful on a population basis, may pro-vide clues to cancer susceptibility in individual families (Kopelovich, 1980).

Multiple polyposis syndromes

These conditions are of considerable interest to the geneticist because they are heritable, with the exception of the Cronkhite-Canada syndrome, a rather enigmatic disorder in which the adenomatosis gastrointestinal polyps are generally considered to be inflammatory. Some of the syndromes with polyposis are complex and have extracolonic features that facilitate diagnosis, such as the Gardner and Peutz-Jegher syndromes.

Table 98.6 Tumours reported in the Gardner syndrome

Colon polyps and adenocarcinoma
Carcinoma of duodenum
Carcinoma of ampulla of Vater
Osteoma and osteosarcoma
Papillary thyroid carcinoma
Adrenal carcinoma
Bladder carcinoma
Fibroma and fibrosarcoma
Lipoma
Leiomyoma
Epidermoid cyst
Ovarian fibroma and carcinoma
Brain tumour
Melanoma
Parotid fibroma

Gardner syndrome

The Gardner syndrome consists of the triad of colon polyps, sebaceous cysts and osteomas, but the gene has multiple pleiotropic effects and tumous of a host of organs have been described (Table 98.6). It is inherited as a quite variable autosomal dominant disorder with complete penetrance (Naylor & Gardner, 1977). The probability of malignant degeneration of the colon polyps is essentially 100% by age 40. While the diagnosis may be difficult to make in childhood, almost all patients have some extracolonic manifestation of the gene by the third decade. Danes (1978) has found increased tetraploidy in epitheial cell cultures taken from tissues known to undergo malignant change in the Gardner syndrome. Cells from benign tumours such as lipomas, cysts and fibromas and skin fibroblasts did not show this phenomenon. The significance of this finding is not at the moment clear.

Some families have been described whose features in part are compatible with the Gardner syndrome but in which other clinical findings are sufficiently different that the authors have felt they were dealing with a distinct entity (Binder et al, 1978). Alternatively, occasional patients with familial polyposis coli have had skin lesions of one sort or another or osteomas prompting the suggestion that the two syndromes are in reality one (MConnell, 1980). This seems unlikely in view of Gardner's elaborate analysis (Naylor & Gardner, 1977) but it illustrates the complexity of adequate nosology when overlapping clinical features are present and the basic genetic lesion is unknown.

Familial polyposis coli

This is the classic autosomal dominant polyposis syndrome in which the colon contains few to literally thousands of adenomatous polyps (Kussin et al, 1979). Gastric polyps also occur but less commonly. Colon polyps have been detected in the first year of life or as late as the eighth decade, but the average age of onset is in the mid-twenties. Patients are generally managed by early colectomy with ileoproctostomy, remaining rectal polyps having been found to regress in some instances. More recent data suggests that the incidence of recurrent rectal cancer is high if rectal polyps are present and low if not, so that the former group must be watched carefully if a conservative surgical approach is adopted (Bess et al, 1980).

Peutz-Jegher syndrome

The buccal and labial pigmentation should alert the clinician to the diagnosis of this condition in which the gastrointestinal polyps are hamartomas and are generally considered benign, although they may cause bleeding or obstruction. Malignant degeneration does occur, however, especially if the polyps are in the stomach and duodenum, although the magnitude of this risk probably is no greater than 5% (Hsu et al, 1979). Of considerable interest is the fact that affected females have an increased risk of sex-cord ovarian tumours (Simpson & Photopoulos, 1976a). Breast and endometrial carcinomas have also been described (Gloor, 1978), and a 6-year-old male with a testicular Sertoli cell tumour has been reported (Cantu et al, 1980).

Juvenile polyposis

In this autosomal dominant condition, the polyps appear in childhood, histologically are usually cystic hamartomas and are benign. Simultaneous adenomatous polyps also have been reported, however, and these may be malignant (Goodman et al, 1979). In some families adenomatous polyps have been found in adults and juvenile polyps in children raising the spectre of age-related, environmentally-induced degenerative changes. Treatment is generally conservative, with caution dictating that more aggressively appearing lesions should be removed under fibroscopic visualization.

Turcot syndrome

This is the only polyposis syndrome known to be inherited as an autosomal recessive (Itoh et al, 1979). The extra colonic feature is a glioma. The condition is quite rare, only a few cases having been reported.

Other syndromes with polyps

Benign colon polyps occur in the Cowden syndrome. In neurofibromatosis and the mucosal neuroma syndrome, gangliomas of the colon may stimulate polyps, but they are virtually never malignant. Colon carcinoma has also been reported in some of the heritable immunodeficiency states, particularly those with absent IgA (Spector et al, 1978).

URINARY TRACT MALIGNANCY

Hypernephroma in families is rare, with fewer than 25 instances having been documented in the literature (Lyons et al, 1977). In some of these families, the affected individuals may have had the von Hippel-Lindau syndrome, a condition in which the incidence of renal cell carcinoma may exceed 20%, and one in which the renal tumour may precede the other more diagnostic features (Richards et al, 1973). Associations of familial renal cell carcinoma with various HLA types have been sought and found, notably with BW17, A2, B12, BW21 and AW30/31 but none of these are convincing, nor have they been established as very useful for predicting which relatives will likewise be affected (Pilepich et al, 1978). One apparently unique family has been described in which ten individuals over 3 generations had either uni- or bilateral hypernephroma (Cohen et al, 1979). Also segregating in this family was a balanced translocation between chromosomes 3 and 8. Five hypernephroma patients carried the translocation and 3 others must have had it according to pedigree analysis. Other sporadic and familial cases of hypernephroma were also studied by the same authors but the chromosomes in all instances were normal. Save for these few families in which the condition behaves like a Mendelian dominant, the heritability of hypernephroma should be considered low.

Familial examples of cancer of the renal pelvis, ureter and bladder are even more scarce and most workers feel these tumours are more directly related to environmental exposure to aromatic hydrocarbons. Only one family with ureteral cancer has been described, a mother and son being affected (Burkland & Juzek, 1966). Genetic factors may play some role in the aetiology of bladder cancer in some families, although the data in these families is perhaps more suggestive of the cancer family syndrome in which the genitourinary malignancy could be considered just one component (Lynch et al, 1979). These lesions are usually transitional cell carcinomas. The recent study of 101 unrelated patients with this tumour suggested a statistically significant association with blood group A and HLA types B5 and CW4 (Herring et al, 1975). Bladder cancer seems to be unusually frequent in elderly relatives of patients with familial retinoblastoma, but the tumours tend to be sarcomatous. In view of scarcity of familial reports, there would seem to be very little risk for lower urinary tract cancer in first degree relatives of an affected individual, unless the family history is striking or a common environmental carcinogen can be identified.

CANCER OF THE RESPIRATORY TRACT

There is little doubt that cigarette smoking is of prime aetiologic importance in bronchogenic carcinoma. Small cell or squamous cell lung tumours are virtually non-existent in non-smokers, save for those exposed to whole body irradiation, to chlormethyl ethyl ether or to uranium ore (Greco & Oldham, 1979). Tokuhata and Lillienfeld (1963) showed more lung cancer in families of lung cancer probands even when there was no smoking history. There is evidence that smoking may act synergistically with other factors which may have at least partial genetic control, such as a tendency to develop chronic obstructive pulmonary disease (Cohen et al, 1977). Alpha-1-antitrypsin phenotypes MZ or ZZ account for some, but not all, differences in tendency toward COPD (Kueppers et al, 1979). The value of aryl hydrocarbon hydroxylase inducibility as a potential marker for lung cancer susceptibility remains in question. In view of the fact that lung cancer is so common in the Western World, the lack of familial aggregation on purely environmental grounds is surprising and perhaps underreported (Mulvihill, 1976). Carcinoma of the larynx should probably be considered together with bronchogenic carcinoma, both on anatomic and epidemiological grounds, since it essentially never appears in non-smokers.

Pulmonary fibrosis, whether idiopathic, caused by chronic infection, or associated with scleroderma seems to predispose to adenocarcinoma of the lung. This tumour may be a facet of the cancer family syndrome, particularly that variety with the breast cancer-sarcoma complex. Bronchial carcinoid is an irregular feature of MEN I, and mucosal neuromas of the bronchi and larnyx may complicate MlEN III.

Nasopharyngeal carcinoma is a peculiar small cell tumour of ill-defined origin that occurs predominantly in Chinese and Alaskan natives. Because of this ethnic predilection, genetic factors must be of some aetiologic importance and must account for some of the recognized familial aggregation (Lanier et al, 1979). That this is not the whole story is supported by the finding that affected individuals have high antibody titres to EB virus, the same virus incriminated in tumour formation in non-genetic Burkitt lymphoma and in X–linked selective immunodeficiency syndrome. These findings suggest that not only tumour induction but tumour type and even site may depend in part on an ethnically distinct immune deficiency state, perhaps polygenic in type (Ho, 1976).

TUMOURS OF THE CENTRAL NERVOUS SYSTEM

The world wide incidence of CNS tumours is about 1/10 000 about 90% of which occur in the brain. The mortality is age-dependent with children doing less well, brain tumours being second only to leukaemia as a cause of death in children under age 15. The implication is that adult lesions are less virulent, more effectively treated or that the patients die of other causes. Most neurologists feel that heredity is not of major importance in the pathogenesis of brain tumours. However, relatives of glioma patients have been estimated to have a 4–10 fold increased risk of the same tumour (von Motz et al, 1977), and for children, the frequency of sib pairs with brain tumours is nine times greater than expected by chance (Miller, 1968). It is not certain how many patients with the hamartoma syndromes such as neurofibromatosis may be included in this sib pair series, since it is possible that relatively pure central forms of these simply inherited conditions exist. That the genetic predisposition is not limited to the CNS is attested by the occurrence in sibs of tumours such as adrenocortical carcinoma, osteogenic sarcoma and leukaemia at a rate much higher than expected (Draper et al, 1977; Meadows et al, 1977). In adults, extraneural primaries are most common in meningioma patients, one series of 76 such individuals harbouring 20 additional malignancies, 12 of which were in the gastrointestinal tract or the lung (Bellur et al, 1979). Another series associated meningiomas with breast carcinoma (Schoenberg, 1975). Some of the patients may be members of cancer families, but pertinent detailed family history is not sufficient to draw conclusions in this regard. Save for a few select families with the cancer family syndrome or with recognized conditions in which CNS tumours occur with unusual frequency, the heritability of brain tumours is likely to be low. Single gene inheritance may be operating in some instances where familial aggregation is particularly striking, but even here multifactorial causation cannot be excluded (Delleman et al, 1978).

Two autosomal recessive conditions in which brain tumours have been reported include the Werner syndrome and ataxia-telangiectasia. Heterozygotes for the latter disorder may also be at increased risk for brain tumours (Swift, 1976). Acoustic neuromas, frequently bilateral, have been reported as an autosomal dominant trait (Young et al, 1970). Perhaps this is an example of a central variant of neurofibromatosis.

Cytogenetic studies of brain tumours have not been rewarding except for meningiomas where about 2/3 of the tumours proper have either a missing 22 chromosome or a 22q− without evidence of translocation (Zarnl and Zang, 1980). As far as is known, familial meningiomas are no more likely to have this cytogenetic alteration than are sporadic tumours.

SKIN

Cancer of the integument is common among light-skinned races. The usual cell types are basal or squamous cell with melanomas being less frequent. Heritable non-syndromic varieties of basal and squamous cell tumours probably exist, but the lesions are relatively common, are for the most part age-dependent and may be aetiologically related to a host of environmental carcinogens. No systematic genetic survey has been undertaken.

Melanoma has been more extensively studied from a genetic point of view. It has been estimated that from 3–11% of all melanomas are heritable as revealed in a review of more than 90 families reported in the literature through 1974 (Gleicher et al, 1979). Despite this the genetics remain unclear, especially since affected children are about twice as likely to have an affected mother than father implicating possible cytoplastic or even intra-uterine effects. A rather interesting lesion, an inherited nevus called the B-K mole syndrome, seems to be inordinately susceptible to malignant transformation, and could account for some, but certainly not all instances of familial melanoma (Clark et al, 1978).

There are a number of genetic disorders in which skin cancer can occur and some of these are listed in Table 98.7.

Table 98.7 Genetic syndromes with basal, squamous cell carcinoma or melanoma

Basal cell nevus syndrome
Dyskeratosis congenita
Hidrotic ectodermal dysplasia
Multiple cylindromas of Brooke
Multiple keratoacanthoma
Flegel disease
Porokeratosis of Mibelli
Albinism
Epidermodysplasia verruciformis
Epidermolysis bullosa dystrophica
Fanconi panmyelopathy
Rothmund-Thompson syndrome
Xeroderma pigmentosum
Neurocutaneous melanosis
B-K mole syndrome
Familial melanoma
Cancer family syndrome

LEUKAEMIA AND LYMPHOMA

Leukaemia is usually considered to be either lymphocytic or non-lymphocytic in type, and either variety may be acute or chronic. Leukaemia may occur at any age, and this factor along with the lack of a universal and precise nosology and the absence of any detailed prospective family studies have hampered genetic investigation. The proportion of cases with a heritable component have been variously estimated from 0–25%. Monozygotic twin concordance is about 25% but this fact must be accepted with reservation, since concordance beyond age 5 is rare and the twins tend to be affected within weeks to months of each other suggesting the possibility of cross-transfusion of a single malignant clone through the common placental circulation. Identical cytogenetic alterations have been found in the leukaemic cell lines in twin pairs studied in detail, and this lends support to the common circulation hypothesis (Chaganti et al, 1979). Risks to sibs in childhood leukaemia are two-four times higher than the population incidence, but the absolute risk under these circumstances is low (Gunz et al, 1975). The risk to adult relatives of these children is unknown. It is possible that the risk will vary also depending on the type of leukaemia.

Acute leukaemia

Acute leukaemia tends to be more a disease of childhood with the lymphocytic form (ALL) predominant in the first five years, and nonlymphocytic leukaemia (ANLL) becoming evident later. In some instances the cell type is so primitive that accurate classification is impossible. A number of impressive pedigrees, some multigenerational, have been published (Gunz et al, 1978; Davidson et al, 1978; Luddy et al, 1978). Consanguinity is generally not impressive, save for one study in Japan (Kurita et al, 1974) and another in a religious and cultural isolate (Feldman et al, 1976). In one instance, X–linked inheritance was suggested, although male-limited autosomal dominant inheritance could not be excluded (Li et al, 1979). Some families have had markers suggested as being predictors of an ultimate leukaemia state. While these putative markers may be useful in an individual family, they are likely to be of little reliability in a population survey. HLA identity has been reported in one sib pair with ALL whose parents both had rheumatoid arthritis (Blattner et al, 1973). Restricted genetic heterogeneity at the HLA loci has been reported in patients with ALL, suggesting that there may be subpopulations at greater than average risk (McSween et al, 1980). Studies of ALL in G6PD heterozygotes has suggested that the disease is both clonal in origin and that it may be heterogeneous in terms of whether it is expressed in stem cells or becomes evident in a more differentiated cell line (Fialkow et al, 1979).

A reasonable interpretation of the available data suggests that perhaps 5% of all cases of acute leukaemia result from an autosomal dominant predisposition, although polygenic inheritance cannot be excluded with certainty. If there is no one else affected in the family the risk to any first degree relative is small. An important caveat is to be certain that the proband does not suffer from a simply inherited genetic disease in which acute leukaemia has been reported (Table 98.8).

Cytogenetic alterations are found in about half the malignant cell lines in acute leukaemia, as reviewed by Rowley (1980) and Sandberg (1980). Although there is considerable variability, the changes are not random. Among the more common abnormalities in ALL are tri-

Table 98.8 Syndromes in which acute leukaemia has been reported

Neurofibromatosis
Ataxia-telangiectasia
Glutathione reductase deficiency
Incontinentia pigmenti
Immune deficiency diseases
Rubenstein-Taybi syndrome
Kostman syndrome
Fanconi anemia
Bloom syndrome
WT syndrome
Shwachman syndrome
Klinefelter syndrome
Poland anomaly
Trisomy 21
Trisomy D
Trisomy 8
Cancer family syndrome
Kaposi sarcoma

somy 8, monosomy 7, and 8–21 translocation, frequently with concomitant loss of a X or Y, the latter change appearing in perhaps 10% of all patients. A 15;17 translocation may herald acute promyelocytic leukaemia. Deletion of the long arm of chromosome 20 (20q−) has been found in a number of histologically unclassifiable myeloproliferative disorders and in polycythemia vera, all of which may terminate in acute leukaemia of one form or another. 5q− and 21q− together or independently have been found in patients with refractory macrocytic anaemia and thrombocytosis, a condition that may well be a preleukaemic state. Generally, the more complex the cytogenetic alteration in acute nonlymphocytic leukaemia the poorer the prognosis, whether in children or adults. In children the cytogenetic changes are less consistent, but the basic patterns tend to be similar.

Less data is available in regard to cytogenetic alterations in ALL, perhaps because the cells do not proliferate well in vitro and are difficult to band. A partial 6q− has been reported most consistently. As with lymphomas, 14q+ is relatively common, the extra chromatin generally being derived via translocation from chromosomes 8 or 11. Deletions of chromosomes also have been noted. Curiously, the Phildelphia (Ph[1]) chromosome, a 22q− configuration most often due to translocation with chromosome 9, has been seen in ALL, although this alteration was previously considered specific for chronic myelogenous leukaemia (CML). Cheson et al (1980) reported a mother and son who developed leukaemia in close temporal proximity. The boy had ALL, the mother CML; both had an associated Ph[1] chromosome. Presumably, the cell lines bearing the abnormal chromosome configuration in any form of acute leukaemia have a selective advantage.

Chronic leukaemia

There is no firm evidence for a genetic aetiology of CML,

only a small number of families having been reported in which more than one member was affected. More than 80% of patients with CML have the Ph^1 chromosome, the cells harbouring this anomaly all having been derived from a single clone (Fialkow, 1977). In families where more than one individual had CML, the Ph^1 chromosome is generally present (Svarch and de la Torre, 1977). CML in children is uncommon and about half the cases are Ph^1 negative. The absence of this chromosome generally portends a poorer prognosis. When Ph^1 positive CML enters an acute phase, a variety of cytogenetic aberrations supervene as with ANLL, a double Ph^1 chromosome configuration being quite common.

The data in regard to genetic factors in chronic lymphocytic leukaemia (CLL) are more substantial. It tends to be more common in elderly individuals and long term survival is not unusual. About 90% of the time the involved lymphocyte is B cell in type, only a few percent being T cells and the remainder non-T, non-B or null cells (Nowell et al, 1980). Familial occurrence of CLL occurs more frequently than expected by chance. Impressive sibship aggregation and apparent two-generation transmission have been seen often enough to implicate genetic factors in aetiology. In one of the earliest reports, 56-year-old identical twin brothers were affected within three months of one another (Dameshek et al, 1929). A follow-up report 28 years later documents the disease in a 53-year-old son of one of the twins (Gunz & Dameshek, 1953).

Exactly what might be inherited is unknown. Immunological abnormalities have been detected in both affected and unaffected family members but they are not always consistent (Cohen et al, 1979). Some family members with CLL may have virtually identical clinical courses with the same morphologic and functional characteristics and the same surface markers (Blattner et al, 1976; Branda et al, 1978) whereas in other families, not only is the immune defect discordant, but the disease may assume a different form; e.g., lymphosarcoma, reticulum cell sarcoma, hairy cell leukaemia or acute leukaemia (Cohen et al, 1979). Some relatives have even had CML. Non-leukaemic malignancies occur commonly in patients with CLL or lymphocytic lymphosarcoma showing an overall incidence of 34.4% (Hyman, 1969). Roughly 40% of these patients developed the other neoplasm before the CLL, the remainder being about equally divided between those whose onset of combined neoplasia was within 3 months and those whose non-leukaemic tumour developed later. In another retrospective series of 102 patients, it was concluded that the overall risk of subsequent malignancy was increased three fold (Mamison & Weinerman, 1975). It is interesting that the families of most patients with CLL contain relatives with non-leukaemic malignancy as well.

The basic genetic lesion would appear to reside in some defect of immune function, perhaps in immune surveillance, in suppressor cell function, or in some subtle alteration that allows for the persistence of an oncogenic antigen. Based on a review of the available pedigrees, it seems reasonable to postulate that 10–15% of patients with CLL have their disease on the basis of a heritable predisposition that behaves in a manner consistent with autosomal dominance. However, in view of the variable clinical presentation in some families, it is also possible that the disease is heterogeneous, comprising both dominant and polygenic forms.

Detailed chromosome data in CLL are not available. The 14q+ marker is relatively common as with lymphomas. Trisomy of number 2 and 18 have also been seen frequently. More detailed evaluation of the chromosome spectrum of T-cell disorders would be of interest. This disease category seems to be clinically heterogenous, ranging from pure CLL to hairy cell leukaemia, Sezary syndrome and so forth.

Lymphoma

Most authorities classify lymphoma as being Hodgkin (HD) or non-Hodgkin in type. The latter not uncommonly occur in families of patients with CLL, and unfortunately, both types of lymphoma may develop in a given family such that the genetic issue is confused (Buehler et al, 1975). Moreover, examination of such families frequently reveals not only the expected immunologic abnormalities in affected relatives, but also nonlymphomatous tumours in some (Escobar and Bixler, 1976; Greco and Mliller, 1978). Whether this simply reflects a more general loss of immune surveillance capability or denotes a type of cancer family syndrome is not clear.

Family studies of HD are fairly extensive (Grufferman et al 1977). The usual aggregation is that of sibs, but parent-child and affected cousins have been reported. In fact, HD has been described in colleagues at work, in teacher-student pairs, in drug addicts, in neighbours, in relatives working in the same environment and rarely even in spouses (Nagel et al, 1978). In one extensive study of sib pairs, Grufferman et al (1977) found 46 sib pairs under age 45 from personal experience and literature review, 30 of whom were concordant for sex. They concluded that both genetic and common environmental factors were important in aetiology. The risk of a relative developing HD has been estimated to be at least three fold higher than the basic age-adjusted population risk (Fraumeni, 1974). HLA studies by and large have not shown an impressive association between HD and any particular allele or haplotype. In 13 families prone to HD, the probands showed an excess of BW35 (Greene et al, 1979). In general, affected sibs tend to be HLA concordant, a finding that suggests to some authors that susceptibility to HD is recessive (Hors et al, 1980). The discovery of multiple affected individuals in consanguineous families would tend to support this hypothesis. However, the numbers studied are small and no firm conclusion can be drawn at present. An occupational exposure to wood and wood products has been suggested to be of aetiologic importance in some families presumably genetically predisposed as evidenced by multiple affected members (Greene et al, 1978).

Lymphomas commonly complicate the heritable immunodeficiency diseases. A peculiar form of lymphoma may be seen in the autosomal recessive Chediak-Higashi syndrome. Abnormalities of chromosome 14 are among the most common cytogenetic alterations seen in lymphomas, including Burkitt lymphoma and lymphomas complicating ataxia-telangiectasia. The marker chromosome is 14q+ with the extra material on the long arm being derived chiefly from chromosomes 8, 11, or from a tendem duplication of 14q. Other cytogenetic alterations have been described but not in sufficient quantity to be diagnostically or prognostically useful.

Multiple myeloma

Multiple myeloma and the related condition, Waldenstrom macroglobulinaemia, are diseases of old age. Familial instances of these conditions are relatively few and two generation occurrence, while uncommon, has been reported (Maldonado & Kyle, 1974). Interestingly, in some unaffected family members benign monoclonal gammopathy has been discovered. A series of twenty asymptomatic monoclonal gammopathy patients has been recently described in which individuals were followed for up to 14 years (Fine et al, 1979). Four cases evolved into malignant disease, two into macroglobulinaemia and two into myeloma, indicating that the appellation 'benign' is not always appropriate. As with many other lymphoreticular malignancies, immunoglobulin abnormalities have also been recorded in unaffected family members. Undoubtedly, both elements; i.e., the presence of paraproteins or immune markers must relate to the basic pathogenetic mechanism, but it is not of all clear that these are primarily genetic. The heritability of myeloma appears to be low, with relatives having no more than a five fold risk of developing malignant lymphoreticular disease at some time of their life. Cytogenetic studies in myeloma have not yet proved rewarding.

Familial histocytosis

This condition has a number of alternative names including familial reticuloendotheliosis, familial Letterer-Siwe disease and erythrophagocytic lymphohistocytosis, the latter being particularly descriptive of the typical heavy, largely perivascular infiltrate found at autopsy. The disease in adults, often termed histiocytic medullary reticulosis, is not known to have a genetic component whereas the childhood form is not only heritable but heterogeneous, both autosomal and X–linked recessive forms having been described. In the autosomal recessive form affected infants fail to thrive, develop anaemia and

neutropenia, occasionally with paradoxic eosinophilia, diarrhoea, hepatosplenomegaly, occasional rash and hyperlipidaemia, and histocytic infiltration of virtually every organ including the central nervous system (Frisell et al, 1977). The condition is usually rapidly progressive. There is some question whether the disorder is truely a malignancy or is a basic immunodeficiency disease with secondary histocytic proliferation (Ladish et al, 1978). Defects in both T and B-cell function have been identified, but it is not clear whether these are primary or secondary. Some affected children have responded, albeit transiently, to immunosuppressive therapy, a seemingly unlikely phenomenon if the disorder is actually a primary immunodeficiency state (Lilleyman, 1980).

The X–linked form is more clearly an immunodeficiency disease and apparently a selective one in that affected males respond inappropriately to EB virus (Hamilton et al, 1980). For reasons as yet unknown, the disease has a number of phenotypes ranging from fatal infectious mononucleosis, through non-Hodgkin and/or Burkitt lymphoma or a- or dysgammaglobulinaemia. Earlier reports of familial intestinal lymphoma and sibs with fatal infectious mononucleosis probably represented this entity. However, not all forms of increased susceptibility to EB virus need be necessarily X–linked. Gut lymphoma has been described in a male and female sib, one aged 51 and the other 54, both of whom had high EB virus titres (Freedlander et al, 1978). Jones et al (1976) have noted a family in which sibs and first cousins were variously affected with nasopharyngeal carcinoma (one with EB virus titre >640), Burkitt lymphoma and myeloma. Polyclonal B-cell lymphoma occurred during the course of EB virus infection in a female child whose parents were first cousins (Robinson et al, 1980). Thus it is conceivable that a number of different genetic types of lymphohistocytosis may exist, the primary lesion most likely being related to altered immunity to EB virus in some cases and to unknown agents in other instances.

IMMUNE DEFICIENCY STATES

It has long been known that patients who have deficient immunity, either on the basis of a genetic defect or because of immunosuppressive and/or cytotoxic therapy have an increased incidence of malignancy. In both types of patients, lymphoma and leukaemia are among the predominant lesions, but tumours in a variety of other sites have been described as well (Penn, 1978). A survey of 267 individuals with genetically determined immunodeficiency diseases (GDID) and malignancy revealed the following: (1) the tumour type in a child with GDID is generally a non-Hodgkin's lymphoma; in an adult, lymphoma and carcinoma occur in about equal proportions;

(2) the lymphomas are mostly lymphoreticular or histocytic with the former being either B- or T-cell more commonly than null type; (3) gastric carcinomas are much more common than expected especially in adolescence and early adult life; (4) in some instances, there are cell patterns that are unique, such as the excess of epithelial malignancies in girls with ataxia-telangiectasia and the association of myelogenous leukaemia in boys with the X–linked Wiscott-Aldrich syndrome (Spector et al, 1978). The incidence of malignancy varies with the GDID being highest with Wiscott-Aldrich syndrome (15.4%), ataxia-telangiectasia (11.7%), selective IgM deficiency (10%) and common variable immunodeficiency, all ages combined (4.3%). A much larger series of patients with Wiscott-Aldrich syndrome recently confirmed the high incidence of cancer in those males, with 36 of 301 individuals (12%) being affected, 30% of whom had either lymphoreticular malignancies or leukaemia (Perry et al, 1980). In view of the suggested increased incidence of malignancies in heterozygotes with ataxia-telangiectasia, it would be of interest to examine the first degree female relatives of boys with Wiscott-Aldrich syndrome to see if any consistent pattern emerged.

REFERENCES

Abramson D H, Ronner H J, Ellsworth R M 1979 Second tumors in nonirradiated bilateral retinoblastoma. American Journal of Opthalmology 87: 624–627

Anderson D E 1974 Genetic study of breast cancer: identification of a high risk group. Cancer 34: 1090–1097

Anderson D E 1977 Breast cancer in females. Cancer 40 (4 Suppl): 1855–60

Anderson D E 1978a Familial cancer and cancer families. Seminars Oncology 5: 11–16

Anderson D E 1980a Risk in families of patients with colon cancer. In: Winawer S, Schottenfeld D, Sherlock P (eds) Colorectal cancer: prevention, epidemiology and screening, Raven Press, New York. p 109–115

Anderson D E 1980b An inherited form of large bowel cancer. Cancer 45: 1103–1107

Andriola M 1976 Nevus unius lateralis and brain tumors. American Journal of Diseases of Children 130: 1259–1261

Annegers J F, Strom H, Decker D G, Dockerty M B, O'Fallon W M 1979 Ovarian cancer. Cancer 43: 723–729

Arce B, Licea M, Hung S, Pardron R 1978 Familial Cushing's syndrome. Acta Endocrinology 87: 139–147

Arlet C F, Lehman A R 1978 Human disorders showing increased sensitivity to the induction of genetic damage. Annual Review of Genetics 12: 95–115

Ashcraft K, Holder T M, Harris D J 1975 Familial presacral teratomas. Birth Defects 11: 143–146

Ashley D J 1969 Oesophageal cancer in Wales. Journal of Medical Genetics 6: 70–75

Auerbach A D, Wolman S R 1978 Carcinogen-induced chromosome breakage in Fanconi's anaemia heterozygous cells. Nature 271: 69–70

Bader J L, Miller R W, Meadows A T, Zimmerman L E, Champion L A A, Voûte P A 1980 Trilateral retinoblastoma. Lancet 2: 582–583

Baird P A, Worth A J 1976 Congenital generalized fibromatosis: an autosomal recessive condition. Clinical Genetics 9: 488–494

Baylin S B, Hsu S H, Gann D S, Smallridge R C, Wells S A Jr 1978 Inherited medullary thyroid carcinoma: a final monoclonal mutation in one of multiple clones of susceptible cells. Science 199: 429–431

Bellur S N, Chandra V, McDonald L W 1979 Association of meningiomas with extra neural primary malignancy. Neurology 29: 1165–1168

Bess M A, Adson M A, Elveback L R, Moertel C G 1980 Rectal cancer following colectomy for polyposis. Archives of Surgery 115: 460–467

Binder M K, Zablen M A, Fleischer D E, Sue D Y, Dwyer R M, Hanelin L 1978 Colon polyps, sebaceous cysts, gastric polyps, and malignant brain tumor in a family. American Journal of Digestive Diseases 23: 460–466 23: 460–466

Blattner W A, Strober W, Muchmore A V, Blaese R M, Broder S, Fraumeni J F Jr 1976 Familial chronic lymphocytic leukemia. Annals of Internal Medicine 84: 554–557 84: 554–557

Blattner W A, Naiman J L, Mann D L, Wimer R S, Dean J S, Fraumeni J F Jr 1978 Immunogenetic determinants of familial acute lymphocytic leukemia. Annals of Internal lledicine 89: 173–176

Blattner W A, Dean J H, Fraumeni J F Jr 1979 Familial lymphoproliferative malignancy: clinical and laboratory follow-up. Annals of Internal Medicine 90: 943–944

Blattner W A, McGuire D B, Mulvihill J J, Lampkin B C, Hanamian J, Fraumeni J F Jr 1979 Genealogy of cancer in a family. Journal of the American Medical Association 241: 259–261

Boden G, Owen O E 1977 Familial glucagonemia – an autosomal dominant disorder. New England Journal of Medicine 296: 534–538

Bolande R P 1977 Childhood tumors and their relationship to birth defects, in Genetics of human cancer. Mulvihill J J, Miller R W, Fraumeni J F Jr (eds) Raven Press, New York. pp 43–75

Bottomly R H, Trainer A L, Condet P T 1971 Chromosome studies in a 'cancer family'. Cancer 28: 519–528

Bove K E, McAdams A J 1976 The nephroblastomatosis complex and its relationship to Wilms tumor: a clinicopathologic study. Perspect Pediatr Pathol 3: 185–223

Branda R F, Ackerman S K, Handwerger B S, Howe R B, Douglas S D 1978 Lymphocyte studies in familial chroma lymphatic leukemia. American Journal of Medicine 64: 508–514

Brodeur G M, Green A A, Hayes F A 1980a Cytogenetic studies of primary human neuroblastomas. In: Evans A E (ed) Advances in Neuroblastoma Research, Raven Press, New York. p 73–80

Brodeur G lM, Caces J, Williams D L, Look A T, Pratt C B 1980b Osteosarcoma, fibrous dysplasia, and a chromosome abnormality in a 3-year-old child. Cancer 46: 1197–1201

Brown E H 1979 Identical twins with twisted benign cystic teratoma of the ovary. American Journal of Obstetrics and Gynecology 134: 879–880

Buehler S K, Firme F, Fodor G, Fraser G R, Marshall W H,

Vaze P 1975 Common variable immunodeficiency, Hodgkin's disease and other malignancies in a New Foundland family. Lancet 1: 195–197

Burkland C E, Juzek R H 1966 Familial occurrence of carcinoma of the uterus. Journal of Urology 96: 697–701

Cantu J M, Rivera H, Ocampo-Campos R, Bedolla N, Cortes-Gallegos V, Gonzalez Mendosa A, Diaz M, Hernandez A 1980 Peutz-Jeghers syndrome with feminizing Sertoli cell tumor. Cancer 46: 223–228

Carney A, Sizemore G W, Tyce G M 1975 Bilateral adrenal medullary hyperplasia in multiple endocrine neoplasia, type 2. Mayo Clinical Proceedings 50: 3–10

Carney J A, Hayles A B 1978 Alimentary tract manifestations of multiple endocrine neoplasia, type 2B. Mayo Clinical Proceedings 52: 543–548

Carney J A, Go V L W, Gordon H, Northcutt R C, Pearse A G E, Sheps S G 1980 Familial pheochromocytoma and islet cell tumor of the pancreas. American Journal of Medicine 68: 515–521

Chan H, Pratt C B 1977 A new familial cancer syndrome? Journal of the National Cancer Institute 58: 205–207

Chaganti R S K, Miller D R, Meyers P A, German J 1979 Cytogenetic evidence of the intrauterine origin of acute leukemia in monozygotic twins. New England Journal of Medicine 300: 1032–1034

Chaussain J L, Lemerle J, Roger M, Canlorbe P, Job J C 1980 Klinefelter syndrome, tumor, and sexual prococity. Journal of Pediatrics 97: 607–609

Chen P C, Lavin M F, Kidson C 1978 Identification of ataxia telangiectasia heterozygote, a cancer prone population. Nature 274: 484–486

Cheson B D, Vananetti S M, Bieskjaer L, Fineman R M 1980 Philadelphia chromosome (Ph^1)-associated leukemias: a family study. Cancer W H Jr, Riemer R R, Greene M, Ainsworth A M, Mastroangelo M J 1978 Origin of familial malignant melanomas from heritable melanocytic lesions. Archives of Dermatology 114: 732–738

Cohen B H, Diamond E L, Graves C G, Kreiss P, Levy D A, Menkes H A, Permutt S, Quaskey S, Tockman M S 1977 A common familial component in lung cancer and chronic obstructive pulmonary disease. Lancet 2: 523–526

Cohen A J, Li F P, Berg S, Marchetto tJ, Tsai S, Jacobs S C, Brown R S 1979 Heredity renal-cell carcinoma associated with a chromosomal translocation. New England Journal of Medicine 301: 592–595

Cohen H J, Shimm D, Paris S A, Buckley C E III, Kremer W B 1979 Hairy cell leukemia-associated familial lymphoproliferate disorder: immunologic abnormalities in unaffected family members. Annals of Internal Medicine 90: 174–179

Colyer R A 1979 Osteogenic sarcoma in siblings. Johns Hopkins Medical Journal 145: 13–135

Conley C L, Misiti J, Laster A J 1980 Genetic factors predisposing to chronic lymphocytic leukemia and to autoimmune disease. Medicine 59: 323–334

Dameshek W, Savitz H A, Arbor B 1929 Chronic lymphatic leukemia in twin brothers age 56. JAMA 92: 1343–1349

Danes B S 1978 Increased in vitro tetraploidy: tissue specific in the heritable colorectal cancer syndromes with polyposis coli. Cancer 41: 2330–2334

Davidson R J L, Walker W, Watt J L, Page B M 1978 Familial erythroleukemia: a cytogenetic and haematologic study. Scandanavian Journal of Haematology 20: 351–359

Delleman J W, DeJong J G Y, Bleeker G M 1978 Meningiomas in five members of a family over two generations, in one member simultaneously with acoustic neurinomas. Neurology 28: 567–570

Devor E J, Buechley R W 1978 Gallbladder cancer in Hispanic New Mexicans. Cancer Genetics and Cytogenetics 1: 139–145

Draper G J, Heaf M M, Wilson L M K 1977 Occurrence of childhood cancer among sibs and estimation of familial risks. Journal of Medical Genetics 14: 81–95

Dumont-Herskowitz R A, Safari H S, Senior B 1978 Ovarian fibromata in four successive generations. Journal of Pediatrics 93: 621–624

Ehrich J H H, Ostertag H, Flatz S, Kamran D 1978 Bilateral Wilms' tumor in Klippel-Trenaunay syndrome. Archives of Disease in Childhood 54: 405 only

Epstein L I, Bixler D, Bennett J E 1970 An incident of familial cancer including 3 cases of osteogenic sarcoma. Cancer 25: 889–891

Escobar V, Bixler D 1976 Familial reticulum cell sarcoma. Birth Defects 12: 151–158

Evans A E, Chatten J, D'Angio G J, Gerson J M, Robinson J, Schnaufer L 1980 A review of 17 IV-S neuroblastoma patients at the children's hosptial of Philadelphia. Cancer 45: 833–839

Feingold M, Gheraodi G, Simons C 1971 Familial neuroblastoma and trisomy 13. American Journal of Diseases of Children 121: 451–452

Feldman J G, Lee S L, Seligman B 1976 Occurrence of acute leukemia in females in a genetically isolated population. Cancer 38: 2548–2550

Fialkow P J 1977 Clonal original stem cell evolution of human tumors, In: Mulvihill J J, Miller R W, Fraumeni J F Jr (eds) Genetics of human cancer, Raven Press, New York. pp 439–453

Fialkow P J, Singer J W, Adamson J W, Berkow R L, Friedman J M, Jacobson R J, Moohr J W 1979 Acute nonlymphocytic leukemia. New England Journal of Medicine 301: 1–5

Fine J M, Laubin P, Muller J Y 1979 The evolution of asymptomatic monoclonal gammapathies. Acta Medica Scandinavica 205: 339–341

Foster J H, Donohue T A, Berman M M 1978 Familial liver-cell adenomas and diabetes mellitus. New England Journal of Medicine 299: 239–241

Francke U, Holmes L B, Atkins L, Riccardi V M 1979 Aniridia-Wilms' tumor association: evidence for specific deletion of 11p13. Cytogenetics and Cell Genetics 24: 185–192

Fraumeni J F Jr, Glass A G 1968 Wilms' tumor and congenital aniridia. JAMA 206: 825–828

Fraumeni, J F Jr, Rosen P J, Hull E W, Barton R F, Shapiro S R, O'Connor J F 1969 Hepatoblastoma in infant sisters. Cancer 24: 1086–1090

Fraumeni J F Jr 1974 Family studies in Hodgkin's disease. Cancer Research 34: 1164–1165

Freedlander E, Kissen L H, McVee J G 1978 Gut lymphoma presenting simultaneously in two siblings. British Medical Journal 1: 80–81

Frisell E, Bjorksten B, Holmgren G, Angstrom T 1977 Familial occurrence of histiocytosis. Clinical Genetics 11: 163–170

Gallo G E 1978 Pathology of 'uninvolved' renal parenchyma in nephroblastima. Pediatric Research 12: 1030 only

Gleiser C F, Schindler A M 1969 Long survival in a male with 18 trisomy syndrome and Wilms' tumor. Pediatrics 44: 111–113

Gentry W C Jr, Reed W B, Siegel J M 1975 Cowden disease. Birth Defects 11: 137–141

Gilbert G, Cleveland W W 1970 Cushing's syndrome in infancy. Pediatrics 46: 217–222

Gleicher N, Cohen C J Deppe G, Ginsberg S B 1979 Familial malignant melanoma of the female genitalia: a case report and review. Obstetrics and Gynecological Surveys 34: 1–15

Gloor E 1978 Un cas de syndrome de Peutz-Jeghers associe a un carcinome mammaire bilateral, a un adenocarcinome du col uterin et des tumeurs des cordons sexuels a tubules anneles bilaterales dans les ovaires. Schweiz Med Wochenschr 108: 717–721

Goodman Z D, Yardley J H, Milligan F D 1979 Pathogenesis of colonic polyps in multiple juvenile polyposis. Cancer 43: 1906–1913

Gorlin R J, Sedano H O 1972 The multiple nevoid basal cell carcinoma syndrome. Birth Defects 7: 140–48

Gorlin R J 1976 Some soft tissue heritable tumors. Birth Defects 12: 7–14

Greco F A, Oldham R K 1979 Current concepts in cancer: small cell lung cancer. New England Journal of Medicine 301: 355–358

Greene M H, Brinton L A, Fraumeni J F Jr, D'Amico R 1978 Familial sporadic Hodgkin's disease associated with occupational wood exposure. Lancet 2: 626–627

Greene M H, Miller R W 1978 Familial non-Hodgkin lymphoma: histologic diversity and relation to other cancers. American Journal of Medical Genetics 1: 437–43

Greene M H, McKeen E A, Li F P, Blattner W A, Fraumeni J F Jr 1979 HLA antigens in familial Hodgkin's disease. International Journal of Cancer 23: 777–780

Grufferman S, Cole P, Smith P G, Lukes R J 1977 Hodgkin's disease in siblings. New England Journal of Meddicine 296: 248–250

Gunz F, Dameshek W 1957 Chronic lymphocyte leukemia in a family, including twin brothers and a son. Journal of the American Medical Association 164: 1323–1324

Gunz F W, Gunz J P, Veale A M O, Chapman C J, Houston I B 1975 Familial leukemia: a study of 909 families. Scandinavian Journal of Haematology 15: 117–131

Gunz F W, Gunz J P, Vincent P C, Bergin M, Johnson F L, Bashir H, Kirk R L 1978 Thirteen cases of leukemia in a family. Journal of the National Cancer Institute 60: 1243–1250

Gustavson H, Gamstorp I, Meruling S 1975 Bilateral teratoma of the testes in two brothers with 47, XXY Klinefelter's syndrome. Clinical Genetics 8: 5–10

Hagstrom R M, Baker T D 1968 Primary hepatocellular carcinoma in three siblings. Cancer 22: 142–150

Hamilton J K, Paquin L A, Sullivan J L, Mauer H S, Cruzi F G, Provisor A J, Steuber C P, Hawkins E, Yawn D, Cornet J A, Clausen K, Finkelstein G Z, Landing B, Grunnet M, Purtillo D T 1980 X–linked lymphoproliferative syndrome registry report. Journal of Pediatrics 96: 669–673

Hapnes S A, Boman H, Skeie S O 1980 Familial angiolipomatosis. Clinical Genetics 17: 202–208

Hariez C, Deminatti M, Agache P, Mennecier M 1968 Une genodysplasie non encore individualisee: la genodermatose sclero-atrophiante et keratodermique des extremities frequemment degenerative. Semaine des hôpitaux de Paris 44: 481–488

Harper P S, Harper R M J, Howel-Evans A 1970 Carcinoma of the oesphagus with tylosis. Quarterly Journal of Medicine 39: 317–333

Harris R E, Lynch H T, Guirgis H 1978 Familial breast cancer: risk to the contralateral breast. Journal of the National Cancer Institute 60: 955–960

Herring D W, Cartwright R A, Williams D RD R 1979 Genetic associations of transitional cell carcinoma. British Journal of Medicine 51: 73–77

Hittner H M, Riccardi V M, Francke V 1979 Aniridia caused by a heritable chromosome 11 deletion. Ophthalmology 86: 1173–1183

Ho H C 1972 Nasopharyngeal carcinoma. Advances in Cancer Research 15: 57–92

Hors J, Steinberg G, Andrieu J M, Jacquillat C, Minev M, Messerschmitt J, Mlilinvaud G, Fumeron F, Dausset J, Bernard J 1980 HLA genotypes in familial Hodgkin's disease: excess of HLA identical sibs. European Journal of Cancer 16: 809–815

Horton W A 1976 Genetics of central nervous system tumors. Birth Defects 12: 91–97

Horton W A, Wong V, Eldridge R 1976 Von Hippel-Lindau disease. Archives of Internal Medicine 136: 769a–777

Howe J W, Manson N 1976 Familial retinoblastoma – a cautionary tale. Journal of Pediatric Ophthalmology 13: 278–282

Hsu S D, Zaharapoulos P, May J T, Costanzi J J 1979 Peutz-Jeghers syndrome with intestinal carcinoma. Cancer 44: 1527–1532

Hulka B S, Fowler W C, Kaufman D G, Grimson D G, Greenberg B G, Hogue C J, Berger G S, Pulliam C C 1980 Estrogen and endometrial cancer: cases and two control groups from North Carolina. American Journal of Obstetrics and Gynecology 137: 92–101

Hull M T, Warfel K A, Muller J, Higgins J T 1979 Familial islet cell tumors in von Hippel-Lindau's disease. Cancer 44: 1523– a1526

Hutchinson W B, Thomas D B, Hamlin W B, Roth G J, Peterson A V, Williams B 1980 Risk of breast cancer in women with benign breast disease. Journal of the National Cancer Institute 65: 13–20

Hyman G A 1969 Increased incidence of neoplasia in association into chronic lymphocytic leukaemia. Scandinavian Journal of Haematology 6: 99–104

Isurugi K, Imao S, Hirose K, Aoki H 1977 Seminoma in Klinefelter's syndrome with 47,XXY, 15+ karyotype. Cancer 39: 2041–2047

Itoh H, Ohsato K, Yao T, Iida M, Watanabe H 1979 Turcot's syndrome and its mode of inheritance. Gut 20: 414–419

Jackson L G, Anderson D E, Schimke R N 1979 Genetics and cancer, In: Jackson L G, Schimke R N (eds) Clinical Genetics, Wiley, New York. pp 85–120

Janson K L, Roberts J A, Varela M 1978 Multiple endocrine adenomatous: in support of the common origin theories. Journal of Urology 119: 161–165

Jensen R D, Norris H J, Fraumeni J F Jr 1974 Familial arrhenoblastoma and thyroid adenoma. Cancer 33: 218–223

Joneas J H, Rioux E, Robitaille R, Wastriaux J P 1976 Multiple cases of lymphoepithelioma and Burkitt's lymphoma in a Canadian family. Bibliotheca Haematologica 43: 224–276

Kahn L B 1977 Vagal body tumor (nonchromaffin paraganglioma, chemodectoma and carotid body-like tumor) with cervical node metastasis and familial association. Cancer 39: 2367–2377

Kaplan C G, Askin F B, Benirschke K 1979 Cytogenetics of extragonadal tumors. Teratology 19: 261–266

Khairi M R, Dexter R N, Burzynski N J, Johnson C C 1975 Mucosal neuroma, pheochromocytoma and medullary thyroid carcinoma: multiple endocrine neoplasia, type 3. Medicine 54: 89–112

King M, Go R C P, Elston R C, Lynch H T, Petrakis N L 1980 Allele increasing susceptibility to human breast cancer may be linked to the glutamatepyruvate transaminase locus. Science 208: 406–408

Knight L A, Gardner H A, Gallie B L 1980 Familial retinoblastoma: segregation of chromosone 13 in four families. American Journal of Human Genetics 32: 194–201

Knudson A G Jr, Strong L C 1972 Mutations and cancer: a model for Wilms' tumor of the kidney. Journal of the National Cancer Institute 48: 313–324

Knudson A G, Strong L C, Anderson D E 1973 Heredity and cancer in Man. Progress in Medical Genetics 9: 113–158

Knudson A G Jr, Meadow A T 1976 Developmental genetics of neuroblastoma. Journal o of the National Cancer Institute 57: 675–682

Knudson A G Jr, Meadows A T 1980 Regression of neuroblastoma IV-S: a genetic hypothesis. New England Journal of Medicine 302: 1254–1256

Kopelovich L 1980 Hereditary adenomatosis of the colon and rectum: recent studies on the nature of cancer promotion and cancer prognosis in vitro, In: Winawer S J, Schottenfeld D, Sherlock P (eds) Colorectal cancer: prevention, epidemiology and screening, Raven Press, New York. pp 97–108

Kueppers F, Miller R D, Gordon H, Hepper N G, Offord K 1977 Familial prevalence of chronic obstructive pulmonary disease in a matched pair study. American Journal of Medicine 63: 336–342

Kurita S, Kamei Y, Ota K 1974 Genetic studies on familial leukemia. Cancer 34: 1098–1101

Kussin S Z, Lipkin M, Winawer S J 1979 Inherited colon cancer: clinical implications. American Journal of Gastroenterology 72: 448–457

Ladish S, Poplack D G, Holiman B, Blaese R M 1978 Immunodeficiency in familial erythrophagocytic lymphohistiocytosis. Lancet 1: 581–583

Land C E 1980 Low-dose radiation – a cause of breast cancer? Cancer 46: 868–873

Lanier A P, Bender T R, Tschopp C F, Dohan p 1979 Nasopharyngeal carcinoma in an Alaskan Eskimo family: report of three cases. Journal of the National Cancer Institute 62: 1121–1124

Lehtola J 1978 Family study of gastric carcinoma with special reference to histologic types. Scandinavian Journal of Gastroenterology 13 (Suppl 5):t3–54

Levin S R, Hofeldt F D, Becker N, Wilson C B, Seymour R, Forsham P H 1974 Hypersomatotropism and acanthosis nigricans in two brothers. Archives of Internal Medicine 134: 365–367

Li F P, 1977 Second malignant tumors after cancer in childhood. Cancer 40: 1899–1902

Li F P, Marchetto D J, Vawter G F 1979 Acute leukemia and preleukemia in eight males in a family: an X–linked disorder? American Journal of Hematology 6: 61–69

Li F P, Corkery J, Canellos G, Neitlich H W 1981 Breast Cancer after Hodgkin's disease in two sisters. Cancer 47: 200–202

Lichtig C 1971 Multiple skin and gastrointestinal haemangiomata (blue rubbers-bleb nevus). Dermatologica 142: 356–362

Lilleyman J S 1980 The treatment of familial erythrophagocytic lymphohistiocytosis. Cancer 46: 468–470

Linquette M, Herlaut M, Laine E, Fossati P, DuPont-LeCompte J 1967 Adenome a prolactive chez une jeune fille dont la niere etait porteuse d'un adenoma hypophysaire avec amenorrhee-galactorrhee. Annales d'endocrinologie 28: 773–776

LiVolsi V A, Feind C R 1976 Parathyroid adenoma and nonmedullary thyroid carcinoma. Cancer 38: 1391–1393

Lovett H E 1976 Family studies in cancer of the colon and rectum. British Journal of Surgery 63: 13–18

Lowell S H, llMathog R H 1979 Head and neck manifestations of Maffucci's syndrome. Archives of Otolaryngology 105: 427–430

Luddy R E Champion L A A, Schwartz A D 1978 A fatal myeloproliferative syndrome in a family with thrombocytopenia and platelet dysfunction. Cancer 41: 1959–1963

Lynch H T, Larsen A L, Magnuson C W, Krush A J 1966 Prostate carcinoma and multiple primary malignancies. Cancer 19: 1891–1897

Lynch H T, Krush A J, Larsen A L 1967 Hereditary and endometrial carcinoma. Southern Medical Journal 60: 231–235

Lynch H T (ed) 1976 Cancer genetics. Springfield, III., Thomas

Lynch H T, Mulcahy G M, Lynch P, Guirgis H, Brodkey F, Lynch J, Maloney K, Rankin L 1976 Genetic factors in breast cancer: a survey. Pathol Ann 11: 77–101

Lynch H T, Harris R E, Lynch P M, Guirgis H A, Lynch J F, Bardawil, W A 1977 Role of heredity in multiple primary cancer. Cancer 40: 1849–1854

Lynch H T, Mulcahy G M, Harris R E, Guigis H A, Lynch J F 1978a Genetic and pathologic findings in a kindred with hereditary sarcoma, breast cancer, brain tumors, leukemia, lung, laryngeal and adrenal cortical carcinoma. Cancer 41: 2055–2064

Lynch H T, Harris R E, Guirgis H A, Maloney K, Carmody L L, Lynch J F 1978b Familial association of breast/ovarian carcinoma. Cancer 41: 1543–1549

Lynch H T, Bardawil W A, Harris R E, Lynch P M, Guirgis H A, Lynch J F 1978c Multiple primary cancers and prolonged survival. Diseases of the Colon and Rectum 21: 165–168

Lynch H T, Walzak M P, Fried R, Domina A H, Lynch J F 1979 Familial factors in bladder carcinoma. Journal of Orology 122: 458–461

Lyons A R, Logan H, Johnston G W 1977 Hypernephroma in two brothers. British Medical Journal 1: 816–817

MacMahon B, Cole P, Brown J B 1975 Factors that influence mammary carcinogenesis. New England Journal of Medicine 292: 974–975

MacSween J M, Fernandez L A, Eastwood S L, Pyesmany A F 1980 Restricted growth heterogeneity in families of patients with acute lymphocytic leukaemia. Tissue Antigens 16: 70–72

Maldonado J E, Kyle R A 1979 Familial myeloma. American Journal of Medicine 57: 875–884

Manusow D, Weinerman B H 1975 Subsequent neoplasia in chronic lymphocytic leukemia. Journal of the American Medical Association 232: 267–-269

Marger D, Urdaneta N, Fisher J J 1975 Breast carcinoma in brothers: case report and a review of 30 cases of male breast cancer. Cancer 36: 458–461

Marx S J, Spiegel A M, Brown F M, Aurbach G O 1977 Family studies in patients with primary parathyroid hyperplasia. American Journal of Medicine 62: 698–706

Matsunaga E 1980 Hereditary retinoblastoma: host resistance and second primary tumors. Journal of the National Cancer Institute 65: 47–51

Mauer H S, Pendergrass W, Borges W, Honig G R 1979 The role of genetic factors in the etiology of Wilms' tumor. Cancer 43: 205–n209

McCarty K S Jr, Barton T K, Peete C H Jr, Creasman W T 1978 Gonadal dysgenesis with adenocarcinoma of the endometrium. Cancer 42: 512–520

McConnell R B 1980 Genetics of familial polyposis, in Colorectal cancer: prevention epidemiology and screening,

Winawer P, Shottenfeld D, Sherlock P (eds), Raven Press, New York. pp 69–71

Meadows A T, Lichtenfeld J L, Koop C E 1974 Wilms' tumor in three children of a woman with congenital hemihypertrophy. New England Journal of Medicine 291: 23–24

Meadows A T, D'Angio G J, Mike V, Banfi A, Harris C, Jenkins R D T, Schwartz A 1977 Patterns of second malignant neoplasms in children. Cancer 40: 1903–1911

Merten D F, Gooding C A, Newton T H, Malamud N 1974 Meningiomas of childhood and adolescence. Journal of Pediatrics 84: 696–750

Miller R W 1968 Deaths from childhood cancer in sibs. New England Journal of Medicine 279: 122–126

Miller R W 1971 Deaths from childhood leukemia and solid tumors among twins and other sibs in the United States, 1960–1967. Journal of the National Cancer Institute 46: 203–209

Moyes C D, Alexander F W 1977 Mucosal neuroma syndrome presenting in a neonate. Developmental Medicine and Child Neurology 19: 518–534

Müller S, Gadner H, Weber B, Vogel M, Riekm H 1978 Wilms' tumor and adrenocortical carcinoma with hemihypertrophy and hamartomas. European Journal of Pediatrics 127: 219–226

Mulvihill J J 1976 Host factors in human lung tumors: an example of ecogenetics in oncology. Journal of the National Cancer Institute. 57: 3–7

Mulvihill J J, Miller R W, Fraumeni J F Jr (eds) 1977a Genetics of Human Cancer. Raven, New York

Mulvihill J J, Gralnick H R, Whang-Peng J, Leventhal B E 1977b Multiple childhood osteosarcomas in an American Indian family with erythroid mastocytosis and skeletal anomalies. Cancer 40: 3115–3122

Mulvihill J J, McKeen E A 1977 Discussion: genetics of multiple primary tumors. Cancer 40: 1867—1871

Nagel G A, Nagel-Studer E, Seiler W, Hofer H O 1973 Malignant lymphoma in 4 of 5 siblings. International Journal of Cancer 22: 675–679

Napoli V M, Campbell W G 1977 Hepatoblasoma in infant sisters and brothers. Cancer 39: 2647 a–2650

Naylor E W, Garder E J 1977 Penetrance and expressivity of the gene responsible for the Gardner syndrome. Clinical Genetics 11: 381–393

Nove J, Little J B, Weichelbaum R R, Nichols W W, Hoffman E 1979 Retinoblastoma, chromosome 13 and in vitro cellular radiosensitivity. Cytogenetics and Cell Genetics 24: 185–192

Nowell P, Daniele R, Rowland D Jr, Finan J 1980 Cytogenetics of chronic B-cell and T-cell leukemia. Cancer Genetics and Cytogenetics 1: 273–280

Ohbayashi A, Okochi K, Mayumi M 1972 Familial clustering of a symptomatic carrier of Australian antigen and patients with chronic liver disease or primary liver cancer. Gastroenterology 62: 617–625

Odell W D, Wolfsen A R 1980 Hormones from tumors: are they ubiquitous? American Medicine 63: 317–318

Parry D M, Mulvihill J J, Miller R W 1979 Sarcomas in a child and her father. American Journal of Diseases of Children 133: 130–132

Pauli R M, Pauli M E, Hale J G 1980 Gardner syndrome and periampillary malignancy. American Journal of Medical Genetics 6: 205–219

Pearse A G E 1977 The diffuse neuroendocrine system and the APUD concept. Medical Biology 55: 115–125

Pilepich M V, Berkman E M, Goodchild N T 1978 HLA typing in familial renal carcinoma. Tissue Antigens 11: 487--488

Penn I 1978 Malignancies associated with immunosuppressive or cytotoxic therapy. Surgery 83: 492–502

Perry S III, Spector B D, Schuman L M, Mandel J S, Anderson V E, McHugh R B, Hanson M R, Fahlstrom S M, Krivit W, Kersey J H 1980 The Wiscott-Aldrich syndrome in the United States and Canada (1892–1979). Journal of Pediatrics 97: 72–78

Petrakis N L 1977 Genetic factors in the etiology of breast cancer. Cancer 39 (6 suppl): 2709–2715

Pohl G, Boeckl O, Galvan G, Salis-Samaden R, Steiner H, Thurner J 1977 Konkordantes medullares Schilddrusen-karzinom bei eineiigen Zwillingen mit diskordantem Phaochromozytom (Sipple-syndrom). Wiener Klinische Wochenschrift 89: 481–484

Pollack R S 1973 Carotid body tumors – idiosyncracies. Oncology 27: 81–91

Raghavan D, Jelihovsky T, Fox R M 1980 Father-son testicular malignancy: does genetic anticipation occur? Cancer 45: 1005–1008

Reimer R R, Fraumeni J F Jr, Ozols R F, Bender R 1977 Pancreatic cancer in father and son. Lancer 1: 911 only

Riccardi V M, Hittner H Ml, Francke U, Pippin S, Hohnquist G P, Kretzer F L, Ferrell R 1979 Partial triplication and deletion of 13q: study of a family presenting with bilateral retinoblastoma. Clinical Genetics 15: 332–345

Riccardi V M, Hittner H M, Francke U, Yunis J J, Ledbetter D, Borges W 1980 The aniridia-Wilms' tumor association: the critical role of chromosome band 11p13. Cancer Genetics and Cytogenetics 2: 131–137

Richards R D, Mebust W K, Schimke R N 1973 A prospective study in von Hippel-Lindau disease. Journal of Urology 110: 27–30

Rimoin D L, Schimke R N Genetic disorders of the endocrine glands, 2nd ed. Plenum, New York. (in press)

Robboy S J, Kaufman R H, Prat J, Welch W R, Gaffey T, Scully R E, Richart R, Fenoglio C M, Verata R, Tilley B C 1979 Pathologic findings in young women enrolled in the National Cooperative Diethylstilbestrol Adenosis (DESAD) project. Obstetrics and Gynecology 53: 309–317

Robinson J E, Brown N B, Andiman W, Holliday K, Francke U, Robert M F, Andersson-Anvret M, Horstmann D, Miller G 1980 Diffuse polyclonal B-cell lymphoma during primary infection with Epstein-Barr virus. New England Journal of Medicine 302: 1293–1297

Rowley J D 1980 Chromosome abnormalities in cancer. Cancer Genetics and Cytogenetics 2: 175–198

Sandberg A 1980 Chromosomes in human cancer and leukemia. Elsevier, New York

San Filippo J S, Holtman J, Day T G, Stone R, Wittliff J L 1979 Gonadal dysgenesis with vulvar carcinoma. Obstetrics and Gynecology 54 387–390

Santos J G, Magalhaes J 1980 Familial gastric polyposis, Journal of Human Genetics 28: 293–297

Schimke R N 1972 The mucosal neuroma syndrome, In: Lyncy H T (ed) Heredity, skin and malignant neoplasm. Medical Exam Pub Co., Flushing, New York. pp 208–219

Schimke R N 1973 Phenotype of malignancy: the mucosal neuroma syndrome. Pediatrics 52: 283–285

Schimke R N 1976 The multiple endocrine adenoma syndrome. Advances in Internal Medicine 21: 249–265

Schimke R N 1977 Tumors of the neural crest system, In: Mulvihill J J, Miller R W, Fraumeni J F Jr (eds) Genetics of human cancer. Raven Press, New York. pp 179–198

Schimke R N 1978 Genetics and cancer in man. Churchill Livingstone, Edinburgh

Schimke R N 1979 The neurocristopathy concept: fact or fiction, In: Advances in neuroblastoma research. Raven Press, New York. pp 13–24

Schimke R N 1981 Genetics and cancer in children: current concepts. In: Kaback M M (ed) Genetic Issues in Pediatric and Obstetric Practice Year Book, Chicago. 413–442

Schimke R N 1980 Genetic syndromes with gastrointestinal cancer, In: Genetics and heterogeneity in common gastrointestinal disease. Academic Press, New York. pp 377–389

Schnall A M, Genuth S M 1976 Multiple endocrine adenomas in a patient with the Maffucci syndrome. American Journal of Medicine 61: 952–956

Schoenberg B S 1975 Nervous system neoplasms and primary malignancies at other sites. Neurology 25: 705–712

Schwartz S S, Rich B H, Lucky A W, Straus F H II, Gonen B, Wolfsdorf J, Thorp F W, Burrington J D, Madden J O, Rubenstein A H, Rosenfield R L 1979 Familial nesidioblastosis: severe neonatal hypoglycaemia in two families. Journal of Pediatrics 95: 44–53

Shinohara M, Komatsu H, Kawamura T, Yokoyama M 1980 Familial testicular teratoma in 2 children: familial report and review of the literature. Journal of Urology 123: 552–555

Simpson J L, Photopoulos G 1976a Hereditary aspects of ovarian and testicular neoplasia. Birth Defects 12: 51–60

Simpson J L, Photopoulos G 1976b The relationship of neoplasia to disorders of abnormal sexual differentiation. Birth Defects 12: 15–50

Skrabenek P 1980 APUD concept: hypothesis or tautology. Medical Hypotheses 6: 437–440

Seeler R A, Israel J N, Royal J E, Kaye C I, Rao S, Abulabam M 1979 Ganglioneuroblastoma and fetal hydantoin-alcohol syndrome. Pediatrics 63: 524–527

Sogge M R, McDonell S D, Cofold P B 1979 The malignant potential of the dysgenetic germ cell in Klinefelter's syndrome. American Journal of Medicine 66. 515–518

Sotelo-Avila C, Gonzalez-Crussi F, Fowler J W 1980 Complete and incomplete forms of the Beckwith-Wiedemann syndrome: their oncogenic potential. Journal of Pediatircs 96: 47–50

Southwick G J, Schwartz R A 1979 The basal cell nevus syndrome. Cancer 44: 2294–2305

Sparkes R S, Muller H, Klisak I 1979 Retinoblastoma with 13q– chromosome deletion associated with maternal paracentric inversion of 13q. Science 203: 1027–1029

Sparkes R S, Sparkes M C, Wilson M G, Towner J W, Benedict W, Murphree A L, Yunis J 1980 Regional assignment of genes for human esterase D and retinoblastoma to chromosome band 13q14. Science 208: 1042–104

Spector B D, Perry G S III, Kersey J H 1978 Genetically determined immunodeficiency disease (GDID) and malignancy: report from the immunodeficiency-cancer registry. Clinics in Immunology and Immunopathology 11: 12–29

Strong L, Riccardi V, Ferrell R, Sparkes R, Ledbetter D, Strobel R, Hass C 1980 Familial retinoblastoma and chromosome 13 deletion transmitted via an insertional translocation. Americal Journal of Human Genetics

Svarch E, de la Torre E 1977 Myelomonocytic leukaemia with a preleukaemic syndrome and a Ph[1] chromosome in monozygotic twins. Archives of Diseases in Childhood 52: 72–74

Swift M, Chen J, Pinkham R 1974 A maximum likelihood method for estimating the disease predisposition of heterozygotes. American Journal of Human Genetics 26: 304–317

Swift M, Caldwell R J, Chase C 1980 Reassessment of cancer predisposition of Fanconi anemia heterozygotes. Journal of the National Cancer Society 65: 863–867

Taylor W F, Myers M, Taylor W R 1980 Extrarenal Wilms' tumor in an infant exposed to intrauterine phenytoin. Lancet 2: 481–482

Thiessen E J 1974 Concerning a familial association between breast cancer and both prostatic and uterine malignancies. Cancer 34: 1102–1107

Tischler A S, Dichter M A, Biales B, DeSellis R A, Wolfe H 1976 Neural properties of cultured human endocrine tumor cells of proposed neural crest origin. Science 192: 902–904

Tokuhata G K, Lilienfeld A M 1963 Familial aggregation of lung cancer in humans. Journal of the National Cancer Institute 30: 289–312

Tragl K H, Mayr W R 1977 Familial islet-cell adenomatosis. Lancet 2: 426–428

Vogel F 1979 Genetics of retinoblastoma. Human Genetics 52: 1–54

Von Metz I P, Bots G T, Enotz L J 1977 Astrocytoma in three sisters. Neurology 27: 1038–1041

Wertelecki W, Fraumeni J F Jr, Mulvihill J J 1970 Nongonadal neoplasia in Turner's syndrome. Cancer 26: 485–488

West R J, Leonard J V 1980 Familial insulin resistance with pineal hyperplasia: metabolic studies and effect of hypophysectomy. Archives of Diseases in Childhood 55: 619–621

Williams E D 1977 Thyroidectomy for genetically determined medullary carcinoma. Lancet 1: 1309–1310

Williams E D 1979 Medullary carcinoma of the thyroid, In: Degroot L J, Cahill G F Jr, Odele W D, Martini L, Potts J T Jr, Nelson D H, Sternberger E, Winegrad A J (eds) Endocrinology, Vol. 2. Grune & Stratton, New York. pp 777–792

Wilson L M, Draper G J 1974 Neuroblastoma, its natural history and prognosis: a study of 487 cases. British Medical Journal 3: 301–307

Yamaguchi K, Kameya T, Abe K 1980 Multiple endocrine neoplasia type I. Clinics in Endocrinology and Metabolism 9: 261–284

Young D F, Eldridge R, Gardner W J 1970 Bilateral acoustic neuromas in a large kindred. Journal of the American Medical Association 214: 347–353

Yunis J, Ramsey N 1978 Retinoblastoma and subband deletion of chromosome 13. American Journal of Diseases of Children 132: 161–163

Yunis J J, Ramsey N 1980 Familial occurrence of the aniridia-Wilms' tumor syndrome with deletion 11p13–14.1. Journal of Pediatrics 96: 1027–1030

Zankl L T, Zang K D 1980 Correlations between clinical and cytogenetical data in 180 human meningiomes. Cancer Genetics and Cytogenetics 1: 351–356

Genetic counselling

R. Skinner

The last few decades have seen a dramatic decrease in the importance of environmental causes of ill-health in developed countries. As a result there has been a sharp increase in the relative importance of genetic and partially genetic disorders as causes of present day morbidity and mortality, particularly amongst children. Many studies in recent years have shown that roughly 30% of admissions to, and between 40 and 50% of deaths occurring in, paediatric hospitals are accounted for by children with genetic disorders or congenital malformations. Genetic diseases are almost always serious, are not curable, and relatively few are amenable to satisfactory modes of treatment. Thus, in the current situation the prevention of this group of diseases remains of paramount importance. At the present time the most effective means of preventing genetic diseases remains the provision of genetic counselling for individuals at risk of having a child with a serious genetic disorder, coupled with prenatal diagnosis where possible.

One of the prime requirements of an effective genetic counselling programme is the comprehensive ascertainment of those individuals in the population who are at risk of having an affected child so that they can be offered genetic advice. There are a number of ways in which such individuals can be ascertained, but these fall mainly into two categories. Population screening is one obvious way of ascertaining people at risk, but such methods are accompanied by many problems, both practical and ethical. The main way in which ascertainment is achieved therefore, is as a result of routine diagnosis, when an individual is found to have a disorder known to be genetic. The families of such individuals can then be screened and advice offered to those at risk of having affected children. This approach can of course be greatly facilitated by the use of a genetic register system designed for this purpose. The intricacies and usage of both population screening and genetic registers for the ascertainment of individuals in need of genetic counselling have been reviewed elsewhere in this text and will therefore not be discussed further here.

Traditionally, genetic counselling has been viewed as the process by which individuals seeking advice are provided with all the information that is required to enable them to make a wholly informed decision on what their future reproductive plans will be. Mainly, therefore, this has taken the form of what has been termed 'factually-oriented' counselling. Recent years, however, have seen increasing recognition of the importance of the many psychological aspects of such counselling. Awareness of the variety of problems which may lessen the degree of communication between counsellor and counsellee, of the feelings of guilt often attendant on the birth of a handicapped child, and of the dynamics of the coping and decision making processes themselves, have led to the trend by most genetic counsellors now to move away from traditional approaches towards what Kessler has described as more 'person-oriented' counselling. This aspect of genetic counselling will be explored towards the end of the chapter when the more basic, factual aspects of the problem have been considered.

BASIC INFORMATION NEEDED FOR GENETIC COUNSELLING

Before a counsellor can embark upon giving definitive genetic advice he must have available to him certain basic, essential information. He must have at least a precise and fully confirmed diagnosis in the index patient, an accurate pedigree of the family, and know the mode of inheritance of the disorder at hand so that the precise risk of occurrence or recurrence can be estimated. Who gathers this information together after the referral of a family to a genetic advisory centre will vary from centre to centre. Although a medically qualified geneticist will certainly be required to evaluate the accuracy of a diagnosis, whether by personal examination of the proband or from scrutiny of the relevant documentation, the family details and pedigree can well be coordinated by another suitably trained member of the team, a nurse, social worker or genetic associate.

A precise diagnosis of the disease in the proband is essential if accurate genetic advice is to be given. This is largely because of the problem of genetic heterogeneity which will be discussed below. Knowing the mode of inheritance of the disease within the family is of course mandatory so that the genetic implications can be assessed and explained. The mode of inheritance may be obvious once the diagnosis is established, if dealing with a well known genetic disorder. If not, it may have to be assessed on the basis of the individual family's pedigree – hence the need for accurate recording of the family data.

When in possession of an established diagnosis and when the mode of inheritance is known, then the counsellor is able to estimate the recurrence risks involved either from first principles in the case of unifactorial disorders (with or without modification by carrier detection tests), or from empirical data in the case of chromosome or multifactorial disorders. These risks can then be explained and explored with those seeking advice.

DIAGNOSTIC PROBLEMS IN GENETIC COUNSELLING

Genetic heterogeneity

One of the major problems for genetic counsellors is the occurrence of *genetic heterogeneity*, which often complicates the establishment of a precise diagnosis. Genetic heterogeneity is the phenomenon whereby certain disorders, though superficially resembling one another at the clinical level, may result from quite different genetic defects. Thus, similar disorders may be caused by different mutations at the same locus or by mutations at different loci and may therefore have quite different modes of inheritance. Congenital methaemoglobinaemia is a good example. Here a very similar clinical appearance can result either from autosomal recessive mutations leading to a reduction in erythrocyte methaemoglobin reductase (the enzyme itself being polymorphic) or from dominant mutations at either the α or β chain loci resulting in a number of different haemoglobinopathies. Other excellent examples of well defined genetic disorders which exhibit marked heterogeneity at both the clinical and genetic levels are the Ehlers-Danlos syndrome, the mucopolysaccharidoses and the various muscular dystrophies. Needless to say, if faced with a child with a mucopolysaccharidosis one's genetic advice to the parents would be quite different if the child proved to have X–linked Hunter syndrome rather than any of the other autosomal recessive forms.

Phenocopies

Another important reason for having an accurate diagnosis is to ensure that the disease in question is genetic in origin. The occurrence of *phenocopies* can give rise to considerable difficulty in genetic counselling. Such conditions, although they mimic genetic disorders, are caused by environmental factors and are therefore unlikely to recur. A frequent example of this problem is microcephaly. Although this congenital malformation may be inherited as an autosomal recessive trait, it may also result from intrauterine exposure of the fetus to teratogens such as rubella, toxoplasmosis or maternal radiation. In addition to intrauterine infections and radiation, a variety of other influences including maternal disease, drug ingestion and mechanical factors in the uterus such as amniotic bands, may also give rise to phenocopies.

The sporadic case

The occurrence of an isolated or *sporadic case* within a family poses a problem familiar to all who are regularly involved in genetic counselling. The small size of modern families makes this a common problem. Here the pedigree information is of no value and the counsellor is entirely dependent on a clinical or laboratory diagnosis to establish the mode of inheritance concerned and the risks to various family members. Many different situations may lead to the occurrence of a sporadic case and all of these must be considered:

(a) The disorder may prove to be non-genetic (or only partially genetic) and therefore have little risk of recurring.

(b) The disorder may be due to a chromosome anomaly which, if neither parent is a healthy carrier, will have only a low risk of recurring.

(c) The disorder may have a multifactorial or polygenic aetiology with a definite, but again usually low or moderate risk of recurrence, the actual risk depending on the condition in question.

(d) The disorder may represent a new dominant mutation within the family with very little risk of recurrence in sibs. Great care must however be taken before reassurance is given to ensure that neither parent is in fact affected and only shows very minimal manifestations.

(e) The individual may have an autosomal recessive condition and be the first affected child born to healthy, unsuspecting heterozygous parents. The recurrence risk then would be 1 in 4.

(f) If the affected individual is a male then the disorder may be an X–linked recessive one. This may either represent a new mutation (more common if it is a lethal disease) or the mother may prove to be a carrier with high risks to further children.

Clearly, accurate genetic advice can only be given if a precise diagnosis is established and the mode of inheritance of the disease is well defined. Only then can true risks of recurrence, either empiric or theoretical, be estimated. Needless to say situations do occur, especially when dealing with complex, multiple malformation syndromes, where a diagnosis cannot be reached and hence genetic advice cannot be given. All genetic counsellors must be prepared on occasion to admit that they cannot give an accurate assessment of the genetic implications for a particular, atypical family; they are not clairvoyant!

Illegitimacy

Anyone drawing up a family's pedigree must be aware of the possibility that illegitimacy may be present in the family and could drastically alter the implications of the situation for the person seeking advice. Often such information is freely given by the mother or implied by a family member. Frequently however this vital fact is not volunteered and can only be suspected in a puzzling situation. Illegitimacy itself does not of course present any difficulty, it is clear knowledge of the true father of a child which is important. Recent studies have indicated that as many as 15% of children in Edinburgh are not the offspring of their putative fathers. Presumably in a more liberal environment an even higher figure could apply.

The problems associated with actual disputes about the true paternity of a child, and methods of resolving them, are comprehensively discussed elsewhere in this text.

GENETIC COUNSELLING IN CHROMOSOME DISORDERS

The pooled data from several series in which chromosome studies have been done, comprising 47 000 consecutive live-born children, have shown that roughly 1 in 150 babies (5.81/1000) has a recognizable chromosomal abnormality (Nielsen, 1975). Of these, 3.75/1000 had an autosomal anomaly, and 2.06/1000 had a sex chromosome anomaly. Thus chromosome anomalies are relatively common and are therefore conditions frequently encountered by most genetic centres.

The vast majority of chromosomal disorders show only a very low risk of recurring within the family, except when a family member is found to be a balanced translocation carrier or when maternal age complicates the issue. In spite of the usual low risks of recurrence involved it is important that every effort be made to identify high risk situations since chromosomal abnormalities are so easily and accurately detected during pregnancy by amniocentesis.

Trisomy 21

The single most common and most important chromosomal disorder from the counselling point of view is Down syndrome. This abnormality occurs in roughly 1 in 700 live-births and is mainly accounted for (95%) by trisomy 21. Its increased frequency amongst the offspring of older mothers is well recognised and must be carefully considered when giving genetic counselling. The now well documented increased risk associated with increased paternal age (when maternal age is kept constant) is of much lesser magnitude. Two main problems associated with trisomy 21 present themselves to the genetic counsellor: the risk to the older mother and the risk to the mother of a previously affected child with trisomy 21.

Table 99.1 lists the maternal age related incidence and risk figures for Down syndrome. From these it can be seen that the risk of having a child with trisomy 21 has already risen above the overall population level by a maternal age of 35 years, increasing gradually up to 40 years and thereafter more rapidly. Data from amniocentesis results suggest a slightly higher risk than that derived from live-birth studies (Table 99.1).

After the birth of one child with trisomy 21, the risk of another such child being born to a couple is higher than the normal risk. This increased risk is more marked in the mothers of both the low and high extremes of maternal age than in mothers with maternal ages of

Table 99.1 Age specific rates of Down syndrome in live-births and at amniocentesis.

Maternal age in years	No. cases per 1000 live-births*	Risk at birth*	Risk of DS at amniocentesis[+]	Risk of any aneuploidy at amniocentesis[+]
35	3.09	1/324	1/222	1/133
36	1.96	1/510	1/204	1/102
37	2.94	1/340	1/130	1/75
38	3.10	1/322	1/110	1/68
39	7.57	1/132	1/76	1/54
40	10.50	1/95	1/83	1/43
41	14.50	1/69	1/43	1/33
42	12.59	1/80	1/30	1/16
43	15.72	1/64	1/56	1/25
44	36.91	1/27	1/18	1/13
45	33.64	1/30	1/30	1/20
46	28.11	1/36	1/12	1/7

* Data from Trimble and Baird 1978.
[+] Data from Ferguson-Smith 1979.

25–35 years. Combined amniocentesis data (Mikkelson, 1979) show the overall risk to be about 0.5% specifically for another child with Down syndrome. After the age of 35 years a woman with a previous affected child would seem to run about twice the normal age specific risk of having a further child with Down syndrome.

Maternal age

It is important to remember that Down syndrome is not the only chromosome anomaly related to maternal age. Trisomies of certain other autosomes (which occur in live-borns) occur more frequently in the offspring of older mothers, as do the XXY and XXX sex chromosome anomalies. The XYY and XO syndromes are however not related to maternal age. At any particular maternal age the risk of having a child with any form of chromosomal aneuploidy is roughly twice the age related risk of having a child with Down syndrome.

Autosomal abnormalities other than trisomy 21

Available data on the recurrence risks for any of these anomalies are scanty. Nevertheless, recurrence seems to be rare except where a familial translocation is involved. Maternal age can however be a complicating factor and should be borne in mind.

Sex chromosome anomalies

Recurrence of any of the sex chromosome anomalies within families is extremely rare and reassurance can be given. The relationship between maternal age and the XXY or XXX syndrome should however be borne in mind.

A common reason for sex chromosome abnormalities to be brought to a genetic counsellor, apart from diagnostic situations and the birth of an affected child, is the detection of a sex chromosome abnormality in a live-birth screening programme or in the products of a spontaneous abortion. In the former situation, the parents are usually anxious to discuss the prognosis of the condition discovered unexpectedly in their apparently healthy offspring. In the latter situation, information is usually wanted about the risk of such an abnormality occurring in any future live-born child.

Chromosomal translocations

The most common translocations encountered by the genetic counsellor are those involving chromosome 21 and D/D group translocations. No matter what the translocation involved, the recurrence risk is small unless one of the parents is a balanced carrier of the translocation. Since such individuals may have a relatively high risk of abnormality in their offspring, it is essential to test all close relatives of a patient with an unbalanced translocation in order to identify unsuspected balanced carriers, so that they can be offered amniocentesis if appropriate.

Table 99.2 Recurrence risk of Down syndrome due to various chromosome aberrations. From Emery A E H (1979) with permission.

Karyotypes Patient	Father	Mother	Chance of recurrence %
Translocation			
D/G	N	C	10–15
	C	N	5
21/22	N	C	10–15
	C	N	5
21/21	C	N	100
	N	C	100
Trisomy 21	N	N	1
Translocation or mosaic	N	N	small

C = carrier; N = normal

Some 4% of all patients with Down syndrome prove to have unbalanced translocations and in about half of them this is familial. Most commonly chromosome 21 is translocated to a D group chromosome, usually chromosome 14 (less commonly 13 or 15). Alternatively it may be translocated to another G group chromosome which may be chromosome 22, or the two 21 chromosomes are translocated onto each other. Table 99.2 shows the risk of live-born chromosomally abnormal children amongst the offspring of balanced carriers of translocations involving chromosome 21.

Balanced D/D group translocations are not uncommon and are usually not associated with unbalanced chromosome defects in live-born offspring (de Grouchy, 1976).

Recurrent spontaneous abortion

Repeated studies of the chromosomes of early spontaneous abortions consistently show a very high rate of chromosome abnormality. This is especially so in those occurring before 12 weeks of gestation when some 60% show abnormalities (Boué & Boué, 1975; Jacobs et al, 1981). Many of the chromosome abnormalities commonly found in abortions do not occur in live-births. Since chromosome anomalies are such a common cause of abortion, there have been several studies of the chromosomes of couples who have had repeated spontaneous abortions. In more than 10% of such couples one partner is found to have a balanced chromosome anomaly (Kaosaar & Mikelsaar, 1973; Kim et al, 1975). It is therefore valuable to do chromosome studies on all couples when no adequate gynaecological reason can be found to account for repeated spontaneous abortions, so that amniocentesis can be considered if appropriate.

GENETIC COUNSELLING IN MULTIFACTORIAL DISORDERS

A multifactorial disorder is presumed to result largely from the additive effect of a number of factors, some undoubtedly genetic and others environmental. Since the genetic component in the aetiology of such conditions is not simple, but results from a combination of many genes, estimation of recurrence risks from first principles is not possible. Nevertheless it is still possible to give reasonably accurate genetic advice by resorting to the use of *empiric risks* of recurrence (see below). Diseases thought to be inherited in this way include most of the commoner birth defects as well as most of the important chronic diseases of later adulthood and thus are frequent problems for the genetic counsellor. It is fortunate, in view of the frequency of these disorders, that almost always the recurrence risks within the family are low.

Empiric risks of recurrence

These are risks of recurrence estimated directly from family data. Thus they provide statistical estimates of recurrence which may be of great value in counselling families with a multifactorial disorder. Empiric risks are available now for many multifactorial conditions, and some of these can be seen in Table 99.3.

The accuracy and usefulness of empiric risk data have been comprehensively reviewed by Carter (1977). He concluded that such data can be extremely accurate and valuable, providing careful attention is paid to several sources of error in its collection and application. Sources of error include the precision of the diagnosis in the proband, accurate collection of family data, random sampling of probands, adequate size of the study group, and appropriateness of the population studied (as risks may vary considerably between populations).

Factors modifying the risks for the individual family

After finding a satisfactory empiric risk estimate for the disorder in question, the genetic counsellor's next move should be to consider whether or not the risk needs to be modified for the particular patient or family seeking advice. Factors which need consideration include the severity of the disorder in the affected individual, the sex of the patient, the presence or not of other affected individuals in the family, parental consanguinity, and any relevant predisposing environmental factors.

Table 99.3 Empiric risks for some common disorders (in per cent). From Emery A E H (1979) with permission.

Disorder	Incidence	Sex ratio M:F	Normal parents having a second affected child	Affected parent having an affected child	Affected parent having a second affected child
Anencephaly	0.20	1:2	5★	–	–
Cleft palate only	0.04	2:3	2	7	15
Cleft lip ± cleft palate	0.10	3:2	4	4	10
Club foot	0.10	2:1	3	3	10
Cong. heart disease (all types)	0.50	–	1–4	1–4	–
Diabetes mellitus (early onset)	0.20	1:1	8	8	10
Dislocation of hip	0.07	1:6	4	4	10
Epilepsy ('idiopathic')	0.50	1:1	5	5	10
Hirschsprung disease	0.02	4:1			
male proband			2	–	–
female proband			8	–	–
Hypospadias (in males)	0.20	–	10	–	–
Manic-depressive psychoses	0.40	2:3	–	10–15	–
Mental retardation ('idiopathic')	0.30 0.50	1:1	3–5	–	–
Profound childhood deafness	0.10	1:1	10	8	–
Pyloric stenosis	0.30	5:1			
male proband			2	4	13
female proband			10	17	38
Renal agenesis (bilat.)	0.01	3:1			
male proband			3	–	–
female proband			7	–	–
Schizophrenia	1–2	1:1	–	16	–
Scoliosis (idiopathic, adolescent)	0.22	1:6	7	5	
Spina bifida	0.30	2:3	5★	3★	–

★ Anencephaly or spina bifida

The degree of severity with which the patient is affected is important as the recurrence risk is likely to increase with increasing severity. Thus the recurrence risk in sibs if the proband has a unilateral cleft lip is about 4%, but is 6% if a bilateral cleft lip is present.

Where the sex ratio of the condition differs significantly from unity, the recurrence risk is likely to be higher when the patient is of the sex less often affected. Thus the risk to sibs of a male proband with congenital pyloric stenosis is 3% whereas to the sibs of an affected female is 8%, the malformation being five times more common in males than in females.

The occurrence of other affected individuals in the family in addition to the proband may significantly increase the risk, especially if a first degree relative is involved. The risk to the sibs of an isolated child with club feet is only 3%, but if one parent is also affected the risk to subsequent children is about 10%.

Lastly, the presence of consanginuity between the parents should be recorded. However, this has little effect on the risk for multifactorial disorders, only increasing it by 1–2%.

GENETIC COUNSELLING IN UNIFACTORIAL DISORDERS

These disorders segregate within affected families according to Mendel's laws and therefore risk figures for various family members can be readily and accurately estimated in most situations. Thus genetic counselling is usually straightforward, provided an accurate diagnosis can be established. The actual risks calculated from pedigree data alone may be modified and made more accurate in a variety of situations. Thus, taking into account the ages of family members may drastically alter the basic risks when dealing with an autosomal dominant disorder of variable or late onset. Similarly, appropriate biochemical investigations may be very valuable in estimating the probable carrier status of an individual, particularly a woman in a family in which an X-linked recessive disorder is segregating (see below).

Mendelian inheritance can be established in a variety of ways, but most commonly this results from knowing the diagnosis, a characteristic pedigree pattern being found even if the diagnosis remains in doubt, or a combination of the diagnosis of a known Mendelian disorder and a compatible pedigree pattern. The recent tendency towards smaller family size may not allow the development of a typical pedigree pattern and therefore isolated cases are frequently encountered.

Autosomal dominant disorders
In families with an autosomal dominant disorder, risks of recurrence can be easily calculated from first princi-

ples. Therefore genetic counselling in such disorders should be relatively simple. However, in practice many factors associated with dominant inheritance may cause great problems in the genetic counselling situation. If an individual is definitely heterozygous for an autosomal dominant gene then there is a 50% risk of transmitting the gene to any offspring, regardless of the sex of the child or the severity of the condition. Problems arise in counselling when the condition has variable or late onset, or when variable expressivity or incomplete penetrance can make it difficult to be sure whether an apparently unaffected member of the family is either truly normal or a heterozygote with minimal or no manifestations of the gene.

When giving genetic counselling in late onset autosomal dominant disorders there is no problem in risk estimation for clearly affected family members, but one of the major problems arising is at what age one can assume an apparently unaffected person to be genetically normal and therefore not about to develop the disease. When data are available on age related occurrence rates, such as those for Huntington chorea, then substantial modification of the basic *a priori* risk for an individual can often be made, particularly if the individual or an apparently unaffected parent is well into middle-age. The other major problem associated with counselling in late onset dominant disorders is that individuals found to be affected may already have families before genetic advice is found to be necessary. Not only does this mean additional individuals at risk, but it is also a situation which proves emotionally very traumatic. Also traumatic are occasions when the counsellor has to indicate that a counsellee is himself at high risk. This may be done so that the counsellee can appreciate the risk of a dominant disorder in his children.

The problems associated with variable expressivity and incomplete penetrance have been discussed elsewhere in this text. It remains merely to emphasize the importance of ensuring that great caution be exercised before full reassurance is given to apparently unaffected family members when variable expressivity or incomplete penetrance is suspected.

The same problem arises in the case of apparently new mutations, great care being required to ensure that neither supposedly normal parent is minimally affected. The lower the fitness of affected individuals the higher is the likelihood that an isolated case has been caused by a new mutation.

Autosomal recessive disorders
The major difficulty in dealing with autosomal recessive disorders is being confident that this is in fact the mode of inheritance in question. So frequently the counsellor is faced (because of small family size) with an isolated case or perhaps two affected sibs, who by chance may

both be male and hence raise the possibility of X–linkage. Usually autosomal recessive inheritance is established by confirmation of the diagnosis of a recognised genetic disorder and perhaps further supported by consanguinity of the parents if it is a rare disease.

Once this mode of inheritance is firmly established counselling is usually straightforward, since recessive conditions seldom show many of the problems of dominant conditions such as variable expression. Certainly heterogeneity may occur, but this is often defined at the biochemical level (often as enzyme kinetic variations) and each different form of the disorder 'runs true' within families, the mode of inheritance remaining unaltered. A frequent query from the parents of children with recessive disorders concerns the genetic implications for both the affected child himself and any normal sibs. In both cases of course the risk to offspring is small pro-

Table 99.4 Carrier detection tests in X-linked disorders.

Disorder	Manifestation in carrier
Anhidrotic ectodermal dysplasia	Sweat pore counts reduced, dental anomalies
Becker muscular dystrophy	↑ serum creatine kinase
Duchenne muscular dystrophy	↑ serum creatine kinase
Choroideraemia	Pigmentary changes in retina
Chronic granulomatous disease (one type)	WBC phagocytosis and nitro blue tetrazolium test abnormal
Diabetes insipidus (nephrogenic)	↓ urinary concentration
Fabry disease (angiokeratoma)	↓ α-galactosidase in skin fibroblasts. Two cell populations demonstrable
G6PD deficiency	↓ erythrocyte G6PD
Haemophilia A	Abnormal ratio of factor VIII to inactive antigen
Haemophilia B	↓ factor IX
Hunter syndrome	↓ iduronosulphate sulphatase in skin fibroblasts. Two cell populations demonstrable
Hypogammaglobulinaemia (Bruton type)	↓ IgG
Lesch-Nyhan syndrome	↓ HGPRT in skin fibroblasts or hair root bulbs. Two populations of cells demonstrable
Lowe (oculo-cerebral-renal) syndrome	Lenticular opacities, aminoaciduria
Ocular albinism	Patchy depigmentation of the retina
Retinitis pigmentosa (X-linked form)	Peripheral pigmentary changes in retina. Abnormal ERG or fluorescein angiography
Vit. D resistant rickets	↓ serum phosphorus
X-linked mental retardation	? fragile X-chromosome (in positive families)
X-linked ichthyosis	Corneal opacities, ↓ steroid sulphatase.

vided their partner does not have the same recessive gene – hence the need to warn against marrying within the family in such situations.

X–linked recessive disorders
As X–linked dominant disorders are few and rare, in practice most of the X–linked disease met by genetic counsellors is X–linked recessive in aetiology.

As in the other unifactorial situations, counselling in X–linked recessive disorders is relatively straightforward, and *a priori* risks can be easily estimated using first principles. However, these disorders do present some interesting counselling problems. The most important is in trying to differentiate between normal women in the family (who are at low risk of having affected children) and healthy heterozygous carriers (whose offspring are at very high risk). It is in these disorders most of all that *a priori* risks can be modified considerably by conditional information (either clinical or biochemical) which can thus drastically alter the risks given at genetic counselling and hence perhaps the whole orientation of the problem for a family. Females heterozygous for X–linked genes show a much greater degree of phenotypic variation than seen with autosomal recessive disorders, which is thought to arise because of Lyonisation.

The carrier state can be demonstrated to different degrees in many situations, either in terms of clinical or biochemical manifestations of the gene, or both. Table 99.4 shows a list of X–linked disorders in which manifestations may be detected in the female heterozygote. Examples of how carrier detection tests are applied can be found in Chapters devoted to the individual disorders. Such tests are particularly useful for the detection of carriers of Duchenne muscular dystrophy.

THE PRACTICAL ASPECTS AND EFFECTIVENESS OF GENETIC COUNSELLING

The process of genetic counselling can reasonably be divided into 4 consecutive phases: an initial phase in which all necessary information is gathered and the diagnosis in the proband established; a phase during which facts about the disease, the genetic implications and the possible options are imparted to and discussed with the counsellee; a phase during which the counsellee evaluates, assimilates and learns to cope with the information given; and finally a phase during which decisions are reached about eventual reproductive choices and adjustment is made to the changed milieu created by genetic counselling.

Essential prelude to genetic counselling
Either at the initial visit or before the prospective counsellee even comes to the genetic centre, a certain amount

of essential ground work needs to be done in preparation for the definitive genetic counselling session or sessions. Primarily, this is required to provide the basic core of information which enables assessment of the prognostic information and recurrence risks to be explained to the counsellee. It also can be used to assimilate valuable indications of the emotional status of the counsellees and their expectations and possible reactions to the counselling situation, which can have such marked influences on the counselling session.

This phase of counselling includes the gathering of information and the diagnostic work-up required to establish and confirm the diagnosis of the condition in question and its mode of inheritance within the family. Usually therefore, a fairly routine series of events takes place in most counselling clinics. These include drawing up an accurate pedigree of both sides of the family, clinical examination of the proband (if alive) and any family members at risk, and performing any appropriate laboratory investigations. If the proband is no longer alive then the appropriate hospital records will have to be found and carefully inspected. Once a diagnosis is established and any necessary tests done then the actual risks for various family members can be estimated.

A prior, sensitive appraisal of the psychological status of the prospective counsellees, and knowledge of any socio-economic or religious factors which may influence their attitude to the situation, can help to make the actual genetic counselling session much more successful. Here also prior warning of the counsellee's expectations from the session can be very helpful since lengthy and detailed explanation of probability estimates for further children are not very relevant if the counsellee has been sterilized already and is concerned about the genetic implications for the children already born in the family.

The type of person who gathers such important pre-counselling information will vary from clinic to clinic. This need not be a physician genetic counsellor, but can just as well be a social worker, health visitor, nurse, psychologist or genetic assistant. Confirmation of the diagnosis in question should however always be the ultimate responsibility of the physician.

The factual content of genetic counselling

Although for most genetic counsellors the emphasis in the counselling situation is shifting very much away from primary concern with the basic facts of the situation to evaluation of the patient's problems and worries in a much wider context, the factual content of the counselling process remains a very important aspect. After all, it is concern about this that has usually motivated the counsellee to seek advice in the first instance. Thus great care must be taken in the evaluation of the facts and their communication to the counsellee. The way in which these facts are presented to the counsellee is de-

termined largely by whether the counselling is to be 'directive' or 'non-directive' in approach. Certainly most counsellors now opt for the latter course in most situations.

Many people involved in genetic counselling would agree that there is a certain amount of basic information that must be included in the counselling process in order for it to be a complete and meaningful experience for the counsellee. Certainly, there should be full discussion of at least the diagnosis and prognosis of the condition in question, the genetic risks involved for that particular individual and the options or courses of action available.

The importance of establishing the correct diagnosis has already been discussed. Of equal importance is the need to divulge and explain this diagnosis to the counsellee and to discuss fully the prognosis of the condition and the nature and availability of treatment. There is much evidence to show that parents are just as much influenced in their decision making by the implications of what has been termed the 'burden' of the disease as they are by the actual genetic risks involved.

Most counsellees come expecting to hear about the genetic risks involved in their particular situation. Thus care must be taken in assessing these risks accurately and in communicating them as clearly as possible. Evidence from many follow-up studies shows that most subjects do remember the level of risk they were told at counselling, although not always in numerical form, but rather whether it was a high or low risk of recurrence. In practical terms therefore great refinement of risk estimation is not relevant (Carter et al, 1971; Emery et al, 1971; Leonard et al, 1972; Emery et al, 1978). The mode in which this type of information is explained to counsellees is also of the utmost importance. Many individuals seen for counselling have little or no concept of probability theory (Pearn, 1973; Lippman-Hand & Fraser, 1979) and thus the skill of a good counsellor is shown by his ability to judge prospective clients and tailor the information and mode of delivery to their particular needs. In this area too, more than any other, the mode of presentation of the information can greatly influence the interpretation of the facts. Although most counsellors would certainly claim to be non-directive in their approach, few would deny that in some situations they do deliver the risk figures in such a way that their clients are left in little doubt about their gravity!

Discussion of the options open to a couple makes the counselling process more comprehensive and relevant, for this is one of the aspects of the problem which will have a profound influence on their decision making. If the occurrence or recurrence risk involved is low then the major decision for a couple is whether it is acceptably low to them in the context of their own circumstances. If, however, the risk is a high one then other factors become more important, such as the availability and limitations of prenatal diagnosis, or of adoption, or perhaps of artificial insemination. For those couples who finally decide that in their circumstances they do not wish to have a child, or further children, then good contraceptive advice is of paramount importance not only as a means of reducing one of the possible sources of marital disharmony which can follow counselling, but also to prevent unplanned, high risk pregnancies occurring, as shown in some of the earlier follow-up studies (Carter et al, 1971; Leonard et al, 1972).

Psychological aspects of counselling

Many so-called 'counselling failures' result from a lack of true communication between counsellor and counsellee. Thus, great thought must be given to the process of communication and the factors affecting it. Poor communication can result from a variety of problems associated with the counsellees. Lack of motivation on their behalf, or overt anxiety or even hostility, can seriously disrupt the counselling relationship. Perhaps the factor most commonly found by counsellors to cause difficulties in effective communication is the educational background of their client, and in particular the client's knowledge of biology (Emery et al, 1979; Antley & Seidenfeld, 1978). The environment in which the counselling takes place can also greatly influence the process, no young person for instance will be as much at ease or as receptive in their own home, overheard by insensitive family members, as in a more detached hospital setting. On the other hand, a particularly independent couple may be more at ease in the privacy of their own home. In relation to communication it must be remembered that not all situations viewed by counsellors to be failures may necessarily be true failures, but may rather represent the counsellee's genuinely felt difference of interpretation of the situation. The prospect of having a blind child may certainly be perceived very differently by a blind counsellee who copes well with life, than by a fully sighted counsellor.

The psychological needs and the issues associated with the genetic counselling process are many and complicated. As well as having to cope and come to terms with emotionally traumatic information, clients need to make decisions on future reproductive plans and may also need to make fundamental alterations to their feelings about themselves and about interpersonal relationships. A knowledge of these various psychological aspects is important for genetic counselling if it is to be of value to the majority of clients. These factors have been reviewed in depth by many authors, including McCollum and Silverberg (1979) and Lippmann-Hand and Fraser (1979).

Much has now been written about the psychodynamics of the coping process, and this has been well reviewed by Falek (1977). Realization that this standard, sequen-

tial process occurs in response to genetic counselling, in the same way that it may follow any other major stressful event such as bereavement, has added greatly to our understanding of many patients' responses at various stages of the counselling process. Thus for counsellees to achieve the goal of psychological homeostasis and be in a position then to make the important decisions that are necessary, they must have experienced the four phases of the coping process known to follow exposure to stressful situations. These four phases are initial shock and denial, anxiety, anger and/or guilt, and depression, all familiar situations to those involved in counselling. Awareness that these phases are the natural course of events, and identification of the phases reached by individual counsellees, can help the counsellor to plan his approach more successfully. It will also allow the astute counsellor to recognize the occasional need for more specialist psychiatric help for a particular client to resolve coping problems before a suitable stage of psychological adjustment to allow decision making can be reached.

When the stage of decision making comes, then too it is important to remember that this is a dynamic process and one which may need skilled guidance from the counsellor. The many factors involved in this area are comprehensively reviewed by Pearn (1979) and Lippman-Hand and Fraser (1979) as are their practical relevance in the genetic counselling situation. The fundamental force at play is the counsellee's basic reproductive drive, but this is subject to modification by a variety of factors depending on individual circumstances and attitudes.

Lastly, with respect to the psychological aspects of counselling, mention must be made of the importance of adequate support and follow-up facilities. Two main areas are important here, firstly adequate follow-up and support by personnel trained in psycho-social counselling can help to lessen the emotional trauma involved, not only in receiving genetic counselling, but also in subsequent readjustments within the family and between the family and the rest of society. Secondly, evidence from many studies indicates that reinforcement of the genetic advice is helpful and necessary in many situations if the counselling process is to be of maximum benefit. There is evidence which suggests that reinforcement of the facts may be particularly indicated in certain situations such as chromosomal disorders and X–linked recessive disorders (Emery et al, 1978).

Effectiveness of genetic counselling

When attention was first focused on the success or effectiveness of genetic counselling rather than its ethical problems, it led to many retrospective studies of individuals who had received genetic counselling (Carter et al, 1971; Leonard et al, 1972; Emery et al, 1972; Emery et al, 1973; Emery et al, 1979; Reynolds et al, 1974). Such studies concentrated largely on the reproductive decisions made after counselling and the accuracy with which counsellees remembered the genetic advice given, as these were relatively simple parameters to quantify. Almost uniformly these studies showed that retention of genetic advice was reasonably good (if not always perfectly accurate in strict numerical terms) and that on the whole the higher the genetic risk, the lower the proportion of counsellees deciding to plan pregnancies. They also highlighted for the first time the importance of the so-called 'burden' of the disorder (emotional as well as financial) in influencing reproductive decisions. Thus, much useful information resulted from such studies, much of which significantly altered the approach of many genetic counsellors.

However, many criticisms have been levelled at such studies. They were said to be biased, since follow-up was often done by the counsellors themselves, not to reflect adequately the changing attitudes during the period of the study, and also to show little of how such information affected individual couples and their decision making. A review of the published studies and their findings is given by Evers-Kiebooms and van den Berghe (1979). The obvious shortcomings of such retrospective studies, as well as increased awareness of the various additional dimensions of the genetic counselling process have stimulated new approaches to evaluating the effectiveness and achievements of counselling. Most studies undertaken now are prospective in design and involve in depth analysis of the psychological aspects of the problem. Many new and excellent books dealing with the theory and practice of genetic counselling explore this area in detail.

REFERENCES

Antley R M, Seidenfeld M J 1978 A detailed description of mother's knowledge before genetic counselling for Down syndrome. American Journal of Medical Genetics 2: 357–364

Boúe A, Boúe J 1975 Chromosome abnormalities and abortions. In: Coutinho B E M, Fuchs F (eds) Physiology and Genetics of Reproduction, Plenum Publishing Corporation, New York

Carter C O 1977 Risk data: How good is empiric information. In: Lubs H A, de la Cruz F (eds) Genetic Counselling, Raven Press, New York. ch 5 p 407

Carter C O, Fraser Roberts J A, Evans K A, Buck A R 1971 Genetic clinic: a follow-up. Lancet i: 281–285

Emery A E H 1979 Elements of Medical Genetics, 5th edn. Churchill Livingstone, Edinburgh

Emery A E H, Watt M S, Clack E R 1972 The effects of genetic counselling in Duchenne muscular dystrophy. Clinical Genetics 3: 147–150

Emery A E H, Watt M S, Clack E R 1973 Social effects of genetic counselling. British Medical Journal 1: 724–726

Emery A E H, Raeburn J A, Skinner R, Holloway S, Lewis P 1979 Prospective study of genetic counselling. British Medical Journal 1: 1253–1256

Evers-Kiebooms G, van den Berghe H 1979 Impact of genetic counselling: a review of published follow-up studies. Clinical Genetics 15: 465–474

Falek A 1977 Use of the coping process to achieve psychological homeostasis in genetic counselling. In: Lubs H A, de la Cruz F (eds) Genetic Counselling, Raven Press, New York. ch 2, p 179

Ferguson-Smith M A 1979 Maternal age specific incidence of chromosome aberrations at amniocentesis. In: Murken J D, Stengel-Rutkowski S, Schwinger E (eds) Prenatal Diagnosis, Stuttgart, Enke. ch 1, p 1

Grouchy J de 1976 Human chromosomes and their anomalies. In: Barltrop D (ed) Aspects of Genetics in Paediatrics, Fellowship of Postgraduate Medicine, Lond. ch 1, p 5

Kaosaar M E, Mikelsaar A-V N 1973 Chromosome investigation in married couples with repeated spontaneous abortions. Humangenetik 17: 277–283

Kessler S 1979 The genetic counsellor as psychotherapist. In: Lappe M, Twiss S B, Capron A, Murray R, Powledge T (eds) Genetic Counselling: facts, values and norms. Plenum Press, Miami

Kim H J et al 1975 Cytogenetics of fetal wastage. New England Journal of Medicine 293: 844–847

Leonard C O, Chase G A, Childs B 1972 Genetic counselling: a consumers' view. New England Journal of Medicine 287: 433–439

Lippman-Hand A, Clarke Fraser F 1979a Genetic counselling: provision and reception of information. American Journal of Medical Genetics 3: 113–127

Lippman-Hand A, Clarke Fraser F 1979b Genetic counselling – the post-counselling period: 11. Making reproductive choices. American Journal of Medical Genetics 4: 73–87

McCollum A T, Silverberg R L 1979 Psychosocial Advocacy. In: Hsia Y E, Hirschhorn K, Silverberg R L, Godmilow L (eds) Counselling in Genetics, Alan R Liss, Inc, New York, ch 11, p 239

Mikkelsen M 1979 Previous child with Down syndrome and other chromosome aberration. In: Murken J D, Stengel-Rutkowski S, Schwinger E (eds) Prenatal Diagnosis, Stuttgart, Enke. ch 2, p 22

Nielsen J 1975 Chromosome examination of newborn children. Purpose and ethical aspects. Humangenetik 26: 215

Pearn J H 1973 Patients' subjective interpretation of risks offered in genetic counselling. Journal of Medical Genetics 10: 129–134

Pearn J H 1979 Decision-making and reproductive choice. In: Hsia Y E, Hirschhorn K, Silverberg R L, Godmilow L (eds) Counselling in Genetics, Alan R Liss Inc., New York, ch 10, p 223

Reynolds B DeV, Puck M H, Robinson A 1974 Genetic counselling: an appraisal. Clinical Genetics 5: 177–187

Trimble B K, Baird P A 1978 Maternal age and Down syndrome: age specific incidence rates by single year intervals. American Journal of Medical Genetics 2: 1–5

100

Newborn genetic screening

R.W. Erbe and G.R. Boss

INTRODUCTION

Genetic screening is a search in a population for persons that possess genotypes which (1) are associated with disease or predispose to disease, (2) may lead to disease in their descendants, or (3) produce other variations not known to be associated with disease (Committee for the Study of Inborn Errors of Metabolism, 1975). Genetic screening thus serves several objectives. First, screening can lead to therapy. Newborn screening aims at the earliest possible recognition of disorders in order to intervene. Sometimes this intervention includes effective treatment to prevent the most serious consequences of the disorder, although such therapy is presently available for only a small proportion of the several thousand known genetic disorders. Second, screening can identify those individuals and couples whose pregnancies are at increased risk for producing offspring with serious genetic abnormalities. With effective therapy so limited the current approach in many instances is towards preventing the birth of affected individuals through genetic counselling including prenatal genetic diagnosis and selective abortion. Such screening is usually directed at reproductive-age persons either prior to or during pregnancy. This approach recognizes the fact that an overwhelming proportion of the genes for lethal, recessively inherited disorders are present in asymptomatic carriers who will continue to give birth to affected offspring unless they are identified prospectively and made aware of their risks and reproductive alternatives. Third, genetic screening can be a source of epidemiological data regarding birth defects.

The primary focus of this chapter is newborn genetic screening for inborn errors of metabolism as is presently performed in the relatively comprehensive programme of the Commonwealth of Massachusetts. The nature and number of newborn screening tests vary widely in different localities and may include some or all of the following: (1) prenatal (maternal) blood, (2) cord blood, (3) newborn nursery blood, (4) newborn follow-up blood and/or (5) newborn follow-up urine. In addition to tests for classical inborn errors of metabolism newborn genetic screening may include tests for some or all of the following genetic disorders: congenital hypothyroidism, haemoglobinopathies, α_1-antitrypsin deficiency, cystic fibrosis, Duchenne muscular dystrophy, hyperlipidaemia, adenosine deaminase deficiency and congenital adrenal hyperplasia.

HISTORICAL ASPECTS

Genetic screening as we know it dates from the 1960s. However, as early as 1908 Sir Archibald Garrod stated that inborn errors of metabolism could be recognized '...by some strikingly unusual appearance of surface tissues or of excreta, by the excretion of some substance which responds to a test habitually applied in the routine of clinical work, or by giving rise to obvious morbid symptoms' (Garrod, 1908). These principles were first applied on a population-wide basis to phenylketonuria (PKU). In 1934 Folling had described the association of phenylketonuria with mental retardation (Folling, 1934) while the possibility that diets low in phenylalanine might prevent the associated mental retardation was suggested subsequently (Tourian & Sidbury, 1978). Although testing for amino acid disorders initially relied on urine (Dent, 1946), it soon became clear that the analysis of blood provided a more effective means for detecting PKU in newborns. In 1962 Guthrie described a bacterial growth inhibition assay for measuring blood phenylalanine concentration that required only a few drops of blood spotted on filter paper and dried (Levy, 1973). After a successful field trial in Massachusetts (MacCready & Hussey, 1964) screening for PKU by the Guthrie assay expanded widely in the United States and abroad at a time when important gaps still existed in knowledge regarding diagnosis and management of PKU (Committee for the Study of Inborn Errors of Metabolism, 1975). Guthrie subsequently introduced microbiological assays to screen for maple syrup urine disease, histidinaemia and galactosaemia (Guthrie, 1964). At about the same time, paper chromatographic methods for urinary amino acid analysis were introduced in several screening programmes (Berry et al, 1959; Efron et al, 1964; Scriver et al, 1964).

Since the mid-1970s, newborn genetic screening for PKU and often other inborn errors has continued on a wide scale in the US and elsewhere mainly using dried blood. Although nearly all states in the US screen for PKU, the programmes in different localities vary rather widely, and it is essential that persons concerned with genetics determine what genetic screening tests are being performed in a particular area. The radioimmunoassay for congenital hypothyroidism developed in 1974 by Dussault has been added to many newborn programmes. Moreover, new tests are still being proposed and introduced.

Screening for genetic disorders other than inborn errors of metabolism was initiated early in the 1970s. Much early experience in carrier screening and counselling was gained from programmes focusing on Tay-Sachs disease. This disorder is almost ideally suited to genetic screening because of its uniformly fatal course, the lack of effective therapy, the potential for accurate carrier state diagnosis, and the availability of valid in utero detection. The programme begun in the Baltimore-Washington area by Kaback (see chapter elsewhere in this volume) provided an early model. Screening was generally preceded by educational programmes which enlisted voluntary community participation and were directed at reproductive-age adults. A number of large-scale programmes began to screen for sickle cell trait and sickle cell anaemia in older children and adults, and several programmes screened newborns for chromosome disorders. In contrast haemoglobinopathy screening programmes were very heterogeneous and many problems arose. Many of the programmes were too small or had little guidance from physicians. Laws that mandated testing and specified the activities of the programmes were passed in several states beginning in 1971. These laws generally made no provision for prior education, informed consent, diagnostic accuracy, or genetic counselling during screening. Although some individuals and groups had spoken out earlier in opposition to PKU screening laws, the public and professional controversies that erupted in response to haemoglobinopathy screening were even more vocal and widespread. Two milestones in the analysis of issues in genetic screening were a short report by the Research Group on Ethical, Social and Legal Issues in Genetic Counselling and Genetic Engineering(1972) and the detailed report by the Committee for the Study of Inborn Errors of Metabolism, National Research Council, National Academy of Sciences (1975). Although the controversies over issues are presently less apparent, some programmes continue to operate with flawed designs and in violation of important principles discussed in these two reports.

NEWBORN METABOLIC SCREENING

Collection of specimens

Many screening programmes in the US and other countries test only newborn blood specimens. Most larger programmes in the US test newborns for disorders in addition to PKU. Only a few laboratories screen via urine specimens, cord blood or prenatal blood specimens.

The specimens and tests used in the programme in Massachusetts are shown in Table 100.1. At delivery blood from the end of the umbilical cord is dropped onto filter paper. The samples are used to test for maternal PKU and maternal histidinaemia by means of the Guthrie bacterial inhibition assays. Newborn whole-blood specimens are collected on filter paper after heel stick after the infant has begun to ingest protein and prior to discharge from the nursery, usually day 3 to 5. Newborn urine specimens from the diaper are collected by the parents on filter paper when the infant is 3 to 4 weeks old using a kit given to them at the time the newborn leaves the hospital. Due to the differences in processing and tests performed, analyses of blood and urine are described separately in the following sections.

Table 100.1 Newborn metabolic screening in Massachusetts (modified from Levy, 1973).

Specimen	Age obtained	Test	Primary disorder
Dried blood (umbilical cord)	Birth	BIA (Phe) BIA (His)	Maternal PKU Maternal histidinaemia
Dried blood (newborn)	3–5 days	BIA (Phe) BIA (Leu) BIA (Met) Paigen test Radioimmunoassay (T$_4$)	PKU MSUD Homocystinuria Galactosaemia Congenital hypothyroidism
Dried urine	3–4 weeks	Efron unidimensional paper chromatography	Aminoacidurias and organic acid disorders

BIA = bacterial inhibition assay of Guthrie

Blood

Analysis of blood specimens

In the laboratory small discs are punched out of the blood-impregnated filter paper. For the Guthrie-type bacterial inhibition tests, the discs are placed on agar gels that contain a test strain of bacteria. The principle of the test is that the inhibition of bacterial growth by a toxic compound can be reversed in a competitive manner by the presence of a structurally similar physiological compound. The Guthrie PKU test uses a strain of *B. subtilis* sensitive to beta-2-thienylalanine. The growth inhibition produced by this compound can be reversed by phenylalanine, phenylpyruvic acid or phenyllactic acid. The bacteria are mixed with agar and the toxic compound and poured into a plate. The disc containing blood (or urine) to be tested is placed on the agar with as many as 150 such discs per plate (Fig. 100.1). The amount of bacterial growth is directly proportional to the amounts of phenylalanine, phenylpyruvic acid or phenyllactic acid present in the blood or other physiological fluid with the actual concentrations estimated by comparison with a series of standards in the centre of the plate. Similar bacterial inhibition assays developed by Guthrie are used in screening programmes to measure the concentrations of leucine for maple syrup urine disease, of histidine for histidinaemia, of methionine for one of the three aetiologies of homocystinuria and of tyrosine for tyrosinaemia (Table 100.2). A bacterial inhibition assay for lysine to detect hyperlysinaemia has not been used in screening. In general the tests devised by Guthrie are sensitive, reliable and not subject to interference by other compounds, not even antibiotics.

Increased concentrations of galactose in physiological fluids can be detected by means of a direct inhibition assay developed by Guthrie in which a galactose-1-phosphate uridyltransferase-deficient strain of *E. coli* is killed when galactose or galactose-1-phosphate or both are present in the specimen being tested. In contrast to the

Table 100.2 Guthrie bacterial inhibition assays.

Compound detected	Disorder
Phenylalanine	Phenylketonuria
	Hyperphenylalaninaemic states
Leucine	Maple syrup urine disease
Histidine	Histidinaemia
Galactose	Galactosaemia
Methionine	Homocystinuria (one type, due to cystathionine synthase deficiency)
	Liver disease
Tyrosine	Tyrosinaemia
	Liver disease

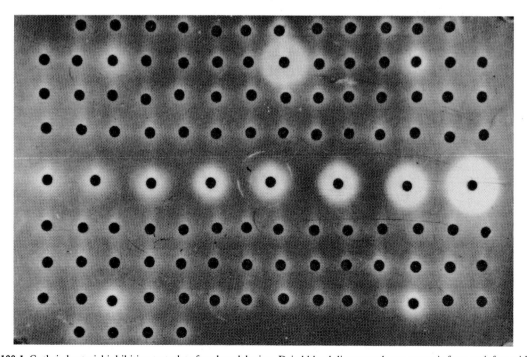

Fig. 100.1 Guthrie bacterial inhibition test plate for phenylalanine. Dried blood disc towards top centre is from an infant with phenylketonuria. The bacterial growth surrounding this disc is in response to a phenylalanine concentration greater than 20 mg/dl. The centre row of discs consists of standard specimens containing concentrations of phenylalanine ranging from 2 mg/dl on the far left to 50 mg/dl on the far right. (Reprinted from Levy (1973) with permission).

Guthrie bacterial inhibition assays noted above, a positive result in the Guthrie test for galactosaemia consists of the absence of bacterial growth around the specimen. A disadvantage of this test is the tendency of the transferase-deficient strain of *E. coli* on which it depends to lose its sensitivity to galactose (Levy & Hammersen, 1978). In contrast, the assay introduced by Paigen et al 1982 uses a strain of *E. coli* blocked in the galactose pathway. In the presence of galactose these bacteria resist lysis by a particular bacteriophage. Like the Guthrie assay discs of dried blood are surrounded on the plate by bacterial growth in direct proportion to the blood galactose concentration. Since it measures both galactose and, when alkaline phosphatase is added, galactose-1-phosphate, this test detects galactosaemia due to transferase deficiency, kinase deficiency or epimerase deficiency and the procedure is technically simple. On the other hand, false positives may occur due to nongalactosaemic liver disease or other causes.

Another useful test employs blood eluted from a dried specimen to measure the activity of the enzyme, galactose-1-phosphate uridyltransferase, the enzyme deficient in classical galactosaemia (Beutler & Baluda, 1966). Similar tests were subsequently devised for other enzymes, notably glucose-6-phosphate dehydrogenase, pyruvate kinase and glutathione reductase. These assays require that the enzymes remain active for several days after the blood has been applied to the filter paper and that enough enzyme activity is present in a drop of blood to permit accurate measurement. The blood is eluted from the filter paper strip and the transferase or other activity measured by means of the fluorescence of NADPH. False positive results are quite frequent in the transferase assay and are often due to inactivation by heat and humidity, a greater problem in warm environments. In view of the relative strengths and weaknesses, it is probably best to combine initial screening by means of a galactose metabolic assay with follow up using the Beutler transferase assay.

Confirmatory tests
It must be emphasized that a single abnormal screening test result does not establish a specific diagnosis. Screening tests usually differ from diagnostic tests in regard to sensitivity, specificity and other important characteristics. The abnormality reflected by the positive screening test result may have more than one possible genetic or nongenetic cause, and the aetiology in each particular case must be ascertained. Moreover, transient abnormalities and artifacts must be distinguished.

Confirmation of PKU, galactosaemia and other inborn errors of metabolism requires additional blood specimens as well as urine testing. If these further tests yield abnormal results, specific diagnostic evaluation must be carried out before an appropriate plan of management can be formulated.

Disorders and conditions detected by newborn blood screening

The estimated frequencies of metabolic disorders or conditions detectable by newborn blood screening are listed in Table 100.3. Although detailed description of these disorders is beyond the scope of this chapter, aspects especially pertinent to screening are considered below.

PKU and hyperphenylalaninaemias
As in many inherited disorders, the detection of a primary abnormality, hyperphenylalaninaemia, requires the consideration of a spectrum of genetic heterogeneity before proper diagnosis and management are possible. The failure to appreciate that several disorders as well as benign metabolic conditions can cause hyperphenylalaninaemia was a serious early problem in newborn metabolic screening (Committee for the Study of Inborn Errors of Metabolism, 1975; Erbe, 1981).

Upon detection of hyperphenylalaninaemia, the several aetiologies that must be distinguished include (1) transient hyperphenylalaninaemia, (2) persistent non-PKU hyperphenylalaninaemia, (3) classical PKU, (4) dihydropteridine reductase deficiency and (5) biopterin synthesis deficiency. The phenylalanine concentration in newborn blood is normally less than 2 mg/dl. The Guthrie bacterial inhibition test is positive when the phenylalanine concentration exceeds 2 mg/dl. The diagnosis of classical PKU is generally assigned when (a) blood phenylalanine concentrations are 20 mg/dl or greater in follow-up specimens while the infant is ingesting a diet normal for age and (b) tyrosine concentration in blood is no greater than 5 mg/dl. Urinary concentrations of phenylalanine and its metabolites, such as orthohydroxyphenylacetic acid, may also be elevated in these infants. When these criteria are met a low-phenylalanine diet should be instituted promptly in order to prevent the mental retardation seen in untreated PKU. The rationale for confirming this diagnosis by a phenylalanine challenge as

Table 100.3 Frequencies of some metabolic disorders and conditions detected by screening newborn blood.

Disorder or condition	Frequency
Hyperphenylalaninaemias	
PKU	1 : 13 000
Other hyperphenylalaninaemia	1 : 20 000
Galactosaemia	1 : 50 000
Maple syrup urine disease	1 : 170 000
Hypermethioninaemia	
(homocystinuria)	1 : 200 000
Hereditary tyrosinaemia	Very low

well as a protocol for that purpose have been recommended for all patients three months after initial diagnosis (O'Flynn et al, 1980).

Classical PKU is due to deficiency of hepatic phenylalanine hydroxylase and must be distinguished from two other types of block in the phenylalanine hydroxylating system which are characterized by hyperphenylalaninaemia with progressive neurological deterioration despite a low phenylalanine diet (Smith et al, 1975; Kaufman et al, 1975). The continued deterioration despite successful lowering of blood phenylalanine concentration by altering the diet has led to the designation 'malignant hyperphenylalaninaemia' for these disorders. In one of these, dihydropteridine reductase (DHPR) deficiency, the regeneration of tetrahydrobiopterin is disrupted, thereby interfering with the conversion of phenylalanine to tyrosine. In addition, the conversion of tyrosine to DOPA and tryptophan to 5-hydroxytryptophan (and to serotonin), are also decreased, thus disrupting neurotransmitter synthesis as one important consequence. Similarly, one or more inherited deficiencies of enzymes in the pathway of biopterin synthesis also cause deficient hydroxylation of these three amino acids. Since the degrees of hyperphenylalaninaemia and the clinical pictures of classical PKU, dihydropteridine reductase deficiency and biopterin synthesis deficiency are similar during the newborn period, accurate diagnosis requires a combination of in vivo and in vitro tests (Scriver & Clow, 1980 a &b). Although phenylalanine hydroxylase activity is measurable only in the liver, dihyropteridine reductase can be assayed in white blood cells and in cultured skin fibroblasts and amniotic fluid cells (Kaufman et al, 1975).

Hyperphenylalaninaemias not due to PKU or defects in tetrahydrobiopterin formation are generally associated with less elevation of the plasma phenylalanine concentration, are transient, disappear in the first months of life, and require no specific therapy (O'Flynn et al, 1980). In most instances the hyperphenylalaninaemia is accompanied by transient hypertyrosinaemia.

It has been emphasized that all hyperphenylalaninaemic subjects identified in newborn screening programmes must be appropriately studied to distinguish those with malignant phenotypes due to blocks in tetrahydrobiopterin generation from the 97–99 per cent of subjects who will either respond to low-phenylalanine diets or who need no treatment (Danks et al, 1979; Scriver & Clow, 1980 a & b).

Although most newborns with PKU have plasma phenylalanine concentrations above 12 mg/dl when first tested, occasional phenylketonuric newborns have much milder elevations on initial testing, especially if prior protein intake is low or the infant is discharged early from the nursery. Accordingly, concerns about possible false negative initial PKU tests were raised and arrangements

for retesting recommended. Sepe et al (1979) surveyed by questionnaire the results of routine follow-up blood screening of infants for PKU in the 13 states that conduct such studies. Some 2 382 300 routine follow-up blood specimens were obtained from infants aged two to six weeks, and 11 of these infants, or 1:217 000, were found to have persistent hyperphenylalaninaemia not detected by the initial newborn screening. Seven of these infants had milder forms of hyperphenylalaninaemia that did not require treatment while four had PKU. This analysis of follow-up blood specimens showed that additional cases of PKU were detected at a frequency of 1:596 000 which increased the cost for each PKU case found to $263 000 or 30 times the $8700 cost of identifying a PKU infant by routine screening. The survey clearly indicated that incomplete testing poses a problem. Based on the observed compliance rate of 80 per cent for initial testing, it was estimated that some 640 000 infants each year in the US are not tested and 54 of these would have PKU.

As another approach to evaluate the effectiveness of newborn PKU screening, subsequently-born sibs of children with PKU or mild hyperphenylalaninaemia were followed prospectively (Meryash et al, 1981). Each of the 16 infants with PKU and one of two with mild hyperphenylalaninaemia had an elevated blood phenylalanine concentration detectable by the Guthrie assay within the first one to two days after birth. This early detection was possible despite the fact that three of the 16 infants had been breast fed and three had ingested neither milk nor formula. It seems likely from these and other studies that the instances of unrecognized cases of PKU result mainly from failure to be screened and from human error.

Maternal PKU can be detected by cord blood or prenatal testing. The importance of this condition stems from the occurrence of mental retardation in the nonphenylketonuric offspring of mothers with PKU. Lenke and Levy (1980) collected data on 524 pregnancies in 155 women having PKU or other forms of hyperphenylalaninaemia. A higher rate of spontaneous abortion was found and, moreover, the 423 live-born offspring showed a marked increase in the frequencies of mental retardation, microcephaly and congenital heart disease. Indeed, of mothers having blood phenylalanine concentrations of 20 mg/dl or greater, one or more of their children was mentally retarded in 95 per cent of instances. It is not clear at present what constitutes appropriate prenatal dietary therapy or whether therapy would prevent fetal damage.

Galactosaemia

At least three disorders of galactose metabolism are detectable in newborn screening. They are appropriate targets for newborn screening because of the need for early intervention. The most frequent of these disorders is classical galactosaemia due to deficiency of galactose-1-phosphate uridyl transferase which is normally present in most tissues including liver, skin fibroblasts and red blood cells (Segal, 1978). In this disorder transferase activity is undetectable and the untreated clinical course is characterized by failure to thrive, jaundice, hepatomegaly and often death in infancy, especially due to *E. coli* sepsis (Levy et al, 1977). Untreated infants who survive develop mental retardation, cirrhosis and cataracts. Early diagnosis can lead to effective treatment and hence screening is needed. Moreover, even when the infant is obviously ill, the correct diagnosis of this rare inborn error of metabolism is made infrequently by the primary physicians so that identification by screening is essential.

Several variant forms of transferase deficiency have been described (Segal, 1978). In the so-called Negro variant, low but detectable levels of transferase activity are present in liver and spleen but not erythrocytes, and the clinical course is milder. Variants such as Rennes and Indiana are associated with some or all of the serious clinical abnormalities, while the Duarte variant is characterized by diminished erythrocyte transferase activity or altered electrophoretic mobility without clinical abnormalities.

The other causes of galactosaemia are galactokinase deficiency and uridine diphosphate galactose-4-epimerase deficiency. These are much less frequent than transferase deficiency galactosaemia. Galactokinase deficiency leads to cataract formation in older untreated patients without other evidence of galactose toxicity while epimerase deficiency appears unassociated with any clinical abnormalities. Treatment of galactosaemia due to either transferase deficiency or galactokinase deficiency aims at rigorous exclusion of galactose from the diet and if instituted early is effective in preventing most or all of the serious clinical abnormalities (Segal, 1978).

Cystathionine β-synthase deficiency

The screening of nearly 20 million newborns by the Guthrie bacterial inhibition assay for methionine has led to the detection of approximately 100 infants with cystathionine synthase deficient homocystinuria. This form of homocystinuria results from an autosomal recessively inherited deficiency of cystathionine β-synthase which condenses L-homocysteine and L-serine to cystathionine using pyridoxal-5'-phosphate as a cofactor. Deficiency of this enzyme may result in clinical abnormalities that include mental retardation, ectopia lentis, vascular obstruction and musculoskeletal abnormalities. Treatment includes a low-methionine diet and pharmacological doses of pyridoxine (Mudd & Levy, 1978).

Some cases of cystathionine synthase deficiency have escaped detection by newborn screening and this has raised concerns about possible slow rises in blood methionine (Levy, 1973). The blood methionine concentration may not exceed normal (2 mg/dl) until after the first week of life in cystathionine synthase deficient infants, whereas elevations of 4 mg/dl or greater detected at 1–2 months of age are usually transient and related to a high-protein diet in healthy infants (Levy, 1973). Other causes of hypermethioninaemia include liver disease, tyrosinaemia (see below) and, very rarely, methionine adenosyltransferase deficiency (Mudd & Levy, 1978). Other important causes of homocystinuria and homocystinaemia are due to defects in the metabolism and use of folates and cobalamins that block the transmethylation of homocysteine to methionine. Thus, although the concentrations of homocystine and related compounds are increased in blood and urine, the concentration of methionine is low or normal, so that transmethylation disorders escape detection by assays that detect hypermethioninaemia.

Maple syrup urine disease

Use of the Guthrie bacterial inhibition assay for leucine has allowed detection of some instances of maple syrup urine disease (MSUD). This disorder results from deficient activity of one or more enzymes involved in the oxidative decarboxylation of the α-keto acid derivatives of leucine, isoleucine and valine (Dancis & Levitz, 1978). Although apparently healthy at birth, the newborn begins to feed poorly by the end of the first week. This is followed by vomiting, lethargy, muscular hypertonicity, seizures, coma and death. A distinctive urinary odour resembling maple syrup accompanies the clinical abnormalities. With dramatic severity, the clinical illness can lead to death before the true nature of the disorder is recognized. Levy (1973) has suggested that MSUD may be underdiagnosed because the acute episode may lead to a fatal delay in submission of the appropriate specimens for screening. Attempts at treatment have involved complicated diets which have been partially successful (Dancis & Levitz, 1978). Several variants of MSUD with milder clinical and biochemical abnormalities have been described (Dancis & Levitz, 1978). A transient elevation (6 mg/dl or greater) of the blood leucine concentration occurs in 0.1–0.2 percent of newborns screened.

Hereditary tyrosinaemia

In at least 1–2 per cent of infants the blood tyrosine concentration exceeds 5 mg/dl at some time during the first three months of life and the frequency is even higher in prematures (Levy, 1973). Accordingly, this is the most frequent amino acid abnormality encountered in screening. Such transient tyrosinaemia usually disappears spontaneously within a few weeks although its disappearance can sometimes be promoted by administering vitamin C or with a low-protein diet (La Du & Gjessing, 1978).

Persistent tyrosinaemia can be caused by at least two inherited disorders. First, hereditary tyrosinaemia is an autosomal recessively inherited disorder in which the primary enzyme defect is unknown. This disorder has been recognized most frequently in the Quebec province of Canada. It is characterized by a complex set of clinical and laboratory abnormalities including hepatosplenomegaly, nodular hepatic cirrhosis often with hepatoma formation, disturbed tyrosine and methionine metabolism with marked *p*-hydroxyphenyllactic aciduria (termed tyrosyluria) and renal tubular defects resulting in hyperphosphaturia, rickets, mellituria, proteinuria and a generalized aminoaciduria of a distinct type (La Du & Gjessing, 1978). Dietary treatment has been attempted with limited success.

The second hereditary disorder is termed persistent tyrosinaemia and has been diagnosed in only a few patients (La Du & Gjessing, 1978). Blood tyrosine concentrations are 20–50 mg/dl on an unrestricted diet. Mental retardation is present in all cases but hepatic and renal disease are absent. Over 1.7 million newborns in six countries were screened without finding a single instance of persistent tyrosinaemia and thus either the frequency is very low or the rise in the blood tyrosine concentration is delayed (Levy, 1973).

Other inherited disorders, particularly transferase deficiency galactosaemia and fructosaemia, also called hereditary fructose intolerance, due to deficient fructose-1-phosphate aldolase, lead to persistent elevation of the blood tyrosine concentration. Both of these disorders elevate blood tyrosine concentration by deleterious effects on hepatic metabolism. Indeed, liver disease of any aetiology can elevate the blood tyrosine concentration and thus either tyrosinaemia or hypermethioninaemia may signal liver disease.

Urine

Analysis of urine specimens

Filter paper urine specimens can be analyzed either by unidimensional paper chromatography (Efron et al 1964; Levy et al, 1980) as in Massachusetts and New South Wales, Australia, or by unidimensional thin-layer chromatography as in Quebec, Canada. In the Massachusetts programme two $\frac{1}{4}$ inch diameter discs are punched out of each filter paper, one of these being analyzed for amino acids by overnight descending chromatography and ninhydrin stain for amino acids while the other is analyzed for methylmalonic acid by six hour ascending chromatography developed with *o*-dianisidine reagent (Levy et al, 1980). Each sheet of chromatography paper accommodates 25 specimens plus appropriate reference standards. The identification, analysis and interpretation of suspected abnormalities have been described in detail (Levy et al, 1980), as have the procedures for follow-up and management.

Confirmatory tests

A variety of confirmatory tests are available depending on the specific disorder or condition suspected. These include spot tests of urine for specific compounds, two-dimensional chromatography, electrophoresis and gas chromatography-mass spectrometry. Tests of blood and specific enzyme assays of fluids or cells may also be appropriate.

Disorders and conditions detected by newborn urine specimens

Parents are requested to submit a filter paper urine sample at age 3–4 weeks in the Massachusetts programme and at age 2 weeks in the Quebec programme (Levy et al, 1980). A major goal in screening urine at a later age than that at which newborn blood was collected was to diminish the frequency of false positives due to transient amino acid disturbances. Several transient amino acid abnormalities remain at 3–4 weeks, especially iminoglycinuria and cystinuria/lysinuria, but these usually disappear by age 3 months. In the Massachusetts programme the compliance rate averages 75 per cent. About one per cent of the specimens are inadequate for testing because, for example, they contain insufficient urine or are contaminated with diaper cream or faeces. Detailed analysis of urine screening of 108 353 newborns in the Massachusetts programme during 1976–1977 showed that (a) 20 per cent had been reanalyzed by unidimensional chromatography, (b) 27 per cent had been further analyzed by some special chromatography procedure, (c) 4 per cent were reanalyzed for methylmalonic acid, (d) 3 per cent were analyzed by two-dimensional sequential paper chromatography and (e) in 2 per cent a repeat sample was sought, half because of specimen inadequacy and half because of a suspected abnormality. Importantly, this expensive reanalysis and retesting failed to detect a single infant with a clinically significant disorder not already strongly suspected from the testing of the original filter paper urine specimen. Indeed, although newborn urine screening provides important epidemiologic and medical information, the failure of the programme as now conducted to identify treatable disorders has led to a question of its worth as a service (Levy et al, 1980). Analysis of the programme in Australia leads to similar conclusions (Wilcken et al, 1980).

The frequencies of some metabolic disorders and conditions detected by screening newborn urine are listed in Table 100.4. In several cases, including instances not listed in the table, newborn urinary screening yields abnormal results but incomplete information is available about the natural history, possible medical significance and management. Examples of such findings of uncertain significance include cystathioninaemia, hyperlysinaemia and sarcosinaemia. Several conditions detected are prob-

Table 100.4 Frequencies of some metabolic disorders and conditions detected by screening newborn urine.

Disorder or condition	Frequency
Cystinuria	1 : 8000
Iminoglycinuria	1 : 12 000
Histidinaemia	1 : 20 000
Hartnup disease	1 : 25 000
Methylmalonic aciduria	1 : 50 000
Cystathioninuria	1 : 70 000
Argininosuccinic aciduria	1 : 90 000
Hyperglycaemia, nonketotic	1 : 180 000
Hyperprolinaemia	1 : 200 000

ably benign including iminoglycinuria, Hartnup amino-aciduria and hyperprolinaemia. Treatable disorders detected by newborn urine screening include argininosuccinic acidaemia, methylmalonic aciduria and the Fanconi syndrome. Three of the disorders or conditions in Table 100.4 involve defects in renal transport rather than inborn errors of metabolism, viz., cystinuria, iminoglycinuria and Hartnup aminoaciduria. In most other disorders involving aminoaciduria an extrarenal metabolic disturbance leads to accumulation in plasma of one or more amino acids which are filtered in amounts that exceed the reabsorption capacity of the nephron.

Certain features of specific conditions and disorders are described briefly in the following sections.

Cystinuria

Cystinuria is the most prevalent of the urinary amino acid abnormalities with a frequency of 1:8000 newborns. Cystinuria is a genetically heterogeneous, autosomal recessively inherited disorder involving defective transport of cystine, lysine, arginine and ornithine by the epithelial cells of the renal tubule and the gastrointestinal tract. These amino acids along with cysteine-homocysteine mixed disulphide are excreted in excessive amounts in urine. Blood amino acid concentrations are not increased. Cystine, the least soluble of all the amino acids, precipitates in urine leading to formation of renal calculi with possible obstruction, infection and loss of renal function. Most cystine renal calculi become clinically apparent during the second and third decades although earlier or later initial presentations occur. Therapeutic approaches aim to prevent renal stone formation and include dietary alterations, alkalinization of urine, high volume fluid intake and the administration of penicillamine (Their & Segal, 1978).

Three genetically distinct types of cystinuria were defined by Rosenberg et al (1966). Heterozygotes for the Type I defect can be detected only by studies of intestinal absorption where they lack active transport of cystine, lysine and arginine. In contrast, urine from heterozygotes for the Type II or Type III defects contains increased amounts of the dibasic amino acids. These heterozygotes differ from each other and from Type I heterozygotes in certain other characteristics as well (Scriver & Rosenberg, 1973). While homozygotes excrete the largest quantities of cystine and dibasic amino acids, detection of the qualitative pattern compatible with cystinuria in the much more numerous Type II or Type III heterozygotes may lead to further testing of a substantial number of newborns (Levy et al, 1980).

Iminoglycinuria

Familial iminoglycinuria is an inborn error of membrane transport with persistent and marked urinary excretion of the imino acids, proline and hydroxyproline, and of glycine without other amino aciduria or altered blood amino acid concentrations. Genetic heterogeneity is suggested since some families with iminoglycinuria also show defective intestinal transport of these amino acids. Adult heterozygotes have no iminoaciduria, and may or may not have hyperglycinuria. The characteristic amino acid pattern in urine is not accompanied by any consistent clinical abnormalities, thus suggesting that familial iminoglycinuria is a benign trait (Scriver, 1978b).

False positives for the iminoglycinuric pattern are frequent in newborns. During the first few months of life newborns and infants frequently excrete imino acids and glycine in easily measurable amounts. This transient iminoglycinuria usually disappears by four to six months of age. False positives for this urinary pattern are also frequent in infants who are ill with a variety of unrelated disorders. Heterozygotes for iminoglycinuria may exhibit the iminoglycinuric pattern during the first year of life, with later disappearance of the imino acids from the urine but persistence of the hyperglycinuria. Thus accurate identification of iminoglycinuria homozygotes requires testing of urine beyond the first year of life.

Histidinaemia

Elevations of the blood histidine concentration in newborns reflect (1) transient elevations, (2) histidinaemia due to autosomal recessively inherited deficiency of L-histidine ammonia lyase or (3), as described in one family, variant or atypical histidinaemia. Transient elevation of the histidine concentration in whole blood to 6 mg/dl or greater occurs once per 200–500 infants tested and, since this is nearly as high as the 8–20 mg/dl seen in infants with histidinaemia, false positive Guthrie screening tests may result. Since increased urinary excretion of histidine and its metabolites is more pronounced than the elevated blood histidine concentration in histidinaemia, urinary screening yields a far lower false-positive rate (Levy, 1973).

The major presently unresolved question regarding histidinaemia is whether this is a benign condition or a serious disorder. Other than possible mental retardation, there are no specific clinical features that characterize histidinaemia (La Du, 1978).

Hartnup disease

Hartnup disease, named for the family in which the condition was first described, is a renal aminoaciduria involving monoamino-, monocarboxylic-amino acids with neutral or aromatic side chains. This characteristic aminoaciduria is the only consistent feature. Renal clearances are increased 5–10 fold for alanine, histidine, isoleucine, leucine, phenylalanine, serine, threonine, tryptophan and tyrosine. Asparagine and glutamine are also excreted in large quantities. The faeces contain increased amounts of the same amino acids. Blood amino acid levels are not increased. The urine also contains increased amounts of tryptophan metabolites produced by intestinal bacteria from unabsorbed tryptophan.

In contrast to the consistent urinary pattern of amino acids, clinical features are intermittent and variable. Indeed, individuals detected by screening are often asymptomatic whereas skin lesions, neurological deficits and psychological changes were described earlier in some patients. Skin lesions resemble those of dietary pellagra and involve the face and extremities. Cerebellar signs may be present but are variable and completely reversible. Symptomatic attacks can be precipitated by sunlight, fever, emotional stress or exposure to sulphonamide drugs and are more likely to occur when the nutritional status is poor. Clinical manifestations tend to become less frequent and milder with increasing age. Attempts at therapy include an adequate diet and supplementation with nicotinic acid. The prognosis for persons with Hartnup disease appears to be good (Jepson, 1978).

Hartnup disease is detected at a frequency of 1:25 000 by screening newborn urine. Transient hyperaminoacidurias of the Hartnup pattern are rare (Levy, 1973). Inheritance of Hartnup disease follows an autosomal recessive pattern and parental consanguinity is increased.

Methylmalonic aciduria

Methylmalonic aciduria is one of the most frequent of the inborn errors of organic acid metabolism and is detected in 1:50 000 newborns (Levy et al, 1980; Coulombe et al, 1981). A special stain is used on the chromatogram of urine to detect methylmalonic acid and other organic acids (Coulombe et al, 1981). Normal metabolism of methylmalonate requires the integrity of a series of apoenzymes, and the absorption and metabolic interconversion of the cobalamin derivatives required by one of these apoenzymes. At least five distinct biochemical bases for methylmalonic aciduria have been identified by means of metabolic and cell complementation studies (Rosenberg, 1978). These include methylmalonyl CoA mutase apoenzyme deficiency, two discrete defects

in the synthesis of adenosylcobalamin and defective synthesis of both adenosylcobalamin and methylcobalamin.

The chemical abnormalities associated with the first four of these defects are similar and include life-threatening or fatal ketoacidosis and hyperammonaemia appearing during the first month of life. Continued episodes of ketoacidosis are associated with failure to thrive, neurological abnormalities including mental retardation, recurrent bacterial and viral infections, osteoporosis, neutropenia, thrombocytopenia and other abnormalities. Clinical abnormalities in patients with defective synthesis of both adenosylcobalamin and methlycobalamin are distinctly different reflecting the disturbances of both methylmalonate and sulphur amino acid metabolism (Rosenberg, 1978). Metabolic studies in patients and in their cultured cells are useful in identifying the existence and nature of these various defects. Pedigree studies suggest an autosomal recessive inheritance but methods for detecting heterozygotes are lacking. Therapy with supplementary cobalamin, including prenatally, was effective in some families (Rosenberg, 1978). A low protein diet and a synthetic formula deficient in methylmalonate and propionate precursors may also be used.

The eight Massachusetts infants detected either prenatally or as neonates illustrate the heterogeneity of observed clinical courses (Coulombe et al, 1981). Two died in the newborn period, two showed a poor clinical and biochemical response to therapy, two responded to treatment and were clinically normal, and two were clinically normal without treatment despite persistence of the methylmalonic aciduria. The last two individuals had clinically normal sibs who also had methylmalonic aciduria and were presumed to have the benign forms similar to the one described by Giorgio et al (1976).

An occasional newborn is found to excrete methylmalonic acid transiently. Such methylmalonic aciduria is mild, not accompanied by clinical abnormalities and is found almost exclusively in breast-fed infants (Coulombe et al, 1981). Methylmalonic aciduria was also described with cobalamin deficiency due to pernicious anaemia or severe nutritional deficiency (Higginbottom et al, 1978). Methylmalonic aciduria accompanied by hyperglycinuria constitutes one form of ketotic hyperglycinaemia (see below).

Cystathioninuria

Cystathioninuria was detected by means of newborn urine screening at a frequency of 1:70 000 in the Massachusetts programme (Levy, 1973) but at over twice that frequency in Australia where a more sensitive method is used (Mudd and Levy, 1978). If appropriate preservation measures are not taken, cystathionine in urine may be converted by bacterial contaminants to homocyst(e)ine thus obscuring the diagnosis. Cystathioninuria, usually of mild degree, can occur transiently in newborns but generally resolves by three months of age. Cystathioninuria also has environmental causes and associations including vitamin B_6 deficiency, liver disorders of several kinds including hepatoblastoma and tumours of neural crest origin.

When cystathioninuria persists and acquired causes are ruled out, an autosomal recessively inherited deficiency of γ-cystathionase should be suspected. This hepatic enzyme uses pyridoxal-5′-phosphate as a cofactor and converts cystathionine to cysteine generating one molecule of α-ketobutyrate. Most individuals with γ-cystathionase deficiency decrease their urinary excretion of cystathionine markedly in response to pharmacological doses of vitamin B_6. These biochemical characteristics are accompanied by no consistent clinical features (Mudd & Levy, 1978). Since cystathioninuria is probably a benign metabolic trait, treatment appears not to be indicated.

Argininosuccinic aciduria
Deficiency of argininosuccinase leads to argininosuccinic aciduria, an autosomal recessively inherited disorder that occurs with a frequency of about 1:90 000 newborns. Although normally not detectable, argininosuccinate in this disorder appears in large amounts in urine, blood and cerebrospinal fluid, and the blood citrulline concentration is often 2 to 3 times normal. The increased concentration of argininosuccinate is generally directly related to protein intake but remains elevated even in the absence of symptoms. The argininosuccinate spot detected by chromatography or electrophoresis of urine is usually accompanied by two additional spots which are the anhidrides of the compound.

As part of the urea cycle, argininosuccinase normally converts argininosuccinate to arginine and fumarate. The activity is widely distributed and can be assayed in liver, erythrocytes, and cultured skin fibroblasts and amniotic fluid cells. The accumulation of argininosuccinate and the hyperammonaemia associated with this and other urea cycle disorders appears to be especially injurious to the immature brain (Shih, 1978). Recently methods have been tested to screen for other urea cycle disorders (Naylor, 1981).

Based on age of presentation and natural history, three forms of argininosuccinic aciduria can be distinguished. The late-onset type occurs most frequently with neurological abnormalities being the main feature. Feeding difficulties and vomiting may appear in infancy, followed later by seizures, intermittent ataxia and frank mental retardation. The two other clinical types exhibit a more rapid and severe course. In the neonatal type feeding problems and lethargy appear soon after birth followed by seizures, respiratory distress, coma and death within the first 10 days of life. Onset in the subacute type is

during infancy with failure to thrive, seizures and hepatomegaly.

Over one-third of the reported patients were detected by routine newborn screening. Possible treatments at that time included a low protein diet, arginine supplementation and administration of sodium benzoate (Batshaw et al, 1981). On the other hand, the practice of obtaining newborn urine at 3–4 weeks of age for analysis may preclude effective treatment of patients with the neonatal type who become acutely ill and die at an earlier age (Levy, 1973).

Hyperglycinaemia
Several pathological forms of hyperglycinuria and hyperglycinaemia must be distinguished from each other and from the hyperglycinuria without hyperglycinaemia, a frequent finding in normal newborns. Infants with both hyperglycinuria and hyperglycinaemia should be evaluated for a group of disorders of organic acid metabolism that give rise to the ketotic hyperglycinaemia syndrome. Although the exact mechanism is unknown, organic acid intermediates that accumulate because of an inborn error of organic acid metabolism apparently produce a secondary block in glycine catabolism that leads to accumulation of glycine from dietary sources and endogenous synthesis. Ketotic hyperglycinaemia presents clinically as an acute, severe illness of infancy with recurrent episodes of ketosis and acidosis often precipitated by protein intake or infection. Infants who survive may show neutropenia, thrombocytopenia, seizures and mental retardation. The most common cause of ketotic hyperglycinaemia syndrome is propionic acidaemia due to propionyl-CoA carboxylase deficiency. The syndrome can also occur with methylmalonic acidaemia, isovaleric acidaemia and a defect in isoleucine metabolism termed β-ketothiolase deficiency. A search for these disorders of organic acid metabolism is essential in any infant with hyperglycinaemia both for diagnostic accuracy and because treatment by dietary alteration is often successful.

Nonketotic hyperglycinaemia is approximately as frequent as ketotic hyperglycinaemia and differs from the latter in several important respects. Although it, too, often presents as an overwhelming illness early in life, ketosis and acidosis are absent as are organic acid intermediates from blood or urine. The glycine concentration is increased 5 or more fold in plasma, cerebrospinal fluid and brain tissue, and 10–20 fold in urine while all other amino acids are normal. As in ketotic hyperglycinaemia, conversion of the C1 of glycine to CO_2 is blocked in vivo but, in contrast to the ketotic forms, conversion of the C2 of glycine to the C3 of serine may also be blocked (Nyhan, 1978). Some patients die in infancy while many of those who survive show severe neurological abnormalities including mental retardation, seizures, opisthotonos, myoclonus and spasticity. Attempts at therapy by several approaches have reduced the plasma glycine concentration but do not cause sustained clinical improvement. In contrast, several infants with hyperglycinaemia but without evident abnormality in organic acid metabolism developed quite normally on unrestricted diets despite having elevated plasma glycine concentration (Levy, 1973). Individuals with these other forms of hyperglycinaemia have normal concentrations of glycine in cerebrospinal fluid and brain despite the fact that their plasma glycine concentration may be as high as the patients with nonketotic hyperglycinaemia. Thus, measurement of glycine concentration in cerebrospinal fluid is an effective means of determining whether or not a hyperglycinaemic patient with neurological abnormalities has glycine encephalopathy (Perry et al, 1975).

Detection by screening is more difficult in hyperglycinuric patients whose acute illness in the neonatal period leads to reduced protein intake and therefore decreased glycine excretion. Under these circumstances the glycinuria may be much less striking and resemble the amounts frequently seen in normal newborns.

Hyperprolinaemia

Hyperprolinaemia is detected by urine screening at a frequency of approximately 1:200 000 and occurs in two forms. Type I hyperprolinaemia due to a deficiency of pyrroline-5-carboxylate reductase or proline oxidase activity is probably an innocent metabolic trait despite suggestions that it is associated with hereditary nephropathy (Scriver, 1978a). Type II hyperprolinaemia due to 1-pyrroline dehydrogenase deficiency leads to more pronounced hyperprolinuria and is probably benign although an association with neurological disease has been suggested (Scriver, 1978a).

Despite the specificity of the inherited block for proline metabolism, hyperprolinaemia results in iminoglycinuria, not to be confused with familial iminoglycinuria described earlier. The increased plasma concentration of proline leads to saturation by proline of the renal transport system shared by the imino acids and glycine so that, in addition to proline, hydroxyproline and glycine also appear in elevated amounts in the urine (Scriver & Rosenberg, 1973).

OTHER NEWBORN SCREENING

Congenital hypothyroidism screening began in 1974 with the introduction by Dussault (Dussault et al, 1975) of a radioimmunoassay procedure applicable to cord blood specimens. Congenital hypothyroidism screening is now part of many programmes and has had the interesting effect of promoting regionalization of screening since the radioimmunoassays used for hypothyroidism are technically more complicated than the tests used for inborn error screening. In this procedure the initial test involves measurement of the newborn blood thyroxine (T_4) concentration. A filter paper disc of dried blood is incubated with radiolabelled T_4, anti-T_4 antibodies and an inhibitor of thyroxine binding globulin. A low blood T_4 concentration leads to greater radioactive T_4 binding by the anti-T_4 antibody and reduced amounts of unbound radioactive T_4. Following separation of the bound and unbound fractions, the measurement of radioactivity in each fraction allows estimation of the blood T_4 concentration. The procedure can be automated and the data analysis completed by computer. Commonly the detection of a T_4 value two standard deviations or more below the mean is followed by measurement of the concentration of thyroid stimulating hormone (TSH) by radioimmunoassay using another disc from the blood sample. When both a low T_4 and an elevated TSH concentration are detected, the newborn's parents and physician are advised regarding the need for additional testing and possibly treatment. This approach requires TSH testing in three percent of newborns and identifies congenital hypothyroidism in approximately 1:4–5000 newborns. Although commonly combined with newborn screening for principally genetic disorders, only a few of the aetiologies of congenital hypothyroidism are Mendelian (Stanbury, 1978; Fisher & Klein, 1981).

Screening newborns for haemoglobinopathy by cord blood haemoglobin electrophoresis (Garrick et al, 1973) is conducted in several programmes. The main objectives of this screening include the early diagnosis of sickle cell anaemia and other serious haemoglobinopathies, the collection of epidemiological data and genetic counselling. Attention is directed at those infants with a sickling disorder, rather than the heterozygotes who are too numerous to be contacted and counselled as part of such programmes. Little detailed information about the effectiveness of newborn haemoglobinopathy screening is available.

Newborn screening for cystic fibrosis has been attempted with limited success using tests of meconium or newborn faecal specimens. More recently Crossley et al (1981) introduced a method that measures the serum immunoreactive trypsin in the blood spot obtained routinely on filter paper. This approach currently appears promising and is being evaluated in a pilot programme. Many obstacles remain, however, to full usefulness in regard to genetic counselling objectives, most notably the lack of a valid test for cystic fibrosis carriers and of a prenatal diagnostic test.

Other programmes considered or begun are screening for α_1-antitrypsin deficiency (Sveger, 1978), Duchenne muscular dystrophy, adenosine deaminase deficiency (Moore & Meurissen, 1974), hyperlipidaemia (Glueck,

1980; Holtzman, 1980) and congenital adrenal hyperplasia. Their ultimate place in newborn screening programmes remains to be established.

ISSUES AND CONCERNS IN SCREENING

Most screening tests are designed to be sensitive in order to minimize false-negative results but these tests may not be specific and they are seldom diagnostic. Accurate and definitive diagnosis requires additional testing in nearly all instances. Since false negative results do occur with every screening procedure, a negative result from screening should not preclude an appropriate evaluation for a disorder suspected clinically.

Screening programmes and procedures should meet a variety of criteria both before they are implemented and continually during their operation (Committee for the Study of Inborn Errors of Metabolism, 1975). These criteria include technical, educational and organizational aspects. A high signal-to-noise ratio is needed to maximize effectiveness and minimize adverse effects. The noise in the system includes the true biological variation of the character being measured in the screened population and the variation within the testing procedure itself. As noted earlier, positive results in a screening test necessitate repeat testing with follow up and additional testing, possibly over a period of weeks or months. These can be expensive in terms of personnel, materials and parental anxiety and inconvenience. The rarer the trait being sought by screening, the higher will be the proportion of false positives.

In addition to normal biological variation and transient abnormalities, confusing artifacts are produced by contamination of blood and urine specimens with microorganisms, drugs used systemically or locally, diaper powder, food supplements and the like. Disentangling these sources of confusion and delay requires great expertise.

Finally, screening programmes should be organized and administered in such a way that they are constantly updated to incorporate the latest technical and medical advances. They must also be responsive to changes in society. The present trends towards the earlier discharge of mother and child from the hospital and the increased numbers of home births provide poignant examples of changes having major potential impact on newborn screening.

REFERENCES

Batshaw M L, Thomas G H, Brusilow S W 1981 New approaches to the diagnosis and treatment of inborn errors of urea synthesis. Pediatrics. 68: 290–297

Berry H K 1959 Procedures for testing urine specimens dried on filter paper. Clinical Chemistry 5: 603–608

Beutler E, Baluda M C 1966 A simple spot screening test for galactosemia. Journal of Laboratory and Clinical Medicine. 68: 137–141

Committee for the Study of Inborn Errors of Metabolism 1975 Genetic Screening: Programs, Principles and Research National Academy of Sciences, Washington, D.C.

Coulombe J T, Shih V E, Levy H L 1981 Massachusetts metabolic disorders screening program. II. Methylmalonic aciduria. Pediatrics 67: 26–31

Crossley J R, Smith P A, Edgar B W, Glucjman P D, Elliott R B 1981 Neonatal screening for cystic fibrosis, using immunoreactive trypsin assay in dried blood spots. Clinica Chimica Acta. 113: 111–124

Dancis J, Levitz M 1978 Abnormalities of branched chain amino acid metabolism. In: Stanbury J B, Wyngaarden J B, Fredrickson D S (eds) The Metabolic Basis of Inherited Disease. 4th edn. McGraw-Hill, New York. ch 20, p 397

Danks D M, Cotton R G H, Schlesinger P 1979 Diagnosis of malignant hyperphenylalaninemia. Archives of Diseases of Childhood 54: 329–330

Dent C E 1946 Detection of amino acids in urine and other fluids. Lancet 2: 637–639

Dussault J H, Coulombe P, Laberge C, Letarte J, Guyda H, Khoury K 1975 Preliminary report on a mass screening program for neonatal hypothyroidism. Journal of Pediatrics 86: 670–674

Efron M L, Young D, Moser H W, MacCready R A 1964 A simple chromatographic screening test for the detection of disorders of amino acid metabolism. New England Journal of Medicine 270: 1378–1383

Erbe R W 1981 Issues in newborn genetic screening. In: Bloom A D, James L S (eds) The Fetus and the the Newborn (Birth Defects Original Article Series, vol 17). Alan R. Liss, New York, p 167

Fisher D A, Klein A H 1981 Thyroid development and disorders of thyroid function in the newborn. New England Journal of Medicine 304: 702–712

Folling A 1934 Uber Ausscheidung von Phenylbrenztraubensaure in den Harn als Stoffwechselanomalie in Verbindung mit Imbezillitat. Hoppe Seyler Zeitschrift Physiologische Chemie 227: 169–176

Garrick M D, Dembure P, Guthrie 1973 Sickle-cell anemia and other hemoglobinopathies. Procedures and strategy for screening employing spots of blood on filter paper as specimens. New England Journal of Medicine 288: 1265–1268

Giorgio A J, Trowbridge M, Boone A W, Patten R S 1976 Methylmalonic aciduria without vitamin B_{12} deficiency in an adult sibship. New England Journal of Medicine 295: 310–313

Glueck C J 1980 Detection of risk factors for coronary artery disease in children: Semmelweis revisted? Pediatrics 66: 834–837

Guthrie R 1964 Routine screening for inborn errors in the newborn: "inhibition assays," "instant bacteria" and multiple tests. International Copenhagen Congress on the Scientific Study of Mental Retardation, Denmark, August 7–14.

Guthrie R, Susi A 1963 A simple phenylalanine method for detecting phenylketonuria in large populations of newborn infants. Pediatrics 32: 338–343

Higginbottom M C, Sweetman L, Nyhan W L 1978 A syndrome of methylmalonic aciduria, homocystinuria, megaloblastic anemia and neurologic abnormalities in a vitamin B_{12}-deficient breast-fed infant of a strict vegetarian. New England Journal of Medicine 299: 317–323

Holtzman N A 1978 Newborn screening for inborn errors of metabolism. Pediatric Clinics of North America 25: 25: 411–421

Holtzman N A 1980 Hyperlipidemia screening and Semmelweis re-revisited. Pediatrics 66: 838–839

Jepson J B 1978 Hartnup disease In: Stanbury J B, Wyngaarden J B, Fredrickson D S (eds) The Metabolic Basis of Inherited Disease. 4th edn. McGraw-Hill, New York. ch 66, p 1563

Kaufman S, Holtzman N A, Milstien S, Butler I J, Krumholz A 1975 Phenylketonuria due to a deficiency of dihydropteridine reductase. New England Journal of Medicine 293: 785–790

La Du B N 1978 Histidinemia. In: Stanbury J B, Wyngaarden J B, Fredrickson D S (eds) The Metabolic Basis of Inherited Disease. 4th edn. Mc-McGraw-Hill, New York. ch 15, p 317

La Du B N, Gjessing L R 1978 Tyrosinosis and tyrosinemia. In: Stanbury J B, Wyngaarden J B, Fredrickson D S (eds) The Metabolic Basis of Inherited Disease. 4th edn. McGraw-Hill, New York. ch 12, p 256

Lenke R R, Levy H L 1980 Maternal phenylketonuria and hyperphenylalaninemia: an international survey of the outcome of untreated pregnancies. New England Journal of Medicine 303: 1202–1208

Levy H L 1973 Genetic screening. In: Harris H, Hirschhorn K (eds) Advances in Human Genetics. Plenum, New York. vol 4, p 1

Levy H L 1977 Screening for genetic disorders in the newborn. In: Altman P L, Katz D D (eds) Human Health and Disease. Federation of American Societies for Experimental Biology, Bethesda p 107

Levy H L, Coulombe J T, Shih V E 1980 Newborn urine screening. In: Bickel H, Guthrie R, Hammersen G (eds) Neonatal Screening for Inborn Errors of Metabolism. Springer-Verlag, Heidelberg. p 89

Levy H L, Hammersen G 1978 Newborn screening for galactosemia and other galactose metabolic defects. Journal of Pediatrics 92: 871–877

Levy H L, Sepe S J, Shih V E, Vawter G F, Klein J O 1977 Sepsis due to Escherichia coli in neonates with galactosemia. New England Journal of Medicine 297: 823–825

MacCready R A, Hussey M G 1964 Newborn phenylketonuria detection program in Massachusetts. American Journal of Public Health 54: 2075–2081

Meryash D L, Levy H L, Guthrie R, Warner R, Bloom S, Carr J R 1981 Prospective study of early neonatal screening for phenylketonuria. New England Journal of Medicine 304: 294–296

Moore E C, Meuwissen H J 1974 Screening for ADA deficiency. Journal of Pediatrics 85: 802–804

Mudd S H, Levy H L 1978 Disorders of transsulfuration. In: Stanbury J B, Wyngaarden J B, Fredrickson D S (eds) The Metabolic Basis of Inherited Disease. 4th edn. McGraw-Hill, New York. ch 23, p 458

Naylor E W 1981 Newborn screening for urea cycle disorders. Pediatrics. 68: 453–457

Nyhan W L 1978 Nonketotic hyperglycinemia. In: Stanbury J B, Wyngaarden J B, Fredrickson D S (eds) The

Metabolic Basis of Inherited Disease. 4th edn. McGraw-Hill, New York. ch 26, p 518

O'Flynn M E, Holtzman N A, Blaskovics M, Azen C, Williamson M L 1980 The diagnosis of phenylketonuria. A report from the collaborative study of children treated for phenylketonuria. American Journal of Diseases of Children 134: 769–774

Paigen K, Pacholec S, Levy H L 1982 A new method of screening neonates for galactosemia and other galactose metabolic defects. Journal of Laboratory and Clinical Investigation 99: 895–907

Perry T L, Urquhart N, MacLean J, Evans M E, Hansen S, Davidson A G F, Applegarth D A, MacLeod P J, Lock J E 1975 Nonketotic hyperglycinemia. Glycine accumulation due to absence of glycine cleavage in brain. New England Journal of Medicine 292: 1269–1273

Research Group on Ethical, Social and Legal Issues in Genetic Counseling and Genetic Engineering 1972 Ethical and social issues in screening for genetic disease. New England Journal of Medicine 286: 1129–1132

Rosenberg L E 1978 Disorders of propionate, methylmalonate, and cobalamin metabolism. In: Stanbury J B, Wyngaarden J B, Fredrickson D S (eds) The Metabolic Basis of Inherited Disease. 4th edn. McGraw-Hill, New York. ch 21, p 411

Schneider J A, Schulman J D, Seegmiller J E 1978 Cystinosis and the Fanconi syndrome. In: Stanbury J B, Wyngaarden J B, Fredrickson D S (eds) The Metabolic Basis of Inherited Disease. 4th edn. McGraw-Hill, New York. ch 72, p 1660

Scriver C R 1978a Disorders of proline and hydroxyproline metabolism. In: Stanbury J B, Wyngaarden J B, Fredrickson D S (eds) The Metabolic Basis of Inherited Disease. 4th edn. McGraw-Hill, New York. ch 17, p 336

Scriver C R 1978b Familial iminoglycinuria. In: Stanbury J B, Wyngaarden J B, Fredrickson D S (eds) The Metabolic Basis of Inherited Disease. 4th edn. McGraw-Hill, New York. ch 68, p 1593

Scriver C R, Clow C L 1980a Phenylketonuria and other phenylalanine hydroxylation mutants in man. Annual Review of Genetics 14: 179–202

Scriver C R, Clow C L 1980b Phenylketonuria: epitome of human biochemical genetics. New England Journal of Medicine 303: 1336–1342 and 1394–1400

Scriver C R, Davies E, Cullen A M 1964 Application of a simple micromethod to the screening of plasma for a variety of aminoacidopathies. Lancet 2: 230–232

Scriver C R, Rosenberg L E 1973 Amino Acid Metabolism and Its Disorders. W.B. Saunders Company, New York

Segals S 1978 Disorders of galactose metabolism. In: Stanbury J B, Wyngaarden J B, Fredrickson D S (eds) The Metabolic Basis of Inherited Disease. 4th edn. McGraw-Hill, New York. ch 8, p 160

Sepe S J, Levy H L, Mount F W 1979 An evaluation of routine follow-up blood screening of infants for phenylketonuria. New England Journal of Medicine 300: 606–609

Shih V E 1978 Urea cycle disorders and other congenital hyperammonemic syndromes. In: Stanbury J B, Wyngaarden J B, Fredrickson D S (eds) The Metabolic Basis of Inherited Disease. 4th edn. McGraw-Hill, New York. ch 18, p 362

Smith I, Clayton B E, Wolff O H 1975 New variant of phenylketonuria with progressive neurological illness unresponsive to phenylalanine restriction. Lancet 1: 1108–1111

Stanbury J B 1978 Familial goiter. In: Stanbury J B,

Wyngaarden J B, Fredrickson D S (eds) The Metabolic
Basis of Inherited Disease. 4th edn. McGraw-Hill, New
York. ch 10, p 206

Sveger T 1978 α_1-Antitrypsin deficiency in early childhood.
Pediatrics 62: 22–25

Their S O, Segal S 1978 Cystinuria. In: Stanbury J B,
Wyngaarden J B, Fredrickson D S (eds) The Metabolic
Basis of Inherited Disease. 4th edn. McGraw-Hill, New
York. ch 67, p 1578

Tourian A Y, Sidbury J B 1978 Phenylketonuria. In:
Stanbury J B, Wyngaarden J B, Fredrickson D S (eds)
The Metabolic Basis of Inherited Disease. 4th edn.
McGraw-Hill, New York. ch 11, p 240

Wilcken B, Smith A, Brown D A 1980 Urine screening for
aminoacidopathies: Is it beneficial? Journal of Pediatrics
97: 492–497

101

Heterozygote screening

M.M. Kaback

INTRODUCTION

The specific biochemical abnormality in more than 100 inborn errors of metabolism in man have now been determined. (Stanbury, et al, 1978; McKusick, 1978). Nearly all are inherited either as autosomal or X–linked recessive disorders. The capability to identify such conditions in relatively easily available tissues from affected individuals permits the rapid and accurate diagnosis of such disorders, minimizing the necessity for complicated and, at times, risk-associated diagnostic procedures. Many of these methods also have been applied to the prenatal detection of such conditions in the fetus during early gestation. This approach has provided a vital new option in genetic counselling for many families. In addition, in some instances, the delineation of the underlying metabolic defect has enabled investigators to develop rational and effective therapies for certain of these disorders (Desnick, 1981).

In addition to the diagnostic and possible therapeutic implications of such discoveries, comparable methodologies have been employed for the detection of heterozygous carriers of many of the recessive traits involved. Accordingly, not only is a striking deficiency of enzymatic activity or metabolic dysfunction evident in the diagnosis of the homozygous or hemizygous state (the affected male with an X–linked recessive disorder), but a distinct quantitative decrease of the same function can be demonstrated in the otherwise normal individual carrying the recessive allele. In some instances variant protein products of the mutant gene can be directly demonstrated by immunological or electrophoretic methods. (Harris & Hopkinson, 1978). This capability to quantify gene dosage, and thereby to identify carriers of recessive traits, has been reported for many, but not all, of the inborn errors of metabolism where the primary defect is known.

It must be emphasized, however, that for many conditions, the accuracy and feasibility of carrier detection is less-than-optimal. Either significant overlap with homozygous normal individuals is evident with the method(s) employed; the procedures are associated with

significant complexity and possible morbidity; or sufficient numbers of obligate heterozygotes (parents of affected children) and normal homozygotes have not been studied as yet to establish the statistical validity of the carrier identification method. These issues will be addressed in detail in subsequent parts of this chapter. It is not the intent of this article to review all of the metabolic disorders known as to their current status re: carrier detection. Rather, specific disorders will be cited solely as examples of the issues being discussed. Other chapters in this volume provide a detailed elaboration of the fundamental inborn errors associated with such conditions.

CARRIER SCREENING IN CLINICAL PRACTICE

When a patient is identified with an inborn error of metabolism or their family history reveals such a disorder in a close blood relative, the question of testing that individual and other family members for heterozygosity should be considered. In many instances where such tests are available and accurate, this can serve to *reduce expressed or hidden anxieties in other family members*. Since most of these disorders are individually rare, it is relatively unlikely that other family members need be too fearful of producing affected offspring. For example, taking a maximum risk situation, an American black individual whose brother or sister is a patient with sickle cell anaemia may be concerned about their having children of their own with this disease. Assuming they reproduce with another black person with *no known* sickle cell anaemia in his or her family – what are the actual risks? The unaffected sib of a person with sickle cell anaemia has two chances in three of having sickle trait (if born of the same parents as the patient with sickle cell anaemia). The approximate overall sickle trait frequency in American blacks is about one in ten. Therefore, the likelihood that the person will be at-risk for sickle cell anaemia in his or her offspring is: $2/3 \times 1/10 = 1/15$. The likelihood that any given pregnancy will result in a child with sickle cell anaemia is $1/4$ of that risk, or 1 in 60. Although these statistics alone can be somewhat comforting, simple carrier detection studies in the appropriate persons can put this question out of the realm of 'calculation', and establish definitively whether either or both individuals are carriers. If both prospective parents are found to be carriers, then comprehensive genetic counselling with a complete discussion of all available options can be initiated. Where at-risk couples are identified, this can lead to *prevention of subsequent intrafamilial cases of disease* – a second major reason to consider carrier testing in such families.

A third rationale relates to *marital counselling*, particularly where consanguinity between prospective parents may exist. In certain situations because of religious, moral, or other concerns; individuals might utilize such information about their carrier status in their decision re: mate selection. Another important consideration for carrier screening is where *artificial insemination* is being considered as an alternative for a couple who have had a child previously with an autosomal recessive disorder. Potential sperm donors should be evaluated (where feasible and practical) by appropriate carrier screening tests to avoid what otherwise could be a most unfortunate tragedy. The author is aware of two children with Tay-Sachs disease (TSD), conceived by artificial insemination, born to two unrelated families who were attempting to have an unaffected child after they had had a previous child with this fatal condition. In another instance, screening three medical students as potential sperm donors for a woman who had been identified previously as a TSD heterozygote, showed one of the three to be a TSD carrier also. Of course, he was excluded as a potential donor. Simply, such screening before the fact, in addition to a thorough family history on all potential sperm donors for other relevant issues, can help to avert tragedy.

CARRIER SCREENING IN INDIVIDUALS OF DEFINED SUBPOPULATION GROUPS

In Table 101.1, a list of relatively 'common' autosomal recessive disorders seen in defined subpopulations in the U.S.A. are presented with data indicating the respective carrier frequencies and newborn disease incidence in those ethnic groups. Gene frequencies and incidence of the disorder may vary considerably in the same ethnic groups in other parts of the world. The fact that selected genetic diseases occur predominately in certain ethnic, religious, or racial groups should not be surprising when one considers the relatively high degree of 'inbreeding' which are predominately seen in defined subpopulations (McKusick, 1978; Ramot, 1974). In addition to inbreeding, in some situations, selective environmental factors may have existed at some point in history which provided a biological (reproductive) advantage to carriers of the recessive gene (e.g. relative resistance to Malaria in individuals who are heterozygous for either sickle haemoglobin, β-thalassaemia, or G6PD deficiency). Because of this selective effect, the gene becomes 'enriched' from one generation to the next in that population.

Because of these populational distributions and the availability of relatively simple, accurate, and inexpensive carrier detection methods for the respective traits, it is conceivable to screen individuals in these groups and identify persons (and more critically, couples) at-risk for homozygous disease in their offspring before affected children have been born to them. With comprehensive genetic counselling, and the important new options which prenatal diagnosis can provide, many 'at-risk' families, so identified through screening such subpopulations, might choose to have only children unaffected with the disorder for which they are found to be at risk.

Perhaps the most effective effort of this nature in the past decade has been the experience with TSD carrier screening and prenatal diagnosis in western countries. (Kaback, 1981). From 1970 (when serum carrier detection methods first were described) to 1980, community-based TSD education-screening-counselling programs have been initiated in Jewish communities throughout North America, as well as in Israel, South Africa, Europe and South America. More than 300 000 Jewish adults have been screened voluntarily and over 13 000 hetero-

Table 101.1 Frequency and incidence estimates for selected autosomal recessive disorders in defined ethnic groups in the U.S.A.

Disease	Ethnic group	Gene frequency	Carrier frequency	'At risk' couple frequency'*	Disease incidence in newborns
Sickle cell anaemia	Blacks	0.040	0.080	1 in 150	1 in 600
Tay-Sachs disease	Ashkenazic Jews	0.016	0.032	1 in 900	1 in 3600
β-Thalassaemia	Greeks, Italians	0.016	0.032	1 in 900	1 in 3600
α-Thalassaemia	S.E. Asians and Chinese	0.020	0.040	1 in 625	1 in 2500
Cystic fibrosis	N. Europeans	0.020	0.040	1 in 625	1 in 2500
Phenylketonuria	Europeans	0.008	0.016	1 in 4000	1 in 16,000

* Likelihood that both members of a couple are heterozygous for the same recessive allele (assuming nonconsanguinity and that both are of the same ethnic group)

zygotes detected. Most critically, 268 couples – none of whom had had affected children previously – have been identified as being at risk for this fatal disorder in their offspring. Over 800 pregnancies at risk for TSD have been monitored by amniocentesis, and the births of nearly 200 infants destined to die with this disorder have been prevented. Recent data indicates that these efforts have contributed to a 60–85% decrease in the incidence of this disorder in Jewish infants through out North America. (Kaback et al, 1981).

Most recently, similar efforts directed at the prevention of β-thalassaemia, through carrier screening and prenatal diagnosis, have been initiated in several European countries and certain areas of North America. Although screening for sickle trait has been initiated in several parts of the world (including the U.S.A.) it is only recently that the option of prenatal diagnostic studies for this disorder has been available. (Kan & Dozy, 1978; Kan & Reid, 1980). The 'positive reproductive alternative' which this option may provide many families could facilitate greatly the extent of carrier screening in many areas. Carrier detection and prenatal diagnostic methods for cystic fibrosis, although still in experimental stages, are likely to lead to broad scale carrier screening among Northern European-derived caucasians in the near future. (Breslow, et al, 1981; Nadler & Walsh, 1980).

It is important to remember that for these relatively 'common' autosomal disorders occurring in defined ethnic groups, there is *usually no known prior history of the disease in either side of the family.* Perhaps, such a positive family history may be present in only about 20% of instances where a child with such a disorder is diagnosed. For this reason, clinicians should consider carrier screening for all individuals in these subpopulational groups where heterozygote detection is readily available. Certainly, such testing and its implications should be discussed thoroughly with the patient – or they can be referred to appropriate regional agencies for such services.

Not only is this considered optimal preventive medicine, but considerable concern has arisen recently regarding the medical-legal implications of failing to do so.

THERAPEUTIC IMPLICATIONS FOR HETEROZYGOTES

Although in most instances heterozygosity for a recessive trait is of no known health consequence to the individual, there are certain conditions in which the heterozygous state may impart certain health hazards.

Accordingly, in heterozygotes for certain conditions, the individual's knowledge of their carrier status may have certain therapeutic or preventive health implications for them. For example, persons with AS haemoglobin (sickle cell trait) should be aware of possible hazards they might incur if exposed to reduced ambient oxygen concentrations, e.g., mountain climbing at high altitude, flying in an unpressurized aircraft above 8000 feet, etc. Also, alerting the anaesthesiologist of the AS trait of their patient prior to gaseous anaesthesia, could avert inadvertent hypoxaemia which might be particularly hazardous to such an individual. Heterozygous individuals for Type II hypercholestrolaemia may be predisposed to premature atherosclerotic degeneration and coronary artery insufficiency. It is believed that appropriate therapy (diet, weight control and/or specific medication) may obviate substantially the increased risk for early myocardial infarction in individuals carrying this dominantly-expressed disorder. In a similar context, persons heterozygous for α-1-antitrypsin deficiency (MZ) clearly are predisposed to chronic obstructive pulmonary disease in early adulthood. Avoidance of tobacco smoke and other noxious inhalants may reduce this risk greatly. Having identified an individual as heterozygous for this genetic mutation, it might be of great practical value for this person to be so counselled and to be guided into appropriate job selection and/or environmentally safe areas, as well as of the particular importance of not smoking.

METHODS AND TISSUES USED IN CARRIER IDENTIFICATION

Depending upon the genetic nature of the condition, its expression in different organ systems, and the availability of appropriate material for examination, a variety of approaches have been employed for the purpose of heterozygote identification. Table 101.2 lists a series of approaches, ranging from physiological studies to genetic linkage analysis which have been utilized in carrier detection for different disorders. The disorders listed are representative only of the different categories of methods used. In some instances, combined techniques are involved for optimal ascertainment of the carrier state. For example, in Duchenne dystrophy, use of biochemical (CPK) and Bayesian methods in combination allow for the best estimation of possible carrier status in certain women. Combined coagulation studies (physiological) with immunoquantitation of Faction VIII is optimal for carrier identification in haemophilia A. Somatic cell methods assessing the enzymatic (HGPRTase) or physiological (^{3}H-hypoxanthine incorporation) properties of clones of skin fibroblast cells have been applied effectively to carrier detection in Lesch-Nyhan syndrome.

In Table 101.3, a compilation is presented of various tissues used for heterozygote detection in representative recessive disorders. In considering carrier screening in

Table 101.2 Methods employed for carrier detection in representative autosomal and X-linked recessive disorders

Approach	Method*	Disorder*
Physiological	Loading test Kinetics	PKU, OTC
Biochemical	Quant. enzyme activity	TSD, MLD
Functional	NBT dye reduction	Chron. gran. dis.
Structural	Hb electrophoresis	Haemoglobinopathies
Somatic cell	Clonal mosaicism	Lesch-Nyhan
Immunological	Quant. immunochem.	Haemophilias
Statistical	Bayesian pedigree analysis	DMD
Genetic linkage	Xg family study	XR-MR

* NBT = Nitro-blue tetrazolium; Xg = X chromosome linked blood group;
PKU = phenylkentonuria; OTC = Ornithine transcarbamylase deficiency;
TSD = Tay-Sachs disease; MLD = Metachromatic leukodystrophy;
DMD = Duchenne muscular dystrophy; XR–MR = X-linked recessive mental retardation

Table 101.3 Tissue used for carrier detection in representative recessive disorders

Tissue	Methods	Disorders*
Serum, plasma	Enzyme assay, immunoquantitation functional assay	TSD, haemophilias
Erythrocytes	Enzyme assay, electrophoresis	G6PD deficiency, haemoglobinopathies
Leukocytes	Enzyme assay, histology, functional tests	Gaucher, Batten, CGD
Cultivated skin fibroblasts	Enzyme assay, cloning	MLD, Hunter
Hair follicles	Enzyme assay/ratio	Lesch-Nyhan, Fabry disease
Tears	Enzyme assay	TSD
Teeth	Vertical banding	Amaelogenesis Imperfecta-XR
Eyes	Fundoscopy	XR-fundal dystrophies, RP
Liver, muscle biopsy	Enzyme assay, cellular histology	OTC, DMD

* TSD = Tay-Sachs disease; CGD = Chronic granulomatous disease;
MLD = Metachromatic leukodystrophy; XR = X-linked recessive;
RP = Retinitis pigmentosum; OTC = Ornithine transcarbamylase deficiency;
DMD = Duchenne muscular dystrophy

any individual (or subpopulation, for that matter) the accessability of appropriate tissue or material for testing very much influences the feasibility and cost of such procedures. In some instances, accurate heterozygote identification can be achieved with such readily available tissues as serum, erythrocytes, or even tears. In other examples cited, optimal carrier detection may require cultured skin fibroblasts or even biopsied liver or muscle tissue. Clearly, whether to conduct such studies in individuals related to an affected person or more generally will be strongly influenced by such considerations.

PROBLEMS IN HETEROZYGOTE DETECTION

Statistical constraints

The great majority of the inborn errors of metabolism alluded to in this chapter are relatively rare conditions. Although in the aggregate it is estimated that perhaps (1%) of all live born infants will, at some time in life,

manifest such a single-gene disorder, there are more than 2000 such disorders now recognized. This poses certain critical problems for carrier identification. The only individuals who are obligatory carriers of an autosomal recessive genetic trait are the biological parents of an affected individual (discounting the 10^{-5} to 10^{-6} possibility of new mutation). Therefore, in the establishment of a carrier identification method, it is critical that a 'significant number' of such obligatory heterozygotes be studied (and control individuals as well) before a statistical validity to the testing method can be assigned. In this regard one must be careful in interpreting many of the research publications in which only small numbers of obligate heterozygotes have been tested and where results suggest that the methods are applicable to carrier detection. Obviously, the larger the samples of obligate carriers and controls studied and the greater the separation observed in the test results between the two groups, the greater the likelihood for significant application of the method to heterozygote identification.

It is a very different matter to study persons who the investigator knows *must be* carriers for a particular trait from that of studying individuals who are complete unknowns. Since all experiences in this context show a *distribution of test results*, both for carriers and controls, the narrowness of each distribution and the degree of separation of one from the other become critical considerations in assigning a statistical probability that any given person's test result falls into one or the other distribution.

Why variability?

One would expect that individuals who are heterozygotes for an autosomal recessive mutation would reflect 50% of the value (whatever the measurement happens to be) of that found in homozygous normal persons. This is clearly not the case. Not only is there variability of test values in heterozygotes, but considerable variation also may be evident in data derived from normals. This may reflect the limitations of the methods employed and/or depict the inherent *biological variability* of such functions. Assuredly, other genetic and environmental factors, may influence any given biological parameter such that a definite range of results are seen in both carriers and in non-carriers. In some instances where, for example, an enzymatic activity measurement is the test employed, there may be levels of activity in heterozygotes distinctly less than 50% of normal. Where the relevant enzyme is comprised of multiple subunits – only one of which is under control of the gene in question – random aggregation of normal and abnormal subunits can result in a wide range of activities in the comprised multimeric enzyme. Other mutations may result in only partial reduction in activity of the respective polypeptide. In this instance, the heterozygote may have near normal activity or activity of the enzyme in question which overlaps considerably with the range of measurements found in non-carriers.

With X–linked conditions, the carrier female, quite characteristically, reflects a broad range of test results extending from clearly normal levels to those seen in affected males. This is predominately a manifestation of the well-known Lyonization effect with X–chromosome linked genes. This biological phenomenon makes carrier determination for such X–linked genes particularly difficult. In fact, heterozygous females who carry X–linked recessive genes are mosaic in the expression of most of the genes in question, with a certain proportion of their somatic cells expressing the normal gene and the remainder reflecting the mutant state. The issue of X–linked disorders and implications for carrier detection are discussed elsewhere in this volume.

Other factors influencing the carrier test

In addition to the consideration that other genes in an individual's constitution might influence the expression of a distant specific gene locus, other biological factors may influence gene expression as well. Such factors as age, pregnancy, and certain illnesses might influence the parameter in question, thereby altering the ability to distinguish carriers from non-carriers. Such issues need to be addressed before wide scale application of a carrier detection method is made.

Genetic heterogeneity is another important consideration in this regard. This means that more than one genetic locus may cause a similar alteration in the test used or in the phenotype observed. If standard haemoglobin electrophoresis is the only parameter used for sickle trait identification, then persons carrying the mutation for haemoglobin-D will be incorrectly identified as AS since S and D haemoglobin electrophorese similarly under standard conditions. In this instance, of course, the adjunct use of other methods such as haemoglobin solubility studies or sickling on deoxygenation will clarify this possible discrepancy.

In some instances, certain environmental factors such as drugs, diet, or other agents could affect biological functions and thereby influence their applicability to carrier detection. Iron deficiency can cause haematological changes which mimic the findings of those seen in heterozygotes for β-thalassaemia. Birth control medications have been shown to reduce the *relative* amount of serum hexosaminidase A, making some women taking 'the pill' appear as carriers for Tay-Sachs disease (Kaback, 1977). These are only two examples, where such determinations can be influenced by external factors resulting in inaccurate carrier identification studies. Certainly, other examples may exist as well.

SENSITIVITY AND SPECIFICITY

With all of the above considerations in mind, and having assessed reasonable numbers of obligate heterozygotes and controls with the method(s) recommended, significant overlap in the distribution of carriers and non-carriers may still remain. Capabilities of any one laboratory may not be comparable with those of others reflecting, perhaps, differences in preferred methodologies or other inherent variables. Thus the ability to identify all true carriers (*sensitivity*) is reflected in the *false negative* frequency with the test employed. The identification of only true carriers (*specificity*), and not other persons with a *false positive* test, is also of paramount importance. The greater the overlap in distributions between carrier and non-carrier, the greater the likelihood for either or both types of misidentification.

In certain instances, even where a defined level of overlap is known to exist, carrier detection studies may still be appropriate. In this context, a test result clearly in the carrier range may indicate, with great likelihood, that the person is heterozygous, whereas a result in the overlap area would be less definitive and leave the possibility of carrier status indeterminate. Similarly, a result at the upper levels of the non-carrier distribution might make the probability of heterozygosity exceedingly small.

Where such difficulties exist, carrier screening is (most definately) best restricted to use only in high risk individuals (close relatives of probands) rather than in more general or subpopulational screening. Only those approaches in which prior studies have proven the statistical reliability and accuracy of the method and its relative ease of applicability should be candidates for possible more general use.

COST AND FEASIBILITY

Where significant morbidity or cost would be involved in performing carrier detection studies (even where the accuracy is optimal), these issues should be considered and discussed with the individual before proceeding. Performing a skin biopsy for cultivation of fibroblast cells may have minimal morbidity, but is quite an expensive endeavor to undertake. For this reason, carrier screening using this approach should only be applicable to the highest risk individuals. Liver or muscle biopsy for such determinations obviously cannot be undertaken lightly. Again, perhaps only brothers and sisters, or aunts and uncles would be at sufficient risk to warrant considering such studies.

AGE FOR CARRIER TESTING

As mentioned previously, for most recessive traits heterozygosity has little if any health consequences for the individual. It is only a matter relevant to his or her reproduction. For this reason, it is the author's opinion that carrier testing is best instituted at a time just prior to, or during, the reproductive age. This has added benefits in that the person's ability to comprehend the meaning of such information is much more likely to be adequate at such an age. For this reason, carrier testing

among children or young teenagers should not be undertaken routinely and should be considered only under very special circumstances. One's level of maturity and background education may be important factors in obviating any possible stigmatization which carrier identification potentially could entail. Simply, parental request to determine the possible carrier status of their child(ren) need not be a sufficient basis to proceed. Rather, a full discussion with the parents as to the lack of health implications and possible psychosocial hazards of testing youngsters may lead to deferral of such studies until a more appropriate time.

CONCLUDING REMARKS

From its very outset a number of complex and important social and ethical issues have been identified with genetic screening. (Hastings Center, 1972; Bergsma, 1974). Such issues as the possible personal, familial, or even more general stigmatization of the identified carrier – maintenance of utmost confidentiality of test results – rigorous protection of the individual's privacy – the informed consent of the tested individual — are but a few of the more important concerns raised. Clearly, the physician must consider all of these matters in his patient interaction where possible genetic testing is being anticipated. These issues notwithstanding, it is the author's opinion that heterozygote testing is likely to increase substantially in the future for many of the reasons cited earlier. With appropriate technical, medical and communicative expertise, the expanded utilization of these new approaches may serve importantly to reduce the individual, familial, and societal burdens associated with many severe, currently untreatable, hereditary disorders.

ACKNOWLEDGEMENTS

This work was supported in part by a contract from the Genetic Disease Section, Maternal and Child Health Branch, State of California, Department of Health, by NIH Research Training Grant No. 5 T32 GM-07414-04 and by grants from the National Tay-Sachs Disease and Allied Disorders Association and from the Gould Family Foundation.

REFERENCES

Bergsma D (ed) 1974 Ethical Social and Legal Dimensions of Screening for Human Genetic Disease, Birth Defects: Original Article Series, Vol. X, March of Dimes Birth Defects Foundation

Breslow V W, McPherson J, Epstein J 1974 Distinguishing homozygous and heterozygous cystic fibrosis fibroblasts from normal cells by differences in sodium transport; New England Journal of Medicine 304: 1

Desnick R J 1981 Treatment of Inherited Metabolic Diseases: An Overview In: Kaback M (ed) Genetic Issues in Pediatric and Obstetrical Practice Year-Book Medical Publishes, New York

Harris H, Hopkinson D A 1978 Handbook of Enzyme Electrophoresis in Human Genetics, North-Holland, Amsterdam

Hastings Center 1972 Ethical and Social issues in screening

for genetic disease, New England Journal of Medicine 286: 1129

Kaback M (ed) 1977 Tay-Sachs Disease: Screening and Prevention, A R Liss Inc, New York

Kaback M M, Greenwald S, Brossman R 1981 Carrier Detection and Prenatal Diagnosis in Tay-Sachs Disease: Experience of the First Decade, Pediatric Research 15: 632A

Kaback M M 1981 Heterozygote Screening and Prenatal Diagnosis in Tay-Sachs Disease: A Worldwide Update, In: Callahan J W, Alexander Lowden J (eds) Lysosomes and Lysosomal Storage Diseases, Raven Press, New York

Kan Y W, Dozy A 1978 Antenatal diagnosis of sickle-cell anemia by DNA analysis of amniotic fluid cells. Lancet ii: 910

Kan Y W, Reid C D, (eds) 1980 Prenatal Approaches to the Diagnosis of Fetal Hemoglobinopathies, US Dept HHS, NIH Publ, No 80–1529, Washington D.C.

McKusick V A 1978 Mendelian Inheritance in Man, 5th edn, Johns Hopkins Press, Baltimore

Nadler H A, Walsh M M 1980 Intrauterine Detection of Cystic Fibrosis; Pediatrics 66: 690

Ramot B (ed) 1974 Genetic Polymorphisms and Diseases in Man; Academic Press, New York

Stanbury J B, Wyngaarden J, Fredrickson D S (eds) 1978 The Metabolic Basis of Inherited Disease 4th edn McGraw-Hill, New York

102

Prenatal diagnosis

J. Charrow and H.L. Nadler

INTRODUCTION

Despite our continually expanding understanding of genetics and genetic disorders, the clinical geneticist often functions as no more than diagnostician and counsellor; the ability to significantly alter the course of many genetic disorders, let alone cure them, is very much limited. The development of reliable methods for prenatal diagnosis and the availability and safety of midtrimester abortion have had tremendous impact on the field of clinical genetics by making it possible to prevent many of these devastating disorders.

Many approaches to prenatal diagnosis have been tried (Table 102.1). Attempts to visualize the fetus radiographically have until recently been disappointing because of the incomplete mineralization of fetal bones early in gestation and the potential hazards of ionizing radiation for the developing organism. Fetography and amniography permit visualization of the fetus but have had limited application. The development of ultrasonographic equipment, however, has made indirect visualization of the fetus early in gestation a commonplace event, and as the resolution of the equipment has improved it has become possible to identify an ever increasing number of malformations *in utero*. Recently, direct visualization of the fetus has become possible through fetoscopy and fetal blood and skin specimens

Table 102.1 Methods for prenatal diagnosis

Invasive	
Amniocentesis	(a) cell free fluid analysis
	(b) uncultivated cells
	(c) cultivated cells
Placentocentesis	
Fetoscopy	(a) fetal visualization
	(b) fetal blood sampling
	(c) fetal skin biopsy
Amniography and fetography	
Non-Invasive	
Analysis of maternal serum and urine	
Ultrasonography	
Radiography	

can be obtained at 16–18 weeks gestation under direct vision. Perhaps the most powerful tool, however, has been amniocentesis, which was first applied to the prenatal determination of fetal sex by Barr body identification in the 1950's (Fuchs & Riis, 1956; Serr et al, 1955). Within 10 years, it was demonstrated that karyotype analysis could be performed on amniotic fluid cells (Steele & Breg, 1966) and the first prenatal diagnosis of a chromosomal abnormality was reported (Jacobson & Barter, 1967). A year later, Nadler (1968) demonstrated the applicability of the technique to the diagnosis of the inborn errors of metabolism.

Prenatal diagnosis is most often applied to the determination of congenital disorders which would result in significant disability, handicap or premature death. It is often assumed that the sole purpose of attempting diagnosis is to permit early termination of the pregnancy (which may be legally done in the U.S.A. prior to 24 weeks gestation) if the fetus is in some way abnormal. There are a handful of disorders, however, in which prenatal diagnosis permits prenatal or early postnatal therapy: the galactose intake of the mother of a galactosemic fetus may be restricted; B_{12} may be given in B_{12} responsive methylmalonic acidemia. Later in pregnancy, erythroblastosis fetalis may be treated by *in utero* blood transfusion if the haemolysis is severe. Antenatal diagnosis may also affect early management of the neonate known to have congenital virilizing adrenal hyperplasia. Where no potential therapy is available, one might be tempted to discourage couples who are opposed to abortion from seeking prenatal diagnosis. It is clear, however, that the information obtained may still have a significant impact even if abortion is not considered. If the fetus is abnormal the parents may ready themselves emotionally and mobilize their support systems in preparation for raising a handicapped child. If the fetus appears normal, the alleviation of anxiety which may be provided is immeasurable. In either event, it is well recognized that parents often act differently than they expected when confronted with the reality of a diagnosis.

It should be clear that prenatal diagnosis is not restricted to genetic disorders, although it is usually the geneticist who is most experienced in this area. It is the diagnosis of congenital conditions rather than solely genetic disorders which are of interest. In fact, monitoring pregnancies for acquired illness has been common obstetric practice for many years (e.g., the measurement of anti-rubella titres) and has been used in counselling couples regarding early termination of pregnancy. Nor is prenatal diagnosis confined to the first 24 weeks of gestation. Maternal oestriol excretion near term may be used as an index of fetal well being. The amniotic fluid lecithin/sphingomyelin ratio is used as an index of fetal maturity in the third trimester. Amniotic fluid spectrophotometry may be used to monitor the degree of haemolysis in erythroblastosis fetalis.

Who, then are the subjects of prenatal diagnosis? Amniocentesis for karyotype analysis in women over the age of 35 is the most common application of a prenatal diagnostic technique. For most disorders, however, it is unfortunately true that it is only after the birth of an affected child that prenatal diagnosis may be attempted in subsequent pregnancies. When there has not been a previously affected child or a family history of a genetic disorder, prenatal diagnosis may be feasible only if (1) a population at risk can be identified; (2) the at risk population can be safely screened for unaffected carriers or for affected pregnancies; and (3) the pregnancies at risk may be monitored and the condition diagnosed with a high degree of reliability prior to 24 weeks gestation. These criteria are fulfilled by unfortunately few conditions: Tay-Sachs disease in Ashkenazi Jews (Kaback, 1977); Sickle cell anaemia in Blacks (Alter et al, 1976) and β-thalassaemia in Mediterranean peoples (Fairweather et al, 1978; Kan et al, 1977). Because the frequency of the respective mutuant allele is sufficiently high in these populations and the means of carrier detection reliable and relatively simple, population screening for carriers can be performed and couples at risk identified. There are a few disorders which are so common that the entire population may be considered to be at risk. Rhesus incompatibility and congenital rubella are two such situations for which screening of all pregnancies has been recommended for many years. In the former, if primary prevention fails, prenatal diagnosis allows prenatal and early postnatal care for the affected individual. In the latter, a change in titre suggesting first trimester infection indicates a high risk for congenital heart disease, deafness and increased neonatal mortality and early termination of the pregnancy may be the preferred course. It has been suggested that neural tube defects (which occur with a frequency of 1–2/1000 in the U.S.A. and 2–3/1000 in the U.K.) are also amenable to population screening by measurement of maternal serum alphafetoprotein. In several areas programmes have already been established to screen all women in the 16th week of pregnancy. Unfortunately, screening for several other common genetic disorders, most notably cystic fibrosis, is not yet possible, although *in utero* diagnosis may now be achieved.

The identification of a pregnancy at high risk for a congenital disorder from among a population at risk is the essential first step in prenatal diagnosis. Equally important is the reliability of the technique used to monitor the pregnancy. As with all diagnostics, the sensitivity and specificity of any test increase with the experience of the laboratory. Experience in this area implies more than technical competence; an appreciation of the full range of normal and an ability to tailor the procedure to the question being asked are both necessary. It is also essential that the diagnosis be verified after birth of the child or the termination of the pregnancy so that the analytical methods can be continually evaluated and improved. Prenatal diagnosis is not simply a laboratory exercise. It is a process which requires identification of pregnancies at risk, genetic counselling, parental education about genetics, procedures and their risks, and emotional support at a time when difficult and sensitive issues are being decided. In addition, follow-up, both for verification of the diagnosis and continued interaction with the parents who are frequently guilt ridden and uncertain of the wisdom of their decisions, cannot be neglected. Support services beyond those of the genetic counselling facility may be required, including social service, clergy and dieticians. Good communication between the geneticist and the referring physician is essential. Lastly, the parents must feel confident that their needs will be met, be they emotional or medical, by a team with expertise in this area.

In genetic counselling and prenatal diagnosis, the subject of 'risks' is discussed frequently. While for many disorders determination of the incidence of a disorder in a population, and understanding the mode of transmission, permit the calculation of a couple's numerical risk, the couple's assessment of the magnitude of this risk (i.e. whether it is perceived to be large or small) necessarily remains subjective. In those disorders for which prenatal diagnosis is possible, the risks of the diagnostic procedure must be considered as well. For the administrator of public health funds, the numerical risk may be evaluated by a cost-benefit analysis. While this approach may be useful for the allocation of fixed resources to public health programmes, it is most often irrelevant to a prospective parent, who sees the risks in terms of 'human' and emotional costs. For this reason the decision reached will vary from couple to couple, even when faced with the same statistics. The childless couple with a history of repeated fetal loss may prefer the risk of a child with a chromosomal abnormality to the increased risk of spontaneous abortion after amniocentesis. On the other hand, the 33 year old woman with 3 healthy children may well prefer the risk of abortion even though it is greater than the odds of having a chromosomally abnormal child. For some people, one alternative is absolutely not acceptable - for example, another child with a devastating illness, and the risk of fetal loss may be preferable no matter how great it is. It is perhaps crudely put, but true, that if one plays the odds, one must be prepared to lose.

While prenatal diagnosis may be attempted throughout gestation, of greatest interest are those studies which may be performed prior to 24 weeks gestation. The following discussion will be restricted to these methods and their applications, risks and indications.

AMNIOCENTESIS

Technique

Transabdominal amniocentesis in combination with ultrasonography is undoubtedly the most widely used technique for prenatal diagnosis because of the wealth of information that can be derived by studying material of fetal origin, namely the amniotic fluid cells and the fluid itself. The amniotic fluid is probably derived from many sources; transudation of maternal serum across the placental membranes, fetal urine and tracheobronchial secretions, and secretion by the amniotic epithelium. The circulation of the fluid and origin of many of its components are still poorly understood. The volume of amniotic fluid increases during gestation to a maximum of approximately 1 litre at 38 weeks and gradually decreases thereafter (Elliot & Inman, 1961). At 15–16 weeks gestation approximately 180–200 ml is present (Wagner & Fuchs, 1962) and the uterus has risen above the pelvic brim and is therefore accessible to a transabdominal approach (Gerbie & Elias, 1980). Although success in obtaining amniotic fluid increases with the duration of gestation, the time needed to complete many of the desired studies on the material obtained dictates that the procedure be performed as early as possible so that termination of the pregnancy, if indicated, may be performed before 24 weeks.

Prior to amniocentesis, ultrasonography (either B-mode or real-time) is extremely useful to (1) verify fetal life; (2) determine gestational age by measurement of the biparietal diameter (BPD); (3) diagnose multiple gestations; (4) determine placental and fetal positions; (5) detect gross fetal malformation or hydatid mole and (6) to detect uterine malformations. If estimation of gestational age by BPD is at variance with that calculated from the last menstrual period, the BPD is used for timing the amniocentesis and interpretation of the derived information. Amniocentesis should be performed by an obstetrician skilled in the technique. Immediately prior to the procedure, the woman is instructed to void and then under strict aseptic conditions, a local anaesthetic is injected into the needle insertion site. A $3\frac{1}{2}$ inch, 20 or 22 gauge spinal needle is then inserted and the stylet removed. A few drops of fluid are discarded to minimize the risk of contaminating the sample with maternal cells; if blood is present in the first drops, and subsequently clears, the bloody aliquot is discarded and 20–30 ml of yellow tinged fluid is gently aspirated, transferred to sterile tubes, and transported at room temperature to the laboratory as quickly as possible. A few drops of fluid may be observed for 'ferning' to insure that the sample is not urine (Elias et al, 1978). In diamniotic twin gestations a water soluble dye (e.g., indigo carmine) is injected after withdrawal of the fluid, the needle removed and reinsertion in the second sac attempted. If colourless fluid is then aspirated it is clear that the first sac has not been re-entered. After the procedure, the woman may return to normal activity and is told to report any cramping or leakage of fluid from the puncture site or vagina.

An adequate specimen is obtained on the first attempt in 99% of women and successful cell cultures established in 98% of fluids delivered to the laboratory immediately and in 87% of specimens received by mail (Golbus et al, 1979). Other groups have reported higher rates for having to repeat the amniocentesis, varying from 10 to 15% (Simpson et al, 1976; NICHD, 1976; Burton et al, 1974). Failure to cell growth has been the most common problem, followed by unsuccessful taps and inconclusive laboratory results.

RISKS

The major risk of amniocentesis is fetal loss. In the NICHD study (1976) the rate of loss (spontaneous abortions, fetal deaths *in utero* and stillbirths) was 3.5% in the subjects and 3.2% in the controls; after adjustment for maternal age, the rates were 3.3 and 3.4%, respectively. No difference in the distribution of fetal loss at various gestational ages was observed. The rate was not increased in women requiring more than 1 needle insertion and was not related to the volume of fluid withdrawn. Ultrasonographic placental localization also did not alter the outcome. A study in the U.K. (Working Party on Amniocentesis, Medical Research Council, 1978) suggested a somewhat higher rate of loss after amniocentesis but the design of the study and composition of the populations complicate interpretation of the data. The increase in risk is generally taken to be on the order of 0.5 %.

Amnionitis occurs after amniocentesis with an estimated frequency of 0.1% (Murken et al, 1979). Rhesus isoimmunization may occur and is of particular concern if the amniotic fluid is bloody. Examination of a Kleihauer-Betke preparation of the maternal blood smear after amniocentesis has been advocated to detect entry of fetal blood cells into the maternal circulation but this method is not sensitive enough to detect small but significant transfusions. Although the routine administration of Rh immune globulin (Rhogam) to Rh negative women after amniocentesis should prevent isoimmunization, controversy over this procedure continues because of the possibility of adverse effects on the fetus. Many centres are now administering a 'micro-dose' (100 micrograms) after the procedure to all Rh negative women who do not have a detectable anti-Rh titre.

Despite much concern about possible injury from fetal puncture at the time of amniocentesis, no evidence for this occurrence was found in the NICHD study. Skin scarring and dimpling (Karp & Hayden, 1977) have been reported, however.

Amniotic fluid leakage and vaginal bleeding occur in less than 1% of women and are usually of no significance. Premature labour pains occurred very infrequently (0.2%) in the NICHD study.

Table 102.2 Disorders of amino acid and organic acid metabolism which may be diagnosed through midtrimester amniocentesis

Disorder	Inheritance	Basis of diagnosis
Argininosuccinic aciduria	AR	amniotic fluid argininosuccinic acid; argininosuccinase
Citrullinaemia	AR	argininosuccinate synthetase
Cystathioninuria	AR	cystathionase
Cystinosis	AR	intracellular cystine
Gamma-glutamyl synthetase deficiency	AR	gamma-glutamyl synthetase
Histidinaemia	AR	histidase
Homocystinuria (B_6 responsive and unresponsive)	AR	cystathionine synthase
3-Hydroxy-3-methylglutaryl CoA lyase deficiency	AR	3-hydroxy-3-methylglutaryl CoA lyase
Hypervalinaemia	AR	valine transaminase
Isovaleric acidaemia	AR	isovaleryl CoA dehydrogenase
β-Ketothiolase deficiency	AR	β-ketothiolase
Maple syrup urine disease (severe and intermittent types)	AR	branched chain ketooacid decarboxylase
β-Methylcrotonic aciduria	AR	β-methylcrotonyl CoA carboxylase
Methylene tetrahydrofolate reductase deficiency	AR	methylene tetrahydrofolate reductase
Methylmalonic acidaemia (B_{12} responsive and unresponsive)	AR	aminiotic fluid methylmalonic acid; methylmalonyl CoA mutase
Methyltetrahydrofolate homocysteine: methyltransferase deficiency	AR	methyltetrahydrofolate homocysteine: methyltransferase deficiency
Multiple carboxylase deficiency	AR	amniotic flud methyl citrate; acyl CoA carboxylases
Ornithinemia	AR	ornithine ketoacid transaminase
5-Oxoprolinuria	AR	glutathione synthetase
Prolidase deficiency	AR	prolidase
Propionic acidaemia	AR	propionyl CoA carboxylase
Pyruvate carboxylase deficiency	AR	pyruvate carboxylase
Pyruvate decarboxylase deficiency	AR	pyruvate decarboxylase
Pyruvate dehydrogenase deficiency	AR	pyruvate dehydrogenase
Saccharopinuria	AR	lysine-ketoglutarate reductase; saccharopine dehydrogenase

Table 102.3 Disorders of carbohydrate metabolism which may be diagnosable through midtrimester amniocentesis

Disorder	Inheritance	Basis of diagnosis
Aspartylglucosaminuria	AR	aspartylglucosaminidase
Fucosidosis	AR	α-fucosidase
Galactokinase deficiency	AR	galactokinase
Galactosaemia	AR	galactose-1-phosphate uridyl transferase
Glucose-6-phosphate dehydrogenase deficiency	X-linked	glucose-6-phosphate dehydrogenase
Glycogen storage diseases		
Type II – Pompe disease	AR	α-1, 4-glucosidase
Type III – Debrancher deficiency	AR	amylo-1, 6-glucosidase
Type IV – Brancher deficiency	AR	amylo-1, 4 to 1, 6-transglucosidase
Type VIII – Phosphorylase kinase deficiency		
	X-linked	phosphorylase kinase
Mannosidosis	AR	α-mannosidase
Phosphohexose isomerase deficiency	AR	phosphohexose isomerase
Sialidosis	AR	glycoprotein neuraminidase

Table 102.4 Disorders of lipid metabolism which may be diagnosable through midtrimester amniocentesis

Disorder	Inheritance	Basis of diagnosis
Cholesterol ester storage disease	AR	acid lipase
Fabry disease	X-linked	α-galactosidase A
Familial hypercholesterolaemia	AD	Defective suppression of 3-hydroxy, 3-methyl glutaryl CoA reductase
Farber disease	AR	ceramidase
Gaucher disease, types I, II, III	AR	glucocerebrosidase
GM₁ gangliosidosis (all types)	AR	α-galactosidase
GM₂ gangliosidosis		
Type I – Tay Sachs disease	AR	hexosaminidase A
Type II – Sandhoff disease	AR	hexosaminidase A and B
Type III – Juvenile type	AR	hexosaminidase A
Adult type	AR	hexosaminidase A
Ichthyosis	X-linked	steroid sulphatase
Krabbe disease (Globoid cell leukodystrophy)	AR	galactocerebrosidase
Metachromatic leukodystrophy (late infantile, juvenile and adult types)		arylsuphatase A
Mucolipidosis		
Type I	AR	glycoprotein neuraminidase
Type II – I-Cell disease	AR	multiple lysosomal hydrolase deficiencies
Type III	AR	multiple lysosomal hydrolase deficiencies
Type IV	AR	? ganglioside neuraminidase, cellular inclusions on electron microscopy
Multiple sulphatase deficiency	AR	multiple sulphatase deficiencies
Niemann-Pick disease, types A, B, C	AR	sphingomyelinase
Refsum disease	AR	phytanic acid α-hydrolase
Wolman disease	AR	acid lipase

Table 102.5 Disorders of mucopolysaccharide metabolism which may be diagnosable through midtrimester amniocentesis

Disorder	Inheritance	Basis of diagnosis
Type I H Hurler syndrome	AR	α-L-iduronidase
Type I S Scheie syndrome	AR	α-L-iduronidase
Type I H/S Hurler/Scheie syndrome	AR	α-L-iduronidase
Type II Hunter syndrome	X-linked	iduronate sulphatase
Type III A Sanfilippo A	AR	heparan-N-sulphatase
Type III B Sanfilippo B	AR	N-acetyl-α-D-glucosaminidase
Type III C Sanfilippo C	AR	acetyl CoA: α-glucosaminide N-acetyl transferase
Type IV Morquio syndrome	AR	N-acetyl galactosamine-6-sulfatase
Type VI Maroteaux-Lamy syndrome	AR	arylsulphatase B
Type VII β-glucuronidase deficiency	AR	β-glucuronidase

Processing of the specimen should begin immediately on arrival in the laboratory. Usually the fluid is centrifuged and the cell free supernatant analyzed for alphafetoprotein. The cells are introduced into tissue culture for subsequent cytogenetic analysis. Other studies are performed as indicated and are discussed in detail below. Tables 102.2–7 list the various disorders which may be diagnosed.

APPLICATIONS

Amniotic fluid analysis
Although analysis of the enzymes, hormones, amino acids and metabolic products that are found in the amniotic fluid have been used for prenatal diagnosis, results are often not reliable and in most instances other more direct procedures exist. Many of these components are derived from multiple sources; in some the origin is unknown. Enzymes may enter the amniotic fluid through secretion by the amnion, from the fetal urine, desquamated intestinal cells, lysis of amniotic fluid cells, and tracheobronchial secretions. Others probably originate in the maternal decidua. It is clear now that for those disorders in which a cellular biochemical defect is known and expressed in amniotic fluid cells, analyses based on these cells are more reliable than those based on cell free fluid.

Tay-Sachs disease has been diagnosed using cell free

Table 102.6 Other enzyme deficiencies which may be diagnosed through midtrimester amniocentesis.

Disorder	Inheritance	Basis of diagnosis
Acatalasaemia	AR	catalase
Adenosine deaminase deficiency	AR	adenosine deaminase
Congenital adrenal hyperplasia (21-hydroxylase deficiency)	AR	amniotic fluid 17-hydroxyprogesterone, linkage analysis by HLA typing
Dihydropteridine reductase deficiency	AR	dihydropteridine reductase
Ehlers-Danlos syndrome		
Type VI	AR	lysyl hydroxylase
Type VII	AR	Procollagen peptidase
Hypophosphatasia	AR	amniotic fluid alkaline phosphatase
Lesch-Nyhan syndrome	X-linked	hypoxanthine-guanine phosphoribosyl transferase
Lysosomal acid phosphatase deficiency	AR	lysosomal acid phosphatase
Nucleoside phosphorylase deficiency	AR	nucleoside phosphorylase
Orotic aciduria	AR	orotidylic pyrophosphoribosyl transferase; orotidylic 5' phosphate decarboxylase
Porphyria		
Acute intermittent porphyria	AD	uroporphyrinogen I synthetase
Congenital erythropoetic porphyria	AR	uroporphyrinogen III cosynthetase
Coproporphyria	AD	coproporphyrinogen oxidase
Protoporphyria	AD	ferrochetalase
Variegate porphyria	AD	protoporphyrinogen oxidase
Sulphite oxidase deficiency	AR	sulphite oxidase

Table 102.7 Miscellaneous disorders which may be diagnosable through midtrimester amniocentesis

Disorder	Inheritance	Basis of diagnosis
Chediak-Higashi disease	AR	amniotic fluid cell inclusions
Chromosomal abnormalities	—	karyotype of amniotic fluid cells
Chromosome instability syndromes		bleomycin induced breaks
Ataxia telangiectasia	AR	sister chromatid exchange
Bloom syndrome	AR	DEB induced chromosome breaks and rearrangements
Fanconi anaemia	AR	
Xeroderma pigmentosum	AR	DNA 'repair' synthesis after UVL exposure
Congenital nephrosis	AR	amniotic fluid alpha-fetoprotein
Cystic fibrosis	AR	amniotic fluid MUGB-reactive proteases
Haemoglobinopathies/thalassaemias	AR	restriction endonuclease mapping, hybridization, linkage analysis
Menkes kinky hair	X-linked	copper accumulation
Myotonic dystrophy	AD	linkage to secretor gene
Neural tube defects	—	amniotic fluid alpha-fetoprotein
Primary pituitary dysgenesis	AR	amniotic fluid prolactin
Tangier disease	AR	amniotic fluid apoA-I

fluid (Schneck et al, 1970; Friedland et al, 1971) as has Hunter syndrome (Liebaers et al, 1977) and hypophosphatasia (Mulivor et al, 1978). The diagnosis of Pompe disease (Type II glycogen storage disease) based on deficient amniotic fluid α-1,4-glucosidase activity has been reported (Nadler & Messina, 1969) but this approach has subsequently been shown to be unreliable (Nadler et al, 1970).

While methylmalonic acidaemia and argininosuccinic aciduria may be recognized by accumulation of metabolites in the amniotic fluid (Morror et al, 1970; Fleisher et al, 1977) not all aminocidurias are amenable to this approach. In phenylketonuria, for example, the placental circulation and maternal metabolism are capable of maintaining normal serum and urine phenylalanine levels *in utero*, and abnormal metabolites are not noted even at birth.

The first attempts to diagnose congenital adrenal hyperplasia were based on 17-ketosteroid and pregnanetriol levels in the amniotic fluid but this approach was subsequently found to be unreliable in midtrimester (Merkatz et al, 1969). Elevated levels of 17-α-hydroxyprogesterone are more consistently associated with the disorder (Milunsky & Tulchinsky, 1977) although HLA typing of amniotic fluid cells will probably supplant this (see below).

Primary pituitary dysgenesis, a rare autosomal recessive disorder in which serum HDL is deficient secondary to a deficiency of ApoA-I, may be diagnosable through detection of low levels of this apoprotein in amniotic fluid (Gebhardt, 1979).

Alpha-fetoprotein and the detection of neural tube defects
Neural tube defects (NTD's) are among the most common of congenital malformations and are discussed in detail elsewhere in this volume. While new surgical techniques have improved morbidity and mortality in these disorders, primary prevention through prenatal diagnosis and abortion has been possible since 1972 by the measurement of midtrimester amniotic fluid alpha-fetoprotein levels (Brock & Sutcliffe, 1972). The subject has been recently reviewed by Crandall et al (1978).

AFP is first detectable in fetal serum 30 days after conception. Early in gestation it is produced in the yolk sac but hepatic synthesis increases steadily and by the end of the first trimester the liver is the major source of the protein. The function of this albumin-like glycoprotein is unknown. Its concentration in fetal serum (Fig 102.1, top) rises until 10–13 weeks is attributed to the increase in fetal size, since the total amount of circulating AFP remains fairly constant, after which it steadily declines (Gitlin &Boesman, 1966). Some of the protein is secreted in the urine and thereby enters the amniotic fluid where its concentration is 1/100th that of the fetal serum at 14 weeks. Amniotic fluid levels decline from about 2 mg/dl at 12–13 weeks to less than 0.5 mg/dl at 20 weeks (Fig. 102.1, middle) and an accurate assessment of gestational age is therefore critical for interpretation of levels (Milunksy & Alpert, 1974; Seller, 1974; Seppälä & Ruoslahti, 1972).

The mechanism by which AFP levels are increased in NTD's is still unclear but its reliability in the detection of open defects has been well established. Recent data indicate that the amniotic fluid AFP is elevated in 98.2% of anencephalic pregnancies (elevation is defined as : 2.5 X the median at 13–15 weeks, 3.0 X the median at 16–18 weeks, 3.5 X the median at 19–21 weeks, and 4.0 X the median at 22–24 weeks)(Second Report of the U.K. Collaborative Study on Alpha-fetoprotein in relation to neural tube defects, 1979). Closed neural tube defects which account for 10–15% of NTD's, often do not have elevated levels and may therefore escape detection. Some of these cases may be diagnosed by ultrasonography if the lesion is specifically sought. Overall, approximately 90% of all NTD's may be detected with the use of amniotic fluid and maternal serum AFP levels and ultrasonography.

Neural tube defects are not the only disorders associated with elevated amniotic fluid AFP levels. In congenital nephrosis of the Finnish type, missed abortion, severe Rh isoimmunization, oesophageal atresia, duo-

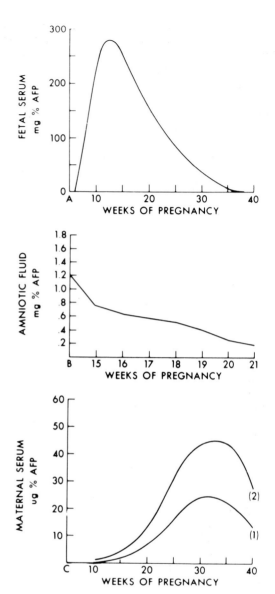

Fig. 102.1 Changes in alpha-fetoprotein concentrations during gestation. *top*, fetal serum (from Gitlin & Boesman, 1966); *middle*, amniotic fluid (from Crandall et al, 1978); *bottom*, maternal serum (from Leighton et al, 1975).

denal atresia, omphalocele, Turner syndrome with cystic hygromas and several chromosomal abnormalities, increased AFP levels have been found (Seppälä & Ruoslahti, 1973 a,b; Guibaud et al, 1973; Whyley et al, 1974; Seppälä, 1973; DeBruijn & Huisjes, 1975). False positive elevations of amniotic fluid AFP may also occur. In the U.K. Collaborative Study, the rate of elevated AFP's without a neural tube defect was 0.8%. One third of these pregnancies subsequently terminated in a spontaneous abortion. Half of the remaining fluids were blood stained. In ⅕ of these pregnancies in which the fluid was clear, infants with serious anomalies were later delivered (3 with exomphalos, 2 with cogenital nephrosis, 1 with microcephaly and oligohydramnios and 1 with Turner syndrome). The resulting 'practical' false positive rate was 0.27%.

Amniotic fluid AFP levels may be measured by several techniques including 'rocket' immunoelectrophoresis and radioimmunoassay (Ruoslahti & Seppälä, 1971). It is essential that the laboratory performing the assay be highly experienced and have established its own normative data as a function of gestational age.

Although the sensitivity of AFP testing for spina bifida and anencephaly is impressive, the false positive rate is approximately the same as the incidence of these malformations. Therefore, since most amniocenteses are done for cytogenetic indications (i.e. where there is no increased risk for a NTD) an elevated amniotic fluid AFP is as likely to be a false positive as it is to be indicative of an NTD. Ultrasonography is often rewarding in confirming the presence of a NTD, but the false negative rate in most centres is unacceptable. A complementary biochemical test would therefore be very welcome.

The presence of acetylcholinesterase activity in cerebrospinal fluid suggested the possibility of detecting open NTD's by measurement of this enzyme in amniotic fluid (Smith et al, 1979). Although experience with this procedure is still limited, the results obtained to date have been very promising and the assay appears to be both sensitive and specific – so much so that the possibility of it replacing AFP has been raised (Zeisel et al, 1980; Amniotic fluid acetylcholinesterase, 1980).

Cystic fibrosis
The potential for the diagnosis of cystic fibrosis (CF) *in utero* by the study of arginine esterase activity is a recent development in the use of cell free amniotic fluid for prenatal diagnosis. Walsh, Rao and Nadler (1980) have demonstrated decreased activity of the benzamidine inhibitable fraction of 4-methylumbelliferylguanidinobenzoate (MUGB) – reactive proteases in midtrimester amniotic fluid from fetuses subsequently shown to have CF. In addition, a specific band of enzyme activity which is normally observed is not seen in CF amniotic fluids after isoelectricfocusing and staining with α-N-Benzoyl-L-arginine ethylester (BAEE) or MUGB (Walsh & Nadler, 1979). When normal amniotic fluid is subjected to gel filtration on Biogel P-150, MUGB activity is found in a peak with MW of 100 000. Similarly analyzed CF amniotic fluids show approximately equal activities in 2 peaks: one with MW 100 000 and the other 50 000 (Nadler & Walsh, 1980b). To date, 13 pregnancies at risk for CF have been prospectively monitored and the outcome of each predicted correctly using these techniques; 10 normal and 3 infants affected with CF have been deliv-

ered (Nadelr & Walsh, 1980 a,c). A large scale prospective study is currently in progress on a research basis to determine the reliability of the tests.

Uncultivated amniotic fluid cells
The first application of amniocenteses to prenatal diagnosis was sex determination by examination for Barr bodies in uncultivated amniotic fluid cells. These fetal cells derive from the amnion itself, desquamatior from the fetal skin, and mucosal surfaces (buccal and vaginal) and from the urine. Contamination of the fluid with maternal blood may, however, result in the presence of leucocytes. Although some of the cells possess some enzymatic activity (Nadler & Gerbie, 1969), many nonviable and serve only to render interpretation of results more difficult. At present there are no reliable enzymatic assays based on uncultivated amniotic fluid cells. Restriction endonuclease mapping has been performed on uncultivated cells but is usually done on cultivated cells.

Cultivated amniotic fluid cells
The number of disorders diagnosable from the study of cultivated amniotic fluid (AF) cells exceeds by far the number possible by using any other prenatal diagnostic tool. Two types of disorders are amenable to diagnosis in this way: cytogenetic abnormalities and genetic defects resulting in abnormalities of the synthesis of specific proteins, many of which (but not all) result in 'inborn errors of metabolism'.

Cytogenetic abnormalities
Approximately 90% of all amniocenteses are performed for cytogenetic analysis. The date presented in Table 102.8, demonstrating the increasing risk of Down syndrome with advancing maternal age is familiar and is the basis of the recommendation that women over the age of 35 consider amniocentesis. Other cytogenetic indications will be discussed later. The fibroblast-like cells obtained at amniocentesis are cultured in any one of a variety of tissue culture media enriched with fetal calf serum and after 2–3 weeks a sufficient number of cells have grown to permit karyotyping. A minimum of 25 cells is examined and the modal chromosome number established. A smaller number of cells is then examined after G-banding to detect minor structural rearrangements. The original fluid specimen should be seeded into at least 2 culture flasks, and samples of each studied.

Sex determination and abnormalities of chromosome number and structure can be determined with 99.4% accuracy (NICHD, 1976; Golbus et al, 1979). There are, however, a number of potential pitfalls in the interpretation of cytogenetic studies. Polyploidy has been observed frequently in amniotic fluid cell cultures and may comprise 4–100% of the cells studied (Milunsky et al, 197C, 1971; Kohn & Robinson, 1970). In most of the

Table 102.8 Incidence of Down syndrome with increasing maternal age (from Hook and Chambers, 1977).

Maternal age	Estimated rate per 1000 live births[a]	Fractional rate
32	1.38	1/725
33	1.69	1/592
34	2.15	1/465
35	2.74	1/365
36	3.49	1/287
37	4.45	1/255
38	5.66	1/177
39	7.21	1/139
40	9.19	1/109
41	11.71	1/85
42	14.91	1/67
43	19.00	1/53
44	24.20	1/41
45	30.84	1/32
46	39.28	1/25
47	50.04	1/20
48	63.75	1/16
49	81.21	1/12

[a] Regression adjusted estimates corrected underreporting.

reported cases, pregnancy has not been terminated and the infants born at term have had normal karyotypes. The origin of the tetraploid cell lines is uncertain but they may derive from the amnion in which tetraploidy may normally occur. Mosaicism is another relatively frequent finding in cultured AF cells, resulting from the appearance of a trisomic clone which may arise in as many as 2–3% of cultures (Peakman et al, 1978, 1979). Although this 'pseudomosaicism' is typically found in only one flask of cells, repeating the amniocentesis is often necessary for confirmation. Detection of true mosaicism is also difficult since the mosaicism may not affect the amniotic fluid cells. Lastly, the recognition of the normal variations in chromosome length, satellite size, or the position of specific bands may be problematic. Karyotype analysis of the parents may be the only means of interpreting unusual findings.

Chromosomal instability syndromes

Several of the 'chromosomal instability' syndromes may be amenable to prenatal diagnosis by midtrimester amniocentesis. For example, in Bloom syndrome an increased frequency of sister chromatid exchanges (SCE's) in phytohaemagglutinin stimulated lymphocytes and cultured fibroblasts is pathognomonic. In at least 4 pregnancies at risk, amniotic fluid cells have been studied for SCE frequencies and no abnormalities found; at birth, all 4 infants were normal (German et al, 1979). In Fanconi anaemia (FA) lymphocytes and fibroblasts from affected children also show spontaneous chromosomal

breaks with specific sensitivity to the mutagen diepoxybutane (DEB). Four pregnancies at risk for FA have now been monitored by this technique and the outcome of each predicted correctly: 3 affected and 1 normal (Auerbach et al, 1979; Auerbach et al, 1980). In ataxia telangiectasia, spontaneous chromosomal breakage has been frequently, but not universally observed. Recently, it has been demonstrated that AT cells may be uniquely sensitive to bleomycin, responding with decreased cell viability and increased chromosomal damage, a 'stress' test which may be applicable to prenatal diagnosis (Cohen & Simpson, 1980). Lastly, Xeroderma pigmentosum has been diagnosed *in utero* by demonstration of decreased radio-active thymidine incorporation (repair synthesis') after exposure of cultivated amniotic fluid cells to ultraviolet light (Ramsay et al, 1974; Halley et al, 1979).

Disorders affecting protein synthesis

These disorders include 3 types of defects (1) structural gene mutations resulting in the synthesis of abnormal and often biologically defective proteins; (2) gene deletions, and (3) regulatory gene mutations resulting in decreased synthesis of a protein. Most of the inborn errors of metabolism fall into the first category and result in the synthesis of catalytically defective enzyme proteins. Theoretically, even if a gene defect were of the 2nd or 3rd type, the result would be the same: decreased enzyme activity. For those enzymes which are expressed in amniotic fluid cells, the measurement of enzyme activity is the basis for prenatal diagnosis. It cannot be overstated, though, that a pre-requisite to accurate diagnosis is the simultaneous use of normal control AF cells by a laboratory experienced in the assay. Published normals are inadequate; not only do assay conditions vary slightly from one lab to another, but the medium in which the cells are cultured and even the number of passages in tissue culture may affect the results. It is preferable, therefore, that the control cells be selected from amniotic fluid cells obtained on the same day for other indications. It is also essential that the fibroblasts from the obligate heterzygotes (i.e. the parents) be assayed prior to attempted prenatal diagnosis, since occasional variants may result in deficient activity in heterozygotes as well as homozygotes or hemizygotes and render the distinction between them impossible.

Numerous autosomal recessive and X–linked enzyme deficiencies may be diagnosed prenatally by assaying amniotic fluid cell activity and are listed in Tables 2–7. For some of the disorders listed, prenatal diagnosis has not yet been attempted, although all are amenable to this approach. Many excellent reviews have been written on this subject (Burton, 1980; Nadler, 1976; Milunsky, 1975) and further details of these disorders are discussed in other sections of this volume. There are, however, many disorders in which the abnormal protein is not expressed in AF cells and other means of diagnosis must be sought.

DNA hybridization

For disorders which are the result of gene deletions it may be possible to detect the deletion itself, rather than the consequent impaired production of a protein. Because the full genetic complement is present in all nucleated cells, amniotic fluid cells may be employed for this type of analysis even if the gene under study is not normally expressed in these cells.

Alpha thalasseaemia has been diagnosed *in utero* using this approach. The specific messenger RNA for the α-globin chain may be isolated from reticulocytes and a complementary strand of radioactive DNA (cDNA) synthesized using a vital reverse transcriptase and radiolabelled bases.

After separation of the strands of isolated DNA, the radioactive cDNA 'probe' should hybridize to the α-globin genes in the single stranded DNA. The newly formed double stranded DNA segments may be removed from the reaction mixutre and the radioactivity in them measured. The amount of radioactivity in these double stranded DNA fragments is a function of the number of α-genes present; in homozygous α-thalassaemia, no hybridization would be expected. This method has been successfully employed in several pregnancies at risk for homozygous α-thalassaemia (Kan et al, 1976; Dozy et al, 1979). It is theoretically applicable to the diagnosis of δβ and β° thalassaemia and hereditary persistence of fetal haemoglobin as well.

Restriction endonuclease analysis

The hybridization technique described above is technically difficult and subject to error (Nathan, 1976). These problems may be obviated by the use of a somewhat different technique, restriction endonuclease analysis. The isolation of bacterial endonucleases which possess recognition sites for specific short nucleotide sequences and cleave the DNA only where that sequence is found has made it possible to construct 'restriction maps' of DNA in any cell (Southern, 1975). The method involves extraction of DNA from the cells under study and incubation of the extracted DNA with the endonuclease, which breaks the nucleotide strands where it encounters a 'restriction site', i.e., the base sequence for which the enzyme is specific. The DNA fragments which are obtained are then subjected to electrophoresis on an agarose gel which separates them according to their size (expressed in 'kilobases' or Kb). A radioactive cDNA 'probe' is then hybridized to the DNA fragments and an autoradiograph prepared. Those fragments which contain the globin genes will appear as dark areas on the autoradiograph. After digestion of human DNA with the endonuclease EcoRI, both copies of the α-gene are found in a fragment approximately 20 Kb in size. In homozygous α-thalassaemia, no hybridization with α-cDNA probes occurs and the 20 Kb fragment is therefore not seen on the autoradiographs. Using a β-cDNA probe, β-thalassaemia, δβ-thalassaemia and hereditary persistence of fetal haemoglobin (in which the β-genes or β and δ genes are deleted) may similarly be detected (Orkin et al, 1978; Dozy et al, 1979). The technique is so sensitive that sufficient DNA may be obtained from uncultivated amniotic fluid cells.

The endonuclease EcoRI recognizes the DNA sequence 5'-GAATTC-3' and cleaves the DNA where this sequence is encountered. This sequence is found in the normal β-globin gene and codes for amino acids 121 and 122 in the β-globin peptide. In haemoglobin O^{Arab} a single base substitution results in the sequence 5'-AAATTC-3' and the substitution of lysine for glutamic acid at position 121 in the β-globin molecule. Because of the single base substitution in the β^{O-Arab} gene, EcoRI does not recognize that area as a restriction site, and digestion with the endonuclease results in a DNA fragment that is larger than normal (Fig. 102.2). Digestion of DNA from subjects with haemoglobin O^{Arab} and hybridization with β-cDNA will show the β gene to be located in an abnormally large DNA fragment (Phillips et al, 1979).

For most of the haemoglobinopathies, however, the base substitutions do not result in loss (or eain) of recognized restriction sites for the available endonucleases. The discovery of polymorphism of the endonuclease restriction sites, however, suggested another approach to the diagnosis of these disorders: Linkage analysis.

Linkage analysis

When 2 genes are linked, it is often possible to determine the nature of the linkage (i.e. attraction or repulsion) within a given family group. If this is achieved, the presence or absence of one gene may be inferred by the presence or absence of the other. When a gene which is not expressed in amniotic fluid cells is linked to a gene which is, linkage analysis may be applicable to prenatal diagnosis.

The simplest application of this approach is in the case of X−linked disorders in which cytogenetic analysis and

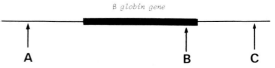

Fig. 102.2 The β-globin gene and EcoRI restriction sites (arrows). Normally the endonuclease will cleave the DNA at all three sites (A, B, C). In haemoglobin O^{Arab}, a single base substitution results in loss of restriction site B, and cleavage occurs only at A and C.

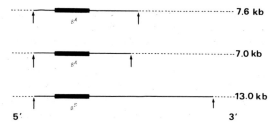

Fig. 102.3 The most common relationships between the β-globin genes and the polymorphic HpaI restriction sites. The arrows indicate where the DNA is cleaved by HpaI.

selective abortion of all male fetuses may be undertaken. Half of the aborted fetuses, however, will not have been affected. For several X-linked and autosomal disorders, including several haemoglobin variants, more refined techniques employing linkage analysis have been developed.

Haemoglobinopathies. Using the endonuclease HpaI on DNA from individuals with haemoglobins A, AS and S, Kan and Dozy (1978a) observed that (1) the β-globin gene was usually found in a 7.6 Kb fragment; (2) in some individuals of African descent, the β-globin gene was in 7.0 or 13.0 Kb fragment instead of the usual 7.6 Kb fragment (i.e. there was polymorphism in the restriction site); (3) the presence of these unusual sized fragments was inherited in a simple Mendelian fashion and; (4) 87%

of the β-genes in Blacks with Sickle Cell disease were found in 13.0 Kb fragments. In Blacks with haemoglobin A only 3% of the β genes were in 13.0 Kb fragments. They also demonstrated the relative positions of the globin gene and the HpaI restriction sites on the DNA (see Fig. 102.3). It is clear that the HpaI site is not directly adjacent to the β-globin gene, but rather, they are linked. They suggested that by taking advantage of this linkage, an individual's haemoglobin type might be determined by restriction analysis.

From Kan and Dozy's data, it was clear that the β^s gene was not always on the 13.0 Kb fragment. In several individuals it was found on the 7.6 Kb fragment. In addition, several patients wth Hgb A were found to have 13.0 Kb fragments. The finding of a 13.0 Kb fragment after restriction analysis with HpaI does not, therefore, necessarily imply the presence of the β^gene. In order to apply restriction analysis to prenatal diagnosis, the size of the DNA fragment to which the β^s gene is linked must be determined *in the family under study*. This can be done only by restriction analysis of the heterozygous parents and at least one other family member. Table 102.9 and Figure 102.4 illustrate the point.

The results of restriction analysis of leucocyte DNA and haemoglobin typing from a hypothetical family who seek prenatal diagnosis for Sickle Cell disease are given in Table 102.9. The parents, II.1 and II.2, are both known

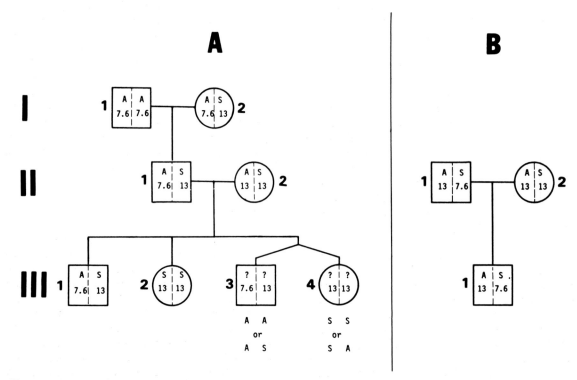

Fig. 102.4 Pedigrees for a hypothetical family seeking prenatal diagnosis for sickle cell disease. Details in text.

Table 102.9 Results of haemoglobin typing and restriction analysis of leucocytes from hypothetical family

Patient	Hgb	Restriction fragments
I.1 Grandfather	A	7.6
I.2 Grandmother		
II.1 Father	A,S	7.6, 13.0
II.2 Mother	A,S	7.6, 13.0
III.1 First child	A,S	13.0
III.2 Second child	A,S	7.6, 13.0
III.3 Amniotic fluid cells Twin A	S	13.0
III.4 Amniotic fluid cells Twin B	?	7.6, 13.0
	?	13.0

carriers and have one heterozygous child (III.1) and one child with sickle cell disease (III.1) Ultrasonography reveals tthat this is a twin gestation and at 16 weeks amniocentesis is performed and specimens are successfully obtained from both amniotic sacs.

If one were to examine the data from only the parents and the first child (III.1) the linkage between the HpaI sites and the β^s could not be established. In Figure 102.4, pedigrees A and B, which show opposite linkages between the β^s gene and the fragments sizes, account for these data equally well. The ambiguity is resolved when the paternal grandparents (I.1, I.2) or the affected child (III.2) are included. It then becomes clear that in both the paternal grandmother and the father, the 13.0 Kb site and the β^s gene are linked, and in the paternal grandfather and the father, the linkage is between 7.6 Kb site and the β^A gene. Since the affected child has only the 13.0 Kb fragment, she must be homozygous for this as well as for the β^S gene, and they must therefore be linked in her and both parents. Even though the linkage can be established in this family, definitive diagnosis is not possible in either twin. In III.3 homozygosity for the β^s gene can be excluded, but $\beta^{S\beta A}$ or $\beta^{A\beta A}$ are possible. In III.4, either $\beta^{S\beta S}$ or $\beta^{S\beta A}$ are possible and even exclusion is not possible although the risk for this child having Sickle Cell disease is now 50% instead of 25%. In this situation, a diagnosis might be reached if a second restriction enzyme with specificity for a different site were employed and the analysis thereby extended.

It should be evident that the method is only applicable to prenatal diagnosis after a family study is performed. The method requires (1) polymorphism of the restriction site for the enzyme being used; (2) a specific probe; (3) the assumption that linkage is tight enough that meiotic cross over will be a rare event. If crossover should occur between the restriction site and the globin gene, the linkage will be reversed and the diagnosis will be in error.

This type of analysis has been successfully applied to the prenatal diagnosis of a variety of haemoglobin var-

iants and α, β^+, β^{oc} and $\delta\beta$-thalassaemias (Orkin et al, 1978; Kan and Dozy, 1978b; Phillips et al, 1979).

Congenital adrenal hyperplasia (21-hydroxylase deficiency). This inborn error is one which is expressed in adrenal cortex cells but not in fibroblast or AF cells. In infancy, the diagnosis may be made by the characteristic alterations in steroid levels, and as already noted, increased levels of 17-α-hydroxyprogesterone levels in amniotic fluid may be found in affected pregnancies. The 21-hydroxylase gene, located on the short arm of chromosome 6, is closely linked to the major histocompatibility (HLA) complex. These genes are sufficiently close together that meiotic crossing over is thought to be an infrequent event. Because the histocompatibility antigens are expressed on amniotic fluid cells, the HLA type of an individual may be determined *in utero*.

The procedure for diagnosis is entirely analogous to that for Sickle Cell disease (Pollack et al, 1979). The HLA haplotypes of the parents and the affected child must be determined in order to establish the linkage of the HLA types to the defective 21-hydroxylase gene. Because of the polymorphisms for each of the 4 HLA loci, establishing the linkage may more easily be achieved than it is in the haemoglobinopathies. Even if an affected child is not available for study, it may be possible to exclude the diagnosis if the fetal HLA type is identical to that of an unaffected sib.

Myotonic dystrophy. The gene for myotonic dystrophy, an autosomal dominant disorder, appears to be linked to the gene determining secretor status (the ability to secrete ABH blood group antigens into body fluids) and in some families this linkage may be used to advantage for prenatal diagnosis (Schrott & Omenn, 1975). Because secretor status is also a dominant trait, the parent affected with myotonic dystrophy must be heterozygous for the analysis to be fruitful. If, in addition, the linkage betweer the 2 genes can be determined by studying other family members, prenatal diagnosis may be performed by determining the presence or absence of ABH blood group antigen in cell free amniotic fluid.

INDICATIONS

The most common indication for midtrimester amniocentesis is advanced maternal age. Even before the chromosomal basis of Down syndrome was recognized, the increase in incidence with advanced maternal age was appreciated (Table 102.8). The frequencies of trisomies 13 and 18 also increase with maternal age. Most centres recommend that women over the age of 35 consider amniocentesis. The combined risk for all chromosomal abnormalities at this age is 1–2%. In addition, after the birth of a child with Down syndrome, the recurrence risk is generally considered to be approximately 1%. The recurrence risks for other autosomal or sex chromosome trisomies are not known. These data have been reviewed in many sources (see Simpson, 1980; Miles & Kaback, 1978).

It has been recently demonstrated that in 20–30% of cases of trisomic Down syndrome, the extra chromosome is of paternal origin. Thus, an effect of paternal age independent of maternal age has been suggested. At present, it appears that the risk for Down syndrome may be twice the expected rate when the father is more than 55 years old; below this age or effect has been detected consistently (Hook, 1980).

Couples in which one member is a carrier of a balanced translocation or other rearrangement are at significantly increase risk of having a chromosomally abnormal child and should be counselled about amniocentesis. The magnitude of the risk varies depending on the specific rearrangement and which parent is the carrier. In general, if the mother has a reciprocal translocation, it is approximately 10%; if the father is the carrier it is 2–3%.

Amniocentesis for sex identification may be indicated in women at risk for X–linked disorders for which specific diagnosis is not possible (e.g. Bruton and Swiss type agammaglobulinaemia, X–linked mental retardation, Duchenne muscular dystrophy).

Amniocentesis may be indicated if a couple is found by screening to be at risk for Tay-Sachs disease or a haemoglobinopathy. Amniocentesis for NTD detection may be indicated in the couple with an affected first degree relative, or after finding elevated maternal serum AFP's on two occasions and after confirmation or gestational age and exclusion of multiple gestation is accomplished ultrasonographically.

Prenatal diagnosis is attempted in other conditions only after the birth of an affected child and is potentially possible for any of the conditions listed in Tables 102.2–7.

FETAL BLOOD SAMPLING

The diagnosis of hereditary disease by analysis of fetal blood has recently become a reality as the technical difficulties of sample collection have been largely overcome. The discovery that adult haemoglobin types are synthesized by fetal reticulocytes (albeit in small amounts) suggested the possibility of prenatal diagnosis of haemoglobinopathies ard provided the stimulus for much of this work (Hollenberg et al, 1971; Kan et al, 1972; Cividalli et al, 1974; Kazazian & Woodhead, 1973). Other disorders are also detectable and are discussed below (Table 102.10). Although many of the haemoglobinopathies may now be diagnosed by restriction analysis of amniotic fluid cells, diagnosis or exclusion is not

Table 102.10 Disorders in which fetal blood samples have been used for diagnosis

Alpha-1-antitrypsin deficiency
Chronic granulomatous disease
Galactosaemia
Haemoglobinopathies
Haemophilia A and B
Homozygous Von Willebrand disease

always possible, and fetal blood analysis, despite the higher risks, may still be indicated.

The haemoglobinopathies may be detected by the measurement of *in vitro* haemoglobin synthesis by fetal reticulocytes. The cells are incubated in medium containing radioactive leucine which is incorporated into the newly produced proteins (primarily globins). The different globin chains (α, β and γ)are separated by ion exchange chromatography or other methods (Fig. 102.5) and the radioactivity in each type of globin chain determined and expressed as the $\beta{:}\gamma$ ratio. The incorporation of radioactivity permits sufficient sensitivity that even the small amounts of β-globin produced are detected. Abnormal β chains are identified by their later elution from the ion exchange column. In β-thalassaemia, the $\beta{:}\gamma$ ratio is lower than normal. The methodology has been reviewed in greater detail in several sources (Alter, 1979, 1980; Leonard & Kazazian, 1978).

Because β-globin production occurs at a very low rate early in gestation, it is essential that fetal blood samples be relatively pure. Contamination of the sample with maternal blood, and the resultant β-chain synthesis by adult reticulocytes, is a potential source of great error. Several methods have been developed to minimize and/or correct this source of variation and will be briefly reviewed.

Maternal reticulocyte production may be suppressed by hypertransfusion of the mother prior to fetal blood sampling. There are many reasons why this undesirable (e.g., risk of hepatitis, transfusion reaction, sensitization to minor blood groups). The procedure therefore usually begins with the assessment of the proportion of cells obtained which are of fetal origin. Advantage may be taken of the fact that the fetal red blood cells are considerably larger (120–160 μm^3) than in the adult (80–95 μm^3). After a blood sample is obtained, it may be immediately analyzed in a particle size distribution analyzer (Coulter channelyzer). If the distribution of cells is primarily in the smaller range, additional samples may be immediately withdrawn. When an adequate specimen is obtained, the precise proportion of fetal cells is determined by preparing a blood smear and counting the percentage of cells remaining after acid elution (Kleihauer-Betke technique). Samples in which there is corsiderable

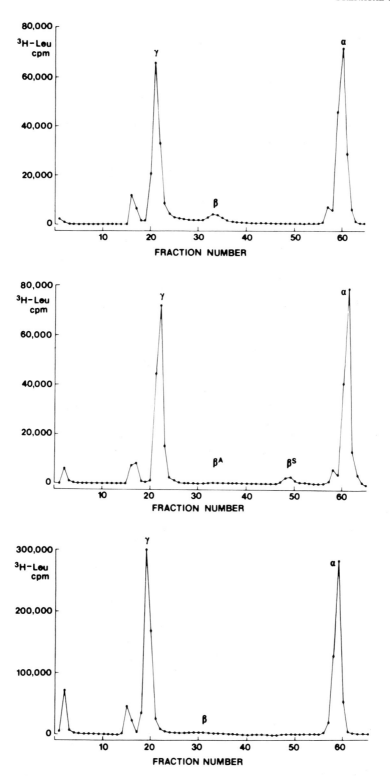

Fig. 102.5 Elution from a CM cellulose ion exchange column of different globin chains produced by fetal reticulocytes. The cells were first incubated with ³H-leucine. *Top*, normal fetus; *middle*, fetus with sickle cell disease; *bottom*, fetus with β-thalassaemia major (from Alter, 1979).

mixing of fetal and maternal cells may be handled in several ways. A mathematical correction of the data based on the proportion of cells which are known to be of maternal origin and the measured leucine incorporation of these cells may be employed. In some instances, the fetal and maternal cells may be physically separated by several techniques: selective agglutination of one population of cells based on differing fetal and maternal blood types, selective haemolysis of maternal cells (which have higher carbonic anhydrase activity) in $NH_4Cl-NH_4HCO_3$ solutions, and separation on the basis of size or density differences in a cell sorter or by velocity or density gradient sendimentation.

Although the procedures are technically demanding and require transfer of the mother to be a centre with the facilities and expertise to perform these procedures, there are still situations in which no alternative means of diagnosis are possible. The blood samples obtained for this analysis may be obtained by one of 2 methods: placentocentesis and fetoscopy.

PLACENTOCENTESIS

This technique (Golbus et al, 1976; Kan et al, 1974), usually performed at 18 weeks gestation, employs direct insertion of a spinal needle into the placenta under ultrasonographic guidance. The needle is manipulated until it is 2–4 mm beneath the amnion. Samples are withdrawn and evaluated as above. The procedure may be performed when the placenta is either anteriorly or posteriorly implanted.

Several potential complications must be considered. The fetal loss rate is now approximately 5%. Puncture of a major vessel is potentially devastating. Amnionitis, Rh isoimmunization and significant fetal-maternal transfusion may occur. Although fetal blood typing may be performed and Rhogam administered to the antibody-negative mother with an Rh-position fetus, iso-immunization could still occur if a fetal-maternal transfusion excuded the capacity of Rhogam to neutralize the cells (estimated to be 15 ml).

FETOSCOPY

Fetoscopy has recently emerged as a promising technique for direct visualization of the fetus. Performed at 17–20 weeks gestation it may be employed for fetal blood sampling under direct visualization when the placenta is posterior or fundal and occasionally even when it is anteriorly located. In addition, fetal skin biopsies may be obtained (Elias, 1980).

The fetoscope, which is approximately 2.7 mm in its outer diameter, consists of a fiberoptic light source and self-focusing lens. A separate channel may be employed for fetal blood sampling. The depth of focus is approximately 2 cm, the viewing angle 55–70 degrees and there is a 2–5 fold magnification factor under most circumstances.

Ultrasonography is essential prior to the procedure for location of the placenta and umbilical cord insertion, determination of the fetal position and selection of an insertion site as well as for confirmation of fetal viability, gestational age, and detection of multiple gestations. In addition, real time ultrasonography is useful for directing and orienting the fetoscope once it is inserted.

Under strict aseptic conditions, the trochar and cannula are inserted through a stab incision under local anaesthesia. The trochar and cannula are advanced into the amniotic cavity, the trochar removed, and the fetoscope inserted through the cannula. Because of the short viewing distance and limited viewing angle, the area seen is usually only 2–4 cm². Positioning of the instrument near the desired fetal part is facilitated with ultrasonography. Fetal blood is obtained through a 27 gauge flexible needle from a placenta. If a biopsy is to be obtained, the cannula is positioned at the desired site (e.g., back, scalp, thorax), the fetoscope removed, the biopsy forceps inserted, and a 2 × 2 mm punch biopsy obtained. With some models, the biopsy forceps may be inserted through a separate channel and the specimen taken under direct vision.

Spontaneous abortion remains an all too frequent complication of the procedure, occurring with an incidence of 5–10%. Premature delivery has occurred in 10% of the cases. The other potential complications are identical to those in placentocentesis.

APPLICATIONS

A large number of disorders may theoretically be diagnosed by fetal blood analysis; only those which have been attempted are shown in Table 102.10 and will be discussed. The methods employed for the diagnosis of the haemoglobinopathies have already been reviewed. In several X–linked disorders (below) specific diagnoses may be achieved on fetal blood specimens. In pregnancies at risk for these disorders, amniocentesis should be performed at 16 weeks for fetal sex determination. Only if the fetus is male should blood sampling be attempted.

The prenatal detection of classic haemophilia A by standard coagulation assays has been complicated by the lability of factor VIII coagulant activity, the presence of tissue thromboplastins in amniotic fluid (which is frequently present in fetal blood samples) and the variable levels of activity which have been reported for normal fetuses. Two antigens are now known to be associated with factor VIII: factor VIII related antigen (VIII-R) which is present in normal and haemophilic plasma and factor VIII coagulant antigen (VIII-C) which is deficient in the plasma of 90% of classic haemophiliacs. Those haemophiliacs with normal VIII-C levels tend to have mild disease. Measurement of the ratio of VIII-C:VIII-R has permitted the correct prenatal diagnosis in several pregnancies at risk. Establishment of the VIII-R level is necessary as an internal control for the variable dilution of the blood samples with amniotic fluid (Firschein et al, 1979). Mibashan et al (1979) have employed fetoscopy and with meticulous attention to the purity of sample collection have succeeded in obtaining fetal blood uncontaminated with maternal blood or amniotic fluid. In their hands, the standard assays for factor VIII and IX were reliable and correctly predicted and the outcome in 4 pregnancies at risk. The measurement of factor VIII-R antigen, which is deficient in von Willebrand disease, has been employed for the prenatal evaluation of a fetus at risk for hemozygosity for this disorder (Hoyer et al, 1979). Alpha-antitrypsin has also been measured in fetal blood in a pregnancy at risk for this autosomal recessive disease (Jeppson et al, 1979).

Chronic granulomatous disease is functional disorder of polymorpho-nuclear leucocytes and monocytes which is usually transmitted as an X-linked trait, although autosomal recessive inheritance has also been observed. 'Stimulated' leucocytes from affected individuals fail to generate superoxide and reduce the dye nitroblue tetrazolium; both phenomena have been successfully monitored in blood samples from an affected fetus (Newburger et al, 1979).

Although galactosaemia may be diagnosed using cultivated amniotic fluid cells, at least one fetus has been evaluated by measurement of the transferase activity in red cells. In this case, prenatal diagnosis was not requested until 20 weeks gestation and amniotic fluid cell studies could not have been completed prior to 24 weeks (Fensom et al, 1979).

The Duchenne type of muscular dystrophy is an X-linked disorder of unknown aetiology. Although successful prenatal diagnosis based or blood creatine phosphokinase (CPK) activity has been reported (Mahoney et al, 1977) the reliability of this method is under serious question (Golbus et al, 1979; Emery et al, 1979).

The histological examination of fetal skin biopsies obtained through fetoscopy has made possible the pre-

natal diagnosis of Harlequin ichthyosis (Elias et al, 1980), epidermolytic hyperkeratosis (congenital bullous ichthyosiform erythroderma) (Golbus et al, 1980) and epidermolysis bullosa letalis (Rodeck et al, 1980) (Table 11).

Direct visualization of fetal parts is extremely difficult, but incombination with ultrasonography several disorders have been detected. Chondroectodermal dysplasia (Ellis van Creveld syndrome) is associated with polydactyly and hypoplastic nails which may be seen at the time of fetoscopy (Mahoney & Hobbins, 1977). A previously undescribed heritable chondrodystrophy has been similarly diagnosed (Carey et al, 1979)

RADIOGRAPHIC METHODS

Midtrimester X-ray examination of the fetus would appear to be the logical means for the diagnosis of malformation ard dwarfism syndromes in which bony abnormalities are manifest at birth. Although mineralization of the fetal skeleton is adequate to permit radiographic visualization, experience with this modality has been disappointing. Several conditions which may be diagnosed radiographically are listed in Table at 102.12. For many of these disorders successful diagnosis has not yet been reported, although they appear amenable to this approach. Notably absent from this list are heterozygous achondroplasia and the Ellis van Creveld syndrome, for which prenatal diagnosis has not been possible by this means. An excellent review of the subject is available (Lachman & Hall, 1979).

Several disorders which are associated with major limb or other anomalies are amenable to diagnosis by radiographic means employing injection of contrast materials at amniocentesis. Two such methods are in use: amniography and fetography.

The injection of a water soluble dye (amniography) opacifies the amniotic cavity and allows visualization of the fetus by contrast. In addition, some of the contrast material is swallowed by the fetus and outlines the gastrointestinal tract. For this reason, amniography has been employed in the evaluation of polyhydramnios and has been used successfully in the diagnosis of achondrogenesis, a variety of gastrointestinal atresias and diaphragmatic hernia.

Fetography employs an oil soluble contrast material

Table 102.11 Disorders which have been diagnosed in fetoscopy

Disorder	Inheritance	Method of diagnosis
Chondroectodermal dysplasia	AR	polydactyly
Epidermolysis bullosa letalis	AR	skin biopsy histology
Epidermolytic hyperkeratosis	AD	skin biopsy histology
Harlequin ichthyosis	AR	skin biopsy histology

Table 102.12 Disorders which may be diagnosable in the second trimester of pregnancy by radiographic means

Disorder	Inheritance
Achondrogenesis, types 1 and 2	AR
Achondroplasia, homozygous	AD
Asphyxiating thoracic dystrophy (Jeune)	AR
Campomelic dysplasia (long limbed)	AR
Campomelic dysplasia (short limbed with cloverleaf skull)	?
Campomelic dysplasia (short limbed, normocephalic)	AR
Chondrodystrophia punctata, rhizomelic type	AR
Chondrodystrophia punctata, dominant type	AD
Cleidocranial dysplasia	AD
Craniometaphaseal dysplasia	AD or AR
Dysosteosclerosis	AR
Dyssegmented dwarfism	?AR
Hypophosphatasia, congenital lethal	AR
Hypophosphatasia tarda	AR
Larsen syndrome	AD, ? AR
Mesomelic dysplasias, some types	AD, AR
Osteoectasia with hyperphosphatasia	AR
Osteogenesis imperfecta congenita (crumpled bone)	AR
Osteogenesis imperfecta, other types if fractures present	AD, AR
Osteopetrosis	AR
Pyknodysostosis	AR
Short-rib polydactyly, I (Saldino-Noonan)	AR
Short-rib polydactyly, II (Majewski)	?
Thanatophoric dysplasia	?
Thanatophoric dysplasia with cloverleaf skull	AR
Thrombocytopenia with absent radii	AR

which adheres to the fetal vernix caseosa and permits visualization of the fetal outline. It may be useful in the recognition of limb length anomalies or major malformations which are externally manifest.

With all radiographic examinations, the risks of exposure to ionizing radiation are a cause for some concern. Although fetal exposures of less than 10 rad do not have a significant impact on the observed rate of congenital malformations (Swartz & Reighling, 1978) the incidence of childhood cancer may be increased by 40% (MacHahon & Hutchison, 1964). The use of contrast material further complicates the risks; a transient impairment of thyroid function has been observed in newborns who are exposed to iodinated contrast media *in utero* (Rodesh et al, 1976).

MATERNAL SERUM AND URINE

Analysis of maternal urine is occasionally of diagnostic value in those disorders in which either an abnormal metabolite or abnormal amounts of a normal metabolite are produced by the fetus, cleared from the fetal circulation through the placenta and excreted by the mother's kidneys. In argininosuccinic aciduria and methylmalonic acidaemia markedly increased amounts of ASA and

MMA, respectively, may be detected in maternal urine by midtrimester. Several other disorders my be amenable to this approach but it should not be relied on for definitive diagnosis.

ALPHA-FETOPROTEIN

The measurement of AFP levels for the detection of neural tube defects is the only prenatal diagnostic technique in current use which is based on maternal serum. The association of elevated maternal serum AFP and neural tube defects, first reported in 1973 (Leek et al, 1973; Brock et al, 1973) has been the basis for the establishment of screening programs both in the U.K. and U.S.A. (Report of the U.K. collaborative study on alpha-fetoprotein in relation to neural tube defects, 1977). Probably only 10% of infants with neural tube defects are born to women who have had a previous child with a NTD or are undergoing amniocentesis for some other reason (Towards the prevention of spina bifida, 1974). It is estimated that with maternal serum AFP screening 80% of open defects may be detected. Despite considerable controversy over the advisability of establishing screening programs in the U.S.A. (Nsdler & Simpson, 1979) it appears inevitable that mass population screening will occur.

The precise mechanisms by which fetal AFP enters the maternal circulation are poorly understood (Origin of Maternal Serum AFP, 1979). Transplacental transfer from fetal to maternal serum can be demonstrated in experimental animals and probably is one source of maternal serum AFP. It is reasonable to suppose that the normal increase in maternal AFP levels as pregnancy continues (Fig. 102.1, bottom) as well as the elevations observed in multiple pregnancies, threatened abortion and some placental lesions, are acquired through this mechanism. The elevation observed maternal serum with NTD's can not be attributed to this, however, since fetal serum levels are normal (Brock, 1974). It seems likely, therefore, that the increased levels in maternal serum in these conditions reflect the elevated concentration in amniotic fluid. This is supported by the finding of elevated maternal serum AFP concentration in other disorders which are known to be associated with increased amniotic fluid AFP: congenital nephrosis, omphalocele and intrauterine death.

One might expect, therefore, a good correlation between amniotic fluid and maternal serum AFP; this has not been the case (Second Report of U.K. Collaborative Study on alpha-fetoprotein in relation to neural tube defects, 1979). The conditions associated with enhanced transplacental transfer occur far more frequently than those associated with elevated amniotic fluid AFP levels. It is likely, therefore, that most elevated maternal serum AFP values will not be indicative of neural tube defects or any other fetal condition in which the amniotic fluid AFP is raised. It is clear that while the amniotic fluid AFP may be diagnostic for neural tube defects, maternal serum AFP certainly is not; at best it may be useful for screening.

In most screening programmes, maternal serum is obtained at 16–18 weeks gestation. If an elevated AFP level is detected, a second sample is obtained. If the second level is elevated, ultrasonography, and, if indicated, amniocentesis are performed. Approximately 7–8% of the screened population may be expected to have an elevated AFP when first tested. On repeat testing this may be reduced to 4–5% of the original population. Incorrect gestational timing will account for 25% of these elevations and multiple gestations for another 15–20%. Of the 2–3% of the original population who undergo amniocentesis, the amniotic fluid AFP will be significantly elevated in approximately 10% (Macri et al, 1979). The risk of a NTD with a confirmed elevation of maternal serum AFP is therefore estimated to be 5–10% varying with the geographic variation in the incidence of the defect.

There are clearly many problems in the development of screening programmes, particularly when most prenatal care is practiced in the private office, as it is in the U.S.A. for screening to be effective it must be performed by 16–18 weeks gestation. A conscientious, reliable and effective means of promptly recalling all women whose initial levels are elevated must be established. Regional laboratories that are experienced in this sensitive assay and that have established reliable normative data and controls must be utilized. Perhaps most problematic, however, is parent education and the potential anxiety that is created when an abnormal level is encountered, particularly since it is only in a few per cent of those women who are initially found to have an elevated AFP that a NTD will be subsequently confirmed.

ULTRASONOGRAPHY

The use of ultrasound for indirect visualization of internal body parts has had tremendous impact in all areas of medicine. While the number of abnormalities which may be diagnosed *in utero* by ultrasonographic examination is still small, this modality is of inestimable value when used in conjunction with other approaches (e.g. prior to amniocentesis, in conjunction with fetoscopy or placentocentesis) and with continual improvement of high resolution equipment ultrasonography will undoubtedly become a primary diagnostic tool for an increasing number of congenital malformations.

The echoes generated by the reflection of the ultrasound waves are generally displayed in one of two ways: B (brightness mode) in which a cross section of the anatomy is created as the transducer is moved across an area, and real-time imaging in which repetitive B-mode images are generated in rapid sequence, allowing the appreciation of motion.

The following discussion will be limited to the use of ultrasonography during the second trimester of pregnancy.

Estimation of fetal size. Despite considerable interest in the early recognition of intrauterine growth retardation this diagnosis can only tentatively be made by ultrasonographic means. Estimation of fetal size is best evaluated by the measurement of the biparietal diameter and fetal abdominal circumference; neither is very reliable in the prediction of fetal weight. The BPD, however, may be used for estimation of the duration of gestation.

Oligo- and polydramnios. Although determination of amniotic fluid volume is theoretically possible, in fact it is difficult, and the recognition of these conditions is most often based on the subjective impression of 'crowding' of the interatuterine contents. The finding of oligohydramnios strongly suggests an impairment of renal function and in the context of a 'positive' family history may be of diagnostic value. Polyhydramnios is associated with fetal anomalies in 20% of the cases. Many of these (anencephaly, spina bifida, obstruction of the esphageal-gastrointestinal tract, intrathoracic cysts, diaphragmatic hernias) may be diagnosable through ultrasonography or other means (e.g. amniography, amniocentesis).

Ascites. Fetal ascites is an ominous finding associated with chylous ascites, urinary tract obstruction, prune belly syndrome and a variety of multiple anomaly syndromes, many of which may be more specifically diagnosed ultrasonographically,

Hydrops fetalis. The ultrasonographic finding of the generalized oedema of hydrops carries a very grave prognosis. Several conditions known to cause this condition (Rh isoimmunization, thalassaemia) may be specifically diagnosed.

Neural tube defects. Anencephaly is most often easily diagnosed and with careful examination of the spine by an experienced examiner, a majority of meningomyeloceles may be detected. In several pregnancies at risk, closed defects associated with normal AFP, however, remains the major diagnostic test for these malformations.

Congenital heart disease. To date there has been little success in the diagnosis of CHD, although one case of tricuspid atresia and hypoplastic right ventricle has been respectively recognized.

Limb anomalies. By comparing measured limb segment lengths to control values, several short limb dwarfism syndromes have now been diagnosed (Ellis var Creveld, campomelic dwarfism) in midtrimester, and the method, though technically difficult, may be applicable to many other disorders. Osteogenesis imperfecta has been diagnosed through the recognition of fetal fractures at 19 weeks gestation.

Many other malformations my be detected by ultrasonographic means in midtrimester and are summarized in Table 102.13. Several excellent reviews have been written (Sabbagha & Shkolnik, 1980; Hobbins et al, 1979).

THE FUTURE

Just as the last 10 years have seen tremendous advances in both the technology and utilization of prenatal diagnostic methods, so may further strides be expected in the next few years. The biochemical basis for many additional disorders will undoubtedly be better understood and applicable both to diagnosis of affected individuals and screening for carriers. It seems likely that a means of identifying carriers for cystic fibrosis will be available and permit identification of couples at risk. Ongoing research on the basis of the cartilage and bone dysplasias may well make biochemical diagnosis a reality. Linkage analysis and restriction endonuclease mapping will prob-

Table 102.13 Abnormalities which may be detected by ultrasonography in the second trimester of pregnancy

Hydrops fetalis
Oligohydramnios
Polyhydramnios
CNS
Anencephaly
Encephalocele
Hydrocephalus
Meningomyelocele
Spina bifida
Chest
Diaphragmatic hernia
Intrathoracic cyst
Pulmonary hypoplasia
Small chest wall (thoracochondrodystrophy, asphyxiating thoracic dystrophy, thanatophoric dwarfism)
Abdomen/GI
Duodenal atresia
Esophageal atresia
Gastroschisis
Omphalocele
Renal/GU
Polycystic or multicystic kidneys (rarely)
Renal agenesis
Urethral obstruction and hydronephrosis
Miscellaneous
Osteogenesis imperfecta with *in utero* fractures
Robert syndrome
Short limbed dwarfism syndromes

ably find wider application in the diagnosis of disorders which are not expressed in amniotic fluid cells.

Methods for fetal visualization are continually improving. Diagnostic ultrasonography will probably be at the forefront as the resolution of equipment and our appreciation of normal improves. We may well be able to diagnose congenital heart disease, the various dwarfism syndromes and several isolated malformations in the near future utilizing this technique.

The identification of Y–chromosome containing cells in maternal blood samples has demonstrated the entry of fetal cells into the maternal circulation as early as 15 weeks gestation. This observation has suggested the possibility of fetal karyotyping using these cells. With the development of fluorescence activated cell sorting methodology, it has become possible to sort leucocytes obtained from maternal blood and to prepare an 'enriched' fraction in which the proportion of cells of fetal origin is approximately ten-fold higher than in the original specimen (Herzenberg et al, 1979). It may be possible to perform cytogenetic studies on the cells in the enriched fraction and thereby obtain a fetal karyotype without amniocentesis (Jores, 1979). Although the contamination of the enriched fraction with maternal cells is considerable and technical problems render it exceedingly difficult to perform cytogenetic studies on these cells, this is an exciting area of investigation which may have tremendous impact or prenatal diagnosis in the future.

The identification of couples at risk for children with birth defects represents probably the greatest challenge in prenatal diagnosis, and one that may be insurmountable prior to the birth of an affected child for most diagnosable disorders. Despite progress in diagnostic capabilities, the vast majority of these rare disorders are first inflicted on the unsuspecting. The availability and capacity of centres for prenatal diagnosis is also a major issue; utilization of these services has increased exponentially in the last ten years as the public has become educated in the risks of advanced maternal age and the possibility of prenatal diagnosis. This trend may be expected to continue. With the establishment of new centres, training of personnel and education of the professional and lay public it may be hoped that the need will be met, the services more efficiently utilized and the likelihood of a defective child being born reduced.

REFERENCES

Alter B P 1979 Prenatal diagnosis of hemoglobinopathies and other hematologic diseases. 95 501–513

Atler B P 1980 Journal of Pediatrics Intrauterine diagnosis of hemoelobinopathies. Seminars in Perinatology 4: 189–198

Alter B P, Modell C B, Fairweather D, Hobbins J C, Mahoney M J, Frigoletto F D, Sherman A S, Nathan D G 1976 Prenatal diagnosis of hemoglobinopathies. New England Journal of Medicine 295: 1437–1443

Amniotic fluid acetylcholinesterase 1980. Lancet 2: 407–408

Auerbach A D, Adler B, Chaganti R S K 1980 Fanconi anemia: Pre-and postnatal diagnosis and carrier detection by a cytogenetic method. Presented at the American Society of Human Genetics (24–27 September) New York City

Auerbach A D, WarburtonD, Bloom A D, Chaeanti R S K 1979 Prenatal detection of the Fanconi anemia gene by cytogenetic methods. American Journal of Human Genetics 31: 77–81

Brock D J H 1974 The molecular nature of alpha-fetoprotein in anencephaly and spina bifida. Clinica Chimica Acta 57: 315–320

Brock D J H, Bolton A E, Monghan J M 1973 Prenatal diagnosis of anencephaly through maternal serum alpha-fetoprotein measurements. Lancet 2: 923–924

Burton B K, 1980 Intrauterine diagnosis of biochemical disorders. Seminars in Perinatology 4: 179–185

Burton B K, Gerbie A B, Nadler H L 1974 Present status of intrauterine diagnosis of genetic defects. American Journal of Obstetrics and Gynecology 118: 718–746

Carey J C, Golbus M S, Filly R A, Hall J G, Sillence D O, Hsia Y T 1979 Prenatal diagnosis of a previously undescribed heritable chondrodystrophy. Presented at the 1979 Birth Defects Conference Chicago

Cividalli G, Nathan D G, Kan Y W, Santamarina B, Frigoletto F 1974 Relation of beta to gamma synthesis during the first trimester: An approach to prenatal diagnosis of thalassemia. Pediatric Research 8:553–560

Cohen M M, Simpson S J 1980 Bleomycin induced chromosome damage in ataxia telangiectasia lymphoblastoid cells. Presented at the American Society of Human Genetics (24–27 September) New York City

Crandall B F, Lebherz T B, Freihube R 1978 Neural tube defects. Maternal serum screening and prenatal diagnosis. Pediatric Clinics of North America 25: 619–629

De Bruijn H W A, Huisjes H J 1975 Omphalocele and raised alpha-fetoprotein in amniotic fluid. Lancet 1: 525–526

Dozy A M, Forman E N, Abuelo D N 1979 Prenatal diagnosis of homozygous α-thalassemi. Journal of the American Medical Association 241: 1610–1612

Elias S 1980 Fetoscopy in prenatal diagnosis. Seminar as in Perinatology 4: 199–205

Elias S, Martin A O, Patel V A, Gerbie A B, Simpson J L 1978 Analysis for amniotic fluid crystallization in second trimester amniocentesis. American Journal of Obstetrics and Gynecology 133: 401–404

Elias S, Mazur M, Sabbagha R, Esterly N, Simpson J L 1980 Prenatal diagnosis of harlequin ichthyosis. Clinical Genetics 17: 275–280

Elliot P M, Inman W N 1961 Volume of liquor amnii in normal and abnormal pregnancy. Lancet 2: 835–840

Emery A E H, Burt D, Dubowitz V, Rocker I, Donnai D, Harris R, Donnai P 1979 Antenatal diagnosis of Duchenne muscular dystrophy. Lancet 1: 847–a849

Fairweather D V I, Modell B, Berdoukas V, Alter B P, Nathan D G, Loukopoulos D, Wood W, Clegg J B, Weatherall D J 1978 Antenatal diagnosis of thalassemia major. British Medical Journal 1: 350–353

Fensom A H, Benson P F, Rodeck C H, Campbell S, Gould J D M 1979 Prenatal diagnosis of a galactosemia heterozygote by fetal blood enzyme assay.

Firschein S I, Hoyer L W, Lazarchik J, Forget B G, Hobbins J C, Clyne L P, Pitlick F A, Muir W A, Merkatz I, Mahoney M J 1979 Prenatal diagnosis of classic hemophilia. New England Journal of Medicine 300: 937–941

Fleisher L D, Rassin D K, Rogers P, Desnick R J, Gaull G E 1977 Arginionosuccinic aciduria – prenatal diagnosis and studies of an affected fetus. Pediatric Research 11: 455

Friedland J, Perle G, Saifera A, Schneck L, Volk B W 1971 Screening for Tay-Sachs disease in utero using amniotic fluid. Proceedings of the Society for Experimental Biology and Medicine 136: 1297–1298

Fuchs F, Riis P 1956 Antenatal sex determination. Nature 177: 330

Gebhardt D O E 1979 Prenatal detection of Tangier Disease. Lancet 2: 754–755

Gerbie A B, Elias S 1980 Technique for midtrimester amniocentesis for prenatal diagnosis. Seminars in Perinatology 4:159–163

German J, Bloom D, Passarge E 1979 Bloom's syndrome. VII. Progress report for 1978. Clinical Genetics 15: 361–1367

Gitlin D, Boesman M 1966 Serum alpha-fetoprotein, albumin and gamma-G-globulin in the human conceptus. Journal of Clinical Investigation 45: 1826–1838

Golbus M S, Kan Y W, Naglich-Craig M 1976 Fetal blood sampling in midtrimester pregnancies. American Journal of Obstetrics and Gynecology 124: 653–655

Golbus M S, Loughman W D, Epstein C J, Halbasch G, Stephens J D, Hall B D 1979 Prenatal genetic diagnosis in 3000 Amniocentesis. New England Journal of Medicine 300: 157–163

Golbus M S, Sagebiel R W, Filly R A, Gindhart T D, Hall J G 1980 Prenatal diagnosis of congenital bullous ichthyosiform erythroderma (epidermolytic hyperkeratosis) by fetal skin biopsy. New England Journal of Medicine 302: 93–a95

Golbus M S, Stephens J D, Mahoney M J, Hobbins J C, Haseltine F P, Caskey C T, Banker B Q 1979 Failure of fetal creatine phosphokinase as a diagnostic indicator of Duchenne muscular dystrophy. New England Journal of Medicine 300: 860–861@Guiband S, Bonnet M, Thoulon J M, Dumont M 1973 Alpha-fetoprotein in amniotic fluid. Lancet 1: 1261

Halley D J J, Keijzer W, Jaspers N G H, Niermeijer M F, Kleijer W J, Boué J, Boué A, Bootsma D 1979 Prenatal diagnosis of xeroderma pigmentosum (group C) using assays of unscheduled DNA synthesis and post replication repair. Clinical Genetics 16: 137–146

Herzenberg L A, Bianchi D W, Schröder J, Cann H M, Iverson G M 1979 Fetal cells in the blood of pregnant women: Detection and enrichment by fluorescence-activated cell sorting. Proceeding of National Academy of Sciences U.S.A. 76: 1453–1455

Hobbins J C, Grannum P A T, Berkowitz R L, Silverman R, Mahoney M J 1979 Ultrasound in the diagnosis of congenital anomalies. American Journal of Obstetrics and Gynecology 134: 331–345

Hollenberg M D, Kaback M M, Kazazian H H Jr 1971 Adult hemoglobin synthesis by reticulocytes from the human fetus at mid trimester. Science 174: 698–702

Hook E B 1980 Genetic counselling delemmas: Down syndrome, paternal age, and recurrence risk after remarriage. American Journal of Medical Genetics 5: 145–151

Hook E B, Chambers G M 1977 Estimated rates of Down syndrome in live births by one year maternal age intervals for mothers aged 20–49 in a New York state study – implications of the risk figures for genetic counselling and cost-benefit analysis of prenatal diagnosis programs. Birth Defects 13: 123–141

Hoyer L W, Lindsten J, Blomback M, Hagenfeldt L, Cordesius E, Stromberg P, Gustavi B 1979 Prenatal evaluation of fetus at risk for severe von Willebrand's disease. Lancet 2: 191–192

Jacobson C B, Barter R H 1967 Intrauterine diagnosis and management of genetic defects. American Journal of Obstetrics and Gynecology 99: 795–805

Jeppsson J O, Franzen B, Sveger T, Cordesius E, Stromberg P, Gustavi B 1979 Prenatal exclusion of alpha-1-antitrypsin deficiency in a high risk fetus. New England Journal of Medicine 300: 1441–1442

Jones O W 1979 Cytogenetic diagnosis. Proceedings of the seventy-eighth Ross conference on pediatric research: Obstetrical decisions and neonatal outcome. San Diego

Kaback M M 1977 Tay-Sachs disease: prenatal diagnosis and heterzygote screening 1969–1976. Pediatric Research 11: 458

Kan Y W, Dozy A M 1978a Polymorphism of DNA sequence adjacent to human β-globin structural gene: Relationship to sickle mutation. Proceedings of the National Academy of Sciences U.S.A. 75: 5631–5635

Kan Y W, Dozy A M 1978b Antenatal diagnosis of sickle-cell anemia by DNA analysis of amniotic fluid cells. Lancet 2: 910–912

Kan Y W, Dozy A M, Alter B P, Frigoletto F D, Nathan D G 1972 Detection of the sickle gene in the human fetus. Potential for intrauterine diagnosis of sickle-cell anemia. New England Journal of Medicine 287: 1–5

Kan Y W, Golbus M S, Dozy A M 1976 Prenatal diagnosis of α-thalassemia. New England Journal of Medicine 295: 1165–1167

Kan Y W, Golbus M S, Trecartin R F, Filly R A, Valenti C, Furbetta M, Cao A 1977 Prenatal diagnosis of β-thalassemia and sickle-cell anemia – experience with 24 cases. Lancet 1: 269–271

Kan Y W, Valenti C, Carnazza V, Guidotti R, Rieder R F 1974 Fetal blood sampling in utero. Lancet 1: 79–80

Karp L E, Hayden P W 1977 Fetal puncture during mid trimester amniocentesis. 49: 115–117

Obstetrics and Gynecology Kazazian H H Jr, Woodhead A P 1973 Hemoglobin A synthesis in the developing fetus. New England Journal of Medicine 289: 58–62

Kohn G, Robinson A 1970 Tetraploidy in cells cultured from amniotic fluid. Lancet 2: 778–779

Lachman R, Hall J G 1979 The radiographic prenatal diagnosis of the generalized bone dysplasias and other skeletal abnormalities. Birth Defects 15: 3–24

Leek A E, Ruoss C F, Kitau M J, Chard T 1973 Raised alpha-fetoprotein in maternal serum with anencephalic pregnancy. Lancet 2 385

Leighton P C, Gordon Y B, Ritau M J, Leek A T, Chard T 1975 Levels of alpha-fetoprotein in maternal blood as a screening test for fetal neural tube defect. Lancet 2: 1012–1015

Leonard C O, Kazazian H H Jr 1978 Prenatal diagnosis of hemoglobinopathies. Pediatric Clinics of North America 25: 631–642

Liebaers I, DiNatale P, Neufeld E 1977 Iduronate sulfatase in amniotic fluid: an aid in the prenatal diagnosis of Hunter syndrome. Journal of Pediatrics 90: 423–425

MacMahon B, Hutchinson G 1964 Prenanal X–ray and childhood cancer: A review. Acta Unio Internat Contra Canc 20: 1172–1174

Macri J N, Haddow J E, Weiss R R 1979 Screening for neural tube defects in the United States. A summary of the Scarborough Confernece. American Journal Of Obstetrics and Gynecology 133: 119–126

Mahoney M J, Hobbins J C 1977 Prenatal diagnosis of chondroectodermal dysplasia (Ellis van Creveld syndrome) with fetoscopy and ultrasound. New England Journal of Medicine 297: 258–260

Mahoney M J, Haseltine F P, Hobbins J C, Banker B Q, Caskey C T, Golbus M S 1977 Prenatal diagnosis of Duchenne's muscular dystrophy. New England Journal of Medicine 297: 968–973

Merkatz I R, New M I, Peterson R E, Seaman M P 1969 Prenatal diagnosis of adrenogenital syndrome by amniocentesis. Journal of Pediatrics 75: 977–982

Mibashan R S, Rodeck C H, Thumptson J K, Edwards R J, Singer J D, White J M, Campbell S 1979 Plasma assay of fetal factors VIII C and IX for prenatal diagnosis of hemophilia. Lancet 1: 1309–1311

Miles J H, Kaback M M 1978 Prenatal diagnosis of hereditary disorders. Pediatric Clinics of North America 25: 593–618

Milunsky A (ed) 1975 The prevention of genetic disease and mental retardation. W B Saunders, Philadelphia

Milunsky A, Alpert E 1974 The value of alpha-fetoprotein in the prenatal diagnosis of neural tube defects. Journal of Pediatrics 84: 889–893

Milunsky A, Tulchinsky D 1977 Prenatal diagnosis of

congenital adrenal hyperplasia due to zl-hydroxylase deficiency. Pediatrics 59: 768–773

Milunsky A, Atkins L, Littlefield J W 1971 Polyploidy in prenatal genetic diagnosis. Journal of Pediatrics 79: 303–305

Miluky A, Littlefield J W, in amniotic fluid cells. Lancet 2: 979

Morrow G, Schwarz R H, Hallock J A, Barness L A 1970 Prenatal detection of methylmalonic acidemia. Journal of Pediatrics 77: 120–123

Mulivor R A, Mennuti M, Zackai E H, Harris H 1978 Prenatal diagnosis of hypophosphatasia: genetic, biochemical and clinical studies. American Journal of Human Genetics 30: 271–282

Murken J A, Stengel-Rutkowski S, Schwinger E 1979 Prenatal Diagnosis. Proceedings of the 3 d European conference of prenatal diagnosis of genetic disorders. Ferdinand Enke Publishers, Stuttgart

Nadler H L 1968 Antenatal detection of hereditary disorders. Pediatrics 42: 912–918

Nadler H L 1976 Prenatal detection of genetic defects. Advances in Pediatrics 22: 1–81

Nadler H L, Gerbie A B 1969 Enzymes in non-cultured amniotic fluid cells. American Journal of Obstetrics and Gynecology 103: 710–712

Nadler H L, Messina A 1969 In utero detection of type II glycogenosis (Pompe's disease).Lancet 2: 1277–1278

Nadler H L, Simpson J L 1979 Maternal serum AFP screening: Promise not yet fulfilled. Obstetrics and Gynecology 54: 333–334

Nadler H L, Walsh M M J 1980a Methylumbelliferylguanidinobenzoate (MUGB) reactive proteases in amniotic fluid (AF): Promising marker for the intrauterine detection of cystic fibrosis (CF). Pediatric Research 14: 525

Nadler H L, Walsh M M J 1980b Prenatal detection of cystic fibrosis on amniotic fluid. Lancet 2: 96–97

Nadler H L, Walsh M M J 1980c Intrauterine detection of cystic fibrosis. Pediatrics 65 (November)

Nadler H L, Bigley R H, Hug G 1970 Prenatal detection of Pompe's disease. Lancet 2:369–370

Nathan D G 1976 Antenatal diagnosis of hemoglobinopathies: An exquisite molecular brew. New England Journal of Medicine 295: 1196–1198

Newburger P E, Cohen H J, Rothchild S B, Hobbins J C, Malawista S E, Mahoney M J 1979 Prenatal diagnosis of chronic granulomatous disease. New England Journal of Medicine 300: 178–181

NICHD National Registry for amniocentesis study group 1976 Mid trimester amniocentesis for prenatal diagnosis: Safety and accuracy. Journal of the American Medical Association 236: 1471–1476

Origin of Maternal Serum AFP 1979 Lancet 2: 9999–1000

Orkin S H, Alter B P, Altay C, Mahoney M J, Lazarus H, Hobbins J C, Nathan D G 1978 Application endonuclease mapping to the analysis and prenatal diagnosis of thalassemias caused by globin gene deletion. New England Journal of Medicine 299: 166–172

Peakman D C, Moreton M F, Corn B J, Robinson A 1978 Chromosomal mosaicism in amniotic fluid cell cultures. Pediatric Research 12: 455

Peakman D C, Moreton M E, Corn B J, Robinson A 1979 Chromosomal mosaicism in amniotic fluid cultures. American Journal of Human Genetics 31: 149–155

Phillips J A III, Scott A F, Kazazian H H Jr, Smith K D, Stetter G, Thomas G H 1979 Prenatal diagnosis of hemoglobinopathies by restriction endonuclease analysis: pregnancies at risk for sickle cell anemia and S-O^{Arab}disease. Johns Hopkins Medical Journal 145: 57–60

Pollack M S, Maurer D, Levine L S, New M I, Pang S, Duchon M, Owens R P, Merkatz I R, Nitowsky H M, Sachs G, Dupont B 1979 Prenatal diagnosis of congenital adrenal hyperplasia (21-hydroxylase deficiency) by HLA typing. Lancet 1: 1107–1108

Ramsay C A, Coltart T M, Blunt S, Pawsey S A, Giannelli F 1974 Prenatal diagnosis of xeroderma pigmentosum, Report of the first successful case. Lancet 2: 1109–1112

Report of U.K. Collaborative Study on alpha-fetoprotein in relation to neural tube defects 1977 Maternal serum AFP measurements in antenatal screening for anencephaly and spina bifida in several early pregnancies. Lancet 1: 1323–1332

Rodeck C H, Eady R A J, Gosden C M 1980 Prenatal diagnosis of epidermolysis bullosa letalis. Lancet 1: 949–952

Rodesch F, Camus M, Ermans A M, Dodion J, Delange F 1976 Adverse effect of amniofetography on fetal thyroid function. American Journal of Obstetrics and Gynecology 126: 723–726

Ruoslahti E, Seppälä M 1971 Studies of carcino-fetal proteins, III. Development of a radioimmunoassay for alpha-fetoprotein in serum of healthy adults. International Journal of Cancer 8: 374–383

Sabbagha R E, Shkolnik A 1980 Ultrasound diagnosis of fetal abnormalities. Seminars in Perinatology 4: 213–227

Schneck L, Friedland J, Valenti C, Adachi M, Amsterdam D, Volk B W 1970 Prenatal diagnosis of Tay-Sachs disease. Lancet 1: 582–583

Schrott H G, Omean G S 1975 dystrophy: opportunities for prentalprediction. Neurology 25: 789–791

Second Report of the U.K. Collaborative Study on alpha-fetoprotein in relation to neural tube defects 1979 Amniotic fluid alpha-fetoprotein measurements in antenatal diagnosis of anencephaly and open spina bifida in early pregnancy. Lancet 2: 651–662

Seller M J 1974 Alpha-fetoprotein and the prenatal diagnosis of neural tube defects. Developmental Medicine and Child Neurology 16: 369–381

Seppälä M 1973 Increased alpha-fetoprotein in amniotic fluid associated with a congenital esophageal atresia of the fetus. Obstetrics and Gynecology 42: 613–614

Seppälä M, Ruoslahti E 1972 Alpha-fetoprotein in amniotic fluid: an index of gestational age. American Journal of Obstetrics and Gynecology 114: 595–598

Seppälä M, Ruoslahti E 1973a Alpha-fetoprotein in antenatal diagnosis. Lancet 1: 155

Seppälä M, Ruoslahti E 1973b Alpha-fetoprotein in Rh negative immunized pregnancies. Obstetrics and Gynecology 42: 701– 706

Serr D M, Sachs L, Danon M 1955 Diagnosis of sex before birth using cells from the amniotic fluid. Bulletin of the Research Council Israel 5B: 137

Simpson J L1980 Antenatal diagnosis of cytogenetic abnormalities. Seminars in Perinatology 4: 165–168

Simpson N E, Dallaire L, Miller J R, Siminovich L, Hamerton J L, Miller J, McKeen C 1976 Prenatal diagnosis of genetic disease in Canada: Report of a collaborative study. Canadian Medical Association Journal 115: 739–748

Smith A D, Wald N J, Cuckle H S, Stirrat G M, Bobrow M, Lagercrantz H 1979 Amniotic fluid acetylcholinesterase as a possible diagnostic test for neural tube defects in early pregnancy. Lancet 1: 685–690

Southern E M 1975 Detection of specific sequences among

DNA fragments separated by gel electrophoresis. Journal of Molecular Biology 98: 503–517

Steele M W, Breg W R Jr 1966 Chromosome analysis of human amniotic fluid cells, Lancet 1: 383–385

Stoll C, Willard D, Czernichow P, Boué J 1978 Prenatal diagnosis of primary pituitary dysgenesis, Lancet 1: 932

Swartz H M, Reichling B A 1978 Hazards of radiation exposure for pregnant women. Journal of the American Medical Association 239: 1907–1908

Towards the prevention of spina bifida 1974 Lancet 1: 907

Wagner G, Fuchs F 1962 Volume of amniotic fluid in the first half of human pregnancy. J Obstet Gynaecol Br Commonw 69: 131–a136

Walsh M M, Nadler H L 1979 Methylumbelliferylguanidinobenzoate reactive proteases in amniotic fluid: possible marker for cystic fibrosis. Lancet 1: 622

Walsh M M J, Rao G J S, Nadler H L 1980 Reaction of 4-methylumbelliferylguanidinobenzoate with proteases in human amniotic fluid. Pediatric Research 14: 353–356

Whyley G A, Ward H, Hardy N R 1974 Alpha-fetoprotein levels in amniotic fluids in pregnancies complicated by Rhesus insoimmunization. Journal of Obstetrics and Gynaecology of the British Commonwealth 81: 459–465

Working Party on amniocentesis, Medical Research Council 1978 An assessment of the hazards of amniocentesis British Hournal of Obstetrics and Gynaecology 85 Suppl 2: 1–41

Zeisel S H, Milunsky A, Blusztajn J K 1980 Prenatal diagnosis of of neural tube defects V. The value of amniotic fluid cholinesterase studies. American Journal of Obstetrics and Gynecology 137: 481–485

103

Genetic registers

P.E. Robertson

INTRODUCTION

The role of preventive medicine is changing in developed countries with alterations in the pattern of disease, and new methods are being found to cope with modern problems. Genetic registers are a development in this field.

In Britain fifty years ago, infection represented the greatest cause of mortality in children (Registrar General's Annual Reports) and the greatest scope for preventive medicine lay in combating this through improving nutrition and hygiene (McKeown et al, 1975). Nowadays genetic factors are becoming increasingly more important in the aetiology of childhood illness (Carter, 1956; Roberts et al, 1970). Youth in Britain no longer 'grows pale and spectre-thin and dies' from consumption (Keats, 1795–1821) but is increasingly likely to do so as the result of a genetic disorder.

Many varieties of genetic disease have been illustrated in the preceding chapters. These all place physical, emotional and financial burdens on the family who has an affected member and the society who has to provide care for them. Tips and Lynch (1963) have described the tensions and conflicts within families of children with genetic defects.

Stevenson (1959) estimated that in Northern Ireland 26.5% of all institutional beds were occupied by persons handicapped by hereditary defects and that 2 per 1000 of the population (other than relatives) were employed full-time in looking after them. Genetic disorders may also place a considerable financial load on afflicted families. It was estimated that in the United States in 1977 (Fink et al, 1977) an average case of Huntington chorea in which the illness lasted for 15 years and required institutional care for the last five years accumulated medical costs varying between 64 000 and 234 000 dollars depending on the type of care provided. The loss in salary, which the person would otherwise have earned over the 15 year period, has been estimated at 150 000 dollars (Commission for the Control of Huntington Disease Report, 1977). These examples illustrate the problems caused by hereditary disease, which would be lessened if the incidence of genetic disease in the population were reduced.

To do this one would need to identify people at high risk of producing a child with a serious genetic disorder and offer genetic counselling in the hope of preventing births of further affected children. It is here that a genetic register may be most useful as a means of practising preventive medicine. There are of course various types of genetic register (Table 103.1). Any register may have several functions, but is more likely to operate efficiently if its aims are specified from the beginning and adhered to strictly, so that similar information is recorded on all registered individuals from the outset (Miller, 1975). Here we shall be concerned with genetic registers designed specifically for the prevention of genetic disease.

Table 103.1 Types of Genetic Register and their functions.

Clinical
Aims – to observe the natural history of genetic disease
– to assess the effects of treatment
– to list patients with a particular disorder so that any new developments in treatment or prenatal diagnosis can be offered quickly to those concerned.

Cytogenetic
Aim – to act as a source of reference so that chromosomal abnormalities can be related to the phenotype of the affected individual.

Epidemiological
Aims – to ascertain the incidence of genetic disease in the population
– where the disease is multifactorial, to assess the possible role of environmental factors.

Monitoring
Aims – to evaluate the effect of genetic counselling or prenatal diagnosis
– to assess the cost of health care in genetic disease.

Preventive
Aim – to reduce the incidence and burden of genetic disease by offering genetic counselling and, where appropriate, prenatal diagnosis to those at high risk of having an affected child.

REGISTERS AND THE PREVENTION OF INHERITED DISEASE

A WHO Scientific Group recommended in 1972 that medical genetics centres should establish registers of genetically determined disorders, so that genetic counselling could be offered to all who would benefit by it (WHO 1972).

Previous studies (Emery & Smith, 1970; Smith, 1970) have shown that the best scope for preventing genetic disease lies with the simply inherited disorders, as it is in these that other family members at high risk of having an affected child may most easily be identified. A register designed for the prevention of genetic disease ideally constitutes a record of all cases of serious genetic disorder in the population of the area which it serves, together with a list of relatives at high risk of producing an affected child and/or becoming affected themselves.

The work of such a register involves ascertaining individuals in the population at high risk of having a child with a serious genetic disorder, assessing the individual's risk and providing genetic counselling, prenatal diagnosis where this is possible, and medical, psychological and social support.

Genetic counselling has often been given retrospectively, that is, to individuals *after* the birth of an affected child. Prospective counselling (*before* the birth of an affected or at-risk child) has not usually been provided through the conventional medical services for relatives at high risk.

Emery and Smith (1970) found that 86% of relatives at high risk of having a child with a serious genetic disorder had not been referred for counselling. Using a genetic register, such relatives may be traced and offered counselling.

Autosomal dominant and X–linked recessive disorders are the most appropriate for a genetic register designed for the prevention of inherited disease. The types of disease included in a register will however, vary from area to area, depending on the prevalence of specific genetic disorders. Table 103.2 illustrates the most common diseases on the Edinburgh register.

OPERATION OF A GENETIC REGISTER

Ascertainment of individuals

Having decided on the type of disorder which will be included on the register, and on the geographical area to be covered, affected individuals within that area must be identified.

This may be done in two ways: *indirectly*, by searching health records for the area, or *directly* by referral of the patient to the genetics centre by the family doctor or hospital practitioner.

Table 103.2 Genetic disorders on the Edinburgh register.

Disorder	% Individuals
Autosomal dominant	
Huntington chorea	21
Polycystic kidney disease	9
Myotonic dystrophy	6
Neurofibromatosis	3
Polyposis coli	2
Retinitis pigmentosa	2
Marfan syndrome	2
X-linked recessive	
Haemophilia A + B	21
Duchenne muscular dystrophy	7
Retinitis pigmentosa	3

Indirect ascertainment

In theory, if all health records can be screened for individuals with genetic disease, then ascertainment should be complete. Types of records suitable for such screening are hospital records, family practitioner and public health records and registers of the physically handicapped.

In practice however, several difficulties arise. It may not be possible to gain access to all health records. They may be incomplete, or out of date. The person's name or address may have changed. The diagnosis may not be sufficiently specific e.g. 'cystic disease of the kidney' covers many more causes of renal cyst than just genetic disorders.

It has been found in Edinburgh that screening health records gives a poor yield of patients suitable for the Register for the Ascertainment and Prevention of Inherited Disease (RAPID).

When RAPID was being established, over 39 000 records were screened. 1205 individuals were identified from the diagnosis as being possible candidates for the register, but eventually only 250 cases of a serious genetic disorder suitable for the register were found and 469 relatives at risk identified. Thus the yield of at risk individuals from indirect ascertainment is very low and makes this form of ascertainment very inefficient.

Direct ascertainment

With direct ascertainment, the individual is referred to the geneticist by his family doctor or hospital consultant, or through special clinics such as haemophilia or neurology, or special schools for the deaf, blind or mentally handicapped.

The extent of the ascertainment naturally depends on the cooperation of the referring physician. However, as far as the patients are concerned this is probably a more satisfactory method. If they are referred directly by their family doctor or other physician, they are aware that they or their children have a hereditary disease, and that counselling is indicated for themselves and other members of the family.

Contacting individuals and other family members

The method of contacting individuals affected by, or at high risk of having a child with, a serious genetic disorder depends on the method of ascertainment.

If the person has been ascertained indirectly, without his knowledge, through searching health records, it is advisable to contact his family doctor to ask his opinion as to the need for genetic counselling and to confirm the diagnosis. It may be that family circumstances are highly inappropriate for counselling and the family doctor is likely to know about such a situation. He may wish to speak to the family himself before they are offered an appointment for genetic counselling and this can be very helpful. It has been suggested in a WHO report that the family doctor be involved whenever possible to augment the information given to a patient by the geneticist and to ensure that continuing support for the patient and his family is available when required (WHO, 1969). If the individual is ascertained directly, the referring doctor will already have discussed the hereditary nature of the disease with him to some extent. He may then be sent an appointment for counselling directly.

Once the individual is seen for counselling, a family history is taken so that other members at high risk of developing, or having a child with, a serious genetic disorder may be identified. Those of child-bearing age with a risk greater than 1 in 10 are thought to be the most suitable for counselling. Children below this age may be recorded, with their parent's consent, for counselling when they reach an appropriate age.

The individual is asked for his permission to contact other members of his family at risk. Once this has been given, each relative's family doctor is also approached as there may be factors unknown to the index case which would make counselling inappropriate. If both the index case and the family doctor agree, the relative is then offered an appointment for counselling.

Figure 103.1 summarises the methods of contact of index cases and their relatives. Some relatives may of course live outside the area covered by the register. In such a situation the index case may inform them of the problem and suggest that they seek counselling in their own area.

Follow-up

Follow-up constitutes an important part in the management of families with genetic problems particularly in the case of relatives at risk who may not be under the care of a physician. It may be divided into short-term and long-term, which have slightly different objectives. Short-term follow-up is carried out within 3 months of the initial counselling session. One of the chief aims here is to ensure that the person has understood and remembers the information given during counselling, and understands what options are available e.g. if prenatal diagnosis is possible. On reflection, there may be further questions about the disease and its implications that were not raised during the first visit. There may be an indication for referral to other medical, family planning or social services.

Long-term follow-up involves maintaining contact with families on the register. Changes of name and address can be recorded. Hook (1975) found in a follow-up study of children seen at a paediatric cardiology clinic that 23% of families had changed their address within 24 months of being seen at the clinic, in an area in New York State which was believed to have a stable population. This illustrates the need for updating the register.

If the family is in regular contact with those running the register, at-risk pregnancies can be identified early, so that appropriate action with regard to prenatal sexing or diagnosis can be taken.

New developments in the management of the condition can be brought to the attention of the family or their doctors. Continued follow-up may also provide emotional support to a family burdened by a chronic progressive disorder. The family can be put in touch with appropriate agencies as the need for help becomes apparent during the course of the disease.

Many of these follow-up functions can be fulfilled by a field worker, usually a trained nurse or health visitor, working with the register. Other problems, perhaps requiring referral for other medical help, are dealt with by a medical geneticist. The best arrangement may be for the field worker to keep in touch with the family and refer them back to the geneticist if it is felt that medical intervention is needed.

A follow-up system also helps to monitor the effect of counselling on the family. Their attitudes to counselling can be discussed and the effect of counselling assessed in terms of the prevention of further cases of the disease, through family limitation or prenatal sexing or diagnosis.

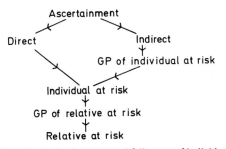

Fig. 103.1 Methods of contact and follow-up of individuals in a genetic register system (from Emery, 1976).

RECORDING OF INFORMATION

Informed consent

A recent Working Party on Genetic Registers (Emery et al, 1978) recommended that no individuals should be included on the register without their full knowledge and approval. It is helpful if the individual signs some type of consent form, such as the one illustrated in Figure 103.2, to show that he gives his consent to be included on the register, knowing the nature and purpose of the information recorded about him or his children.

Storage of information

This may be done manually on record cards or the information may be computerised. When planning the form of storage, the nature of the information and the eventual size of the register should be taken into consideration. Manual storage is suitable for a small register with a limited amount of data, but if the information is more extensive, computerisation is probably easier.

Naturally the type of data stored will vary with the function of the register. A preventive register, designed to offer a counselling service to families at high risk of inherited disease, needs only to store identifying information on the individual, the doctors immediately concerned with his care, the disease from which he or his children are at risk, and the dates when follow-up visits

University Department of Human Genetics,

Western General Hospital,

Edinburgh.

I .... of ....

....

give the Department of Human Genetics at the Western General Hospital,

Edinburgh my consent to record details of myself and/or my children

....

in the Genetic Register System (RAPID) held in the Department.

I understand

(a) that the information includes medical and genetic details

(b) that it is computerised

(c) that it is strictly confidential and that access is limited to the
     medical staff concerned with my condition.

                              Signed ....

                              Date   ....

I also give the Department of Human Genetics my consent to contact my

relatives concerning the genetic disorder in my family.

                              Signed ....

                              Date   ....

Fig. 103.2 Consent form used in the Edinburgh RAPID system.

are required. Such a system may be extended to include other genetic data, as in the Indiana Medical Genetics Acquisition and Data Transmission System (MEGADATS) which in addition to family details stores cytogenetic and biochemical data (Merritt et al, 1975).

In the Edinburgh RAPID register, details are recorded concisely on a clinical card, and then transferred to a computer using punched cards. The clinical record card is illustrated in Figure 103.3.

COMPUTERISATION

Computerisation greatly facilitates the running of a genetic register. If records are computerised, information can be retrieved quickly and accurately.

If for example a new method of prenatal diagnosis becomes available for one of the conditions included on the register, all those of childbearing age who might like to be informed of such a development can be quickly identified. The computer can also deliver lists at regular intervals of people who are due for follow-up visits, or children who are due for counselling at sixteen or eighteen years; this is particularly useful as children may be very young when the family is first seen, and under a manual system it is difficult to ensure that an appointment will be sent out in perhaps fifteen years time, whereas this can easily be done through the computer. Technical details of a computer program suitable for a genetic register have been published (Moores & Emery, 1976).

The computer may also be used to estimate the genetic risk to various family members using such programs as PEDIG and RISKMF (Conneally & Heuch, 1974; Smith, 1972).

CONFIDENTIALITY

The nature of the information stored in a genetic register demands that strict attention be paid to confidentiality and that there is no unauthorised access.

If a manual system is used, there should be some physical security for the records, such as a locked cabinet. If the register is computerised, the computer itself can be used to protect the confidentiality of the information which it contains (HMSO, 1975). The program can be arranged so that the information is coded, and/or a password is required to gain access. Several passwords can be incorporated to give access to different levels of information so that the clinician dealing with a family has access to all the genetic and medical information, while a field worker may only retrieve pedigree data to facilitate the tracing of relatives (Emery et al, 1974). If cytogenetic or other technical data are held on the register, research

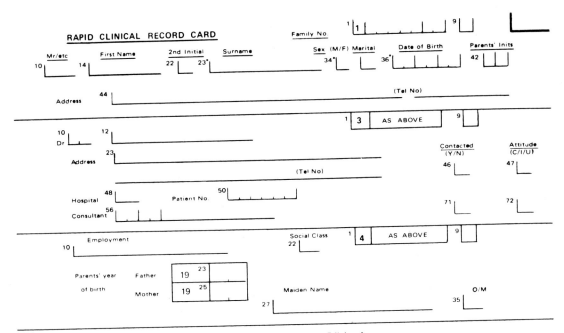

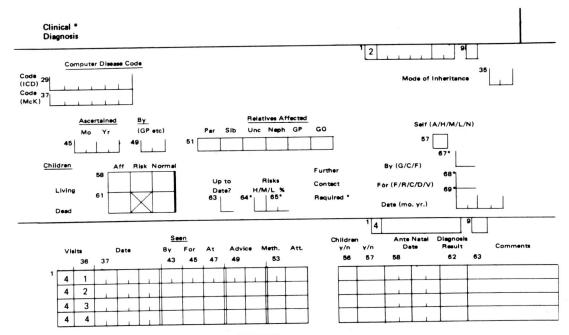

Fig. 103.3 Clinical record card used in the Edinburgh RAPID system.

workers may be given access to this without knowing the identity of the individuals concerned (Merritt et al, 1975). It has been suggested that a small dedicated mini-computer is the most suitable for a genetic register, as it is easier with such equipment to maintain confidentiality and to ensure that access is strictly limited (Emery et al, 1978).

SIZE OF AREA TO BE COVERED BY A REGISTER

The necessity to maintain contact with families on a register limits the size of the area which can be covered. It might seem reasonable to establish registers on a national basis, so that family members living in different parts of a country may all be included on the same register, but this can lead to practical problems. If the register covers too large an area, it is difficult to ensure that all the information recorded is accurate and up-to-date. It is also difficult to maintain confidentiality if many people are involved in feeding in and retrieving information from the system.

Registers covering a smaller area have the advantage that personal contact can be maintained between individuals on the register and those who run it, and breaches of security are less likely. Arranging genetic counselling for family members who live in other parts of the country can be a problem. However, this can be overcome if genetic centres in different parts of the country can collaborate; especially if similar forms of registers are used so that information can easily be exchanged (Emery et al, 1978).

Local conditions with regard to population density and siting of genetic centres will of course determine the size of the area for which the register provides a service. In Britain the area covered by a Health Board Region has been thought to be appropriate, as most medical specialist services are based on this.

The registers established in Edinburgh and Belfast cover populations of 750 000 and 1 500 000 respectively.

EFFICACY OF PREVENTIVE GENETIC REGISTERS

The first of these registers was established in Edinburgh in 1970, and has only been fully operational since 1976. It is thus too early to assess the effect of counselling through the register system in preventing genetic handicap in families known to be at risk. The proportion of cases theoretically preventable by genetic counselling and prenatal diagnosis has been calculated (Emery, 1978). In autosomal dominant disorders, the proportion preventable depends on the biological fitness of the parent who is affected. In X–linked recessive conditions, 66% could be prevented by parental screening, 12% by prospective counselling and 10% by retrospective counselling. Several studies have been made of the response of individuals to retrospective genetic counselling. In these (summarised by Emery, 1978) it was found that between 59% and 90% of those at high risk of having affected children were deterred by the risk.

A prospective study of individuals seen at a genetic clinic with a variety of genetic disorders (Emery et al, 1979) showed that 46% of individuals given a high risk were deterred from having children immediately after counselling and 53% were deterred two years later. The effect of a genetic register in reducing the incidence of inherited disease in the population remains to be seen, but the approach certainly seems feasible. It is to be hoped that by the end of the twentieth century genetic counselling will have played a major part in reducing the incidence of genetic disease comparable to the part played by improving public health measures in reducing infectious disease at the beginning of the century.

REFERENCES

Carter C O 1956 Changing patterns in the cause of death at the Hospital for Sick Children. Great Ormond Street Journal 11: 65–68

Commission for the Control of Huntington Disease Report 1977 U.S. Department of Health, Education and Welfare. National Institutes of Health, Bethesda, Maryland 78-1501: Vol 1, p 56–57

Conneally P M, Heuch I 1974 A computer program to determine genetic risks – a simplified version of PEDIG. American Journal of Human Genetics 26: 773–775

Emery A E H 1976 A computerized 'at risk' register for genetic disease. In: Turnbull A C, Woodford F P (eds) Prevention of handicap through antenatal care. North-Holland, Amsterdam p 13–19

Emery A E H 1978 Prevention of genetic disease. In:

Weatherall D J (ed) Advanced Medicine 14, Pitman Medical, London p 118–127

Emery A E H, Smith C 1970 Ascertainment and prevention of genetic disease. British Medical Journal 3: 636–637

Emery A E H, Elliott D, Moores M, Smith C 1974 A genetic register system (RAPID). Journal of Medical Genetics 11: 145–151

Emery A E H, Brough C, Crawfurd M, Harper P, Harris R, Oakshott G 1978 A report on genetic registers. Journal of Medical Genetics 15: 435–442

Emery A E H, Raeburn J A, Skinner R, Holloway S, Lewis P 1979 Prospective study of genetic counselling. British Medical Journal 1: 1253–1256

Fink A, Kosekoff J, Lewis C 1977 A study of the resources available to Huntington's disease patients, families and health care providers. UCLA Health Services Research Centre Report HS-2015

HMSO 1975 Computers and privacy. HMSO London Cmnd 6353

Hook E B 1975 Types of genetic registers. In: Emery A E H, Miller J R (eds) Registers for the detection and prevention of genetic disease, Stratton Intercontinental, New York p 22

Keats J 1795–1821 Ode to a Nightingale

McKeown T, Record R G, Turner R D 1975 An interpretation of the decline of mortality in England and Wales during the twentieth century. Population Studies 29: 391–422

Merritt A D, Kang K W, Conneally P M, Gersting J M, Rigo T 1975 MEGADATS. In: Emery A E H, Miller J R (eds) Registers for the detection and prevention of genetic disease, Stratton Intercontinental, New York p 31–51

Miller J R 1975 Some uses of genetic registers. In: Emery A E H, Miller J R (eds) Registers for the detection and prevention of genetic disease, Stratton Intercontinental, New York p 6

Moores H M, Emery A E H 1976 RAPID. Inter-University Research Councils Report Series, Edinburgh Regional Computing Centre

Registrar General's annual reports for England, Wales and Scotland. HMSO London and Edinburgh

Roberts D F, Chavez J, Court S D M 1970 The genetic component in child mortality. Archives of Disease in Childhood 45 (239): 33–38

Smith C 1970 Ascertaining those at risk in the prevention and treatment of genetic disease. In: Emery A E H (ed) Modern trends in human genetics, Butterworth, London Vol 1, p 350–369

Smith C 1972 Computer programme to estimate recurrence risks for multifactorial familial disease. British Medical Journal 1: 495–497

Stevenson A C 1959 The load of hereditary defects in human populations. Radiation Research Suppl 1: 306–325

Tips R L, Lynch H T 1963 The impact of genetic counselling on the family milieu. Journal of the American Medical Association 184: 183–186

WHO 1969 Genetic Counselling. Technical Report Series no 416, WHO Geneva

WHO 1972 Genetic disorders: prevention, treatment and rehabilitation. Technical report series no 497, WHO Geneva

104

Treatment of genetic diseases

L. J. Shapiro

INTRODUCTION

It is a commonly held misconception by workers in fields other than human genetics that genetic diseases are inherently untreatable. Both historical perspective and recent experience clearly indicate the fallacy of this point of view. Advances in basic science laboratories continue to rapidly add powerful ammunition to the genetically oriented physician's armamentarium. With the rapid developments in biochemistry and molecular biology, in particular, the future for sophisticated intervention is very bright indeed.

The traditional medical model provides for delineation of new disease entities followed by studies of their epidemiology, aetiology, pathogenesis, prevention, and therapy. This is no less true of genetically determined disorders than it is of infectious illnesses. Since there are such a large number of genetic diseases, it would be impractical for a limited consideration such as this chapter, to be totally comprehensive. Accordingly, specific discussions of modalities of therapy of each of the conditions described in this text is best left for the relevant chapter and author. What will be attempted is a general overview of strategies in the therapy of genetically determined illnesses.

General considerations of the *management* of genetic disease can be divided into areas of prevention, treatment, and cure. Prevention of genetic disease is, of course, well within our grasp and is being practised around the world on a daily basis. This most often consists of genetic and reproductive counselling for individuals at high risk of producing offspring with inherited illnesses, and prenatal diagnosis, when possible. It may take into its structure, prospective screening of either probands or clinically normal carriers of mutant genes. Such strategies have been shown to be very effective in reducing the total burden of genetic disease upon the population as a whole as well as upon individual families. Cure of a medical condition requires the application of some therapeutic modality which can irrevocably alter the course of an illness and return the patient to a normal state of health and well being. In the context of genetic

diseases, this clearly implies effecting a fundamental change in the structure of DNA which would be both permanent and heritable. At present, this notion may seem a bit far-fetched, but spectacular advances in the fundamental biological sciences of the past decade makes such speculations much less futuristic than they once were.

It is inherent in the medical genetics paradigm that virtually all disease results from an interaction of environmental factors and hereditary predispositions (Stern, 1973). Thus, while few would dispute that phenylketonuria is a genetic illness, it is only of pathological consequence in the context of an environment which provides dietary phenylalanine in excess of the subject's ability to metabolize it, and through appropriate environmental intervention, the adverse impact of the mutant gene can be lessened. Similarly, it has been pointed out that a fractured long bone is usually the result of some environmental stress, but susceptibility to such factors may be substantially modified by genetic predisposition as in the case of osteogenesis imperfecta, or Gaucher disease. The goal of treatment of genetic disease can perhaps be codified as an attempt to create an equilibrium between inherited factors and environmental influences which allow the individual to live as full and healthy a life as possible.

DIRECT ALTERATION OF THE GENOME

As alluded to above, the ultimate approach in therapy of genetic diseases would be to directly alter defective genetic material and render the nucleotide sequence of the individual 'normal'. It is obvious that there is no truly 'normal' state of the genome. Each individual on this planet is thought to be genetically unique (except, of course, for identical twins). Estimates of human polymorphism continue to increase with progressive sophistication of methods of detection (Vogel & Motulsky, 1979). Only a small fraction of this genetic variability is harmful and, of course, the definition of which forms of polymorphism are deleterious are to some degree, subjective.

Table 104.1 Strategies of therapy for genetic diseases

I. *Direct alteration of the genome*
1. Site specific mutagenesis
2. Synthetic polynucleotides
3. Use of cloned, normal genes
4. Use of novel artificial sequences

II. *Introduction of replicating, functional DNA into cells or intact organisms*
1. Transformation
   (a) With selection in vitro
   (b) With selection in the whole animal
   (c) Cotransformation of non-selectable markers
2. Transduction with viral vectors
3. Microinjection
   (a) Into individual somatic cells
   (b) Into fertilized eggs

III. *Replacement of missing gene products*
1. Peptide hormones
2. Circulating plasma components
3. Lysosomal enzymes
   (a) Purified enzymes
      (i) Targeting strategies
      (ii) Erythrocyte entrapment
      (iii) Liposome entrapment
   (b) Organ/cell transplantation as a source of enzyme

IV. *Enzyme induction/augmentation*
1. Induction
2. Stabilization of labile enzymes
3. Cofactor supplementation
   (a) In defective cofactor transport or metabolism
   (b) In defective apoenzyme interaction
4. Stimulation of alternative pathways?

V. *Limitation of toxic substrate accumulation*
1. Dietary restriction
2. Enternal or extracorporeal enzymes
3. Plasmaphoresis/dialysis/affinity binding
4. Surgical bypass
5. Chelation
6. Alternative excretion pathways
7. Enhanced solubility
8. Metabolic inhibitors

VI. *Endproduct replacement*
VII. *Avoidance of noxious agents*
1. Common environmental exposures
2. Pharmacogenetic polymorphisms

VIII. *Correction of the consequences of mutant genes*
1. Replacement of damaged or non-functional tissues
   (a) Transfusion
   (b) Bone marrow transplantation
   (c) Organ transplantation
   (d) Dialysis
   (e) Artificial organs
2. Plastic, reconstructive, orthopedic and other surgical intervention
3. Drugs e.g. antibiotics, digitalis, diuretics, etc., etc.

The precise molecular defect in a number of human disorders has been elucidated. This has been most notable in the case of the haemoglobinopathies and the thalassaemias, however, knowledge of other conditions will undoubtedly follow suit. Once the relevant nucleotide substitutions, deletions, additions, etc., are identified, a number of strategies for correction of such defects can begin to take shape. Several approaches for direct alteration of the genome can be envisioned. These would include site specific mutagenesis, replacement of defective sequences with synthetic oligonucleotides, and the introduction of cloned normal genes into the homologous chromosomal location of the mutant recipient (Razin et al, 1978; Hutchison et al, 1978; Riggs & Itakura, 1979). None of these forms of intervention has yet been shown feasible in experimental systems. However, introduction of functional, replicating DNA into foreign recipient cells in vitro has been accomplished (Wigler et al, 1978). Cloned genes have been inserted into a variety of cell types and substantial evidence indicates that such genes become integrated into stable chromosomal sites, are replicated with the host cellular DNA, and may function (Robins et al, 1981). The donor DNA may be derived from animals with considerable species divergence from the recipient cell line. Most often, these experiments have utilized a selectable genetic marker to facilitate identification of a rare transformational event. Such genes as the hypoxanthine guanine phosphoribosyl transferase, adenosine phosphoribosyl transferase, and thymidine kinase (mammalian or viral) genes have been studied in these systems (Pellicer et al, 1980). Recently, transformation of bone marrow cells has been followed by selection of the relevant cell population in an intact animal. Cline and coworkers (1980) treated mice with a drug, methotrexate, following transplantation of donor marrow cells which had been exposed to a cloned dihydrofolate reductase gene. The successfully transformed cells had a selective advantage in the treated mice, and multiplied to populate their marrow.

A modification of this strategy entails cotransformation of a gene which confers a selective advantage with another cloned gene of interest for which selective techniques do not exist. The genes may be physically linked (Mantei et al, 1979), or simply mixed together. It appears from the available experimental data that both molecules may enter isolated cells, replicate in tandem and be selectively retained (Wigler et al, 1979). Other techniques for introducing genetic information into cultured cells have also been validated such as the insertion of a gene into the SV 40 or other viral genomes and infecting a suitable host cell (Mulligan & Berg, 1980). Finally, direct injection of cloned genes into cultured somatic cells (Anderson et al, 1980) and even developing mouse eggs (Gordon et al, 1980) has been shown to be a workable, albeit tedious way to accomplish similar ends. It is of note that in the initial mouse embryo experiments, a small percentage of animals showed persistence of a viral thymidine kinase gene into adult life, although gene expression was not detected. However, later experiments have in fact established chromosomal integration, germ cell transmission and expression of the introduced genes in such mice (Brinster, et al, 1981; E. Wagner, et al, 1981; T. Wagner et al, 1981).

The recent advances in synthetic polynucleotide chemistry previously described also hold importance for entirely new directions in gene therapy. In addition to permitting the production of abundant amounts of genetic material, this technology could permit the generation of new nucleotide sequences not previously encountered in nature, which would direct the production of a new gene product with novel properties which might have some beneficial therapeutic effect. In this way, peptides and enzymes could be custom designed. Clearly such applications are far in the future, but the synthesis of hybrid proteins combining antibody or receptor domains with enzymatic active sites, etc., could be envisioned.

At present, procedures exist, at least in theory, for isolating, cloning, and modifying virtually any gene of interest. The problems which remain are to devise ways to efficiently and reliably introduce this information into a large percentage of cells of interest in a predetermined chromosomal location. This will probably be necessary to ensure that appropriate regulatory input and modification are achieved. Much work will be needed before precise tissue specific and developmentally programmed regulation of expression of foreign genes can be accomplished. Accurate control of gene activity will probably turn out to be the most difficult aspect of gene therapy.

REPLACEMENT OF MISSING GENE PRODUCTS

The next level at which attempts may be made to deal with mutant genes and their deleterious effect is at the level of replacement of missing gene products. This type of therapy has already been accomplished for several disorders in which it is feasible to isolate and prepare adequate amounts of the relevant protein. For purposes of considerations of this sort, it does not matter a great deal if the actual nature and location of the mutation is known. If the end result is an inadequate supply of some important protein or polypeptide gene product, in theory, this sort of attack is strategically sound. Where the proteins and polypeptides under consideration are found in the circulation, it seems reasonable to expect that administration of purified proteins into the same compartment should result in a salutory effect. Of course, various forms of diabetes have been treated with exogenous insulin for many decades. On the imminent horizon, is the potential for treating such conditions with purified human insulin produced by recombinant DNA techniques (Goeddel et al, 1979). In a similar fashion,

human growth hormone isolated from pituitary glands has been utilized in many hundreds of patients for the therapy of growth hormone deficiency (Raben, 1958) (Chapter 82) and preparations of increasing purity of antihaemophiliac globulin (factor VIII) have been utilized in clinical practice for many years (Pool & Shannon, 1965) (Chapter 76). The use of immunoglobulin preparations in immunodeficiency states, and plasma therapy to treat children with deficiencies of complement components has a similar theoretical basis (Rosen & Merler, 1978; Ruddy & Austen, 1978). (Chapters 78 and 79)

In recent years, attention has been directed toward the possibility of enzyme replacement for a host of other kinds of disorders. Of particular note are efforts to treat the lysosomal storage diseases by such a route (Desnick et al, 1973; Rietra et al, 1974; Desnick, 1980). Ever since the identification of lysosomal storage diseases, the elucidation of their aetiology, and the demonstration that one cannot modulate substrate accumulation by dietary manipulation, such kinds of approaches have seemed particularly attractive. When correction of abnormal metabolic patterns in cell cultures from patients with lysosomal storage of mucopolysaccharides was achieved by Neufeld and her collaborators (1974), the possibility of delivering enzyme to this subcellular compartment seemed particularly feasible. Much work has been done over the ensuing years in an effort to bring these theories to fruition. A number of human experiments have been performed with enzyme prepared from a variety of sources including fungi, bovine liver, and human tissues. It is relatively apparent, that human sources will be preferable in order to avoid significant immunological consequences.

More recently, it has become clear that bulk endocytosis is a relatively inefficient way to deliver enzyme into the lysosomal compartment. Much more efficient pathways exist which make use of receptor mediated binding of ligands at the cell surface, the aggregation of these receptors, and resultant pinocytosis into the cell (Neufeld, 1981; Sly et al, 1981). A number of attempts are currently underway to utilize this newer knowledge to develop strategies of enhancing uptake of enzyme into lysosomes and utilizing tissue specificity of some of these receptors to target lysosomal enzymes to organs of primary pathology. Studies in several laboratories have clearly indicated that the carbohydrate portions of circulating or infused lysosomal enzymes (which all seem to be glycoproteins) substantially influence the length of time these molecules spend in the circulation and the specific tissue which effects their uptake. Selecting appropriate lysosomal enzyme preparations and modifying some of them in vitro (e.g. by addition of receptor recognized ligands) will become an increasingly important part of experimental design.

A very substantial problem remains in dealing with those conditions involving neuronal storage of macromolecules. The blood brain barrier is a formidable obstacle to be negotiated, however, a number of experimental approaches are currently being studied in an effort to create a treatment modality capable of temporarily disrupting the blood brain barrier without undue physiologic consequences (Ratazzi et al, 1981). In this regard, use of the rapidly expanding number of animal models of storage diseases identified in recent years should be of considerable utility.

Other forms of packaging of enzymes are also being investigated and attempts to immobilize enzymes within autologous erythrocyte ghosts, or to entrap them within liposomes which can then have their lipid or surface properties altered to gain specificity of enzyme uptake are currently being evaluated in a number of laboratories (Desnick & Grabowski, 1981). Concern about liposome entrapped enzyme has recently been expressed, however. Some studies suggest that liposome entrapment may actually enhance immunogenicity of injected enzymes acting similarly to lipid based immunologic adjuvants (Tyrell et al, 1976; Belchetz et al, 1977).

In spite of all of these theoretical and practical difficulties, experimental progress continues to be rapid, both in the animal models and in very limited clinical trials. Fabry disease (Brady et al, 1973; Desnick et al, 1979), Gaucher disease (Brady et al, 1974; Beutler et al, 1980; Belchetz et al, 1977), and Pompe disease (De Barsy et al, 1973; Tyrell et al, 1976; Williams & Murray, 1980) have been particularly singled out for study and a variety of data have accrued from these efforts. At present, it is difficult to evaluate the ultimate role of this type of therapy. Eventually, recombinant DNA technology may play a large role in such therapy since many injected enzymes have a very short half-life and large doses of enzyme may be required to eliminate the substantial stores of pathological material which have accrued over a number of years in many patients. Such requirements severely tax current technologies for isolating and purifying enzyme protein molecules, but may be overcome through bacterial production.

An alternative method of supplying missing gene products is to attempt organ or cellular transplantation. This notion differs from the strategy which will be mentioned below of merely replacing missing or damaged organs in that the goal of treatment is to engraft functional tissue in the hope that it will continue to produce and export a missing gene product which can then be taken up by relevant tissues so that it may function. Renal allografts, liver transplantation, splenic transplantation, lymphocyte infusions and subcutaneous fibroblast transplantation have all been attempted. Varying degrees of success have been noted (Desnick & Grabowski, 1981).

INDUCTION, STABILIZATION, AND ENHANCEMENT OF ENZYME ACTIVITY

Another approach which is sometimes feasible in the treatment of genetic disorders is the induction or augmentation of activity of an enzyme or other gene product whose function is rate limiting. For example, in patients with certain forms of chronic unconjugated hyperbilirubinaemia (Crigler-Najjar syndrome, Type II) activity of the rate limiting enzyme hepatic glucuronyl transferase can be substantially increased by therapy with phenobarbital (Yaffe, et al, 1966). This enhanced enzyme activity may be sufficient to lower the levels of unconjugated bilirubin to a range which is acceptable for normal growth and development, although the exact mechanism by which phenobarbital acts in these patients is still under study.

Several inborn errors of metabolism have been recognized in which apparently functional enzymes are produced, but in which diminished enzyme stability leads to insufficient activity under certain circumstances. The best studied and most frequently encountered example of this is the common black A- variant of red cell glucose-6-phosphate dehydrogenase deficiency. One treatment strategy which has not been systematically pursued, is to attempt to enhance stability of such labile enzymes. A model worthy of further study may be the effect of divalent cations on the activity of α-mannosidase in certain patients with mannosidosis (Grabowski et al, 1980).

Acquisition of new knowledge regarding metabolic pathways has facilitated the development of treatment for a whole new class of inborn errors of metabolism in recent years. This is a group of conditions which has come to be known as the vitamin responsive inborn errors of metabolism (Rosenberg, 1976). Vitamins are, of course, essential dietary constituents which frequently subserve the function of coenzymes or cofactors in various enzymatically catalyzed reactions. The utilization of vitamin cofactors is often a complex process and so there are numerous opportunities for genetically determined defects to be manifested. Abberant absorbtion, transport, cellular uptake, and metabolism to active forms have all been recognized. Similarly, mutations in apoenzymes which alter affinity for cofactor may be the basis for significant disease. In an increasing number of such disorders, supplementation with supraphysiologic doses of the relevant vitamin, in concert with other metabolic measures, often produces substantial clinical benefits. Supplying the vitamin in adequate amounts as in a suitable chemical form may thus permit such patients to overcome marginal affinities of relevant enzymes or transport-carrier proteins. As knowledge of reaction mechanisms increases, it seems likely that other conditions will emerge as candidates for similar types of treatment.

Another strategy in the treatment of inborn errors of metabolism is the amelioration of the effects of a mutant gene through stimulation of alternate biochemical pathways. Examples of such efforts include treatment of certain methemoglobinemic states with methylene blue (Schwartz & Jaffe, 1978). In some of these patients, insufficient reductive power is generated by red blood cell NADH dehydrogenase to maintain haemoglobin iron in the Fe* state. This defect may be circumvented by the action of methylene blue which can activate the NADPH dehydrogenase pathway to stimulate methaemoglobin reduction. Another possible example of this approach is the use of thiamine therapy in pyruvate carboxylase deficiency. Apparently, some subjects with difficulty in pyruvate metabolism as a result of this defect can augment their metabolism of pyruvate via the pyruvate dehydrogenase reaction which is enhanced by thiamine administration (Brunette et al, 1972). Again, acquisition of further knowledge about regulatory aspects of intermediary metabolism may facilitate similar attempts at treatment of still other diseases.

LIMITATION OF SUBSTRATE ACCUMULATION

In many genetic disorders, accumulation of low molecular weight substrates both in tissues and extracellular fluids is thought to be pathogenetically involved in the disease process. Either a metabolite immediately proximal to a geneticaly determined metabolic block may be at fault, or some derivative metabolite thereof. Although enzyme replacement might be desirable for such patients, in most instances it is not technically feasible. Other strategies may, however, be employed to reduce the level of the toxic metabolite. The classic and most common example of this therapeutic strategy is the treatment of phenylketonuria by dietary restriction of phenylalanine intake (Bickel et al, 1953) (Chapter 88). Similar kinds of treatment have been performed in a whole host of other disturbances of amino acid metabolism, organic acid metabolism, and carbohydrate metabolism (Stanbury et al, 1978). In most instances, therapy must be carefully constructed and balanced so as not to unduly deplete the patient of essential amino acids or other nutrients. Since the degree of genetic defect may be variable from patient to patient, and requirements and endogenous supply of precursors may be altered by a variety of physiological stimuli, therapy most often has to be carefully individualized and carefully monitored. Dietary intake must be titrated to the needs of the patient and often requires the concerted efforts of skilled professionals in a wide variety of disciplines. Nonetheless, successful therapy of phenylketonuria and galactosaemia, and other disorders represents a major and dramatic medical success. Future directions in therapy may well employ alternative strategies at control of substrate levels or substrate depletion. The use of immobilized or microencapsulated enzyme for haemoprofusion has been frequently suggested (Chang, 1973). Recently, a proposal has been made that oral administration of microencapsulated bacterial enzymes such as phenylalanine ammonia lyase could be of use in metabolizing within the gut potentially deleterious metabolites prior to their absorption (Hoskins et al, 1980). A modification of the dietary restriction approach is the provision of well tolerated analogues of essential nutrients. Patients with urea cycle disorders have a very limited capacity to dispose of waste nitrogen, but an ongoing need for the carbon skeletons of essential amino acids. For this reason, it was anticipated that α keto acid analogues of the essential amino acids would provide these needed nutrients without the cost of further nitrogen and could even act as a nitrogen 'sink' as a result of analogue transamination. Although such treatment is not completely effective, substantial biochemical benefit can be demonstrated (Brusilow et al, 1979). (Chapter 88)

SUBSTRATE DEPLETION

Other strategies designed to deplete circulating substrate levels have also been employed for those low molecular weight substances which can be efficiently removed by dialysis. Peritoneal and haemodialysis, and exchange transfusion have been utilized successfully in the acute management of a number of disorders of amino acid and organic acid metabolism (Danks, 1976; Donn et al, 1979; Wiegand et al, 1980). For larger molecules with poorer dialysis clearance, plasmaphoresis and/or 'affinity binding' may be contemplated. Removal of lipid substrates such as phytanic acid in Refsum disease (Gibberd, 1979) and ceramide trihexoside in Fabry disease have been demonstrated (Desnick & Grabowski, 1981). Elimination of low density lipoprotein by exposing plasma to a heparin-agarose matrix has also been reported in type II hypercholesterolaemia (Lupien et al, 1976), and haemoperfusion over albumin-agarose columns has been studied for the removal of bilirubin from a variety of experimental animals (Scharschmidt et al, 1977). In a similar fashion, transfusion of enzyme containing red blood cells from normal donors to patients with combined immunodeficiency due to adenosine deaminase deficiency appears to exert a beneficial effect via reduction of the toxic substrates adenosine and deoxyadenosine (Hirschhorn, 1980).

Enhanced elimination or excretion of potentially toxic substrates is another approach which may be utilized in therapy. Wilson disease may be very successfully managed by chelation and removal of stored copper following administration of d-penicillamine (Walshe, 1956). (Chapter 92) Patients with haemochromotosis can be somewhat successfully treated through administration of iron chelating agents (Pollycove, 1978) (Chapter 93). Enhanced urinary excretion of urates in the treatment of patients with gout is frequently accomplished with drugs such as probenicid, salicylate, and sulphinpyrazone which exhibit striking uricosuric properties (Wyngaarden & Kelly, 1978) (Chapter 90).

Recently, considerable improvement in the therapy of urea cycle disorders has been accomplished through providing alternative means for waste nitrogen excretion in affected patients. In infants with inborn errors of the urea cycle in whom enzymatic defects render them unable to efficiently convert ammonia to urea, the administration of sodium benzoate or phenylacetate appears to provide them an effective alternative means of excreting waste nitrogen as hippuric acid or phenylacetylglutamate respectively (Batshaw et al, 1981).

In some instances, altering the biophysical properties of substrates through pharmacologic means can ameliorate symptoms of a disease. An example of this approach is therapy of patients with cystinuria with d-penicillamine. Due to an inherited transport defect, such patients excrete massive amounts of cystine in their urine. The limited solubility of cystine leads to precipitation and urolithiasis. Treatment with d-penicillamine has proven very effective. Penicillamine and cysteine can form a mixed disulphide which is much more soluble than cystine and so obviate these problems (Crawhall et al, 1964). Penicillamine can even be used to dissolve stones that are already in existence.

One final means occasionally used to control aberrant substrate levels is the use of suitable metabolic inhibitors. For example, hyperuricaemia occurring in certain disorders of purine metabolism can be modulated by administration of the xanthine oxidase inhibitor, allopurinol. Use of this drug will lower serum uric acid levels (Wyngaarden & Kelley, 1978) and urinary excretion, although levels of the much more soluble hypoxanthine and xanthine may increase.

In limited instances, surgical therapy may anatomically reroute substates in a fashion which reduces their accumulation in target tissues. This is the rationale for the historic use of protocaval shunts in type I glycogen storage disease, done in an effort to reroute glucose from the intestinal circulation around the liver where it would be taken up and irreversibly trapped (Riddell et al, 1966). Similarly, intestinal bypass can limit enterohepatic circulation of cholesterol in homozygous type II hypercholesterolemic patients (Moore et al, 1973) (Chapter 69).

END PRODUCT REPLACEMENT

In another large group of inherited metabolic disorders, disease manifestations appear to be due to insufficient production of some end product of a metabolic reaction.

Examples of such conditions are the various adrenogenital syndromes resulting from impaired steroidogenesis, or the heritable forms of hypothyroidism. In both situations, supplementation with the end product of the metabolic pathway (either corticosteroids, mineralocorticoids, or thyroid hormone) virtually completely ameliorates symptoms. Thyroid administration restores metabolic integrity to the patient with congenital hypothyroidism and administration of appropriate steroid therapy to patients with the adrenogenital syndrome not only obviates symptoms of glucocorticoid or mineralocorticoid deficiency but provides the needed feedback inhibition of the hypothalamic-pituitary axis so that stimulation of adrenal production of androgens or other deleterious steroids is reduced.

Occasionally the end product which is in short supply is not a hormone, but an important metabolite. In such situations, repletion of the relevant molecule is beneficial. As an example, a number of genetic disorders are known which impair action of one of the four irreversible reactions in gluconeogenesis. Frequent supplementation of adequate glucose can prevent the ravages of acute and chronic hypoglycaemia in such subjects.

AVOIDANCE OF NOXIOUS ENVIRONMENTAL AGENTS

In contrast to individuals subject to dietary substrate overload as in the aminoacidopathies, some patients with heritable illnesses can have their symptoms precipitated by exposure to relatively less ubiquitous environmental agents. For such people, careful avoidance of noxious effectors can be very important. Patients with certain porphyrias need to assiduously avoid contact with barbiturates and other provocative stimuli (Meyer & Schmid, 1978) (Chapter 50). Sunlight can be quite harmful to other porphyric patients or, for example, to xeroderma pigmentosa patients who readily get solar induced malignancies. Patients with unusual pharmacogenetic traits also need to carefully avoid certain drugs as exemplified by the effects of succinylcholine in patients with pseudocholinesterase deficiency (Goedde, 1971), or ingestion of fava beans or many drugs in patients with G6PD deficiency (Beutler, 1978) (Chapter 75).

CORRECTION OF THE CONSEQUENCES OF MUTANT GENES

For many inherited illnesses, primary or even secondary treatment cannot yet be accomplished. The inborn errors of metabolism have received perhaps a disproportionate share of the discussion so far. This is the case for several very obvious reasons. In these metabolic diseases, the fundamental genetic defect can be known, or at least, inferred and direct forms of treatment employed. The bulk of the remainder of genetic diseases are probably inborn errors of metabolism, too, and would respond to similar therapeutic strategies if only we knew the primary abberations in these conditions. In the absence of such knowledge, however, useful medical intervention can still occur via efforts to correct the consequences of mutant genes. Replacement of damaged, absent, or non-functional tissues is being attempted with increasing frequency. Transfusion of normal blood to patients with poorly functioning haemoglobins is an everyday event. Bone marrow transplantation may become practical for such patients as technology improves, and at present is useful for selected patients with heritable aplastic anaemias or malignancies. Organ transplantation (renal, hepatic, corneal, cardiac, etc.) have all been attempted in patients with genetic illnesses which have wrecked havoc with one or more organ systems. Haemodialysis and the ultimate use of artificial organs (e.g. artificial pancreas, heart) can also be of use in appropriately selected individuals. Plastic, reconstructive, orthopedic, and other surgical procedures may similarly be of benefit in patients with a wide variety of genetic diseases. Finally, the entire modern day pharmacopea of antibiotics, digitalis, diuretics, etc., etc., etc., can have an incredibly positive effect on genetic illnesses to an extent just as great as in environmentally determined conditions. One of many examples that could be cited is the major improvement in quality of life and longevity for patients with cystic fibrosis as a result of the use of pancreatic enzymes, respiratory physiotherapy, expectorants, antibiotics, digitalis, diuretics and the like.

CONCLUSIONS*

It should be apparent that the enhanced understanding of normal and abnormal metabolic and physiological processes brought about by intensive research of the past several decades has changed the outlook for patients with many inherited diseases. With adequate discourse between basic science laboratories and clinicians at the bedside, the pace of development of new forms of therapy shows promising signs of further acceleration.

When dealing with families affected by major genetically determined illnesses, a variety of psychological responses are frequently observed. One major recurring theme is the feeling such individuals often have of isolation from the medical mainstream. They feel that the rarity of their condition or their child's illness mitigates against aggressive interest in the medical community. Unfortunately, this perception is frequently reinforced by medical practitioners with a similarly pessimistic view. It is important to share, both with colleagues and patients, the important advances which have been made and the considerable efforts which continue to be expended, all of which justify cautious optimism for the future.

---

* In the discussions just concluded, a substantial degree of editorial selectivity has been employed. The examples of therapeutic efforts described were selected to indicate strategies with which genetic disease treatment may be approached. No effort was made to be comprehensive and references were selected primarily from recent publications.

REFERENCES

Anderson W F, Killow L, Sanders Haigh L, Kretchmer P J, Diacumakos E G 1980 Thymidine kinase and human globin genes microinjected into mouse fibroblasts: replication and expression. Proceeding of the National Academy of Sciences USA 77: 5399–5403

Batshaw M L, Thomas G H, Brusilow S W 1981 New approaches to the diagnosis and treatment of inborn errors of urea synthesis. Pediatrics 68: 290–297

Belchetz P E, Braidman I P, Crawley J C W, Gregoriadis G 1977 Treatment of Gaucher's disease with liposome-entrapped glucocerebroside: β-glucosidase. Lancet 2: 116–117

Beutler E 1983 Glucose -6- phosphate dehydrogenase deficiency. In: Stanbury J B, Wyngaarden J B, Fredrickson D S (eds) Metabolic basis of inherited disease, 5th edn. McGraw-Hill, New York. pp 1629–1653

Beutler E, Dale, G L, Guinto E, Kuhl W 1977 Enzyme replacement therapy in Gaucher's disease: Preliminary clinical trial of a new enzyme preparation. Proceedings of the National Academy of Sciences USA 74: 4620–4623

Bickel H, Gerrard A J, Hickman E M 1953 Influence of phenylalanine intake on phenylketonuria. Lancet ii: 812

Brady R O, Tallman J F, Johnson W G, Gal A E, Leahy W R, Quirk J M, Dekaban A S 1973 Replacement therapy for inherited enzyme deficiency: Use of purified ceramidetrihexosidase in Fabry's disease. New England Journal of Medicine 289: 9–14

Brady R O, Pentchev P G, Gal A E, Hibbert S R, Dekaban A S 1974 Replacement therapy for inherited enzymatic deficiency: Use of purified glucocerebrosidase in Gaucher's disease. New England Journal of Medicine 291: 989–993

Brinster R L, Chen H Y, Trumbauer M, Senear A W, Warren R, Palmiter R D 1981 Somatic expression of herpes thymidine kinase in mice following injection of a fusion gene into eggs. Cell 27: 223–231

Brunette M G, Delvin E, Hazel B, Scriver C R 1972 Thiamine-responsive lactic acidosis in a patient with deficient low-Km pyruvate carboxylase activity in liver. Pediatrics 50: 707–711

Brusilow S W, Valle D L, Batshaw M L 1979 New pathways of nitrogen excretion in inborn errors of urea synthesis. Lancet 2: 452–454

Chang T M S 1973 Immobilization of enzymes, adsorbents or both within semipermeable microcapsules for clinical and experimental treatment of metabolic-related disorders. In: Desnick R J, Bernlohr R W, Krivit W (eds) Enzyme therapy in genetic diseases. Williams & Wilkins, Baltimore. pp 66–76

Cline M J, Stang H, Mercola K, Morse L, Ruprecht R, Browne J, Salser W 1980 Gene transfer in intact animals. Nature 284: 422–427

Crawhall J C, Scowen E F, Watts R W E 1964 Further observations on use of D-penicillamine in cystinuria. British Medical Journal 1: 1411–1413

Danks D M 1976 Plan of management for newborn babies in whom metabolic disease is anticipated or suspected. Clinical Perinatology 3: 251–259

DeBarsy T, Jacquemin P, Van Hoof F, Hers H G 1973 Enzyme replacement in Pompe's disease: An attempt with purified human α-glucosidase. In: Desnick R J, Bernlohr R, Krivit W (eds) Enzyme therapy in genetic diseases. Williams and Wilkins, Baltimore. pp 184–190

Desnick R J, Grabowski G A 1981 Advances in the treatment of inherited metabolic diseases. Advances in Human Genetics 11: 281–370

Desnick R J, Bernlohr R W, Krivit W (eds) 1973 Enzyme Therapy in Genetic Diseases. Williams and Wilkins, Baltimore

Desnick R J (ed) 1980 Enzyme Therapy in Genetic Diseases: 2. Alan R Liss, New York

Desnick R J, Dean K J, Grabowski G A, Bishop D F, Sweeley C C 1979 Enzyme therapy in Fabry disease: Differential in vivo plasma clearance and metabolic effectiveness of plasma and splenic α-galactosidase. Proceeding of the National Academy of Sciences USA 76: 5326–5330

Donn S M, Swartz R D, Thoene J G 1979 Comparison of exchange transfusion, peritoneal dialysis, and hemodialysis for the treatment of hyper ammonemia in an anuric newborn infant. Journal of Pediatrics 95: 67–70

Gibberd F B, Page N G R, Billimoria J D, Retsas S 1979 Heredopathia atactica polyneuritiformia (Refsum's disease) treated by diet and plasma exchange. Lancet 1: 575–576

Goedde H W, Atland K 1971 Suxamethoniam sensitivity. Annals of the New York Academy of Sciences 179: 695–703

Goeddel D V, Kleid D G, Bolivar F, Heyneker H L, Yansura D G, Crea R, Hirose T, Kraszewski A, Itakura K, Riggs A D 1979 Expression in Escherichia coli of chemically synthesized genes for human insulin. Proceeding of the National Academy of Sciences USA 76: 106–110

Gordon J W, Scangus G A, Plotkin D J, Barbosa J A, Ruddle F H 1980 Genetic transformation of mouse embryos by microinjection of purified DNA. Proceedings of the National Academy of Sciences USA 77: 7380–7384

Grabowski G A, Walling L, Desnick R J 1980 Human mannosidosis: In vitro and in vivo studies of cofactor supplementation. In: Desnick R J (ed) Enzyme therapy in genetic diseases: 2. Alan R Liss, New York. pp 319–334

Hirschorn R 1980 Treatment of genetic diseases by allotransplantation. In: Desnick R J (ed) Enzyme therapy in genetic diseases: 2. Alan R Liss, New York. pp 429–444

Hoskins J A, Jack G, Peiris R J D, Starr D J T, Wade H E, Wright E C, Stern J 1980 Enzymatic control of phenylalanine intake in phenylketonuria. Lancet 1: 392

Hutchinson C A, Phillips S, Edgell M H, Gillams S, Jahnke P, Smith M 1978 Mutagenesis at a specific position in a DNA sequence. Journal of Biological Chemistry 253: 6551–6560

Lupien P J, Moorjani S, Awad J 1976 A new approach to the management of familial hypercholesterolemias: Removal of plasma-cholesterol based on the principal of affinity chromatography. Lancet 1: 1261

Mantei N, Boll W, Weissman C 1979 Rabbit β-globin mRNA

production in mouse L-cells transformed with cloned rabbit β-globin chromosomal DNA. Nature 281: 40–43

Meyer U A, Schmid R 1978 Diseases of porphyrin and heme metabolism. In: Stanbury J B, Wyngaarden J B, Fredrickson D S (eds) Metabolic basis of inherited disease, 4th edn. McGraw-Hill, New York. pp 1106–1220

Moore R B, Varco R L, Buchwald H 1973 Metabolic surgery in the hyperlipoproteinemias. American Journal of Cardiology 31: 148–157

Mulligan R C, Borg P 1980 Expressions of a bacterial gene in mammalian cells. Science 209: 1422–1427

Neufeld E F 1974 The biochemical basis for mucopolysaccharidoses and mucolipidoses. Progress in Medical Genetics X: 81–101

Neufeld E F 1981 Recognition and processing of lysosomal enzymes in cultured fibroblasts. In: Callahan J W, Lowden J A (eds) Lysosomes and Lysosomal Storage Diseases. Raven Press, New York. pp 115–130

Pellicer A, Robins D, Wold B, Sweet R, Jackson J, Lowy I, Roberts J M, Sim G K, Silverstein S, Axel R 1980 Altering genotype and phenotype by DNA-mediated gene transfer. Science 209: 1414–1421

Pollycove M 1978 Hemochromatosis. In: Stanbury J B, Wyngaarden J B, Fredrickson D S (eds) Metabolic basis of inherited disease, 4th edn. McGraw-Hill, New York. pp 1127–1164

Pool J G, Shannon A E 1965 Production of high potency concentrates of antihemophilic globulin in a closed bag system assay in vitro and in vivo. New England Journal of Medicine 273: 1443–1447

Raben M S 1958 Treatment of a pituitary disease with human growth hormone. Journal of Clinical Endocrinology and Metabolism 18: 901–903

Ratazzi M C, Appel A M, Baker H J, Nester J 1981 Toward enzyme replacement in GM₂ gangliosidosis: inhibition of hepatic uptake and induction of CNS uptake of human β-hexosaminidase in the cat. In: Callahan J W, Lowden J A (eds) Lysosomes and lysosomal storage diseases. Raven Press, New York. pp 405–424

Riddell A G, Davies R P, Clark A D 1966 Portacaval transposition in the treatment of glycogen storage disease. Lancet 2: 1146–1148

Rietra P J G M, van der Bergh F A J T M, Tager J M 1974 Recent developments in enzyme replacement therapy of lysosomal storage disease. In: Tager J M, Hooghwinkel G J M, Daems T (eds) Enzyme therapy in lysosomal storage diseases. North-Holland, Amsterdam. p 53

Riggs A D, Itakura K 1979 Synthetic DNA and Medicine. American Journal of Human Genetics 31: 531–538

Robins D M, Ripley S, Henderson A S, Axel R 1981 Transforming DNA integrates into the host chromosome. Cell 23: 29–39

Rosen F S 1983 Genetic defects in gamma globulin synthesis. In: Stanbury J B, Wyngaarden J B, Fredrickson D S (eds) Metabolic basis of inherited disease, 5th ed. McGraw-Hill, New York. pp 1726–1736

Rosenberg L E 1976 Vitamin responsive inherited metabolic disorders. In: Harris H, Hirschhorn K (eds) Advances in human genetics, Vol 6, Plenum Press, New York. pp 1–74

Ruddy S, Austen K F 1978 Inherited abnormalities of the complement system. In: Stanbury J B, Wyngaarden J B, Fredrickson D S (eds) Metabolic Basis of Inherited Disease, 4th edn. McGraw-Hill, New York. pp 1726–1736

Ruzin A, Hiruse T, Itakura K, Riggs A D 1978 Efficient correction of a mutation by use of a chemically synthesized DNA. Proceeding of the National Academy of Science USA 75: 4268–4270

Scharschmidt B F, Martin J F, Shapiro L J, Plotz P H, Beck P D 1977 Hemoperfusion through albumin-conjugated agarose gel for the treatment of neonatal jaundice in premature rhesus monkeys. Journal of Laboratory and Clinical Medicine 89: 101–109

Schwartz J M, Jaffe E R 1978 Heriditary methemoglobinemia with deficiency of NAON dehydrogenase. In: Stanbury J B, Wyngaarden J B, Fredrickson D S (eds) Metabolic basis of inherited disease, 4th edn. McGraw-Hill, New York. pp 1452–1464

Sly W S, Natowicz M, Gonzalez-Noriega A, Grubb J H, Fischer H D, 1981 The role of the mannose-6-phosphate recognition marker and its reception in the uptake and intracellular transport of lysosomal enzymes. In: Callahan J W, Lowden J A (eds) Lysosomes and lysosomal storage diseases. Raven Press, New York. pp 131–146

Stanbury J B, Wyngaarden J B, Fredrickson D S (eds) 1978 The Metabolic basis of inherited disease, 4th edn. McGraw-Hill, New York

Stern Curt 1973 Principles of Human Genetics, 3rd edn. W H Freeman & Co, San Francisco

Tyrell D A, Ryman B E, Kieton B R, Dubovitz V 1976 Use of liposomes in treating type II glycogenosis. British Medical Journal 12: 88

Vogel F, Motulsky A G 1979 Human genetics, problems and approaches. Springer-Verlag, New York. pp 372–381

Wagner E, Steward T, Mintz B 1981 The human β-globin gene and a functional viral thymidine kinase gene in developing mice. Proceedings of the National Academy of Sciences USA 78: 5016–5020

Wagner T E, Hoppe P C, Jollick J D, Scholl D R, Hodinka R L, Gault J B (1981) Microinjection of a rabbit β-globin gene into zygotes and its subsequent expression in adult mice and their offspring. Proceedings of the National Academy of Sciences USA 78: 6376–6380

Walshe, J M, 1956 Penicillamine, a new oral therapy for Wilson's disease. American Journal of Medicine 21: 487–495

Wiegand C, Thompson T, Bock G H, Mathis R K, Kjellstrand C M, Mauer S M 1980 The management of life-threatening hyperammonemia: a comparison of several therapeutic modalities. Journal of Pediatrics 96: 142–144

Wigler M, Pellicer A, Silverstein S, Axel R 1978 Biochemical transfer of single-copy eucaryotic genes using total cellular DNA as donor. Cell 14: 725–731

Wigler M, Sweet R, Sim G K, Wold B, Pellicer A, Lacy E, Maniatis T Silverstein S, Axel R 1979 Transformation of mammalian cells with genes from procaryotes and eucaryotes. Cell 16: 777–785

Williams J C, Murray A K 1980 Enzyme replacement in Pompe disease with an α-glucosidase low density lipoprotein complex. In: Desnick R J (ed) Enzyme therapy in genetic diseases: 2. Alan R Liss, New York. pp 415–423

Wyngaarden J B, Kelly W N 1983 Gout. In: Stanbury J B, Wyngaarden J B, Fredrickson D S (eds) Metabolic basis of inherited disease, 5th edn. McGraw-Hill, New York. pp 1043–1114

Yaffe S J, Levy G, Matsuzawa T, Baliah T 1966 Enhancement of glucuronide-conjugating capacity in a hyperbilirubinemic infant due to apparent enzyme induction by phenobarbital. New England Journal of Medicine 275: 1461–1466

105

Parentage testing

B.A. Myhre

The establishment of parentage by scientific means is a necessary adjunct to the fields of genetics, clinical medicine, anthropology, and law. The study has expanded to the point that it now is possible to establish with a relatively large degree of certainty the parentage of a child or an inheritance pattern in an entire family.

The usual methods employ genetic markers to trace the inheritance, but before these markers can be used, they must meet several requirements.

1. The markers should be associated into a system which is proven to be genetically transmissable and uninfluenced by non-genetic factors.
2. The system should be studied sufficiently so that most of the common alleles have been found and their inheritance patterns confirmed.
3. Sufficient laboratory tests should be performed to show the reproducibility of the results of the test system.
4. Adequate numbers of families should be found so that inheritance patterns and possible variants will be known.
5. The presence and identification of the major amorphic genes should be determined.
6. Enough anthropological studies should have been performed to assure that the system is found worldwide, and is not confined to one small sector of population.
7. Adequate time should have passed so that the system is generally accepted as valid by most of the scientific community, and has been challenged in court sufficiently that there is a body of legal evidence pertaining to it.

Once these criteria have been met, the genetic marker systems can be used for all inheritance studies including legal ones. Here they are employed to establish paternity in child support cases (Myhre, 1975; Lee, 1975) to establish maternity (Weiner, 1959) and paternity in kidnapping or mixed baby cases, even for stain analysis in murder and rape cases (Culliford, 1971).

There are several points which delay the use of new evidence in the courts. The United States Courts have traditionally been slow in accepting evidence based on scientific tests until the tests have survived a rather rigorous examination by experts in the laboratory and in court. This delay was compounded by the fact that these courts, until recently, have felt that almost anyone who is licensed to practice medicine should be acceptable as an expert in the field of parentage testing; therefore, until about 10 years ago, only the ABO, Rh and MNSs systems were acceptable. Today, this attitude is rapidly changing. New tests are being accepted with less rigorous legal (although no less scientific) proof, and now it is being acknowledged that not all licensed practitioners of medicine are authorities in the field of parentage testing, nor are all authorities in parentage testing necessarily practitioners of medicine (AMA, ABA Committee, 1976; Weiner & Socha, 1976). The European Courts made this jump a long time ago, and thus parentage testing is more advanced in the European Countries. (Henningsen, 1969). However, a note of caution has been sounded by Sussman (1978) who urges considerable conservatism in adopting the newest and latest technics just because they are new, and feels many should be studied further.

Because of the limitation of the use of blood grouping in the United States to the ABO, Rh, and MN groups, only about 50% of the falsely accused males could be excluded. It is interesting to note that even with this low rate, Sussman and Schatkin (1973) were able to demonstrate non-paternity in 10% of non-contested paternity cases who took part in their study. However, in 1975 the passage of P.L. −93647 required each state to develop an appropriate plan for the determination of paternity. This allowed many more scientifically acceptable blood groups to be introduced as evidence and encouraged the courts to press more aggressively in the establishment of paternity, and to obtain child support by the father in many cases. At the same time, a large number of new genetic marker systems were being found, and this allowed more discrimination. When ABO grouping is done alone the chance of excluding a falsely accused male is about 0.17 (Polesky, 1975). When Rh and MN are added to this, the chances rise to 0.5309. If 10 or more systems are tested, the chances of exclusion rise to 90% or better. At the same time, the probability of inclusion similarly rises if the accused male is not excluded. Therefore we see that at about the same time the courts became more liberal in accepting new systems, the systems were available to use.

RED CELL ANTIGENS

The time honoured method for establishing parentage is through the use of red cell antigens. Red cell studies mainly use agglutination methods to show reactivity. A red cell suspension is mixed with a known antiserum, and the resulting mixture is tested for agglutination. If it is seen, the results are positive. The major advantages of this method are that it is traditional and well known to all. The disadvantages are that it is slow, expensive of labour, and requires that a unique antiserum be used for the detection of each red cell antigen, regardless of whether it is rare or common. There is therefore, a great tendency to test only for the more common antigens, and not to test for the rarer ones which occur less frequently. Table 105.1 lists most of the red cell groups now being used and lists some of their characteristics.

As can be seen, the ABO, Rh and MN systems do have the attributes that make them useful. The Kell system, even though the gene frequencies are badly skewed, is compensated by the availability of strong, avid antisera and thus becomes helpful in some cases. The Duffy and Kidd systems are useful even though the antisera are not always available, and the very common Duffy amorphic gene which is found in blacks, can cause confusion to the unwary. Some times this gene can be detected by titration studies (Sussman, 1960). The Lewis and P systems are cursed with unstable antigens and weak antisera which will probably always prevent them from being dependable systems used in parentage testing.

Although a number of other red cell antigen systems can be studied, most of them suffer from a lack of one or more of the attributes which have been listed in this table. Therefore, the usual red cell systems used for parentage testing are ABO (including A_1 and A_2) Rh (including C^w and D^u), Kell, Kidd, Duffy, Lutheran and MNSs. One should note that subgroups should also be tested (Sussman, 1965). In addition some laboratories test for the other alleles of the Kell system (Kp and Js) and the Xg group. Few laboratories rely on the P and Lewis system but may use them for ancillary information, and not as a basis for a sole exclusion. The inheritance of all these systems is too much to cover in this brief report, but the reader should consult such texts as Race and Sanger (1975), Sussman (1976), Polesky (1975), and Dodd (1977) for further details.

ENZYME AND SERUM GROUPS

Today, one of the areas of parentage testing that is showing the greatest progress is that of red cell enzymes, and serum groups as determined by electrophoretic methods. These have added an immense amount of knowledge to genetic inheritance due to their ease of performance, interpretation, and reproducibility. The basic technic is simple. A sample of serum or a red cell haemolysate is placed on some carrier such as a cellulose acetate membrane or a starch gel block and a direct electric current is placed across the carrier. The different proteins migrate along the carrier at a rate which is dependent on their electrical charge. The proteins are stained and examined by visible or ultra-violet light. The migration rate is measured and compared to standards. From this comparison, the genetic types of the proteins are determined. The patterns are usually clear and easy to read. Further, the membranes can be dried and stored as permanent records. There is a final advantage – with enzyme and serum groups, rare variants are demonstrated on the same gel or membrane as are the usual types, the only

Table 105.1 List of red cell groups used for establishing parentage (Adapted from Myhre, 1975)

Blood group	Stable antigens	Good antisera	Balanced gene frequency	Multiple alleles	Known genetics	Use in testing
ABO	+	+	+	+	+	Good
Rh	+	+	+	+	+	Good
MNSs	+	?	+	+	+	Fairly good
Kell	+	+	0	+	+	Sometime helpful
Duffy	(1)	+	+	+	+	Good
Kidd	+	0	+	+	+	Sometimes helpful
Lutheran	+	0	0	+	+	In rare cases
Lewis	0	0	0	0	?	Rarely
P	0	?	0	0	+	Little use
Xg	+	+	(2)	0	+	Occasionally

(1) Silent genes in blacks
(2) Useful for daughters only

difference being their migration rate. Therefore, rare variants are found with no extra labour. The examination for rare variants is not at all impractical if one does not have to look specifically for each one. If one assumes that a rare variant is found 1 in 1000 times in a system (a not unreasonable assumption) then if one is testing 10 systems, a rare variant in one of the systems will occur 1 in 100 times. If this variant is passed on to the child, parentage is relatively assured. For all of these reasons, the electrophoretically demonstrated systems are becoming popular. The most common groups being studied are phosphoglucomutase (PGM), adenylate kinase (AK), erythrocyte acid phosphatase (EAP), esterase D (EsD), 6-phosphogluconate dehydrogenase (6-PGD), adenosine deaminase (ADA), glyoxalase I (GLO-I) and group specific component (Gc). Most of these systems are rather straightforward to use and do have fairly balanced gene frequencies. (Grunbaum et al, 1980)

OTHER SERUM GROUPS

Other serum groups are determined by inhibition methods (e.g. Gm, and Km) and they too have been reported to be useful in paternity testing (Sebring et al, 1979). The method of detection uses an interesting neutralization method. A detection system is made by coating red cells with a human antiserum (usually anti Rh). These coated red cells can be agglutinated by some sera taken from patients with rheumatoid arthritis. A specific rheumatoid serum has been picked so that it will react with human gamma globulin of a specific type. If it reacts with the gamma globulin, it will not react with the coating on the red cells, therefore these cells will not be agglutinated. In use, the client's serum is mixed with the specific rheumatoid serum. If it is of the correct type, the client's serum will neutralize the rheumatoid serum so that it will not agglutinate the coated cells. The major limiting factor to this system is that there are not very many laboratories who have the capability of performing these studies (Polesky & Krause, 1977). Other wise the method is good, the reactions fairly specific, a number of antigens exist, and gene frequencies are fairly evenly distributed.

HLA

By far the single most popular group for parentage testing today is the HLA system. This is determined by reacting known antisera with the lymphocytes of the person to be tested with the addition of complement. After an incubation period, the lymphocytes are placed in a dye. If the cells are alive, they are stained only slightly with the dye, while if dead, the cell nuclei stain strongly. The system, in its simplest state is represented as 4 genetic loci, 2 of which are usually tested. A large series of alleles (getting larger daily) occupy these loci. The multiplicity of antigens, the general widespread distribution of all the antigens, and the presence of a strong reaction in vitro, all help this system to be very useful. This system has been used extensively (Jeannet et al, 1972; Speiser et al, 1974; Terasaki, 1977–8; Terasaki et al, 1978) and its proponents are most enthusiastic. However, it should be regarded as only one other system for parentage testing, and not the total answer to the question. Its use as inclusive evidence has been challenged on legal grounds (Jaffe, 1977–8). The major drawback to the HLA system is that currently, commercial reagents are infrequently available, and therefore, there maybe a problem obtaining enough of the not-so-common reagents. Further the method is expensive to set up and represents a major commitment of money and time. For these reasons most HLA typing is being done in a few larger centers, but this may well change in the near future.

OTHER DEVELOPING METHODS

A final system which is just being considered is the study of chromosomal banding (Matsunaga, 1973; Schwinger, 1974). This system looks as if it also will be a powerful tool in the study of parentage, but it is still too new to have passed the test of legal acceptance and therefore must still be regarded as being in the investigational phase at this time. Already problems have been documented (Nakagome et al, 1977).

There are many other genetic markers which could be used for various studies but before they can be acceptable, they still must meet the requirements listed at the beginning of this chapter. Not all of the blood group systems studied will satisfy all of these criteria, but if one of these is missing, it may be balanced by some outstanding characteristic in another area. Therefore, we expect to see more genetic factors being used in the determination of paternity.

METHODS OF EXCLUSION

Traditionally parentage testing was reported as an exclusion only, since the courts would only accept exclusions of parentage and would not accept inclusions. Indeed most state laws stipulate this today. Two types of exclusions are usually reported.
1. A direct or first degree exclusion is characterized by the child having a blood group antigen not possessed by either parent. For example, the mother is group O, the putative father is A, and the child is group B. In this case the B gene could not have

been given by either parent and parentage is thus disproved. Since there are almost no exceptions to this rule, a single first degree exclusion is usually considered adequate evidence for non-parentage.

2. An indirect or second degree exclusion is characterized by the child not having an antigen that it should have received if its father or mother is homozygous for this antigen. For example, the mother is rhrh, the putative father is Rh_1Rh_1. The child should be $rhRh_1$ if the father is homozygous. This is a much less solid exclusion since it implies that there is a true knowledge of the homozygosity of either of the parents. A large number of exceptions to this rule can be seen immediately. Any amorphic gene, a gene deletion, or an unexpressed gene all can leave an unexpressed antigen on the other chromosome. Therefore, an indirect exclusion is only a suggestion of non-parentage and not the proof that a direct one is. For this reason, few laboratories base a statement of non-paternity on one indirect exclusion alone. If studies have been done for the known alternate alleles, (for example – Mg in the MN system) more reliability can be placed on this type exclusion, but most laboratories still feel that a minimum number of indirect exclusions are needed to exclude parentage with some confidence.

In the interpretation of exclusion of parentage, the following genetic abnormalities must be considered since they can produce spurious or confusing results:

1. Suppressor genes or non-expressed genes, e.g.: Bombay in the ABO system
2. Silent alleles, e.g.: C^w in the Rh system
3. Linked phenotypes, e.g.: Linked AB in the ABO system
4. Mutations
5. Recombinations
6. Deletions, e.g.: D—In the Rh system
7. Rare variants
8. Variables in the strength of the antigen being tested, e.g.: D^u in the Rh system.

If all these abnormalities have not been considered, then exclusion of parentage cannot be seriously entertained – especially if the exclusion is an indirect one.

INCLUSION OF PATERNITY

Today, there is great interest in reporting the statistical probability of inclusion of parentage. As long as courts held that only exclusions could be reported, (and those in only a small group of systems) then there was little need for calculating inclusion percentages. But as the number of genetic markers which can be used has risen the possibility of deriving a meaningful inclusion per-centage has increased. Today, three basic systems are used for reporting percentages. All have their champions, and one is not yet considered the best of all. All methods of inclusion must be based on studying the maximum of number of systems available. If only a few systems are studied, then the inclusion percentage must of necessity be low.

1. The simplest method is to multiply together the gene frequencies of each gene presumably inherited by the child from the father. The final product shows the occurrence of all the factors totaled. This value (although small) does not mean too much. Gene pools do not father children, people do. Therefore, the calculated percentage of the concurrence of genes only shows the incidence of the specific set of antigens in that population. It does not give any true value of the possibility of parentage in that person.

2. In the second method one calculates for each system the total percentage of all the parents whose phenotypes are such that they are excluded from being the parent of the child. This percentage is then subtracted from 1 to derive how many individuals could have conceived the child. This figure will only show the portion of the population that could have conceived the child, and will not give the probability of parentage. Further, it makes no differentiation as to whether the putative parent is homozygous or heterozygous. For this reason, it also is not too helpful.

3. The system now being used most is that employing the so-called paternity index. In this method, a numerical fraction is derived in which the numerator is the probability of the non-excluded father contributing the gene to the child. In a 2 allele system in which both alleles can be detected, this figure would be 1 if the putative father were homozygous, and 0.5 if the child were heterozygous. If the system includes an amorphic gene, appropriate calculations would have to be made to account for this possibility. The denominator is the probability of a random member of the race contributing the gene (gene frequency). This fraction, expressed as a decimal, is the paternity index (P.I.). The paternity index of each genetic system is multiplied by the next P.I. to derive the total P.I. This final P.I. is divided by P.I. +1 to determine the probability of inclusion. This system appears to be the best because it does provide a result which is weighted depending on the homozygosity or the heterozygosity of the putative father. The articles by Walker (1978) and Lee (1980), present a more detailed account of this method. The finest set of tables for calculating these percentages are those of Hummel but they are not too easy to find. They

also have a disadvantage that the gene frequencies used are those of European whites only. Therefore, if other races are involved it is best to calculate one's own (Grunbaum et al, 1980).

EXPERTISE

One of the most important fundamentals involved in paternity testing is to remember that the client is not only asking for the tests to be done, but in addition, he needs an opinion as to the interpretation of the results, the validity of the methods, the probability of error, etc. The person supervising the performance of the tests should be an expert in the field – should have knowledge of the genetics involved, know the vagaries of the antisera being used, and should have had sufficient experience in giving court testimony that the client's case is presented in the fairest possible light. The expert should also be aware of the pitfalls in paternity testing so that the evidence will be credible in court. Wiener (1972) has stated these requirements very clearly and succinctly.

MISCELLANEOUS POINTS

The use of scientific technics in parentage testing is necessary and useful, but some points should be remembered. We deal in parentage testing with highly motivated individuals with much to gain or lose financially, socially, and emotionally, depending on the results of the tests. Therefore, in addition to the science involved in parentage testing there are some practical aspects which cannot be overlooked. At the time of testing, all parties must be identified and the chain of evidence established so that there is no possibility of the specimens or results being altered. It is best if possible to have all subjects identify each other. If that is not possible enough identification should be produced to be certain that one is drawing blood samples from the right persons, and that one can positively identify them from the witness stand several years in the future. A photograph, or a drivers license with an attached picture usually is adequate, especially if the photograph is signed at the time of the blood being drawn. If there is any doubt about the identity of the baby, footprinting facilities should be available. A transfusion history should be taken of both mother and child. Sussman (1957) has reported a case in which the previous exchange transfusion of the child rendered the results incorrect. After being drawn, the specimens should be stored in an area where they are safe and cannot be tampered with, until the testing is done. At the time of testing, positive and negative controls should be run to make certain that the reagents are working properly, and a list of the lot numbers of all reagents should be kept. The laboratory director should confirm personally all exclusion results; so that at the time of testimony, he may be able to say, that he personally supervised and confirmed all meaningful tests. The case files themselves should also be stored in a safe place; since one may have to refer to them for the next four or five years. Lastly, all details should be recorded, no matter how trivial, and these comments should be stored with the file. In this manner, there will be few surprises presented during testimony.

BIBLIOGRAPHY

AMA-ABA Committee 1976 Joint AMA-ABA Guidelines: present status of serologic testing in problems of disputed parentage. Family Law Quarterly X: 247–85

Boorman K E, Dodd B E, Lincoln P J 1977 Blood grouping serology 5th edn. Churchill Livingstone, Edinburgh pp 393–419

Culliford B J 1971 The Examination and typing of bloodstains in the crime laboratory, US Dept of Justice, Law Enforc Assist Admin, US Govt Print Office

Grunbaum B W, Selvin S, Myhre B A, Pace N 1980 Distribution of gene frequencies and discrimination probabilitie for 22 human blood genetic systems in four racial groups, Journal of Forensic Science 25: 428–44

Henningsen K 1969 On the application of blood tests to legal cases of disputed paternity. Revue Transfusion XII: 137–58

Hummel K, Ihm P, Schmidt V, Stuttgartgustayfischerverlag, Biostatistical Opinion of Parentage: Based upon the results of blood group tests, Vol. 1

Jaffee L R 1978–79 Comment on the judicial use of HLA paternity test results and other statistical evidence: A response to Terasaki. Journal of Family Law 17: 457–85

Jeannet M, Hassig A, Bernheim J 1972 Use of the HLA antigen system in disputed paternity cases. Vox Sanguinis 23: 197–200

Lee C L 1975 Current status of paternity testing. Family Law Quarterly IX: 615–33

Lee C L 1980 Numerical expression of paternity test results using predetermined indexes. American Journal of Clinical Pathology 73: 522–36

Matsunaga E 1973 Investigation of disputed paternity, theoretical and practical aspects, Japan. Journal of Legal Medicine 27: 419–31

Myhre B A 1975 The use of red cell antigens for the determination of disputed parentage. In: Walker R W A seminar on polymorphisms in human blood. American Association of Blood Banks, Washington DC pp 13–25

Nakagome Y, Kitagawa T, Linuma K, Matsunaga E, Shinoda T, Ando T 1977 Pitfalls in the use of chromosome variants for paternity dispute cases. Human Genetics 37: 255–60

Polesky H F 1975 Paternity testing. American Journal of Clinical Pathology

Polesky H F, Krause H D 1977 Blood typing in disputed paternity cases-capabilities of American laboratories. Transfusion 17: 521–4

Race R R, Sanger R 1975 Blood groups in man. 6th Edn
Blackwell Scientific Publications, Oxford p 659

Schwinger V E 1974 Markerchromosomen in der
vaterschaftsbegutachtung. Beitraege zur Gerichtlichen
Medizin 32: 163–6

Sebring E S, Polesky H F, Schanfield M S 1979 Gm and Km
allotypes in disputed parentage. American Journal of
Clinical Pathology 71: 281–5

Speiser P, Mayr W R, Pacher M, Pausch V, Bieier I, Metzer
G, Groer K 1974 Exclusion of paternity in the HLA system
without testing the deceased accused man. Vox Sanguinis
27: 379–81

Sussman L N 1965 Titration and scoring in disputed
parentage. Transfusion 5: 248–53

Sussman L N 1960 Pitfalls of paternity blood grouping tests.
American Journal of Clinical Pathology 33: 406–15

Sussman L N (Ed) 1976 Paternity testing by blood grouping.
2nd Edn Charles C Thomas, Springfield. Ill

Sussman L N 1978 Letter to the Editor. Paternity blood
grouping tests using legally unacceptable testing systems.
American Journal of Clinical Pathology 69: 649

Sussman L N, Solomon R 1973 Another pitfall in blood
group testing for non-parernity. Transfusion 13: 231–2,
1973

Sussman L N, Schatkin S B 1957 Blood-grouping tests in
undisputed paternity proceedings. Journal of the American
Medical Association 164: 249–50

Terasaki P 1977–8, Resolution by HLA testing of 1000
paternity cases not excluded by ABO testing. Journal of
Family Law 16: 543

Terasaki P, Gjertson D, Bernoco D, Perdue S, Mickey M R,
Bond J 1978 Twins with two different fathers identified by
HLA. New England Journal of Medicine 299: 590–2

Walker R 1978 Probability in the analysis of paternity test
results. In: Silvers H (Ed) Paternity testing. American
Association of Blood Banks, Washington DC

Wiener A S 1959 Application of blood grouping tests in cases
of disputed maternity. Journal of Forensic Science
4: 351–61

Wiener A S 1972 Problems and pitfalls in blood grouping
tests for non-parentage IV. Qualifications of experts.

Wiener A S, Socha W W 1976 Methods available for solving
mediolega problems of disputed parentage. Journal of
Forensic Science 21: 42–64

Index   *Volumes 1 and 2*

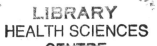